ANNUAL REVIEW OF
PHYSIOLOGY

ANNUAL REVIEW OF PHYSIOLOGY

VOLUME 52, 1990

JOSEPH F. HOFFMAN, *Editor*

Yale University School of Medicine

PAUL De WEER, *Associate Editor*

Washington University School of Medicine

ANNUAL REVIEW INC.   4139 EL CAMINO WAY,   P.O. Box 10139   PALO ALTO, CALIFORNIA 94303-0897

R̶ ANNUAL REVIEWS INC.
    Palo Alto, California, USA

International Standard Serial Number: 0066–4278
International Standard Book Number: 0–8243–0352-0
Library of Congress Catalog Card Number: 39-15404

Annual Review and publication titles are registered trademarks of Annual Reviews
Inc.

⊗   The paper used in this publication meets the minimum requirements of American National Standard for Information Sciences—Permanence of Paper for Printed
Library Materials, ANSI Z39.48-1984.

Annual Reviews Inc. and the Editors of its publications assume no responsibility
for the statements expressed by the contributors to this *Review*.

Typesetting by Kachina Typesetting Inc., Tempe, Arizona; John Olson, President
Typesetting Coordinator, Janis Hoffman

PREFACE

The *Annual Review of Physiology* presents current surveys of the various traditional and emerging fields of physiology together with coverage of closely related developing areas considered relevant to the interests of physiologists. The format of this series, beginning with Volume 41, has been to divide the corpus of physiology into sections, defined primarily by organ systems, together with general and comparative physiology. Each section has its own editor, and since coverage in any year is necessarily limited, the subject matter of each section is organized around a central theme that changes each year. This thematic organization also applies to the topics and fields reviewed in the special sections. Because of the expanding scope of all aspects of physiology, as well as the merging at the cellular and molecular levels, we have developed intersectional themes that extend beyond yet incorporate the special interests of each section. The subjects and numbers of these common themes necessarily vary yearly and to the extent possible include new aspects of whole animal physiology. A highlight of each volume remains the prefatory chapter written by an acknowledged authority but with a new focus on perspectives and trends in the author's special fields rather than a philosophical/historical focus as in the past.

My association with the *Annual Review of Physiology* began with Volume 41 (1981) as a member of the Editorial Committee, and I was honored to accept the editorship in 1988. In no small measure the continued success of this series is due to the insight, judgment, and leadership of our past editors the most recent of whom is Robert M. Berne. The Editorial Committee joins me in acknowledging his many accomplishments on behalf of the *Annual Review of Physiology* and in thanking him for his past service. I personally take this opportunity to acknowledge his studied and enjoyable contributions in the Brillat-Savarin tradition to taste.

Joseph F. Hoffman
Editor

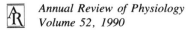

Annual Review of Physiology
Volume 52, 1990

CONTENTS

PERSPECTIVES

Mechanisms Regulating the Reactions of Human Hemoglobin
with Oxygen and Carbon Monoxide, *M. F. Perutz*   1

COMPARATIVE PHYSIOLOGY

Donald C. Jackson, Section Editor

Ca^{2+}-Activated Cell Volume Recovery Mechanisms, *Sidney K.
Pierce and Alexander D. Politis*   27

An Emerging Role for a Cardiac Peptide Hormone in Fish
Osmoregulation, *David H. Evans*   43

Respiratory and Ionic Regulation in Invertebrates Exposed to
Water and Air, *J. P. Truchot*   61

Unusual Aspects of Calcium Metabolism in Aquatic Animals,
James N. Cameron   77

RESPIRATORY PHYSIOLOGY

John A. Clements, Section Editor

The Serous Cell, *Carol B. Basbaum, Berthold Jany,
Walter E. Finkbeiner*   97

Regulation of Cl^- and K^+ Channels in Airway Epithelium,
J. D. McCann and M. J. Welsh   115

The Physiology of Cilia and Mucociliary Interactions, *Peter
Satir and Michael A. Sleigh*   137

Goblet Cell Secretion and Mucogenesis, *Pedro Verdugo*   157

Immunoglobulin Secretion in the Airways, *R. P. Daniele*   177

See also

    Hemoglobin Mechanisms   1

    Amphibious Invertebrates   61

    The Gastric H,K-ATPase   321

    Free Radicals and Infarct Size   487

    Myocardial Respiratory Control   523

Secretion from Endothelium   661
Proximal Tubule Volume Regulation   709
Nuclear Receptors   823
Reverse Genetics   841

NEUROPHYSIOLOGY

Arthur M. Brown, Section Editor

Ionic Channels and Their Regulation by G Protein Subunits,
   Arthur M. Brown and Lutz Birnbaumer   197

G Proteins and Potassium Currents in Neurons, *David A. Brown*   215

G Protein Modulation of Calcium Currents in Neurons, *Annette
   C. Dolphin*   243

Regulation of Cardiac L-Type Calcium Current by
   Phosphorylation and G Proteins, *Wolfgang Trautwein and
   Jürgen Hescheler*   257

Role of G Proteins in Calcium Channel Modulation, *G. Schultz,
   W. Rosenthal, J. Hescheler, and W. Trautwein*   275

G Protein-Mediated Regulation of K^+ Channels in Heart, *Gabor
   Szabo and Angela S. Otero*   293

See also

   Airway Epithelial Cl^- and K^+ Channels   115
   Ion Channels in Lymphocytes   415
   G Protein in Exocytosis   607

GASTROINTESTINAL PHYSIOLOGY

George Sachs, Section Editor

Electrophysiology of the Parietal Cell, *Jeffrey R. Demarest and
   Donald D. F. Loo*   307

The Mechanism and Structure of the Gastric H,K-ATPase, *Edd
   C. Rabon and Michael A. Reuben*   321

Permeable Cell Models in Stimulus-Secretion Coupling,
   S. J. Hersey and A. Perez   345

See also

   Cardiac Calcium Current Regulation   257
   G Proteins and Ca^{2+} Channels   275
   Anion Exchange in Leukocytes   381
   Ion Channels in Lymphocytes   415
   Ca in Platelets   431
   $[Ca^{2+}]_i$ Transients in Heart   467

viii   CONTENTS   (*continued*)

Ca^{2+} Dependence of Protein Synthesis   577

G Protein in Exocytosis   591

Exocytosis   607

Secretory Vesicle Proteins   647

Secretion from Endothelium   661

Smooth Muscle   857

Caged Divalent Cations   897

SPECIAL TOPIC: ION MOVEMENTS IN LEUKOCYTES

Introduction, *Louis Simchowitz, Section Editor*   363

Role of Ion Movements in Neutrophil Activation, *Ramadan I.
Sha'afi and Thaddeus F. P. Molski*   365

Functional Analysis of the Modes of Anion Transport in
Neutrophils and HL-60 Cells, *Louis Simchowitz and
James A. Bibb*   381

Ionic Mechanisms of Cell Volume Regulation in Leukocytes,
Sergio Grinstein and J. Kevin Foskett   399

Ion Channels and Signal Transduction in Lymphocytes, *Richard
S. Lewis and Michael D. Cahalan*   415

Calcium Signaling in Human Platelets, *T. J. Rink and
S. O. Sage*   431

See also

Volume Recovery Mechanisms   27

Airway Epithelial Cl$^-$ and K$^+$ Channels   115

G Proteins and Ca^{2+} Channels   275

Parietal Cell Electrophysiology   307

Permeable Cells   345

Free Radicals and Infarct Size   487

Reperfusion Injury   561

G Protein in Exocytosis   591

Secretion from Endothelium   661

Kidney Cell Volume Regulation   761

CARDIOVASCULAR PHYSIOLOGY

Howard E. Morgan, Section Editor

Ca^{2+} as a Second Messenger Within Mitochondria of the Heart
and Other Tissues, *J. G. McCormack and R. M. Denton*   451

Cytoplasmic Ca^{2+} in Mammalian Ventricle: Dynamic Control by
Cellular Processes, *G. Wier*   467

Free Radicals and Their Involvement During Long-Term
Myocardial Ischemia and Reperfusion, *J. M. Downey*   487

Load and Length Regulation of Cardiac Energetics, *George
Cooper, IV*   505

Control of Mitochondrial Respiration in the Heart In Vivo,
F. W. Heineman and R. S. Balaban   523

Mechanisms of Calcium^{2+} Overload in Reperfused Ischemic
Myocardium, *Masato Tani*   543

Modulation of Leukocyte-Mediated Myocardial Reperfusion
Injury, *Benedict R. Lucchesi*   561

Calcium-Dependent Regulation of Protein Synthesis in Intact
Mammalian Cells, *Charles O. Brostrom and
Margaret A. Brostrom*   577

See also

    Cardiac Calcium Current Regulation   257
    G Proteins and Ca^{2+} Channels   275
    G Proteins and Neural K Currents   293
    Ca in Platelets   431
    Smooth Muscle   857
    Caged Compounds and Contraction   875
    Caged Divalent Cations   897

CELL AND MOLECULAR PHYSIOLOGY

Paul De Weer, Section Editor

G$_E$: A GTP-Binding Protein Mediating Exocytosis,
B. D. Gomperts   591

Exocytosis, *W. Almers*   607

Pathways to Regulated Exocytosis in Neurons, *Pietro De
Camilli and Reinhard Jahn*   625

Secretory Vesicle-Associated Proteins and Their Role in
Exocytosis, *Robert D. Burgoyne*   647

Stimulus-Secretion Coupling in Vascular Endothelial Cells,
Andrew C. Newby and Andrew H. Henderson   661

Viral and Cellular Membrane Fusion Proteins, *Judith M. White*   675

See also

    Airway Epithelial Cl$^-$ and K$^+$ Channels   115
    Cilia and Mucociliary Transport   137
    Ionic Channels and G Proteins   197
    G Proteins and Neural K Currents   215

G Proteins and Neuronal Ca Currents   243
Cardiac Calcium Current Regulation   257
G Proteins and Ca^{2+} Channels   275
G Proteins in Heart   293
Parietal Cell Electrophysiology   307
The Gastric H,K-ATPase   321
Permeable Cells   345
Ions and Neutrophils   365
Anion Exchange in Leukocytes   381
Leukocyte Volume Regulation   399
Ion Channels in Lymphocytes   415
Ca in Platelets   431
Role of Ca^{2+} in Mitochondria   451
$[Ca^{2+}]_i$ Transients in Heart   467
Free Radicals and Infarct Size   487
Load Regulation of Energetics   505
Myocardial Respiratory Control   523
Proximal Tubule Volume Regulation   709
Kidney Cell Volume Regulation   761
Caged Divalent Cations   897

RENAL AND ELECTROLYTE PHYSIOLOGY

Erich E. Windhager, Section Editor

Renal Effects of Atrial Natriuretic Factor, *Martin G. Cogan*   699
Transepithelial Osmolality Differences, Hydraulic Conductivities,
    and Volume Absorption in the Proximal Tubule,
    James A. Schafer   709
Regulation of the Predominant Renal Medullary Organic Solutes
    In Vivo, *S. D. Wolff and R. S. Balaban*   727
Renal Action of Atrial Natriuretic Peptide: Regulation of
    Collecting Duct Sodium and Water Transport, *Mark L. Zeidel*   747
Cell Volume Regulation in the Nephron, *Chahrzad
    Montrose-Rafizadeh and William B. Guggino*   761

See also

Volume Recovery Mechanisms   27
Fish Atriopeptin   43
Leukocyte Volume Regulation   399

ENDOCRINOLOGY

Michael G. Rosenfeld, Section Editor

A Family of POU-Domain and PIT-1 Tissue-Specific
Transcription Factors in Pituitary and Neuroendocrine
Development, *Holly A. Ingraham, Vivian R. Albert, Ruoping
Chen, E. Brian Crenshaw, III, Harry P. Elsholtz, Xi He,
Michael S. Kapiloff, Harry J. Mangalam, Larry W. Swanson,
Maurice N. Treacy, Michael G. Rosenfeld* 773

Somatostatin Gene Expression, *O. M. Andrisani, J. E. Dixon* ... 793

Regulation of Rat Inhibin Synthesis in the Rat Ovary, *Teresa K.
Woodruff and Kelly E. Mayo* 807

Gene Regulation by Receptors Binding Lipid-Soluble
Substances, *Cary Weinberger and David J. Bradley* 823

Reverse Genetics Using Transgenic Mice, *Carlisle P. Landel,
Shizhong Chen, and Glen A. Evans* 841

See also

Fish Atriopeptin 43

G Protein in Exocytosis 591

Exocytosis 607

Regulated Exocytosis in Neurons 625

Secretory Vesicle Proteins 647

Secretion from Endothelium 661

Membrane Fusion Proteins 675

ANF and Renal Function 699

ANP and the Collecting Duct 747

SPECIAL TOPIC: CAGED COMPOUNDS IN CELLULAR PHYSIOLOGY

Introduction, *Jack H. Kaplan, Section Editor* 853

Flash Photolysis Studies of Excitation-Contraction Coupling,
Regulation, and Contraction in Smooth Muscle, *Andrew P.
Somlyo and Avril V. Somlyo* 857

Caged Compounds and Striated Muscle Contraction, *Earl
Homsher and Neil C. Millar* 875

Photochemical Manipulation of Divalent Cation Levels,
Jack H. Kaplan 897

INDEXES

Subject Index 915

Cumulative Index of Contributing Authors, Volumes 48–52 931

Cumulative Index of Chapter Titles, Volumes 48–52 934

OTHER REVIEWS OF INTEREST TO PHYSIOLOGISTS

From the *Annual Review of Biochemistry*, Volume 59 (1990):

Occluded Cations in Active Transport, I. M. Glynn, S. J. D. Karlish
Microtubule Motors, R. B. Vallee
The Mitochondrial Protein Import Apparatus, N. Pfanner, W. Neupert
Clathrin and Associated Assembly and Disassembly Proteins, J. H. Keen
Cadherins: A Molecular Family Important in Selective Cell-Cell Adhesion,
    M. Takeichi
*cAMP-Dependent Protein Kinase: Framework for a Diverse Family of
    Regulatory Enzymes*, S. S. Taylor, J. A. Buechler, W. Yonemoto
Biochemical Aspects of Obesity, H. Lardy, E. Shrago
Intermediates in the Reactions of Small Folding Proteins, P. S. Kim,
    R. L. Baldwin
Structural Patterns of Protein Folding, C. Chothia
Antibody-Antigen Complexes, D. R. Davies, E. A. Padlan, S. Sheriff
The Bacterial Phosphoenolpyruvate: Glycose Phosphotransferase System,
    N. D. Meadow, D. K. Fox, S. Roseman

From the *Annual Review of Medicine*, Volume 41 (1990):

Atrial Natriuretic Factor in Edematous Disorders, R. J. Cody
Cellular Mechanism for Ischemic Ventricular Arrhythmias, L. H. Opie,
    W. T. Clusin
Insulin Receptor Structure and Function in Normal and Pathologic Conditions,
    A. B. Becker, R. A. Roth
The Gut as an Endocrine Organ, J. DelValle, T. Yamada
Intestinal Malabsorption Syndromes, T. A. Brasitus, M. D. Sitrin
Digestion and Absorption of Dietary Protein, R. H. Erickson, Y. S. Kim
Preserving Renal Function by Revascularization, M. J. Schreiber, Jr.,
    M. A. Pohl, A. C. Novick
Molecular Mechanisms of Diuretic Agents, J. Breyer, H. R. Jacobson
Effects of Calcium Channel Blockers on Renal Function, L.Chan,
    R. W. Schrier
*Treatment of the Anemia of Chronic Renal Failure with Recombinant
    Human Erythropoietin*, J. W. Admason, J. W. Eschbach

Fom the *Annual Review of Neuroscience,* Volume 13 (1990):

Neurotransmitters in the Mammalian Circadian System, B. Rusak, K. G. Bina
Calcium Channels in Vertebrate Cells, P. Hess
Ion Channels in Vertebrate Glia, B. A. Barres, L. L. Y. Chun, D. P. Corey

From the *Annual Review of Pharmacology & Toxicology,* Volume 30 (1989):

Molecular Characterization of Opioid Receptors, H. H. Loh, A. P. Smith
G Proteins in Signal Transduction, L. Birnbaumer
Conformational and Structural Considerations in Oxytocin-Receptor Binding and Biological Activity, V. J. Hruby, M.-S. Chow, D. D. Smith

For the convenience of readers, a detachable order form/envelope is bound into the back of this volume.

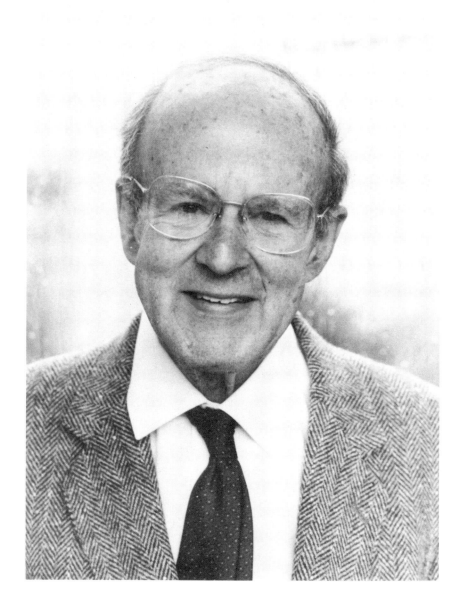

Max Perutz

Annu. Rev. Physiol. 1990. 52:1–25

MECHANISMS REGULATING THE REACTIONS OF HUMAN HEMOGLOBIN WITH OXYGEN AND CARBON MONOXIDE

M. F. Perutz[1]

Medical Research Council Laboratory of Molecular Biology, Hills Road, Cambridge, England CB2 2QH

KEY WORDS: allostery, oxygen equilibria, stereochemistry, drug-binding, mutant hemoglobins

PERSPECTIVES AND SUMMARY

The reactions of hemoglobin with oxygen and carbon monoxide are subject to regulation by the heme and the residues surrounding it and by the effectors, also known as heterotropic ligands (H^+, Cl^-, CO_2 and 2,3-diphospho-glycerate), that regulate the equilibrium between its two forms, the oxy or R-structure with high, and the deoxy or T-structure with low oxygen affinity. The stereochemical mechanisms of regulation have been studied for many years by a variety of methods. What is new since the subject had last been surveyed in *Annual Review of Biochemistry* (38) is determination of the crystal structures at resolutions sufficient to resolve individual atoms of the heme and its surroundings; such structures have now been determined for deoxy, oxy, and carbonmonoxyhemoglobin, and for several analogues of

[1]Portions of this review are adapted from "Mechanisms of Cooperativity and Allosteric Regulation in Proteins" © by *Quarterly Review of Biophysics* and Cambridge University Press and are preprinted here by permission of the publisher.

transition states in the reaction with oxygen and carbon monoxide. In the past much useful information about the stereochemical mechanism of hemoglobin has come from the study of abnormal human hemoglobins. Now that the genes for the α and β chains of hemoglobin and for the single chain of myoglobin have been cloned in *E. coli,* directed mutagenesis has provided new tools for probing the reactions of these proteins with ligands. Finally, an (unsuccessful) search for possible antisickling drugs has led to the discovery of a family of compounds that are more powerful allosteric effectors than the natural one, 2,3-diphosphoglycerate (DPG), and that combine with sites that are far removed from the diphosphoglycerate binding site.

In this review I shall describe the new insights into the allosteric mechanism provided by X-ray analysis at high resolution, or perhaps I should say, the refinement of the mechanism I proposed in 1970 (36). I then suggested that combination of the heme iron with oxygen or carbon monoxide is accompanied by a shift of the iron atom and its attached histidine relative to the porphyrin. That shift causes changes in the tertiary structure of the subunits that lead to a rearrangement of the subunits from the quaternary deoxy or T, to the oxy or R-structure. I proposed that the low oxygen affinity of the T-structure is due to additional bonds between the four subunits that take the form of hydrogen bonds between groups of opposite charge, also known as salt bridges, and that these bonds oppose the movement of the iron that is needed for the binding of oxygen. On oxygenation these salt bridges are broken, with the release of the hydrogen ions that are linked to the Bohr effect.

All these proposals have been confirmed, but certain aspects of my mechanism have remained unresolved. The structure of deoxyhemoglobin showed that the ligand sites in the β-subunits are obstructed by the distal valines, which suggests that no ligands can bind, but chemical studies showed that the oxygen affinity of the β-hemes in the T-structure is only slightly less than that of the α-hemes. X-ray analysis of a transition state analogue has now resolved this apparent contradiction. Another puzzle concerned the transmission of stereochemical effects from the hemes to the salt bridges. I proposed a system of levers that turned out to be wrong, but none of the studies of transition state analogues have suggested what the right mechanism could be. The partition coefficients of hemoglobin, and especially of myoglobin between oxygen and carbon monoxide, are much smaller than that of free heme. This difference is vital because one mole of carbon monoxide is produced endogenously for each mole of porphyrin broken down and would otherwise block the transport of oxygen. Directed mutagenesis has shown how myoglobin and the α-subunit discriminate between oxygen and carbon monoxide, but has left the mechanism of discrimination by the β-subunits obscure.

INTRODUCTION

Common Features of Hemoglobins

All hemoglobins have similar structures. The globin chain has a characteristic fold that envelops the heme in a deep pocket with its hydrophobic edges inside and its propionates facing the solvent. The chain is made up of seven or eight α-helical segments and an equal number of nonhelical ones placed at the corners between them and at the ends of the chain (Figure 1). According to a notation introduced by Watson & Kendrew (49), the helices are named A to

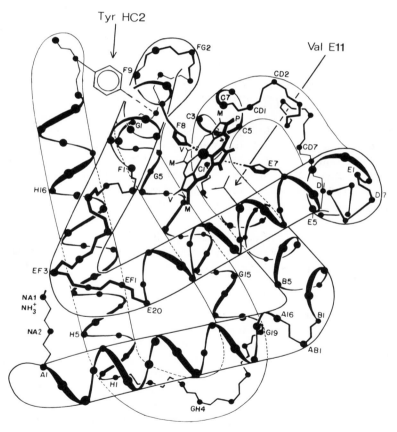

Figure 1   Tertiary structure of β-chains of human hemoglobin, typical of hemoglobins and myoglobins of all other species. The figure also shows the proximal and distal histidines, marked F8 and E7, the distal valine E11, and the tyrosine HC2 that ties down the C-terminus by its hydrogen bond to the main chain carbonyl of valine FG5.

H, starting from the amino end; the nonhelical segments that lie between helices are named AB, BC, CD, and so on. The nonhelical segments at the ends of the chain are called NA and HC. Residues within each segment are numbered from the amino end. A1, A2, CD1, CD2, and so on. Evolution has conserved this fold of the chain despite great divergence of the sequence: the only residues common to all hemoglobins are the proximal histidine F8 and the phenylalanine CD1, which wedges the heme into its pocket. Most, but not all, globins also have a histidine on the distal (oxygen) side of the heme. Ionized residues are excluded from the interior of the globin chains, which is filled largely by hydrocarbon side chains, but some serines and threonines also occur there. The proximal and distal histidines (also called the heme-linked histidines) are potentially polar, but the proximal histidine does not ionize, and the pK_a of the distal one is so low (~ 5.5) that the fraction ionized in vivo is negligible.

REACTION WITH OXYGEN AND CHANGE OF QUATERNARY STRUCTURE

Hemoglobin combines with oxygen and carbon monoxide cooperatively. This cooperativity arises not primarily by any direct interaction between the active sites, but mainly by a change in equilibrium between the two alternative structures, T and R, at successive steps of ligand binding. The degree of cooperativity is expressed as the slope n at the midpoint of the a plot of log $p(O_2)$ against log $y/1-y$, where y is the fractional saturation with oxygen or carbon monoxide. Cooperativity ensures that most of the molecules are either fully oxygenated or fully deoxygenated. This has first been demonstrated directly by Perella & his collaborators who devised a method of trapping the intermediates in the reaction of hemoglobin with carbon monoxide (33, 34) (Figure 2).

The oxygen affinity of the R-structure is slightly larger than the average one of free α- and β-subunits; that of the T-structure is lower by the equivalent of the free energy of cooperativity. The oxygen equilibrium can be described by the oxygen association constants K_T and K_R, usually expressed in (mm Hg)$^{-1}$, and by the equilibrium constant $L_o = [T]/[R]$ in the absence of oxygen. Imai has shown empirically that log K_T/K_R = A $-$ 0.25 log L_o, where A is a constant, which leaves K_R and K_T as the only independent variables. K_T varies over a wide range as a function of $[H^+]$, $[Cl^-]$, $[CO_2]$ and [DPG]; K_R varies as a function of $[H^+]$ below pH7, but is little affected by the other ligands. (1, 3, 5, 10, 13, 17, 38, 41).

The T- and R-structures differ in the arrangement of the four subunits, referred to as the quaternary structure, and the conformation of the subunits, referred to as the tertiary structure. The quaternary R $\rightarrow$ T transition consists

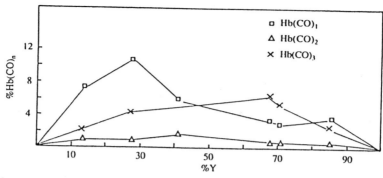

Figure 2   Observed distribution of intermediates in the reaction of hemoglobin with CO as a function of percentage saturation with CO. The reaction showed a Hill's coefficient of 3.0. The concentration of intermediates was obtained after quenching the reaction of two solutions expelled into a mixing chamber from two separate syringes. Either one syringe was filled with deoxy and the other with carbonylhemoglobin, or one was filled with partially oxidized carbonylhemoglobin and the other with a solution of dithionite. After mixing the solution was expelled into a cryochamber at $-25°C$ containing a tenfold molar excess of ferricyanide in an equal mixture of phosphate buffer and ethyleneglycol. Salt and ferricyanide were removed, and the different species separated by isoelectric focusing at $-25°C$. Contrary to the claims of Gill et al (16), the triligated species is significantly populated. The diligated species are nearly all of the type $\alpha(CO)\beta(CO)\alpha\beta$ (from Perrella et al, 33, 34).

of a rotation of the dimer $\alpha_1\beta_1$ relative to the dimer $\alpha_2\beta_2$ by 12–15° and a translation of one dimer relative to the other by 0.8Å. The $\alpha\beta$ dimers move relative to each other at the symmetry-related contacts $\alpha_1\beta_2$ and $\alpha_2\beta_1$ and at the contacts $\alpha_1\alpha_2$ and $\beta_1\beta_2$; the contacts $\alpha_1\beta_1$ and $\alpha_2\beta_2$ remain rigid (Figure 3).

The key questions for the understanding of hemoglobin function are these: how does the reaction with oxygen affect the stereochemistry at and around the heme so as to trigger the transition from the T- to the R-structure? What are the constraints of the T-structure and how do they lower the oxygen affinity? By what mechanisms do the heterotropic ligands influence the oxygen affinity? Single crystal X-ray analyses of deoxy and oxyhemoglobin, and of analogues of intermediates in the reactions with oxygen or carbon monoxide, together with chemical, spectroscopic, and magnetic studies have furnished some of the answers.

STRUCTURAL MECHANISM

Changes in the Allosteric Core

Figure 4 summarizes the stereochemistry of the hemes in deoxyhemoglobin, oxyhemoglobin, and in two intermediates. In deoxyhemoglobin the iron is high spin ferrous (S=2) and five-coordinated. The iron atoms are displaced

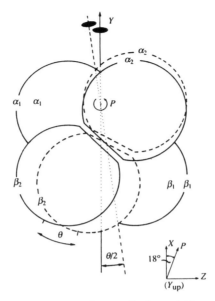

Figure 3   Change of quaternary structure of mammalian hemoglobin on transition from deoxy or T *(full lines)* to oxy or R *(broken lines)*. The dimer $\alpha_2\beta_2$ turns by $\theta = 13°$ about the P axis; this entails a rotation of the dyad symmetry axis Y by $\theta/2 = 6.5°$. If the four subunits were identical, P would have to coincide with X (from Baldwin & Chothia, 4).

---------->

Figure 4   Change of allosteric core on-going from deoxy-T via oxy-T to oxy-R and from there via deoxy-R back to deoxy-T. The vertical bars indicate the distance of N_ϵ of the proximal histidine F8 from the mean plane of the porphyrin nitrogens and carbons (excluding β and γ carbons of the side chains). The horizontal bar gives the $Fe-N_{porphyrin}$ distance, and the figure to the right of the iron atoms in the lower two diagrams the displacement of the iron from the plane of the porphyrin nitrogens. L_o is the allosteric constant in the absence of oxygen, K_T and K_R are the association constants with oxygen of the T- and R-structures, and K_m is the mean oxygen association constant. Note that the porphyrin is flat only in oxy-R and that the proximal histidine tilts relative to the heme normal in the T-structures. Note also the water molecule attached to the distal histidine in deoxy. The bottom diagram illustrates how the flattening of the porphyrin on-going from deoxy to oxy exerts a leverage on leucine FG3 and valine FG5, which lie at the switching contact between the two structures. (from Perutz et al, 41). The differences in heme geometry between deoxyhemoglobins in the T- and R-structures shown here are closely similar to those found between sterically hindered 2-methyl- and unhindered 1-methylimidazole iron porphyrin complexes (Momenteau et al, 29).

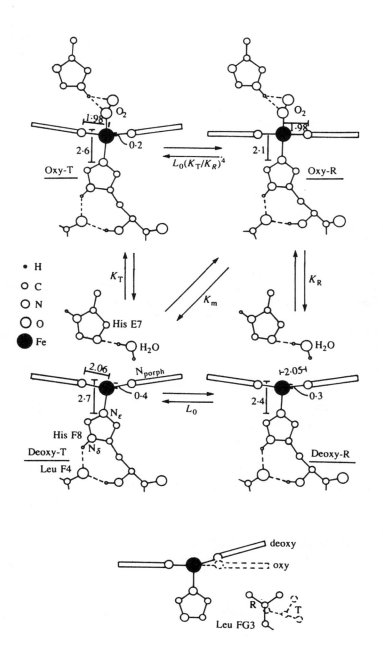

from the planes of the porphyrin nitrogens, and the porphyrins are domed. On oxygenation the iron becomes low spin ferrous (S=0) and six-coordinated. The porphyrins flatten, and the Fe-$N_{porphyrin}$ bond lengths contract from 2.06 to 1.98Å, thus moving the iron atoms towards the porphyrin planes (36, 38). As a result the proximal histidines come 0.5–0.6Å closer to the porphyrin planes in oxy than in deoxyhemoglobin. Do these movements trigger the allosteric transitions between the R- and T-structures, and if so, how are the transitions initiated?

Semi-liganded derivatives in the T-structure show that on combination of oxygen or carbon monoxide with the α-hemes the irons move by 0.15Å toward the plane of the porphyrin nitrogens, while the doming of the pyrroles is preserved. The movements of the irons are transmitted to the proximal histidines and their adjoining residues, while the bulk of the protein remains unperturbed. Thus perturbations are confined to what Gelin et al (15) have called the "allosteric core". On loss of iron-linked H_2O and reduction of the irons of a ferric hemoglobin in the R-structure, the iron atoms move away from the plane of the porphyrin nitrogens by 0.2Å, and the porphyrins become domed; the movements are transmitted not just to the proximal histidines and their adjoining residues, but also to the $\alpha_1\beta_2$ and $\alpha_2\beta_1$ contacts that shift a short way towards their positions in the T-structure (25, 41).

There have been suggestions that the hydrogen bonds between N_δ of His F8 and the carbonyl of Leu F4 play a part in the allosteric mechanism. The lengths of these bonds may change in transition states, but they remain the same in deoxyhemoglobin and oxyhemoglobin. There has also been a suggestion that changes in charge transfer interactions between the porphyrin and Phe CD1 contribute to the free energy of cooperativity, but the distance between the phenylalanine side chain and the porphyrin is too large (3.8–4.1Å) for such interactions to occur. We are thus left with the distances of the Fes and the proximal histidines from the porphyrin as the only determinants of the allosteric equilibrium visible in the α-subunits. In the β-subunits, displacement of the distal valine relative to the heme is necessary in the T-structure before oxygen can bind. In the R-structure this steric hindrance is absent.

Changes in the Globin Chains

THE α-SUBUNITS   Since the $\alpha_1\beta_1$ contact undergoes no significant changes during the R → T transition, the atoms at this contact can serve as a reference frame for changes in tertiary structure elsewhere; except for residues G1–4 and H18–21, the B, G, and H helices were also found to be static. The largest movements relative to either of these frames occur in helix F, in segment FG, and in residues G1–4, H18–21, and HC1–3. Figure 5 shows the heme environment of deoxyhemoglobin superimposed on that of oxyhemoglobin. It

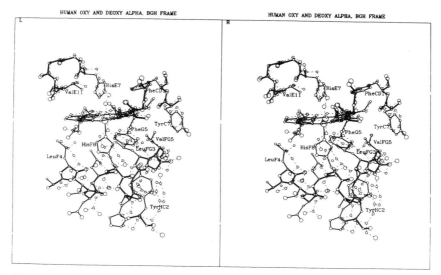

HUMAN OXY AND DEOXY ALPHA, BGH FRAME

HUMAN OXY AND DEOXY ALPHA, BGH FRAME

Figure 5   Change of tertiary structure near the α-heme on-going from deoxy-T *(full lines)* to oxy-R *(broken lines)*. Note how the proximal histidine straightens and moves closer to the porphyrin, carrying the residues in helix F with it (from Perutz et al, 41).

can be seen that on oxygenation helix Fα shifts towards the heme and to the right and carries the FG segment with it. In deoxyhemoglobin the imidazole of His F8 is tilted relative to the heme normal; in oxyhemoglobin the shift of helix F relative to deoxyhemoglobin aligns it with the heme normal. Taking as a reference frame residues F1–8 to which the heme is attached, the heme flattens and turns clockwise by 10°; the motion of its right-hand edge pushes down Leu FG3(91)α and Val FG5(93)α, which form part of the $\alpha_1\beta_2$ contact where the quaternary switch occurs (Figure 4). In the T-structure the N- and C- termini form the hydrogen bonds shown in Figures 6–8. In the R-structure these hydrogen bonds are broken, and the terminal residues are seen only at a low level of electron density, which implies that they are mobile.

THE β-SUBUNITS   Figure 9 shows that on oxygenation helix F moves towards the heme and in the direction of the FG segment, carrying that segment with it and aligning His F8 with the heme normal. The movement of F and FG is transmitted to residue G1 and dissipated beyond G5. The center of the heme moves farther into its pocket along a line linking porphyrin N_1 to N_3, and the heme rotates about an axis close to the line linking N_2 to N_4. Referred to residues F1 to F6, the iron stays still and the porphyrin becomes coplanar with it. In the T-structure, CγH_3 of Val E11(67) obstructs the ligand site at the iron; in the oxygenated R-structure that obstruction is cleared by a

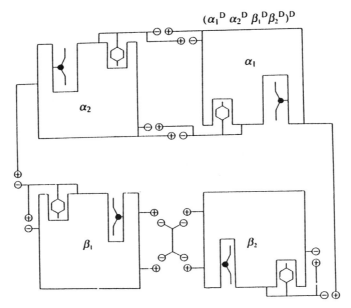

$(\alpha_1{}^D \alpha_2{}^D \beta_1{}^D \beta_2{}^D)^D$

α_1

α_2

β_1

β_2

Figure 6 Diagrammatic representation of salt bridges in the T-structure. Those at the top link the C-terminal Arg HC3(141)α_2 to Asp H9(126)α_1 and Lys H10(127)α_1. The others link the C-terminal His HC3 (146)β_1 to Asp FG1 (94)β_1 and Lys C5(40)α_2. The bridge between the β-subunits represents 2,3-diphosphoglycerate (from Perutz, 36).

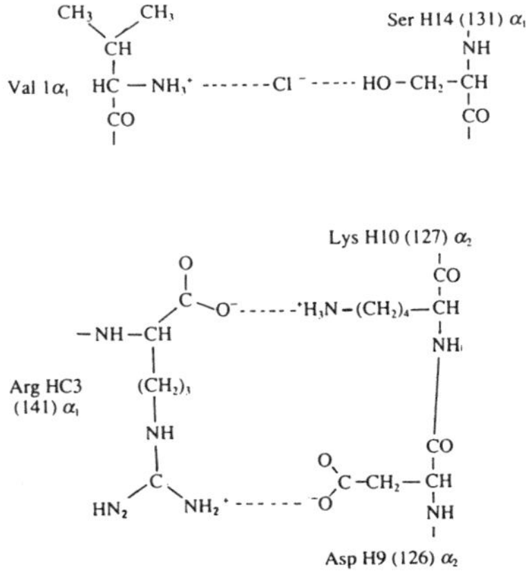

$$CH_3 \quad CH_3$$
$$\backslash \,/$$
$$CH$$
$$|$$
$$\text{Val 1}\alpha_1 \quad HC-NH_3{}^+ \text{-------} Cl^- \text{-----} HO-CH_2-CH \quad \begin{array}{l}\text{Ser H14 (131) }\alpha_1\\ | \\ NH \end{array}$$
$$| \qquad\qquad\qquad\qquad\qquad\qquad\qquad |$$
$$CO \qquad\qquad\qquad\qquad\qquad\qquad\qquad CO$$
$$| \qquad\qquad\qquad\qquad\qquad\qquad\qquad |$$

Lys H10 (127) α_2

$$\begin{array}{l} CO \\ | \end{array}$$
$$-NH-CH \quad \overset{O}{\overset{\|}{C}}-O^- \text{------} {}^+H_3N-(CH_2)_4-CH$$
$$| \qquad\qquad\qquad\qquad\qquad\qquad NH_3$$
$$\begin{array}{l}\text{Arg HC3}\\ \text{(141) }\alpha_1\end{array} \quad (CH_2)_3$$
$$|$$
$$NH \qquad\qquad\qquad\qquad\qquad CO$$
$$| \qquad\qquad\qquad\qquad\qquad |$$
$$\overset{}{\underset{HN_2}{C}} \overset{\;}{\underset{NH_2{}^+}{}} \text{-----} \overset{O}{\underset{O}{\overset{\backslash}{C}}} -CH_2-CH$$
$$\qquad\qquad\qquad\qquad\qquad\qquad NH$$
$$\qquad\qquad\qquad\qquad \text{Asp H9 (126) }\alpha_2$$

Figure 7 Salt bridges between the α-chains in the T-structure.

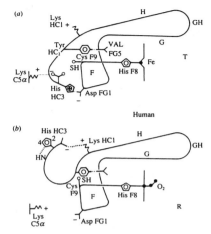

Figure 8   Change in conformation of histidine HC3 (146)β and cysteine F9 (93)β on-going from the T- to the R-structure. In the T-structure the imidazole of the histidine donates a hydrogen bond to Asp FG1 and is positively charged (pK$_a$ = 8.0). Its carboxylate accepts a hydrogen bond from Lys C5α. The SH is *cis* to CO and points away from the heme. In the R-structure the imidazole accepts a hydrogen bond from the histidine's main chain NH and has a pK$_a$ of 7.1 or below; and the C-terminal carboxylate accepts a weak hydrogen bond from Lys HC1. The SH group is *cis* to NH and in contact with Tyr HC2.

concerted shift of helices D and E and the CD segment together with the beginning of helix B, away from and across the heme.

The C-terminal histidines form different sets of hydrogen bonds in the T- and R-structures, and as a result their pK$_a$s drop on oxygenation. The conformation of the reactive sulfhydryl groups of Cys F9(93)β also changes (figure 8) (41).

In the T-structure the two β-subunits form a binding site for 2,3-diphosphoglycerate (Figure 10). In the R-structure the gap between the two β-chains becomes too narrow to accommodate it.

THE HETEROTROPIC LIGANDS

According to allosteric theory the low oxygen affinity of the T- as compared to that of the R-structure arises from increased energy and/or number of bonds between the subunits (31). The contact areas and the number of bonds between segments Cα_1 and FGβ_2 and between segments Cβ_2 and FGα_1 are about equal in the R- and T-structures (4); the C-terminal residues and DPG, on the other hand, form 14 salt bridges between the subunits that are absent in the R-structure (Figures 6–9). The bond energies of the four pairs of salt bridges made by the C-terminal residues have been measured. Those formed by the C-terminal histidines and histidines H21 (143) of the β-chains together contribute 7.6 kcal mol^{-1} (26), and those formed by arginine HC3 (141)α

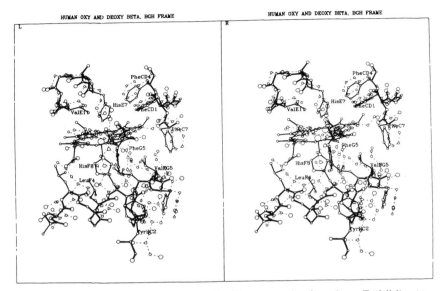

Figure 9   Change of tertiary structure near the β-heme on-going from deoxy-T *(full lines)* to oxy-R *(broken lines)*. Note how the heme moves to the right into the heme pocket, and the distal valine and histidine make way for the bound oxygen (from Perutz et al, 41).

contribute at least 4 kcal mol⁻1, which leaves only 300 cal mol^{-1} per salt bridge to be contributed by the remaining eight salt bridges, sufficient to account for the total free energy of cooperativity of 14.4 kcal/tetramer, because a salt bridge contributes usually at least 1 kcal mol^{-1} (14). Absence of any of the bridges raises K_T and lowers L. The salt bridges keep the subunits rigidly in the tertiary deoxy structure and hinder the movement of the iron atoms into the planes of the porphyrin nitrogens and the flattening of the porphyrins themselves. This hindrance manifests itself in spectroscopic and magnetic differences between liganded hemoglobins in the two quaternary structures; these have recently been reviewed (41).

All the heterotropic ligands lower the oxygen affinity by forming additional hydrogen bonds that specifically stabilize and constrain the T-structure. The most important heterotropic ligands are protons. The linkage of proton uptake to oxygen release, and vice versa, is known as the Bohr effect. For each mole of oxygen released at pH7.4 and 25°C, human Hb takes up 0.2 moles H^+ in a deionized solution, 0.5 moles H^+ in 0.1 M Cl^-, and 0.7 moles H^+ in the presence of a molar excess of DPG (19, 39). The identity of the residues that take up protons has been determined by X-ray crystallographic and chemical studies of normal and mutant hemoglobins. In deionized solutions all the protons are taken up by His HC3(146)β, which donates a hydrogen bond to Asp FG1(94)β in the T-structure and accepts a hydrogen bond from its own

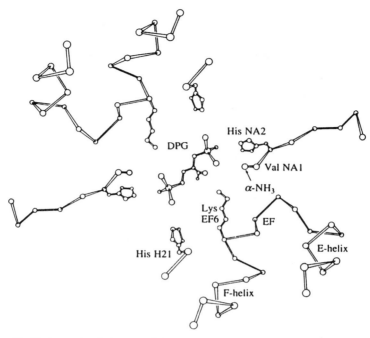

Figure 10 Hydrogen bonds between 2,3-diphosphoglycerate; and cationic groups of the β-chains in the T-structure. In the R-structure the gap between the EF corners closes and the N-termini move apart (from Arnone, 2).

main chain NH in the R-structure (Figure 8). In consequence its pK_a rises from 7.1 or less in oxyhemoglobin to 8.0 in deoxyhemoglobin (20, 27). The binding of Cl^- by the T-structure raises the pK_as of Val NA1(1)α (Figure 7) and Lys EF6(82)β, which contribute an additional 0.28 moles H^+ to the Bohr effect. DPG enters a cleft flanked by the N-termini and helices H of the β-chains and forms hydrogen bonds with Val NA1(1), His NA2(2), Lys EF6(82), and His H21(143) (Figure 10). The rise in pK_as of their cationic groups contributes 0.33 moles H^+ to the Bohr effect (19). Carbon dioxide forms carbamino groups with Val NA1(1)α and β, and these in turn make hydrogen bonds with cationic groups of the globin. All the groups that bind heterotropic ligands are at some distance from the hemes, consistent with Monod et al's prediction (30) that "no direct interaction need occur between the substrate of the (allosteric) protein and the regulatory metabolite which controls its activity".

In 0.1 M Tris HCl + 0.1 M NaCl at pH 7.4 and 21.5°C, the first mole of oxygen taken up releases 0.64($\pm$7) moles H^+, the second and third mole of oxygen combined release 1.62($\pm$27) moles H^+, and the fourth mole of oxygen releases only 0.05($\pm$6) moles H^+ (8). How is their release related to the allosteric transition from T to R? Allosteric theory allows the equilibrium constant $L_i = [T]/[R]$ at the ith step of oxygenation to be calculated from $L_i = L_o (K_R/K_T)^i$. Under the above non-physiologic conditions $L_1 = 8.7 \times 10^4 \times 0.0073 = 635$ (3, 17). Thus more than a quarter of the Bohr protons are discharged before 1/600 of the Hb molecules have switched from T to R, which implies that the hydrogen bonds responsible for H^+ discharge must break in the T-structure. The bulk of the protons are released in the T $\rightarrow$ R transition that takes place mostly at the second and third oxygenation steps. After the third oxygenation step $L_3 = 0.034$, which leaves a little more than 1/30 of the Hb molecules in the T-structure, roughly equivalent to the fraction of 1/20 of the protons discharged at the fourth oxygenation step.

EFFECTS OF ABNORMAL HEMOGLOBINS ON RESPIRATORY FUNCTION

Study of the abnormal human hemoglobins has taught us a great deal about the respiratory function. The $\alpha_1 \beta_2$ contact acts as a two-way switch between the T- and R-structures. Each position of the switch is stabilized by a different set of hydrogen bonds. Disruption of any bond that specifically stabilizes the R-structure lowers the oxygen affinity and raises the allosteric constant L, and disruption of any bond that stabilizes the T-structure does the reverse. For example, hemoglobin Kansas [Asn G4(102)$\beta\rightarrow$Thr] has a low oxygen affinity and low Hill's coefficient because the R-structure is destabilized (Figure 11), while hemoglobin Kempsey [Asp G1(99)$\rightarrow$Asn] has a high oxygen

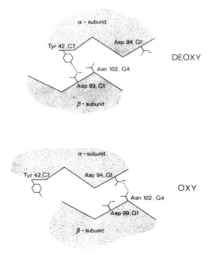

Figure 11   The $\alpha_1\beta_2$ contact as a two-way switch, showing alternative hydrogen bonds stabilizing the deoxy-T and oxy-R structures.

Springer et al (46, 47) have studied the protection of the heme iron from oxidation by replacing the distal histidine in sperm whale myoglobin by ten different amino acid residues and shaking the deoxygenated myoglobin solutions in air in 75 mM potassium phosphate + 25 mM EDTA pH 7.0 at 37°C. All replacements reduced the oxygen affinity and accelerated autoxidation. Phenylalanine, methionine, and arginine produced the smallest accelerations (~50-fold); aspartate the largest (350-fold).

How can these results be interpreted? Paradoxically, combination with oxygen protects the heme iron from oxidation, as can be shown by performing the same experiments at several atmospheres of pure oxygen. Apparently oxidation occurs in that fraction of molecules that is deoxygenated at any one moment. The larger that fraction is at atmospheric oxygen pressure, the faster myoglobin autoxidizes. For example, replacement of the distal histidine by phenylalanine reduced the oxygen affinity 170-fold, so that a larger fraction of myoglobin molecules will have remained deoxygenated at atmospheric oxygen pressure and therefore have become autoxidized. However, this can be only part of the explanation, because the replacement of histidine by glycine reduces the oxygen affinity merely elevenfold, yet accelerates autoxidation over a hundredfold.

Autoxidation is catalyzed by protons, hence the 350-fold acceleration by aspartate. I suggest that the distal histidine protects the ferrous heme iron by acting as a proton trap. The distal histidine has a pK_a of about 5.5; at neutral pH it is protonated only at N_s, which faces the solvent. Any proton entering the heme pocket of deoxymyoglobin would be bound by N_ϵ, and simultaneously N_δ would release its proton to the solvent. When the histidine side chain swings out of the heme pocket, the protons would interchange, restoring the previous state. No other amino acid side chain could function in this way. Evolution is a brilliant chemist.

HEMOGLOBIN AS A DRUG RECEPTOR

In a search for compounds that might prevent the aggregation of deoxyhemoglobin S in patients with sickle cell anemia, two anti-lipidemic drugs, clofibric acid and its analogue bezafibrate, were found to lower the oxygen affinity of hemoglobin. X-ray analysis of crystals grown in the presence of these compounds showed that they combine with deoxy, but not with oxyhemoglobin. They stabilize the T-structure by combining with sites in the central cavity that are about 20Å away from the DPG binding sites; their effects and that of DPG on the allosteric equilibrium are additive (40).

This discovery led Lalezari to synthesize a family of new compounds related to, but more active than bezafibrate (24, 50); one of these, which has the formula shown in Figure 13, has turned out to be the most powerful

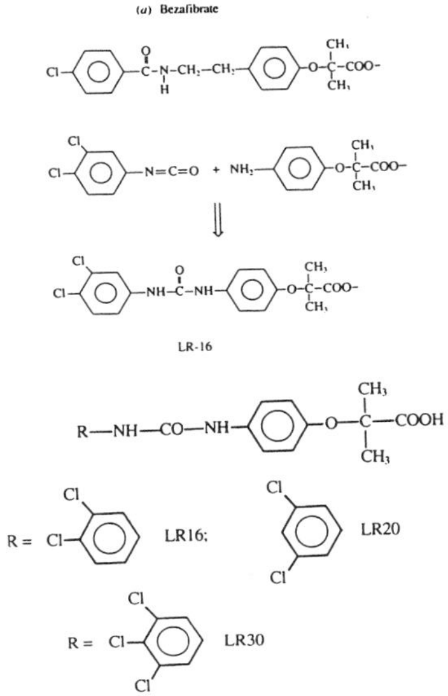

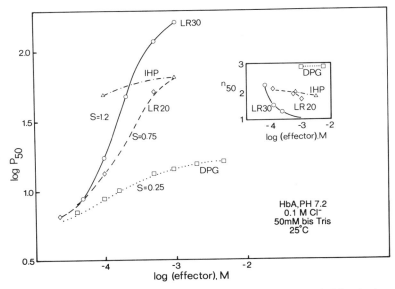

Figure 13   Novel allosteric effectors of hemoglobin: bezafibrate, an anti-lipidemic drug, and compounds derived from it by Dr. I. Lalezari (50).

Figure 14   Effect on partial pressure of oxygen at half-saturation (P_{50}) of 2,3-diphosphoglycerate (DPG), inositol hexaphosphate (IHP) and two of Dr. Lalezari's synthetic effectors LR20 and LR30. The inset shows their effect on Hill's coefficient at half-saturation. At 1mM LR30 the hemoglobin is only half-saturated at 2 × atmospheric oxygen pressure and its Hill's coefficient is near unity because the allosteric constant L is very large. (50).

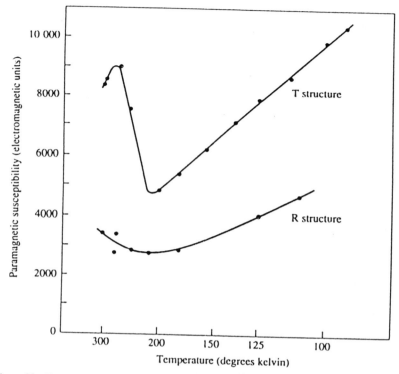

Figure 15   Temperature dependence of paramagnetic susceptibility of carp azidemethemoglobin in the R- and T-structures. Below about 200°K the susceptibility rises with falling temperature in accordance with Curie's law. Above that temperature a thermal equilibrium between a high and a low spin form masks that behavior, since the high spin form gains stability with rising tempera- ture. It has longer Fe-N bond distances than the low spin form. Tension at the heme in the T-structure therefore shifts the equilibrium towards higher spin (from Messana et al 28).

allosteric effector yet found. At an effector concentration equimolar to heme and at pH6, it lowers the oxygen affinity of solutions of human hemoglobin to a level found until now only in fish hemoglobins that exhibit a Root effect i.e. a drastic drop in oxygen affinity below pH7 (Figure 14). In such fish hemoglobins, the tension on the heme in the T-structure that is associated with the low oxygen affinity has been demonstrated directly. In azidemethemoglo- bin the iron is in a thermal equilibrium between two different spin states that are characterized by different lengths of the iron nitrogen bonds; they are longer in the high spin than in the low spin state. In azidemethemoglobin of trout, transition from the R- to the T-structure induces a transition to higher spin, equivalent to a stretching of the Fe-N bonds (28, 37). This is manifested by an increase in paramagnetic susceptibility equivalent to a change in free

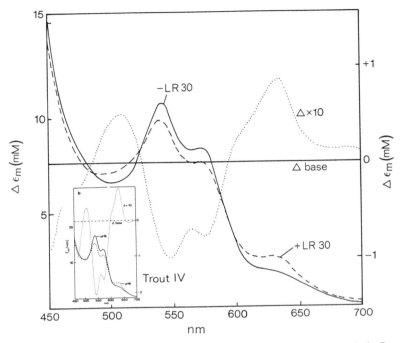

Figure 16 Optical absorption spectra of human and trout IV azidemethemoglobin in the R- and T-structures, showing the rise in intensity of the high spin bands at 500 and 630 nm and the fall of the low spin bands at 540 and 570 nm. *Full lines:* T-structure; *broken lines:* R-structure; *dotted lines:* difference spectra 10 × enlarged (50).

energy of 1 kcal/mol (Figure 15) and also by a change in optical spectra that show a rise in intensity of the high spin bands at 500 and 630 nm and a drop in intensity of the low spin bands at 540 and 570 nm. Until recently it was not possible to induce this transition in human azidemethemoglobin (43), but combination with the powerful new synthetic effector induced a difference spectrum identical to that of trout hemoglobin, which demonstrates that the hemes are under tension also in human hemoglobin in the liganded T-state (Figure 16).

X-ray analysis and oxygen equilibria show that four molecules of the effector combine with one molecule of human deoxyhemoglobin both in the crystal and in solution. One pair of symmetry-related binding sites is close to those of bezafibrate; the other pair is nearly at right angles to the first (Figure 17). The four trichlorobenzene moieties form a parallel stack. Their close packing seems to dominate their mode of binding. The combination of human

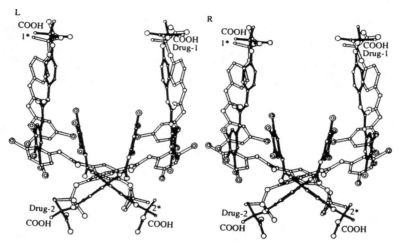

Figure 17 Arrangement of the two effectors LR20 and LR 30 in the central cavity of hemoglobin. The vertical pairs lie mainly between the two α-chains in sites that overlap those of bezafibrate. The other pairs occupy positions not taken up by bezafibrate, and the sites of the 3,5-dichloro derivative (LR20, open bonds) differ from those occupied by the 3,4,5-trichloro derivative (LR30, shaded bonds). The four trichlorobenzene moieties form a close-packed parallel stack right in the center of the hemoglobin molecule, while the dichlorobenzene moieties stack in separate pairs. (50).

deoxyhemoglobin with the effectors induced no stereochemical changes at the allosteric core that were visible at 2.5Å resolution, and they produced a decrease of the Fe-N$_\epsilon$ stretching frequency by only 1–2cm^{-1} (T. Kitagawa, private communication). Only in the liganded T-structure do the effectors make themselves felt strongly at the hemes.

The work on drug binding by hemoglobin has led to generalizations that are relevant to the binding of effectors, transmitters, and drugs to other proteins. The stereochemistry of binding is determined by the available van der Waals space and, within that space, by interactions of a wide range of polarity, from strong hydrogen bonds between ionized groups of opposite charge to weak interactions between aromatic quadrupoles, and non-polar interactions between aliphatic hydrocarbons. The detailed stereochemistry is governed by a tendency to maximize the sum of the energy of electrostatic interactions, for example by aligning effectors relative to the protein so that the mutual polarizabilities are maximized. Drugs may influence the allosteric equilibrium of a protein receptor in the same direction as the natural effector even though they are chemically unrelated to it because proteins may offer a variety of binding sites not used in nature (40).

Literature Cited

1. Angel, W.-L., Karplus, M., Poyart, C., Burseaux, E. 1988. Analysis of proton release in oxygen binding by haemoglobin: implications for the cooperative mechanism. *Biochemistry* 27:1285–1301

2. Arnone, A. 1972. X-ray diffraction study of binding of 2,3-diphosphoglycerate to human deoxyhaemoglobin. *Nature* 237:146–49

3. Baldwin, J. M. 1975. Structure and function of haemoglobin. *Progr. Biophys. Mol. Biol.* 29:225–320

4. Baldwin, J. M., Chothia, C. 1979. Haemoglobin: the structural changes related to ligand binding and its allosteric mechanism. *J. Mol. Biol.* 129:183–91

5. Bunn, H. F., Forget, G. B. 1985. *Hemoglobin, molecular and clinical aspects.* Philadelphia: Saunders. 690 pp.

6. Bolognesi, M., Cannillo, E., Ascenzi, P., Giacometti, G. M. Merli, A., et al 1982. Reactivity of ferric *Aplysia* and sperm whale myoglobins towards imidazole: X-ray and binding study. *J. Molec. Biol.* 158:301–15

7. Calhoun, D. B., Vanderkooi, J. M., Woodrow, G. V. III, Englander, S. W. 1983. Penetration of dioxygen into proteins studied by quenching of phosphorescence and fluorescence. *Biochemistry* 22:1526–32

8. Chu, A. H., Turner, B. W., Ackers, G. K. 1984. Effects of protons on the oxygen-linked subassembly in human haemoglobin. *Biochemistry* 23:604–17

9. Dalvit, C., Wright, P. E. 1987. Assignment of resonances in the ^1H nuclear magnetic resonance spectrum of the carbonmonoxide complex of sperm whale myoglobin by phase-sensitive two-dimensional techniques. *J. Mol. Biol.* 194:313–27

9a. Derewenda, Z., Dodson, G., Emsley, P., Harris, D., Nagai, K., Perutz, M. F., Renaud, J.-P. 1989. The stereochemistry of CO binding to normal human adult and Cowtown haemoglobin. *J. Molec. Biol.* In press

10. Dickerson, R. E., Geis, I. 1983. *Hemoglobin: structure, function, evolution, pathology.* Menlo Park: Cummings. 176 pp.

11. Elber, R., Karplus, M. 1989. Molecular dynamics simulations of myoglobin. In press

12. Englander, S. W., Kallenbach, N. R. 1984. Hydrogen exchange and structural dynamics of proteins and nucleic acids. *Q. Rev. Biophys.* 16:521–65

13. Fermi, G., Perutz, M. F. 1981. *Atlas of Molecular Structures in Biology: Haemoglobin & Myoglobin.* Oxford: Clarendon. 104 pp.

14. Fersht, A. R., Leatherbarrow, R. J., Wells, T. N. C. 1986. Structure and activity of the tyrosyl-tRNA synthetase: the hydrogen bond in catalysis and specificity. *Phil. Trans. Roy. Soc. A* 317:305–20

15. Gelin, R. G., Lee, A. W.-M., Karplus, M. 1983. Hemoglobin tertiary structural change on ligand binding. Its role in the cooperative mechanism. *J. Mol. Biol.* 171:489–559

16. Gill, S. J., di Cera, E., Doyle, M. L., Roberts, C. H. 1988. New twists of an old story: hemoglobin. *Trends. Biochem Sci.* 13:465–67

17. Imai, K. 1982. *Allosteric Effects in Haemoglobin* Cambridge: Cambridge Univ. Press. 275 pp.

18. Johnson, K. A., Olson, J. S., Phillips, G. N. Jr. 1989. Structure of myoglobinethyl isocyanide: histidine as a swinging door for ligand entry. *J. Mol. Biol.* 207:459–60

19. Kilmartin, J. V. 1974. Influence of DPG on the Bohr effect of human haemoglobin. *FEBS Letts.* 38:147–48

20. Kilmartin, J. V., Breen, J. J., Roberts, G. C. K., Ho, C. 1973. Direct measurement of the pK values of an alkaline Bohr group in human haemoglobin. *Proc. Nat. Acad. Sci. USA* 70:1246–49

21. Kim, K., Fettinger, J., Sessler, J. L., Cyr, M., Hugdahl, J., et al. 1989. Structural characterization of a sterically encumbered iron (II) porphyrin CO complex. *J. Amer. Chem. Soc.* 111:403–5

22. Kuriyan, J., Wilz, S., Karplus, M., Petsko, G. A. 1986. X-ray structure and refinement of carbonmonoxy (FeII)-myoglobin at 1.5Å resolution. *J. Mol. Biol.* 192:133–54

23. Lakowicz, J. R., Weber, G. 1973. Quenching of protein fluorescence by oxygen. Detection of structural fluctuations in proteins on the nanosecond time scale. *Biochemistry* 12:4171–79

24. Lalezari, I., Rahbar, S., Lalezari, P., Fermi, G., Perutz, M. F. 1988. LR16, a compound with potent effects on the oxygen affinity of hemoglobin, on blood cholesterol, and on low density lipoprotein. *Proc. Nat. Acad. Sci. USA* 85:6117–21

25. Liddington, R., Derewenda, Z., Dodson, G., Harris, D. 1988. Structure of liganded T-state of haemoglobin identities the origin of cooperative oxygen binding. *Nature* 331:725–28

26. Louie, G., Tran, T., Englander, J. J., Englander, S. W. 1988. Allosteric energy at the hemoglobin β-chain C-terminus studied by hydrogen exchange. *J. Mol. Biol.* 201:755–64

27. Matsukawa, S., Itatani, Y., Mawatari, K., Shimokawa, Y., Yoneyama, Y. 1978. Quantitative evaluation for the role β-146 His and β-143 His residues in the Bohr effect of human haemoglobin in the presence of 0.1M chloride ion. *J. Biol. Chem.* 259:11479–86

28. Messana, C., Cerdonio, M., Shenkin, P., Noble, R. W., Fermi, G., et al 1978. Influence of quaternary structure of the globin on thermal spin equilibria in different methaemoglobin derivatives. *Biochemistry* 17:3652–62

29. Momenteau, M., Scheidt, W. R., Eigenbrot, C. W., Reed, C. A. 1988. A deoxymyoglobin model with a sterically unhindered axial imidazole. *J. Am. Chem. Soc.* 110:1207–15

30. Monod, J., Changeux, J. P., Jacob, F. 1963. Allosteric proteins and molecular control systems. *J. Mol. Biol.* 6:306–29

31. Monod, J., Wyman, J., Changeux, J. P. 1965. On the nature of allosteric transitions: a plausible model. *J. Mol. Biol.* 12:88–118

32. Olson, J. S., Mathews, A. J., Rohlfs, R. J., Springer, B. A., Edelberg, K. D., et al 1988. The role of the distal histidine in myoglobin and haemoglobin. *Nature,* 336:265–66

33. Perrella, M., Sabionedda, L., Lamaja, M., Rossi-Bernardi, L. 1986. The intermediate compounds between human hemoglobin and carbon monoxide at equilibrium and during approach to equilibrium. *J. Biol. Chem.* 261:8391–96

34. Perrella, M., Colosimo, A., Benazzi, L., Samaja, M., Rossi-Bernardi, L. 1988. Intermediate compounds between hemoglobin and carbonmonoxide under equilibrium conditions. *Symp. Oxygen Binding Heme Proteins,* Asilomar, Pacific Grove, Calif.

35. Perutz, M. F., Mathews, F. S. 1966. An X-ray study of azide methaemoglobin. *J. Mol. Biol.* 21:199–202

36. Perutz, M. F. 1970. Stereochemistry of cooperative effects in haemoglobin. *Nature* 228:726–39

37. Perutz, M. F., Sanders, J. K. M., Chenery, D. H., Noble, R. W., Pennelly, R. R., et al 1978. Interactions between the quaternary structure of the globin and the spin state of the heme in ferric mixed

NOTE ADDED IN PROOF

50. Lalezari, I., Lalezari, P., Poyart, C., Marden, M., Kister, J., et al. 1990. *Biochemistry* In press

spin derivatives of hemoglobin. *Biochemistry* 17:3640–52

38. Perutz, M. F. 1979. Regulation of oxygen affinity of hemoglobin: influence of structure of the globin on the heme. *Annu. Rev. Biochem.* 48:327–86

39. Perutz, M. F., Kilmartin, J. V., Nishikura, K., Fogg, J. H., Butler, P. J. G., et al. 1980. Identification of residues contributing to the Bohr effect of human haemoglobin. *J. Mol. Biol.* 138:649–70

40. Perutz, M. F., Fermi, G., Abraham, D. J., Poyart, C., Bursaux, E. 1986. Hemoglobin as a receptor of drugs and peptides: X-ray studies of the stereochemistry of binding. *J. Amer. Chem. Soc.* 108:1064–78

41. Perutz, M. F., Fermi, G., Luisi, B., Shaanan, B., Liddington, R. C. 1987. Stereochemistry of cooperative effects in hemoglobin. *Acc. Chem. Res.* 20:309–21

42. Phillips, S. E. V., Schoenborn, B. P. 1981. Neutron diffraction reveals oxygen-histidine hydrogen bond in myoglobin. *Nature* 292:81–82

43. Philo, S., Dreyer, U. 1985. Quaternary structure has little influence on spin states in mixed-spin human methemoglobins. *Biochemistry* 24:2985–91

44. Ringe, D., Petsko, G. E., Kerr, D. E., de Montellano, F. R. O. 1984. Reaction of myoglobin with phenylhydrazine—a molecular doorstop. *Biochemistry* 23:2–4

45. Shaanan, B. 1983. Structure of human oxyhaemoglobin at 2.1Å resolution. *J. Mol. Biol.* 171:31–50

46. Springer, B. A., Egeberg, K. D., Sligar, S. G., Rohlfs, R. J., Mathews, A. J., et al. 1989. Discrimination between oxygen and carbonmonoxide and inhibition of autodixation by myoglobin. *J. Biol. Chem.* 264:3057–60

47. Springer, B. A., Egeberg, K. D., Sligar, S. G., Rohlfs, R. J., Mathews, A. J., et al. 1989. Site-directed mutagenesis of sperm whale myoglobin: role of His E7 and Val E11 in ligand binding. *J. Biol. Chem.* In press

48. Szabo, A. 1978. The kinetics of haemoglobin and transition state theory. *Proc. Nat. Acad. Sci. USA* 75:2108–11

49. Watson, H. C., Kendrew, J. C. 1961. Comparison between the amino-acid sequences of sperm whale myoglobin and of human haemoglobin. *Nature* 190:670–72

Annu. Rev. Physiol. 1990. 52:27–42

Ca²⁺-ACTIVATED CELL VOLUME RECOVERY MECHANISMS

Sidney K. Pierce[1] and Alexander D. Politis[2]

Department of Zoology, University of Maryland, College Park, Maryland 20742

KEY WORDS: volume regulation, osmoregulation, calmodulin, stretch-activated channels, cytoskeleton

INTRODUCTION

Cellular swelling occurs in response to a hypoosmotic stress. All cells seem to have some capacity to counteract this swelling by a mechanism that regulates the intracellular concentrations of certain osmotically active particles called osmolytes. The osmolytes are of two main types, inorganic ions and small molecular weight organic compounds. Most of the existing literature indicates that ionic osmolytes, usually some combination of K^+ or (less often) Na^+, with Cl^-, predominate the volume recovery mechanism in cells from animals that do not routinely encounter high (perhaps to a maximum of 300–400 mosm/kg H_2O, hereafter designated mosm) external osmotic concentrations. In addition, most of the literature also indicates that organic osmolytes, usually free amino acids or quaternary ammonium compounds, are the major osmolytes in cells from organisms that normally encounter either a higher or wider variation in external osmotic pressure. Marine and estuarine animals are the usual examples of this latter type. Available data, although as yet too limited to permit firm generalizations, suggest that the cells that regulate volume with ions often have an organic osmolyte component [Ehrlich ascites cells (26), mammalian brain and heart (58, 59), mammalian kidney (3, 24,

[1]Center of Marine Biotechnology, 600 E. Lombard Street, Baltimore, Maryland

[2]Uniformed Services University of the Health Sciences, Department of Microbiology, 4301 Jones Bridge Road, Bethesda, Maryland 20814

0066-4278/90/0315-0027$02.00

68), Madin-Darby canine kidney (MDCK) cells (50)], which becomes increasingly important as external osmotic concentrations rise above 300–400 mosm. Apparently, once intracellular salt concentrations rise above this range of osmotic concentrations, the salts begin to cause structural perturbations of the intracellular proteins. As a result cells have turned to other types of osmolytes at higher osmotic concentrations (see 69, for a review of this phenomenon). Even below 300–400 mosm, organic osmolytes may play an important, albeit usually ignored, role in osmoregulation by the cells of terrestrial animals. For example, the free amino acid concentration in MDCK cells exceeds that of intracellular Cl^- (50). In cells from the rat kidney tubule, ionic osmolytes can not account for 100–650 mosm of the osmolyte pool, much of which consists of small molecular weight molecules such as amino acids, glycine betaine, sorbitol, and glycerophosphorylcholine (24). Similarly it has recently been recognized that the cells of several marine animals [*Glycera* red coelomocyte (12), *Cancer* walking leg muscle (36), *Noetia* red blood cell (57), *Limulus* heart (63)] have an ionic component to volume recovery that complements organic osmolyte regulation. In these marine invertebrate cell types the release of ionic and organic osmolytes occurs with very distinct time courses. The ions leave the cells immediately upon application of the hypoosmotic stress, followed later by the organic osmolytes (36, 57, 63). These data clearly suggest that combined, coordinated inorganic and organic osmolyte regulation may be a common feature to all cells, but we need to test the matter in a wider array of cell types.

ROLE OF Ca^{2+} IN CELL VOLUME RECOVERY

Both extracellular and intracellular $[Ca^{2+}]$ are too low in animals to be useful as osmolytes. However it is well established that Ca^{2+} affects volume recovery of cells following a hypoosmotic stress. In many cases removal of extracellular Ca^{2+} blocks volume recovery by somehow preventing osmolyte efflux. In other instances the volume recovery process is not sensitive to $[Ca^{2+}]_o$, but changes in $[Ca^{2+}]_i$ alter volume recovery following hypoosmotic stress, again by altering the pattern of osmolyte efflux. Only one report (50) indicates that cell volume recovery from a hypoosmotic stress was insensitive to Ca^{2+}. MDCK cells that had been incubated for up to four hr in Ca^{2+}-free medium containing EGTA and the divalent cation ionophore, A23187, recovered volume with a normal osmolyte efflux. However another report (1) found that volume recovery in MDCK cells was indeed Ca^{2+}-sensitive and that different MDCK cell lines showed different sensitivities to A23187, perhaps explaining the earlier (50) result.

Whether or not the volume recovery from hypoosmotic stress is sensitive to

$[Ca^{2+}]_o$ or only $[Ca^{2+}]_i$, the divalent cation causes its effect by altering transport of at least one of the two general types of osmolytes. First, in many of the terrestrial vertebrate cell types the volume recovery from a hypoosmotic stress is accomplished by an efflux of K^+ and Cl^-. In some of these cell types the K^+ and Cl^- conductances are separate [for example, frog urinary bladder cells (13), human lymphocytes (22), human intestinal epithelial cells (25), Ehrlich ascites cells (28), Chinese hamster ovary cells (52)], in others the K^+ movements are Cl^--dependent [for example, red blood cells from *Amphiuma* (5), human (30), sheep (33), dog (41), duck (55), and *Necturus* gall bladder epithelial cells (32)]. Coupled or not, alterations in $[Ca^{2+}]$ change the volume-regulating K^+ and Cl^- effluxes. Most of the data indicate that Ca^{2+} specifically affects the K^+ movement, because quinine, a drug that inhibits Ca^{2+}-dependent K^+ transport, blocks or reduces cell volume recovery (18, 22, 25, 27, 50) (Figure 1). There is less evidence for an effect of Ca^{2+} on Cl^- efflux. Volume regulatory Cl^- conductances are still activated in response to hypoosmotic stress in Ca^{2+}-depleted human lymphocytes (22) and Ca^{2+}-depleted human gut epithelial cells (25). On the other hand, A23187 promotes Cl^- loss from hypoosmotically stressed Ehrlich ascites cells (27). Only one of the above studies has considered the possibility of Ca^{2+} effects on the organic osmolyte side of cell volume recovery. The MDCK cells, whose pattern of volume regulation was not affected by Ca^{2+}, not surprisingly also showed no effect of Ca^{2+} on either ion or amino acid regulation following hypoosmotic stress (50).

The second type of Ca^{2+} effect on osmolyte regulation occurs in cells of marine animals in which the amino acid efflux is altered by variation in $[Ca^{2+}]_o$. Although marine animal cell types recently have been studied less broadly than the cells from terrestrial animals, the following picture is emerging. Following a hypoosmotic stress the cells of marine animals rapidly lost K^+ or Na^+, both accompanied by Cl^- (reviewed by 42; more recently 12, 15, 36, 57). This rapid ionic efflux undoubtedly prevented lysis and initiated the volume recovery. However these same studies found that at time periods ranging from a few minutes to hours following the ionic response, depending upon the cell type, an efflux of amino acids or glycine betaine occurred that sustained the volume recovery. In one case the depleted ion levels partially returned toward pre-stress levels (63) as the efflux of organic oxmolytes continued. In Ca^{2+}-depleted media, volume recovery from hypoosmotic stress was blocked or reduced in molluscan *(Noetia)* red blood cells. The inorganic ion reduction occurred normally, but the efflux of amino acids was markedly reduced (2, 57). In contrast to the terrestrial cell types cited above, the ionic portions of volume recovery were not affected by the divalent cation in the *Noetia* cell (57).

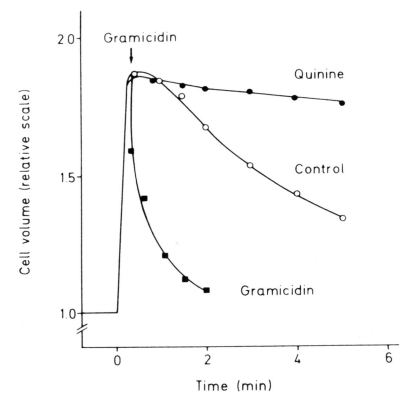

Figure 1 The role of the Ca^{2+}-dependent K^+ channel in volume recovery from a hypoosmotic stress by Ehrlich ascites cells. The Na^+ in all the experimental media has been replaced with choline, and Ca^{2+} is present at 1mM throughout. At time 0 the one batch of cells was exposed to the Na^+-free hypotonic medium containing quinine (which blocks the Ca^{2+}-dependent K^+ channel), which prevented volume recovery. Another batch was exposed to a Na^+-free hypotonic medium (control) and recovered volume normally. A third batch was exposed to the Na^+-free hypotonic medium to which gramacidin had been added. Volume recovery in this latter batch was potentiated, indicating that the K^+ permeability of these cells is rate-limiting during the recovery. This figure was reprinted from (27) with permission.

In summary, the available data indicate that Ca^{2+} is undoubtedly involved in the regulation of inorganic osmolytes in the cells of terrestrial vertebrates, but perhaps not of marine invertebrates. Conversely, Ca^{2+} has a major effect on the regulation of amino acid osmolytes in the cells of marine invertebrates, but there are almost no data on the organic osmolytes in terrestrial vertebrate cell types. Whether or not these differences are phylogenetic or simply reflect lack of appropriate study is not clear at this point.

Regardless of the phyletic source of the cell type, virtually all of the above studies came to the conclusion that Ca^{2+} was involved in the initiation or regulation of the volume recovery mechanism, but the nature of the role was not clear.

Calcium has several sites of action that mediate a variety of cellular functions. As a result, several possibilities exist that might explain the basis of Ca^{2+} action on hypoosmotic volume recovery. Indeed, after several years of investigation into the matter, evidence has accumulated pointing to more than one regulatory system.

SITE OF Ca^{2+} ACTION

A change in $[Ca^{2+}]_o$ might exert its effect at an extracellular site or an intracellular site or both. Most studies have come to the conclusion, often based on experiments that have altered $[Ca^{2+}]_i$ with A23187 (see above), that the site of Ca^{2+} action is at some intracellular location. In addition, volume recovery in the *Noetia* cell could be titrated by $[Ca^{2+}]_o$ in the presence of the calcium ionophore, ionomycin (Figure 2). In spite of this conclusion only a few attempts to demonstrate changes in $[Ca^{2+}]_i$ during the volume recovery have been reported. Of those, one (49) found no change (using quin-2) in $[Ca^{2+}]_i$ in lymphocytes following a hypoosmotic stress, although volume recovery in these cells was altered and K^+ loss (measured as ^{86}Rb) reduced by a Ca^{2+}-depleted medium (22). On the other hand, cell swelling of *Amphiuma* red cells caused an increase in $[Ca^{2+}]_i$, measured with Arsenazo III (6). Two other studies, using ^{45}Ca flux (67, 44), found that hypoosmotic stress produced an increase in $[Ca^{2+}]_i$. First, the rate of ^{45}Ca uptake by isolated toad bladder cells increased almost threefold following hypoosmotic stress, and measurements with quin-2 similarly indicated $[Ca^{2+}]_i$ increases (67). Second, a net influx of ^{45}Ca occurred into both polychaete *(Glycera)* red coelomocytes and *Noetia* erythrocytes immediately following exposure of the cells to a hypoosmotic stress. The influx was initiated by the hypoosmotic stress rather than by the reduced ion concentrations because a hypoionic solution made isotonic with sucrose did not produce Ca^{2+} influx into either invertebrate cell type (44). Thus in the few cell types where the measurement has been made, with the exception of the lymphocyte, $[Ca^{2+}]_i$ increases rapidly following a hypoosmotic stress. In addition, in the toad bladder cells, the *Noetia* and *Glycera* red cells, the source of the increased $[Ca^{2+}]_i$ was extracellular Ca^{2+}.

These few studies may ultimately prove to be exceptions as other cell types with external Ca^{2+}-sensitive volume regulatory mechanisms are tested. However at present the site of Ca^{2+} action seems to be an intracellular one, regardless of whether the Ca^{2+} source is in the extracellular fluids or from intracellular stores.

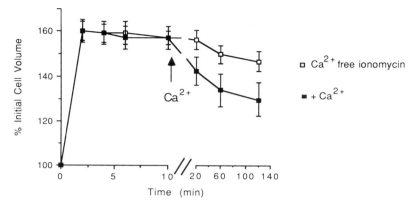

Figure 2 The effects of the calcium ionophore, ionomycin, on volume recovery by the *Noetia* erythrocyte. At time 0 the cells, taken from animals adapted to sea water, were split into two batches and exposed to a Ca^{2+}-free hypoosmotic medium containing 0.05 μM ionomycin (Ca^{2+}-free ionomycin), which produced the swelling. After 10 min the medium was changed on one batch from the Ca^{2+}-free solution to a hypoosmotic ionomycin solution containing Ca^{2+} (*+ Ca^{2+}, closed squares*), while the other batch was maintained in the Ca^{2+}-free solution (*open squares*). The arrow indicates point of the Ca^{2+} addition. Following Ca^{2+} return volume recovery began immediately.

Ca^{2+}-ACTIVATED VOLUME RECOVERY MECHANISMS—SOME POSSIBILITIES

Calmodulin

While sensitivity to Ca^{2+} is a trait common among cell volume recovery mechanisms, the actual mechanism may be different from cell type to cell type. For example, two groups of antipsychotic drugs, the phenothiazines and the diphenylbutylpiperidines, are well-known calmodulin inhibitors and affect the volume recovery of several cell types. Trifluoperazine, chlorpromazine (phenothiazines), and pimozide (diphenylbutylpiperidine) all blocked volume recovery as well as Ca^{2+}-induced volume changes in human lymphocytes (21, 22). The effect of these calmodulin antagonists was due to a blockade of osmolyte efflux, K^+ (measured as $^{86}Rb^+$) in this case. In Ehrlich ascites cells where volume recovery is also accomplished by a Ca^{2+}-sensitive activation of separate K^+ and Cl^- pathways, both of the conductances were inhibited by pimozide (27). In addition, pimozide reduced the taurine efflux under isosmotic conditions (anisosmotic conditions were not tested) from Ehrlich ascites cells (31). Both chlorpromazine and trifluoperazine reduced the Ca^{2+}-regulated K^+-H^+ exchange used by osmotically swollen *Amphiuma* red blood cells for volume recovery (6). Trifluoperazine prevented KCl-regulated (quinidine-inhibited) volume recovery in *Necturus* gall bladder epithelial cells (18). Finally, cell volume recovery from hypoosmotic stress in the *Noetia* red cell is also blocked by phenothiazines. However unlike the vertebrate cell types, K^+ regulation in this invertebrate cell was not the target of the drugs. Instead, amino acid efflux was reduced by both chlorpromazine and trifluoperazine (44).

All of these results may indicate that calmodulin is involved in volume recovery from hypoosmotic stress, but this interpretation must be viewed with caution. While the phenothiazines are well-known calmodulin blockers, they are also nonspecific. In addition to the calmodulin effects, these compounds are local anesthetics, exerting membrane effects that do not involve calmodulin (39). They also block protein kinase C, itself a Ca^{2+}-activated enzyme (29, 37, 54) and, at least in some secretory cells, interfere with voltage-sensitive Ca^{2+} channels (10, 20, 66). These alternate effects have not generally been ruled out in volume recovery studies. However the sulfoxide derivatives of the phenothiazines, which retain the anesthetic properties of the parent drug, but at low doses do not block calmodulin (see for instance, 38, 61), had no effect on cell volume recovery of either human lymphocytes (22) or the *Noetia* red blood cell (43). In addition, the hypoosmotically initiated ^{45}Ca influx into the molluscan red blood cell proceeds unabated in the presence of either trifluoperazine or chlorpromazine. Therefore, in these two cell types the anesthetic effects of the phenothiazines do not seem to be involved in the blockade of volume recovery and, in addition, in the *Noetia* red cell, the drugs did not inhibit Ca^{2+} entry (44). Finally, there are fewer data yet on the issue of protein kinase C and volume recovery from hypoosmotic stress. In the clam red blood cells volume recovery was potentiated by a phorbol ester (TPA) known to stimulate protein kinase C activity (43). However the potentiation was produced by an alteration in K^+ regulation, rather than in the Ca^{2+}-sensitive amino acid efflux. TPA also had an effect on human lymphocytes during hyperosmotic stress where Ca^{2+}-sensitive Na^+-H^+ exchange was stimulated by the drug (23). Na^+-H^+ exchange is not the same volume recovery mechanism that the lymphocyte uses in hypoosmotic stress, so while protein kinase C may be involved during recovery from hyperosmotic stress, the involvement of that enzyme in the Ca^{2+}-mediated responses to low osmotic concentrations is not established.

Altogether the pharmacological data from both terrestrial and marine animals suggest that calmodulin may be activated by the changes in $[Ca^{2+}]_i$ caused, in turn, by hypoosmotic stress. However the *Noetia* red cell is the only type where the other known targets of the phenothiazines have been ruled out. While this comparative pharmacology is not an entirely sufficient demonstration, calmodulin activation after the Ca^{2+} influx initiated by the hypoosmotic stress is still a viable hypothesis.

Cytoskeleton

Some evidence suggests that changes in the organization of the cytoskeleton occur that are, at least temporally, associated with cell volume recovery following a hypoosmotic stress. For instance, volume recovery of rat liver cells swollen by exposure to cold was prevented by the microfilament disrupting drug, cytochalasin (62). The volume recovery of hypoosmotically stressed *Necturus* gall bladder cells was reduced by 75% with cytochalasin B treatment. Colchicine had no effect, thereby eliminating microtubules in the response (16–18). Cytochalasin B also inhibited the volume recovery of hypoosmotically stressed *Carcinus maenas* axons without effecting the usual K^+ reduction (amino acids were not measured) (19). On the other hand, cytochalasin D, which specifically inhibits actin polymerization, potentiated cell volume recovery by *Noetia* red blood cells. In this case, the amino acid efflux was stimulated by the cytochalasin, but as in the crab axon, K^+ regulation was normal (56). The amount of sedimentable actin in the *Noetia* cytoskeleton declines following hypoosmotic stress in a manner coincident with the onset of amino acid efflux (Figure 3) following the Ca^{2+} influx. The change in actin was inhibited by both Ca^{2+}-depleted medium and trifluoperazine (56).

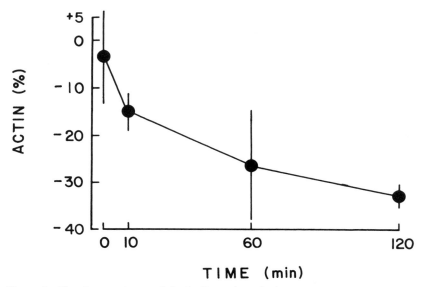

Figure 3 The decrease in cytoskeletal oligomeric actin in *Noetia* red cells following a hypoosmotic stress. At time 0 red cells isolated from animals adapted to sea water were exposed to a hypoosmotic stress. At the intervals indicated, cells were removed in an actin-stabilizing buffer, and the actin quantified by densitometry of SDS-polyacrylamide gels. After two hr of hypoosmotic stress, the amount of polymerized cytoskeletal actin had decreased by 30%. This figure is reprinted from (56) with permission.

Cytochalasin B also stimulated an isosmotic volume reduction in MDCK cells, mimicking the effect produced by exposure to dibutryl cyclic AMP. The isosmotic volume reduction in the MDCK cells is associated with a condensation of F-actin fibers within the cytoskeleton into dense bundles, which can be seen optically (34, 35).

There is not yet a cohesive picture of how the cytoskeleton is involved in cell volume regulation. However in all cases, disruption of microfilaments either inhibits or potentiates volume recovery depending upon the cell type, and in the clam red cell, the cytoskeletal actin changes that are coincident with volume recovery from hypoosmotic stress are $[Ca^{2+}]_i$-sensitive and blocked by calmodulin inhibitors.

Protein Phosphorylation

Calcium-activated calmodulin directly stimulates the activity of some enzymes responsible for physiologic processes, for example the plasma membrane Ca^{2+} pump (7). However, Ca^{2+}-activated calmodulin often influences cellular physiology by regulating enzymes that control the degree of phosphorylation of specific proteins (11). Therefore, if calmodulin is involved in volume recovery from hypoosmotic stress, it may exert control by protein phosphorylation. Indeed, recent investigations have found that the phosphorylation of at least two proteins associated with the nucleated ghosts of *Noetia* blood cells is stimulated following hypoosmotic stress (Figure 4). This stimulation of phosphorylation is markedly reduced in the absence of the osmotic stress, in Ca^{2+}-free medium or in the presence of the phenothiazines (45). In addition, activation of Na^+-H^+ transport by hyperosmotically stimulated human lymphocytes is associated with phosphorylation of at least one membrane protein (23).

Calcium-activated calmodulin can also influence protein phosphorylation by stimulating phosphodiesterase, or adenylate cyclase, and thereby altering cellular cyclic AMP levels. Indeed, cyclic AMP has been implicated in volume recovery of a few cell types. For example, cyclic AMP seems to be partially involved in the Na^+ regulation that precedes glycine betaine loss from hypoosmotically stimulated *Limulus* walking leg muscle (14). In this case the portion of the ionic regulation stimulated by cyclic AMP was inhibited by ouabain, while most of the hypoosmotically induced Na^+ loss was independent of ouabain. Thus in the *Limulus* cells the second messenger effect seems to be on the Na^+ pump and is not a major part of the volume recovery mechanism. Cyclic AMP has also been implicated in isosmotic volume reductions by MDCK cells. Exposure to dibutryl cyclic AMP caused a volume reduction and a reorganization of F-actin in these cells (34, 35). However the matter has not been tested under hypoosmotic stress in the MDCK cells and cyclic AMP is well known to cause shape changes in various

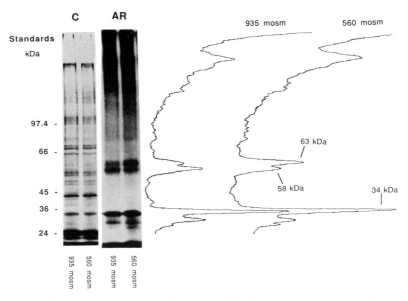

Figure 4 Two proteins show increased phosphorylation in nucleated ghosts from *Noetia* red cells following hypoosmotic stress. Whole cells were incubated in ^{32}P for two hr and then subjected to hypoosmotic stress. After the stress, ghosts were prepared, proteins extracted, SDS-polyacrylamide gels run with the extract, and autoradiographs prepared from the gels. The numbered column on the right indicates the position of molecular weight markers along the first two Coomassie Blue stained lanes (*C*). The corresponding autoradiographs (*AR*) indicate a single band at 58 kd that was always phosphorylated by the same amount regardless of the osmotic stimulus. Two other bands (34 and 63 kd) always showed an increased phosphorylation following hypoosmotic stress. Other bands are visible on the autoradiograph, but their occurrence was not consistent in other gels. The densitometric scans of the autoradiographs are reproduced on the right side of the figure. This figure is reproduced from (45).

cell types (see for example, 46, 64) in situations that do not involve external osmotic pressure changes. Therefore it is not clear that cyclic AMP plays a role in volume recovery from hypoosmotic stress.

VOLUME-SENSITIVE SIGNAL TRANSDUCTION MECHANISMS

One of the more intriguing, but not well studied, aspects of the volume recovery mechanism is the means by which the environmental signal produces a biological response. While almost all studies agree that Ca^{2+} is involved in the initiation of the volume recovery mechanism, the link between alteration of external osmotic concentration and $[Ca^{2+}]_i$ is not known. However some possibilities are obvious. A change in external osmotic concentration results in several perturbations, any of which might be the stimulus for the intracellular $[Ca^{2+}]$ change: the osmotic change itself, the accompanying external ionic dilution, and both the cellular swelling and the intracellular dilution produced by the osmotic influx of water.

In those cell types where the source of the increased free $[Ca^{2+}]_i$ is the external Ca^{2+}, there is some evidence that Ca^{2+} entry into the cell is by means of a stretch-activated channel. For example, patch-clamped membranes from *Necturus* choroid plexus epithelium contain a cation-selective Ca^{2+} channel and a Ca^{2+} and voltage-activated K^+ channel that are normally closed. The K^+ channels are activated by internal Ca^{2+} and a membrane stretch. The Ca^{2+} channel could be opened only by applying a negative pressure to the patch pipette or by applying a hypoosmotic stress. Thus the hypothesis is that the osmotic stress mechanically stretches the cell membrane, which activates the Ca^{2+} channel and permits Ca^{2+} entry. The K^+ channel is activated by the stretch and the increased free $[Ca^{2+}]_i$, thereby permitting the volume regulating efflux of K^+ (9) (Figure 5). An analogous situation may occur with amino acid efflux from the *Noetia* blood cells where amino acid efflux does not occur without an osmotic stress and Ca^{2+} influx, and the influx does not occur without the osmotic stimulus (44, 45, 57). In addition, the evidence indicating that stretch-activated channels are coupled with the cytoskeleton (51) may eventually help explain the effect of the cytoskeletal reorganizations that have been seen following hypoosmotic stress (see above). Finally, cultured opossum kidney epithelial cells also have osmotically activated membrane channels that are permeable to Na^+, K^+, and Cl^- (60). These channels are distinct from the osmotically activated, Ca^2-dependent K^+ channel that is also present (60) and may represent a route for Cl^- loss following the osmotic stress. However the channels are open for much shorter periods than the Ca^{2+}-dependent K^+ channel. The patch current evoked by their opening returns to the resting state within ten min, while opening the Ca^{2+}-dependent K^+ channel results in a large membrane depolarization that is sustained for much longer (60).

The membrane potential of many cell types depolarizes immediately (sometimes preceded by a brief hyperpolarization) following a hypoosmotic stress (4, 8, 22, 40, 47, 48, 53, 65). These electrical changes do not occur if the external ionic concentrations are lowered isosmotically (8, 47), and they seem to result from the activation of volume-sensitive conductive pathways (22, 53). These electrical events occur in cell types with volume recovery mechanisms that are only sensitive to $[Ca^{2+}]_i$ as well as in those that respond to extracellular Ca^{2+}. The steps between hypoosmotic stress and elevations in $[Ca^{2+}]_i$ in those cell types insensitive to $[Ca^{2+}]_o$ are not yet obvious, but the occurrence of these osmotically induced electrical changes suggest the pres-

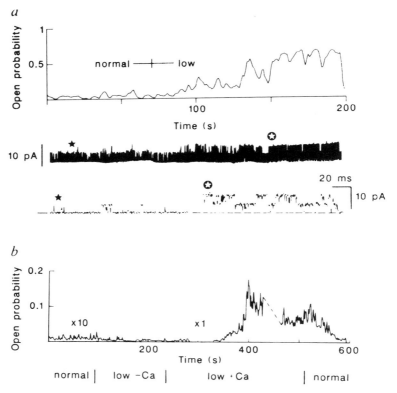

Figure 5 The activity of the stretch-activated, Ca^{2+}-dependent K^+ channel in cells from *Necturus* choroid plexus. The top graph (*a*) demonstrates the increased K^+ channel opening following a change from normal to low tonicity (with Ca^{2+} present). The probabilities plotted here were obtained from the patch current shown in the trace immediately below the graph. The lower trace shows the patch current from the corresponding starred regions at an expanded time scale. The lower graph (*b*) demonstrates the Ca^{2+} requirement for K^+ channel opening. The patch was bathed in normal tonicity medium and, at the mark, exposed to Ca^{2+}-free low tonicity medium (low-Ca). At the second mark, the medium was changed to low tonicity medium containing Ca^{2+} (low + Ca). Note the scale amplification at that point as well as the increase in open probability. At the last mark, the medium was returned to normal tonicity. This figure was reproduced from (9) with permission.

ence of stretch-sensitive channels for ions other than Ca^{2+} which might provide the signal producing the intracellular Ca^{2+} change.

Lastly, factors other than altered ion conductances might also induce a release of intracellular Ca^{2+} in those cell types insensitive to $[Ca^{2+}]_o$. The osmotic influx of water resulting from the imposition of the hypoosmotic stress, together with cell swelling and membrane stretching, must also concomitantly dilute the cytoplasmic milieu. This dilution itself could easily alter intracellular Ca^{2+} homeostasis sufficiently to produce a release of the divalent cation from intracellular stores, a possibility that remains to be investigated.

CONCLUSIONS

Clearly $[Ca^{2+}]_i$ is involved in the recovery of cell volume following hypoosmotic stress. The divalent cation is involved in the regulation of inorganic osmolyte efflux from the cells of terrestrial animals and the organic osmolyte efflux from marine animal cell types. This apparent dichotomy may only be the result of lack of testing for both osmolyte types in each cell type, or may represent a real phyletic difference. In any case, it seems clear that the type of osmolyte transporting system regulated by Ca^{2+} is dependent upon the cell type.

The existing data indicate that the site of Ca^{2+} action is located intracellularly, and calmodulin has been implicated pharmacologically in the process in several cell types. The biochemical target for Ca^{2+}-activated calmodulin in the volume recovery mechanism is not yet known. However, recent (albeit limited) evidence has correlated Ca^{2+}-sensitive alterations in both protein phosphorylation and the cytoskeleton with cell volume recovery and osmolyte efflux. These results may lead to the identification and characterization of the molecules involved in the control of the volume recovery mechanism. Finally, the imposition of a hypoosmotic stress activates one or more types of previously unrecognized, stretch-activated ion (and perhaps other kinds) channels in the cell membrane. The characterizations of the channels most likely will be important contributions to the understanding of the transduction mechanism producing osmolyte efflux in response to hypoosmotic stress.

Literature Cited

1. Allen, J. C., Mills, J. W. 1988. Two lines of MDCK epithelial cells with different volume and ion responses to calcium ionophore A23187. *In Vitro Cell. Dev. Biol.* 24:588–92
2. Amende, L. M., Pierce, S. K. 1980. Free amino acid mediated volume regulation of isolated *Noetia ponderosa* red blood cells: Control by Ca^{2+} and ATP. *J. Comp. Physiol.* 138:291–98
3. Bagnasco, S., Balaban, R., Fales, H. M., Yang, Y-M., Burg, M. 1986. Predominate osmotically active organic solutes in rat and rabbit renal medullas. *J. Biol. Chem.* 261:5872–77
4. Beres, L., Pierce, S. K. 1981. The effects of salinity stress on the electrophysiological properties of *Mya are-*

naria neurons. *J. Comp. Physiol.* 144: 165–73
5. Cala, P. M. 1983. Volume regulation by *Amphiuma* red blood cells: the role of Ca^{2+} as a modulator of alkali metal/H^+ exchange. *J. Gen. Physiol.* 82:761–84
6. Cala, P. M., Mandel, L. J., Murphy, E. 1986. Volume regulation by *Amphiuma* red blood cells: cytosolic free Ca and alkali metal-H exchange. *Am. J. Physiol.* 250:C423–C429
7. Carafoli, E. 1987. Intracellular calcium homeostasis. *Annu. Rev. Biochem.* 56: 395–433
8. Carlson, A. D., Pichon, Y., Treherne, J. E. 1978. Effects of osmotic stress on the electrical activities of the giant axon

of a marine osmoconformer, *Sabella penicillus*. *J. Exp. Biol.* 75:237–51

9. Christensen, O. 1987. Mediation of cell volume regulation by Ca^{2+} influx through stretch-activated channels. *Nature* 330:66–68

10. Clapham, D. E., Neher, E. 1984. Trifluoperazine reduces inward ionic currents and secretion by separate mechanisms in bovine chromaffin cells. *J. Physiol.* 353:541–64

11. Cohen, P. 1982. The role of protein phosphorylation in neural and hormonal control of cellular activity. *Nature* 296:613–20

12. Costa, C. J., Pierce, S. K. 1983. Volume regulation in the red coelomocytes of *Glycera dibranchiata*: An interaction of amino acid and K^+ effluxes. *J. Comp. Physiol. B* 151:133–44

13. Davis, W. C., Finn, A. L. 1987. Interactions of sodium transport, cell volume, and calcium in frog urinary bladder. *J. Gen. Physiol.* 89:687–702

14. Edwards, S. C. 1984. *Neurohormonal involvement of octopamine in cell volume regulation in* Limulus polyphemus. PhD thesis. Univ. Maryland, College Park. 78 pp.

15. Edwards, S. C., Pierce, S. K. 1986. Octopamine potentiates intracellular Na^+ and Cl^- reductions during cell volume regulation in *Limulus* exposed to hypoosmotic stress. *J. Comp. Physiol. B* 156:481–89

16. Foskett, J. K., Spring, K. R. 1983. Control of epithelial cell volume regulation. *J. Gen. Physiol.* 82:21a

17. Foskett, J. K., Spring, K. R. 1984. Ca and microfilaments in epithelial cell volume regulation. *Fed. Proc.* 43:447

18. Foskett, J. K., Spring, K. R. 1985. Involvement of calcium and cytoskeleton in gall bladder epithelial cell volume regulation. *Am. J. Physiol.* 248:C27–C36

19. Gilles, R., Delpire, E., Duchene, C., Cornet, M., Pequeux, A. 1986. The effect of cytochalasin B on the volume regulation response of isolated axons of the green crab *Carcinus maenas* submitted to hypo-osmotic media. *Comp. Biochem. Physiol. A* 85:523–25

20. Greenberg, D. A., Carpenter, C. L., Messing, R. O. 1987. Interaction of calmodulin inhibitors and protein kinase C inhibitors with voltage-dependant calcium channels. *Brain Res.* 404:401–4

21. Grinstein, S., Cohen, S., Sarkadi, B., Rothstein, A. 1983. Induction of ^{83}Rb fluxes by Ca^{2+} and volume changes in thymocytes and their isolated membranes. *J. Cell. Physiol.* 116:352–62

22. Grinstein, S., Dupre, A., Rothstein, A. 1982. Volume regulation by human lymphocytes. Role of calcium. *J. Gen. Physiol.* 79:849–68

23. Grinstein, S., Goetz-Smith, J. D., Stewart, D., Beresford, B. J., Mellors, A. 1986. Protein phosphorylation during activation of Na^+/H^+ exchange by phorbol esters and by osmotic shrinking. *J. Biol. Chem.* 261:8009–8016

24. Gullans, S. R., Blumenfeld, J. D., Balschi, J. A., Kaleta, M., Brenner, R. M., et al. 1988. Accumulation of major organic osmolytes in rat renal inner medulla in dehydration. *Am. J. Physiol.* 255:F626–F634

25. Hazama, A., Okada, Y. 1988. Ca^{2+} sensitivity of volume-regulatory K^+ and Cl^- channels in cultured human epithelial cells. *J. Physiol.* 402:687–702

26. Hoffmann, E. K., Lambert, I. H. 1983. Amino acid transport and cell volume regulation in Ehrlich ascites tumour cells. *J. Physiol.* 338:613–25

27. Hoffmann, E. K., Lambert, I. H., Simonsen, L. O. 1986. Separate, Ca^{2+}-activated K^+ and Cl^- transport pathways in Ehrlich ascites tumor cells. *J. Membr. Biol.* 91:227–44

28. Hoffmann, E. K., Simonsen, L. O., Lambert, I. H. 1984. Volume-induced increase of K^+ and Cl^- permeabilities in Ehrlich ascites tumor cells. Role of internal Ca^{2+}. *J. Membr. Biol.* 78:211–22

29. Kaczmarek, L. K. 1986. Phorbol esters, protein phosphorylation and the regulation of neuronal ion channels. *J. Exp. Biol.* 134:375–92

30. Kaji, D. 1986. Volume-sensitive K transport in human erythrocytes. *J. Gen. Physiol.* 88:719–38

31. Lambert, I. H. 1985. Taurine transport in Ehrlich ascites tumour cells. Specificity and chloride dependence. *Mol. Physiol.* 7:323–31

32. Larson, M., Spring, K. R. 1984. Volume regulation by *Necturus* gallbladder: basolateral KCl exit. *J. Membr. Biol.* 81:219–32

33. Lauf, P. K., Mangor-Jensen, A. 1984. Effects of A23187 and Ca^{2+} on volume- and thiol-stimulated, ouabain-resistant K^+Cl^- fluxes in low K^+ sheep erythrocytes. *Biochem. Biophys. Res. Commun.* 125:790–96

34. Mills, J. W., Lubin, M. 1986. Effect of adenosine 3',5'-cyclic monophosphate on volume and cytoskeleton of MDCK cells. *Am. J. Physiol.* 250:C319–C324

35. Mills, J. W., Skiest, D. J. 1985. Role of cyclic AMP and the cytoskeleton in volume control in MDCK cells. *Mol. Physiol.* 8:247–62

36. Moran, W. M., Pierce, S. K. 1984. The mechanism of crustacean salinity tolerance: cell volume regulation by K^+ and glycine fluxes. *Mar. Biol.* 81:41–46

37. Mori, T., Takai, Y., Minakuchi, B. Yu., Nishizuka, Y. 1980. Inhibitory action of chlorpromazine, dibucaine, and other phospholipid-interacting drugs on calcium activated, phospholipid-dependent protein kinase. *J. Biol. Chem.* 255:8378–80

38. Nelson, G. A., Andrews, M. L., Karnovsky, M. J. 1983. Control of cell shape by calmodulin. *J. Cell. Biol.* 96:730–35

39. Norman, J. A., Drummond, A. H., Moser, P. 1979. Inhibition of calcium-dependent, regulator-stimulated phosphodiesterase activity by neuroleptic drugs is unrelated to their clinical efficacy. *Mol. Pharmacol.* 16:1089–1094

40. Parker, H. T., Pierce, S. K. 1985. Comparative electrical properties of identified neurons in *Elysia chlorotica* before and after low salinity acclimation. *Comp. Biochem. Physiol. A* 82:367–72

41. Parker, J. C. 1988. Volume-activated transport systems in dog red blood cells. *Comp. Biochem. Physiol. A* 90:539–42

42. Pierce, S. K. 1982. Invertebrate cell volume control mechanisms: a coordinated use of intracellular amino acid and inorganic ions as osmotic solute. *Biol. Bull.* 163:405–19

43. Pierce, S. K., Politis, A. D., Cronkite, D. C., Rowland, L. M., Smith, L. H. Jr. 1989. Evidence of calmodulin involvement in cell volume recovery following hypoosmotic stress. *Cell Calcium* 10:159–69

44. Pierce, S. K., Politis, A. D., Smith, L. H. Jr., Rowland, L. M. 1988. A Ca^{2+} influx in response to hypo-osmotic stress may alter osmolyte permeability by a phenothiazine-sensitive mechanism. *Cell Calcium* 9:129–40

45. Politis, A. D. 1988. *The mechanism of cell volume recovery: Ca^{2+} influx, calmodulin activation and protein phosphorylation.* PhD thesis, Univ. Maryland, College Park. 68 pp.

46. Porter, K. R., Puck, T. T., Hsie, A. W., Kelley, D. 1974. An electron microscopy study of the effects of dibutyryl cyclic AMP on Chinese hamster ovary cells. *Cell.* 2:145–62

47. Prior, D. J., Pierce, S. K. 1981. Adaptation and tolerance of invertebrate nervous systems to osmotic stress. *J. Exp. Zool.* 215:237–45

48. Quinn, R. H. 1988. *The basis of membrane depolarization during hypoosmotic stress.* PhD thesis, Univ. Maryland, College Park. 63 pp.

49. Rink, T. J., Sanchez, A., Grinstein, S., Rothstein, A. 1983. Volume restoration in osmotically swollen lymphocytes does not involve changes in free Ca^{2+} concentration. *Biochim. Biophys. Acta* 762:593–96

50. Roy, G., Sauve, R. 1987. Effect of anisotonic media on volume, ion and amino acid content and membrane potential of kidney cells (MDCK) in culture. *J. Membr. Biol.* 100:83–96

51. Sachs, F. 1987. Baroreceptor mechanisms at the cellular level. *Fed. Proc.* 46:12–16

52. Sarkadi, B., Attisano, L., Grinstein, S., Buchwals, M., Rothstein, A. 1984. Volume regulation of Chinese hamster ovary cells in anisosmotic media. *Biochim. Biophys. Acta* 774:159–68

53. Sakadi, B., Mack, E., Rothstein, A. 1984. Ionic events during the volume response of human peripheral blood lymphocytes to hypotonic media. I. Distinction between volume activated Cl^- and K^+ conductance pathways. *J. Gen. Physiol.* 83:497–512

54. Schatzman, R. C., Wise, B. C., Kuo, J. F. 1981. Phospholipid-sensitive, calcium-dependent protein kinase: Inhibition by antipsychotic drugs. *Biochem. Biophys. Res. Commun.* 98:669–76

55. Schmidt, W. F. III, McManus, T. J. 1977. Ouabain-insensitive salt and water movements in duck red cells. I. Kinetics of cation transport under hypotonic conditions. *J. Gen. Physiol.* 49:849–66

56. Smith, L. H. Jr. 1985. *Osmolyte permeability in* Noetia ponderosa *erythrocytes during hypoosmotic stress: control by Ca^{2+} and the cytoskeleton.* PhD thesis. Univ. Maryland, College Park. 84 pp.

57. Smith, L. H. Jr., Pierce, S. K. 1987. Cell volume regulation by molluscan erythrocytes during hypoosmotic stress: Ca^{2+} effects on ionic and organic osmolyte effluxes. *Biol. Bull.* 172:407–18

58. Thurston, J. H., Hauharn, R. E., Dirco, J. A. 1980. Taurine: A role in osmotic regulation of mammalian brain and possible clinical significance. *Life Sci.* 26:1561–68

59. Thurston, J. H., Hauhart, R. E., Naccarato, E. G. 1981. Taurine: Possible role in osmotic regulation of the mammalian heart. *Science* 214:1373–74

60. Ubl, J., Murer, H., Kolb, H.-A. 1988. Ion channels activated by osmotic and mechanical stress in membranes of opossum kidney cells. *J. Membr. Biol.* 104:223–32

61. Van Eldik, L. J., Zendegui, J. G., Marshak, D. R., Watterson, D. M. 1982. Calcium binding proteins and the molecular basis of calcium action. *Int. Rev. Cytol.* 77:1–61

62. Van Rossum, G., D., V., Russo, M. A. 1981. Ouabain-resistant mechanism of volume control and the ultrastructural organization of liver slices recovering from swelling in vitro. *J. Memb. Biol.* 59:191–209

63. Warren, M. K., Pierce, S. K. 1982. Two cell volume regulatory systems in the *Limulus* myocardium: An interaction of ions and quaternary ammonium compounds. *Biol. Bull.* 163:504–6

64. Willingham, M. C., Pastan, I. 1975. Cyclic AMP and cell morphology in cultured fibroblasts: effects on cell shape, microfilament and microtubule distribution, and orientation to the substratum. *J. Cell Biol.* 67:146–59

65. Wilmer, P. G. 1978. Volume regulation and solute balance in the nervous tissue of an osmoconforming bivalve *(Mytilus edulis). J. Exp. Biol.* 77:157–79

66. Wolfe, S. E., Brostrom, M. A. 1986. Mechanisms of action of inhibitors of prolactin secretion in GH_3 cells. II. Blockade of voltage-dependent Ca^{2+} channels. *Mol. Pharmacol.* 29:420–26

67. Wong, S. M. E., Chase, H. S. Jr. 1986. Role of intracellular calcium in cellular volume regulation. *Am. J. Physiol.* 250: C841–C852

68. Yancey, P. H. 1988. Osmotic effectors in kidneys of xeric and mesic rodents: corticomedullary distributions and changes with water availability. *J. Comp. Physiol. B* 158:369–80

69. Yancey, P. H., Clark, M. E., Hand, S. C., Bowlus, R. D., Somero, G. N. 1982. Living with water-stress: Evolution of osmolyte systems. *Science* 217: 1214–22

Annu. Rev. Physiol. 1990. 52:43–60

AN EMERGING ROLE FOR A CARDIAC PEPTIDE HORMONE IN FISH OSMOREGULATION

David H. Evans

Department of Zoology, University of Florida, Gainesville, Florida 32611 and Mount Desert Island Biological Laboratory, Salsbury Cove, Maine 04672

KEY WORDS: fish endocrinology, cardiac hormone, teleosts, kidney, gill

INTRODUCTION

Since the demonstration that atrial extracts produced a massive, rapid diuresis and natriuresis in rats (21), there has been intense interest in the role of a cardiac hormone in fluid homeostasis in mammals. Subsequently, the relevant hormone (atrial natriuretic peptide or atriopeptin, hereafter referred to as AP) has been isolated, sequenced, and synthesized; and its gene has been isolated, cloned, and mapped on chromosome 1 in humans (see 47 for a recent review). Despite some uncertainty about the actual role that atriopeptin may play in normal fluid homeostasis in mammals (49–51, 125), it is clear that atriopeptin is a potent vasodilator in a variety of pre-contracted blood vessels and produces natriuresis by increasing glomerular filtration and decreasing tubular sodium reabsorption, as well as by inhibiting the release of aldosterone, ADH, and possibly renin.

Investigation of a putative role for atriopeptin in fluid homeostasis in non-mammalian vertebrates is only now beginning. Fishes, in particular, have chronic problems of salt and water balance because of the ionic and osmotic gradients present across their thin branchial epithelia. Specifically, marine teleost fishes face chronic dehydration and salt loading, while freshwater teleosts confront volume loading and salt depletion. Marine chondrichthyan

43

0066-4278/90/0315-0043$02.00

fishes face salt loading and hypervolemia because of a slight hypertonicity compared to sea water, produced by high blood levels ($\sim$ 350mmol/l) of urea and trimethylamine oxide ($\sim$ 70 mmol/l), in addition to NaCl concentrations about 50% those of sea water (28). Thus one might suspect a priori that a cardiac peptide hormone may play some role in fish osmoregulation. The intent of this short review is to describe recent studies that support this proposition, in the context of relevant literature on the role of atriopeptin in mammalian fluid balance, as well as the hormonal control of fish osmoregulation.

PHYSIOLOGIC EFFECTS OF ATRIOPEPTIN IN MAMMALS

The physiology, biochemistry, pharmacology, and molecular biology of AP have been reviewed extensively in the last few years (e.g. 2, 8, 14–17, 47, 69, 83, 87, 110). References supporting general statements in the present review can be found in these sources; recent or unique primary sources will be referenced only for specific points. The circulating form of AP is now generally agreed to be an $\sim$ 3-kd C-terminal, 28 amino acid fragment (termed AP_{99-126}) from a 126 amino acid prohormone that is synthesized and stored in vesicles in cardiocytes in both the atria and ventricles of numerous mammals including man. Immunoreactive AP can be extracted from heart tissue, with 1–100 μg/g generally found in the atria and 1–10 ng/g in the ventricles. Ventricular synthesis and secretion of AP is relatively higher in fetal mammals and stimulated by various cardiac pathologies (e.g. congestive heart failure), but always is less than atrial production (85, 127). Plasma concentrations of immunoreactive AP in unstressed mammals are in the range of 10–200 pg/ml (3–70 pM/l). The common intracellular second messenger in the array of tissues sensitive to AP is cyclic GMP, with cyclic AMP often being inhibited (73). It appears, however, that the AP inhibition of aldosterone secretion may not be mediated by cyclic GMP (73, 80).

Vascular Smooth Muscle

Atriopeptin is a potent dilator of mammalian arteries that have been preconstricted with factors such as angiotensin II, α-adrenergic agonists, and K^+. The vascular endothelium is not necessary for this effect. Efficacy of this inhibition of constriction varies widely, but generally is demonstrated by EC_{50s} in the range of 0.1 to 10 nM. Preconstriction in vitro seems to be critical, so the vasodilatory action of AP is generally thought to be antagonistic rather than direct (8, 47, 129). It has been shown that AP stimulates the Na-K-2Cl cotransporter in vascular smooth muscle, but does not affect other sites such as Na/K and Na/H exchanges. However the role of this cotransport system in vascular tension is unknown (98).

Kidney

The diuretic and natriuretic effects of AP on the mammalian kidney appear to be secondary to both an increase in glomerular filtration (because of pre-glomerular vasodilation, post-glomerular vasoconstriction, and an increase in glomerular permeability) and inhibition of Na^+ reabsorption in renal tubules. The site of reduced Na^+ uptake is somewhat debatable, but it is generally considered to be mainly in the distal nephron, specifically in the inner medullary collecting duct (e.g. 3, 5, 74, 132), probably via inhibition of an amiloride-sensitive Na^+ channel (133). It is still unclear whether AP also can inhibit Na^+ reabsorption in the proximal tubule (compare 46 and 75). Finally, some have proposed that the natriuresis is at least partially the result of redistribution of blood flow, washing out the medullary osmotic gradient (e.g. 3, 12).

Renin-Angiotensin System

In addition to direct effects on vascular diameter and renal filtration and transport, AP can produce vasodilation and natriuresis secondarily by inhibiting the release of hormones of the renin-angiotensin system (RAS) that are vasoconstrictive (angiotensin II) and anti-natriuretic (aldosterone) (e.g. 3, 47). It is not clear if the AP-induced fall in renin secretion is secondary to direct effect on the juxtaglomerular cells (e.g. 55, 56), or merely an adjunct to alterations in renal blood flow (e.g. 24), but AP has been shown to be a potent, direct inhibitor of the release of aldosterone from the glomerulosa cells of the adrenal cortex (e.g. 3, 82). Cortisol secretion may also be inhibited by AP (86).

Central Nervous System

There is increasing evidence that atriopeptin may be a very important hormone (neurotransmitter?) in the brain and may exert many of its effects via the central nervous system (61, 111). In fact it appears that the AP resident in the brain (termed brain natriuretic peptide, BNP), which is 26 amino acids long, has a similar, but distinct, sequence from circulating AP (124). Brain levels of immunoreactive AP are generally found to be 1–10 ng/g tissue (62). Receptors for AP are numerous in the diencephalic regions associated with the control of cardiovascular and osmoregulatory function, and it now appears that centrally administrated AP can inhibit ADH release directly (111, 112). Other effects of AP in the mammalian brain include: inhibition of the dipsogenic action of dehydration or angiotensin II injection, and inhibition of the secretion of prolactin, LH, and ACTH, but not TSH or GH (61, 112).

CONTROL OF ATRIOPEPTIN SECRETION IN MAMMALS

The dominant direct stimulus for secretion of AP seems to be atrial stretch (e.g. 47), which can be produced by either volume loading or an increase in salt intake, which results in an increase in plasma volume. Hormonal secretagogues are glucocorticoids (e.g. 88) and thyroid hormone (T_3, T_4; 44), which apparently act directly on the AP gene (44, 45). Mineralocorticoids, both α- and β-adrenergic agonists, and cholinergic agonists have been found to also stimulate AP secretion, but the effects may be indirect via hemodynamic changes (47). There is some evidence that increased plasma [Na^+] itself may stimulate AP release from isolated atrial (1, 48) or hypothalamic (115) fragments, but hypernatremia in vivo is associated with hypervolemia, which itself would stimulate release of AP (47).

FISH OSMOREGULATION

Recent reviews of various aspects of fish (teleost and elasmobranch) osmoregulation include: (22, 28, 30, 63, 64, 102, 104, 105, 131). Fish species will be referred to by their common name; genera and species are given in the original papers.

Freshwater Teleosts

Since the plasma NaCl content of fishes in fresh water is distinctly above that of the environment ($\sim$ 150 mM vs $<$ 1 mM), they face chronic, potential hypervolemia and hyponatremia (hypochloremia). These osmotic and ionic gradients are across the relatively thin, highly vascularized gill epithelium characteristic of the group (60, 71). It is now well established (see 28) that volume control is maintained by excretion of relatively copious volumes of dilute urine, with needed salts extracted in the distal tubule, collecting duct, and urinary bladder, when present. Required NaCl is extracted from the medium by the gill epithelium via the parallel antiports Na/H (NH_4) and Cl/HCO_3, which also function in acid-base regulation (31) and possibly ammonia excretion (33).

Seawater Teleosts

In sea water, teleosts face chronic, potential hypovolemia and hypernatremia (hyperchloremia) because they reside in a hyperosmotic environment containing approximately 500 mM NaCl. Volume is maintained by oral ingestion of the medium, followed by intestinal uptake of water secondary to the active extraction of salt via a Na-K-2Cl cotransport system (84). Urinary loss of water is kept to a minimum by very low glomerular filtration rates; in fact some marine teleosts are actually aglomerular (see 28, 57), and urine is formed by NaCl secretion (probably Na-K-2Cl cotransport) in the proximal tubule. This salt secretory system is apparently also resident in the proximal tubule of glomerular fishes and other vertebrates (11). Urine volume is also reduced by uptake of water from the urine in the urinary bladder, when present. The net influx of salt across the intestinal epithelium, as well as any salt that enters across the gills down the electrochemical gradient (which may be minor for Na^+ in some species; 29) is balanced by gill extrusion via Na-K-Cl (probably 2Cl) cotransport (131). Marine teleosts usually do not produce hypernatric (hyperchloric) urine, despite the presence of a NaCl secretory step in the proximal tubule (11). Isotopically measured Na^+ and Cl^- fluxes across marine teleosts are two orders of magnitude greater than those seen in freshwater teleosts, which indicates that the branchial epithelium is considerably more permeable to salts in seawater teleosts than freshwater teleosts (28).

Euryhaline Teleosts

Significant numbers of species of teleosts are termed euryhaline because they are capable of osmoregulation in both marine and brackish/freshwater salinities (see review by Evans, 30). Entry into lower salinities by marine species requires stimulation of renal water loss, increased renal and urinary bladder salt reabsorption, cessation of oral ingestion of the medium, decreased intestinal uptake of salt and water, cessation of branchial salt extrusion, and reduction in branchial permeability to ions. Salt uptake mechanisms may be stimulated, but they are already present because of their use in acid-base regulation, even in marine species (30, 31). Entry of fresh or brackish water species into the marine environment (more rarely seen) would require opposite physiologic alterations.

Seawater Elasmobranchs

The sharks, skates, and rays are slightly hyperosmotic to sea water because of the retention of urea and trimethylamine oxide, which accounts for some 40% of the plasma solutes. Thus GFRs and urine flows in elasmobranchs may approach those described for freshwater teleosts. Elasmobranchs do not ingest sea water (28). Plasma NaCl concentrations are approximately 50% those in the surrounding sea water, so despite relatively low gill salt permeability, elasmobranchs face chronic hypernatremia (hyperchloremia) (28). Excess NaCl is excreted through rectal salt glands via Na-K-2Cl cotransport (27), although similar transporters are apparently present in the shark gill epithelium and may also play a role in NaCl secretion (35).

HORMONAL CONTROL OF FISH OSMOREGULATION

Various aspects of the hormonal control of fish osmoregulation have been reviewed recently (30, 40, 70, 99), but it is clear that even a moderately detailed synthesis is still lacking.

Freshwater Teleosts

Rather surprisingly, it appears that arginine vasotocin (AVT) and prolactin are important modulators of osmoregulation in fresh water, where fishes are volume-loaded and salt-depleted. AVT, rather than arginine vasopressin (AVP), is the vasoactive neurohypophysial peptide in fishes (113). It produces vasoconstriction of branchial vessels (e.g. 10) as well as increased dorsal aortic pressure (134), which suggests vasoconstriction of systemic vessels as well. Constriction of branchial vessels could theoretically limit osmotic uptake of water in fresh water, but one might argue that it would also be effective in limiting branchial osmotic loss in marine teleosts, thus suggesting that AVT might be important to osmoregulation in either salinity. Contrary to the antidiuretic response of tetrapods to either AVT or AVP, AVT usually produces diuresis in teleost fishes (99), except for a few studies that have shown antidiuresis produced by low concentrations, but diuresis at higher concentrations (e.g. 4). Pang (99) has suggested that the usual diuresis in fishes is best explained by differential receptor sensitivity, with highly sensitive systemic receptors overcoming less sensitive, pre-glomerular receptors that normally produce antidiuretic vasoconstriction. The increased systemic pressures would then produce diuresis in response to AVT. Renal tubular sites of action for AVT have not been proposed (99, 100), and fish lack the loop of Henle (e.g. 57) and therefore cannot produce a concentrated urine by water withdrawal in the collecting duct.

Prolactin appears to be one of the most versatile fish hormones and is generally considered to be the dominant osmoregulatory hormone in freshwater fishes (40, 58). Indeed, it has long been known that various species of teleosts can only survive in fresh water if their pituitary is intact, or prolactin is injected (76). Prolactin reduces branchial salt and possibly water permeability, inhibits branchial salt extrusion, intestinal salt uptake, and urinary bladder water permeability, but stimulates urinary bladder Na^+ uptake (58). In many cases the response to prolactin seems to be mediated by morphologic changes and is therefore probably more important during chronic, rather than acute, osmotic stress (40). Immunoreactive prolactin levels in plasma increase when various species of euryhaline teleosts are acclimated to fresh water (e.g. 58).

Other hormones that inhibit salt secretion across the fish gill epithelium and therefore may be important in freshwater osmoregulation include: α-adrenergic agonists (42, 81), somatostatin (41), and urotensin II (79). There has been no clear demonstration of hormonal control of active salt uptake by the gill epithelium of freshwater fishes, but there is some indication that stimulation of β-adrenoceptors in the gill epithelium may enhance Na^+ uptake (103).

Seawater Teleosts

The drinking reflex in marine fishes is apparently controlled by angiotensin II, as it is in mammals (37). Injection of angiotensin II into four marine species stimulated oral ingestion of the medium (9, 18, 78). In addition, injection of the angiotensin I converting enzyme inhibitors, captopril or SQ 20881, attenuated the drinking response in two of these species (6, 78). However the actual role of angiotensin II in stimulating drinking may be species specific because neither SQ 20881 nor the angiotensin II antagonist saralasin inhibited the baseline or hemorrhage-stimulated drinking by two other marine teleosts (9). Injection of angiotensin II did not stimulate drinking in two freshwater teleosts (9), but did in another (95). There is more consistent evidence that the renin-angiotensin system (RAS) may be involved in maintaining blood pressure in teleosts. Graded hemorrhage of the marine toadfish produced a graded increase in plasma renin activity, and injection of angiotensin II into the eel increased blood pressure. This suggests that the RAS is activated in response to hypovolemia that occurs chronically in teleosts in the marine environment (see 90). However sodium depletion produced by adapting teleosts to hypoosmotic salinities did not stimulate the RAS (89), which indicates that the primary sensory stimulus for the RAS system in fishes may be hypovolemia, rather than reduced blood osmolarity. Injection of synthetic angiotensin II into unanesthetized eels was followed by diuresis, but only at vasopressor doses (91), and no diuresis was demonstrated in aglomerular toadfish (134), which suggests that diuresis was secondary to vascular, rather than tubular, events. In fact, angiotensin II produced antidiuresis (by reducing GFR) in both freshwater- and seawater-adapted trout when blood pressures were maintained constant by norepinephrine infusion (13). It is clear that more data are needed before the role of the RAS in fish osmoregulation is fully understood. Nevertheless, the extant data are consistent with the proposition that the RAS functions in fishes primarily to control blood pressure and volume, by dipsogenesis, vasoconstriction, and antidiuresis, in the face of the dehydrating effects of the marine environment. A role for the RAS in marine fishes is supported by the fact that plasma renin activities or angiotension II concentrations are usually elevated in sea water (e.g. 54, 128).

Aldosterone is present in at least some species of teleosts, but its secretion in a single freshwater species is apparently not stimulated by injection of renin, angiotensin II, ACTH, Na^+ depletion, Na^+ loading, or moderate hemorrhage (109). Its role in fish osmoregulation is unknown. The glucocorticoid cortisol is the dominant adrenal (actually interrenal) steroid in fishes, but its secretion is apparently not coupled to that of renin (66, 92). A variety of studies have demonstrated that plasma cortisol levels increase when euryhaline teleosts are transferred to sea water (e.g. 38, 66), or even when the stenohaline carp is transferred to 45% sea water (53). Cortisol stimulates intestinal ion and water absorption(59), gill salt extrusion (40), and urinary bladder salt and water reabsorption (77). However the effects on these tissues appear to be via differentiation of the respective epithelium, rather than a direct effect on the transport itself (40). Various studies have demonstrated that cortisol secretion in teleosts is under the control of ACTH (52, 77, 101) as it is in other vertebrates.

Other neurohumoral agents, which have been found to stimulate salt extrusion by the gill epithelium and therefore may play roles in teleost osmoregulation in sea water, include: β-adrenergic agonists (23), vasoactive intestinal peptide (VIP; 42), and glucagon (42).

Seawater Elasmobranchs

The hormonal control of elasmobranch osmoregulation is poorly studied, with the major exception of the rectal gland. Salt secretion by the gland is controlled by a variety of hormones and neurotransmitters. The primary stimulant appears to be either VIP (123) or another peptide from the gut termed rectin (116). Adenosine has also been found to be an effective stimulant at concentrations above 10^{-5} M (65), but an inhibitor at lower concentrations (39). Somatostatin inhibits the stimulatory action of both VIP and adenosine (117). Angiotensin II is vasoconstrictive in elasmobranchs, but acts via release of catecholamines in the periphery (19, 97).

EVIDENCE FOR A ROLE OF ATRIOPEPTIN IN FISH OSMOREGULATION

In the past four years a small literature has emerged that suggests strongly that fish hearts (and brains) produce a vasoactive and natriuretic factor, that this factor probably has substantial structural homology with the mammalian peptide, and that its secretion is affected by alternations in osmoregulation.

Electron dense granules have been described in cardiac tissue from hagfish (106), elasmobranchs (121), and teleosts (126), and immunoreactivity with antibodies raised against mammalian AP is also present in all three groups (20, 106–108). This suggests structural similarity between a putative fish AP and the mammalian hormone, a conclusion supported by recent physiologic studies (see below), as well as an autoradiographic study demonstrating binding sites for AP in the kidney and aorta of the hagfish (68).

Mammalian AP was diuretic and natriuretic in the freshwater trout

$(AP_{101-126})$ (25) and the marine aglomerular toadfish $(AP_{103-126})$ (72), but in both studies extremely high doses (10–60 μg/kg; $\sim 10^{-7}$ to 10^{-6} M) had to be used. The fact that effects were seen in an aglomerular species demonstrates directly that tubular effects can produce natriuresis without glomerular intervention. In the trout the stimulation of Na^+ excretion was more than twice the diuretic effect, suggesting that salt secretion is more important than water balance when AP is injected. The dogfish shark kidney was unresponsive to AP $(AP_{103-125}$; 2 μg/kg) when the shark was acclimated to sea water (130), but injection of the same dose 24 hr after transfer to 70% sea water stimulated urinary excretion of Cl^- significantly (119).

Mammalian AP is also vasoactive in fish blood vessels. Injection into the dorsal aorta of the trout produced an increase in blood pressure in that vessel (25), but injection into the coeliac artery of the toadfish reduced the BP in that vessel (72), which suggests that the increase in the dorsal aortic BP in the trout may have been secondary to vasodilation of the gill vasculature rather than systemic vasoconstriction. This is supported by the fact that isolated vascular rings from the trout (96) and the toadfish, as well as the perfused gills of the toadfish (34), vasodilated in response to mammalian AP $(AP_{101-126})$. In both studies the apparent EC$_{50}$ of the response was in the nanomolar range, similar to that described for mammalian vessels (see above). We have found a similar EC$_{50}$ for the vasodilatory action of mammalian AP $(AP_{101-126})$ on isolated ventral aortic rings from the dogfish shark (35a). Solomon et al (120) found a somewhat higher EC$_{50}$ in the same system, but they used a more truncated peptide $(AP_{103-125})$ and preconstricted the rings with carbachol. It is of interest to note that neither the dogfish nor toadfish aortic ring required preconstriction to demonstrate the vasodilatory action of mammalian AP, contrary to the situation in mammalian vascular preparations. It is unclear what adaptive role vasodilation of either the ventral aorta or branchial vasculature would have for either teleosts or elasmobranchs. Increased branchial perfusion would presumably exacerbate the osmotic loss of water in marine teleosts and the osmotic gain of water in marine elasmobranchs and freshwater teleosts. It would therefore appear to be maladaptive (except for possibly the elasmobranchs), unless one proposes that increased perfusion would stimulate relevant branchial ionic transport steps.

Recent studies have also shown that mammalian AP can have significant effects on at least three epithelia that are involved in osmoregulation in marine fishes. O'Grady et al (94) demonstrated that mammalian AP $(AP_{103-126})$ could produce significant inhibition of the Na-K-2Cl cotransport system that drives the necessary extraction of water from the intestine of the seawater-adapted flounder. The EC$_{50}$ of the inhibition was 7 nM, certainly in the range described for mammalian systems. This and a subsequent study (93) also demonstrated that cyclic GMP was the intracellular second messenger in this effect, as it is in mammalian systems (see above). Surprisingly, another study has shown clearly that mammalian AP can have the opposite effect on the same cotransporter in the gill epithelium (114). In this case, the stimulation of Na-K-2Cl had an EC_{50} slightly less than 10 nM ($AP_{103-125}$). In both systems (93, 114), tetrodotoxin did not inhibit the AP response, suggesting that nerve activity was not involved. This finding of a direct effect of mammalian AP on these epithelia (consistent with effects on mammalian epithelia) is to be contrasted with the unique finding that mammalian AP ($AP_{103-125}$) could stimulate Na-K-2Cl-driven Cl^- and water secretion by the shark rectal gland (121) indirectly by stimulation of the release of VIP from nerves in the rectal gland itself (118).

These effects of AP on three epithelia involved in osmoregulation in sea water fishes are also somewhat difficult to put into a single model of proposed function for AP in fishes. Certainly stimulation of gill and rectal gland salt secretion is of some importance for the regulation of plasma salt content in sea water, as is inhibition of intestinal salt uptake in teleosts. Intestinal salt uptake, however, is also the driving force for retrieving needed water from the ingested sea water in hypovolemic marine teleosts. So one might consider that AP inhibition of this step would be maladaptive for osmoregulation, despite the apparent importance for salt regulation by marine teleosts. Moreover, since a primary stimulus for elasmobranch rectal gland secretion appears to be volume expansion (122), one might also propose that AP stimulation of the gland is a volume-regulatory, rather than a salt-regulatory, mechanism.

Some of these studies also have shown that fish cardiac (and brain) extracts can produce physiologic responses in fishes and mammals. Cardiac extracts were vasoactive, diuretic, and natriuretic in the trout (25, 96) and toadfish (72). In the trout the renal response to ventricular extracts was substantially greater than the response to atrial extracts. Ventricular extracts were substantially more effective in relaxing the ventral aortic rings from the toadfish (apparent EC_{50} of 6 mg of ventricle vs 12 mg of atrium; 34). This preparation was also sensitive to extracts from toadfish brain (apparent EC_{50} of 2 mg), but the maximal relaxation produced by brain extracts was only 50% of that produced by either atrial or ventricular extracts. Atrial and ventricular extracts from trout, shark, and hagfish were also able to relax precontracted helical strips from rabbit aortae (107). Whole heart extracts from the chub produced diuresis and natriuresis, but not an increase in GFR or fall in systemic BP, when injected into rats (126).

Very recent studies (26, 31a, 34, 43, 126) have determined that immunoreactive AP (AP_{ir}) could be demonstrated in plasma and cardiac and brain tissue of various fish species by using antibodies raised against mammalian (usually human) AP. Levels of AP_{ir} in the plasma were in the same range (10–200 pg/ml) as those found in mammals; however cardiac and brain concentrations were usually less than 1 ng/g tissue (31a), significantly less than that described for mammals (see above). Since extracts from the same tissues displayed significant vasoactivity (34), it appears that the fish tissue prohormone may be structurally inaccessible to the antibody raised against mammalian AP. Apparent ventricular AP_{ir} was significantly below atrial AP_{ir} but fish atrial:ventricular content is on the order of $4:1$ vs $>1000:1$ in normotensive mammals (31a, and see above). In addition, cultured chub ventricular cells secreted AP_{ir} at the same rate as cultured atrial cells and substantially faster than either rat or mouse cultured ventricular cells (7). These two studies strongly suggest that ventricular synthesis and secretion may be substantial (corroborating the physiologic data) in the lower vertebrates, as it is in neonatal and hypertensive mammals (e.g. 47), an interesting case of "ontogeny recapitulating phylogeny." The fact that AP_{ir} can be demonstrated in plasma and tissues from the hagfish, shark and stingray, and teleosts (31a, 34) indicates that AP was probably present in the earliest vertebrates. The finding of AP_{ir} in the hagfish plasma (34) and heart and brain (31a, 106), as well as apparent AP binding sites in the aorta and kidney of hagfish (68), is especially interesting since these modern agnathan fishes are isotonic to sea water and quite stenohaline (28). It is, therefore, unclear what volume or salt homeostasis problems these fish actually might face and what function AP might have in their physiology.

The demonstration of AP immunoreactivity in fish plasma and tissues does not in itself demonstrate a function for a putative fish AP in osmoregulation. It is now clear, however, that osmotic perturbations change AP_{ir} in fishes. It has now been shown in five species of marine teleosts that acclimation to reduced salinities is associated with a significant reduction in plasma AP_{ir} (34, 43), which suggests that salt- rather than volume-loading may be the major stimulus for AP secretion in teleosts. This conclusion is supported by the fact that the euryhaline freshwater chub increased its plasma AP_{ir} when acclimated to approximately isotonic saline (126). Cardiac and brain AP_{ir} was also reduced concomitant with salinity reduction in the toadfish (43) and sculpin (31a).

The physiologic, immunologic, and autoradiographic cross-reactivity between a putative fish AP (and its receptors) and mammalian AP (and its receptors) suggest structural homologies. The fact that human AP co-eluted with immunoreactive extracts from chub atria and ventricles on an HPLC acetonitrile gradient (7) supports this conclusion.

SUMMARY AND CONCLUSIONS

It is clear from the extant literature that various fish groups face chronic osmoregulatory problems that depend on the surrounding salinity. Their physiologic and hormonal responses are largely those seen in the mammals, but their terrestrial descendants have lost osmoregulatory structures such as gills and rectal glands and depend primarily on renal function. A data base is now emerging that strongly suggests that a putative atriopeptin plays a role in osmoregulation in fishes. This conclusion is supported by the fact that heterologous AP produces relevant physiologic responses (e.g. natriuresis, vasodilation, stimulation, or inhibition of Na^+ secretion by intestine, gills, and rectal gland) in both teleosts and elasmobranchs. Moreover, cardiac and brain extracts from fish can produce similar effects in both fishes and mammals, and these tissues from various fish groups contain immunoreactive AP, as does plasma. Both physiologic and immunologic evidence suggests that the ventricle may be a significant source of AP in fishes, contrary to the situation in mammals. Finally, osmotic perturbations result in a change in plasma and tissue AP_{ir} levels. The finding that plasma AP_{ir} levels increase in sea water, and that heterologous AP stimulates salt secretion by the teleost gill and shark rectal gland, and inhibits salt uptake by the teleost intestine, suggests that AP may primarily play a role in salt, rather than fluid, secretion in fishes. The fact that in mammals AP inhibits prolactin secretion, but is itself stimulated by cortisol, supports this conclusion, since prolactin is generally considered to be the dominant osmoregulatory hormone in freshwater fishes, and cortisol serves this function in marine fishes. In addition, if AP inhibits brain AVT release in fishes, as it apparently inhibits vasopressin release in mammals, this also would be adaptive in marine fishes since AVT in fishes is diuretic, rather than antidiuretic. Interactions between AP and these hormones (prolactin, cortisol, and ATV) have not been studied in fishes to date, but these theoretical interactions do lend support to the hypothesis that AP may function primarily in salt homeostasis in fishes. At least one potential hormonal interaction counters this argument, however. Atriopeptin is known to inhibit the production and effects of angiotensin II in mammals, and since this hormone is apparently dipsogenic in fishes, it may play a critical role in osmoregulation in sea water.

Finally, it is of some historical interest that in Keys' (67) original description of the eel heart-gill perfusion system in 1931 he commented that gill resistance remained constant for hours only if the heart itself was perfused. Perfusion through the bulbous arteriosus or ventral aorta resulted in increasing gill resistance and loss of fluid from the preparation. He wrote: "(one) explanation which offers itself is that the perfusion medium derives a hormone, or hormones, from the heart which acts to preserve capillary tone." There is increasing evidence nearly sixty years later that Keys' proposal may have been prescient. It is clear that the role(s) atriopeptin may play in fishes and other nonmammalian vertebrates represents an interesting area for future research in the comparative physiology of vertebrate osmoregulation. As has been true of comparative studies in the past, such investigations may give us better insight into the fundamental roles of atriopeptin in mammalian osmoregulation, as well as insight into the evolution of the structure and function of this interesting peptide hormone.

ACKNOWLEDGMENTS

The author's work has been supported recently by NSF PCM-8302621 and DCB-8801572, NIEHS EHS-P30-ES03828 to the Center for Membrane Toxicity Studies at the Mount Desert Island Biological Laboratory, as well as the University of Florida, Division of Sponsored Research and Interdisciplinary Center for Biotechnology Research. Appreciation is expressed to Rick Solomon who first suggested that it might be interesting to examine the effects of AP on fish gill hemodynamics, and Bill Marshall who reminded me of Ancel Keys' paper.

NOTE ADDED IN PROOF

Epstein et al (25a) recently found that transfer of the American eel from sea water to fresh water for 24 hr did not alter plasma AP concentration, despite a significant increase in body weight and fall in plasma Na^+ levels. Moreover, the plasma AP concentrations of eels acclimated to fresh water did not differ significantly from those in eels acclimated to sea water. Y. Takei (personal communication) has recently sequenced the Japanese eel cardiac AP; it is 27 amino acids long, 17 of which are homologous to the human AP sequence. The brain AP from killifish has also recently been sequenced (D. Price, B. Dunn, personal communication); it is 22 amino acids long, shares 14 amino acids with porcine brain natriuretic peptide (124), and ends with a C-terminal cysteine in the cystine ring, which characterizes all atriopeptins. Both of these newly described sequences share the Asp-Arg-Ile-Gly (DRIG) sequence found inside the cystine ring in all atriopeptins. Finally, K. Karnaky, J. Valentich, M. Currie (personal communication) have recently shown that 10^{-7} M AP (rat AP $_{101-126}$) stimulated chloride-dependent bumetanide-sensitive short-circuit current in monolayer cultures of dogfish shark rectal gland epithelial cells. 20 mM procaine did not inhibit this effect, which suggests that AP directly activates chloride secretion by these cells exclusive of any neural release of VIP, which is necessary for stimulation in the intact gland (118).

Literature Cited

1. Arjamaa, O., Vuolteenaho, O. 1985. Sodium ion stimulates the release of atrial natriuretic polypeptides (ANP) from rat atria. *Biochem. Biophys. Res. Commun.* 132:375–81
2. Atlas, S. A. 1986. Atrial natriuretic factor: A new hormone of cardiac origin. *Recent Prog. Horm. Res.* 42:207–49
3. Atlas, S. A., Maack, T. 1987. Effects of atrial natriuretic factor on the kidney and the renin-angiotensin-aldosterone system. See Ref. 110, pp. 107–43
4. Babiker, M. M., Rankin, J. C. 1978. Neurohypophysial hormonal control of kidney function in the European eel (*Anguilla anguilla* L.) adapted to seawater or freshwater. *J. Endocrinol.* 76:347–58
5. Ballerman, B. J., Dunn, B. R., Mendez, R. E., Zeidel, M. L., Seifter, J. L., et al. 1987. Renal actions of atrial natriuretic peptides. See Ref. 83, pp. 83–92
6. Balment, R. J., Carrick, S. 1985. Endogenous renin-angiotensin system and drinking behavior in flounder. *Am. J. Physiol.* 248:R157–60
7. Baranowski, R. L., Westenfelder, C. 1989. Secretion of atrial natriuretic peptide (ANP) from fish atrial and ventricu-

lar myocytes in tissue culture. *Life Sci.* 44:187–91

8. Baxter, J. D., Lewicki, J. S., Gardner, D G. 1988. Atrial natriuretic peptide. *Biotechnology* 6:529–46

9. Beasley, D., Shier, D. N., Malvin, R. L., Smith, G. 1986. Angiotensin-stimulated drinking in marine fish. *Am. J. Physiol.* 250:R1034–38

10. Bennett, M. B., Rankin, J. C. 1986. The effects of neurohypophysial hormones on the vascular resistance of the isolated, perfused gill of the European eel, *Anguilla anguilla* L. *Gen. Comp. Endocrinol.* 64:60–66

11. Beyenbach, K. W. 1986. Secretory NaCl and volume flow in renal tubles. *Am. J. Physiol.* 250:R753–63

12. Borenstein, H. B., Cupples, W. A., Sonnenberg, H. A., Veress, A. T. 1983. The effect of a natriuretic atrial extract on renal haemodynamics and urinary excretion in anaesthetized rats. *J. Physiol.* 334:133–40

13. Brown, J. A., Oliver, J. A., Henderson, I. W., Jackson, B. A. 1980. Angiotensin and single nephron glomerular function in the trout *Salmo gairdneri*. *Am. J. Physiol.* 239:R509–14

14. Buckalew, V. M., Morris, M., Hamilton, R. W. 1987. Atrial natriuretic factor. *Adv. Int. Med.* 32:1–26

15. Cantin, M., Genest, J. 1985. The heart and the atrial natriuretic factor. *Endocr. Rev.* 6:107–27

16. Cantin, M., Genest, J. 1987. The heart as an endocrine gland. *Hypertension* 10:118–21

17. Cantin, M., Thibault, G., Ding, J., Gutkowska, J., Garcia, R., et al. 1987. Natriuretic factors, The whole heart as an endocrine gland. *Nucl. Med. Biol.* 14:313–22

18. Carrick, S., Balment, R. J. 1983. The renin-angiotensin system and drinking in the euryhaline flounder, *Platichthys flesus*. *Gen Comp. Endocrinol.* 51:423–33

19. Carroll, R. G. 1981. Vascular response of the dogfish and sculpin to angiotensin II. *Am. J. Physiol.* 240:R139–48

20. Chapeau, C., Gutkowska, J., Schiller, P. W., Milne, R. W., Thibault, G., et al. 1985. Localization of immunoreactive synthetic atrial natriuretic factor (ANF) in the heart of various animal species. *J. Histochem. Cytochem.* 33:541–50

21. De Bold, A. J., Borenstein, H. B., Veress, A. T., Sonnenberg, S. 1981. A rapid and potent natriuretic response to intravenous injection of atrial myocardial extract in rats. *Life Sci.* 39:89–94

22. de Renzis, G., Bornancin, M. 1984. Ion transport and gill ATPases. In *Fish Physiology*, ed. W. S. Hoar, D. J. Randall, 10B:65–104. Orlando: Academic. 416 pp.

23. Degnan, K. J., Zadunaisky, J. 1979. Open-circuit sodium and chloride fluxes across isolated opercular epithelia from the teleost *Fundulus heteroclitus*. *J. Physiol.* 294:483–95

24. Deray, G., Branch, R. A., Herzer, W. A., Ohnishi, A., Jackson, E. A. 1987. Effects of atrial natriuretic factor on hormone-induced renin release. *Hypertension* 9:513–17

25. Duff, D. W., Olson, K. R. 1986. Trout vascular and renal responses to atrial natriuretic factor and heart extracts. *Am. J. Physiol.* 251:R639–42

26. Epstein, F. H., Clark, B., Taylor, M., Silva, P., Dick, L., et al. 1988. Atrial natriuretic peptide (ANP) assayed in plasma of *Squalus acanthias*. *Bull. Mt. Desert Isl. Biol. Lab.* 27:72–73

27. Epstein, F. H., Stoff, J. S., Silva, P. 1983. Mechanism and control of hyperosmotic NaCl-rich secretion by the rectal gland of *Squalus acanthias*. *J. Exp Biol.* 106:25–41

28. Evans, D. H. 1979. Fish. In *Comparative Physiology of Osmoregulation in Animals*, ed. G. M. O. Maloiy, 1: 305–70. Orlando: Academic. 677 pp.

29. Evans, D. H. 1980. Kinetic studies of ion transport by fish gill epithelium. *Am. J. Physiol.* 238:R224–30

30. Evans, D H. 1984. The roles of gill permeability and transport mechanisms in euryhalinity. See Ref. 22, pp. 10B:239–83

31. Evans, D. H. 1986. The role of branchial and dermal epithelia in acid-base regulation in aquatic vertebrates. In *Acid-Base Regulation in Animals*, ed. N. Heisler, pp. 139–72. Amsterdam: Elsevier-North Holland. 492 pp.

31a. Evans, D. H. 1989. Immunoreactive atriopeptin in plasma and tissues of fishes: The effect of salinity change. *Bull. Mt. Desert Isl. Biol. Lab.* 28:39–41

32. Deleted in proof

33. Evans, D. H., Cameron, J. N. 1986. Gill ammonia transport. *J. Exp. Zool.* 239:17–23

34. Evans, D. H. Chipouras, E., Payne, J. A. 1989. Immunoreactive atriopeptin in the plasma of fishes: Its potential role in gill hemodynamics. *Am. J. Physiol.* In press

35. Evans, D. H., More, K. 1988. Modes of ammonia transport across the gill epithelium of the dogfish pup *(Squalus acanthias)*. *J. Exp. Biol.* 138:375–97

35a. Evans, D. H., Weingarten, K. E. 1989. Vasoactive effects of adenosine, vasoactive intestinal peptide, and atriopeptin on ventral aortic rings from the shark, *Squalus acanthias*. *Bull. Mt. Desert Isl. Biol. Lab.* 28:4–5

36. Deleted in proof

37. Fitzsimons, J. T. 1985. Physiology and pathophysiology of thirst and sodium appetite. In *The Kidney: Physiology and Pathophysiology,* ed. D. W. Seldin, G. Giebisch, II:885–901. New York: Raven. 1293 pp.

38. Forrest, J. N. Jr., Mackay, W. C., Gallagher, B., Epstein, F. H. 1973. Plasma cortisol response to saltwater adaptation in the American eel, *Anguilla anguilla. Am. J. Physiol.* 224:714–17

39. Forrest, J. N. Jr., Rieck, D., Murdaugh, A. 1980. Evidence for a ribose specific adenosine receptor (Ra) mediating stimulation of chloride secretion in the rectal gland of *Squalus acanthias. Bull. Mt. Desert Isl. Biol. Lab.* 20:152–55

40. Foskett, J. K., Bern, H. A., Machen, T. E., Conner, M. 1983. Chloride cells and the hormonal control of fish osmoregulation. *J. Exp. Biol.* 106:255–81

41. Foskett, J. K., Hubbard, G. M. 1981. Hormonal control of chloride secretion by teleost opercular membrane. *Ann. NY Acad. Sci.* 372:643

42. Foskett, J. K., Hubbard, G. M., Machen, T. E., Bern, H. A. 1982. Effects of epinephrine, glucagon and vasoactive intestinal polypeptide on chloride secretion by teleost opercular membrane. *J. Comp. Physiol. B* 146:27–34

43. Galli, S. M., Evans, D. H., Kimura, B., Phillips, M. I. 1988. Changes in plasma and brain levels of atrial natriuretic peptide in fish adapting to fresh water and sea water. *FASEB J.* 2:A524

44. Gardner, D. G., Gertz, B. J., Hane, S. 1987. Thyroid hormone increases ANP mRNA accumulation in vivo and in vitro. *Mol. Endocrinol.* 1:260–65

45. Gardner, D. G., Hane, S., Trachewsky, D., Schenk, D., Baxter, J. D. 1986. Atrial natriuretic peptide mRNA is regulated by glucocorticoids in vivo. *Biochem. Biophys. Res. Commun.* 139:1047–54

46. Garvin, J. L. 1989. ANF inhibits transport in the isolated, perfused rat proximal straight tubule (PST). *FASEB J.* 3:A247

47. Genest, J., Cantin, M. 1988. The atrial natriuretic factor: Its physiology and biochemistry. *Rev. Physiol. Biochem. Pharmacol.* 110:2–147

48. Gibbs, D. M. 1987. Non-calcium dependent modulation of in vitro atrial natriuretic factor release by extracellular osmolality. *Endocrinology* 120:194–97

49. Goetz, K. L. 1988. Effects of atrial peptides and atrial stretch receptors on hemodynamics and renal function. See Ref. 87, pp. 127–38

50. Goetz, K. L. 1988. Physiology and pathophysiology of atrial peptides. *Am. J. Physiol.* 254:E1–15

51. Greenwald, J. E., Sakata, M., Michener, M. L., Sides, S. D., Needleman, P. 1988. Is atriopeptin a physiological or pathophysiological substance? Studies in the autoimmune rat. *J. Clin. Invest.* 81:1036–41

52. Gupta, O. P., Lahlou, B., Botella, J., Porthe-Nibelle, J. 1985. In vivo and in vitro studies on the release of cortisol from interrenal tissue in trout. I. Effects of ACTH and prostaglandins. *Exp. Biol.* 43:201–12

53. Hegab, S. A., Hanke, W. 1984. The significance of cortisol for osmoregulation in carp *(Cyprinus carpio)* and tilapia *(Sarotherodon mossambicus). Gen. Comp. Endocrinol.* 54:409–17

54. Henderson, I. W., Hazon, N., Hughes, K. 1985. Hormones, ionic regulation and kidney function in fishes. In *Physiological Adaptations of Marine Animals,* ed. M. S. Laverack, 34:245–65. Cambridge: Company of Biologists. 265 pp.

55. Henrich, W. L., McAllister, E. A., Smith, P. B., Lipton, J., Campbell, W. B. 1987. Direct inhibitory effect of atriopeptin III on renin release in primate kidney. *Life Sci.* 41:259–64

56. Henrich, W. L., McAllister, E. A., Smith, P. B., Campbell, W. B. 1988. Guanosine 3',5'-cyclic monophosphate as a mediator of inhibition of renin release. *Am. J. Physiol.* 255:F474–78

57. Hickman, C. P. Jr. 1969. The kidney. In *Fish Physiology,* ed. W. S. Hoar, D. J. Randall, I:91–239. New York: Academic. 416 pp.

58. Hirano, T. 1986. The spectrum of prolactin action in teleosts. In *Comparative Endocrinology: Developments and Directions,* ed. C. L. Ralph, pp. 53–74. New York: Liss. 367 pp.

59. Hirano, T., Morisawa, M., Ando, M., Utida, S. 1975. Adaptive changes in ion and water transport mechanism in the eel intestine. In *Intestinal Ion Transport,* ed. J. W. L. Robinson, pp. 301–17. London: MTP. 268 pp.

60. Hughes, G. M. 1984. General anatomy of the gills. See Ref. 22, pp. 1–72

61. Imura, H., Nakao, K. 1988. Atrial natriuretic peptide in the central nervous

system and its possible function. See Ref. 87, pp. 205–15

62. Inagami, T., Imada, T., Tanaka, I., Takayanagi, R., Natuse, M., et al. 1987. Tissue distribution of atrial natriuretic factor and determination of its concentration. See Ref. 83, pp. 39–52

63. Isaia, J. 1984. Water and nonelectrolyte permeation. See Ref. 22, pp. 1–38

64. Karnaky, K. J. Jr. 1986. Structure and function of the chloride cell of *Fundulus heteroclitus* and other teleosts. *Am. Zool.* 26:209–24

65. Kelley, G., Gifford, D. R., Forrest, J. N. Jr. 1983. Stimulation and inhibition of adenlyate cyclase in the rectal gland of *Squalus acanthias. Bull. Mt. Desert Isl. Biol. Lab.* 23:86–88

66. Kenyon, C. J., McKeever, A., Oliver, J. A., Henderson, I. W. 1985. Control of renal and adrenocortical function by the renin-angiotensin system in two euryhaline teleost fishes. *Gen. Comp. Endocrinol.* 58:93–100

67. Keys, A. B. 1931. The heart-gill preparation of the eel and its perfusion for the study of a natural membrane in situ. *Z. Vergl. Physiol.* 15:352–63

68. Kloas, W., Flugge, G., Fuchs, E., Stolte, H. 1988. Binding sites for atrial natriuretic peptide in the kidney and aorta of the hagfish *(Myxine glutinosa). Comp. Biochem. Physiol. A* 91:685–88

69. Kramer, H. J. 1988. Atrial natriuretic hormones. *Gen. Pharmacol.* 19:7478–753

70. Lahlou, B. 1980. Les hormones dans l'osmoregulation des poissons. In *Environmental Physiology of Fishes,* ed. M. A. Ali, pp. 201–40. New York: Plenum. 723 pp.

71. Laurent, P. 1984. Gill internal morphology. See Ref. 22, pp. 73–183

72. Lee, J., Malvin, R. L. 1987. Natriuretic response to homologous heart extract in aglomerular toadfish. *Am. J. Physiol.* 252:R1055–58

73. Leitman, D. C., Murad, F. 1988. Atrial natriuretic factor receptor heterogeneity and stimulation of particulate granulate cyclase and cyclic GMP accumulation. See Ref. 110, pp. 79–105

74. Light, D. B., Schwiebert, E. M., Karlson, K. H., Stanton, B. A. 1989. Atrial natriuretic peptide inhibits a cation channel in renal inner medullary collecting duct cells. *Science* 243:383–85

75. Liu, F., Cogan, M. G. 1988. Atrial natriuretic factor does not inhibit basal or angiotensin II-stimulated proximal transport. *Am. J. Physiol.* 255:F434–37

76. Loretz, C. A., Bern, H. A. 1982. Pro-

lactin and osmoregulation in vertebrates. An update. *Neuroendocrinology* 35: 292–304

77. Loretz, C. A., Bern, H. A. 1983. Control of ion transport by *Gillichthys mirabilis* urinary bladder. *Am. J. Physiol.* 245:R45–52

78. Malvin, R. L., Schiff, D., Eiger, S. 1980. Angiotensin and drinking rates in the euryhaline killifish. *Am. J. Physiol.* 239:R31–34

79. Marshall, W. S., Bern, H. A. 1979. Teleostean urophysics: urotensin II and ion transport across the isolated skin of a marine teleost. *Science* 204:519–21

80. Matsuoka, H., Ishii, M., Hirata, Y., Atarashi, K., Sugimoto, T., et al. 1987. Evidence for lack of a role of cGMP in effect of α-hANP on aldosterone inhibition. *Am. J. Physiol.* 252:E643–47

81. May, S. A., Baratz, K. H., Key, S. Z., Degnan, K. J. 1984. Characterization of the adrenergic receptors regulating chloride secretion by the opercular epithelium. *J. Comp. Physiol. B* 154: 343–48

82. Mulrow, P. J., Franco-Saenz, R., Atarashi, K., Takagi, M., Takagi, M. 1987. Effect of atrial peptides on the adrenal cortex. See Ref. 83, pp. 93–109

83. Mulrow, P. J., Schrier, R., eds. 1987. *Atrial Hormones and Other Natriuretic Factors.* Clin. Physiol. Ser. Bethesda, MD: Am. Physiol. Soc. 178 pp.

84. Musch, M. W., Orellana, S. A., Kimberg, L. S., Field, M., Halm, D. R., et al. 1982. Na-K-Cl cotransport in the intestine of a marine teleost. *Nature* 300:351–54

85. Nakao, K., Imura, K. 1988. Biosynthesis, secretion and effect of atrial natriuretic polypeptide (ANP) in congestive heart failure (CHF). See Ref. 87, pp. 241–59

86. Naruse, M., Obana, K., Naruse, K., Yamaguchi, H., Demura, H., et al. 1987. Atrial natriuretic polypeptide inhibits cortisol secretion as well as aldosterone secretion in vitro from human adrenal tissue. *J. Clin. Endocrinol. Metab.* 64:10–16

87. Needleman, P., ed. 1988. *Biological and Molecular Aspects of Atrial Factors.* UCLA Symp. Mol. Cell. Biol. (N S), Vol. 81. New York: Liss. 282 pp.

88. Nemer, M., Argentin, S., Lavigne, J. P., Chamberland, M., Drouin, J. 1987. Glucocorticoid regulation of pronatriodilatin gene expression. *J. Cell. Biochem. A* 11:121

89. Nishimura, H. 1980. Comparative endocrinology of renin and angiotensin. In *The Renin-Angiotensin System,* ed. J.

A. Johnson, R. R. Anderson, pp. 29–77. New York: Plenum. 219 pp.

90. Nishimura, H., Bailey, J. R. 1982. Intrarenal renin-angiotensin system in primitive vertebrates. *Kidney Int.* 22 (Suppl. 12):S185–92

91. Nishimura, H., Sawyer, W. H. 1976. Vasopressor, diuretic, and natriuretic responses to angiotensins by the American eel, *Anguilla anguilla. Gen. Comp. Endocrinol.* 29:337–48

92. Nishimura, H., Sawyer, W. H., Nigelli, R. F. 1976. Renin, cortisol and plasma volume in marine teleosts fishes adapted to dilute media. *J. Endocrinol.* 70:47–59

93. O'Grady, S. M. 1989. Cyclic nucleotide-mediated effects of ANF and VIP on flounder intestinal ion transport. *Am. J. Physiol.* 256:C142–46

94. O'Grady, S. M., Field, M., Nash, N. T., Rao, M. C. 1985. Atrial natriuretic factor inhibits Na-K-Cl cotransport in teleost intestine. *Am. J. Physiol.* 249:C531–34

95. Okawara, Y., Kobayashi, H. 1988. Enhancement of water intake by captopril (SQ14225), an angiotensin I-converting enzyme inhibitor, in the goldfish, *Carassius auratus. Gen. Comp. Endocrinol.* 69:114–18

96. Olson, K. R., Meisheri, K. D. 1989. Effects of atrial natriuretic factor on isolated arteries and perfused organs of trout. *Am. J. Physiol.* 256:R10–18

97. Opdyke, D. F., Carroll, R. G., Keller, N. E., Taylor, A. A. 1981. Angiotensin II releases catecholamines in dogfish. *Comp. Biochem. Physiol. C* 70:131–36

98. Owen, N. E., O'Connell, M. E., Bush, E. N., Holleman, W. 1988. Effect of atrial natriuretic factor on sodium transport in vascular smooth muscle cells. See Ref. 87, pp. 173–84

99. Pang, P. K. T. 1983. Evolution of control of epithelial transport in vertebrates. *J. Exp. Biol.* 106:283–99

100. Pang, P. K. T., Furspan, P. B., Sawyer, W. H. 1983. Evolution of neurohypophyseal hormone actions in vertebrates. *Am. Zool.* 23:655–62

101. Parwez, I., Goswami, S. V., Sundararaj, B. I. 1984. Effects of hypophysectomy on some osmoregulatory parameters of the catfish, *Heteropneustes fossilis* (Bloch). *J. Exp. Zool.* 229:375–81

102. Payan, P., Girard, J. P., Mayer-Gostan, N. 1984. Branchial ion movements in teleosts: The roles of respiratory and chloride cells. See Ref. 22, pp. 39–63

103. Payan, P., Matty, A. J., Maetz, J. 1977. A study of the sodium pump in the perfused head preparation of the trout *Salmo gairdneri* in freshwater. *J. Comp. Physiol.* 104:33–48

104. Potts, W. T. W. 1984. Transepithelial potentials in fish gills. See Ref. 22, pp. 105–28

105. Rankin, J. C., Bolis, L. 1984. Hormonal control of water movement across the gills. See Ref. 22, pp. 177–201

106. Reinecke, M., Betzler, D., Forssmann, W. G. 1987. Immunocytochemistry of cardiac polypeptide hormones (Cardiodilatin/atrial natriuretic polypeptide) in brain and hearts of *Myxine glutinosa* (Cyclostomata). *Histochemistry* 86:233–39

107. Reinecke, M., Betzler, D., Forssmann, W. G., Thorndyke, M., Askensten, U., et al. 1987. Electromicroscopical, immunohistochemical, immunocytochemical and biological evidence for the occurrence of cardiac hormones (ANP/CDD) in chondrichthyes. *Histochemistry* 87:531–38

108. Reinecke, M., Nehls, M., Forssmann, W. B. 1985. Phylogenetic aspects of cardiac hormones as revealed by immunocytochemistry, electronmicroscopy, and bioassay. *Peptides* 6(Suppl. 3):321–31

109. Reinking, L. N. 1983. Aldosterone response to renin, angiotensin, ACTH, hemorrhage and sodium depletion in a freshwater teleost, *Catostomus macrocheilus. Comp. Biochem. Physiol. A* 74:873–80

110. Rosenblatt, M., Jacobs, J. W., eds. 1987. *Atrial Natriuretic Factor.* Endocrinol. Metab. Clin. North Am. Vol. 16, No. 1. Philadelphia: Saunders. 228 pp.

111. Samson, W. K. 1987. Atrial natriuretic factor and the central nervous system. See Ref. 110, 145–61

112. Samson, W. K. 1988. Hypothalamic actions of the atrial factors to alter hormone secretion from both the anterior and posterior pituitary. See Ref. 87, pp. 217–30

113. Sawyer, R. H. 1977. Evolution of neurohypophysial hormones and their receptors. *Fed. Proc.* 36:1842–47

114. Scheide, J. I., Zadunaisky, J. A. 1988. Effect of atriopeptin II on isolated opercular epithelium of *Fundulus heteroclitus. Am. J. Physiol.* 254:R27–32

115. Shibasaki, T., Naruse, M., Narus, K., Yamauchi, N., Sim, Y. S., et al. 1988. Effect of sodium ion on atrial natriuretic factor release from rat hypothalamic fragments. *Life Sci.* 42:1173–80

116. Shuttleworth, T. J., Thorndyke, M. C. 1984. An endogenous peptide stimulates secretory activity in the elasmobranch rectal gland. *Science* 225:319–21

117. Silva, P., Stoff, J. S., Leone, D. R., Epstein, F. H. 1985. Mode of action of somatostatin to inhibit secretion by shark rectal glands. *Am. J. Physiol.* 249:R329–34

118. Silva, P., Stoff, J. S., Solomon, R. J., Lear, S., Kniaz, D., et al. 1987. Atrial natriuretic peptide stimulates salt secretion by shark rectal gland by releasing VIP. *Am. J. Physiol.* 252:F99–F103

119. Solomon, R., Dubey, A., Silva, P., Epstein, F. 1988. Effect of atrial natriuretic peptide on renal function in *Squalus acanthias. Bull. Mt. Desert Isl. Biol. Lab.* 27:18–21

120. Solomon, R. J., Solomon, G., Silva, P., Epstein, F. H. 1985. The effect of atriopeptin and cardiac extracts on the ventral aorta of *Squalus acanthias. Bull. Mt. Desert Isl. Biol. Lab.* 25:146–49

121. Solomon, R., Taylor, M., Dorsey, D., Silva, P., Epstein, F. H. 1985. Atriopeptin stimulation of rectal gland in *Squalus acanthias. Am. J. Physiol.* 249:R348–54

122. Solomon, R., Taylor, M., Sheth, S., Silva, P., Epstein, F. H. 1985. Primary role of volume expansion in stimulation of rectal gland function. *Am. J. Physiol.* 248:R638–40

123. Stoff, J. S., Rosa, R., Hallac, R., Silva, P., Epstein, F. H. 1979. Hormonal regulation of active chloride transport in the dogfish rectal gland. *Am. J. Physiol.* 237:138–44

124. Sudoh, T., Kangawa, K., Minamino, N., Matsuo, H. 1988. A new natriuretic peptide in porcine brain. *Nature* 332:78–81

125. Trippodo, N. C. 1987. An update on the physiology of atrial natriuretic factor. *Hypertension* 10 (Suppl. I):I122–27

126. Westenfelder, C., Birch, F. M., Baranowski, R. L., Rosenfeld, M. J., Shiozawa, D. K., et al. 1988. Atrial natriuretic factor and salt adaptation in the teleost fish *Gila atraria. Am. J. Physiol.* 255:F1281–86

127. Wiegand, R. C., Day, M. L., Rodi, C. P., Schwartz, D., Needleman, P. 1987. Atriopeptin expression in the ventricle. See Ref. 83, pp. 33–38

128. Wilson, J. X. 1984. The renin-angiotensin system in nonmammalian vertebrates. *Endocr. Rev.* 5:45–61

129. Winquist, R. J. 1985. The relaxant effects of atrial natriuretic factor on vascular smooth muscle. *Life Sci.* 37:1081–87

130. Yakota, S. D., Benyajati, S. 1986. Regulation of glomerular filtration rate in a marine elasmobranch, the dogfish *(Squalus acanthias). Bull. Mt. Desert Isl. Biol. Lab.* 26:87–90

131. Zadunaisky, J. A. 1984. The chloride cell: The active transport of chloride and the paracellular pathways. See Ref. 22, pp. 129–76

132. Zeidel, M. L., Brenner, B. M. 1987. Actions of atrial natriuretic peptides on the kidney. *Semin. Nephrol.* 7:91–97

133. Zeidel, M. L., Seifter, J. L., Lear, S., Brenner, B. M., Silva, P. 1986. Atrial peptides inhibit oxygen consumption in kidney medullary collecting duct cells. *Am. J. Physiol.* 251:F379–83

134. Zucker, A., Nishimura. H. 1981. Renal responses to vasoactive hormones in the aglomerular toadfish, *Opsanus tau. Gen. Comp. Endocrinol.* 43:1–9

Annu. Rev. Physiol. 1990. 52:61–76

RESPIRATORY AND IONIC REGULATION IN INVERTEBRATES EXPOSED TO BOTH WATER AND AIR

J. P. Truchot

Laboratoire de Neurobiologie et Physiologie Comparées, CNRS-Université de Bordeaux I, 33120 Arcachon, France

KEY WORDS: amphibious life, invertebrates, gas exchange, acid-base balance, ionic regulation

INTRODUCTION

Transition from aquatic to aerial life is a major event that probably took place several times during animal evolution, but was often far from complete. A great number of forms, particularly invertebrates, now occupy ecological niches at the water-air interface and remain able to thrive, at least temporarily, in both media. Due to very contrasted physical properties, successful life in water and in air requires many different physiologic characteristics (22–24). Accordingly, a variety of specific adaptations have been recognized in animals exposed to both water and air. The present review focuses on those adaptations concerned with respiratory and ionic regulations.

THE NATURE OF THE PROBLEMS

Physical Properties of Aquatic and Aerial Environments

Respiratory gases, oxygen and carbon dioxide, have very different properties in water and in air. Primarily there is the ratio of the increment of gas

61

0066-4278/90/0315-0061$02.00

concentration (C) to the corresponding increment of gas partial pressure (P), the so-called capacitance coefficient $\beta = \Delta C/\Delta P$ (54). β_{O_2} is much higher in air than in water. As a consequence, at any given P_{O_2}, air contains 20 to 40 times more oxygen per unit volume than water. Conversely, β_{CO_2} is of the same order of magnitude in both media and thus is much higher than β_{O_2} in water. Furthermore, as a consequence of the gas law, O_2 and CO_2 capacitance coefficients have the same value, $1/RT$, in a gas phase. Another important point is that gas diffusion coefficients (D) as well as Krogh's constants of diffusion $(D \cdot \beta)$ are roughly 10^6 and 10^4 times higher for O_2 and CO_2 respectively, in air compared to water (22, 69). All this makes O_2 more readily available in air than in water and as a result, convective flow of medium across the respiratory surfaces must be higher in water than in air. However, because of the high convection and the comparable CO_2 capacitance coefficient in the two media, CO_2 elimination requires much smaller P_{CO_2} gradients in water than in air, and internal P_{CO_2} values are consequently low in water breathers. Thus, acute transition from water to air breathing induces hypercapnia and acidosis.

Air is a strongly dehydrating environment for intertidal dwellers. Because they periodically experience immersion in water, most of the invertebrates living at the water-air interface can not be fully adapted to a terrestrial existence. They have retained a moist, water permeable skin and are consequently exposed to the threat of dessication when in air. Evaporative water loss depends on the saturation deficit that increases with temperature at a given relative humidity. All these factors are highly variable spatially at the water-air interface and offer a large choice of microhabitats to suit particular needs. In addition residual water stores may be available, but their ionic and osmotic characteristics may differ from those of the nearby aquatic habitats. In other words, while respiratory constraints depending on physical properties of gases in both media are hardly avoidable, those linked to water and ion balance may be largely offset by adaptive behavior of intertidal animals.

The Various Patterns of Using Both Media

Extensive literature exists about the natural history of invertebrate animals living at the interface between water and air, and a brief account of the physiologic problems encountered by these animals is given below.

Periodic exposure to air on a predictable time basis is the rule for true intertidal animals. Most of them are basically designed for water breathing and can withstand only short-term air exposure. In fact, several types of behavior can be recognized among them. Some species isolate themselves from air as completely as possible by burrowing into the substratum or closing their shell or operculum. Others are able to use the aerial environment for respiratory gas exchange but must suffer some degree of dessication. Finally, some seek residual water to avoid permanent air exposure, but can spontaneously leave the aquatic medium when it becomes oxygen-depleted. Similar behavior is also found in freshwater animals, with the difference that such habitats usually dry out on a much less regular time basis than the intertidal zone.

Another category of invertebrates live permanently under water but are mostly dependent on the aerial environment for gas exchange. Good examples are found among freshwater pulmonate snails (e.g. *Lymnaea, Planorbis*) that breathe on a renewable gas store in their lung, but are completely dependent on the aquatic medium for water and ion exchange.

A number of brachyuran and anomuran crabs exhibit various degrees of terrestrialness. Most of the so-called land crabs are, in fact, air breathers and use either their gills or the gill cavity lining for gas exchange. But many also require periodic visits to water to rehydrate or replenish the water stores in the gill cavity or in the shell. Also most species return to water to spawn.

RESPIRATORY GAS EXCHANGE IN WATER AND IN AIR

Aerobic vs Anaerobic Metabolism in Air-Exposed Intertidal Invertebrates

It is commonly held that intertidal animals have two major respiratory options when exposed to air at low tide (11, 49): either to isolate themselves completely from the atmosphere and rely on anaerobic pathways for energy production, or to maintain gas exchange in air to support aerobic metabolism. There are, in fact, very few precisely documented examples of complete suppression of oxygen uptake in air at low tide. This appears to occur only under special conditions in some low shore species normally experiencing short exposure durations, e.g. the mussel *Mytilus edulis,* when starved or pre-acclimated to permanent immersion in the laboratory (74, 75). Most midshore intertidal invertebrates probably behave as facultative anaerobes, simultaneously using various fermentative pathways as well as aerobic metabolism when exposed to air. Anaerobic energy production is demonstrated in two ways. First, accumulation of anaerobic endproducts has been extensively documented in many species (51, 74). Second, calorimetric studies have shown that total heat dissipation in many cases greatly exceeds that accounted for by the oxygen used when in air (58). Partitioning of energy production between aerobic and anaerobic pathways appears highly variable according to species and environmental or trophic conditions. Such variability is usually credited with having an energetic significance. Most intertidal species utilize anaerobic pathways that lead to multiple endproducts such as alanine, succinate, and propionate. These pathways produce energy more efficiently than glycolysis in terms of ATP equivalents per mole of substrate and, because they lack a Pasteur effect (26), the metabolic level can be markedly depressed, an advantageous energy-saving measure during the inactive, food-restricted emersion period (49).

A convenient way to evaluate the ability of intertidal invertebrates to breathe air is to measure the air/water oxygen consumption ratio. An extensive compilation of such ratios can be found for intertidal molluscs in a recent review (49), and a more limited number of representative examples is shown in Table 1. From these values, it appears as a general rule that the higher the level of the shore where the animal thrives the greater its reliance upon air breathing. Low shore species have low air/water ratios and correspondingly accumulate anaerobic endproducts when exposed to air. Conversely, many high shore animals do not rely on anaerobic metabolism and are able to breathe in air as well as in water during natural exposure periods. Some high shore species even have considerably depressed respiratory rates when in water (Table 1). Such differences can often be explained by the nature of the respiratory organs, ecological conditions, or behavior (49). But it is particularly worth noting that for a given species or shore level, the reliance on air breathing is much dependent on the degree to which conditions of emersion affect dessication rates. Increased water loss always reduces air breathing. It

Table 1 Some representative examples of air/water oxygen consumption ratios in intertidal animals

Species[a]	Temperature (°C) (air and water)	Oxygen consumption Air/water ratio	References
Pollicipes polymerus (gooseneck barnacle)	10	5.0	52
Littorina rudis (littorine snail)	17.5	2.6	66
Patella vulgata (limpet)	10	2.34	41
Monodonta turbinata (trochid snail)	20	1.18	40
Carcinus maenas (shore crab)	15	1.18	62
Gibbula rarilineata (trochid snail)	20	0.76	40
Geukensia demissa (ribbed mussel)	20–23	0.66	7
Cerastoderma edule (common cockle)	10	0.28	74
Mytilus edulis (common mussel)	10	0.04	74

[a] Species roughly listed from high to low shore position in the intertidal zone.

is thus interesting to analyze how intertidal invertebrates can manage efficient aerobic energy production while limiting water loss when in air.

Dual Breathing: Some Morphological and Behavioral Adaptations

Most intertidal bivalves do not keep the shell tightly closed during air exposure. Rather, they periodically separate the valves, which exposes the mantle edge to the atmosphere, a behavior known as shell gaping (45). The pallial cavity can either remain filled with water or be partially occupied by an air space, which is ventilated by valve movements in some species (48, 49). The respiratory significance of shell gaping has been repeatedly demonstrated. The ability to gape correlates with high air/water O_2 consumption ratios. Whereas pallial fluid P_{O_2} rapidly decrease to zero in valve-clamped bivalves, it reaches steady-state levels between 15 and 40 torr in free gaping animals, which indicates that O_2 diffuses across the shell gape (4, 45). Accessibility of the tissues to gases in gaping bivalves is also clear from data that show labeling in various metabolites in cockles and mussels exposed to a $^{14}CO_2$-containing atmosphere (1). How shell gaping is regulated is poorly known. Body fluid pH increases in *Mytilus* during periodic bouts of gaping, probably because of CO_2 washout. This has led to the hypothesis that shell gaping is stimulated by decreased pH (76), which allows CO_2 escape and more efficient buffering of acidic endproducts by calcium carbonate in the shell. This interpretation, however, conflicts with observations that indicate the incidence of gaping is reduced after long-term emersion when both water loss and anaerobic endproducts accumulation are increased (49).

Barnacles are sessile crustaceans inhabiting intertidal and subtidal rocky areas. When exposed, high shore barnacles exhibit a small, diamond-shaped opening between the opercular valves called the micropylar aperture or pneumostome (2, 28). In fact, water is expelled from the mantle cavity upon emersion, and periodic opening and closing of the pneumostome allow gas to enter, mainly by diffusion. Several observations have shown that this behavior, which is not found in low shore or subtidal barnacles, is carefully regulated to ensure aerial respiration while avoiding excessive water loss. In a barnacle population the percentage of open pneumostomes is directly related to atmospheric humidity and inversely related to the time of exposure or to the evaporative weight loss. Analysis of gas bubbles expelled at reimmersion shows that oxygen depletion is more marked, and thus micropylar opening is less frequent for barnacles exposed to dry air compared to those in a wet atmosphere (28). Interestingly, the pneumostome tends to open more frequently in hypoxic gas (2), which suggests that both O_2 availability and dehydration stress are regulatory factors. Aerobic metabolism, in fact, prevails during natural short exposure, but longer periods induce lactate accumulation, which indicates that reliance upon air breathing ceases when excessive dehydration must be prevented.

Dual breathing is very common among decapod crustaceans. Many intertidal crabs are unimodal dual breathers using their gills for aerial gas exchange. Upon emersion, most of the water is drained away from the gill chamber, which is ventilated in air using the scaphognathites (62). Some species of the families Grapsidae and Ocypodidae, however, are able to retain gill water that is recirculated externally over the carapace for the purposes of aeration and for evaporative cooling (35). As the terrestrialness in land crabs increases, the reduction of the gills, which probably limits evaporative water loss, is accompanied by development of accessory exchange surfaces at the branchial chamber lining. These so-called lungs may be ventilated either continuously by the scaphognathites, or even tidally by thoracic movements, i.e. as in *Holthuisana transversa* (31).

Blood Oxygen Levels and Limitations of Gas Exchange

Even though O_2 availability is greater in air than in water, the gas exchange performance of invertebrates living at the water-air interface varies to a large extent, according to species and media. Table 2 illustrates several examples of blood oxygen levels of these animals. Some species such as true land crabs and a few high shore intertidal animals seem better designed for air breathing

Table 2 Oxygen partial pressures in arterial blood of invertebrates breathing either in well-aerated water or in normoxic air

Species	Temperature (°C) (water and air)	Arterial O_2 partial pressure (Torr)		References
		In water	In air	
Intertidal[a]				
Pollicipes polymerus	10	42	50	52
Carcinus maenas	15	75	19	62
Carcinus maenas	20	101	41	25
Cancer productus	10	59	21	19
Geukensia demissa	20–23	43	29	7
Mytilus edulis	12	44	25	43
Cryptochiton stelleri	10	85	29	53
Freshwater				
Austropotamobius pallipes	15	33	11	64
Terrestrial				
Gecarcinus Lateralis	25	17	80	59, 60
Holthuisana transversa	25	18	56	29, 30
Pseudotelphusa garmani	25	27	120–140	42

[a] Intertidal species roughly listed from high to low shore position in the intertidal zone

and have Pa_{O_2} levels higher in air than in water. Conversely, most mid- or low shore intertidal animals exhibit lower Pa_{O_2} values when breathing air, while arterial P_{CO_2} is at the same time increased, thus indicating CO_2 retention in air. In the latter case, many factors depending on species, respiratory organs, or particular behavior can account for gas exchange limitation in air. As stressed above, low water O_2 levels are maintained in the mantle cavity of gaping bivalves, which should result in greatly reduced P_{O_2} in body fluids. In decapod crustaceans using their gills for air breathing, strong diffusion limitations could arise from reduced gas exchange area because of gill collapse or retention of water in the intralamellar spaces. Possible perfusion limitations have also been suggested as a result of either reduced cardiac output or increased perfusion resistance in the gill (18).

Control of Ventilation and Circulation

Adequate ventilatory and circulatory levels are required for efficient oxygen uptake and transfer during air exposure. While ventilation obviously ceases in the water-filled mantle cavity of gaping bivalves and emersed gastropods, many intertidal crabs actively ventilate their gill chamber when in air. Ventilatory patterns, however, change greatly upon emersion. Primarily water-breathing species such as *Carcinus maenas* typically exhibit a reduction in ventilatory frequency and/or a shift from continuous to intermittent activity (18, 25). Very low extraction coefficients (2–3%), however, indicate that the ventilatory flow rate is not strongly depressed in air, as could be expected from a much greater oxygen availability. This probably relates to the poor oxygenation of the arterial hemolymph (see above), which maintains a strong ventilatory drive. Recently it was shown that *Carcinus* exposed to a hyperoxic atmosphere hypoventilates as its Pa_{O_2} increases and conversely hyperventilates when its Pa_{O_2} decreases in hypoxic air, thereby demonstrating that a typical O_2-chemosensitivity is retained when breathing air (25). Apparently CO_2-ventilatory drive is weak or absent in primary water-breathing crabs, either in water or in air (3), but exists in true terrestrial crabs such as *Gecarcinus lateralis* (14) or *Holthuisana transversa* (30).

Circulatory responses during air exposure are poorly documented. Typically, bradycardia develops in molluscs (49) and in decapod crustaceans (18), although there are exceptions. But corresponding changes in cardiac output are variable (Table 3). An intertidal crab such as *Carcinus maenas* exhibits an increased cardiac output when in air, which compensates for decreased arterial oxygen content and allows for maintenance of a completely aerobic metabolism (62). Conversely, in a subtidal species such as *Cancer productus*, cardiac output is considerably decreased in air, which correlates with a low air/water O_2 consumption ratio and a partial reliance upon anaerobic metabolism, which leads to lactate accumulation (19, 20). *Gecarcinus lateralis*, a

Table 3 Gas exchange performance in water and in air for three crab species

Species		Temperature (°C)	Oxygen consumption (μmol/kg·min)	Arterial O$_2$ partial pressure (Torr)	Cardiac output (ml/kg·min)	Blood lactate (mmol/l)	References
Cancer productus	Water	10	12.6	57	59	0.9	19, 20
(Subtidal)	Air	10	3.3	10	47	8.8	
Carcinus maenas	Water	15	37	75	118	3.05	62
(Intertidal)	Air	15	43	19	203	3.74	
Gecarcinus	Water	25	18.0	17	70	2.34	59, 60
lateralis	Air	25	34.3	80.5	137	1.38	
(Terrestrial)							

mostly air breathing terrestrial crab, by contrast shows depressed cardiac output and arterial P_{O_2} when submerged in water (59, 60).

An interesting circulatory adjustment has been recently described in the amphibious crab *Holthuisana transversa*, which has retained gills for aquatic gas exchange but also breathes in air by a tidally ventilated lung (65). Venous return is distributed in parallel between gill and lung areas. Studies using labeled microspheres have clearly shown than venous blood is directed preferentially to the gills during aquatic respiration and to the lungs during aerial respiration. Full development of the change in venous blood distribution takes hours and the mechanisms accounting for it are unclear. But, conceivably, partitioning of appropriate chemoreceptors between the two pathways could explain why amphibious crabs exhibit ventilatory controls primarily based on oxygen in water and on carbon dioxide in air.

Escape Behavior from Hypoxic Water

Residual water on the shore may be used as refuges by intertidal invertebrates to avoid dessication at low tide. However, microhabitats such as tide pools or burrow waters often exhibit large and rapid variations of respiratory conditions. In rockpools densely populated with plants and animals for example, dissolved oxygen accumulates during the day when photosynthesis is active but may become largely exhausted at night, and CO_2 and pH vary accordingly (70, 71). A number of species exposed to such conditions are known to spontaneously leave hypoxic water to breathe air. Such is the case for burrowing thalassinid shrimps (39), freshwater crayfish (47, 64), and the shore crab *Carcinus maenas* (61). In shallow hypoxic water, the shore crab raises the anterior border of its cephalothorax above the water level and reverses respiratory pumping, which causes air to bubble through the water retained in the gill chamber. This behavior appears carefully regulated, triggered at well-defined threshold P_{O_2} values in water, and results in increased oxygen levels not only in the gill water but also in the postbranchial blood. Simultaneous tachycardia suggests that oxygen delivery to the tissues is most likely enhanced (63, 73).

REGULATION OF ACID-BASE BALANCE

Blood P_{CO_2} and pH in Water Breathers vs Air Breathers

A comparison of blood P_{CO_2} levels among animals shows that values recorded in water breathers are invariably lower than in air breathers (69). This basic relationship results from the fact that water is a very efficient sink for metabolic CO_2 because of (*a*) a high CO_2 capacitance coefficient and (*b*) huge ventilatory flow rates needed to extract oxygen from the aquatic medium. However, extracellular pH values are not radically different in water breathers and in air breathers when considered at the same body temperature. This is because extracellular HCO_3^- concentrations are set at a higher level in air breathers than water breathers, thus maintaining a roughly identical $[HCO_3^-]/$ dissolved CO_2 ratio (56). The fact that similar pH values prevail at the same body temperature in all animals irrespective of the respiratory medium probably relates to the necessity of preserving the electrical charge state and thus the conformation and function of macromolecules (57).

Acid-Base Balance at the Transition from Water to Air Breathing

Because the range of P_{CO_2} values experienced by a given animal primarily depends on the respiratory medium, invertebrates living at the water-air interface must be exposed to particularly large excursions of their P_{CO_2} levels and acid-base balance. Accumulation of acidic endproducts can promote a metabolic acidosis, but the most typical response is a hypercapnic acidosis, which, in fact, has been observed upon air exposure in all forms tested to date: crabs (11, 20, 62, 67); bivalves (8, 43); cirripeds (52). In crabs the usually rapid increase in blood P_{CO_2} at emersion is followed more slowly by a compensatory buildup of bicarbonate. Compensation of emersion acidosis in *Carcinus* takes much longer than the usual emersion durations in the field, but observations on *Cancer productus* suggest that compensation could be more effective in nature than in the laboratory, especially if the crab is buried in a moist substrate (21). A switch to water breathing at reimmersion conversely induces rapid CO_2 washout with a transient hypocapnic alkalosis that is quickly offset by a rapid decrease of bicarbonate concentration (67). Such a rapidly compensated "immersion hypocapnia" is also observed in *Cardisoma carnifex,* a terrestrial crab with well-developed gills (15).

Although air exposure always leads to hypercapnia, P_{CO_2} levels recorded in emersed invertebrates are in most cases much lower than those prevailing in true air breathers. This probably relates to a diffusion limitation of O_2 uptake, which results in poorly oxygenated blood and a higher than usual ventilatory activity in air. Indeed, a recent study in *Carcinus* showed that crabs exposed to a hyperoxic atmosphere had reduced ventilation and higher hemolymph P_{CO_2} than in normoxic air (25). Diffusion limitation, however, can not explain the observation that hemolymph P_{CO_2} is also low in the land crab *Pseudotelphusa garmani,* despite a very efficient lung and high P_{O_2} levels in arterial blood (42; see Table 2).

Possible Mechanisms Accounting for Acid-Base Compensations

Branchial ionic exchanges most probably ensure compensation of various acid-base disturbances in aquatic animals (27, 69). Reduction of hemolymph bicarbonate compensating for reimmersion alkalosis in the shore crab *Carcinus maenas* correlates with a concomitant outflux of alkaline equivalents (68), which indicates that these branchial mechanisms are switched on at the transition from air to water breathing. During air exposure however, the branchial route can hardly be used and several studies indicate that at least in crabs, the capacity for urine acidification is poor (15, 68, 69). Thus buffering of the acid load brought about by elevated P_{co_2} must take place inside the organism. Tissue buffers may be involved (15, 68), but the major source of bicarbonate accounting for the compensation of emersion acidosis is probably the shell in molluscs (13) and the calcified exoskeleton in decapod crustaceans (17). This is indirectly indicated by many reports showing that Ca^{2+} concentration increases in the hemolymph during the compensatory phase, particularly in terrestrial crabs (36). A direct proof of calcium carbonate mobilization has been provided for the crab *Callinectes sapidus,* but the contribution of the carapace was found relatively small in this primarily aquatic species (16).

Another potential sink for acidic equivalents during the compensation of emersion acidosis is the water retained in the gill cavity when in air. A recent laboratory study (12) concluded that branchial water stores were too small to contribute significantly in three species of intertidal crabs. If, however, they can be replenished, which is usually the case in the field, their role may become significant (79).

IONIC REGULATION AND MAINTENANCE OF HYDROMINERAL BALANCE

Dessication Rates and Integumental Water Permeability

Dehydration stress is certainly a major problem for invertebrates during air exposure. Evaporative water loss obviously depends on many factors such as temperature, relative humidity, and so on. Also the extent to which the moist integument or the gills are protected from the atmosphere varies considerably among species, in relation with particular behaviors such as those allowing air breathing (see above). Nevertheless, a general relationship emerges from numerous studies. Dessication rates are always found to be lower in invertebrates living at the water-air interface than in related fully aquatic animals. For intertidal animals such as molluscs, barnacles, crabs, and so on, the rate of water loss in air correlates closely with the vertical distribution on the shore; the higher the zonation level, and therefore the longer the duration of air exposure at low tide, the smaller is the ratio of water loss (50, 72). In addition to morphological and behavioral adaptations, several physiologic characteristics may explain such differences. Integumental water permeability in air is reduced in amphibious and terrestrial crabs compared to aquatic species (5, 37). Also in terrestrial crabs, urinary flow rate is considerably decreased during dehydration, mainly because of a reduction of filtration processes indicated by lowered inulin clearance values (33, 34).

Amphibious invertebrates not only exhibit low dessication rates, but they are also particularly resistant to dehydration. For example, while aquatic crabs usually tolerate no more than a 12–14% loss of total body water, intertidal and terrestrial crabs can withstand up to 20–40% body water loss (38, 44). Similar relationships hold for many other intertidal animals (50).

The Role of Gill or Shell Water Stores

Many invertebrates retain variable amounts of water when exposed to air, for example in the pallial cavity in molluscs, the gill chamber in some crustaceans, or the home shell in hermit crabs. These water stores not only serve respiratory and perhaps acid-base regulatory purposes as discussed above, but they also have a prominent role in water conservation and ionic regulation. Several studies in molluscs (9) and crustaceans (10, 80) have shown that these water stores are progressively depleted and become concentrated during air exposure, while hemolymph composition is minimally affected. This indicates that evaporative water loss mainly originates from these external water stores and thereby limits the effects of dessication on body fluid osmolality.

Uptake of Interstitial Water

Some crabs exposed to air on a damp substratum can compensate for evaporative water loss by taking up interstitial water. This is made possible by rows or tufts of setae located near the ventral apertures of the gill chamber. When closely applied to the substratum, these structures can conduct water by capillarity. The occurrence of this behavior is usually correlated with the degree of dehydration. In *Gecarcinus lateralis,* water apparently travels to the gills over the setose surfaces of two diverticula of the pericardial cavity known as the pericardial sacs (6). In the ghost crab *Ocypode quadrata,* water uptake from poorly hydrated sand is aided by a strong gill chamber depression caused by scaphognathite beating (77). In both cases water is probably absorbed at the gills. Similar mechanisms seems to operate in the soldier crab *Mictyris longicarpus,* which, in addition, uses gill water to collect organic detritus for food (55).

Ion Conservation Mechanisms in Land Crabs

There are probably two groups of semi-terrestrial and terrestrial crabs, those originating from the sea and those from freshwater habitats. The former have retained high hemolymph osmolalities but typically hypoosmoregulate when in sea water. The tendency to become hypoosmoregulators generally increases with increasing terrestrialness (32). When in air, these terrestrial crabs need to replenish their body water in order to compensate for evaporative losses, but the water available inland may often be more dilute than sea water. Furthermore, some of them live or take refuge in burrows containing essentially freshwater (79). Since crabs, unlike crayfish, can not produce dilute urine (46), the high flow rate of isosmotic urine needed for water balance in these conditions could result in salt depletion unless urine salts are reclaimed by specific mechanisms. Salt recovery from isosmotic urine appears to occur in the ghost crab *Ocypode quadrata* (78). When artificially loaded in air with a hypoosmotic solution, this animal produces a dilute final excretory product from isosmotic urine. Where this occurs is not established, but is probably the gills.

CONCLUDING REMARKS

There are many natural history studies of invertebrates living at the interface between water and air, but too few address the problems, in physiologic terms, that such animals have had to solve in order to survive in this environment. Many species, in fact, are hardly amenable to experimental work because of their small size. Also physiologic processes at the organ level often seem, at first glance, hidden behind an amazing diversity of morphologies and behavior, which apparently discourages generalizations about regulatory and adaptational features. Yet recent studies have shown that many physiologic responses attributable to the contrasted properties of water and air are found not only in vertebrates, but also in invertebrates living at the interface between both media. Because most are not yet fully adapted to a terrestrial existence, these creatures can provide a rich choice of models for exploring the transition from life in water to life on land.

Literature Cited

1. Ahmad, T. A., Chaplin, H. E. 1977. The intermediary metabolism of *Mytilus edulis* (L.) and *Cerastoderma edule* (L.) during exposure to the atmosphere. *Biochem. Soc. Trans.* 5:1320–23
2. Barnes, H. D., Finlayson, D. M., Piatigorsky, J. 1963. The effect of dessication on the behavior, survival and general metabolism of three common cirripeds. *J. Anim. Ecol.* 32:233–52
3. Batterton, C. V., Cameron, J. N. 1978. Characteristics of resting ventilation and responses to hypoxia, hypercapnia, and emersion in the blue crab *Callinectes sapidus* (Rathbun). *J. Exp. Zool.* 203: 403–18
4. Bayne, B. L., Bayne, C. J., Carefoot, T. C., Thompson, R. J. 1976. The phys-

iological ecology of *Mytilus californianus* Conrad. 2. Adaptations to low oxygen tension and air exposure. *Oecologia* 22:229–50
5. Bliss, D. E. 1968. Transition from water to land in decapod crustaceans. *Am. Zool.* 8:355–92
6. Bliss, D. E. 1979. From sea to tree: saga of a land crab. *Am. Zool.* 19:385–410
7. Booth, C. E., Mangum, C. P. 1978. Oxygen uptake and transport in the lamellibranch mollusc *Modiolus demissus*. *Physiol. Zool.* 51:27–32
8. Booth, C. E., McDonald, D. G., Walsh, P. J. 1984. Acid-base balance in the sea mussel, *Mytilus edulis*. Effects of hypoxia and air exposure on hemolymph

acid-base status. *Mar. Biol. Lett.* 5:347–58

9. Boyle, P. R., Sillar, M., Bryceson, K. 1979. Water balance and the mantle cavity fluid of *Nucella lapillus* (L.) (Mollusca: Prosobranchia). *J. Exp. Mar. Biol. Ecol.* 40:41–51

10. Burggren, W. W., McMahon, B. R. 1981. Hemolymph oxygen transport, acid-base status, and hydromineral regulation during dehydration in three terrestrial crabs, *Cardisoma, Birgus* and *Coenobita. J. Exp. Zool.* 218:53–64

11. Burnett, L. E. 1988. Physiological responses to air esposure: acid-base balance and the role of branchial water stores. *Am. Zool.* 28:125–35

12. Burnett, L. E., McMahon, B. R. 1987. Gas exchange, hemolymph acid-base status, and the role of branchial water stores during air exposure in three littoral crab species. *Physiol. Zool.* 60:27–36

13. Burton, R. F. 1983. Ionic regulation and water balance. In *The Mollusca, Physiology*, Vol. 5. Pt. 2. ed. A. S. M. Saleuddin, K. M. Wilbur, pp. 291–352. London:Academic

14. Cameron, J. N. 1975. Aerial gas exchange in the terrestrial brachyura *Gecarcinus lateralis* and *Cardisoma guanhumi. Comp. Biochem. Physiol.* 50A:129–34

15. Cameron, J. N. 1981. Acid-base responses to changes in CO_2 in two Pacific crabs: the coconut crab, *Birgus latro,* and a mangrove crab, *Cardisoma carnifex. J. Exp. Zool.* 218:65–73

16. Cameron, J. N. 1985. Compensation of hypercapnic acidosis in the aquatic blue crab, *Callinectes sapidus:* the predominance of external sea water over carapace carbonate as the proton sink. *J. Exp. Biol.* 114:197–206

17. Cameron, J. N. 1986. Acid-base equilibria in invertebrates. In *Acid-base Regulation in Animals,* ed. N. Heisler, pp. 357–94. Amsterdam: Elsevier

18. deFur, P. L. 1988. Systemic respiratory adaptations to air exposure in intertidal decapod crustaceans. *Am. Zool.* 28:115–24

19. deFur, P. L., McMahon, B. R. 1984. Physiological compensation to short-term air exposure in red rock crabs, *Cancer productus* Randall, from littoral and sublittoral habitats. I. Oxygen uptake and transport. *Physiol. Zool.* 57:137–50

20. deFur, P. L., McMahon, B. R. 1984. Physiological compensation to short-term air exposure in red rock crabs, *Cancer productus* Randall, from littoral and sublittoral habitats. II. Acid-base balance. *Physiol. Zool.* 57:151–60

21. deFur, P. L., McMahon, B. R., Booth, C. E. 1983. Analysis of hemolymph oxygen levels and acid-base status during emersion 'in situ' in the Red Rock Crab, *Cancer productus. Biol. Bull.* 165:582–90

22. Dejours, P. 1981. *Principles of Comparative Respiratory Physiology.* Amsterdam: Elsevier. 265 pp. 2nd ed.

23. Dejours, P. 1988. *Respiration in Water and in Air. Adaptations—Regulation—Evolution.* Amsterdam: Elsevier. 179 pp.

24. Dejours, P., Bolis, L., Taylor, C. R., Weibel, E. R., eds. 1987. *Comparative Physiology: Life in Water and on Land.* Padova: Liviana. 556 pp.

25. Dejours, P., Truchot, J. P. 1988. Respiration of the emersed shore crab at variable ambient oxygenation. *J. Comp. Physiol.* B 158:387–91

26. deZwaan, A. 1977. Anaerobic energy metabolism in bivalve molluscs. In *Oceanography and Marine Biology. An Annual Review,* ed. H. Barnes, pp. 103–87. Aberdeen: Aberdeen University

27. Evans, D. H. 1986. The role of branchial and dermal epithelia in acid-base regulation in aquatic vertebrates. In *Acid-base Regulation in Animals,* ed. N. Heisler, pp. 139–72. Amsterdam: Elsevier

28. Grainger, F., Newell, G. E. 1965. Aerial respiration in *Balanus belanoides. J. Mar. Biol. Assoc. UK* 45:469–79

29. Greenaway, P., Bonaventura, J., Taylor, H. H. 1983. Aquatic gas exchange in the freshwater/land crab, *Holthuisana transversa. J. Exp. Biol.* 103:225–36

30. Greenaway, P., Taylor, H. H., Bonaventura, J. 1983. Aerial gas exchange in Australian freshwater/land crabs of the genus *Holthuisana. J. Exp. Biol.* 103:237–51

31. Greenaway, P., Taylor, H. H. 1976. Aerial gas exchange in Australian arid-zone crab *Paratelphusa transversa* Von Martens. *Nature* 262:711–13

32. Gross, W. J. 1964. Trends in water and salt regulation among aquatic and amphibious crabs. *Biol. Bull.* 127:447–66

33. Harris, R. R. 1977. Urine production rate and water balance in the terrestrial crabs *Gecarcinus lateralis* and *Cardisoma guanhumi. J. Exp. Biol.* 68:57–67

34. Harris, R. R., Kormanik, G. A. 1981. Salt and water balance and antennal gland function in three Pacific species of terrestrial crabs *(Gecarcoidea lalandii, Cardisoma carnifex, Birgus latro).* II.

The effects of dessication. *J. Exp. Zool.* 218:107–16

35. Hawkins, A. J. S., Jones, M. B. 1982. Gill area and ventilation in two mud crabs, *Helice crassa* Dana (Grapsidae) and *Macrophthalmus hirtipes* (Jacquinot) (Ocypodidae) in relation to habitat. *J. Exp. Mar. Biol. Ecol.* 60:103–18

36. Henry, R. P., Kormanik, G. A., Smatresk, N. J., Cameron, J. N. 1981. The role of CaCO$_3$ dissolution as a source of HCO$^-_3$ for the buffering of hypercapnic acidosis in aquatic and terrestrial decapod crustaceans. *J. Exp. Biol.* 94:269–74

37. Herreid, C. F. II 1969. Integumental permeability of crabs and adaptation to land. *Comp. Biochem. Physiol.* 29:425–29

38. Herreid, C. F. II 1969. Water loss of crabs from different habitats. *Comp. Biochem. Physiol.* 28:829–39

39. Hill, B. 1981. Respiratory adaptations of three species of *Upogebia* (Thalassinidea, Crustacea) with special reference to low tide periods. *Biol. Bull.* 160:272–79

40. Houlihan, D. F., Innes, A. J. 1982. Respiration in air and water of four Mediterranean trochids. *J. Exp. Mar. Biol. Ecol.* 57:35–54

41. Houlihan, D. F., Newton, J. R. L. 1978. Respiration of *Patella vulgata* on the shore. In *Physiology and Behaviour of Marine Organisms*, ed. D. S. McLusky, A. J. Berry, pp. 39–46. Oxford: Pergamon

42. Innes, A. J., Taylor, E. W. 1986. The evolution of air-breathing in crustaceans: a functional analysis of branchial, cutaneous and pulmonary gas exchange. *Comp. Biochem. Physiol.* 85A:621–37

43. Jokumsen, A., Fyhn, H. J. 1982. The influence of aerial exposure upon respiratory and osmotic properties of haemolymph from two intertidal mussels, *Mytilus edulis* L. and *Modiolus modiolus* L. *J. Exp. Mar. Biol. Ecol.* 61:189–203

44. Jones, M. B., Greenwood, J. G. 1982. Water loss of a porcelain crab, *Petrolisthes elongatus* (Milne Edwards, 1837) (Decapoda Anomura) during atmospheric exposure. *Comp. Biochem. Physiol.* 72A:631–36

45. Lent, C. M. 1968. Air-gaping by the ribbed mussel, *Modiolus demissus* (Dillwyn): effects and adaptive significance. *Biol. Bull.* 134:60–73

46. Mantel, L. H., Farmer, L. L. 1983. Osmotic and ionic regulation. In *The Biology of Crustacea, Internal Anatomy and Physiological Regulation*, Vol. 5.

ed. L. H. Mantel, pp. 54–161. New York: Academic

47. McMahon, B. R., Wilkes, P. R. H. 1983. Emergence responses and aerial ventilation in normoxic and hypoxic crayfish *Orconectes rusticus*. *Physiol. Zool.* 56:133–41

48. McMahon, R. F. 1983. Dessication resistance and use of the mantle cavity for aerial respiration in the mangrove bivalve mollusc, *Geloina erosa*. *Am. Zool.* 23:938

49. McMahon, R. F. 1988. Respiratory response to periodic emergence in intertidal molluscs. *Am. Zool.* 28:97–114

50. Newell, R. C. 1979. *Biology of Intertidal Animals.* Faversham Kent England: Mar. Ecol. Surv.

51. Nicchita, C. V., Ellington, W. R. 1983. Energy metabolism during air exposure and recovery in the high intertidal bivalve mollusc *Geukensia demissa granosissima* and the subtidal bivalve mollusc *Modiolus squamosus*. *Biol. Bull.* 165:708–22

52. Petersen, J. A., Fyhn, H. J., Johansen, K. 1974. Ecophysiological studies of an intertidal crustacean, *Pollicipes polymerus* (Cirripedia Lepadomorpha): aquatic and aerial respiration. *J. Exp. Biol.* 61:309–20

53. Petersen, J. A., Johansen, K. 1973. Gas exchange in the giant cradle *Cryptochiton stelleri* (Middendorf). *J. Exp. Mar. Biol. Ecol.* 12:27–43

54. Piiper, J., Dejours, P., Haab, P., Rahn, H. 1971. Concepts and basic quantities in gas exchange physiology. *Respir. Physiol.* 13:292–304

55. Quinn, R. H. 1980. Mechanisms for obtaining water for flotation feeding in the soldier crab, *Mictyris longicarpus* Latreille, 1806 (Decapoda Mictyridae). *J. Exp. Mar. Biol. Ecol.* 43:49–60

56. Rahn, H. 1967. Gas transport from the external environment to the cell. In *Development of the Lung. Ciba Foundation Symposium*, ed. A. V. S. de Reuck, R. Porter, pp. 3–23. London: Churchill

57. Reeves, R. B. 1977. The interaction of body temperature and acid-base balance in ectothermic vertebrates. *Annu. Rev. Physiol.* 39:559–86

58. Shick, J. M., Widdows, J., Gnaiger, E. 1988. Calorimetric studies of behavior, metabolism and energetics of sessile intertidal animals. *Am. Zool.* 28:161–81

59. Taylor, A. C., Davies, P. S. 1981. Respiration in the land crab, *Gecarcinus lateralis*. *J. Exp. Biol.* 93:197–208

60. Taylor, A. C., Davies, P. S. 1982. Aquatic respiration in the land crab,

Gecarcinus lateralis (Freminville). *Comp. Biochem. Physiol.* 72A:683–88

61. Taylor, E. W., Butler, P. J. 1973. The behaviour and physiological responses of the shore crab *Carcinus maenas* during changes of environmental oxygen tensions. *Neth. J. Sea Res.* 7:496–505

62. Taylor, E. W., Butler, P. J. 1978. Aquatic and aerial respiration in the shore crab, *Carcinus maenas* (L.), acclimated to 15°C. *J. Comp. Physiol.* B127:315–23

63. Taylor, E. W., Butler, P. J., Sherlock, P. J. 1973. The respiratory and cardiovascular changes associated with the emersion response of *Carcinus maenas* (L.) during environmental hypoxia. *J. Comp. Physiol.* 86:95–115

64. Taylor, E. W., Wheatly, M. G. 1980. Ventilation, heart rate and respiratory gas exchange in the crayfish *Austropotamobius pallipes* (Lereboullet) submerged in normoxic water and following 3 h exposure in air at 15°C. *J. Comp. Physiol.* B138:67–78

65. Taylor, H. H., Greenaway, P. 1984. The role of the gills and the branchiostegites in gas exchange in a bimodally breathing crab, *Holthuisana transversa*: evidence for a facultative change in the distribution of the respiratory circulation. *J. Exp. Biol.* 111:103–21

66. Toulmond, A. 1967. Etude de la consommation d'oxygène en fonction du poids, dans l'air et dans l'eau, chez quatre espèces du genre *Littorina* (Gasteropoda, Prosobranchiata). *C. R. Hebd. Séances Acad. Sci. Paris Série D* 264: 636–38

67. Truchot, J. P. 1975. Blood acid-base changes during experimental emersion and reimmersion of the intertidal crab, *Carcinus maenas* (L.). *Respir. Physiol.* 23:351–60

68. Truchot, J. P. 1979. Mechanisms of the compensation of blood respiratory acid-base disturbances in the shore crab, *Carcinus maenas* (L.). *J. Exp. Zool.* 210: 407–16

69. Truchot, J. P. 1987. *Comparative Aspects of Extracellular Acid-base Balance*. Berlin: Springer. 248 pp.

70. Truchot, J. P. 1988. Problems of acid-base balance in rapidly changing intertidal environments. *Am. Zool.* 28:55–64

71. Truchot, J. P., Duhamel-Jouve, A. 1980. Oxygen and carbon dioxide in the marine intertidal environment: diurnal and tidal changes in rockpools. *Respir. Physiol.* 39:241–54

72. Vernberg, W. B., Vernberg, F. J. 1972. *Environmental Physiology of Marine Animals*. Berlin: Springer. 346 pp.

73. Wheatly, M. G., Taylor, E. W. 1979. Oxygen levels, acid-base status and heart rate during emersion of the shore crab into air. *J. Comp. Physiol.* B132: 305–11

74. Widdows, J., Bayne, B. L., Livingstone, D. R., Newell, R. I. E., Donkin, P. 1979. Physiological and biochemical responses of bivalve molluscs to exposure to air. *Comp. Biochem. Physiol.* 62A:301–8

75. Widdows, J., Shick, J. M. 1985. Physiological responses of *Mytilus edulis* and *Cardium edule* to aerial exposure. *Mar. Biol.* 85:217–32

76. Wijsman, T. C. M. 1975. pH fluctuations in *Mytilus edulis* L. in relation to shell movements under aerobic and anaerobic conditions. In *Proceedings of the 9th European Marine Biology Symposium*, ed. H. Barnes, pp. 139–49. Aberdeen: Aberdeen University

77. Wolcott, T. G. 1976. Uptake of soil capillary water by ghost crabs. *Nature* 264:756–57

78. Wolcott, T. G., Wolcott, D. L. 1985. Extrarenal modification of urine for ion conservation in ghost crabs, *Ocypode quadrata* (Fabricius). *J. Exp. Mar. Biol. Ecol.* 91:93–107

79. Wood, C. M., Boutilier, R. G. 1985. Osmoregulation, ionic exchanges, blood chemistry, and nitrogenous waste excretion in the land crab *Cardisoma carnifex*: a field and laboratory study. *Biol. Bull.* 169:267–90

80. Wood, C. M., Boutilier, R. G. 1986. The physiology of dehydration stress in the land crab, *Cardisoma carnifex*: respiration, ionoregulation, acid-base balance and nitrogenous waste excretion. *J. Exp. Biol.* 126:271–96

Annu. Rev. Physiol. 1990. 52:77–95

UNUSUAL ASPECTS OF CALCIUM METABOLISM IN AQUATIC ANIMALS

James N. Cameron

The University of Texas, Marine Science Institute, Port Aransas, Texas 78373

KEY WORDS: calcification, homeostasis, skeleton, invertebrate, molt

INTRODUCTION

Calcium constitutes about 3.6% of the earth's crust, and is the fifth most abundant element. Moderately soluble, calcium is an abundant component of both natural waters and of the extracellular fluids of animals. Seawater contains 400mg L^{-1} (10 mM L^{-1}) of calcium; fresh waters vary considerably, from a few millimolar in hard waters to the micromolar range in very soft waters, especially in boggy areas where humic acids and other organic substances act as effective chelators.

In biological fluids the abundance and function of calcium differ sharply between the intra- and extracellular environments. Many marine animals classified as osmoconformers have calcium concentrations in blood and other extracellular fluids that are very similar to the surrounding seawater, i.e. about 10 mM L^{-1}. Among the osmoregulators, calcium concentrations are generally lower, but still in the millimolar range. Typical values for animals in brackish water are 2–8 mM L^{-1} (96). The same sort of range is found in the higher vertebrates, with human plasma regulated at about 2.6 mM L^{-1}. The free calcium ion activity in the intracellular environment, however, is three to four orders of magnitude lower, averaging 0.1–1 μM L^{-1} (94). The total calcium is much higher, but most of the calcium present is chemically bound

77

0066-4278/90/0315-0077$02.00

to proteins, phospholipids, or other cellular components. The typical animal cell, then, maintains a standing calcium gradient between inside and out of between 1000 and 10,000 to 1. The typical cell has an inside potential of a few tens of millivolts negative, so calcium is far out of electrochemical equilibrium. Since the passive (inward) permeability of calcium is never quite zero, the steady-state gradients must be maintained by an energy-requiring (active transport) process, the "calcium pump" (32, 57, 75, 105).

Teleologically speaking it is difficult to say why the free intracellular calcium activity must be maintained at such a low level, but there is considerable evidence that sharp increases in the free intracellular calcium activity are a prime factor in cell death (48, 94). At a much more subtle level, calcium is known to exert a powerful influence on a multitude of cell processes, both as an immediate effector and as a second messenger. Indeed, so ubiquitous is the intracellular influence of calcium that it prompted one scientist to remark "Calcium does everything." These intracellular aspects of calcium regulation have received a great deal of attention over the past few decades and have been reviewed extensively (32, 42, 47, 49, 57, 66, 75, 119, 141). For the present article I shall consider these to be usual functions of calcium, and will deal no further with them.

An intriguing aspect of the biochemistry of calcium is that while small changes in an extremely low free calcium concentration inside of cells can produce very large effects on cellular processes, animals at the same time carry out various processes involving calcium at several orders of magnitude higher concentration. Many of these involve the mineral compounds of calcium, principally calcium carbonate ($CaCO_3 \cdot xH_2O$), calcium phosphate ($Ca_3(PO_4)_2$), and hydroxyapatite, a complex crystal usually given as $3Ca_3(PO_4)_2 \cdot Ca(OH)_2$. These minerals are employed for structural strength of the skeleton, for enclosing eggs, and for hardening of teeth and claws. They may also serve as buffer reservoirs in certain circumstances, and formation of such deposits has acid-base consequences. Calcium has a marked effect on the permeability of certain epithelia, notably the gills of aquatic animals. And finally, the chemistry of calcium is in some ways similar to other divalent metal ions, many of which are toxic. These largely extracellular aspects of calcium chemistry and physiology provide the focus of the necessarily selective review that follows.

CALCIUM CHEMISTRY

The many inorganic salts of calcium differ considerably in their solubility in water. Calcium chloride is a deliquescent salt, of essentially infinite solubility, whereas calcium carbonate and calcium sulfate are only slightly soluble at room temperature and pressure. A dissolved salt in equilibrium with its solid phase, i.e. in saturated solution, is characterized by a solubility product calculated as the product of the concentrations of anion and cation. The smaller the solubility product, the less soluble the salt is in the solvent. For calcium carbonate, the solubility product is on the order of 10^{-8} M (21, 134). This is interesting, since a typical marine invertebrate has an extracellular calcium concentration of 5–15 mM and carbonate concentrations in the 5×10^{-5} M range, which yield an ionic product around 5×10^{-7} M, higher than the predicted saturation value.

As discussed by Burton (22–24), this apparent paradox is due to several chemical complications. The first consideration is that calcium binds to proteins and, in the blood of invertebrates, to hemocyanin (20, 85, e.g.), thus reducing its free ionic activity. Calcium also enters into the formation of various ion pairs, such as $CaHCO_3^+$, further reducing its free activity (23). Finally, the small concentrations of phosphate (especially pyrophosphate) ion present act as a crystal poison, inhibiting nucleation of calcium carbonate (6). Addition of finely ground calcite to invertebrate blood generally causes precipitation (22). The equilibrium of free ionic calcium with other compounds in blood is depicted in Figure 1, and makes the point that predicting the chemical behavior of calcium in physiologic solutions is a far from trivial task.

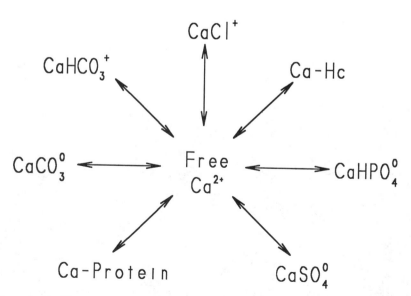

Figure 1 Equilibrium relationships for calcium ion in a complex physiologic electrolyte solution. The formation of many of the ion pairs becomes significant in calculating ion products (Hc = hemacyanin).

In addition to the formation of ion pairs, calcium also participates in two important equilibrium systems that are relevant both to mineralization and acid-base homeostasis. In forming the $CaHCO_3^+$ ion pair and in the formation of $CaCO_3$, calcium influences the carbonic acid buffer system. Removal of calcium from the system by precipitation of carbonate also shifts the carbonic acid equilibrium toward the acid side, which results in excess H^+ ions (Figure 2). Similarly, the formation of calcium phosphate results in a shift of the phosphoric acid buffer system. Alkalinization of either of these systems tends to favor the formation of the mineral precipitates, and acidification of either will reverse the process.

CALCIUM AS A STRUCTURAL ELEMENT

For any material to serve as a mechanical strengthener in the skeleton, it must meet several criteria. It must be reasonably abundant, nontoxic, and have a phase transition that lies within a physiologically controllable range. This last point is perhaps the most critical; potassium salts would not be suitable, since in order to precipitate most of them, concentrations would have to be raised to the molar range. Similarly, barium would not be very suitable, since it precipitates in the micromolar range at physiological pH, is not as abundant, and would have to be strongly acidified to be redissolved. It is not surprising, then, that calcium is the universal cation in the structural salts of animals. Magnesium is incorporated to a lesser extent in many animals, as is strontium

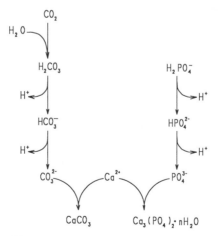

Figure 2 The relationship of calcium to the equilibrium reactions of carbonic acid and phosphoric acid. Precipitation of calcium salts affects the equilibrium distribution of ionic species and the acid-base status.

(31, 113–116, 122–124, 142–143). Strontium fails the abundance test, however, and magnesium is usually maintained at low concentrations in physiologic fluids for other reasons. Whereas calcium is the cation present in structural salts, the anion is not always the same.

Invertebrates

In the invertebrates, and indeed in many plants, carbonate is the anion of choice (31, 113, 114, 122, 137, 143). All that is necessary for calcium carbonate to precipitate is a slight increase in concentration, probably removal of phosphate and other crystal poisons, and often a mild alkalinization (which increases the carbonate concentration). In most cases there is also an organic matrix in which the calcification occurs. Lamina of chitin and proteins, for example, form a quasi-template for crystal formation in crustaceans, calcified insect cuticles, echinoderms, molluscs, trematodes, and others (1, 8, 16, 35–38, 40, 41, 45, 68–70, 74, 91, 103, 109–112, 120, 124, 127, 132, 133, 135–140, 142, 143, 145, 147). There is some evidence that the organic materials provide nucleation sites and orientation for the crystal materials, but, of course, the organic matrix also serves to improve the mechanical properties of the resulting composite (2, 41, 100, 138).

Evidently it is necessary to keep the microenvironment of calcium carbonate more alkaline than the extracellular fluids. In the blue crab, for example, the fluid contained in the carapace behaves as a separate compartment whose pH is kept about 0.5 unit higher than blood over a wide temperature (and pH) range (141; Figure 3). It would appear advantageous for the extrapallial fluid of molluscs to be similarly alkaline in order to maintain the appropriate solubility product (22), but a compilation of the data shows no marked difference between blood and extrapallial fluid pH (114). Carbonate skeletons are also protected from the external seawater by an epicuticle of low permeability, although aquatic forms generally lack the waxy layers found in insects (2, 117).

Vertebrates

In vertebrate bone mineral, the anionic complement is quite different, consisting mostly of phosphate with only a minor component of carbonate (131). The predominant crystalline salt in bone is hydroxyapatite, $3Ca_3(PO_4)_2 \cdot Ca(OH)_2$, but titration or acidification of bone shows a significant carbonate content not accounted for by this formula (12, 26, 95). One advantage of phosphate is that the solubility product is much lower, so alkalinization is not required. A drawback is that the supply of phosphate is much more limited; most animals obtain phosphate from their diet, and concentrations in natural waters are very low. Some carbonaceous structures still occur in the vertebrates, such as the

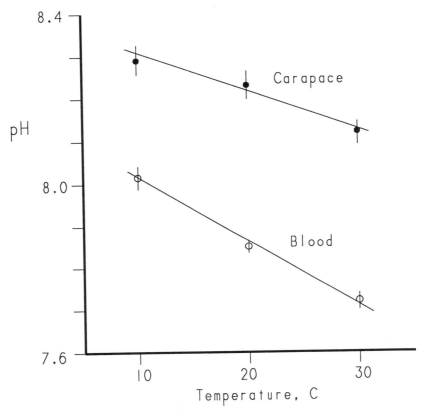

Figure 3   The relationship between extracellular (blood) pH and the pH of the carapace fluid compartment in the blue crab over the temperature range of 10 to 30°C [re-drawn from Wood & Cameron, (144)].

concretions in the endolymphatic sacs of toads (125), but these are more the exception.

One is tempted to speculate that the shift from carbonate to phosphate during evolution was related to the change from an external skeleton to an internal one. An important difference is that the internal skeleton is retained for the life of the animal and can grow with the animal, whereas external skeletons are less permanent. Even if they are not totally shed for growth, they wear and dissolve away and generally require a higher replacement rate. The abundance of carbonate may have been more important that the penalties of keeping it alkaline and protected.

Miscellaneous Calcified Structures

Besides the skeleton there are a number of other structures that are calcified, including tendons, teeth, and eggs. The eggs of birds are the most familiar examples, but other animals, including reptiles, some groups of worms, and molluscs, also protect their eggs with varying degrees of calcification (112, 142, 143). Structural strength and protection is provided by calcified scales in certain groups of fish (50, 89) and reptiles, the plastron of turtles and spicules of many invertebrate groups. Teeth are permanent in some groups of animals, such as man, but are continually replaced in rodents, many reptiles, and fish (including sharks). Various sorts of tooth-like structures in the invertebrates are calcified, and some of these may be replaced frequently or continuously. Certain sensory structures are calcified, usually to provide either mass or stiffness. Some examples are the otoliths and Weberian ossicles of fish, the statocysts of crustaceans, and the middle ear bones of mammals.

THE MECHANISM OF CALCIFICATION

A priori it would appear that there are two possible routes for calcium transport during calcification: transcellular or paracellular; and that transport might be of either free calcium ions, complexes, or granular precipitates of various kinds. The evidence from various species and tissues is incomplete and to some extent contradictory, but it seems safe to state that the mechanism of calcification is not really known for any tissue.

The question of whether calcium transport is likely to be transcellular may be addressed using data on the carapace composition of the blue crab, transport rates during the calcification phase after molt, and a simple model. The intermolt carapace contains an average of 25 mg calcium per cm^2 (J. N. Cameron, unpublished data). This total is deposited in about five days following molt, and from transport rates published by Cameron & Wood (31), a typical peak value appears to be 1.4 nM mm^{-2} min^{-1} at 24 hr after molt, in the range reported for other calcifying tissues (Table 1). Using an average epithelial thickness of $10 \mu m$, the intracellular volume underlying 1 mm^2 is 10^{-5} ml. The simplest possible model assumes that calcium enters at one surface of the epithelium and travels in a linear fashion to the other side, where it is immediately excreted (Figure 4). In a steady-state, the residence time (t) for a calcium ion in the cell is related to the flux (F) and the rise in intracellular concentration (ΔC) by: $t = \Delta C/F$, where ΔC is in nM ml^{-1} and the flux is in nM sec^{-1} ml^{-1}. Assuming (generously) that the intracellular concentration could rise by $10 \mu M$ L^{-1} without killing the cell, and using the data given above, the residence time would be 0.4 msec! Longer residence times require greater concentration changes. The entire intracellular compartment would have to be in furious motion in order for calcium to traverse the cell at such a rate. Studies of secretory ameloblasts (involved in enamel formation in teeth) have shown that calcium crosses the epithelium in perhaps 20–30 sec (90), about five orders of magnitude slower, so even if the data employed in this simple model are considerably in error, there is still little likelihood that free calcium is transported via the intracellular compartment. The protein secreted by the ameloblasts into the enamel layer does clearly originate intracellularly, and components of the protein have been shown to have a cell transit or residence time of around 20–30 min (136).

If transepithelial calcium transport is not channeled through the cells, then some sort of paracellular pathway must exist, capable of sustaining the rates of transport observed. Any such paracellular model must include (very) leaky junctions between the adjacent epithelial cells, plus a driving mechanism for calcium. The latter could be either an electrical gradient generated by the epithelium, or a standing concentration gradient along the length of the basolateral spaces (55). A third intriguing possibility has been suggested by Reith (98, 99), namely that calcium may be transported from basolateral to apical surfaces by the cell membrane itself. This proposal is based on the known ability of phospholipids to act both as calcium binding agents and as ionophores (126, 147) and on histochemical observations of calcium on or in the membranes in actively transporting ameloblasts (99). Reith at first proposed that following calcium binding, transport could be accomplished by membrane fluidity (98), for which there is some independent evidence (34, 106). He has suggested more recently that some sort of saltatory mechanism

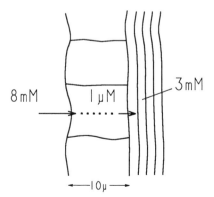

Figure 4 A schematic representation of the simplest possible model for transcellular calcium transport in a calcifying tissue. The bulk calcium concentration of blood is assumed to be 8 mM/L, of the carapace fluid 3 mM/L, and of the intracellular compartment 1 μM (model discussed in text).

Table 1 Calcium fluxes in calcifying systems[a]

System	Ca flux, nM cm^{-2} h^{-1}
Plant	
Coccolithus	130
Molluscs	
Helix uterus	3,000
Anguispira uterus	30,000
Argopecten mantle	80
Crustaceans	
Astacus epithelium	400–2500
Carcinus epithelium *in vitro*	
Influx	18–300
Efflux	13–50
Callinectes sapidus in vivo	8,400
Bird	
Hen oviduct	20,000

[a] Modified from Wilbur's compilation (142), plus *Callinectes* data calculated from References 30, 31.

along the membrane could also be responsible without the requirement of membrane fluidity (99). This proposal has the appeal of getting around the difficulties with maintaining free intracellular calcium in the face of massive transport requirements, but poses additional ones, such as how so much calcium would be moved past the cell junctions.

Part of the gradient for calcium movement may be provided by the H^+ transport that is required along with the formation of carbonates or phosphates (29, 111, 112, 114). Constant pumping of H^+ out of the microenvironment in which calcification is occurring will help maintain a low ion product and favor continued movement of calcium across the epithelium. Actually, similar questions about the pathway for H^+ movement may be raised; how can such a large H^+ flux transit the cytoplasm without causing large disruptions of intracellular pH? The answer is no doubt complex, but intracellular buffering is generally in the range of 30–60 mM/pH, whereas the effective calcium buffering is orders of magnitude less. Also, high activity of carbonic anhydrase appears to be associated with mineralizing tissues (56, 72, 80, 148), and one of its functions may be in reducing local pH gradients by facilitating either equilibration of the buffers or diffusion (66, 71).

Finally, many calcifying tissues have high activity of both Ca-activated ATPases (3, 4, 7, 30, 53, 87, 92, 128) and of alkaline phosphatase (83, 87, 92, 93, 104, 108), but the exact physiologic functions of either are not clear. There is some evidence that alkaline phosphatase is involved in providing phosphate for mineralization in mammalian tissues (93, 108). This is consistent with the low activity found in calcifying crab carapace (J. N. Cameron, unpublished data), a tissue which does not transport phosphate to any appreciable extent (31). Calcium-activated ATPases normally are associated with intracellular calcium regulation rather than transepithelial transport, but Ca-ATPase activity, nonetheless, rises by fivefold during the post-molt calcification in the blue crab (30) and is present in high activity during calcium resorption in the digestive tract of the terrestrial amphipod *Orchestia* (87). The significance of these findings for the mechanism of calcification is presently unclear.

The overall process of calcification requires more than just the transepithelial step. For the post-molt crab, calcification requires transport of H^+, HCO_3^-, and Ca^{2+} across the gills, convective transport by the blood between the gills and the calcifying tissue sites, a series of transport steps at the epithelium, and the appropriate chemical reactions in the cuticle (Figure 5; 29, 30, 58, 60–64, 81, 87, 88, 101–103, 118, 122, 123, 127, 128, 132, 138). Calcium entry at the gills appears to be passive, with both H^+ and HCO_3^- actively transported (29). At the calcifying epithelium we do not have much information except that the calcium movement is probably via a paracellular pathway (see above).

SKELETAL CALCIUM AS A BUFFER

Both calcium phosphate and calcium carbonate can act as buffers, and a number of studies have addressed the question of whether skeletal calcium salts in fact contribute physiologic buffering in response to various acid-base

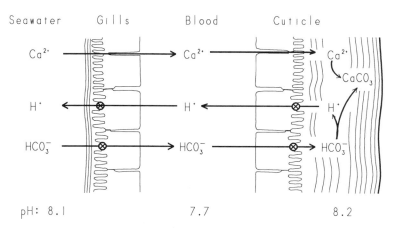

Figure 5 A model of ion movements during the calcifying stage in a crab after molt. The movement of calcium is shown as through a paracellular route; other processes presumed to be active, but assignment of the active process to one cell surface or another is arbitrary [modified from Cameron (30)].

disturbances. Dugal (46) was the first to show that extracellular calcium concentration rose in a mollusc during prolonged anoxia, which presumably caused acidosis. Some work on molluscs has indicated that the rate of shell deposition or dissolution can be related to the acid-base status of the animal (54), but not all agree, and the evidence is not conclusive (22, 44). In crustaceans the results depend upon whether the animal is terrestrial or aquatic. In the marine blue crab even a fairly severe acidosis does not result in significant dissolution of the skeletal carbonates; in this case the exchanges of ions with the seawater across the gills are sufficiently rapid and effective as to obviate participation of the skeleton (28). In terrestrial crabs, however, the skeletal carbonates do participate in buffering to a significant extent (73). Whether this shell buffering occurs under normal circumstances is not clear, but it could certainly proceed for a considerable length of time without compromising structural integrity, since the carbonate pool in the exoskeleton is roughly 500 times larger than that of all other body fluid pools (31).

Similar studies on vertebrates have shown that there is some physiologic buffering by the skeletal mineral salts, but it is generally much less than buffering provided by other mechanisms. In fish, for example, there was no appreciable flux of phosphate out of the bone pool in response to hypercapnic acidosis (27). In mammals chronic acidosis does produce a loss of calcium from bone, but the principal reaction appears to be with bone carbonates, and much less with the phosphates (12, 13, 19, 25, 26, 82).

Anoxic Hibernation in the Turtle

An interesting and unusual situation in hibernating turtles has been described by Jackson, Ultsch & colleagues (76–79, 129, 130). One of the common pond turtles of North America, the painted turtle (*Chrysemys picta*), spends the winter at the bottom of shallow ponds that often go anoxic early in the winter. The turtles can tolerate cold anaerobiosis for periods of three months or more in the laboratory. During this prolonged acidosis, lactate rises gradually from its normal concentration of less than 2 mM to nearly 150 mM, calcium rises from about 4 to nearly 35 mM, and magnesium increases from about 2 to 13 mM (76). The source of this additional calcium and magnesium is clearly the mineral reserves of bone and plastron. The CO_2 from acidification of the mineral salts is apparently excreted across the skin to the water, since the P_{CO_2} is not unduly elevated, and [HCO_3^-] is strongly depressed (77). The free calcium activity rises much less than the total calcium concentration because of formation of the calcium-lactate ion pair and probably because of increased calcium binding by plasma proteins. Nevertheless the activities of calcium and magnesium reach levels that in normal animals adversely affect cardiac contractility. The effects of acidosis and hypercalcemia oppose each other, however, which allows the turtle's heart to maintain contractility under these unusual conditions (146).

CALCIUM ACCUMULATIONS

Calcium-containing concretions are found in the tissues of many different animal groups including trematodes, annelids, molluscs, and crustaceans (9, 111-116, 142–143). These share certain features: they are usually intracellular, contained either within plasma membrane vesicles or mitochondria; they are usually laminar in section, with an organic matrix similar to that seen in extracellular structures; and frequently they incorporate other materials besides calcium salts. In some cases their function may be to remove toxic metals, with calcium only an incidental by-product. In other cases their function is clearly storage, and in some further cases the function is not known (see reviews 113–115, 142, 143). As with transepithelial transport, questions are posed about how they are formed, but here a transmembrane Ca-ATPase system appears to be an adequate explanation.

One particularly interesting example of calcium concretions occurs in the gills of freshwater mussels of the family Unionidae. These concretions may make up as much as 50% of the dry weight of the gills and are more than 75% dry weight inorganic salts, principally calcium phosphate (97, 111, 112). The concretions serve as a store for reproduction: the larvae are able to develop a complete calcium carbonate shell inside the gill channels of the parent. Completion of this larval shell development depletes the concretions, which are then built up again for the next reproductive season (111, 112).

CALCIUM AND EPITHELIAL PERMEABILITY

Amateur aquarists have long known that many marine tropical fish may be kept in fresh water as long as the calcium concentration is kept elevated. Many subsequent studies have demonstrated that there is a direct relationship between calcium concentration and the permeability of the gills (33, 39); at low calcium concentration marine fish typically lose salts more rapidly than they can take them up [see review by Maetz, (84)]. Similar effects of calcium are seen on many epithelia, and these effects appear to result from a direct effect on calcium on the cell junctional complexes (11, 18).

CONTROL OF CALCIUM IN INVERTEBRATES

There is not a great deal of evidence that extracellular calcium concentrations are controlled to any appreciable extent in the marine invertebrates. The majority have concentrations near that of the ambient seawater (96), especially if electrical gradients and activity differences are taken into account. During the post-molt period crabs have blood calcium concentrations considerably below the seawater (30, 65, 67, 121), but this may reflect a steady-state due to rapid removal from the blood by calcification rather than a change in a regulated concentration. Unlike the vertebrates, there are no known calcium hormones in crustaceans, but some recent reports of calcitonin-like immunoreactivity from crustaceans are intriguing (5, 51, 59). Future work will have to show first of all whether this is really a calcitonin, and secondly whether its function in the invertebrates is to regulate calcium (107).

There is some evidence that (neuro)hormones influence calcification (10). Dillaman et al (43) reported apparent changes in neurosecretory cells in the brain of a mollusc during a shell repair period, and McWhinnie et al (86) discussed general aspects of calcium in the molt cycle. Also, the rapid initiation of calcification in the post-molt crab suggests a hormonal signal, although none has yet been found (30). As with most topics in invertebrate endocrinology, very little is known and much remains to be studied.

CONCLUSIONS

The biochemistry of calcium seems to be divided into micro and macro functions. A wide variety of intracellular processes are influenced or controlled by micromolar concentrations of calcium, and a carefully regulated calcium pumping system serves to protect the intracellular calcium regime. Many other processes, however, involve calcium at several orders of magnitude higher concentration. These include the formation, repair, and protection of the skeleton; the formation of calcium storage granules of various kinds; regulation of epithelial permeability; and mobilization of calcium salts as buffers. These latter processes are mainly extracellular, and must involve a different set of controls and transport processes whose affinities differ by several orders of magnitude. The mechanism of calcification remains mysterious for all animals, and the whole area of calcium metabolism and regulation is almost unexplored in the invertebrate world. The rapid advances of the past decade in endocrinology and molecular technique should set the stage for a productive period of research in the future.

Literature Cited

1. Addadi, L., Weiner, S. 1985. Interactions between acidic proteins and crystals: stereochemical requirements in biomineralization. *Proc. Natl. Acad. Sci. USA* 82:4100–14
2. Andersen, S. O. 1985. Sclerotization and tanning of the cuticle. In *Comprehensive Insect Physiology, Biochemistry and Toxicology*, ed. G. A. Kerkut, 3:59–74. Oxford: Pergamon
3. Ando, T., Fujimoto, K., Mayahara, H., Miyajima, H., Ogawa, K. 1981. A new one-step method for the histochemistry and cytochemistry of Ca^{++}-ATPase activity. *Acta Histochem. Cytochem.* 14:705–26
4. Appleton, J., Morris, D. C. 1979. The use of the potassium pyroantimonate-osmium method as a means of identifying and localizing calcium at the ultrastructural level in the cells of calcifying systems. *J. Histochem. Cytochem.* 27:676–80
5. Arlot-Bonnemains, Y., Fouchereau-Peron, M., Moukhtar, M. S., Milhaud, G. 1983. Characterization of target organs for calcitonin in lower and higher vertebrates. *Comp. Biochem. Physiol.* 76A:377–80
6. Bachra, B. N., Trautz, O., Simon, S. L. 1963. Precipitation of calcium carbonates and phosphates under physiological

conditions. I. Spontaneous precipitation of calcium carbonates and phosphates under physiological conditions. *Arch. Biochem. Biophys.* 103:124–38

7. Bambauer, H. J., Ueno, S., Umar, H., Ueck, M. 1984. Ultracytochemical localization of Ca^{++}-ATPase activity in pituicytes of the neurohypophysis of the guinea pig. *Cell Tissue Res.* 237:491–97

8. Becker, G. L., Chen, C. H., Greenwalt, J. W., Lehninger, A. L. 1974. Calcium phosphate granules in the hepatopancreas of the blue crab *Callinectes sapidus. J. Cell Biol.* 61:316–26

9. Becker, G. L., Termine, J. D., Eanes, E. D. 1976. Comparative studies of intra mitochondrial and extramitochondrial calcium phosphates from the hepatopancreas of the blue crab *Callinectes sapidus. Calcif. Tissue Res.* 21:105–13

10. Bellon-Humbert, C., Van-Herp, F., Van Wormhoudt, A. 1984. Localisation immunocytochimique de neuropeptides et d'amines biogenes dan le pedoncle oculaire de la crevette *Palaemon serratus* (Pennant, 1977). *Ann. Soc. Roy. Zool. Belg.* 114:164 (Suppl.)

11. Bentzel, C. J., Martinez, M., Hainan, B., Fromm, M. J., Hegel, U. 1982. Morphological and physiological factors determining transjunctional fluxes. In *The Paracellular Pathway,* ed. S. E. Bradley, E. F. Purcell, pp. 375–383. New York: Josiah Macy

12. Bettice, J. A. 1984. Skeletal carbon dioxide stores during metabolic acidosis. *Amer. J. Physiol.* 247:F326–30

13. Bettice, J. A., Gamble, J. L. Jr. 1975. Skeletal buffering of acute metabolic acidosis. *Amer. J. Physiol.* 229:1619–24

14. Bikle, D. D., Zolock, D. T., Morrissey, R. L., Herman, R. H. 1978. Independence of 1,25-dihyroxyvitamin D_3-mediated calcium transport from *de novo* RNA and protein synthesis. *J. Biol. Chem.* 253:484–88

15. Brehe, J. E., Fleming,, W. R. 1976. Calcium mobilization from acellular bone and effects of hypophysectomy on calcium metabolism in *Fundulus kansae. J. Comp. Physiol.* 110:159–69

16. Brown, B. E. 1982. The form and function of metal-containing "granules" in invertebrate tissues. *Biol. Rev.* 57:621–67

17. Bubel, A. 1983. A fine structural study of the calcareous opercular plate and associated cells in a polychaete annelid. *Tissue Cell* 15:457–76

18. Bullivant, S. 1982. Tight junction structure and development. In *The Paracellular Pathway,* ed. S. E. Bradley, E. F.

Purcell, pp. 13–31. New York: Josiah Macy

19. Burnell, J. M. 1971. Changes in bone sodium and carbonate in metabolic acidosis and alkalosis in the dog. *J. Clin. Invest.* 50:327–31

20. Burton, R. F. 1972. The binding of alkaline earth ions by the haemocyanin of *Helix pomatia L. Comp. Biochem. Physiol.* 41A:555–65

21. Burton, R. F. 1973. The significance of ionic concentrations in the internal media of animals. *Biol. Rev.* 48:195–231

22. Burton, R. F. 1976. Calcium metabolism and acid-base balance in *Helix pomatia.* In *Perspectives in Experimental Biology,* ed. P. S. Davies, pp. 7–16. Oxford: Pergamon

23. Burton, R. F. 1983. Inorganic ion pairs in physiology: Significance and quantitation. *Comp. Biochem. Physiol.* 74A:781–85

24. Burton, R. F., Mathie, R. T. 1975. Calcium and pH homeostasis in the snail *(Helix pomatia):* Effects of CO_2 and $CaCl_2$ infusion. *Experentia* 31:543–44

25. Bushinsky, D. A., Krieger, N. S., Geisser, D. I., Grossman, E. B., Coe, F. L. 1983. Effects of pH on bone calcium and proton fluxes *in vitro. Amer. J. Physiol.* 245:F204–9

26. Bushinsky, D. A., Lechleider, R. J. 1987. Mechanism of proton-induced bone calcium release: calcium carbonate dissolution. *Amer. J. Physiol.* 253: F998–F1005

27. Cameron, J. N. 1985a. The bone compartment in a teleost fish, *Ictalurus punctatus:* Size, composition, and acid-base response to hypercapnia. *J. Exp. Biol.* 117:307–18

28. Cameron, J. N. 1985b. Compensation of hypercapnic acidosis in the aquatic Blue Crab, *Callinectes sapidus:* The predominance of external seawater over carapace carbonate as the proton sink. *J. Exp. Biol.* 114:197–206

29. Cameron, J. N. 1985c. Post-moult calcification in the blue crab *(Callinectes sapidus):* relationships between apparent net H^+ excretion, calcium and bicarbonate. *J. Exp. Biol.* 119:275–86

30. Cameron, J. N. 1989. Post-moult calcification in the blue crab, *Callinectes sapidus:* Timing and mechanism. *J. Exp. Biol.* 143:285–304

31. Cameron, J. N., Wood, C. M. 1985. Apparent net H^+ excretion and CO_2 dynamics accompanying carapace mineralization in the Blue Crab, *(Callinectes sapidus)* following moulting. *J. Exp. Biol.* 114:181–96

32. Carafoli, E. 1982. *Membrane Transport of Calcium.* New York: Academic. 268 pp.

33. Carrier, J. C., Evans, D. H. 1976. The role of environmental calcium in freshwater survival of the marine teleost *Lagodon rhomboides. J. Exp. Biol.* 65:529–38

34. Charon, N. W., Lawrence, C. W., O'Brien, S. 1981. Movement of antibody coated latex beads attached to the spirochete *Leptospira interrogans. Proc. Nat. Acad. Sci. USA* 78:7166–70

35. Chockalingham, S. 1971. Studies on the enzymes associated with calcification of the cuticle of the hermit crab *Clibanarius olivaceous. Mar. Biol.* 10:169–82

36. Constantz, B., Weiner, S. 1988. Acidic macromolecules associated with the mineral phase of scleractinian corals. *J. Exp. Zool.* 248:253–58

37. Crenshaw, M. A., Neff, J. M. 1969. Decalcification at the mantle-shell interface in molluscs. *Amer. Zool.* 9:881–89

38. Currey, J. D., Nash, A., Bonfield, W. 1982. Calcified cuticle in the stomatopod smashing limb. *J. Materials Sci.* 17:1939–44

39. Cuthbert, A. W., Maetz, J. 1972. The effects of calcium and magnesium on sodium fluxes through the gills of *Carassius auratus. J. Physiol.* 221:633–44

40. Degens, E. T., Carey, F. G., Spencer, D. W. 1967. Amino-acids and amino-sugars in calcified tissues of portunid crabs. *Nature* 216:601–3

41. Dendinger, J. E., Alterman, A. 1983. Mechanical properties in relation to chemical constituents of postmolt cuticle of the blue crab, *Callinectes sapidus. Comp. Biochem. Physiol.* 75A:421–24

42. Dieter, P., Marme, D. 1988. The history of calcium-binding proteins. In *Calcium-binding Proteins,* ed. M. P. Thompson, 1:1–9. Boca Raton:CRC Press

43. Dillaman, R. M., Saleuddin, A. S. M., Jones, G. M. 1976. Neurosecretion and shell regeneration in *Helisoma duryi* (Mollusca:Pulmonata). *Can. J. Zool.* 54:1771–78

44. Dotterweich, H., Elssner, F. 1935. Die Mobilisierung des Schalankalkes fur die Reaktionsregulation der Muscheln. *Biol. Zbl.* 55:138–63

45. Drach, P. 1937. Morphogenese de la mosaique cristalline externe dans le squelette teentaire des decapodes brachyoures. *C. r. hebd. Seanc. Acad. Sci. Paris.* 205:1173–76

46. Dugal, L.-P. 1939. The use of calcareous shell to buffer the products of anaerobic glycolysis in *Venus mercenaria. J. Cell. Comp. Physiol.* 13:235–51

47. Ebashi, S., Endo, M., Imahori, K., Kakiuchi, S., Nishizuka, Y., eds. 1984. *Calcium Regulation in Biological Systems.* Orlando: Academic. 260 pp.

48. Farber, J. L. 1981. The role of calcium in cell death. *Life Sci.* 29:1289–95

49. Flaim, S. F., Zelis, R., eds. 1982. *Calcium Blockers: Mechanism of Action and Clinical Applications.* Baltimore/Munich: Urban & Schwarzenburg. 303 pp.

50. Flik, G., Perry, S. F. 1989. Cortisol stimulates whole body calcium uptake and the branchial calcium pump in freshwater rainbow trout. *J. Endocrinol.* 120:75–82

51. Fouchereau-Peron, M., Arlot-Bonnemains, Y., Milhaud, G., Moukhtar, M. S. 1987. Immunoreactive salmon calcitonin-like molecule in crustaceans: high concentrations in *Nephrops norvegicus. Gen. Comp. Endocrinol.* 65:179–83

52. Fouchereau-Peron, M., Moukhtar, M. S., le Gal, Y., Milhaud, G. 1981. Demonstration of specific receptors for calcitonin in isolated trout gill cells. *Comp. Biochem. Physiol.* 68A:417–21

53. Fox, F. R., Ranga Rao, K. 1978. Characteristics of a calcium ion activated ATPase from the hepatopancreas of the blue crab *Callinectes sapidus. Comp. Biochem. Physiol.* 59B:327–32

54. Frick, W. 1965. Der Kalziumstoffwechsel bei Helix pomatia unter dem Einfluss wechselnder Kohlensäureatmosphären. *Mitt. Zool. Mus. Berlin* 41:95–120

55. Fromter, E., Diamond, J. M. 1972. Route of passive ion permeation in epithelia. *Nature (New Biology)* 235:9–13

56. Giraud, M.-M. 1981. Carbonic anhydrase activity in the integument of the crab *Carcinus maenas* during the intermolt cycle. *Comp. Biochem. Physiol.* 69A:381–87

57. Godfraind-DeBecker, A., Godfraind, T. 1980. Calcium transport system: a comparative study in different cells. *Int. Rev. Cytol.* 67:141–70

58. Graf, F. 1978. Les sources de calcium pour les crustaces venant de muer. *Arch. Zool. Exp. Gen.* 119:143–61

59. Graf, F., Fouchereau-Peron, F., Van-Wormhoudt, A., Meyran, J.-C. 1989. Variations of calcitonin-like immunoreactivity in the crustacean *Orchestia cavimana* during a molt cycle. *Gen. Comp. Endocrinol.* 73:80–84

60. Graf, F., Meyran, J.-C. 1983. Premolt

calcium secretion in midgut posterior caeca of the crustacean *Orchestia:* ultrastructure of the epithelium. *J. Morphol.* 177:1–23

61. Graf, F., Meyran, J.-C. 1985. Calcium reabsorption in the posterior caeca of the midgut in a terrestrial crustacean, *Orchestia cavimana. Cell Tissue Res.* 242:83–95

62. Greenaway, P. 1974. Calcium balance at the postmoult stage of the freshwater crayfish *Austropotamobius pallipes* (Lereboullet). *J. Exp. Biol.* 61:35–45

63. Greenaway, P. 1983. Uptake of calcium at the postmoult stage by the marine crabs *Callinectes sapidus* and *Carcinus maenas. Comp. Biochem. Physiol.* 75A:181–84

64. Greenaway, P. 1985. Calcium balance and moulting in the crustacea. *Biol. Rev.* 60:425–54

65. Guderley, H. 1977. Muscle and hypodermal ion concentrations in *Cancer magister:* changes with the molt cycle. *Comp. Biochem. Physiol.* 56A:155–59

66. Gutknecht, J. 1977. Exchange diffusion of inorganic anions through lipid bilayer membranes. *Physiologist* 20(4):39 (Abst.)

67. Haefner, P. A. Jr. 1964. Hemolymph calcium fluctuations as related to environmental salinity during ecdysis of the blue crab, *Callinectes sapidus* Rathbun. *Physiol. Zool.* 37:247–58

68. Hegdahl, T., Gustavsen, F., Silness, J. 1977. The structure and mineralization of the carapace of the crab *(Cancer pagurus* L.). 2. The exocuticle. *Zool. Scripta* 6:101–5

69. Hegdahl, T., Gustavsen, F., Silness, J. 1977. The structure and mineralization of the carapace of the crab *(Cancer pagurus* L.). 3. The epicuticle. *Zool. Scripta* 6:215–20

70. Hegdahl, T., Silness, J., Gustavsen, F. 1977. The structure and mineralization of the carapace of the crab *(Cancer pagurus* L.). 1. The endocuticle. *Zool. Scripta* 6:89–99

71. Henry, R. P. 1988. Multiple functions of carbonic anhydrase in the crustacean gill. *J. Exp. Zool.* 248:19–24

72. Henry, R. P., Kormanik, G. A. 1985. Carbonic anhydrase activity and calcium deposition during the molt cycle of the blue crab *Callinectes sapidus. J. Crust. Biol.* 5:234–41

73. Henry, R. P., Kormanik, G. A., Smatresk, N. J., Cameron, J. N. 1981. The role of $CaCO_3$ dissolution as a source of HCO_3^- for buffering hypercapnic acido-

sis in aquatic and terrestrial decapod crustaceans. *J. Exp. Biol.* 94:269–74

74. Hopkin, S. P., Nott, J. A. 1979. Some observations on concentrically structured, intracellular granules in the hepatopancreas of the shore crab *Carcinus maenas* (L.). *J. Mar. Biol. Assoc. UK* 59:867–77

75. Inesi, G. 1985. Mechanism of calcium transport. *Annu. Rev. Physiol.* 47:573–602

76. Jackson, D. C., Heisler, N. 1982. Plasma ion balance of submerged anoxic turtles at 3°C: the role of calcium lactate formation. *Respir. Physiol.* 49:159–74

77. Jackson, D. C., Heisler, N. 1983. Intracellular and extracellular acid-base and electrolyte status of submerged anoxic turtles at 3°C. *Respir. Physiol.* 53:187–202

78. Jackson, D. C., Herbert, C. V., Ultsch, G. R. 1984. The comparative physiology of diving in North American freshwater turtles. II. Plasma ion balance during prolonged anoxia. *Physiol. Zool.* 57:632–40

79. Jackson, D. C., Ultsch, G. R. 1982. Long-term submergence at 3°C of the turtle, *Chrysemys picta bellii,* in normoxic and severely hypoxic water. II. Extracellular ionic responses to extreme lactic acidosis. *J. Exp. Biol.* 96:29–43

80. Kingsley, R. J., Watabe, N. 1987. Role of carbonic anhydrase in calcification in the Gorgonian *Leptogorgia virgulata. J. Exp. Zool.* 241:171–80

81. Kleinholz, L. H. 1941. Molting and calcium deposition in decapod crustaceans. *J. Cell. Comp. Physiol.* 18:101–7

82. Lemann, J. Jr., Litzow, J. R., Lennon, E. J. 1966. The effects of chronic acid loads in normal man: further evidence for the participation of bone mineral in the defense against chronic metabolic acidosis. *J. Clin. Invest.* 45:1608–14

83. Linde, A. 1981. On enzymes associated with biological calcification. In *The Chemistry and Biology of Mineralized Connective Tissues,* ed. A. Viess, pp. 559–70. New York: Elsevier North-Holland

84. Maetz, J. 1974. Aspects of adaptation to hypo-osmotic and hyperosmotic environments. In *Biochemical and Biophysical Perspectives in Marine Biology,* ed. D. C. Malins, J. R. Sargent, 1:1–167. London/New York: Academic

85. Mangum, C. P., Lykkeboe, G. 1979. The influence of inorganic ions and pH on the oxygenation properties of the blood in the gastropod mollusc *Busycon*

canaliculatum. J. Exp. Zool. 207:417–30

86. McWhinnie, M. A., Cahoon, M. O., Johanneck, R. 1969. Hormonal effects on calcium metabolism in Crustacea. *Amer. Zool.* 9:841–55

87. Meyran, J. C., Graf, F. 1986. Ultrahistochemical localization of Na^+-K^+ATPase, Ca^{2+}-ATPase and alkaline phosphatase activity in a calcium-transporting epithelium of a crustacean during moulting. *Histochemistry* 85:313–20

88. Meyran, J.-C., Graf, F., Nicaise, G. 1984. Calcium pathway through a mineralizing epithelium in the crustacean *Orchestia* in pre-molt: ultrastructural cytochemistry and X-ray microanalysis. *Tissue Cell* 16:269–86

89. Mugiya, Y., Watabe, N. 1977. Studies on fish scale formation and resorption. II. Effects of estradiol on calcium homeostasis and skeletal tissue resorption in the goldfish, *Carassius auratus*, and the killifish, *Fundulus heteroclitus*. *Comp. Biochem. Physiol.* 57A:197–202

90. Munhoz, C. O. G., LeBlond, C. P. 1974. Deposition of calcium phosphate into dentin and enamel as shown by radioautography of sections of incisor teeth following injection of ^{45}Ca into rats. *Calcif. Tiss. Res.* 15:221–35

91. Neff, J. M. 1972. Ultrastructure of the outer epithelium of the mantle in the clam *Mercenaria mercenaria* in relation to calcification of the shell. *Tissue Cell* 4:591–600

92. Nys, Y., De Laage, S. 1984. Effects of suppression of eggshell calcification and of 1,25 $(OH)_2D_3$ on Mg^{2+}, Ca^{2+} and $Mg^{2+}HCO_3^-$ ATPase, alkaline phosphatase, carbonic anhydrase and Ca BP levels. I. The laying hen uterus. *Comp. Biochem. Physiol.* 78A:833–38

93. Orams, H. 1981. Ultrastructural sites of alkaline phosphatase activity during amelogenesis in forming rodent incisors. In *The Chemistry and Biology of Mineralized Connective Tissues*, ed. A. Veis, pp. 571–75. New York: Elsevier North-Holland.

94. Poenie, M., Tsien, R. Y., Schmitt-Verhulst, A.-M. 1987. Sequential activation and lethal hit measured by $[Ca^{2+}]_i$ in individual cytolytic T cells and targets. *EMBO J.* 6:2223–2232.

95. Poyart, C. E., Bursaux, E., Freminet, A. 1975. The bone CO_2 compartment: evidence for a bicarbonate pool. *Respir. Physiol.* 25:84–99

96. Prosser, C. L., ed. 1973. *Comparative Animal Physiology*, Philadelphia: Saunders. 966 pp. 3rd ed.

97. Pynnonen, K., Holwerda, D. A., Zandee, D. I. 1987. Occurrence of calcium concretions in various tissues of freshwater mussels, and their capacity for cadmium sequestration. *Aquatic Toxicol.* 10:101–14

98. Reith, E. J. 1983. A model for transcellular transport of calcium based on membrane fluidity and movement of calcium carriers within the more fluid microdomains of the plasma membrane. *Calcif. Tissue Int.* 35:129–34

99. Reith, E. J., Boyde, A. 1985. The pyroantimonate reaction and transcellular transport of calcium in rat molar enamel organs. *Histochemistry* 83:539–43

100. Reynolds, S. E. 1985. Hormonal control of cuticle mechanical properties. In *Comprehensive Insect Physiology, Biochemistry and Toxicology*, ed. G. A. Kerkut, 8:335–51. Oxford: Pergamon

101. Robertson, J. D. 1937. Some features of the calcium metabolism of the shore crab (*Carcinus maenus* Pennant). *Proc. Roy. Soc. B* 124:162–82

102. Roer, R. D. 1980. Mechanisms of resorption and deposition of calcium in the carapace of the crab *Carcinus maenas. J. Exp. Biol.* 88:205–18

103. Roer, R., Dillaman, R. M. 1984. The structure and calcification of the crustacean cuticle. *Amer. Zool.* 24:893–909

104. Salomon, C. D. 1974. A fine structural study of the extracellular activity of alkaline phosphatase and its role in calcification. *Calcif. Tissue Res.* 15:201–12

105. Schatzmann, H. J. 1982. The plasma membrane calcium pump of erythrocytes and other animal cells. In *Membrane Transport of Calcium*, ed. E. Carafoli, pp. 41–108. London: Academic

106. Schmidt, C. F., Barenholz, Y., Thompson, T. E. 1977. A nuclear magnetic resonance study of sphingomyelin in bilayer systems. *Biochem.* 16:2649–56

107. Sellem, E., Graf, F., Meyran, J.-C. 1989. Some effects of salmon calcitonin on calcium metabolism in the crustacean *Orchestia* during the molt cycle. *J. Exp. Zool.* 249:177–81

108. Shapiro, I. M., Golub, E. E. 1981. Alkaline phosphatases: a link between phosphate metabolism and mineralization. In *The Chemistry and Biology of Mineralized Connective Tissues*, ed. A. Veis, pp. 553–57. New York: Elsevier North-Holland

109. Shimizu, M., Yamada, J. 1976. Light

and electron microscope observations of the regenerating test in the sea urchin, *Strongylocentrotus intermedius*. In *Mechanisms of Mineralization in the Invertebrates and Plants,* ed. N. Watabe, K. M. Wilbur, pp. 261–81. Columbia: Univ. S.C. Press

110. Sikes, C. S., Wheeler, A. P. 1986. The organic matrix from oyster shell as a regulator of calcification in vivo. *Biol. Bull.* 170:494–505

111. Silverman, H., Steffens, W. L., Dietz, T. H. 1983. Calcium concentrations in the gills of a freshwater mussel serve as a calcium reservoir during periods of hypoxia. *J. Exp. Zool.* 227:177–90

112. Silverman, H., Steffens, W. L., Dietz, T. H. 1985. Calcium from extracellular concretions in the gills of freshwater Unionid mussels is mobilized during reproduction. *J. Exp. Zool.* 236:137–48

113. Simkiss, K. 1976. Intracellular and extracellular routes in biomineralization. In *Calcium in Biological Systems,* ed. C. J. Duncan. Symp. Soc. Exp. Biol. 30:423–44

114. Simkiss, K. 1976. Cellular aspects of calcification. In *Mechanisms of Mineralization in the Invertebrates and Plants,* ed. N. Watabe, K. M. Wilbur, pp. 1–32. Columbia: Univ. S.C. Press

115. Simkiss, K. 1979. Metal ions in cells. *Endeavour* 3:2–6

116. Simkiss, K. 1980. Detoxification, calcification and the intracellular storage of ions. In *The Mechanism of Biomineralization in Animals and Plants,* ed. M. Omori, N. Watabe, pp. 13–18. Tokyo: Tokai Univ. Press

117. Stevenson, J. R. 1985. Dynamics of the integument. In *Biology of the Crustacea,* ed. D. E. Bliss, L. H. Mantel, 9:1–42. Orlando: Academic

118. Tang, C.-M., Presser, F., Morad, M. 1988. Amiloride selectively blocks low threshold (T) calcium channel. *Science* 240:213–15

119. Taylor, C. W. 1985. Calcium regulation in vertebrates: an overview. *Comp. Biochem. Physiol.* 82A:249–56

120. Towe, K. M. 1972. Invertebrate shell structure and the organic matrix concept. *Biomineralization* 4:2–14

121. Towle, D. W., Mangum, C. P. 1985. Ionic regulation and transport ATPase activities during the molt cycle in the blue crab *Callinectes sapidus. J. Crust. Biol.* 5:216–22

122. Travis, D. F. 1963. Structural features of mineralization from tissue to macromolecular levels of organization in Decapod Crustacea. *Ann. N. Y. Acad. Sci.* 109:177–245

123. Travis, D. F. 1965. The deposition of skeletal structures in the Crustacea. V. The histomorphological and histochemical changes associated with the development and calcification of the branchial exoskeleton in the crayfish, *Orconectes virilis* Hagen. *Acta Histochem.* 20:193–222

124. Travis, D. F., Friberg, U. 1963. The deposition of skeletal structures in the Crustacea. VI. Microradiographic studies of the exoskeleton of the crayfish *Orconectes virilis* Hagen. *J. Ultrastruct. Res.* 9:285–301

125. Tufts, B. L., Toews, D. P. 1985. Partitioning of regulatory sites in *Bufo marinus* during hypercapnia. *J. Exp. Biol.* 119:199–209

126. Tyson, C. A., Vande Zande, H., Green, D. E. 1976. Phospholipids as ionophores. *J. Biol. Chem.* 251:1326–32

127. Ueno, M. 1980. Calcium transport in crayfish gastrolith disc: morphology of gastrolith disc and ultrahistochemical demonstration of calcium. *J. Exp. Zool.* 213:161–171

128. Ueno, M., Mizuhira, V. 1984. Calcium transport mechanism in crayfish gastrolith epithelium correlated with the molting cycle. II. Cytochemical demonstration of Ca^{2+}-ATPase and Mg^{2+}-ATPase. *Histochemistry* 80:213–17

129. Ultsch, G. R., Herbert, C. V., Jackson, D. C. 1984. The comparative physiology of diving in North American freshwater turtles. I. Submergence tolerance, gas exchange, and acid-base balance. *Physiol. Zool.* 57:620–31

130. Ultsch, G. R., Jackson, D. C. 1982. Long-term submergence at 3°C of the turtle, *Chrysemys picta bellii,* in normoxic and severely hypoxic water. I. Survival, gas exchange and acid-base status. *J. Exp. Biol.* 96:11–28

131. Urist, M. R. 1976. Biogenesis of bone: Calcium and phosphorous in the skeleton and blood in vertebrate evolulation. In *Handbook of Physiology, Endocrinology,* 7:183–213. Bethesda: Amer. Physiol. Soc.

132. Vigh, D. A., Dendinger, J. E. 1982. Temporal relationships of postmolt deposition of calcium, magnesium, chitin and protein in the cuticle of the Atlantic Blue Crab, *Callinectes sapidus* Rathbun. *Comp. Biochem. Physiol.* 72A:365–69

133. Watabe, N., Blackwelder, P. L. 1980. Ultrastructure and calcium localization in the mantle epithelium of freshwater gastropod *Pomacea paludosa* during shell regeneration. In *The Mechanism of Biomineralization in Animals and*

Plants, ed. M. Omori, N. Watabe, pp. 131–144. Tokyo: Tokai Univ. Press

134. Weast, A. C. 1971. *Handbook of Chemistry and Physics,* Cleveland: CRC Press 51st ed.

135. Weiner, S., Traub, W., Lowenstein, H. A. 1983. Organic matrix in calcified exoskeletons. In *Biomineralization and Biological Metal Accumulation,* ed. P. Westbroek, E. W. de Jong, pp. 205–224. The Netherlands: Reidel

136. Weinstock, A., Leblond, C. P. 1971. Elaboration of the matrix glycoprotein of enamel by the secretory ameloblasts of the rat incisor by radioautography after galactose ^{3}H injections. *J. Cell Biol.* 51:26–51

137. Welinder, B. S. 1974. The crustacean cuticle- I. Studies on the composition of the cuticle. *Comp. Biochem. Physiol.* 47A:779–87

138. Welinder, B. S. 1975. The crustacean cuticle- II. Deposition of organic and inorganic material in the cuticle of *Astacus fluviatilis* in the period after moulting. *Comp. Biochem. Physiol.* 51B:409–16

139. Wheeler, A. P., Rusenko, K. W., George, J. W., Sikes, C. S. 1985. Calcium binding by molluscan organic matrix: effects of ionic strength and relevance to biomineralization. *Amer. Zool.* 25(4):50A

140. Wheeler, A. P., Sikes, C. S. 1984. Regulation of carbonate calcification by organic matrix. *Amer. Zool.* 24:933–44

141. White, B. A., Bancroft, C. 1987. Regulation of gene expression by calcium. In *Calcium and Cell Function,* ed. W. Y. Cheung, 7:109–132. Orlando: Academic

142. Wilbur, K. M. 1980. Cells, crystals and skeletons. In *The mechanism of Biomineralization in Animals and Plants,* ed. M. Omori, N. Watabe, pp. 3–17. Tokyo: Tokai Univ. Press

143. Wilbur, K. M. 1984. Many minerals, several phyla, and a few considerations. *Amer. Zool.* 24:839–45

144. Wood, C. M., Cameron, J. N. 1985. Temperature and the physiology of intracellular and extracellular acid-base regulation in the Blue Crab *Callinectes sapidus. J. Exp. Biol.* 114:151–79

145. Worms, D., Weiner, S. 1986. Mollusk shell organic matrix: Fourier transform infrared study of the acidic macromolecules. *J. Exp. Zool.* 237:11–20

146. Yee, H. F. Jr., Jackson, D. C. 1984. The effects of different types of acidosis and extracellular calcium on the mechanical activity of turtle atria. *J. Comp. Physiol. B* 154:385–92

147. Yaari, A. M., Brown, C. E. 1985. Role of lipids in mineralization: an experimental model for membrane transport of calcium and inorganic phosphate. In *Calcium in Biological Systems,* ed. R. P. Rubin, G. B. Weiss, J. W. Putney, Jr., pp. 6235–29. New York: Plenum

148. Yule, A. B., Crisp, D. J., Cotton, I. H. 1982. The action of acetazolamide on calcification in juvenile *Balanus balanoides. Mar. Biol. Lett.* 3:273–88

Annu. Rev. Physiol. 1990. 52:97–113

THE SEROUS CELL

Carol B. Basbaum[1], Berthold Jany, and Walter E. Finkbeiner[2]

Cardiovascular Research Institute and the[1] Departments of Anatomy and[2] Pathology, University of California, San Francisco

KEY WORDS: tracheobronchial cells, respiratory mucus, airway secretion, respiratory epithelium, tracheobronchial glands

INTRODUCTION

The large representation of serous cells in human airway glands (serous cell volume 61%; mucous cell volume 39%) (87, 88) shows that evolutionary pressures have favored the development and persistence of this cell type. What adaptive function justifies their abundance? First, they are the primary defensive cell of the mucosa. They are the regular army, discharging bactericidal compounds that deal efficiently with mundane pathogens (50, 61, 14, 13, 20, 21). Second, at least in experimental airway injury, serous cells are stem cells for the renewal of the epithelium (26), and they may be capable of direct conversion to mucous cells (52).

In the current technological climate, the time is ripe to take advantage of molecular tools to define the essential features of serous cells as serous cells and serous cells as progenitor cells. The first necessity is to define the biochemical phenotype of serous cells, since this will direct attention to marker genes whose activation essentially defines the serous cell. For phenotype conversion to occur, these genes would have to be inactivated just as the marker genes for other phenotypes become activated.

In this review, we will first describe our current view of the serous phenotype based on analyses of tissue sections and short term organ cultures. Next, we will describe newer data obtained from serous cells maintained in homogeneous culture. Finally, we will review a molecular genetic approach that is providing evidence for the idea that serous cells may transdifferentiate to become mucous cells.

SEROUS CELL PHENOTYPE

The mature serous cell somewhat resembles an immobilized neutrophil, for like the neutrophil, the serous cell is the source of proteins that act as endogenous antibiotics. Unlike the neutrophil, however, the serous cell also produces one or more protease inhibitors (30, 69, 70), which protect the airway surface from the destructive effects of bacterial and neutrophil proteases. A surprisingly large number of serous cell proteins are cationic in nature. Probably not by chance, serous cells also produce large polyanions (4, 74). This general pattern mimics that pattern found in mucous cells (see P. Verdugo, this volume), as well as in many other secretory cells (see below). Insofar as secretory granules contain molecules of opposing charge in the appropriate stoichiometry, ionic interactions within the granules will shield charges, reduce Donnan potential, and permit condensation of large amounts of secretory product in a small space (see Verdugo, this volume; 88a).

Distribution and Appearance of Serous Cells

Serous cells of the tracheobronchial tree may occur in the surface epithelium, submucosal glands, or both, depending on species. They are not present in bronchioles or alveoli. In humans, serous cells exist in the surface epithelium before (45) but not after (67) birth. After birth they are confined to the submucosal glands, where they comprise approximately 60% (87, 88) of the gland volume in healthy individuals. In bronchitics, this proportion declines, as mucous cells make up progressively more of the gland volume (87, 88).

Serous cells are prevalent in the surface epithelium of pathogen-free rodents (45), in animals lacking submucosal glands (73, 76), and in the human fetus (45). Basally, the cells rest on the basement membrane, with their apices projecting slightly into the airway lumen (Figure 1). They have irregularly-shaped basally oriented nuclei, a perinuclear zone containing rough endoplasmic reticulum (RER), and a well-developed Golgi apparataus. The apical portion of the cells contains variable numbers of electron dense secretory granules, 600 nm in diameter (43).

In the glands, serous cells are pyramidal in shape and have small round nuclei in the basal region of the cell (Figure 2). Their supranuclear cytoplasm is rich in RER and Golgi apparatus. The apical portion of the cell contains numerous secretory granules (68). The granules are electron dense and range between 100–1800 nm. Adjacent granules remain clearly separated (68).

The electron density and periodic acid-Schiff staining (PAS) of granules of serous cells in the glands and surface epithelium suggest that the cells are of the same phenotype, but this is not yet proven. Extremely little immunocytochemical data is available to define the specific products of the superficial serous cells and compare them with those in the glands. Recently it

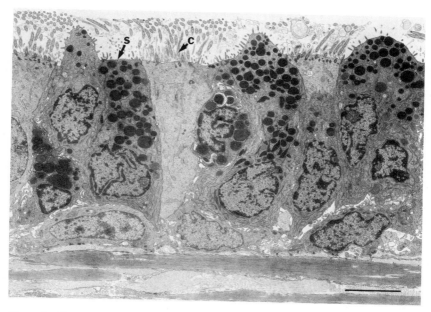

Figure 1   Electron micrograph of rat tracheal epithelium showing epithelial serous *(S)* and ciliated *(C)* cells. Bar = 5 μm.

was reported that nonciliated cells in the surface epithelium of the human bronchi and bronchioles contain both lysozyme- and low molecular weight bronchial inhibitor (antileukoprotease)-like immunoreactivity (31). If the reactive cells, indeed, correspond to serous cells, this would be the first evidence that serous cells of the glands and surface epithelium are similar biochemically as well as morphologically.

Proteins of the Serous Cell

Although mucin is the predominent protein in respiratory tract fluid, nonmucin proteins are present in significant quantities. It has been observed through various techniques that the cell of origin of most of these nonmucin proteins is the serous cell.

LYSOZYME   One of the first proteins recognized as a product of the airway submucosal gland serous cell was lysozyme. Lysozyme is a cationic protein (14 kd) with enzymatic activity that hydrolyzes 1,4 β linkages between N-acetylmuramic acid and N-acetyl-D-glucosamine in the bacterial cell wall. This lytic process is bactericidal and hence protects against infection by bacteria entering with the inspired air. Lysozyme is found not only in respira-

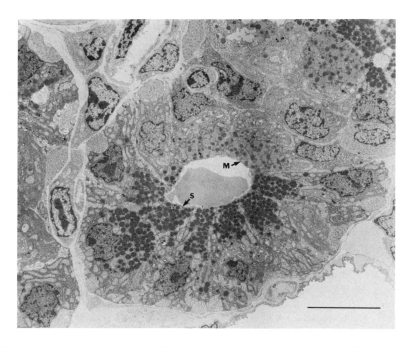

Figure 2   Electron micrograph of a ferret tracheal gland acinus showing serous *(S)* and mucous *(M)* gland cells. Bar = 10 μm. From Basbaum, C. B. 1986. *Clinics Chest Med.* 7:231–237. Reproduced with permission.

tory tract fluid, but also in the secretions protecting most of the body surfaces, and it is found in the secretions of the mammary, salivary, and lacrimal glands, as well as in the specific granules of neutrophils. Im-munocytochemical studies show that lysozyme is present in tracheobronchial submucosal gland serous cell granules (50, 61, 14, 85, 95). Biochemical methods have also been used to demonstrate the release of lysozyme from both the mucosa and submucosa of human airways (51).

LACTOFERRIN   Another of the cationic proteins of the serous cell is lac-toferrin. This iron-binding protein, M_r 70–75 kd, was initially discovered in bovine and human milk and was later detected in many of the secretions protecting body surfaces, including bronchial, lacrimal, salivary, and nasal secretions as well as in the specific granules of neutrophils (63, 64). In tracheobronchial tissue, lactoferrin is found in the secretory granules of submcosal gland serous cells (62, 13). Although the physiologic role of lactoferrin in the airways is not known, two theories exist (22). The first, or bacteriostatic theory, is that sequestering of iron by lactoferrin in the respiratory fluid reduces the growth of iron-dependent bacteria through iron-deprivation. The second, or mucoprotective theory, is that lactoferrin prevents iron-catalysed degradation of mucus glycoproteins.

SECRETORY IgA   Secretory IgA is the major form of immunoglobulin present in respiratory tract fluid as well as in most other external body fluids (94, 93, 91, 92). Although serous cells themselves do not produce antibodies, they synthesize the glycoprotein receptor (secretory component) that binds IgA released by interstitial plasma cells. The receptor is located on the basolateral surface of the serous cell (34) and mediates the internalization and transport of IgA through the cell. The IgA receptor complex (termed secretory IgA) is secreted into the gland lumen and transported via ducts to the airway lumen.

PEROXIDASE   Peroxidases are a family of enzymes that catalyze the reduction of hydrogen peroxide to water by electron donors. In combination with hydrogen peroxide and either thiocyanate or halide ions, peroxidases are active against bacteria, viruses, fungi, and mycoplasma. Like lysozyme and lactoferrin, peroxidase plays a defensive role against infectious agents. Peroxidase is detected by a cytochemical method involving incubation of tissue sections with the substrate diaminobenzidine in the presence of H_2O_2. During the reaction, the substrate is oxidized to an insoluble, indamine polymer visible by light microscopy. Reacted with osmium tetroxide, the product is also visible by electron microscopy. Peroxidase has been reported in the submucosal gland serous cells of a variety of species including man (W. Finkbeiner, C. Basbaum, unpublished observations) as well as in the tracheal lumen and epithelial secretory cells of rodents (20, 21).

ANTILEUKOPROTEASE   Antileukoprotease (bronchial inhibitor) is another cationic protein of the serous cell. It is one of two currently recognized protease inhibitors in airway secretion, (the other being alpha$_1$ proteinase inhibitor). Antileukoprotease is a 12 kd, acid stable molecule, not present in the bloodstream, that is responsible for at least 70% of the total inhibiting capacity of bronchial lavage fluid against neutrophil proteases. Immunocytochemical studies shows that the low molecular weight protease inhibitor is present in granules of serous gland cells in intra- and extrapulmonary airways. (30, 69, 70).

PROLINE RICH PROTEINS   Proline rich proteins (PRP) are products of a multigene gene family originally found to be expressed in salivary glands. These molecules, carrying either positive or negative net charges, have been isolated from human parotid saliva (9, 49). Their primary structure is characterized by the presence of multiple tandem repeats. Using an antibody directed against salivary PRP, Warner & Azen detected PRP in serous cells of nasal, laryngeal, and tracheobronchial submocosal glands (97). Although the function of PRP in respiratory tract fluid is not known, it has been observed that modulation of the concentration of PRP in bronchial fluid influences mucus viscosity (2). This may occur either by direct interaction with gel forming mucins or indirectly by chelating Ca or other ions. This is consistent with the general view that small proteins may alter the physical properties of the mucus gel by their interactions with mucin aggregates (82).

ALBUMIN   Albumin is a 68 kd major serum protein responsible for binding and transport of numerous biologically active molecules. The role of albumin in mucus hydration has been recently demonstrated (1). The major site of albumin synthesis is the liver (33). The presence of albumin in the lung and other non-liver tissues has been attributed to serum transudation from local vessels (48, 58). Recent work (72, 96) using molecular hybridization techniques, however, has revealed the presence of functional albumin RNA in non-liver sources including the kidney, pancreas, lung, heart, and intestine. In analyzing the ^{35}S-methionine labeled proteins synthesized by serous cell cultures, we noticed a prominent band of M_r 67 kd. We analyzed this protein by fast performance liquid chromatography (FPLC) and tested it for immunologic cross-reactivity with bovine albumin. Based on its size, charge, and immunologic cross-reactivity, we identified it as an albumin-like protein. Recent reports (98) indicate that preformed albumin is also actively transported by airway epithelial cells to the airway lumen. The relative contributions of de novo albumin production vs the transport of albumin from blood transudates is currently under investigation.

OTHER PROTEINS   Culture of serous cells has provided an opportunity to identify secretory proteins of the serous cell not yet recognized. Taking advantage of this, we have metabolically labeled both cultured cells and finely dissected glands with ^{35}S-methionine. Stimulation of both cells and intact glands with secretagogues such as isoproterenol causes certain protein bands to be significantly enriched in the medium of stimulated cells and glands. Further studies of this type may lead us to recognize the existence of previously unidentified serous cell proteins.

High Molecular Weight Glycoconjugates of the Serous Cell

Although the name serous denotes cells containing serum-type proteins, it has long been recognized that serous cells of the respiratory tract, like those in the pancreas (79) and parotid gland (39), contain significant amounts of polysaccharide. An apparent paradox surrounds the composition of the serous cell glycoconjugates, since they had been found, on one hand, to be Alcian Blue negative, and on the other, to contain large amounts of ^{35}S. These two findings are inconsistent because the presence of large amounts of sulfate normally renders a molecule so acidic that its negative charge density makes it reactive with Alcian Blue dye. Despite their synthesis of sulfated proteoglycans, serous cells react poorly with Alcian Blue.

The discovery that serous cells contain cationic proteins (50, 13, 14, 30) provides a possible explanation for the above paradox. According to Mowry (71), the complexing of polysaccharides with divalent cations causes them to lose their affinity for Alcian Blue. The same may occur naturally in the granules of serous cells.

The coexistence of proteoglycan and cationic proteins has already been described for secretion granules of the pituitary (99), adrenal medulla (60), and pancreas (79, 89). It has been postulated that ionic interactions between cationic proteins and large polyanions occur in secretory granules (89) to reduce the osmotic activity of granule contents, thus excluding water from the granule without the need for energy-dependent pumping mechanisms. It has also been proposed that cationic shielding of secreted polyanions is necessary to induce their condensation via a polymer gel transition process (96a).

The establishment of homogeneous cultures of airway serous gland cells from the cow made possible a detailed analysis of the glycoconjugates secreted by this cell type. To do this, we pulse-labeled cells with ^{35}S or ^{14}C glucosamine and then stimulated them with isoproterenol to release their products into culture medium. We have analyzed these products by gel filtration chromatography, thin layer chromatography, and electrophoresis (3, 74). Under dissociative conditions, the glycoconjugates elute in both the void and included volumes of Sepharose Cl-4B. Based on chemical analysis and specific enzyme digestions, the material eluting in the void volume contains hyaluronic acid, chondroitin sulfate proteoglycans, and trace amounts of O-linked glycoproteins. The material eluting in the included volume includes heparan sulfate, in addition to chondroitin sulfate, and asparagine-linked glycoproteins with complex type glycans. Based on the analysis of cultured cells, it appears that proteoglycans and hyaluronic acid account for the major part of the carbohydrate secreted by serous cells.

Since cells in culture may show abnormalities including the production of unusual glycoconjugates, we sought to determine whether the glycoconjugates observed in culture were also present in vivo. To do this, we used immunocytochemistry to demonstrate the existence of chondroitin sulfate proteoglycan in secretory granules of submucosal glands in frozen sections of the cow and human trachea (25). Not only were we able to detect the expected granular staining pattern in these cells, but we also observed that chondroitin sulfate was released by a receptor-mediated mechanism when glands in organ culture were stimulated with bethanechol or isoproterenol (25).

Consistent with the notion that proteoglycans are natural secretory products of airway serous cells, Bhaskar et al have reported the presence of proteoglycans including chondroitin and dermatan sulfate in bronchial lavage fluid and organ culture medium from healthy airways of dogs and humans (10, 11). Proteoglycans have also been detected in sputum samples from patients with cystic fibrosis (55). The results of recent studies show that mucin core protein is absent from serous cells (75). Thus, the sulfate taken up by these cells (53) is likely associated with nonmucin glycoconjugates, presumably proteoglycans.

As we approach a consensus that proteoglycans are authentic products of the serous cell, the question is raised of their fate and function in the mucus gel. Has evolution programmed serous cells to produce proteoglycans solely to package cationic proteins within the cell, or do proteoglycans play an important role even after secretion? What is certain is that proteoglycans find their way into respiratory secretions and must make a place for themselves among a tangled network of mucin molecules. As hydration of polymer networks is driven by Donnan potential, the high charge density of proteoglycans due to heavy sulfation provides a more readily hydrated network than that provided by mucins. Serous and mucous cells may control the properties of the mucus gel by regulating the ratio between secreted proteoglycans and mucins.

Regulation of Secretion from the Serous Cell

A phenotypic feature no less important than secretory granule content is the cellular machinery that equips a cell to respond to its environment. In this category are receptors and second messengers that mediate stimulus secretion coupling. Because serous cells exist with mucous cells in mixed glands, it has been difficult to obtain detailed information on their individual receptors and second messengers. Much of the original analysis of airway secretion was performed on the serous/mucous gland as a mixed organ. Results of these studies [reviewed in (4)] constitute an essential background to understanding serous cell function. In addition, through morphological dissection methods (5), the use of lysozyme as a biochemical marker (95), and more recently analysis of serous cells in culture (27, 28), we have obtained more specific information about serous cell physiology.

RECEPTORS   Although the mixed serous-mucous bovine tracheal gland is responsive to alpha- and beta-adrenergic as well as cholinergic activation, the serous cell line obtained from these glands is directly responsive only to beta-adrenergic agonists. Cholinergic receptors are not present on this line of cultured serous cells, as evaluated by quinuclidinylbenzilate (QNB) binding studies (M. Madison, C. Basbaum, unpublished data).

In view of the almost inevitable loss of function because of dedifferentiation in culture, the serous cells seem to retain a relatively large number of functional receptors. We have detected several receptors for cyclooxygenase products (84), which presumably mediate serous cell secretion during inflammatory reactions initiated by diverse insults. The secretory potency of the prostaglandins, evaluated by their ability to cause significant augmentation of the release of ^{35}S-labeled glycoconjugates, shows the following rank order: $PGE_1 = PGE_2 > PGA_1 > PGD_2$. PGE_1 and PGE_2 more than doubled the secretory rate of the cultured serous cells, whereas PGA_1 and PGD_2 produced somewhat smaller effects. The other prostaglandins (e.g. $PGF_2\alpha$) produced negligible effects on the cultured serous cells (84).

Not only do the serous cells contain prostaglandin receptors, but they are also sensitive to several other inflammatory mediators. For example, we have found dose-dependent excitatory responses to bradykinin (C. Sommerhoff, unpublished results) and histamine. The histamine effect, mediated through H_2 receptors, is consistent with previous evidence obtained by Shelhamer et al (81) in human airway explants. A surprising finding in the serous cell cultures was that degranulation supernatant from mastocytoma cells produced a much larger secretory response than expected from its histamine concentration alone. Subsequent studies revealed that this response was attributable to the mast cell protease, chymase (83).

Recently we explored the beta-adrenergic receptor of the serous cell in some detail (59). To define its subtype, we performed functional and radioligand binding studies in parallel. We metabolically labeled the cells with Na_2SO_4, then in pulse-chase experiments, we observed the relative potency of a variety of adrenergic agonists in releasing macromolecular ^{35}S from the cells. The rank order of potency was isoproterenol > epinephrine > norepinephrine, consistent with the presence of a β_2-adrenergic receptor. These data were supported by radioligand binding studies using ^{125}(iodo)cyanopindolol (^{125}I-CYP) (24) to identify beta-adrenergic receptors. ^{125}I-CYP binding to membrane particulates prepared from cultured serous cells was saturable and of high affinity (equilibrium dissociation constant 20 +/− 3 pM, mean +/− S E M n=6) and was antagonized stereoselectively by propranolol. Adrenergic agonists competed for ^{125}I-CYP binding sites with a rank order of potency characteristic of the β_2-adrenergic receptor subtype. Further, a specific β_2-adrenergic receptor antagonist, ICI 118.551, competed for a single class of ICYP binding sites with high affinity. This demonstrates that the secretory response of cultured tracheal gland cells to β-adrenergic agonists is mediated by β-adrenergic receptors of the β_2 subtype. The preferred natural agonist for this type of receptor is the circulating catecholamine, epinephrine, which suggests that serous cells may be strongly influenced by release of this substance from the adrenal medulla (18, 1a).

cAMP AND PHOSPHOPROTEINS OF THE SEROUS CELL   Isoproterenol stimulation of the β_2 receptor in cultured serous cells elicits a dose-dependent elevation of the level of intracellular cAMP (28). Further, the secretory response to isoproterenol is potentiated by inhibiting the degradation of cAMP within the cell. These findings strongly suggest that cAMP functions as a second messenger in the serous cell secretory pathway, probably acting through stimulation of cAMP-dependent protein kinases. The isoproterenol-cAMP-protein kinase pathway has already been demonstrated for in situ secretory cells of the cat trachea (57).

Cellular effects of cAMP are generally mediated through the activity of protein kinases and their phosphoprotein substrates (8). Based on previous work in other cells, the kinases and their substrates are likely to play a key role in secretion (23, 35). For example, three parotid phosphoproteins undergo changes in phosphorylation state because of adrenergic stimulation (^{32}P is increased in two, M_r 27 and 14 kd, and decreased in one, M_r 13.6 kd), and these changes are correlated with increases in cAMP-dependent kinase activity as well as augmentation of amylase secretion (7). One particular phosphoprotein, by virtue of its rapid kinetics, could be rate determining for secretion in both the parotid and submandibular glands (78). This is a 26-kd phosphoprotein that is dephosphorylated with a time course similar to that of inactivation of endogenous cAMP-dependent protein kinase activity following β-adrenergic blockade. Such a protein may transfer cAMP-mediated signals to molecules within the cell that directly mediate membrane fusion and exocytosis. Proteins whose phosphorylation levels are modulated by secretagogues are also being examined for their potential to participate actively in exocytosis in the exocrine pancreas (16, 32, 54, 56).

In the airway serous cell, we recently performed experiments analyzing changes in the phosphorylation state of proteins mediated by exogenous cAMP (28). Two membrane proteins M_r, 49 kd and 55 kd showed cAMP-dependent phosphorylation. The rate of phosphorylation of at least 13 cytosolic proteins was altered by cAMP. The phosphorylation rate of 11 proteins (approximate M_r 170, 162, 145, 120, 118, 84, 75, 47, 39, 25, 23) was increased by cAMP. We also observed a prominent reduction in the phosphorylation state of two cytosolic protein bands at approximately 49 and 55 kd.

It is too soon to assign roles to these recently discovered phosphoproteins. However, we know that beta-adrenergic stimulation has multiple effects on exocrine gland cells. These include the regulation of exocytosis (86) as well as the regulation of growth and differentiation (6, 15, 86). It is likely that all of the β-adrenergic effects are mediated by cAMP, protein kinase, and phosphoproteins. We are now taking the initial steps toward deciphering the specific elements of this regulatory pathway.

SEROUS CELLS IN INJURED AIRWAYS

Models of airway injury have been developed primarily in rodents. Since the respiratory epithelium of rodents is rich in serous cells, it has provided the opportunity to observe the responses of these cells to various forms of injury.

Injury models include exposure of rodent airways to cigarette smoke (65, 47), sulfur dioxide (52), NO_2 (26), isoproterenol (12), neutrophil elastase (21), and marijuana smoke (37). Depending on the injury, plastic changes involving hypertrophy, hyperplasia, or apparent transdifferentiation of epithelial cells may occur. Of specific interest is the observation that serous cells are the predominent dividing cell in rat airways one hour after exposure to NO_2 and thus play a major tole in renewal of the airway epithelium (26).

Evidence has been cited to indicate a second possible role for serous cells in the injured epithelium. Lamb & Reid pointed out that the number of mucous cells appearing after SO_2 injury exceeded that expected from the observed rate of mitosis. This was particularly marked in distal airways (52). This means that the increased number of mucous cells present after injury could not be accounted for by mucous cell division. The concomitant decrease in serous cells (42) and the appearance of transitional cells with both mucous and serous granules (44, 46, 80) suggest that conversion of serous to mucous cells at least partly accounted for mucous metaplasia.

Although intriguing, this hypothesis has not been adequately tested during the two decades since the original studies were performed. Two recent developments now make it possible to perform the relevant experiments. The first is the improvement in breeding conditions that make it possible to obtain pathogen-free rats that essentially lack mucous cells in the tracheobronchial tree (38, 77). If mucous metaplasia could be induced in such animals, the hypothesis that new mucous cells arose from previously existing nonmucous cell types would be reinforced. The second development, i.e. the isolation of a cDNA probe encoding airway mucin (40), should make possible in situ hybridization experiments by which to detect after injury cell type(s) that simultaneously retain morphological features of their original phenotype and have initiated mucin gene transcription.

We have recently shown that pathogen-free rats lacking mucous cells (except in upper tracheal glands) develop mucous metaplasia in the surface epithelium throughout the tracheobronchial tree in response to SO_2 (41). Loss of serous cells occurs concomitantly. This indicates that preexisting mucous cells are not an essential element of mucous metaplasia and suggests that serous cells may give rise to new mucous cells, either by mitosis and redifferentiation or direct phenotype conversion.

To obtain more precise information about the cell and molecular changes underlying mucous metaplasia, we have performed experiments with a cDNA corresponding to a portion of the airway mucin core protein (40). In these experiments, we monitored levels of mucin mRNA expression in rat airways, and found that steady-state levels of mucin mRNA increased eight to ninefold from a barely detectable baseline signal after SO_2 exposure. Since mucous cells were virtually absent in the rat airway epithelium before exposure, the increase could not have been a by-product of mucous cell proliferation. Based on these data, we conclude that preexisting cells of a nonmucous phenotype initiate mucin gene transcription in response to extracellular signals related to SO_2 exposure. Since mucin mRNA levels rose significantly before mucous metaplasia was apparent morphologically, initiation of mucin gene transcription may be a primary event leading to mucous metaplasia and hypersecretion. With the same mucin probe, we are currently analyzing rat airways by in situ hybridization. The results of these studies should definitively show whether serous and/or other cell types are the precursors of mucous cells in mucous metaplasia.

CONCLUSION

The biochemical phenotype of the serous cell has been partly defined. It is a cell that secretes antibacterial proteins and anti-proteases, many of which are cationic in nature. Its other major products are sulfated proteoglycans and hyaluronic acid, all of which are polyanions likely to play a role in the storage and release of the cationic proteins. Because the overall charge density on serous cell proteoglycans is higher than that on mucins, the products of serous cells may tend to be more watery. Serous and mucous cells may control the properties of the mucus gel by regulating the ratio between secreted proteoglycans and mucins.

Serous cells in the respiratory epithelium of rodents play a special role in the response to injury. They are progenitor cells for renewal of the airway epithelium, providing increased numbers of cells by mitosis. Using an airway mucin cDNA probe to monitor rat airway mucin mRNA levels, we found that mucin mRNA levels rise in resonse to injury, preceding a loss of serous and gain of mucous cells. In situ hybridization analysis using the mucin probe will permit a direct test of the hypothesis that mucous cells are formed by serous cell transdifferentiation.

Literature Cited

1. Aitken, M., Verdugo, P. 1989. Donnan mechanism of mucin release and conditioning in goblet cells: the role of polyions. In *Mucus and Related Topics,* ed. E. N. Chandler, New York: Plenum

1a. Ariens, E. J., Simonis, A. M. 1983. Physiological and pharmacological aspects of adrenergic receptor classification. *Biochem. Pharmacol.* 32:1539–45

2. Bailleul, V., Richet, C., Hayem, A., Degand, P. 1977. Proprietes rheologiques des secretions bronchiques: mise en evidence et role de polypeptides riches en proline (PRP). *Clin. Chim. Acta* 74:115–23

3. Basbaum, C. B., Paul, A., Finkbeiner, W. E., Mergey, M., Vessiere, D., Picard, J. 1985. Biochemical characterization of glycoconjugates secreted by bovine tracheal gland cells in culture. *J. Cell Biol.* 101:232a (Abstr.)

4. Basbaum, C. B., Finkbeiner, W. E. 1989. Mucus producing cells of the airway. In *Lung Biology in Health and Disease. Pulmonary Cell Biology,* ed. D. Massaro. pp. 37–39. New York: Dekker, 1431 pp.

5. Basbaum, C. B., Ueki, I., Brezina, L., Nadel, J. A. 1981. Tracheal submucosal gland serous cells stimulated in vitro with adrenergic and cholinergic agonists: a morphometric study. *Cell Tissue Res.* 220:481–98

6. Baskerville, A. 1976. The development and persistence of bronchial gland hypertrophy and goblet cell hyperplasia in the pig after injection of isoprenaline. *J. Pathol.* 119:35–47

7. Baum, B., Freiberg, J. M., Ito, H., Roth, G. S., Filburn, C. R. 1981. β-adrenergic regulation of protein phosphorylation and its relationship to exocrine secretion in dispersed rat parotid gland acinar cells. *J. Biol. Chem.* 256:9731–36

8. Beavo, J. Bechtel, P., Krebs, E. 1974. Activation of protein kinase by physiological concentrations of cAMP. *Proc. Natl. Acad. Sci. USA* 71:3580–83

9. Bennick, A., Connell, G. E. 1971. Purification and partial characterization of four proteins from human parotid saliva. *Biochem. J.* 123:455–64

10. Bhaskar, K. R., O'Sullivan, D. D., Seltzer, J., Rossing, T. H., Drazen, J. M., Reid, L. M. 1985. Density gradient study of bronchial mucus aspirates from healthy volunteers (smokers and non-smokers) and from patients with tracheostomy. *Exp. Lung Res.* 9:289–308

11. Bhaskar, K. R., O'Sullivan, D. D., Seltzer, J., Rossing, T. H., Drazen, J. M., Reid, L. M. 1986. Density gradient analysis of secretions produced in vitro by human and canine airway mucosa: identification of lipids and proteoglycans in such secretions. *Exp. Lung Res.* 10:401–22

12. Bolduc, P., Reid, L. 1978. The effect of isoprenaline and pilocarpine on mitotic index and goblet cell number in rat respiratory epithelium. *Br. J. Exp. Pathol.* 59:311–18

13. Bowes, D., Clark, A. E., Corrin, B. 1981. Ultrastructural localization of lactoferrin and glycoprotein in human bronchial glands. *Thorax* 36:108–15

14. Bowes, D., Corrin, B. 1977. Ultrastructural immunocytochemical localisation of lysozyme in human bronchial glands. *Thorax* 32:163–70

15. Burke, G. T., Barka, T. 1978. Beta-adrenergic receptors and adenylate cyclase in hypertrophic and hyperplastic rat salivary glands. *Biochim. Biophys. Acta* 539:54–61

16. Burnham, D. B., Williams, J. A. 1982. Effect of carbachol, cholecystokinin and insulin on protein phosphorylation in isolated pancreatic acini. *J. Biol. Chem.* 257:10523–28

17. Carp, H., Janoff, A. 1980. Inactivation of bronchial mucous proteinase inhibitor by cigarette smoke and phagocyte-derived oxidants. *Exp. Lung Res.* 1:225–37

18. Carstairs, R., Nimmo, A., Barnes, P. J. 1985. Autoradiographic visualization of β-adrenoceptor subtypes in human lung. *Am. Rev. Respir. Dis.* 132:5541–57

19. Christensen, T. G., Blanchard, G. C., Nolley, G., Hayes, J. A. 1981. Ultrastructural localization of endogenous peroxidase in the lower respiratory tract of the guinea pig. *Cell Tissue Res.* 214:407–15

20. Christensen, T. G., Hayes, J. A. 1982. Endogenous peroxidase in the conducting airways of hamsters. *Am. Rev. Respir. Dis.* 125:341–46

21. Christensen, T. G., Korthy, A. L., Snider, G. L., Hayes, J. A. 1977. Irreversible bronchial goblet cell metaplasia in hamsters with elastase-induced panacinar emphysema. *J. Clin. Invest.* 59:397–404

22. Clamp, J. R., Creeth, J. M. 1984. Some non-mucin components of mucus and their possible biological roles. In *Mucous and Mucosa,* ed. J. Nugent, M.

O'Conner, pp. 121–36. London: Pitman. 246 pp.

23. Cohen, P. 1982. The role of protein phosphorylation in the neural and hormonal control of cellular activity. *Nature* 296:613–20

24. Engel, G., Hoyer, D., Berthold, R., Wagner, H. 1981. ^{125}I-CYP, a new ligand for β-adrenoceptors: identification and quantitation of subclasses of β-adrenoceptors in guinea pig. *Naunyn Schmiedebergs Arch Pharmakol.* 317:277–85

25. Escudier, E., Forsberg, L. S., Basbaum, C. B. 1988. Chondroitin sulfate is a secretory product of tracheal gland serous cells in vivo as well as in culture. *J. Cell Biol.* 105:330a (Abstr.)

26. Evans, M. J., Shami, S. G., Cabral-Anderson, L. J., Dekker, N. P. 1986. Role of nonciliated cells in renewal of the bronchial epithelium of rats exposed to NO_2. *Am. J. Pathol.* 123:126–33

27. Finkbeiner, W. E., Nadel, J. A., Basbaum, C. B. 1986. Establishment and characterization of a cell line derived from bovine tracheal glands. *In Vitro Cell Develop. Biol.* 22:561–67

28. Finkbeiner, W. E., Widdicombe, J. H., Hu, L., Basbaum, C. B. 1989. Regulation of secretion in bovine tracheal serous cells: role of cAMP and cAMP-dependent protein kinase. *Am. J. Physiol.*

29. Forstner, G., Shih, M., Lukie, B. 1973. Cyclic AMP and intestinal glycoprotein synthesis: the effect of β-adrenergic agents, theophylline, and dibutyryl cyclic AMP. *Can. J. Physiol. Pharmacol.* 51:122–29

30. Franken, C., Kramps, J. A., Meijer, C. J. L. M., Dijkman, J. H. 1980. Localization of a low-molecular-weight inhibitor in the respiratory tract. *Bull. Eur. Physiopathol. Respir.* 16:231–36

31. Franken, C., Meijer, C. J. L. M., Dijkman, J. H. 1989. Tissue distribution of antileukoprotease and lysozyme in humans. *J. Histochem. Cytochem.* 37:493–98

32. Freedman, S. D., Jamieson, J. D. 1982. Hormone-induced protein phosphorylation. III. Regulation of the phosphorylation of the secretagogue-responsive 29,000-dalton proteins by both Ca^{2+} and cAMP in vitro. *J. Cell Biol.* 95:918–23

33. Gitlin, D., Gitlin, J. D. 1975. Fetal and neonatal development of human plasma proteins. In *The plasma proteins,* ed. F. W. Putman, pp. 263–319. New York: Academic. 436 pp.

34. Goodman, M. R., Link, D. W., Brown, W. R., Nakane, P. K. 1981. Ul-

trastructural evidence of transport of secretory IgA across bronchial epithelium. *Am. Rev. Respir. Dis.* 123:115–19

35. Greengard, P. 1978. Phosphorylated proteins as physiological effectors. *Science* 99:146–52

36. Hay, D. I. 1973. The interaction of human parotid salivary proteins with hydroxyapatite. *Arch. Oral Biol.* 18:1517–29

37. Hayashi, M., Sornberger, G. C., Huber, G. L. 1980. A morphometric analysis of the male and female tracheal epithelium after experimental exposure to marijuana smoke. *Lab. Invest.* 42:65–69

38. Hung, H.-T., Haskell, A., McDonald, D. 1989. Respiratory infections potentiate neurogenic inflammation in the rat trachea: a study of changes in vascular permeability and epithelial cells. *Anat. Embryol.* In press

39. Iversen, J. M., Keller, P. J., Kauffman, D. L., Robinovitch, M. R. 1987. The presence of chondroitin sulfate in parotid secretory granules and saliva of the rat. *Cell Tissue Res.* 250:221–26

40. Jany, B., Gallup, M., Gum, J., Kim, Y., Basbaum, C. 1989. Molecular cloning of human airway mucin. *Eur. J. Respir. Med.* (Abstr.) In press

41. Jany, B., Gallup, M., Gum, J., Kim, Y., Basbaum, C. 1989. Mucin gene expression in experimental airway hypersecretion. *Am. Rev. Resp. Dis.* (Abst.) In press

42. Jeffery, P. K., Ayers, M., Rogers, D. F. 1982. The mechanisms and control of bronchial mucous cell hyperplasia. *Chest* 5:27S–29S

43. Jeffery, P. K., Reid, L. M. 1975. New observations of rat airway epithelium: a quantitative and electron microscopic study. *J. Anat.* 120:295–320

44. Jeffery, P. K., Reid, L. 1977. The respiratory mucous membrane. In *Respiratory Defense Mechanisms,* ed. J. D. Brain, D. F. Proctor, L. Reid, pp. 193–245. New York: Dekker. 1216 pp.

45. Jeffery, P. K., Reid, L. 1977. Ultrastructure of airway epithelium and submucosal gland during development. In *Lung Biology in Health and Disease. Development of the Lung,* ed. W. A. Hodson, pp. 87–134. New York: Dekker, 646 pp.

46. Jeffery, P. K., Reid, L. 1981. The effect of tobacco smoke, with or without phenylmethyloxadiozole (PMO), on rat bronchial epithelium: a light and electron microscopic study. *J. Pathol.* 133:341–59

47. Jones, R., Bolduc, P. Reid, L. 1973. Goblet cell glycoprotein and tracheal

gland hypertrophy in rat airways: the effects of tobacco smoke with or without the anti-inflammatory agent phenylmethyloxadiazole. *Br. J. Exp. Pathol.* 54:229–39

48. Kauffman, D. L., Keller, P. J. 1979. The basic proline-rich proteins in human parotid saliva from a single subject. *Arch. Oral Biol.* 24:249–56

49. Kaliner, M., Shelhamer, J. H., Borson, B., Nadel, J. A., Patow, C., Marom, Z. 1986. Human respiratory mucus. *Am. Rev. Resp. Dis.* 134:612–24

50. Klockars, M., Reitamo, S. 1975. Tissue distribution of lysozyme in man. *J. Histochem. Cytochem.* 23:932–40

51. Konstan, M. W., Chen, P. W., Sherman, J. M., Thomassen, M. J., Wood, R. E., Boat, T. F. 1981. Human lung lysozyme: sources and properties. *Am. Rev. Respir. Dis.* 123:120–24

52. Lamb, D., Reid, L. 1968. Mitotic rates, goblet cell increase and histochemical changes in mucus in rat bronchial epithelium during exposure to sulphur dioxide. *J. Pathol. Bacteriol.* 96:97–111

53. Lamb, D., Reid, L. 1970. Histochemical and autoradiographic investigation of the serous cells of the human bronchial glands. *J. Pathol.* 100:127–38

54. Lambert, M., Camus, J., Christophe, J. 1974. Phosphorylation of protein components of isolated zymogen granule membranes from the rat pancreas, *FEBS Lett.* 49:228–32

55. Le Treut, A., Lamblin, G., Leray, G., Guenet, L., Filliat, M., Roussel, P. 1984. Identification of degraded proteoglycans in the sputum of patients suffering from chronic bronchial hypersecretion. In *Cystic Fibrosis Horizons,* ed. D. Lawson, pp. 347 (Abstr.). New York: Wiley. 446 pp.

56. Lewis, D. S., Ronzio, R. A. 1979. An assessment of the role of protein kinase and zymogen granule phosphorylation during secretion by the rat exocrine pancreas. *Biochem. Biophys. Acta* 583:422–33

57. Liedtke, C. S., Rudolph, T., Boat, T. 1983. β-adrenergic modulation of mucin secretion in cat trachea. *Am. J. Physiol.* 244 *(Cell Physiol.)* 13:C391–98

58. Lopez-Vidriero, M. T., Das, I., Reid, L. M. 1977. Airway secretion: source, biochemical and rheological properties. In *Respiratory Defense Mechanisms,* ed. J. D. Brain, D. F. Proctor, L. Reid, pp. 289–356. New York: Dekker. 1216 pp.

59. Madison, J. M., Basbaum, C. B., Brown, J. K., Finkbeiner, W. E. Characterization of β-adrenergic receptors in cultured bovine tracheal gland cells. *Am. J. Physiol.* 256 *(Cell Physiol.)* 25:C310–14

60. Margolis, R. U., Margolis, R. K. 1973. Isolation of chondroitin sulfate and glycopeptides from chromaffin of adrenal medulla. *Biochem. Pharmacol.* 22: 2195–97

61. Mason, D. Y., Taylor, C. R. 1975. The distribution of muramidase (lysozyme) in human tissues. *J. Clin. Res.* 28:124–32

62. Masson, P. L., Heremans, J. F., Prignot, J. J., Wauters, G. 1966. Immunohistochemical localisation and bacteriostatic properties of an iron binding protein from bronchial mucus. *Thorax* 1:538

63. Masson, P. L. 1970. La lactoferrine, proteine des secretions externes et des leucoytes neutrophiles. PhD thesis. Univer. Catholique de Lauvain, Arcia, Bruxelles.

64. Masson, P. L., Heremans, J. F., Shonn, E. 1969. Lactoferrin, an iron-binding protein in neutrophilic leukocytes. *J. Exp. Med.* 130:643–58

65. Mawdesley-Thomas, L. E., Healey, P., Barry, D. H. 1971. Experimental bronchitis in animals due to suphur dioxide and cigarette smoke. An automated quantitative study. In *Inhaled Particles III,* ed. W. H. Walton, pp. 509–25. Surrey, England: Gresham. 1090 pp.

66. McCarthy, C., Reid, L. 1964. Intracellular mucopolysaccharides in the normal human bronchial tree. *Q. J. Exp. Physiol.* 49:85–94

67. McDowell, E., Barrett, L. A., Glavin, F., Harris, C., Trump, B. F. 1978. The respiratory epithelium. I. Human bronchus. *J. Natl. Canc. Inst.* 61: 539–49

68. Meyrick, B., Reid, L. 1970. Ultrastructure of cells in the human bronchial submucosal glands. *J. Anat.* 107: 281–99

69. Mooren, H. W. D., Kramps, J. A., Franken, C., Meijer, C. J. L. M., Dijkman, J. H. 1983. Localization of a low-molecular-weight bronchial protease inhibitor in the peripheral human lung. *Thorax* 38:180–83

70. Mooren, H. W. D., Meijer, C. J. L. M., Kramps, J. A., Franken, C., Dijkman, J. 1982. Ultrastructural localization of the low molecular weight bronchial protease inhibitor in human bronchial glands. *J. Histochem. Cytochem.* 30: 1130–34

71. Mowry, R. W., Scott, J. E. 1967. Observations on the basophilia of amyloids. *Histochemie* 10:8–32

72. Nahon, J. L. 1987. The regulation of

albumin and α-feto protein gene expression in mammals. *Biochimie* 69:445–59

73. Pack, R. J., Al-Ugaily, L. H., Morris, G., Widdicombe, J. G. 1980. The distribution and structure of cells in the tracheal epithelium of the mouse. *Cell Tissue Res.* 208:65–84

74. Paul, A., Picard, J., Mergey, M., Vessiere, D., Finkbeiner, W., Basbaum, C. 1988. Glycoconjugates secreted by bovine tracheal serous cells in culture. *Arch. Biochem. Biophys.* 260:57–84

75. Perini, J.-M., Marianne, T., Lafitte, J.-J., Lamblin, G., Roussel, P., Mazzuca, M. 1989. Use of an antiserum against deglycosylated human mucins for cellular localization of their peptide precursors: antigenic similarities between bronchial and intestinal mucins. *J. Histochem. Cytochem.* 37:869–75

76. Phipps, R. J., Richardson, P. S., Corfield, A., Gallagher, J. T., Jeffery, P. K., et al. 1977. A physiological, biochemical and histological study of goose tracheal mucin and its secretion. *Philos. Trans. R. Soc. London (Biol.)* 279:513–40

77. Plopper, C. G., Mariassy, A. T., Wilson, D. W., Alley, J. L., Nishio, S. G. Nettesheim, P. 1983. Comparison of nonciliated tracheal epithelial cells in six mammalian species: ultrastructure and population densities. *Exp. Lung Res.* 5:281–94

78. Quissell, D., Deisher, L., Barzen, K. 1985. The rate-determining step in cAMP-mediated exocytosis in the parotid and submandibular glands appears to involve analogous 26kD integral membrane phosphoproteins. *Proc. Natl. Acad. Sci. USA* 82:3237–41

79. Reggio, H. A., Palade, G. E. 1978. Sulfated compounds in the zymogen granules of the guinea pig pancreas. *J. Cell Biol.* 77:288–314

80. Reid, L. M., Jones, R. 1980. Mucous membrane of respiratory epithelium. *Environ. Health Perspect.* 35:113–20

81. Shelhamer, J. H., Marom, Z., Kaliner, M. 1980. Immunologic and neuropharmacologic stimulation of mucous glycoprotein release from human airways in vitro. *J. Clin. Invest.* 66:1400–8

82. Snyder, C. E., Nadziejko, C. E., Herp, A. 1982. Binding of basic proteins to glycoproteins in human bronchial secretions. *Int. J. Biochem.* 14:895–98

83. Sommerhoff, C. P., Finkbeiner, W. E., Nadel, J. A., Basbaum, C. B. 1987. Prostaglandin D_2 and prostaglandin E_2 stimulate ^{35}S-labeled macromolecule secretion from cultured bovine tracheal gland serous cells. *Am. Rev. Respir. Dis.* 135:A363 (Abstr.)

84. Sommerhoff, C. P., Caughey, C. H., Finkbeiner, W. E., Lazarus, S. C., Basbaum, C. B., Nadel, J. A. 1989. Mast cell chymase: a potent secretagogue for airway gland serous cells. *J. Immunol.* 142:2450–56

85. Spicer, S. S., Frayser, R. 1977. Immunocytochemical localization of lysozymes in respiratory and other tissues. *Lab. Invest.* 36:282–95

86. Sturgess, J., Reid, L. 1973. The effect of isoprenaline and pilocarpine on (a) bronchial mucus-secreting tissue and (b) pancreas, salivary glands, heart, thymus, liver and spleen. *Br. J. Exp. Path.* 54:388–403

87. Takizawa, T., Thurlbeck, W. M. 1971. A comparative study of four methods of assessing the morphologic changes in chronic bronchitis. *Am. Rev. Respir. Dis.* 103:774–83

88. Takizawa, T., Thurlbeck, W. M. 1971. Muscle and mucous gland size in the major bronchi of patients with chronic bronchitis, asthma, and asthmatic bronchitis. *Am. Rev. Respir. Dis.* 104:331–36

88a. Tam. Y., Verdugo, P. 1981. Control of mucus hydration as a Donnan equilibrium process. *Nature* 292:340–42

89. Tartakoff, A., Greene, L. J., Palade, G. E. 1974. Studies on the guinea pig pancreas. *J. Biol. Chem.* 249:7420–31

90. Thurlbeck, W. M. 1976. *Chronic Airflow Obstruction in Lung Disease*. Philadelphia: Saunders. 456 pp.

91. Tomasi, T. B. Jr., 1976. *The Immune System of Secretions*. Englewood Cliffs, NJ: Prentice-Hall, 161 pp.

92. Tomasi, T. B., Bienenstock, J. 1968. Secretory immunoglobulins. *Adv. Immunol.* 9:1–96

93. Tomasi, T. B. Jr., Grey, H. M. 1972. Structure and function of immunoglobulin. A. *Prog. Allergy* 16:81–213

94. Tomasi, T. B. Jr., Tan, E. M., Solomon, A., Prendergast, R. A. 1965. Characteristics of an immune system common to certain external secretions. *J. Exp. Med.* 121:101–24

95. Tom-Moy, M., Basbaum, C. B., Nadel, J. A. 1983. Localization and release of lysozyme from ferret trachea: effects of adrenergic and cholinergic drugs. *Cell Tissue Res.* 228:549–62

96. Tratner, I., Nahon, J. L., Sala-Trepat, J. M. 1988. Differences in methylation patterns of the α-fetoprotein and albumin genes in hepatic and non hepatic developing rat tissues. *Nucleic Acids Res.* 16:2749–64

96a. Verdugo, P. 1986. Polymer gel phase transition: a novel mechanism of product storage and release in secretion. *Biophys. J.* 49:231a.

97. Warner, T. F., Azen, E. A. 1984. Proline-rich proteins are present in serous cells of submucosal glands in the respiratory tract. *Am. Rev. Respir. Dis.* 130:115–18

98. Webber, S. E., Widdicombe, J. G. 1988. The transport of albumin and dextran across the ferret isolated trachea *in vitro. J. Physiol.* 396:93P (Abstr.)

99. Zanini, A., Giannattasio, G., Nussdorfer, G., Margolis, R. K., Margolis, R. U., Meldolesi, J. 1980. Molecular organization of prolactin granules. II. Characterization of glycosaminoglycans and glycoproteins of the bovine prolactin matrix. *J. Cell. Biol.* 86:260–72

Annu. Rev. Physiol. 1990. 52:115–35

REGULATION OF Cl⁻ AND K⁺ CHANNELS IN AIRWAY EPITHELIUM

J. D. McCann and M. J. Welsh

Howard Hughes Medical Institute, Departments of Internal Medicine and Physiology and Biophysics, University of Iowa College of Medicine, Iowa City, Iowa 52242

KEY WORDS: secretion, cAMP, cell calcium, phosphorylation, cystic fibrosis

INTRODUCTION

Electrolyte transport by airway epithelia controls the quantity and composition of the respiratory tract fluid, thereby contributing to normal mucociliary clearance. Airway epithelia have the capacity for both active sodium (Na^+) absorption from the mucosal surface to the submucosal surface and for active chloride (Cl^-) secretion from the submucosal to the mucosal surface. The relative contributions of Cl^- secretion and Na^+ absorption to overall transport vary, depending on the neuro-humoral environment, the airway region, and the species. In this review, we focus on Cl^- secretion. We do not attempt to provide an inclusive summary, instead we emphasize recent work.

Electrolyte Transport by Airway Epithelia

Transepithelial Cl^- secretion is made possible by segregation of ion channels, cotransporters, and pumps to either the cell's apical or basolateral membrane. Figure 1 shows a model that describes the mechanism of Cl^- secretion by airway epithelia and by several other Cl^- secreting epithelia (35).

At the basolateral membrane, Cl^- enters the cell on an electrically neutral Na^+-coupled cotransporter. The identity of the transporter is not certain in any Cl^- secreting epithelia and may, in fact, differ from one cell type to another. It is likely, however, to be either a Na^+-Cl^- cotransporter or a

0066/4278/90/0315-0115$02.00

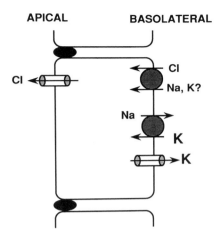

Figure 1   Model of the mechanism of Cl⁻ secretion by airway epithelial cells. See text for details.

$Na^+/K^+/2Cl^-$ cotransporter. The cotransporter uses the energy in the transmembrane Na^+ gradient to accumulate Cl^- within the cell above electrochemical equilibrium. Cl^- then leaves the cell passively across the apical membrane and moves down a favorable electrochemical gradient through an apical membrane Cl^- channel. The Na^+ gradient that drives Cl^- uptake is maintained by the Na^+-K^+-ATPase located on the basolateral membrane. The basolateral membrane also contains a K^+ channel that recycles the K^+ that enters the cell at the basolateral membrane.

Coordination of Apical and Basolateral Transport

Consideration of the model shown in Figure 1 indicates that when a hormone or neurotransmitter stimulates the rate of transepithelial Cl^- secretion, transporters on both sides of the cell must be activated in a coordinated manner to produce secretion. This is particularly evident for coupling activation of a basolateral membrane K^+ channel to activation of the apical Cl^- channel. Activation of a K^+ channel solves two problems faced by the Cl^- secreting cell (22, 35). First, when secretion is stimulated, K^+ will accumulate in the cell because of K^+ entry on the Na^+-K^+-ATPase and possibly on the Cl^- cotransporter. Activation of basolateral K^+ channels allows K^+ to efflux from the cell, which prevents changes in cell volume. Second, stimulation of secretion opens Cl^- channels in the apical membrane, which shifts the cell's voltage toward the Cl^- chemical gradient and diminishes the driving force for Cl^- exit. Activation of basolateral K^+ channels hyperpolarizes the cell thereby maintaining the driving force for Cl^- exit across the apical membrane.

In this review we focus on the regulation of apical Cl^- and basolateral K^+ channels. We first discuss the evidence that shows that they are coordinately regulated, then describe the regulation of each channel individually, and finally discuss the mechanisms by which their activation may be coordinated.

EVIDENCE THAT STIMULATION OF TRANSEPITHELIAL Cl^- SECRETION ACTIVATES K^+ AND Cl^- CHANNELS

Secretagogues Increase Apical and Basolateral Membrane Conductance

Studies with intracellular microelectrodes clearly establish that agents that stimulate Cl^- secretion activate an apical Cl^- conductance (23, 24, 38, 39): (a) secretagogues increase apical membrane conductance; (b) they increase the voltage changes produced by mucosal Cl^- substitutions; and (c) the Cl^- concentration gradient becomes the predominant determinant of apical electromotive force (EMF). Likewise, secretagogues activate a basolateral K^+ conductance (23, 25, 28, 38, 39): (a) secretagogues increase basolateral conductance; and (b) ion substitutions suggest that the predominant conductance is to K^+. Since the intracellular activity of K^+ and Cl^- remain relatively constant during secretion, the changes in electrical parameters caused by secretagogues are consistent only with coordinate activation of an apical Cl^- conductance and a basolateral K^+ conductance.

The sequence of change in the apical Cl^- and basolateral K^+ conductance has been most extensively studied in canine tracheal epithelium. In the native epithelium, epinephrine first causes an increase in apical Cl^- conductance and then an increase in basolateral K^+ conductance (38, 39). In contrast, in the cultured epithelium, epinephrine produces the reverse sequence of changes: first basolateral K^+ conductance increases and then apical Cl^- conductance increases (31). These differences may result from differences in the density of hormone receptors or from quantitative differences in the second messengers. In any case, the important point is that both membrane conductances increase. These results have also been obtained with addition of membrane permeant cAMP analogues and a variety of other hormones and neurotransmitters that have receptors either on the apical or basolateral membrane. Thus it appears that second messengers regulate both the apical and basolateral membrane conductances.

Apical Cl^- and Basolateral K^+ Conductances Are Required for Transepithelial Cl^- Secretion

The use of transport inhibitors has shown that both apical Cl^- and basolateral K^+ channels are required to support transepithelial secretion. At present no highly specific inhibitors of the apical Cl^- conductance have been reported.

Nonetheless, several carboxylic acid analogues including anthracene-9-carboxylic acid, diphenylamine-2-carboxylate (DPC), and 5-nitro-2-(3-phenylpropylamino)-benzoate (NPPB) reversibly decrease transepithelial conductance, inhibit apical membrane Cl^- conductance, and inhibit Cl^- secretion (17, 29, 33).

Evidence that the basolateral K^+ conductance is required for secretion comes from the observation that Ba^{2+} decreases the basolateral membrane K^+ permeability and inhibits Cl^- secretion (25, 27). In addition, an increase in submucosal K^+ concentration depolarizes the cell and inhibits Cl^- secretion, thus demonstrating that the basolateral K^+ conductance is responsible for maintaining the negative intracellular voltage and thereby the driving force for Cl^- exit across the apical membrane (28).

REGULATION OF APICAL MEMBRANE Cl^- CHANNELS

Identification of Apical Membrane Cl^- Channels

Our current understanding of the regulation of Cl^- channels comes from studies that employ a variety of techniques, including studies of epithelia in Ussing Chambers, microelectrode impalements, isotope flux studies, and investigations using the patch-clamp technique. At the single-channel level a characteristic feature of airway epithelial Cl^- channels is their outwardly rectifying current-voltage relationship in the presence of symmetrical Cl^- concentrations (8, 32, 33); Figure 2 shows an example. Evidence that this

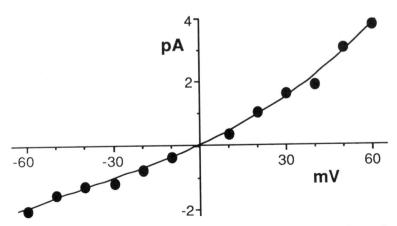

Figure 2 Current-voltage relationship of an apical membrane Cl^- channel from a human airway epithelial cell. Data are from an excised, inside-out patch bathed in symmetrical 140 mM NaCl solutions.

outwardly rectifying Cl⁻ channel is responsible for the apical membrane Cl⁻ conductance is (a) in cell-attached patches, it is activated by hormones and neurotransmitters that increase apical Cl⁻ conductance; (b) it has an anion selectivity sequence of $SCN^- > I^- > Cl^- = Br^- > F^-$, which is the same as the anion permeability sequence of the apical membrane (M. Welsh, unpublished observation); (c) it is blocked by carboxylic acid analogues that also block the apical Cl⁻ conductance; (d) it is found in patches of membrane obtained from confluent sheets of cells where only the apical membrane was accessible to the recording pipet [in contrast the basolateral K⁺ channel was not observed in the apical membrane of confluent sheets of cells (37)]; and (e) its regulation is altered in cystic fibrosis cells (8, 36) in which the apical membrane is Cl⁻ impermeable (11, 12, 41). Activation[1] of this channel in the cell-attached recording mode by addition of hormones and neurotransmitters to the bath solution and activation of the apical Cl⁻ conductance by addition of agonists to the basolateral solution clearly indicated that the apical membrane Cl⁻ channel is activated by an intracellular second messenger.

Another low conductance, anion selective channel has been reported in airway epithelial cells (8) but, as yet, its significance in Cl⁻ secretion is not certain.

When studied with the whole-cell patch-clamp technique (17, 20), Cl⁻ channel currents showed conductive properties similar to those described in single-channel studies: (a) the instantaneous current-voltage relationship rectified in the outward direction in the presence of symmetrical Cl⁻ solutions; (b) in the presence of Cl⁻ concentration gradients, currents reversed near E^{Cl} and were not altered significantly by cations; and (c) agents that inhibit the apical membrane Cl⁻ conductance inhibited Cl⁻ currents. Currents carried by the outwardly rectifying Cl⁻ channel are the predominant Cl⁻ conductive pathway in the cell membrane (17, 20).

Activation of Cl⁻ Channels in Excised, Cell-Free Membrane Patches

In early studies of the Cl⁻ channel, it was observed that after membrane patches were ripped off the cell, Cl⁻ channels activated in previously quiescent patches (8, 32, 33). Later it was found that on some occasions channels activated immediately after excision of the patch, independent of what voltage was maintained across the patch. More frequently, however, channels remained in an inactivated state until the membrane was depolarized to relatively large voltages (+80 to +140 mV) (14, 21). Once activated by depolarization, channels remained in the activated state even when membrane voltage

---

[1]The Cl⁻ channel functions in at least two modes. We refer to an inactivated channel as one that is unstimulated or quiescent and is always in the closed state. An activated channel is one that has been stimulated and spontaneously flickers back and forth between the open and closed state.

was returned to less depolarizing values. A similar phenomenon has been observed when bath temperature is increased from 23°C to 37°C.

The mechanisms responsible for Cl⁻ channel activation by patch excision, by depolarization, and by an increase in bath temperature are uncertain. These phenomena are only observed in excised patches; similar maneuvers do not activate channels in cell-attached patches. These results led to speculation that the channel might be maintained in an inactivated state by an intracellular inhibitor; excision of the membrane patch could relieve the inhibition by altering the interactions between the channel and the inhibitor or by allowing an inhibitor to diffuse from the channel. An alternative possibility is that these maneuvers may somehow physically alter channel conformation, thereby causing it to remain in an activated state. An understanding of these "nonphysiologic" mechanisms of channel activation may provide further insights into the structure and regulation of the channel. In any case, the observation that the large membrane depolarizations activated channels allowed investigators to use depolarization as a tool to determine if a Cl⁻ channel was present in a membrane patch (14, 21).

In contrast to the studies in excised patches, in whole-cell patches depolarization did not appear to activate Cl⁻ channels. Instead, the steady-state and nonsteady-state kinetics indicate that current flows through ion channels that are open at hyperpolarizing voltages and close with depolarization (17, 20). In excised patches, the effect of voltage on open-state probability (P_o) is less certain. In canine tracheal epithelium, P_o usually decreases at depolarizing voltages. In human airway epithelium, P_o sometimes decreases, sometimes increases, and sometimes is unchanged with depolarization. Further work will be required to learn how voltage affects P_o, with particular attention paid to the mechanism of channel activation and the effect of voltage during steady-state (long duration) recording conditions. In any case, studies in the intact epithelium suggest that apical Cl⁻ conductance is not significantly voltage-dependent (30).

Activation of Cl⁻ Channels by cAMP-Dependent Protein Kinase

There is substantial circumstantial evidence that cAMP is an intracellular second messenger that regulates the Cl⁻ channel; many agonists that stimulate Cl⁻ secretion increase cellular levels of cAMP (15, 26), and addition of poorly metabolized, membrane permeant analogues of cAMP stimulate Cl⁻ secretion (1).

In many cells, the biologic effects of cAMP result from activation of cAMP-dependent protein kinase (PKA), which results in phosphorylation of target proteins. To determine if PKA regulates the Cl⁻ channel, investigators used excised, inside-out patches of membrane and added a purified catalytic subunit of PKA plus ATP to the internal (cytosolic) surface (14, 21). Figure 3 shows an example of the results. In the top traces, the channel was in an inactive state; it did not open. Subsequent addition of PKA plus ATP activated the channel, as shown in the bottom traces. Activation required the addition of both ATP and PKA; neither alone was sufficient. Moreover, addition of a boiled catalytic subunit failed to activate Cl⁻ channels. Similar results were obtained with studies of whole-cell Cl⁻ currents; addition of forskolin (20) or a catalytic subunit of PKA (17) increased the outwardly rectifying Cl⁻ current.

Those results showed that addition of PKA plus ATP mimicked the effect of secretagogues, such as β-adrenergic agonists and exogenous cAMP, in regulating Cl⁻ channels. Thus it appears that the Cl⁻ channel or a regulatory protein closely associated with the channel is phosphorylated and results in channel activation.

Activation of Cl⁻ Channels by Protein Kinase C

Protein kinase C (PKC) may play an important role in regulating ion channels in several types of cells. Studies in canine airway epithelium used the membrane permeant activator of PKC, phorbol 12-myristate 13-acetate (PMA), to suggest that PKC might regulate secretion (4, 34). Addition of PMA to cell monolayers caused complex effects on Cl⁻ secretion; PMA caused a transient stimulation of secretion, but then inhibited the secretory response to subsequent addition of a membrane permeant cAMP analogue. An assay of Cl⁻ channel function in the intact cell, ¹²⁵I⁻ efflux (5), provided

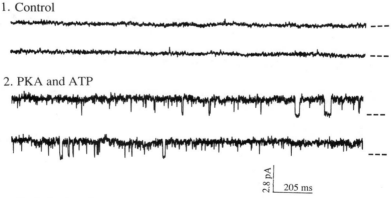

1. Control

2. PKA and ATP

2.8 pA | 205 ms

Figure 3 Activation of a Cl⁻ channel by PKA. Example from excised, inside-out patch from normal human airway epithelial cell. The current level when channel is closed is shown by the dashed line. Holding voltage was −40 mV, and tracings were obtained at +40 mV: (*1*) control; (*2*) catalytic subunit of PKA and ATP (1 mM) added to the internal surface. From (14) with permission.

similar results (13); PMA increased $^{125}I^-$ efflux, but the degree of stimulation was smaller than that produced by agents that increase cellular levels of cAMP. In contrast, addition of PMA before cAMP attenuated the cAMP-induced $^{125}I^-$ efflux.

Those results suggested that PKC might either stimulate or inhibit the Cl^- channel, depending on the physiologic status of the cell. Because those studies did not allow the transport effects to be localized to the Cl^- channel, and because PMA may have effects on secretion other than those mediated by PKC, PKC was added to the cytosolic surface of excised patches (13, 10). Phosphorylation requires the presence of PKC (PKC was highly purified from rat or mouse brain or partially purified from canine tracheal epithelium with similar results), phosphatidylserine (the membrane patch served as a source of phospholipid), and a diacylglycerol or tumor-promoting phorbol ester [dioctanoylglycerol (DiC8), diolein, or PMA were used with similar results]. Some forms of PKC also require Ca^{2+}; therefore experiments were performed at either a low (<10 nM) or a high (1 mM) $[Ca^{2+}]$.

Figure 4 shows the effect of adding PKC at a low $[Ca^{2+}]$. Under baseline conditions, no channels were activated in the patch. When PKC, PMA, and ATP were added to the solution bathing the internal surface of the patch, a channel activated and flickered back and forth between the open and closed state (10, 13). Activation of Cl^- channels required the presence of PKC, ATP, and a diacylglycerol or PMA; addition of any two alone was insufficient

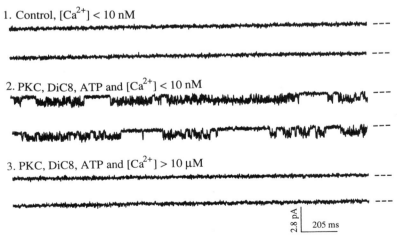

Figure 4   PKC activation of a Cl^- channel at low Ca^{2+} (<10 nM). Membrane voltage was −40 mV throughout. (*1*) Control; (*2*) PKC, DiC8 (1 μg/ml), and ATP (1 mM) were added to the internal solution and the channel activated; (*3*) internal Ca^{2+} was increased to > 10 μM by addition of $CaCl_2$ to the bath and the channel inactivated. From (13) with permission.

to activate the channel. Activation occurred an average of 126 sec after addition of all three agents. In contrast, channels did not activate during 480 sec of observation in paired-patches not exposed to PKC. These observations indicate that PKC phosphorylates and activates the channel at a low $[Ca^{2+}]$. As shown in Figure 5, the observation that cystic fibrosis channels can not be activated by either PKA or PKC at low Ca^{2+} concentration (10, 13, 14, 21) suggests that both enzymes might regulate the Cl⁻ channel at the same phosphorylation site.

Inactivation of Cl⁻ Channels by Protein Kinase C

In contrast to the effect at a low $[Ca^{2+}]$, at a high $[Ca^{2+}]$, PKC inactivated Cl⁻ channels (13). Figure 4 shows that when internal Ca^{2+} was increased to a value greater than 10 μM, channels that had been activated by PKC at a low $[Ca^{2+}]$ inactivated. Thus at a high $[Ca^{2+}]$, PKC had an effect opposite to that observed at a low $[Ca^{2+}]$.

When channels were activated by membrane depolarization, as shown in Figure 6, they spontaneously flickered between the open and closed states. Addition of ATP and then PMA did not alter channel kinetics. However, on addition of PKC to the ATP and PMA containing solution, the channel inactivated (13). Studies of the effect of PMA on Cl⁻ secretion (4, 34) and $^{125}I^-$ efflux (13) suggest an interaction between the effect of PKA and PKC. This was borne out in single channel studies; channels that were first activated by phorphorylation with catalytic subunit of PKA and ATP were inactivated by subsequent addition of PKC plus DiC8 at 1 μM Ca^{2+}. Finally, addition of PKC at a high $[Ca^{2+}]$ (1 μM) prevented activation by depolarization (13).

Inactivation required the addition of PKC, PMA or a diacylglycerol, ATP,

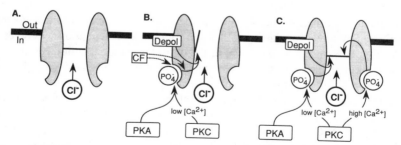

Figure 5 Model of Cl⁻ channel regulation. For the sake of clarity we refer to the channel as a single entity, but it may consist of multiple subunits and associated proteins. Inner and outer surfaces of the membrane are indicated in (A). Channel is defined as inactivated when the gate is closed (A and C), and activated when it is open (B). The gate may involve different molecular steps. Depol refers to strong membrane depolarization (approximately +100 to +140 mV). At high Ca^{2+} concentration, PKC may also phosphorylate the low Ca^{2+} site. From (13) with permission.

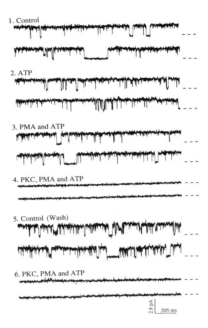

Figure 6   PKC inactivation of a depolarization-activated Cl$^-$ channel at 1 μM Ca^{2+}. Holding voltage was -40 mV, and tracings were obtained at $+40$ mV. After channel was activated by depolarization, recordings were made under the following conditions: (*1*) control, no additions; (*2*) ATP (1 mM); (*3*) PMA (100 nM) and ATP; (*4*) PKC, PMA, and ATP; (*5*) control conditions following removal of PKC, PMA, and ATP from the internal solution; (*6*) readdition of PKC, PMA, and ATP. From (*13*) with permission.

and a high [Ca^{2+}] (1μM). These results suggest that at a high [Ca^{2+}], PKC phosphorylates the channel causing it to inactivate. The results can not be explained by down-regulation of PKC. In some cases inactivation was reversible (Figure 6, *panel 5*). Removal of the phosphorylation solution resulted in reactivation. These results suggest that a membrane-associated phosphatase has access to the channel in the membrane patch.

There are several possible ways to explain the dual effects of PKC on the Cl$^-$ channel: different responses may be due to an effect of Ca^{2+} on the channel, on PKC, or on the interaction between the two. As shown in Figure 5, it appears that the channel has two different phosphorylation sites (one activating and one inactivating), and Ca^{2+} might determine which site is phosphorylated. This could occur in several ways. First, Ca^{2+} might change channel conformation making different sites accessible to PKC. Second, the Ca^{2+}-dependence of PKC might be influenced by the nature of the substrate, so that one phosphorylation site might not require Ca^{2+} for an effect. Third, the interaction of PKC with the membrane might be Ca^{2+} dependent; in the absence of Ca^{2+}, PKC might phosphorylate an extrinsic site on the channel, and in the presence of Ca^{2+}, PKC might phosphorylate a site on the channel associated with the membrane. Alternatively, different effects of PKC could be caused by isozymes that phosphorylate different sites: a Ca^{2+}-independent form that activates the channel and a Ca^{2+}-dependent form that inactivates the channel. This is possible because the purified PKC preparations probably contain more than one isozyme. In any case, each of these alternatives require that PKC show substrate specificity for two different phosphorylation sites on the channel.

Activation of Cl⁻ Channels by an Increase in [Ca²⁺]ᶜ

The first indication that $[Ca^{2+}]_c$ might regulate Cl⁻ channels came from the observation that addition of the Ca^{2+} ionophore, A23187, stimulated Cl⁻ secretion (2). Although part of this effect appears to result from stimulation of arachidonic acid metabolism with subsequent prostaglandin production and thereby an increase in cellular levels of cAMP (6, 34, 40), the effect of A23187 cannot be entirely explained by activation of the cAMP system, especially in human airway epithelia (5, 6, 34, 40, 42). In native canine airway epithelia most of the secretory response to A23187 is abolished by the prostaglandin synthesis inhibitor, indomethacin, whereas in cultured epithelia the response is only attenuated.

In recent studies the rate of $^{125}I^-$ efflux from intact cells was measured to assess the effect of Ca^{2+} on the Cl⁻ channel (5). I⁻ is an excellent tracer for Cl⁻ since it is not secreted across the epithelium, but is conducted by the outwardly rectifying apical membrane Cl⁻ channel. In a series of studies, A23187 was observed to increase $^{125}I^-$ efflux; however the time course of increase in efflux did not parallel the time course of changes in $[Ca^{2+}]_c$; a transient increase in $[Ca^{2+}]_c$ was sufficient to induce a long lasting increase in $^{125}I^-$ efflux. Those findings suggest that Ca^{2+} does not regulate the Cl⁻ channel directly.

In excised membrane patches, an increase in the $[Ca^{2+}]$ bathing the internal surface of the patch did not alter the probability that the Cl⁻ channel was in the open state, nor did it activate Cl⁻ channels (5, 7, 32). These results also suggest that Ca^{2+} does not directly regulate the Cl⁻ channel. Thus Ca^{2+} may interact with some intracellular regulatory factor thereby activating the channel indirectly. Such a factor might be lost (or altered) when a patch of membrane is excised from the cell preventing investigators from observing an effect of Ca^{2+}. What is that factor? It does not appear to be PKA; several possible alternatives include the Ca^{2+}/calmodulin-dependent protein kinase, a Ca^{2+}-dependent phosphatase, or a Ca^{2+}-dependent protease. Further work will be required to resolve this important issue.

Activation of Chloride Channels by Hypotonic Bathing Solution

Decreasing the osmolarity of the bath solution caused activation of Cl⁻ channels studied in the whole-cell patch-clamp mode (17). Figure 7 shows an example in which bath NaCl concentration was reduced from 135 to 90 mM. The increase in current occurred despite a reduction in the chemical gradient for outward Cl⁻ current. (Note that in the absence of a change in Cl⁻ permeability, a reduction in external Cl⁻ concentration would decrease outward current.) When extracellular NaCl concentration was returned to 135 mM, there was initially a small increase in Cl⁻ current followed by a reduction to baseline values. The initial transient increase in outward current likely results from an increase in the chemical gradient for outward Cl⁻ current, and the secondary reduction back to baseline is due to a decrease in Cl⁻ permeability. Activation of Cl⁻ channels resulted from an osmotic gradient across the plasma membrane; the effect was not dependent on the

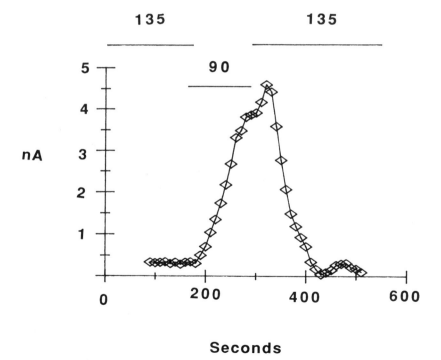

Figure 7 Effect of reducing extracellular osmolarity on whole-cell Cl⁻ channel current. Where indicated the bath NaCl concentration was reduced from 135 to 90 mM and then returned to 135 mM. Adapted from (17).

solute or the absolute value of osmolarity. Changes in osmolarity also stimulate Cl⁻ secretion by cells grown as monolayers on permeable supports. Reduction of the bath osmolarity caused by decreasing the NaCl concentration from 135 to 90 mM transiently doubled the short-circuit current. Stimulation of transepithelial current resulted from a reduction of osmolarity rather than a reduction of NaCl concentration because maintenance of osmolarity with sucrose prevented the increase in current. Moreover, the results can not be explained by diffusion voltages because Cl⁻ concentration was reduced symmetrically in both mucosal and submucosal solutions. The data suggest stimulation of active transport because current increased even though the Cl⁻ concentration decreased. The current was transient, most likely, as a result of cell volume regulatory mechanisms that restore cell volume, even in the presence of altered extracellular osmolarity. Several studies (17) indicate that the increase in short-circuit current resulted from stimulation of Cl⁻ secretion; Cl⁻-free solutions, Cl⁻ channel blockers, and the Cl⁻ cotransport inhibitor bumetanide all inhibit the change in short-circuit current produced by altering the extracellular osmolarity.

The decrease in extracellular osmolarity most likely activated Cl⁻ channels by causing cell swelling. These findings are also consistent with reports that large increases in basolateral K⁺ concentration increase apical Cl⁻ conductance and stimulate Cl⁻ secretion (30); an increase in basolateral K⁺ concentration may have also caused cell swelling. The mechanism by which swelling activates the channel is unknown. Changes in cellular levels of cAMP or an increase in intracellular $[Ca^{2+}]_c$ do not appear to be the second messengers that regulate the Cl⁻ channel in response to a reduction in bath osmolarity. It is tempting to suggest that an interaction of the cell cytoskeleton with the channel may be responsible.

REGULATION OF BASOLATERAL MEMBRANE K⁺

Identification of Airway Epithelial K⁺ Channels

In addition to the study of basolateral membrane conductance with intracellular microelectrodes, the function of K⁺ channels has been assessed with measurements of ⁸⁶Rb⁺ efflux and with the single-channel patch-clamp technique. In cell-attached and excised patches of membrane, a low conductance K⁺ channel was observed (37). Figure 8 shows a characteristic feature of this channel; it has an inwardly rectifying current-voltage relationship even in the presence of symmetrical K⁺ concentrations. Single-channel conductance was approximately 25 pS at negative voltage with symmetrical 135 mM KCl solutions. This channel is highly selective for K⁺ over both anions and Na⁺ as determined from measurements of changes in reversal potential.

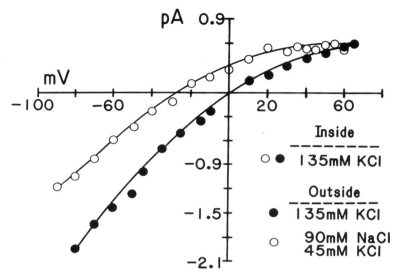

Figure 8 Current-voltage relationship of a basolateral membrane membrane K^+ channel (the K_{CLIC} channel) from a canine airway epithelial cell. Data are from excised, inside-out patches. Internal solution contained 135 mM KCl and external solution contained either 135 mM KCl *(closed circles)* or 45 mM KCl *(open circles)*.

When the K^+ channel is studied in the cell-attached mode, secretagogues such as epinephrine and isoproterenol increase open channel probability. After addition of epinephrine, K^+ channel activity often increased transiently and then decreased toward basal level. Activation of this channel by a secretagogue suggests that it is a channel responsible for basolateral membrane K^+ conductance. The observation that this channel was found in patches from isolated cells and from cells at the edge of a cluster of confluent cells, but not in the apical membrane of cells that had grown to confluency, suggests that it is localized on the basolateral membrane in confluent cells (and therefore is not accessible to the pipette).

An additional marker of the low conductance, inwardly rectifying K^+ channel is charybdotoxin (ChTX). ChTX is a minor component of *Leiurus quinquestriatus hebraeus* scorpion venom that has been observed to inhibit some types of Ca^{2+}-activated K^+ channels (3, 9, 19). ChTX has been shown to inhibit the inwardly rectifying K^+ channel by two types of studies (18, 18a). ChTX inhibits $^{86}Rb^+$ efflux from cultured airway epithelial cells with half-maximal inhibition at 10 nM. More direct evidence came from the observation that application of ChTX to the external surface of patches of membrane containing K^+ channels blocked the channel. As observed with other Ca^{2+}-activated K^+ channels, ChTX block was reversible.

Activation of K⁺ Channels by Internal Ca^{2+}

Evidence that the K⁺ channel in airway epithelial cells was regulated by Ca^{2+} came from several studies. The Ca^{2+} ionophore, A23187, stimulated $^{86}Rb^{+}$ efflux with a time course that paralleled changes in Ca^{2+} under a variety of conditions (18, 18a). This Ca^{2+}-stimulated $^{86}Rb^{+}$ efflux was entirely blocked by ChTX.

Studies of the K⁺ channel with cell-attached patches (37) showed that in nonstimulated cells the channel was quiescent. Addition of the Ca^{2+} ionophore, A23187, activated the channel and such activation was dependent upon the $[Ca^{2+}]$ in the bath solution. In excised, inside-out patches, the channel was also regulated by the $[Ca^{2+}]$ bathing the cytosolic surface of the channel. As shown in Figure 9, at a $[Ca^{2+}]_c$ of 250 nM the channel was rarely open and at 1000 nM the channel was primarily in the open state.

To distinguish this channel from other Ca^{2+}-activated K⁺ channels, it is referred to as the K_{CLIC} channel. CLIC is an acronym that denotes the channel's properties: ChTX-sensitive, low conductance, inwardly rectifying, and Ca^{2+}-activated.

This channel showed no appreciable regulation by voltage in single-channel studies (37) or in the intact epithelium (30). Regulation by Ca^{2+}, but not by voltage, is an unusual property for K⁺ channels, in general, and may be a

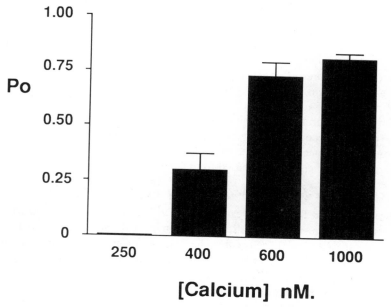

Figure 9   Effect of bath $[Ca^{2+}]$ on open channel probability (P_o) of the basolateral K⁺ channel (the K_{CLIC} channel). Data are mean of 5 excised, inside-out patches.

property particular to K^+ channels in epithelia. Attempts to activate the channel with PKA under conditions that activate the apical membrane Cl^- channel produce no change in open-state probability.

COORDINATED ACTIVATION OF APICAL CHLORIDE CHANNELS AND BASOLATERAL K^+ CHANNELS

Addition of a secretagogue, such as isoproterenol, increases cellular levels of cAMP, thereby activating apical Cl^- channels by PKA-dependent phosphorylation. Basolateral K_{CLIC} channels, however, were activated by Ca^{2+}, not by PKA. This raises the question of how activation of the two channels is coordinated. Measurements of $[Ca^{2+}]_c$ provide some insight.

Secretagogues Increase $[Ca^{2+}]_c$

Studies of intracellular $[Ca^{2+}]_c$ have relied on the use of two primary messengers: the inflammatory peptide bradykinin and the β-adrenergic agonist, isoproterenol. In canine airway epithelium, isoproterenol stimulates cAMP accumulation, but does not alter inositol phosphate production. In contrast, bradykinin stimulates inositol phosphate production but, in the presence of indomethacin, does not alter cellular levels of cAMP (16). Thus the effects of the two agents are mediated via different intracellular second messengers.

$[Ca^{2+}]_c$ was measured using the fluorescent indicator Fura-2 and a fluorescent microscope imaging system (16). Not surprisingly, addition of bradykinin caused an acute but transient increase in $[Ca^{2+}]_c$. Interestingly, isoproterenol also increased $[Ca^{2+}]_c$. Figure 10 summarizes the results. The effect of isoproterenol was mediated by the β-adrenergic receptor and was mimicked by addition of exogenous cAMP analogues. Those studies suggest that $[Ca^{2+}]_c$ was increased because of release of Ca^{2+} from intracellular stores by two different second messenger systems: inositol trisphosphate and cAMP. At present the intracellular source of the Ca^{2+} released by cAMP is uncertain; it is not certain whether it is released from the inositol phosphate-sensitive store.

Secretagogue-Induced Activation of K^+ Channels

The observation that cAMP can release Ca^{2+} from intracellular stores suggests a mechanism for parallel regulation of Cl^- and K^+ channels. An increase in cAMP could cause phosphorylation-dependent activation of apical Cl^- channels and concomitantly release Ca^{2+} from intracellular stores, thereby activating basolateral K^+ channels.

Evidence that isoproterenol and cAMP can stimulate K_{CLIC} channels by releasing Ca^{2+} from intracellular stores was obtained from studies of $^{86}Rb^+$ efflux (18). The time course of activation of $^{86}Rb^+$ efflux paralleled the time

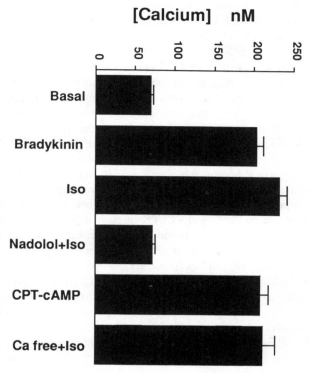

Figure 10   Effect of agonists on $[Ca^{2+}]_c$. Values were obtained under basal conditions and after addition of bradykinin (2 μM), isoproterenol (1 μM), isoproterenol plus nadolol (10 μM), CPT-cAMP (8-(4-chlorophenylthio) adenosine 3' 5'-cyclic monophosphate) (200 μM), and isoproterenol in a Ca^{2+}-free (100 nM) bath solution. Adapted from (16).

course of changes in $[Ca^{2+}]_c$. Both isoproterenol (or cAMP) and A23187 stimulated $^{86}Rb^+$ efflux in a Ca^{2+}-dependent manner. Depletion of cell Ca^{2+} blocked the response. In addition, increasing the intracellular Ca^{2+} buffering capacity with the Ca^{2+} chelator, BAPTA-AM, caused a dose-dependent inhibition of the effect of both cAMP and A23187. ChTX blocked the increase in $^{86}Rb^+$ efflux produced by both Ca^{2+} and cAMP, which suggests an effect on the same channel.

While the results discussed above are consistent with the hypothesis that cAMP, via elevation of $[Ca^{2+}]_c$, couples the apical and basolateral membrane channels, the hypothesis was questioned because cAMP causes only a transient increase in $[Ca^{2+}]_c$, whereas cAMP causes a sustained increase in Cl⁻ secretion and basolateral K⁺ conductance. An understanding of the role of K_{CLIC} channels in transepithelial Cl⁻ secretion came from studies that used charybdotoxin as a probe of K_{CLIC} channel function in the intact epithelium (18, 18a). ChTX inhibited A23187-stimulated Cl^- secretion and $^{86}Rb^+$ efflux at the same concentrations. Those results indicate that the K_{CLIC} channel is required for Ca^{2+}-stimulated Cl^- secretion.

To investigate the function of K_{CLIC} channels in cAMP-stimulated secretion, isoproterenol was added to monolayers and caused a biphasic increase in Cl^- secretion. The time course of the initial transient component of Cl^- secretion correlated with the time course of the isoproterenol-induced increase in $[Ca^{2+}]_c$. The time course of the second component correlated with the time course of isoproterenol induced increase in cAMP. Submucosal ChTX inhibited the initial transient component, but not the prolonged component of secretion; submucosal barium inhibited the sustained component. These results suggest that isoproterenol-induced secretion was dependent upon activation of two types of K^+ channels: the K_{CLIC} channel, which was stimulated initially in response to Ca^{2+}, and a ChTX-insensitive K^+ channel, which was stimulated during sustained secretion. That conclusion was supported by measurement of $^{86}Rb^+$ efflux from cell monolayers; both A23187 and isoproterenol stimulated $^{86}Rb^+$ efflux from the cells into the submucosal solution. The A23187-induced efflux was inhibited by ChTX, but the isoproterenol-induced efflux was only slightly attenuated (18, 18a). Those findings suggest the presence of another Ca^{2+}-insensitive, ChTX-insensitive basolateral membrane K^+ channel.

The data suggest that the ChTX-insensitive basolateral K^+ channel is not present, or is not activated by hormonal stimuli, in cells grown on impermeable support. Thus it was not observed in patch-clamp studies, or in the $^{86}Rb^+$ efflux assay, when cells were studied on impermeable supports. At the present time, the stimuli that cause expression of the ChTX-insensitive K^+ channel are unknown; they might result from an interaction between the cell and the permeable support. Another question concerns the regulation of the ChTX-insensitive channel. As indicated above, the data suggest that it is not regulated by Ca^{2+}. Thus cAMP-dependent regulation would provide the most straight-forward mechanism to directly regulate this channel. The presence of two basolateral membrane K^+ channels regulated by two different mediators provides another mechanism for controlling Cl^- secretion and allows a precise coupling between activation of the channels at the two opposite sides of the cell.

SUMMARY

Stimulation of transepithelial Cl^- secretion by the airway epithelium requires activation of channels at the two opposite sides of the cell: the apical and basolateral membranes. At the apical membrane, the Cl^- channel is regulated by phosphorylation with PKA and PKC. At the basolateral membrane, the

K_{CLIC} channel is regulated by $[Ca^{2+}]_c$. Addition of a secretagogue that increases cellular levels of cAMP also causes release of Ca^{2+} from intracellular stores. The Ca^{2+} may then regulate basolateral membrane K_{CLIC} channels. The cAMP-induced increase in $[Ca^{2+}]_c$ and activation of the K_{CLIC} channel is transient, however, whereas activation of the Cl⁻ channel and stimulation of secretion is a more sustained response. Those results suggest that the presence of a second Ca^{2+}-independent K⁺ channel located at the basolateral membrane, which is only expressed in cells grown on permeable supports.

ACKNOWLEDGMENTS

Work from the authors' laboratory contained in this review was supported by grants from the National Institutes of Health (HL 29851 and HL 42385) and the Cystic Fibrosis Foundation. J. D. McCann is supported by the March of Dimes Birth Defects Foundation. We wish to thank Theresa Mayhew for excellent secretarial assistance.

Literature Cited

1. Al Bazaaz, F. J., Al-Awqati, Q. 1981. Role of cAMP in regulation of chloride secretion by canine tracheal mucosa. *Am. Rev. Respir. Dis.* 123:295–98
2. Al Bazaaz, F. J., Jayaram, T. 1981. Ion transport by canine tracheal mucosa, effect of elevation of cellular calcium. *Exp. Lung Res.* 2:121–30
3. Anderson, C. S., MacKinnon, R., Smith, C., Miller, C. 1988. Charybdotoxin block of single Ca^{2+}-activated K⁺ channels. *J. Gen. Physiol.* 92:317–33
4. Barthelson, R. A., Jacoby, D. B., Widdicombe, H. J. 1987. Regulation of chloride secretion in dog tracheal epithelium by protein kinase C. *Am. J. Physiol.* 253 (*Cell Physiol.* 22):C802–8
5. Clancy, J. P., Li, M., McCann, J. D., Welsh, M. J. 1989. Calcium regulation of airway epithelial chloride channels. *FASEB J.* 3:A562
6. Eling, T. E., Danilowicz, R. M., Henke, D. C., Sivarajah, D. C., Yankaskas, J. R., et al. 1986. Arachidonic acid metabolism by canine tracheal epithelial cells. Product formation and relationship to chloride secretion. *J. Biol. Chem.* 261:12841–49
7. Frizzell, R. A. 1987. Cystic fibrosis: a disease of ion channels? *Perspect. Dis., Trends Neurosci.* 10(5):190–93
8. Frizzell, R. A., Rechkemmer, G., Shoemaker, R. L. 1986. Altered regulation of airway epithelial cell chloride channels in cystic fibrosis. *Science* 233:558–60
9. Gimenez-Gallego, G., Navia, M. A., Reuben, J. P., Katz, G. M., Kaczorowski, G. J., et al. 1988. Purification, sequence, and model structure of charybdotoxin, a potent selective inhibitor of calcium-activated potassium channels. *Proc. Natl. Acad. Sci. USA* 85:3329–33
10. Hwang, T. C., Lu, L., Zeitlin, P. L., Gruenert, D. C., Huganir, R. C., et al. 1989. Cl⁻ channels in CF: Lack of activation by protein kinase C and cAMP-dependent protein kinase. *Science* 244:1351–53
11. Knowles, M. R., Gatzy, J., Boucher, R. 1983. Relative ion permeability of normal and cystic fibrosis nasal epithelium. *J. Clin. Invest.* 71:1410–17
12. Knowles, M. R., Stutts, J. J., Spock, A., Fischer, N. L., Gatzy, J. T., et al. 1983. Abnormal ion permeation through cystic fibrosis respiratory epithelium. *Science* 221:1067–70
13. Li, M., McCann J. D., Anderson M. A., Clancy J. P., Liedtke, C. M., et al. 1989. Regulation of chloride channels by protein kinase C in normal and cystic fibrosis airway epithelia. *Science* 244:1353–56
14. Li, M., McCann, J. D., Liedtke, C. M. Nairn, A. C., Greengard, P., et al. 1988. Cyclic AMP-dependent protein kinase opens chloride channels in normal but not cystic fibrosis airway epithelium. *Nature* 331:358–60
15. Liedtke, C. M., Tandler, B. 1984. Physiological responsiveness of isolated rab-

bit tracheal epithelial cells. *Am. J. Physiol.* 247 (*Cell Physiol.* 16):C441–49

16. McCann, J. D., Bhalla, R. C., Welsh, M. J. 1989. Release of intracellular calcium by two different second messengers in airway epithelium. *Am. J. Physiol. (Lung Cell Mol. Physiol.)* 257:L116–24

17. McCann, J. D., Li, M., Welsh, M. J. 1989. Identification and regulation of whole-cell chloride currents in airway epithelium. *J. Gen. Physiol.* In press

18. McCann, J. D., Matsuda, J., Garcia, M., Kaczorowski, G., Welsh, M. J. 1989. Basolateral K$^+$ channels in airway epithelia: I Regulation by Ca^{2+} and block by charybdotoxin. *Am. J. Physiol. (Lung Cell. Mol. Physiol.)* In press

18a. McCann, J. D., Welsh, M. J. 1989. Basolateral K$^+$ channels in airway epithelia: II Role in Cl$^-$ secretion and evidence for two types of K$^+$ channel. *Am. J. Physiol. (Lung Cell. Mol. Physiol.)* In press

19. Moczydlowski, E., Lucchesi, K., Ravindran, A. 1988. An emerging pharmacology of peptide toxins targeted against potassium channels. *J. Membr. Biol.* 105:95–111

20. Schoppa, N., Shorofsky, S. R., Jow, F., Nelson, D. J. 1989. Voltage-gated chloride currents in cultured canine tracheal epithelial cells. *J. Membr. Biol.* 108:73–90

21. Schoumacher, R. A., Shoemaker, R. L., Halm, D. R., Tallant, E. A., Wallace, R. W., et al. 1987. Phosphorylation fails to activate chloride channels from cystic fibrosis airway cells. *Nature* 330:752–54

22. Schultz, S. G. 1981. Homocellular regulatory mechanisms in sodium-transporting epithelia: Avoidance of extinction by "flush-through". *Am. J. Physiol.* 241:F579–90

23. Shorofsky, S. R., Field, M., Fozzard, H. A. 1983. Electrophysiology of Cl secretion in canine trachea. *J. Membr. Biol.* 72:105–15

24. Shorofsky, S. R., Field M., Fozzard, H. A. 1984. Mechanism of Cl secretion in canine trachea: Changes in intracellular chloride activity with secretion. *J. Membr. Biol.* 81:1–8

25. Smith, P. L., Frizzell, R. A. 1984. Chloride secretion by canine tracheal epithelium: IV. Basolateral membrane K permeability parallels secretion rate. *J. Membr. Biol.* 77:187–99

26. Smith, P. L., Welsh, M. J., Stoff, J. W., Frizzell, R. A. 1982. Chloride secretion by canine tracheal epithelium.

I. Role of intracellular cAMP levels. *J. Membr. Biol.* 70:217–26

27. Welsh, M. J. 1983. Barium inhibition of basolateral membrane potassium conductance in tracheal epithelium. *Am. J. Physiol.* 244(*Renal Fluid Electrolyte Physiol.* 13):F639–45

28. Welsh, M. J. 1983. Evidence for basolateral membrane potassium conductance in canine tracheal epithelium. *Am. J. Physiol.* 244 (*Cell Physiol.* 13):C377–84

29. Welsh, M. J. 1984. Anthracene-9-carboxylic acid inhibits an apical membrane chloride conductance in canine tracheal epithelium. *J. Membr. Biol.* 78:61–71

30. Welsh, M. J. 1985. Basolateral membrane potassium conductance is independent of sodium pump activity and membrane voltage in canine tracheal epithelium. *J. Membr. Biol.* 84:25–33

31. Welsh, M. J. 1986. Adrenergic regulation of ion transport by primary cultures of canine tracheal epithelium: Cellular electrophysiology. *J. Membr. Biol.* 91:121–28

32. Welsh, M. J. 1986. An apical-membrane chloride channel in human tracheal epithelium. *Science* 232:1648–50

33. Welsh, M. J. 1986. Single apical membrane anion channels in primary cultures of canine tracheal epithelium. *Pflügers Arch.* 407:S116–22

34. Welsh, M. J. 1987. Effect of phorbol ester and calcium ionophore on chloride secretion in canine tracheal epithelium. *Am. J. Physiol.* 253 (*Cell Physiol.* 22):C828–34

35. Welsh, M. J. 1987. Electrolyte transport by airway epithelia. *Physiol. Rev.* 67:1143–84

36. Welsh, M. J., Liedtke, C. M. 1986. Chloride and potassium channels in cystic fibrosis airway epithelia. *Nature* 322:467–70

37. Welsh, M. J., McCann, J. D. 1985. Intracellular calcium regulates basolateral potassium channels in a chloride secreting epithelium. *Proc. Natl. Acad. Sci. USA* 82:8823–26

38. Welsh, M. J., Smith, P. L., Frizzell, R. A. 1982. Chloride secretion by canine tracheal epithelium: II. The cellular electrical potential profile. *J. Membr. Biol.* 70:227–38

39. Welsh, M. J., Smith, P. L., Frizzell, R. A. 1983. Chloride secretion by canine tracheal epithelium: III. Membrane resistances and electromotive forces. *J. Membr. Biol.* 71:209–18

40. Widdicombe, J. H. 1986. Cystic fibrosis and beta-adrenergic response of airway epithelial cell cultures. *Am. J. Physiol.* 251(*Reg. Integr. Comp. Physiol.* 20): R818–22

41. Widdicombe, J. H., Welsh, M. J., Finkbeiner, W. E. 1985. Cystic fibrosis decreases the apical membrane chloride permeability of monolayers cultured from cells of tracheal epithelium. *Proc. Natl. Acad. Sci., USA* 82:6167–71

42. Willumsen, N. J., Boucher, R. C. 1989. Activation of an apical Cl⁻ conductance by Ca²⁺ ionophores in cystic fibrosis airway epithelia. *Am. J. Physiol.* 256 (*Cell Physiol.* 25):C226–33

Annu. Rev. Physiol. 1990. 52:137–55

THE PHYSIOLOGY OF CILIA AND MUCOCILIARY INTERACTIONS

Peter Satir

Department of Anatomy and Structural Biology, Albert Einstein College of Medicine, Bronx, New York

Michael A. Sleigh

Department of Biology, University of Southhampton, United Kingdom

KEY WORDS: respiratory epithelium, mucus, ciliary motility, signal transduction, dynein

INTRODUCTION

Mucociliary transport in the respiratory tract is necessary for health and normal function of the tissue, particularly in resistance to respiratory infection. Transport depends upon the characteristics of the cilia and the thin layers of fluid and mucus that form the interface between the respiratory epithelium and air. Understanding of the basic processes involved in mucociliary clearance requires a clear picture of how cilia generate motion, of how the respiratory epithelium controls and coordinates this motion, and of how the cilia interact with periciliary fluid and with mucus. Recent progress has been made because the cell biology and biophysics of ciliary motility studied with a variety of classic nonmammalian systems has proven applicable to mammalian ciliated epithelial function. Genetic approaches to ciliary function have also been uncovered both in human 'immotile cilia syndrome' (1, 75, 45) and in other systems. Because of the complexity of ciliary structure and composition, mutations in many different pathways can produce immotility or abnormal beat. Although such approaches support and augment the functional conclusions discussed here (cf 64), detailed discussion is beyond the scope of this article. This article will review features of the physiology of cilia and

0066-4278/90/0315-0137$02.00

ciliated tissues derived from basic studies and the application of such approaches to mucociliary transport in the respiratory tract. Pertinent earlier reviews include (59, 64, 87, 70).

STRUCTURE AND FUNCTION OF CILIA

Structure and Biochemistry of the Axoneme

Respiratory cilia are virtually identical in structure and closely related in biochemistry to motile cilia of nonmammalian cells. The cilium is an extension of the free cell surface, whose motor is a tubulin-based axoneme. The axoneme is surrounded by a specialized extension of the cell membrane. Axonemal composition and response are studied directly by removing the membrane via detergent treatment, after severing the axoneme from the cell. Although preparations of tracheal cilia of vertebrates (24) including mammals (16, 44, 26) are available, many of the details reported below relate to nonvertebrate axonemes.

AXONEMAL MICROTUBULES   The nine outer doublet microtubules and two single central pair microtubules of the $9+2$ axoneme are constructed mainly from heterodimers of α and β-tubulin, arranged in protofilaments. The doublet microtubules consist of subfiber A comprised of 13 protofilaments upon which subfiber B (10–11 protofilaments) assembles. The α-tubulin is acetylated as is true for many long-lived stable microtubules. Some portion of the doublet, probably the midwall common to both subfibers, is composed of tektin, an intermediate-filament-like protein that resists detergent extraction (cf 89).

In mammalian cells, assembly of the axoneme occurs in a fixed pattern at the cell surface above basal bodies (15). The basal body or centriole is also an organizational site for cytoplasmic microtubules. Although the same pool of tubulin may be used, axonemal assembly is fundamentally different from assembly of cytoplasmic microtubules in two related respects: (a) assembly occurs directly on the basal body microtubules, (b) complex doublets—rather than single tubes—are eventually polymerized. Like other microtubules, axonemal doublets are polarized such that the fast polymerizing (+) end is most distal to the basal body, which corresponds to the tip of the axoneme. Doublet stability probably relies on multiple interactions with other axonemal proteins, of which there are several hundred in two-dimensional gels (34); doublet length is probably controlled or at least influenced by capping structures (13) and by specific membrane interactions. Most axonemes of mammalian respiratory cells grow to about 5–10 μm in length; human respiratory cilia are about 6 μm. Length is under genetic control. Indeed, if too long, the axoneme is less effective in mucociliary transport (2) (see below). At the tip, the doublets simplify and only subfiber A is seen. In mammalian cilia, all nine subfiber As insert into a disc that usually forms the cytoplasmic surface of a transmembrane complex—the ciliary crown.

Near its base, the axoneme is also connected to a special transmembrane complex, the ciliary necklace. Just above the necklace region, there is a zone where Ca^{2+} shock produces severing of the axoneme, possibly by activating a calcium contractile protein localized to this region.

DYNEIN STRUCTURE AND MECHANOCHEMISTRY   Dynein structure and mechanochemistry are reviewed by Warner et al (90). Ciliary dynein is a two- or three-headed bouquet-like molecule of molecular weight 1–2 million daltons (31). Each head contains a heavy chain ATPase of 4–500 kd. The molecule also contains polypeptides of lower molecular weight (intermediate and light chains). Dynein isolated from tracheal cilia is two-headed (27) and resembles sea urchin flagellar dynein. Dynein extracted from bovine or porcine tracheal cilia sediments at 18–19S and at 12S (26, 44), and appears comparable in polypeptide composition to nonmammalian dynein.

As assembled on the axonemal microtubules, the dynein molecule is compacted into an arm. Although there is controversy regarding the exact in situ appearance of the arms, a model consistent with most of the structural evidence has been constructed (5, 63). Each arm projects across the interdoublet gap and is attached, more or less permanently after assembly, to subfiber A of one microtubule (conventionally, N) with at least one head projecting toward and capable of attaching to subfiber B of the next doublet (N+1).

Dynein is a (−) end microtubule motor; that is, it moves the structure to which it is attached in an ATP-insensitive manner (e.g. subfiber A of doublet N) toward the base of the axoneme. By Newton's third law, the microtubule along which the dynein walks by its ATP-sensitive heads (e.g. subfiber B of doublet N+1) moves in a (+) direction toward the tip of the axoneme. Microtubule movement generated by dynein has been studied in sliding axonemes (77, 53, 78, 18) or completely in vitro by using isolated dynein attached to glass and taxol-stabilized microtubules (81, 46). A single-head fragment of dynein is sufficient to give motility (51, 82). Although the polarity of force generation by mammalian ciliary dynein is still undetermined, cytoplasmic dynein from mammalian epithelial or nerve cells (47, 89) translocates vesicles and microtubules with the usual polarity.

PERIODIC LINKS   Two types of linkages integrate the individual microtubules into a functioning axoneme: radial and circumferential. The radial spokes connect the doublet microtubules to the central pair complex. They are a self-assembling, multipolypeptide structure (34) consisting of a cylindrical stalk and an expanded spoke head. They usually occur in groups of three (37) (S1–S3) along subfiber A with a 96 nm period and spacings of S1–S2 of 32 nm; S2–S3, 24 nm; S3–S1, 40 nm. Their function is incompletely understood, but they probably act to limit microtubule sliding of active doublets by converting such sliding into bending; they may help to maintain proper spacing of the doublets. They may also be involved in the activation or inhibition of dynein arm cycling on a specific doublet. Mutants of motile cilia whose spoke assembly is defective are paralyzed, and their axonemal arrays may collapse (74), but restoration of motility does not require restoration of spoke activity (30).

The circumferential linkages connect adjacent doublets. One type of interdoublet link persists after near total extraction of dynein arms by high salt (88, 21). These links are paired, one pair per spoke group. They lie near the base of the inner arm and are relatively inextensible, probably breaking and reforming as the doublets move past one another. In the absence of dynein, they are sufficient to hold the axoneme together. There may be more than one type of circumferential link.

THREE-DIMENSIONAL RECONSTRUCTION OF THE AXONEME   A major activity of the past decade has been reconstruction of the axoneme in three-dimensions at resolution better than 10 nm. Data for such reconstruction have been derived from negative stain electron micrographs (3, 6, 5), thin section images (63), freeze-etch replicas (21), and provisionally from frozen, hydrated specimens (40). Reconstructions differ somewhat depending on the technique used to generate the data. Computer modeling provides for consistency of structure from different perspectives and rapid comparison of models. Tomographic reconstruction is also useful (37). For most of its length, axonemal structure is repetitive; only the tip and base vary significantly. The basic repeat of 96 nm contains four outer arms per doublet, four (63), or possibly three (21, 52), inner arms per doublet, one spoke group, six central sheath projections, and one pair of nonelastic interdoublet links per doublet. This can be considered the unit of motile activity of the axoneme.

The Axonemal Basis of Motility

CURRENT STATUS OF THE SLIDING MICROTUBULE MODEL   It is firmly established that axonemal motility is based on microtubule sliding as a consequence of the mechanochemistry of the dynein arms (65, 31, 90, 10). In vitro sliding of microtubules in isolated, partially digested axonemes (77) has been demonstrated directly for vertebrate sperm (93) and for mammalian tracheal and oviduct cilia (16). Dentler & LeCluyse (14) have reinvestigated the geometrical consequences of sliding for mammalian tracheal cilia, whose tip structure differs from that of invertebrate cilia. Axonemes are reactivated with ATP and bends vs tip configuration studied, using the equation of Satir (60). The results indicate that the relationship of sliding to bending may be more complex for tracheal cilia, where the subfiber As of all nine doublets end in a cap, than for invertebrate cilia. Bend formation may require the generation of compensating bends and axonemal twisting as a consequence of sliding.

THE SWITCH POINT HYPOTHESIS   Since the axoneme is a cylinder, and all dynein arms produce sliding with a single polarity, in order to produce motion, some asynchrony of arm activity must be present. A simple hypothesis—the switch point hypothesis—assumes that half of the doublets of the axoneme have active arms when the axoneme is moving in its effective stroke and that the other half has active arms during the return stroke (62). Activity then switches from one set of arms to another during a ciliary beat and back again at the beginning of the next beat. With slight modifications, this model can be used to correlate specific doublet activity with ciliary beat form. The model has some important features.

Translocation rates imply a non-cycling state of the dynein arm   Translocation rates of microtubules on dynein in vitro or in sliding assays after protease digestion in the axoneme are comparable to sliding rates for microtubules in the intact axoneme i. e. $\simeq 10$ μm/sec (78, 46). However, maximum displacement of a doublet by sliding in the intact axoneme is only $\simeq 0.1$–0.4 μm per half beat (61). According to the switch point hypothesis, in an axoneme beating at a frequency of 50 Hz, arms on doublet N in the active half of the axoneme would switch off after 10 msec and would become non-cycling and refractory for $\simeq 10$ msec before resuming activity. During this refractory period, the doublet would move passively in the opposite direction. This implies that the dynein arm exists in two states: cycling and non-cycling. Spungin et al (71) have produced negative stain images with two differently appearing arm distributions, one which may correspond to cycling arms and one to the non-cycling state. In preliminary reports, R. D. Vale & colleagues (personal communication) note that in vitro translocation by axonemal dyneins is discontinuous with periods of apparent inactivity and consequently, reversed movement of the microtubules being propelled.

Two switches   There are at least two different axonemal switches. One of these turns the arms of one set of doublets on and off, the other turns the complementary set on and off. When one switch is blocked, the cilia will come to rest in one specific position, no matter where in the beat cycle the block is applied (49). Blocking the second switch will lead to ciliary arrest in a second position. In mussel gill cilia (86) one arrest position is near the beginning of the effective stroke and the second is near the beginning of the recovery stroke, and the two positions have been labeled 'hands up' and 'hands down' respectively. If the blocking agent is changed, cilia can be moved from one arrest position to another without restarting beat (49).

Radial spoke function   The switch point hypothesis provides a rationale for the importance of the radial spokes and central complex of 9+2 axonemes. The opposite acting halves of the axoneme are determined by those doublets whose spokes interact with one central microtubule (cm) and its projections and not the other. These correspond to doublets 1–4 that interact with cm 3 to move the axoneme to the hands up position (62) and doublets 6–9 that interact with cm 8 to move the axoneme to the hands down position. Presumably, coordinated spoke-central sheath attachment in the active half of the axoneme is used to regulate sliding and convert sliding into bending. In axonemes where mutations in spoke or central sheath proteins produce immotility, the sliding system is intact and operational. Dynein arm activity along a doublet is regulated in a redundant manner, so that the spoke-central sheath signal can be bypassed by appropriate modifications in other controls. In metazoan cilia, the position of the central pair seems fixed (80, 18) but in protistan axonemes, the central pair may rotate (42) either as a causal factor in switching of arm activity in the axoneme, or as a consequence of such switching.

Timing and comparative physiology   Although ciliary structure, biochemistry, and mechanism of motility have been conserved during animal evolution, cilia from different organisms or cilia and sperm tails from the same organism have quite disparate beat phenotypes. Moreover, ciliary beat is under cellular control. For example, respiratory ciliary beat frequency can be slowed down (79) or speeded up (57). Other cilia—especially of swimming cells—can drastically change their beat form so that the cell swims backwards (cf 33) or turns toward a chemotatic stimulus (9). These changes are readily explained by the switch point hypothesis if the timing of the switches controls beat form of the axoneme. Where dynein arms are actively sliding for equal times in the two half-axonemes (while the opposite half is inactive), the bends generated would be symmetrical; where timing was unequal, the principal bend would correspond to the longer on time, the reverse bend to the shorter, since:

$$\Delta\, l_p = k_1\, \alpha_p \simeq k_2 t_p \qquad \text{and} \qquad\qquad 1.$$

$$\Delta\, l_r = k_1\, \alpha_r \simeq k_2 t_r \qquad \text{where} \qquad\qquad 2.$$

$\Delta\, l_{p,r}$ is the amount of sliding of a given doublet during the principal or reverse bend, respectively, which is proportional to $t_{p,r}$, the on time of dynein arm activity of that doublet, and to $\alpha_{p,r}$, the amount of bend generated (60, 61).

Evidence for asynchronous doublet activity has been summarized by Satir (62). One important finding is that reactivation of hamster sperm flagella by local application of ATP generates a predictable pattern of bending, depending on initial position and consistent with activation of doublets 1–4 or 6–9 (95). Sliding restricted to specific subsets of doublets has been seen directly in ctenophore macrocilia (80). In some cases doublets 9, 1, 2 were consistently extruded after reactivation of these axonemes; in others 5–7 were extruded. Identical patterns have recently been shown in mussel gill axonemes (36); the former pattern occurs when ATP reactivates tethered protease-treated hands down cilia, while the latter occurs in hands up cilia. Sale (50) has also shown that in sea urchin axonemes arrested in a specific position, ATP addition permits one subset of doublets, probably 5–7, to slide away from the remainder of the axoneme. These consistent observations in diverse ciliated cells support the universality of the switch point mechanism.

Qualifications and remaining problems   Several modifications of the switch point hypothesis may be necessary to fit actual beat form. In particular, (*a*) all arms along a particular doublet may not activate synchronously, but rather in progression with bend propagation, and (*b*) the arms on all doublets within a half axoneme may not activate simultaneously, but rather with a defined phase relationship. In this way, one could envision nine separate activation events rather than two. This might be particularly useful in explaining helical beat in certain sperm tails. Some experimental evidence suggesting that these modifications may be necessary has been provided by Sugino & Machemer (76). Another qualification is that axonemal bending may sometimes arise by mechanisms different from axonemal sliding or at least the sliding that is necessary for cyclic bending (17).

The switch point hypothesis does not specify the manner of bend propagation during beat, yet major studies indicate that there are extensive feedback systems in the axoneme relating bend generation and bend propagation (19, 11, cf also 66), and propagation must be understood as part of the description of the axonemal mechanism. Furthermore, the nature of the intrinsic oscillator of arm activity that underlies the switching is unspecified so that it is unclear whether the intrinsic switching of this oscillator is mechanically as well as biochemically controlled. Curvature control models, where physical forces regulate arm activity, are successful to a point, particularly in explaining wave propagation along sperm tails (11). There are very limited possibilities of biochemical controls of arm activity because of time constraints, and also because the controls must be fully operative in the presence of only ATP and simple ionic buffers without other non-axonemal constitutents. One possibility is that the non-cycling state of the arm is intrinsically part of each mechanochemical event. The length of this non-cycling state might be influenced by ATP concentration alone or by phosphorylation of some specific dynein constituents, much as the 'latch state' of smooth muscle is influenced by phosphorylation of myosin. Changes in the phosphorylation state could easily be supposed to influence the intrinsic arm cycle in various ways (62).

MECHANISMS OF PROPULSION BY CILIA

Water Transport and Hydrodynamic Considerations

The propulsion of water by cilia is a low Reynolds number phenomenon, where viscous forces are more important than inertial forces. Reynolds number (Re) for a cilium can be defined by:

$$\text{Re} = \frac{\text{fluid density}}{\text{fluid viscosity}} \times \omega L r \qquad \qquad 3.$$

where ω = angular frequency, L = ciliary length, and r = ciliary radius. Re for a cilium is low because the linear dimensions of cilia are so small. A capture zone of water is dragged along around the cilium as it moves, and in the absence of any appreciable inertial effects, the motion of the water stops as soon as the cilium stops moving. This is evolutionarily significant, since it permits rapid behavioral responses of ciliated cells by switching off ciliary motility. The propulsive effect of the cilium on the water is about twice as high when the motion of the cilium is perpendicular to its long axis as when its motion is parallel to the long axis (cf 29) and, the faster the cilium moves, the faster the water in the capture zone moves. The water tends to adhere to the cell membrane, at the scale of size of the cilium, opposing the tendency of the moving cilium to propel the fluid; the extent of the fluid zone carried around the cilium is limited near the base and increases towards the ciliary tip; the radius of the capture zone at any point along the cilium is approximately half the height of that point above the cell surface (7). During a typical beat cycle, the cilium moves through a large angle in an effective stroke, moving fairly quickly and perpendicular to its long axis, but it moves more slowly along its axis in an unrolling motion close to the cell surface in the recovery stroke. A net movement of water occurs because a larger volume of water is moved to one side in the effective stroke and a smaller volume is carried back in the recovery stroke; indeed, the volume of water carried in the recovery stroke is reduced further because the cilium tends to bend low to one side or the other, close to the cell surface, in this stroke. In the absence of inertial forces, it is easier to think of water being scooped across the cell surface by a ciliary power stroke than being swept along, as if by an oar.

The rate of propulsion of water by a cilium, therefore, depends on ciliary length and beat frequency. The force generated by a cilium is related to the number of active dynein arms and to ciliary length, but stiffness depends upon passive mechanical properties such as the Young modulus of the axoneme, as well as on active dynein arm attachment (29). Efficiency in transmitting force to the surrounding water during the effective stroke will be lost if the cilium is not stiff enough to remain reasonably straight. Such loss can be reduced by cooperation between adjacent cilia, which either stand so close together that they form compound structures or beat in close coordination in metachronal waves where each cilium provides some mutual assistance to the motion of neighboring cilia.

The formation of metachronal waves is usually important in water propulsion. Adjacent cilia experience forces of viscous interaction if their zones of captured water overlap one another as they move. The strength of this viscous-mechanical interaction between cilia depends on their positions relative to the beat direction and their separation relative to their length (69). Interactions between adjacent cilia in the plane of the effective stroke tend to result in synchrony of beating, whereas interactions perpendicular to this plane produce metachrony, with metachronal waves moving in the direction towards which the cilium swings sideways in the recovery stroke. It must be emphasized that metachronism is a property of hydrodynamic coupling between closely packed, relatively synchronously beating axonemes, and it can be reconstituted in single cells (33) or on respiratory epithelial cells (91) after detergent treatment when membraneless axonemes are reactivated by Mg^{2+}-ATP.

The importance of metachronism to water propulsion is that at any instant there are adjacent cilia involved in different stages of their effective stroke; each cilium does not accelerate water from rest during its effective stroke, but adds impetus to water already being moved by adjacent cilia. A continuous flow can therefore be maintained at a level (near 1 mm s^{-1}), which approaches the ciliary tip speed, and the lack of inertial momentum is overcome by use of continuously overlapping viscous paddles. In most ciliary systems specialized for water propulsion, the cilia form narrow bands perpendicular to the water flow. Because the propulsion of water by a cilium is only a local viscous phenomenon, only a shallow zone of water some two cilium lengths deep is transported across the ciliated surface (7); the total volume transported is therefore small, unless the surface is extensive, with many ciliary tracts in parallel. The overall propulsive effect depends upon the arrangement of the cilia, their metachronal relationships and pattern of beating, as well as on ciliary length and beat frequency.

Mucus Transport

Mucus is a non-Newtonian, viscoelastic fluid. It is secreted in concentrated form and rapidly hydrates to a remarkable extent (83), and then only very slowly disperses in water (38). When mucus is secreted onto a ciliated epithelium and hydrates, it spreads as droplets or strings that may coalesce into larger rafts or sheets that are carried along by the cilia at the level of the ciliary tips above a layer of periciliary fluid (cf 39, 58). The ciliary tips penetrate the mucus during their effective stroke, but move beneath it in their recovery stroke. The cilia experience a strong resistance to movement at their extreme tips when they penetrate a mucous layer, and because of their limited stiffness they can only provide effective propulsion of the mucus if they are very short (usually 5–7 μm). The length of mucus-propelling cilia is a compromise between the need to shorten the cilium to minimize backward bending when the cilium meets mucus at its tip and the need to lengthen the cilium both to maximize tip speed at a reasonable beat frequency and to maximize the difference in height between power and recovery strokes (68). Because the cilia are short, the tip speed achievable at the common beat frequencies of 12–20 Hz is modest, at around 600–1000 μm s^{-1} in the absence of mucus. While the effective stroke propels the overlying mucus forward, the underlying periciliary fluid merely oscillates to and fro during the beat cycle. Metachronal coordination of the cilia maintains a continuous forward thrust on the mucus, and the presence of several or many metachronal waves under a raft of mucus spreads the propulsive effect so that the whole raft moves as a unit.

Movement and Coordination of Respiratory Tract Cilia

Between beat cycles, respiratory tract cilia normally rest in the hands down position (58, 35). The beat cycle therefore begins with a recovery stroke. Bending begins at the cilium base and propagates up the shaft. At the same time the cilium is drawn backwards and sideways in a clockwise sweep (as seen from above), moving through 180° until it is inclined in the opposite direction from its starting position. From here it performs an effective stroke, in a plane perpendicular to the cell surface that brings it back to the rest position.

The cilia are packed closely together on mucus-propelling epithelia, and in spite of their short length, the cilia interact with their neighbors as they beat. This interaction results in metachronal coordination, as in water propelling cilia but, because the beat cycle has a rest phase and commences with a recovery stroke, the form of metachronism is a little different. As a cilium commences its recovery stroke and moves backwards and sideways, it presses against other cilia at that side and excites them to commence their recovery stroke (58); these then excite others, and so on. This recruitment of cilia into a coordinated wave proceeds, and the wave moves across a few ciliated cells before it dies away (58, 35), presumably because of a break in the ciliated surface (at a cell boundary, perhaps) sufficient to disrupt transmission of excitation to commence a recovery stroke. If cilia are beating at low frequencies the waves tend to cover a small area and propagate across only 2 or 3 cells, but cilia that beat more vigorously form longer metachronal waves that propagate for longer distances. Because the ciliary beat is not as regularly rhythmic, and the cilia do not have such tightly coupled coordination, the metachronal waves of mucus-propelling cilia are less conspicuous than those of water propelling cilia. The metachronal waves on respiratory epithelia do not sweep across the surface in long lines, but appear as numerous transient islands in a sea of quiescent resting cilia (58).

Mucociliary Transport

Mucus propulsion rates seldom exceed 200 μm s^{-1}, but this speed is relatively independent of the load, apparently because of the recruitment of additional cilia into the propulsive parts of metachronal waves when necessary. This can happen automatically because when cilia in their stroke encounter increased resistance from the mucus and slow down, the cilia following behind will catch them up and add their propulsive force to the effort exerted by the wave until the mucus is pressed forward. In fact, once the mucus is moving, it will be kept in motion by the simultaneous action of numerous cilia, with rather larger numbers of cilia active at any instant if the load is higher. Any cilium whose power stroke is prolonged by reduced speed of swing may show a shortened rest phase in compensation.

Mucus is an incipient gel composed principally of a macromolecular meshwork of glycoprotein molecules in a watery fluid (38, 39, 12). This composition permits it to show slow distortion by viscous flow over a time scale of the order of many seconds, but to act as a relatively solid elastic structure at the size and time scales of the propulsive swing of a cilium (20, 67). Thus, while a cilium penetrates and pushes forward a section of a mucus sheet, energy is stored elastically in the mucus, and the mucus will recoil slowly, if allowed to, unless other cilia propel it further forward; normally the latter occurs and sustained forces are transmitted laterally to regions of the mucus sheet that are not directly propelled.

During propulsion, with mucus moving at about 200 μm s^{-1}, a cilium commencing its effective stroke will swing upwards with a tip speed faster than the mucus flow, the tip will penetrate the mucus, engage in the elastic gel and be slowed down somewhat so it transmits force to the mucus. As the stroke continues, the ciliary tip moves downwards once more towards the cell surface and its speed falls below that of the mucus, so that the mucus is pulled away from the ciliary tip (70). During the ensuing rest phase the cilia are bent low, with tips pointing in the direction of mucus flow; they do not interfere with forward flow of the mucus, but could provide roughness restricting reverse flow. The cilia complete their recovery stroke beneath the mucus. Not only is the effective stroke well matched to mucus propulsion, but other features of the beat cycle are also well adapted for this function.

When mucus is present, it can only be transported if the depth of the periciliary layer is within certain limits. If the periciliary layer is too deep, the cilia will not penetrate the mucus and will be ineffective in mucus propulsion; normally, however, the cilia will propel away surplus periciliary fluid beneath the mucus and bring mucus within the reach of cilia to recommence propulsion. If the periciliary layer becomes too shallow, the cilia will be prevented from completing their beat and mucus propulsion will stop; in this case it is assumed that additional fluid will be released from the epithelium as part of the regulation of fluid flux achieved by chloride secretion and sodium absorption (41, 92). In the absence of mucus the depth of the layer of periciliary fluid is thought to be maintained by capillary action between the shafts of the close set cilia (39).

Cilia on the frog palate cease activity if unstimulated, and mucus secretion stops, but if a particle is dropped onto the ciliated surface, it becomes surrounded by mucus, the cilia are stimulated to beat in its vicinity, and the patch of mucus gets carried away along a strip of epithelium that is stimulated by its presence (72). Stimulation with a wire probe also induces ciliary beating. In mammals, some cilia on unstimulated epithelia appear to continue to beat, albeit slowly, even in the absence of mucus, but can be stimulated to beat more rapidly by mechanical stimulation (55). Because of the recruitment mechanism of the respiratory tract cilia (see above), local mechanical stimulation of a few cilia, physiologically related to the presence of mucus, will initiate coordinated mucociliary transport. In addition to a local activation of beating in response to mechanical stimulation, a more general activation of the cilia may be promoted by nervous or hormonal mechanisms.

CILIATED EPITHELIAL CELLS AND THE MECHANISM OF CILIARY RESPONSE

Ciliated Cell Organization in Relation to Ciliary Function

In discussing ciliary activity of the respiratory tract, it is instructive to consider the organization of the apical cell surface of a ciliated epithelial cell in detail. The organization is conservative, possibly because it is useful in influencing cytoskeletal orientation throughout the cytoplasm for vesicular trafficking (cf 89). In the primitive condition, a single motile cilium is surrounded by a ring of microvilli, but epithelial cells, where transport efficiency of water or mucus seems important, are often multiciliated. Multiciliarity requires an unusual form of organellogenesis (15).

The pattern of organization of the apical surface has been carefully studied in an invertebrate epithelium (48), and a similar organization is found in tracheal epithelium (25, 4, 22). On a single, fully differentiated, 5–10 μm long cell, up to about 200 cilia are arranged in a hexagonally-packed semi-crystalline array, where each cilium is surrounding by six shorter (ca 1–3 μm long) microvilli. The microvilli form at the vertices of a grid of microtubules and actin-based microfilaments that form two trabeculae that underlie the apical cell surface and are integrated into an actin-containing contractile belt, the belt desmosome, at the lateral cell surface. Fodrin has been identified in the web of filaments between basal bodies (32); intermediate filaments are also components of this area. Each basal body is also underpinned by striated rootlets. All these interconnections lead to a mechanically integrated cell cortex where contractile and elastic elements act to resist distortions at the basal end of the beating cilia (28). The epithelial cells are in mechanical communication with other cell types and with one another at their actin-containing belt and in ionic contact via gap junctions (49, 54). In cell cultures of respiratory epithelium, both ciliated and nonciliated cells are electrically coupled, so that changes in ion concentrations or small messenger molecules in one cell spread through the epithelium for short distances (54).

Mechanism of the Mechanosensitive Response

The ciliated cells of the respiratory tract epithelium are mechanosensitive. When the cell surfaces or cilia of cultured ciliated epithelial cells from rabbit trachea are stimulated with a small glass microneedle, beat frequency increases by 20% or more in a transitory manner (55). The ciliary responses are lost if extracellular Ca^{2+} is removed and restored when Ca^{2+} is replaced. Further, beat frequency is increased if the Ca^{2+}-ionophore A23187 is added under similar circumstances (57). After ionophore stimulation, mechanical stimulation results in little or no additional increase in beat frequency. Thus ionophore stimulation and mechanical stimulation are thought to work by an identical mechanism, namely an increase in cytoplasmic Ca^{2+} concentration, caused by Ca^{2+} entering the cell from the exterior. Mechanical stimulation, which physiologically is initiated by the presence of mucus (72), probably permits extracellular Ca^{2+} to enter via cell membrane channels. The Ca^{2+} channel blocker verapamil, albeit at high concentration, added in the presence of external Ca^{2+} inhibits the response to microneedle stimulation. An increase in Ca^{2+} concentration in the cytoplasm can be visualized if the epithelium has previously been loaded with dyes, such as fura-2 (56). The spread of increase in Ca^{2+} from the point of stimulation to adjacent cells can also be directly visualized.

In ciliated unicellular organisms and invertebrates, mechanosensitive cell membrane channels induce depolarization to which voltage-gated Ca^{2+} channels in the ciliary membrane itself respond, by opening to permit Ca^{2+} entry around the axoneme. The time course of this response is rapid compared to that of the response of respiratory cell cilia (55), and it may be that voltage-gated ciliary Ca^{2+} channels are absent or reduced in number in the respiratory tract ciliary membranes. Then, mechanical stimulation might let Ca^{2+} only into the cell body proper, so that the increase in concentration around the axonemes would be slow. Ca^{2+} apparently acts directly on the axoneme, as can be demonstrated with permeabilized cells of respiratory tract epithelia (85) as well as with similar preparations of invertebrate or protistan cilia (33).

The mechanism of Ca^{2+} interaction within the axoneme is probably mediated by calmodulin (CaM) that acts as an axonemal Ca^{2+} sensor. Some CaM is firmly bound to the axoneme, and the addition of CaM antagonists reverses Ca^{2+} responses in permeabilized cells (62, 43, 85). In relation to the switch point hypothesis discussed above, formation of Ca^{2+}-CaM complexes could activate appropriate kinases or phosphatases that might affect the timing of arm activity.

Mechanisms of Hormonally Based Responses

Ciliary beat frequency is increased in human and other species upon application of some neurotransmitters and certain adrenergic or cholinergic drugs (cf 57, 94). In particular, β-adrenergic compounds, such as isoproterenol, increase beat frequency of mammalian respiratory cilia in vivo and in vitro. The effect probably occurs through β-adrenergic receptors, since propranolol, a β-antagonist, blocks the response (84). Although β-adrenergic drugs will stimulate an increase in beat frequency when applied to either the ciliated surface or the basal (serosal) surface of the tissue, stimulation is primarily at the latter (94). Cholinergic drugs, however, may stimulate the ciliated surface slightly more effectively. β-adrenergic receptors act via a signal transduction pathway involving G proteins that activate adenylate cyclase to raise intracellular cAMP. Presumably, serotonin increases the beat frequency of invertebrate cilia by comparable mechanisms (73).

cAMP like Ca^{2+} probably acts directly on the axonemes (62, 73). For example, cAMP applied directly to ATP-reactivated permeabilized paramecia causes the cells to swim faster (8). The effect is most likely achieved through phosphorylation of specific axonemal polypeptides, mediated by cAMP-dependent kinases built into the axonemal structure. Hamasaki et al (23) have recently identified a 29-kd polypeptide in paramecium axonemes that responds appropriately to increases in cAMP around the reactivated permeabilized cells. This polypeptide is extracted by procedures that extract dynein arms and might be a regulatory dynein light chain. This result has not yet been demonstrated in other species.

Tamaoki et al (79) have shown that in cultured rabbit tracheal epithelium, ciliary beat frequency is suppressed by adenosine and related substances. A high affinity receptor for adenosine, the A_1 receptor, inhibits adenylate cyclase activity in tissues. In the presence of adenosine, the intracellular cAMP of the respiratory epithelium is decreased; the decreases in beat frequency and cAMP are reversed by 8-phenyltheophylline, an adenosine receptor antagonist. Adenosine-modulated ciliary inhibition may be regulated by uptake or catabolism of adenosine.

Integration of Stimuli

The normal quiescence of most respiratory cilia at the end of the effective stroke may be due to the fall of intracellular cAMP below a critical level, which temporarily reduces phosphorylation of a critical axonemal polypeptide such that one of the axonemal switches (discussed above) is temporarily inhibited. Mechanical stimulation at the apical surface of the cell by mucus impinging on the cilia would elevate cytoplasmic and axonemal Ca^{2+} and overcome the block, thus leading to beat in quiescent cilia and increasing beat frequency in beating cilia. This local response would have a limited spread from cell to cell and would be dependent on mucus load (57). Alternatively, hormonal or neurotransmitter-based stimulation, mainly at the basal side of the epithelium, would result in an increase in intracellular cAMP. This would lead to a more global response, a generally increased number of beating cilia throughout the epithelium, independent of mucus load and local factors. Sanderson & Dirksen (57) have demonstrated that the beat frequency response of tracheal cilia to isoproterenol and mechanical stimulation are additive. This suggests that there is dual control (57) where Ca^{2+} and cAMP influence the axoneme via independent pathways—that is, Ca^{2+}-CaM does not primarily activate an adenylate cyclase, and cAMP does not work, for example, by releasing intracellular stores of Ca^{2+}. It seems likely that, as in other organisms, both agents will work directly on axonemal polypeptides, probably via changes in their phosphorylation patterns.

In a beating cilium, the switch point hypothesis suggests that during each beat every arm is temporarily converted to a non-cycling state and that this occurs asynchronously in opposite half axonemes. A simple, although not unique, explanation of dual control consistent with the switch point hypothesis may be that cAMP-dependent changes in phosphorylation of axonemal components or of dynein regulatory light chains control the rate of progression from non-cycling to cycling state of the dynein arm, while Ca^{2+}-CaM dependent changes in phosphorylation control the reverse step, namely the conversion of cycling to non-cycling state. In respiratory cilia, increases in either messenger would work to increase the appropriate rate constant and to increase beat frequency; in other cilia, this may not necessarily be the case, even though the axonemal locus of action might be identical. If changes in phosphorylation of axonemal components are a key to our deeper understanding of the control of ciliary movement and to further exploration of this or similar hypotheses, we need to know more specifically which polypeptides change phosphorylation levels under conditions where ciliary behavior is clearly understood in respiratory cilia and in a variety of model systems.

ACKNOWLEDGMENT

A portion of this work was supported by a grant from the United States Public Health Service (HL22560). We thank M. Ann Holland for help with the manuscript.

Literature Cited

1. Afzelius, B. A. 1979. The immotile-cilia syndrome and other ciliary diseases. *Int. Rev. Exp. Pathol.* 19:1–43
2. Afzelius, B. A., Gargani, G., Romano, C. 1985. Abnormal length of cilia as a possible cause of defective mucociliary clearance. *Eur. J. Respir. Dis.* 66:173–80
3. Amos, L. A., Linck, R. W., Klug, A. 1976. Molecular structure of flagellar microtubules. In *Cell Motility*. ed. R. Goldman, T. Pollard, J. L. Rosenbaum, pp. 847–67. New York: Cold Spring Harbor Lab.
4. Arima, T., Shibata, Y., Yamamoto, T. 1985. Three dimensional visualization of basal body structure and some cytoskeletal components in the apical zone of tracheal ciliated cells. *J. Ultrastruct. Res.* 93:61–70
5. Avolio, J., Glazzard, A. N., Holwill, M. E. J., Satir, P. 1986. Structures attached to doublet microtubules of cilia: computer modeling of thin section and negative stained stereo images. *Proc. Natl. Acad. Sci. USA* 83:4804–8
6. Avolio, J., Lebduska, S., Satir, P. 1984. Dynein arm substructure and the orientation of arm-microtubule attachments. *J. Mol. Biol.* 173:389–401
7. Blake, J. R., Sleigh, M. A. 1974. Mechanics of ciliary locomotion. *Biol. Rev.* 49:85–125
8. Bonini, N. M., Nelson, D. L. 1988. Differential regulation of Paramecium ciliary motility by cAMP and cGMP. *J. Cell Biol.* 106:1615–23
9. Brokaw, C. J. 1979. Calcium induced asymmetrical beating of Triton-demembranated sea urchin sperm flagella. *J. Cell Biol.* 82:401–11
10. Brokaw, C. J. 1989. Direct measurements of sliding between outer doublet microtubules in swimming sperm flagella. *Science* 243:1593–96
11. Brokaw, C. J. 1989. Operational regulation of the flagellar oscillator. See Ref. 90, pp. 267–79
12. Carlstedt, I., Sheehan, J. K. 1984. Macromolecular properties and polymeric structure of mucus glycoproteins. Ciba Foundation Symp. 109:157–72
13. Dentler, W. L. 1981. Microtubule-membrane interactions in cilia and flagella. *Int. Rev. Cytol.* 72:1–47
14. Dentler, W. L., LeCluyse, E. L. 1982. Microtubule capping structures at the tips of tracheal cilia: Evidence for their firm attachment during ciliary bend formation and the restriction of microtubule sliding. *Cell Motil.* 2:549–72
15. Dirksen, E. R. 1982. Ciliary basal body morphogenesis: the early events. *Soc. Exp. Biol. Symp.* 35:439–63
16. Dirksen, E. R., Zeira, M. 1981. Microtubule sliding in cilia of the rabbit trachea and oviduct. *Cell Motil.* 1:247–60
17. Eshel, D., Brokaw, C. J. 1987. New evidence for a "biased baseline" mechanism for calcium-regulated asymmetry of flagellar bending. *Cell Motil. Cytoskel.* 7:160–68
18. Fox, L. A., Sale, W. S. 1987. Direction of force generated by the inner row of dynein arms on flagellar microtubules. *J. Cell Biol.* 105:1781–87
19. Gibbons, I. R. 1982. Sliding and bending in sea urchin sperm flagella. *Soc. Exp. Biol. Symp.* 35:225–87
20. Gilboa, A., Silberberg, A. 1976. *In situ* rheological characterization of epithelial mucus. *Biorheology* 13:59–65
21. Goodenough, U. W., Heuser, J. E. 1989. Structure of the soluble and in situ ciliary dyneins visualized by quick-freeze deep etch microscopy. See Ref. 90, pp. 121–40
22. Gordon, R. E. 1982. Three dimensional organization of microtubules and microfilaments of the basal body apparatus of

ciliated respiratory epithelium. *Cell Motil.* 4:385–91

23. Hamasaki, T., Murtaugh, T., Satir, B. H., Satir, P. 1989. *In vitro* phosphorylation of paramecium axonemes and permeabilized cells. *Cell Motil. Cytoskel.* 12:1–11

24. Hard, R., Cypher, C., Schabtach, E. 1988. Isolation and reactivation of highly coupled newt lung cilia. *Cell Motil. Cytoskel.* 10:271–84

25. Hard, R., Reider, C. 1983. Microciliary transport in newt lungs. The ultrastructure of the ciliary apparatus in isolated epithelial sheets and in functional Triton-extracted models. *Tissue Cell* 15:227–43

26. Hastie, A. T., Dicker, D. T., Hingley, S. T., Kueppers, F., Higgins, M. L., Weinbaum, G. 1986. Isolation of cilia from porcine tracheal epithelium and extraction of dynein arms. *Cell Motil. Cytoskel.* 6:25–34

27. Hastie, A. T., Marchese-Ragona, S. P., Johnson, K. A., Wall, J. S. 1988. Structure and mass of mammalian respiratory ciliary outer arm 19S dynein. *Cell Motil. Cytoskel.* 11:157–66

28. Holley, M. C. 1984. The ciliary basal apparatus is adapted to the structure and mechanics of the epithelium. *Tissue Cell* 16:287–310

29. Holwill, M. E. J., Satir, P. 1987. Generation of propulsive forces by cilia and flagella. In *Cytomechanics: The mechanical basis of cell form and structure,* ed. J. Bereiter-Hahn, O. R. Anderson, W. E. Reif, pp. 120–30. Berlin: Springer-Verlag

30. Huang, B., Ramanis, Z., Luck, D. J. L. 1982. Suppressor mutations in *Chlamydomonas* reveal a regulatory mechanism for flagellar function. *Cell* 28:115–24

31. Johnson, K. A. 1985. Pathway of the microtubule-dynein ATPase and the structure of dynein: a comparison with actomyosin. *Annu. Rev. Biophys. Chem.* 14:161–88

32. Kobayashi, N., Hirokawa, N. 1988. Cytoskeletal architecture and immunocytochemical localization of fodrin in the terminal web of the ciliated epithelial cell. *Cell Motil. Cytoskel.* 11: 167–77

33. Lieberman, S. J., Hamasaki, T., Satir, P. 1988. Ultrastructure and motion analysis of permeabilized Paramecium capable of motility and regulation of motility. *Cell Motil. Cytoskel.* 9:73–84

34. Luck, D. J. L. 1984. Genetic and biochemical dissection of the eucaryotic flagellum. *J. Cell Biol.* 98:789–94

35. Marino, M. R., Aiello, E. 1982. Cinemicrographic analysis of beat dynamics of human respiratory cilia. *Cell Motil. Suppl.* 1:35–39

36. Matsuoka, T., P. Satir. 1988. Splitting the ciliary axoneme: patterns that support the 'switch point' model of ciliary activity. *Biophys. J.* 53:29a

37. McEwen, B. F., Radermacher, M., Rieder, C. L., Frank, J. 1986. Tomographic three-dimensional reconstruction of cilia ultrastructure from thick sections. *Proc. Nat. Acad. Sci. USA* 83:9040–44

38. Meyer, F. A., Silberberg, A. 1978. Structure and function of mucus. *Ciba Found. Symp.* 54:203–18

39. Meyer, F. A., Silberberg, A. 1980. The rheology and molecular organization of epithelial mucus. *Biorheology* 17:163–68

40. Murray, J. M. 1989. Electron microscopy of microtubule crosslinking structures. See Ref. 90, pp. 257–65

41. Nadel, J. A., Davis, B., Phipps, R. J. 1979. Control of mucus secretion and ion transport in airways. *Annu. Rev. Physiol.* 41:369–81

42. Omoto, C. K., Whitman, G. B. 1981. Functionally significant central-pair rotation in a primitive eukaryote. *Nature* 290:708–10

43. Otter, T. 1989. Calmodulin and the control of flagellar movement. See Ref. 90, pp. 281–98

44. Pallini, V., Bugnoli, M., Mencarelli, C., Scapigliati, G. 1982. Biochemical properties of ciliary, flagellar, and cytoplasmic dyneins. *Soc. Exp. Biol. Symp.* 35:339–52

45. Palmblad, J., Mossberg, B., Afzelius, B. A. 1984. Ultrastructural, cellular and clinical features of the immotile cilia syndrome. *Annu. Rev. Med.* 35:481–92

46. Paschal, B. M., King, S. M., Moss, A. G., Collins, C. A., Vallee, R. B., Witman, G. B. 1987. Isolated flagella outer arm dynein translocates brain microtubules in vitro. *Nature* 330:672–74

47. Paschal, B. M., Shpetner, H. S., Vallee, R. B. 1987. MAP 1C is a microtubule-activated ATPase which translocates microtubules *in vitro* and has dynein-like properties. *J. Cell Biol.* 105:1273–82

48. Reed, W., Avolio, J., Satir, P. 1984. The cytoskeleton of the apical border of the lateral cells of freshwater mussel gill: structural integration of microtubule and actin filament based organelles. *J. Cell Sci.* 68:1–33

49. Reed, W., Satir, P. 1986. Spreading ciliary arrest in a mussel gill epithelium:

characterization by quick fixation. *J. Cell Physiol.* 126:191–205

50. Sale, W. S. 1986. The axonemal axis and Ca^{2+}-induced asymmetry of active microtubule sliding in sea urchin sperm tails. *J. Cell Biol.* 102:2042–52

51. Sale, W. S., Fox, L. A. 1988. The isolated β-heavy chain subunit of dynein translocates microtubules *in vitro*. *J. Cell Biol.* 107:1793–97

52. Sale, W. S., Fox, L. A., Milgram, S. L. 1989. Composition and organization of the inner row dynein arms. See Ref. 90, pp. 89–102

53. Sale, W. S., Satir, P. 1977. Direction of active sliding of microtubules in Tetrahymena cilia. *Proc. Natl. Acad. Sci. USA.* 74:2045–49

54. Sanderson, M. J., Chow, I., Dirksen, E. R. 1988. Intercellular communication between ciliated cells in culture. *Am. J. Physiol.* 254 *(Cell Physiol.* 23):C63–74

55. Sanderson, M. J., Dirksen, E. R. 1986. Mechanosensitivity of cultured ciliated cells from the mammalian respiratory tract: implications for the regulation of mucociliary clearance. *Proc. Natl. Acad. Sci. USA.* 83:7302–6

56. Sanderson, M. J., Dirksen, E. R. 1988. Intracellular calcium is elevated during mechanosensitivity and intercellular communication between ciliated cells. *J. Cell Biol.* 107:20a

57. Sanderson, M. J., Dirksen, E. R. 1989. Mechanosensitive and beta-adrenergic control of the ciliary beat frequencies of mammalian respiratory tract cells in culture. *Am. Rev. Respir. Dis.* 139:432–40

58. Sanderson, M. J., Sleigh, M. A. 1981. Ciliary activity of cultured rabbit tracheal epithelium: beat pattern and metachrony. *J. Cell Sci.* 47:331–47

59. Sanderson, M. J., Sleigh, M. A. 1982. The function of respiratory tract cilia. In *The Lung and Its Environment* ed. G. Bonsignore, G. Cumming, pp. 81–120. New York: Plenum

60. Satir, P. 1968. Studies on cilia: III. Further studies on the cilium tip and a "sliding filament" model of ciliary motility. *J. Cell Biol.* 39:77–94

61. Satir, P. 1982. Mechanisms and controls of microtubule sliding in cilia. *Soc. Exp. Biol. Symp.* 35:172–201

62. Satir, P. 1985. Switching mechanisms in control of ciliary motility. *Mod. Cell Biol.* 4:1–46

63. Satir, P. 1989. Structural analaysis of the dynein crossbridge cycle. See Ref. 90, pp. 219–34

64. Satir, P., Dirksen, E. R. 1985. Function-structure correlations in cilia from

the mammalian respiratory tract. In *Handbook of Physiology—Respiratory System I.* ed. A. P. Fishman, pp. 473–94. Bethesda: Am. Physiol. Soc.

65. Satir, P., Wais-Steider, J., Lebduska, S., Nasr, A., Avolio, J. 1981. The mechanochemical cycle of the dynein arm. *Cell Motil.* 1:303–27

66. Sato, F., Mogami, Y., Baba, S. A. 1988. Flagellar quiescence and transience of inactivation induced by rapid pH drop. *Cell Motil. Cytoskel.* 10:374–79

67. Silberberg, A. 1983. Biorheological matching: mucociliary interaction and epithelial clearance. *Biorheology* 20: 215–22

68. Sleigh, M. A. 1982. Movement and coordination of tracheal cilia and the relation of these to mucus transport. *Cell Motil. Suppl.* 1:19–24

69. Sleigh, M. A. 1984. The integrated activity of cilia: function and coordination. *J. Protozool.* 31:16–21

70. Sleigh, M. A., Blake, J. R., Liron, N. 1988. The propulsion of mucus by cilia, *Am. Rev. Respir. Dis.* 137:726–41

71. Spungin, B., Avolio, J., Arden, S., Satir, P. 1987. Dynein arm attachment probed with a non-hydrolyzable ATP analog: structural evidence of patterns of activity. *J. Mol. Biol.* 197:671–77

72. Spungin, B., Silberberg, A. 1984. Stimulation of mucus secretion, ciliary activity and transport in frog palate epithelium. *Am. J. Physiol.* 247:C299–308

73. Stephens, R. E., Stommel, E. W. 1989. Role of cyclic adenosine monophosphate in ciliary and flagellar motility. See Ref. 90, pp. 299–316

74. Sturgess, J. M., Chao, J., Wong, J., Aspin, N., Turner, J. A. P. 1979. Cilia with defective radial spokes: a cause of human respiratory disease. *N. Engl. J. Med.* 300:53–56

75. Sturgess, J. M., Thompson, M. W., Czegledy-Nagy, E., Turner, J. A. 1986. Genetic aspects of immotile cilia syndrome. *Am. J. Med. Genet.* 25:149–60

76. Sugino, K., Machemer, H. 1988. The ciliary cycle during hyperpolarization-induced activity: an analysis of axonemal functional parameters. *Cell Motil. Cytoskel.* 11:275–90

77. Summers, K. E., Gibbons, I. R. 1971. Adenosine triphosphate-induced sliding of tubules in trypsin-treated flagella of sea-urchin sperm. *Proc. Natl. Acad. Sci. USA.* 68:3092–96

78. Takahashi, K., Shingyoji, C., Kamimura, S. 1982. Microtubule sliding in reactivated flagella. *Soc. Exp. Biol. Symp.* 35:159–77

79. Tamaoki, J., Kondo, M., Takizawa, T. 1989. Adenosine-mediated cyclic AMP-dependent inhibition of ciliary activity in rabbit tracheal epithelium. *Am. Rev. Respir. Dis.* 139:441–45

80. Tamm, S. L., Tamm, S. 1984. Alternate patterns of doublet microtubule sliding in ATP-disintegrated macrocilia of the ctenophore Beroë. *J. Cell Biol.* 99:1364–71

81. Vale, R. D. and Toyoshima, Y. Y. 1988. Rotation and translocation of microtubules *in vitro* induced by dyneins from *Tetrahymena* cilia. *Cell* 52:459–69

82. Vale, R. D., Toyoshima, Y. Y., Tang, W.-J. Y, Gibbons, I. R. 1988. Dynein induced microtubule movement *in vitro*. *Cell Motil. Cytoskel.* 11:194

83. Verdugo, P. 1984. Hydration kinetics of exocytosed mucins in cultured secretory cells of the rabbit trachea: a new model. *Ciba Found. Symp.* 109:212–25

84. Verdugo, P., Johnson, N. T., Tamm, P. Y. 1980. β-adrenergic stimulation of respiratory ciliary activity. *J. Appl. Physiol.* 48:868–71

85. Verdugo, P., Raess, B. V., Villalon, M. 1983. The role of calmodulin in the regulation of ciliary movement in mammalian epithelial cilia. *J. Submicro. Cytol.* 15:95–96

86. Wais-Steider, J., Satir, P. 1979. Effect of vanadate on gill cilia: switching mechanism in ciliary beat. *J. Supramolec. Struct.* 11:339–47

87. Wanner, A. 1986. Mucociliary clearance in the trachea. *Clin. Chest Med.* 7:247–58

88. Warner, F. D. 1983. Organization of interdoublet links in *Tetrahymena* cilia. *Cell Motil.* 3:321–32

89. Warner, F. D., McIntosh, J. R., eds. 1989. *Cell Movement* Vol. 2. New York: Liss. 478 pp.

90. Warner, F. D., Satir, P., Gibbons, I. R., eds. 1989. *Cell Movement* Vol. 1. New York: Liss. 337 pp.

91. Weaver, A., Hard, R. 1985. Newt lung ciliated cell models: effect of MgATP on beat frequency and waveforms. *Cell Motil.* 5:377–92

92. Widdicombe, J. H. 1984. Fluid transport across airway epithelia. *Ciba Found. Symp.* 109:109–20

93. Woolley, D. M., Brammall, A. 1987. Direction of sliding and relative sliding velocities within trypsinized sperm axonemes of *Gallus domesticus*. *J. Cell Sci.* 88:361–71

94. Wong, L. B., Miller, I. F., Yeats, D. B. 1988. Regulation of ciliary beat frequency by autonomic mechanisms: *in vitro*. *J. Appl. Physiol.* 65:1895–901

95. Yeung, C. N., Woolley, D. M. 1983. Localized reactivation of the principal piece of demembranated hamster sperm by iontophoretic application of ATP. *J. Submicro. Cytol.* 15:327–31

Annu. Rev. Physiol. 1990. 52:157–76

GOBLET CELLS SECRETION AND MUCOGENESIS

Pedro Verdugo

Center for Bioengineering and Department of Biological Structure, University of Washington, Seattle, Washington 98195

KEY WORDS: Donnan equilibrium, exocytosis, gel, mucus, reptative diffusion

INTRODUCTION

In the final discussions of the last Ciba Symposium on Mucus and Mucosa (London, 1984), I voiced my impression that, in this gelatinous drama of mucus formation, several scripts were looking for characters, and some characters were looking for roles. Now, four years later, we have been able to locate a few of the missing characters and see them play their parts. Some, like the serous cell, are telling a potentially fascinating new story. A new polymer thread is being tentatively introduced into this already tangled scene of the mucus matrix (see review by Basbaum, this volume). Other cells, like goblet cells, are sticking to their old role of producing mucin, but are giving up some of their best-guarded secrets on how to store and release such gigantic molecules. We are also starting to realize that perhaps some characters can play not one, but several roles at the same time. For instance, mucous cells in vitro can not only produce mucin, but can also produce proteoglycans.

Are we hearing the true scripts? Or is the culture shock, the isolation of these cells from their natural habitat, forcing them to play subsidiary roles? The whole picture of airway physiology is rapidly changing. Much remains to be learned, including perhaps the painful lesson that some of our most cherished passages in the old play are being swiftly rewritten.

The mucosa of the airways is an organ. Its overall function results from the integrated action of several types of effector cells. Although the organ's

157

principal function—mucociliary clearance—has been extensively investigated, the specific physiologic role of each of the constitutent cellular components, particularly of secretory cells, remains largely unexplored.

Mucociliary clearance involves the coordinated action of at least three generic cellular functions: force generation, ion and water exchange, and secretory function. It operates as a conveyer in which ciliated cells provide the driving force, and mucus performs as a sticky fluidic belt that collects and disposes of foreign particles. Performance depends on the physiologic control of the ciliated cell and on the regulation of the rheological properties of the mucus blanket. Mucus rheology, the most critical and least understood determinant in pulmonary clearance, is controlled by various types of secretory cells, which produce the macromolecules that form the matrix of the mucus gel, and also by ion and water exchange cells (mainly ciliated cells), which modulate the hydration of these macromolecules.

This brief review concerns one of the cellular effectors of the airway mucosa, the respiratory goblet cell. We examine its role in the formation of mucus. The approach will be mechanistic rather than phenomenological, seeking to decipher more than to describe the literature. The focus will be on polymer physics and on the biophysics of mucus and goblet cells, rather than on their biochemistry and morphology. Extensive reports on these latter subjects can be found elsewhere (7, 26, 28, 54, 55). First we will visit the subject of mucus and mucin structure and function, not as a guest of the molecular or cellular anatomist, but as a guest of the molecular and cellular physiologist. Short discussions of the physicochemistry of mucus hydration will follow and bring us to a final focus on the goblet cell and its role in mucogenesis.

MACROMOLECULAR CONFORMATION OF THE MUCUS POLYMER GEL

Respiratory mucus is a heterogeneous mixture of different secretions that form a hydrophilic, viscoelastic polymer gel. It contains about 95% water, electrolytes—including Na^+, which is the major constituent, K^+, Mg^{2+}, and Ca^{2+}—and organic compounds, including carbohydrates, amino acids, and serum proteins, as well as secreted soluble proteins and lipids. The characteristic viscoelastic properties of mucus are directly or indirectly determined by the presence of very high molecular weight sugar-rich polymers, including mucous glycoproteins, and perhaps also proteoglycans. (6, 22, 41).

It had been thought that following exocytosis the secretions of different cells blended to produce a gel of suitable viscoelasticity. For instance, it was supposed that serous cells produced a serous, watery secretion which, when mixed with a presumed highly viscous secretion from mucus cells, resulted in a gel of graded viscoelasticity. However, recent findings indicate that the material inside the serous secretory granule might not be a watery fluid since it contains proteoglycans, which are exceedingly large polymers that must be condensed inside the granule space (4). Furthermore, mucous cells, and perhaps other secretory cells, release their secretions in a densely condensed form. Upon exocytosis the secretory product undergoes massive swelling, and it is only after this hydration step that mucins are mixed and annealed to form a viscoelastic gel (61). Hence, the rheological properties of mucus are probably not determined by directly blending secretions of different fluidity, but by controlling the transepithelial movement of water and ions that hydrate the different secretory products (57).

Mucus, like other polymer gels, consists of a polymer matrix and a solvent. The solvent is water, and the matrix is composed of several polymer species assembled to form a random, three-dimensional network. The principal components in the mucus matrix are a family of very high molecular weight polyionic polymers called mucins, which are secreted by goblet cells and mucous cells of the submucosal glands. However, mucins may not be the sole macromolecular component. Although proteoglycans have not been routinely detected by standard analytical methods, recent experiments have reported the finding of proteoglycans in normal mucus (6). Complementary observations that proteoglycans are secreted by serous cells in vitro have been reported by several groups. [This material has been recently reviewed by Basbaum & Finkbeiner (4).] These findings raise the engaging prospect that this second family of very high molecular weight polyionic, sugar-rich polymers might also be an important structural element of the mucus polymer matrix. Nevertheless, the presence of proteoglycans in respiratory mucus and the interpretation of their release by secretory cells in culture still needs further examination (3).

The rheological properties of polymer gels are primarily determined by the macromolecular configuration in which the polymer chains are assembled and interconnected in the gel's matrix and also by the conformation (size, shape), the length, the flexibility, and the concentration of their constituent polymers (15, 16). However, for the past twenty years the dominant theories of mucus molecular structure and function have been based on indirect evidence obtained after biochemical demolition of the mucus macromolecular polymer network, when the native conformation is no longer preserved.

The Disulfide-Bonded Network Model

Cleaving of s:s bonds results in the dispersion of the mucus gel. This observation led to the idea that mucin chains are covalently cross-linked, forming a three-dimensional random polymer matrix that is held together by s:s bonds (20). The viscoelastic properties of gels containing a cross-linked polymer matrix depend on the degree of cross-linking among polymer chains (16). In the case of mucus, it was thought that hormonal influences would control mucus rheology by modulating the degree of disulfide bonding among the mucin chains produced by secretory cells. The idea of a disulfide-bonded network was initially proposed for mucus of the cervix (20), but was soon extended, with minor variations, to respiratory and gastrointestinal mucus (45). However the high molecular weight of mucins imposes enormous constraints on analytical methods. Biochemical fractionation techniques destroy the mucus quaternary structure, which is precisely the level of molecular organization at which inter-chain cross-linking should be verified. At present there seems to be some consensus on the limitations of a purely biochemical characterization of mucus structure (3). The concept of mucus macromolecular architecture obtained by destructive analytical methods is only an inferential reconstruction built on indirect evidence.

Striking new theories in the field of polymer gel physics and the introduction of novel spectroscopic methods have recently furnished a sound theoretical foundation, as well as a battery of powerful nondestructive techniques, both to understand and to investigate further the physics of polymer gels (13, 14, 15, 60). The application of these ideas and methods to the study of mucus and mucin secretion is creating a surprisingly different picture of mucus architecture. It is also providing a solid physical theory for understanding and guiding future research in this area (36, 39, 48, 65).

The Entangled-Network Model

Molecules in solution exhibit random diffusional motion that depends on their shape and their mutual interactions. For instance, in cross-linked polymer networks, translational motion along the axis of the polymer chains (reptative diffusion) is restricted by the presence of cross-links. Diffusion is local, confined only to the section of polymer between cross-links. Conversely, in tangled polymer networks, both local and translational diffusion can occur (14, 15). Measurements of translational (reptative) diffusion of mucin chains in intact mucus samples, by use of laser photon correlation spectroscopy, gave the first direct indication that mucins are probably not held together by covalent cross-links among polymer chains; instead, these results suggested that mucin polymers must be entangled, forming a loosely woven, random polymer network (36, 65). This new molecular model implies that mucins must be linear polymers that are held together by inter-chain tangles or by low energy bonds, rather than by covalent cross-links (36, 65). An implicit feature of this molecular model is that the disulfide bonds must be in the protein backbone of the polymers rather than as inter-chain cross-links. (see Figure 1.)

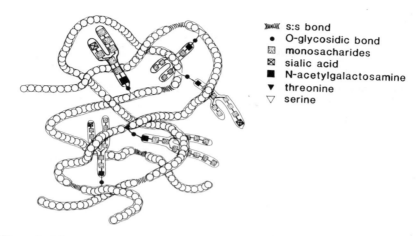

Figure 1 Schematic diagram of the mucus polymer gel. Notice the entangled nature of the polymer network and the presence of s : s bonds in the protein backbone of the mucin polymer.

ANNEALING OF MUCUS   The characteristic annealing of one mucus gel to another can be easily explained by the notion of a tangled polymer network. The reptation of polymer chains beyond the gel boundaries allows gels containing entangled polymer networks to readily undergo annealing when put in contact with other gels. Conversely, annealing does not take place between polymer gels containing a cross-linked matrix because polymer chains are locked in their corresponding networks and cannot undergo translational (reptative) diffusion. Since mucins are released from secretory cells in small, discrete granular quanta, if these polymers were cross-linked mucus would remain as a divisible aggregate of small individual gels rather than as a cohesive gel. Although the annealing properties of mucus have long been recognized, if not emphasized, their significance in ruling out the idea of a cross-linked topology for the mucus polymer network has been inexplicably overlooked.

DISPERSION BY CLEAVING OF S:S BONDS   According to the entangled network model, the dispersion of mucus induced by the cleaving of s : s bonds is caused by the shortening of the mucin chains, which can drastically destabilize the polymer network. Dispersion of tangled network gels depends on reptative diffusion of the polymer chains that randomly walk away from each other. As diffusional times are proportional to the second power of chain length, the stability of tangled polymer gels is proportional to the square of the average polymer length (15). Therefore, small changes in mucin length can result in strikingly faster (or slower) mucus dispersion. Variations in mucin chain length can readily explain why mucus from different sources can exhibit diverse resistances to dispersion.

HYDRATION AND MUCUS RHEOLOGY   Like mucus, synthetic gels built of a tangled polymer network exhibit characteristically non-Newtonian behavior. Their rheological properties are primarily dependent upon tangle density (14, 15). Since tangle concentration decreases exponentially with the gel's volume, the principal factor controlling mucus rheology is mucus hydration. This argument not only has a simple theoretical basis, but it also has a critical physiologic significance and has been validated experimentally (37, 57). The mechanisms that control mucus hydration will be discussed in the section on Donnan equilibrium.

THE MUCIN POLYMER

Structure and Properties

With the revelation of the tangled nature of the mucus polymer network, it is now feasible to identify the features of the mucin polymer chains that are important for determining the physicochemical and rheological properties of the mucus gel: namely, their size, shape, and charge. A brief description of primary structure introduces the subject.

PRIMARY STRUCTURE   Mucins are highly heterogeneous glycoproteins consisting of a filamentous protein core to which short polysaccharide side chains are attached. The peptide core amounts to about 20% of the polymer by weight, and the remaining 80% is carbohydrate. The core includes regions that are densely glycosylated (70–80%) and also naked regions (20–30%) that contain cysteine residues and are susceptible to cleavage (7, 8, 9, 28, 31, 53).

Oligosaccharide side chains are linked to the core by O-glycosidic bonds between threonine and serine on the backbone and N-acetylgalactosamine on the sugar chains. Side chains are 2 to 20 monosaccharides long, can be linear or branched, vary vastly in composition, and are often sulfated, and/or contain sialic terminals. The latter two give mucins their characteristic polyionic properties.

CONFORMATIONAL STRUCTURE   Because of their gigantic molecular size and complex interweaving, mucins are difficult to isolate intact. Procedures for their separation and purification yield broadly polydisperse mixtures of polymer chains. Different analytical procedures yield correspondingly different polymer moieties. Thus the search for a basic mucin building block has remained unresolved (11, 45, 46). Silberberg has recently made the interesting observation that there is a proportional log/log relationship between the radius of gyration and the molecular weight of mucins of different size and origin. This is a characteristic feature of a linear random coil. Based on the estimation of the size of the Kuhn statistical elements that make the polymer chain, Silberberg further postulates a mucin subunit of 150 nm, with a radius of gyration of about 40 nm, and a molecular weight of 0.5 MD. Longer polymer chains would result from the association of subunits (52).

The use of gentler preparative techniques, together with the application of electron microscopy, and nondestructive spectroscopic methods, have permitted a better definition of the conformation of mucins. Fascinating images of mucin polymers captured using rotary shadowing by Harding et al (21), Slayter et al (53), and more recently Sheehan et al (49) reveal unequivocally that mucins, regardless of their origin (respiratory, gastrointestinal, or reproductive tracts), are linear polymers that can reach up to 4–6 μm in length. The notion of a linear conformation for mucins had also been inferred from studies in intact mucus using laser photon correlation spectroscopy (36, 65, 9). However the rotary-shadowed images furnish direct and objective validation for the linear molecular model for mucin proposed by Carlstedt & Sheehan (9).

Measurements of respiratory mucins based on light scattering indicate a hydrodynamic radius of gyration on the order of 270 nm (9). The discrepancy between the hydrodynamic dimensions and the micron-plus dimensions detected by electron microscopy (49, 53) suggests that, in solution, the mucin polymer may be a very flexible random coil.

POLYIONIC PROPERTIES   The presence of sulfate residues and sialic terminals gives mucins their strong polyanionic properties. Although histochemical methods suggest broad variations in the acidity of respiratory mucins, isoelectric focusing methods show that these molecules are consistently acidic, with a pI of 2.7–2.8 (22, 29, 50). An important corollary of this observation is that at near-neutral pH, mucins behave like highly charged negative polyions. Thus, owing to their polyanionic properties, both the molecular conformation of the mucin polymer and the viscoelastic properties of mucus are drastically affected by cations. For instance, Ca^{2+} has been shown to decrease the hydrodynamic radius of respiratory mucins (56) and also to increase the elastic storage modulus of respiratory and digestive mucus gels (17, 38). However, as discussed later, the most significant effect of the polyanionic change of mucins is in the control of hydration in the mucus gel.

In summary, mucins are highly charged thread-like polymers of gigantic molecular dimensions, with a flexible random coil conformation in solution.

DONNAN EQUILIBRIUM AND THE CONTROL OF MUCUS HYDRATION

The rheological properties of gels built of a tangled polymer network are predominantly determined by the tangle density. Since the concentration of tangles decreases with the square of the gel's volume, hydration turns out to be a highly efficient vehicle for the physiologic control of mucus rheology (37, 57). The implication here is that the mucin matrix may be secreted as a condensed polymer network and become a hydrogel (the mucus gel) only after swelling. Since the degree of hydration determines the rheological properties, by modulating the degree of hydration of the polymer network, the mucosa can readily control mucus rheology (57). The questions we address in this section are: What drives mucus hydration? And what are the physicochemical and physiologic mechanisms that modulate this process?

Physicochemical and Physiologic Mechanisms

SWELLING OF GELS   Polymer hydrogels swell when immersed in water. Swelling dynamics are governed by osmotic forces. Because of the large molecular size of the networking polymers, the osmotic drive is small, and swelling is slow (16). However in gels containing a polyionic network, swelling is not driven by simple osmosis, but primarily by the fixed polyionic charges of the polymer chains. Since tangles prevent the polyionic chains from migrating out of the gel, the polymer matrix virtually functions as its own semipermeable membrane. Swelling, in this case, is not governed by simple osmosis, but by a Donnan equilibrium process (12, 30).

SWELLING OF MUCUS AND DONNAN EQUILIBRIUM   The demonstration that mucus swelling had the characteristic features of a Donnan equilibrium revealed a paradigm of remarkably broad physiologic significance (57). A Donnan process can explain the mechanisms that control mucus rheology and also the molecular mechanisms of product release in exocytosis (57, 61). The latter facet will be discussed in the next section.

A direct implication of the Donnan properties of mucus is that in the airways, mucus does not remain static, but undergoes a continuous change regulated by its rate of hydration. Mucins are released as condensed products; they swell and anneal to form transportable mucus, and finally they disperse. Since mucus hydration is governed by a Donnan equilibrium, the polyionic charges of the mucins and other polyions furnish the driving force for swelling. This force is balanced by the effect of free ions and polycations that can penetrate the polymer network and neutralize the fixed polyanionic charges of mucin or other polyanions. Consequently, the concentration of small polyionic proteins (albumin, lysozyme, proline rich protein, and so forth), the pH, and the ionic strength of the fluid on the airways surface can readily modulate the swelling rate of the mucus gel. The characteristic Donnan effect of pH, ionic strength, and albumin on mucus hydration has been experimentally validated (1, 57).

Recent work by Widdicombe (66) indicates that the electrolytic composition of the airways liquid is not constant. In particular, Na^+, Cl^-, and Ca^{2+} concentrations can vary under the influence of pharmacological mediators. His observations also suggest that a homeostatic mechanism to control trans-epithelial pH must be present in the mucosa. The finding that albumin is not only actively transported but perhaps also synthesized (25a) by the epithelium and that albumin transport is affected by autonomic mediators suggests a significant role for this polyion in the control of mucus hydration. Consequently, by controlling the secretion of mucins, pH, and the transepithelial movement of electrolytes, polyelectrolytes, and water the respiratory mucosa can broadly modulate the amount of mucus as well as the rate of mucus swelling and its rheology.

PATHOLOGY OF MUCUS   Abnormal mucus can result from inadequate or excessive mucin hydration. However, regardless of the amount of surface water available for mucus swelling, if the concentration of ions or polyelectrolytes in the airway liquid is elevated, the fixed polyionic charges in the mucins will be neutralized. Donnan potential will decrease or disappear, and mucus swelling will be slow and inefficient. As the effect of fixed polyions weakens, mucus swelling is still present, but it is driven by exceedingly small residual osmotic forces produced by the large mucin polymers. The result is a highly viscous, poorly transportable mucus. Conversely, low ionic concentration in the surface epithelial fluid should result in rapid swelling and once again a poorly transportable, but thin and watery mucus.

We know now that a deficiency of the epithelial hydroelectrolytic exchange system is present in cystic fibrosis. However the logical link between the characteristic thick mucus found in this illness and the defective control of Cl^- channels had been missing (43). Here again the Donnan equilibrium makes specific and verifiable predictions to explain the various physicochemical mechanisms that can result in defective hydration of the mucus in these patients (1, 61, 63). In fact, studies on Donnan swelling of mucus published in 1981 accurately anticipated that the thick mucus found in cystic fibrosis might result from defective hydration because of an altered ionic composition of the fluid on the mucosal surface (57).

The respiratory mucosa is equipped with a battery of ion channels and pumps to effectively control the hydroelectrolytic environment of the luminal surface of the epithelium. Both absorption and secretion of salt take place at the surface epithelium (18). However the significance of such a powerful ion and water exchanger and its responsiveness to neurotransmitters or hormonal mediators remains speculative. Emphasis has been placed on the importance of the regulation of fluid volume that would control the width of the periciliary fluid layer (32). However, experimental information to support this popular yet untested idea is not available, and more recent evidence contradicts this notion (67). The notion of a Donnan mechanism for regulating mucus swelling clearly explains the need and the significance of a well-tuned hydroelectrolytic exchanger in the airways and provides verifiable predictions to further investigate this system.

Because of similarities of size, shape, and polyanionic properties between mucins and proteoglycans, a Donnan mechanism of swelling of gels containing the latter is clearly possible. Proteoglycans have a higher charge density than mucins. Thus given equal ionic composition of the hydrating fluid on the epithelial surface, Donnan swelling predicts that proteoglycans would form gels of higher water content. This is in line with the observation that if serous cells would release proteoglycans (4), their secretions might result in less viscous, more watery mucus.

THE GOBLET CELL

Structure and Function

MORPHOLOGY   Goblet cells take their name from the characteristic, but perhaps artifactual, goblet shape they exhibit in chemically fixed tissue. They are among various cellular types found on the epithelial lining of the respiratory, gastrointestinal, and reproductive tracts. In the airway, goblet cells are one of the secretory cell types that synthesize and release specific components that comprise the mucus. Morphological studies suggest that the contribution of goblet cells to the production of mucin is probably less than that of submucosal mucous gland secretion. However the number of goblet cells is increased by metaplasia in chronic bronchitis, asthma, and cystic fibrosis (44). Thus their relative role in secretory function is probably enhanced in chronic airway diseases.

Optical microscopy of chemically fixed and sectioned goblet cells reveals that the material that fills their apical end is typically PAS (periodic acid-Schiff) and/or AB (Alcian blue) positive, indicating the presence of reacted dialdehydes or acidic sugar groups. In TEM, the apical portion appears filled with large, often coalescent, membrane-bound secretory granules which in SEM give a characteristic domed profile to their luminal surface. Secretory granules vary in number and in electron density. The basal portion of the goblet cell includes a large vesicular nucleus, surrounded by an electron-dense cytoplasm containing a granular endoplasmic reticulum and mitochondria (26, 55).

Cryosubstitution of quick-frozen mucosa reveals a different picture of goblet cells, which suggests that chemical fixation may render a fairly artifactual image. Preliminary studies conducted in my laboratory in quick-frozen trachea of rabbit show remarkable similarities with the images obtained by Sandoz et al (47) in goblet cells of mouse colon and quail oviduct. One of the most striking differences from images obtained by chemical fixation is that secretory granules are smaller, electron dense, and do not coalesce. Since the apical portion is not dilated by expanded secretory granules, there is no apical bulging, and the goblet cell is not goblet but cylindrical-shaped.

CELL FUNCTION   The function of goblet and other respiratory cells in the production of mucus has been approached histochemically, immunocytochemically, and biochemically (4). However the single most difficult problem in the study of goblet cell function has been the development of an experimental model in which secretory products and secretory responses can be unequivocally associated with goblet cells, and not with other secretory (or nonsecretory) cells of the mucosa (3). In this section, I will restrict the discussion to progress achieved using isolated preparations of respiratory goblet cells in vitro.

MUCIN SECRETION IN CULTURED CELLS   Tissue culture methods to grow cells that produce mucin-like materials have long been established. However unequivocal identification of the cultured cells has, with few exceptions, not been achieved (4, 19). Among the few well-characterized in vitro models are the cultured epithelial monolayers from hamster trachea enriched in surface secretory cells (for review see Kim & Brody, 33). Although these cells have not been identified by specific immunocytochemical probes, they produce high molecular weight mucins indistinguishable from the mucins produced in vivo, as judged by size, charge, and carbohydrate composition. Pulse-chase labeling experiments using ^{3}H-glucosamine show that two pools of mucins are released by these cultures, one by membrane shedding (the constitutive-nonregulated pathway) and the other via granule exocytosis (regulated pathway). These cells share most of the stimulating influences, including irritants such as sulfur dioxide, smoke, ammonia (33), and proteases (35), that increase secretory activity in goblet cells in vivo and in organ culture. The secretagogue effect of bacterial proteases on goblet cells depends upon specific proteolytic activity of these enzymes (35). The same dependency was also observed in cultured goblet cells from the hamster trachea. In these cells, however, proteases released surface glycoproteins rather than exocytosed mucins (33). In addition, hamster cultured cells have been found unresponsive to adrenergic or to cholinergic agonists, prostaglandins, leukotrienes, and to the calcium ionophore A23187 (33). A problem with these tissue cultures that remains unresolved is that, depending upon the substrate on which the cells are grown and the culture medium, goblet cells can produce not only mucins, but also proteoglycans (34). The significance of these results is difficult to interpret. It certainly means that surface secretory cells have the potential to synthesize both of these polymers. However, the extent to which the culture conditions facilitate the expression of a phenotype that is not normally expressed in vivo is not known. It may be that the production of proteoglycans is a reflection of immaturity (27). Or is it that goblet cells can normally also produce proteoglycans in situ (6)? Perhaps the procedures for isolation and maintenance of pure-bred cellular lineages of the airway may have some built-in flaw. That is, we do not know if areas of functional overlap exist between different cell types. Morphological diversity does not necessarily imply functional uniqueness in these apparently different, yet closely related, sister cells. However, in view of the remarkable success in establishing a high-yield cell line to harvest mature intestinal goblet cells (40), the prospect for an equivalent line of respiratory goblet cells remains a reasonable goal.

A convenient alternative to primary cultures is the isolation of surface epithelium from cat trachea (35). This preparation yields epithelial sheets enriched in goblet cells that conserve their secretory activity. These cells incorporate radiolabeled precursors into newly synthesized high molecular weight mucins. The labeled mucins are resistant to hyaluronidase degradation and are more sialated, and less sulfated, than mucins from glandular secretions (51).

In summary, pulse-chase experiments in isolated goblet cells are telling a story that is quite consistent with what we know from previous studies in situ. These cells produce high molecular weight acidic mucins and respond directly to irritative stimulation rather than to humoral secretagogues. The finding that these cells have both regulated and unregulated constitutive pathways for mucin release is novel, but its functional significance is difficult to interpret. The observation that these cells can express more than one phenotype for polymer synthesis is disconcerting (34) and reemphasizes the need to further investigate cellular differentiation in the airways.

Mucin Exocytosis

Tissue culture techniques for growing primary cultures of goblet cells from rabbit tracheal epithelium have been developed in our laboratory (61). Both the cultured cells and their secretions were identified immunocytochemically, using specific monoclonal antibodies (5). A major limitation for biochemical studies is that the yield of these cultures is rather small. Nevertheless, these goblet cells have proven to be a fascinating experimental model for studying the molecular mechanisms of mucin storage and release in secretion.

SWELLING KINETICS IN MUCIN SECRETION   The release of secretory products from goblet cells in vitro is almost identical to that observed in mast cells (69). The secretory material undergoes dramatic swelling as it is exocytosed. This outcome was envisioned by previous findings of Donnan swelling of mucus (57). However, we did not expect to be able to resolve this process optically. Neither did we expect to be able to quantitatively measure, by video-enhanced microscopy, the swelling of newly released granules from goblet cells. Thus we return to the discussion of Donnan swelling in polyionic gels. The premise we examine here is that if the mucin polymer network is expanded by swelling (to form the mucus gel), then it must start from a condensed state within the secretory granule. Two questions follow: What is the molecular mechanism of decondensation during exocytosis? Conversely, what is the mechanism of condensation of mucin in secretory granules?

The finding that during exocytotic swelling the radius of the secreted material follows a first order kinetic gave the first clue that the swelling of the exocytosed mucin is governed by Tanaka's linear theory of swelling of gels (59). Although this finding should not have come as a surprise, it was fascinating to verify that a theory formulated and validated in artificial polymer gels could also rule the swelling of a natural polymer gel during exocytosis in living cells. Tanaka's theory further predicts that a linear relationship should exist between the square of the final radius of the swelling exocytosed mucin and the characteristic time of swelling (the reciprocal of the kinetic constant). The slope of this line has the dimensions of a diffusion ($D = r^2/\tau/[cm^2/sec]$), and represents the diffusivity of the polymer network in the solvent (59). A most valuable hint came out of these experiments (61); the apparent diffusion of the mucin network during exocytosis was about one order of magnitude faster than the diffusions we had measured using laser photon correlation spectroscopy in fully swollen gels of respiratory and cervical mucus (36, 65). This remarkable discrepancy signifies that the expansion of the mucin network during exocytosis results primarily from charge repulsion of the mucin polyionic residues rather than from simple diffusional motions (1, 61, 63).

MUCIN CONDENSATION   The counter argument, which brings us to the next question, is the following: If electrostatic interactions drive the explosive expansion of the granule during exocytosis, what stops these forces from preventing the condensation of the polyanionic mucin network within the granule? The search for a cationic shielding agent to screen the polyanionic charges in the mucins brought us to the verification that Ca^{2+} is present in large amounts in a broad number of secretory granules, including mucin secretory granules (25, 64). Thus intragranular Ca^{2+} probably functions as a shielding cation to screen the polyanionic residues of mucins and allows their condensation. Conversely, when the cationic shield is lost the mutual repulsion of the polyionic charges will quickly drive the expansion of the mucin network. This idea is further supported by observations where Ca^{2+} release from exocytosed granules was retarded by increased extracellular Ca^{2+} concentration. Variations from 1 to 4 mM Ca^{2+} in the extracellular medium were sufficient to decrease by 70 to 85% the diffusivity of goblet cell mucins during exocytosis (63). These experiments also have an interesting physiologic significance, since Ca^{2+} is known to be increased in the mucus of cystic fibrosis patients (42). Increased Ca^{2+} may be one of the factors that prevents normal mucus swelling in these patients.

THE JACK-IN-THE-BOX MECHANISM FOR EXOCYTOSIS   The above observations provided the foundation for what we have called the "jack-in-the-box" mechanism of exocytosis (see Figure 2). This notion proposes that inside the granules mucins are condensed and their polyionic charges are screened by Ca^{2+}. Exocytosis could be mediated by the opening of a pore (see review Almers, this volume). Once a waterway between intragranular and extracellular space is established, shielding cations are released and water enters into the granule. As charge shielding is lost, charge repulsion among polyionic chains rapidly expands the polymer network, driving the swelling, the consecutive expansion of the pore, and the release of the secreted mucins (63).

A remarkable feature of this idea is that it can explain exocytosis not only in goblet cells, but also in other secretory cells. The notion that swelling might steer exocytosis had been considered in the past. The swelling was thought to be driven by osmosis (24). However the observed rates of swelling in goblet cells (61), and particularly in mucus granules from terrestrial gastropods (64), are clearly incompatible with a simple osmotic drive. In giant secretory granules of the slug *Ariolimax columbianus,* a 400- to 600-fold volumetric expansion takes place in about 20 msec. Even faster rates of release have been observed in the exocytotic discharge of nematocyst in *Hydra* (23). These rates of granular expansion are far too fast to be explained by simple os-

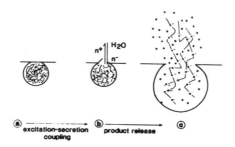

Figure 2   Schematic representation of the jack-in-the-box model for product release in secretion. The secretory granule first docks to the plasma membrane (*a*). Exocytosis is initiated by the opening of a membrane pore (*b*). A waterway between intragranular and extracellular space allows the diffusion of shielding cations and inflow of water into the granule. The loss of charge shielding brings about a catastrophic reaction whereby the polymer network undergoes phase transition, and charge repulsion drives a rapid hydration of the polyionic network release of secretory product (*c*).

mosis, and our evidence suggests that they are probably driven by electrostatic interaction.

The fundamental element necessary to generalize the jack-in-the-box model is the existence within secretory granules of a condensed, shielded polymeric polyion. The release of the shielding species triggers the rapid swelling of the granule's contents, driving its release. Whereas in mucin granules mucin is the condensed polyanion and Ca^{2+} is the shielding cation (64), in mast cell granules heparin is the condensed polyanion and histamine and perhaps K^+ are the shielding cations (70). The corresponding pair in serous cells could be the polyanionic proteoglycan, and perhaps lyzosyme could function as the shielding polycation (see review by Basbaum, this volume). In chromaffin granules, chromogranin A is the condensed polyanion, and H^+, ATP, or perhaps catecholamines are the shielding cations (68). In the parathyroid, the condensed polyanion is the acidic protein I (SP-I), and the cation is Ca^{2+} (10). Acidic proteins similar to SP-I have been found in the thyroid, anterior pituitary, pancreatic islets, celiac and mesenteric ganglia, and the gastric antrum (10), although their companion screening cations or polycations have not yet been identified. Although it has been long proposed that the presence of counterionic species in secretory granules could decrease osmotic activity by promoting the formation of macromolecular aggregates (60a), the function of this family of polyanionic proteins as molecular electrostatic springs that drive exocytosis had not been previously considered.

Thus the basic molecular components for a jack-in-the-box mechanism for product release in exocytosis seem to be present in a large number of secretory cells. The idea of a preloaded energy storage system to drive exocytosis assigns specific roles to both polyions and shielding cations and suggests verifiable propositions for investigating the molecular mechanisms of product storage and release in secretion.

The notion that the driving energy for product release in exocytosis is stored in a condensed polyion inside the granule can also explain why chemical fixation might result in grossly expanded granules. If, for instance, the rate of cross-linking of the fixative is slower than the rate of expansion of intragranular polyions, the granules will look bigger in chemically fixed secretory cells, as compared to quick-frozen specimens.

POLYMER GEL PHASE TRANSITION IN SECRETION   The release of cationic shielding is necessary for mucin condensation, and its release could trigger decondensation in exocytosis. However charge shielding is not sufficient to account for the condensation of the polymer lattice inside the granule. Preliminary evidence suggests that the molecular mechanism of mucin condensation is probably a polymer gel phase transition phenomenon (62).

Depending upon the chemical environment, polymer hydrogels can exist in either of two phases: a condensed phase or an expanded hydrated phase. The volume ratios between these two phases can reach up to several-hundred-fold. The transition of one phase to the other is a critical phenomenon (58). Experiments in isolated demembranated giant mucin granules from *Ariolimax columbianus* show that the intragranular polymer network can indeed undergo reversible phase transition, with volume changes ranging from 400- to 600-fold (62). Based on this evidence, we have proposed that the molecular mechanism of condensation/decondensation of mucin in secretion might be a polymer gel phase transition phenomenon. This hypothesis predicts the existence of one or more intragranular organic species that should behave as nonsolvents for mucins (phosphoglycerol, inositols?). The role of these species would be to stabilize mucin condensation by increasing polymer-polymer (mucin-mucins) affinity over polymer-solvent (mucin-water) affinity. While stored within secretory granules, mucin would be condensed and undergo a critical transition to an expanded hydrated phase upon exocytosis (62). The critical point at which phase transition takes place is determined by the charge density of the polyionic polymer stored in the granule; the degree of electrostatic shielding of the polyionic charges; and the dialectric constant of the nonsolvent species. Pathology of exocytosis could result from defects in any of those factors. For instance, a deficiency in mucins sulphation could lead to a decrease in charge density, with a corresponding increase in the tendency of the mucin to remain condensed and thus inhibit exocytosis.

The triggering of exocytosis by phase transition could result from changes of one or more of the following: increase intragranular water content; release of cations (including H^+) or polycations from the granule to the extracellular space; variations in the dialectric constant of the nonsolvent (by phosphorylation-dephosphorylation); or even changes in the transgranular electrical potential.

CONCLUSIONS

This review was not intended to be a quest for answers, but to furnish a general scaffolding, to build new insight, and to draft new questions. It comes at the dawn of a fascinating renaissance of fresh methods and ideas in airways physiology. However the understanding of airways secretion has remained elusive. The development of techniques to isolate and differentiate the various cell lines of the airways epithelium is still in its early stages. Respiratory secretory cells in culture can have confusing patterns of differentiation and exhibit phenotypic expressions that might not be present in normal cells in situ. Cultured respiratory goblet cells have not yet revealed much about the molecular mechanisms of mucin biosynthesis. They are also giving mixed messages with their aptitude to secrete proteoglycans. However they have disclosed some enticing new facets of what seems to be a general mechanism of product storage and release in exocytosis. Secretory granules always appear to contain a condensed, polyionic polymer network. Their polyionic charges are shielded by counterions. Upon release this network undergoes a phase transition to an expanded hydrated phase. The process could be triggered by the release of the shielding species via a membrane pore. As polyionic charges become unshielded, a jack-in-the-box mechanism is turned on, whereby the polyions unfold driving the exocytotic release of the granular content.

Membrane biophysics is yielding a rich new understanding of the physiology and pathology of water and ion exchange functions in the respiratory mucosa. The biophysics of polymer gels may provide the next set of conceptual tools to understand the other key component in mucus function, that is, how secretory cells control mucus rheology. Based on the Donnan swelling mechanism, mucus rheology could be mainly regulated by both the exchange of ions and water across the respiratory epithelium and by the control of the amount of secreted mucin. Are there any other physiologic controls operating via secretory cells? The Donnan model predicts two additional mechanisms that might function in secretory cells to control mucus rheology. One is the regulation of charge density and chain length of the mucin polymers. The other is the control of secretion of polycationic proteins. Lower charge density makes slower swelling gels. Longer polymers and increased secretion of polycations also make mucins swell more slowly, thus resulting in a mucus that remains harder for a longer time. Some of these effects have been experimentally verified. However none of the potential controls have been systematically investigated, and their validation remains as homework for the future.

ACKNOWLEDGMENTS

This work was supported by grant HL 38494 from National Institutes of Health, United States Public Health Service; and grant R 010 7 01 from the Cystic Fibrosis Foundation. The author thanks Lynn Langley for her technical assistance and Martha Mathiason for the word processing of the manuscript.

NOTE ADDED IN PROOF

Triggering of exocytosis   Secretory granules of mast cells of the mutant beige mice can undergo multiple granular-plasma membrane fusions (pore flickering) without exocytosis (2). This observation, together with the recent verification that exocytosed heparin granules can be reversibly recondensed by histamine thus showing the characteristic features of a critical phenomena (71), implies that the mechanisms that control granular-plasma membrane fusion must be different from those that trigger phase transition and product release in exocytosis. In this case, the opening of a pore between the intragranular space and the extracellular space, could allow the escape of the charge shielding cationic heparin from the granule and the inflow of water into the granule. Although these two events could activate phase transition of the heparin network contained in these granules, they do not unequivocally lead to polymer gel phase transition. According to polymer gel theory, other factors, as those listed in page 172, could also control the triggering of phase transition and exocytosis either individually or else collectively, thus operating as a redundant system.

Literature Cited

1. Aitken, M. L., Verdugo, P. 1989. Donnan mechanism of mucin release and conditioning in goblet cells: the role of polyions. In *Mucus and Related Topics,* ed. E. N. Chantler, pp. 1–8. New York: Plenum
2. Alvarez de Toledo, G., Fernandez, J. M. 1988. The events lending to secretory granule fusion. In *Cell Physiology of the Blood,* ed. R. B. Gunn, J. C. Parker, pp. 334–44. New York: Rockefeller Univ. Press
3. Basbaum, C., Carlson, D., Davidson, E., Verdugo, P., Gail, D. B. 1988. Cellular mechanisms of airway secretion. *Am. Rev. Respir. Dis.* 137:479–85
4. Basbaum, C. B., Finkbeiner, W. E. 1988. Airway secretion: a cell-specific analysis. *Horm. Metabol. Res.* 20:661–67
5. Basbaum, C. B., Mann, J. K., Chow, A. W., Finkbeiner, W. E. 1984. Monoclonal antibodies as probes for unique antigens in secretory cells of mixed exocrine organs. *Proc. Natl. Acad. Sci. USA* 81:4419–23
6. Bhaskar, K. R., O'Sullivan, D. D., Seltzer, J., Rossing, T. H., Drazen, J. M., Reid, L. M. 1985. Density gradient study of bronchial mucus aspirates from healthy volunteers (smokers and nonsmokers) and from patients with tracheostomy. *Exp. Lung. Res.* 9:289–308
7. Boat, T. F., Cheng, P. W. 1980. Biochemistry of airway mucus secretions. *Fed. Proc. Fed. Am. Soc. Exp. Biol.* 39:3067–73
8. Boat, T. F., Cheng, P. W., Iyer, R. N., Carlson, D. M., Polony, I. 1976. Human respiratory tract secretions. *Arch. Biochem. Biophys.* 177:95–104
9. Carlstedt, I., Sheehan, J. K. 1984. Macromolecular properties and polymeric structure of mucus glycoproteins. In *Mucus and Mucosa* (Ciba Found. Symp.), ed. J. Nugent, M. O'Connor, 109:157–166. London: Pitman
10. Cohen, D. V., Morrissey, J. J., Hamilton, J. W., Shofstall, R. E., Smardo, F. L., Chu, L. H. 1981. Isolation and partial characterization of secretory protein I from bovine parathyroid glands. *Biochemistry* 20:4135–40
11. Creeth, J. M., Bhaskar, K. R., Horton, J. R., Das, L., Lopez-Vidriero, M. T., Reid, L. 1977. The separation and characterization of bronchial glycoproteins by density-gradient methods. *Biochem. J.* 167:557–69
12. Donnan, F. G. 1924. The theory of membrane equilibria. *Chem. Rev.* 1:73–90
13. Dubin, S. B., Lunacek, J. H., Benedek, G. B. 1967. Observations of spectrum of light scattered by solutions of biological macromolecules. *Proc. Natl. Acad. Sci. USA* 45:1164–76
14. Edwards, S. F. 1986. The theory of macromolecular networks. *Biorheology* 23:589–603
15. Edwards, S. F., Grant, J. W. V. 1973. The effect of entanglements on viscosity of a polymer melt. *J. Phys. A.* 6:1171–80
16. Flory, P. J. 1969. Rubber elasticity. In *Principles of Polymer Chemistry,* ed. P. J. Flory, pp. 432–493. Ithaca/London: Cornell Univ. Press
17. Forstner, J. F., Forstner, G. G. 1975. Calcium binding to intestinal goblet cell mucin. *Biochim. Biophys. Acta* 386:283–92
18. Frizzell, R. A. 1988. Role of absorptive and secretory processes in hydration of the airway surface. *Am. Rev. Respir. Dis.* 138:S3–S6
19. Gail, D. B., Lenfant, C. J. M. 1983. Cells of the lung: biology and clinical implications. *Am. Rev. Respir. Dis.* 127:366–87
20. Gibbons, R. A., Mattner, P. E. 1966. Some aspects of the chemistry of cervical mucus. *Int. J. Fertil.* 11:366–379
21. Harding, S. E., Rowe, A. J., Creeth, J. M. 1983. Further evidence for a flexible and highly expanded spheroidal model

for mucus glycoproteins in solution. *Biochem. J.* 209:893–96

22. Havez, R., Roussel, P. 1976. Bronchial mucus: physical and biochemical features. In *Bronchial Asthma: Mechanisms and Therapeutics,* ed. E. B. Weiss, M. S. Sega, pp. 409–422. Boston: Little, Brown

23. Holstein, T., Tardent, P. 1984. An ultrahigh-speed analysis of exocytosis: nematocyst discharge. *Science* 223:830–33

24. Holz, R. W. 1986. The role of osmotic forces in exocytosis from adrenal chromaffin cells. *Annu. Rev. Physiol.* 48: 175–89

25. Izutsu, K., Johnson, D., Schubert, M., Wang, E., Ramsey, B., et al. 1985. Electron microprobe analysis of human labial gland secretory granules in cystic fibrosis. *J. Clin. Invest.* 75: 1951–56

25a. Jacquot, J., Goldstein, G., Sommerhoff, C. P., Benali, R., Puchelle, E., Basbaum, C. B. 1988. Synthesis and secretion of an albumin-like protein by cultured bronchial tracheal serous cells. *Biophys. Biochem. Res. Comm.* 155: 857–62

26. Jeffery, P. K. 1983. Morphologic features of airway surface epithelial cells and glands. *Am. Rev. Respir. Dis.* 128:S14–S20

27. Jetten, A. M. 1987. Regulation of differentiation of airway epithelial cells. *Chest* 91:222–35

28. Kaliner, M. A., Borson, D. B., Nadel, J. A., Shelhamer, J. H., Patow, C. A., Marom, Z. 1988. Respiratory mucus. In *The Airways. Neural Control in Health and Disease,* ed. M. A. Kaliner, P. J. Barnes, pp. 575–593. New York: Dekker

29. Kaliner, M., Marom, Z., Patow, C., Shelhamer, J. 1984. Human respiratory mucus. *J. Allergy Clin. Immunol.* 73: 318–23

30. Katchalsky, A., Lifson, S., Eisenberg, H. J. 1951. Equation of swelling for polyelectrolyte gels. *J. Polymer Sci.* 7: 571–74

31. Kent , P. W. 1978. Chemical aspects of tracheal glycoproteins. In *Symposium on Respiratory Tract Mucus,* (Ciba Found. Symp. New Ser.), ed. J. Nuget, M. O'Connor, 54:155–67. London: Pitman

32. Kilburn, K. H. 1968. A hypothesis for pulmonary clearance and its implications. *Am. Rev. Respir. Dis.* 98:449–63

33. Kim, K. C., Brody, J. S. 1989. Use of primary cell culture to study regulation of airway surface epithelial mucus secretion. In *Mucus and Related Topics,* ed. E. N. Chantler, New York: Plenum

34. Kim, K. C., Opaskar-Hincman, H., Bhaskar, K. R. 1989. Secretions from primary hamster tracheal surface epithelial cells in culture: mucin-like glycoproteins, proteoglycans and lipids. *Exp. Lung Res.* 15:299–314

35. Klinger, J. D., Tandler, B., Liedtke, C. M., Boat, T. F. 1984. Proteinases of *Pseudomonas auruginosa* evoke mucin release by tracheal epithelium. *J. Clin. Invest.* 74:1669–78

36. Lee, W. I., Verdugo, P., Blandau, R. J. 1977. Molecular arrangement of cervical mucus: a re-evaluation based on laser scattering spectroscopy. *Gynec. Invest.* 8:254–66

37. Litt, M., Wolf, D. P., Khan, M. A. 1977. Functional aspects of mucus rheology. *Adv. Exp. Med. Biol.* 89:91–102

38. Marriott, C., Shih, C. K., Litt, M. 1979. Changes in the gel properties of tracheal mucus induced by divalent cations. *Biorheology* 16:331–37

39. Nossal, R. 1987. Dynamic light scattering methods for biorheology. *Biorheology* 24:577–84

40. Phillips, T. E., Huet, C., Bilbo, P. R., Podolsky, D. K., Louvard, D., Neutra, M. R. 1988. Human intestinal goblet cells in monolayer culture: characterization of a mucus-secreting subclone derived from the HT29 colon adenocarcinoma cell line. *Gastroenterology* 94: 1390–1403

41. Potter, J. L., Matthews, L. W., Lemm, J., Spector, S. 1963. Human pulmonary secretions in health and disease. *Ann. NY Acad. Sci.* 106:692–708

42. Potter, J. L., Matthews, L. W., Spector, S., Lemm, J. 1967. Studies on pulmonary secretions. II. Osmolality and the ionic environment of pulmonary secretions from patients with cystic fibrosis, bronchiectasis, and laryngectomy. *Am. Rev. Respir. Dis.* 96:83–97

43. Rechkemmer, G. R. 1988. The molecular biology of chloride secretion in epithelia. *Am. Rev. Respir. Dis.* 138: S7–S9

44. Reid, L. 1960. Measurement of the bronchial mucous gland layer: a diagnostic yardstick in chronic bronchitis. *Thorax* 15:132–41

45. Roberts, G. P. 1976. The role of disulfate bonds in maintaining the gel structure of bronchial mucus. *Arch. Biochem. Biophys.* 173:528–37

46. Roberts, G. P. 1978. Chemical aspects

of respiratory mucus. *Br. Med. Bull.* 34: 39–41

47. Sandoz, D., Nicholas, G., Laine, M. C. 1985. Two mucous cell types revisited after quick-freezing and cryosubstitution. *Biol. Cell* 54:79–88

48. Sheehan, J. K., Carlstedt, I. 1984. Hydrodynamic properties of human cervical-mucus glycoproteins in 6M-guanidinium chloride. *Biochem. J.* 217: 93–101

49. Sheehan, J. K., Oates, K., Carlstedt, I. 1986. Electron microscopy of cervical, gastric, and bronchial mucus glycoproteins. *Biochem. J.* 239:147–53

50. Shelhamer, J. H., Marom, Z., Logun, C., Kaliner, M. 1984. Human respiratory mucous glycoproteins. *Exp. Lung Res.* 7:149–62

51. Sherman, J. M. Jr., Hasse, B., Carr, T., Tandler, B. 1988. Goblet cell isolation from cat trachea: a comparison of methods. *Exp. Lung Res.* 14:375–85

52. Silberberg, A. 1987. A model for mucus glycoprotein structure. *Biorheology* 24: 605–14

53. Slayter, H. S., Lamblin, G., Le Treut, A., Galabert, C., Houdret, N., et al. 1984. Complex structure of human bronchial mucus glycoprotein. *Eur. J. Biochem.* 142:209–18

54. Spicer, S. S., Schulte, B. A., Thomopoulos, G. N. 1983. Histochemical properties of the respiratory tract epithelium in different species. *Am. Rev. Respir. Dis.* 128:S20–26

55. St. George, J. A., Harkema, J. R., Hyde, D. M., Plopper, C. G. 1988. Cell populations and structure-function relationships of cells in the airways. In *Toxicology of the Lung*, ed. D. E. Gardner, J. D. Crapo, E. J. Massaro, pp. 71–102. New York: Raven

56. Steiner, C. A., Litt, M., Nossal, R. 1984. Effect of Ca^{++} on the structure and rheology of canine tracheal mucin. *Biorheology* 21:235–52

57. Tam, P. Y., Verdugo, P. 1981. Control of mucus hydration as a Donnan equilibrium process. *Nature* 292:340–42

58. Tanaka, T. 1981. Gels. *Sci. Am.* 244:124–38

59. Tanaka, T., Fillmore, D. J. 1979. Kinetic of swelling of gel. *J. Chem. Phys.* 70:1214–18

60. Tanaka, T., Hocker, L. O., Benedek, G. B. 1973. Spectrum of light scattered from viscoelastic gel. *J. Chem. Phy.* 59:5151–59

60a. Tartakoff, A., Greene, L. J., Palade, G. E. 1974. Studies on the guinea pig pancreas. *J. Biol. Chem.* 249:7420–31

61. Verdugo, P. 1984. Hydration kinetics of exocytosed mucins in cultured secretory cells of the rabbit trachea: a new model. In *Mucus and Mucosa* (Ciba Found. Symp.), ed. J. Nuget, M. O'Connor, 109:212–234. London: Pitman

62. Verdugo, P. 1986. Polymer gel phase transition: a novel mechanism of product storage and release in mucin secretion. *Biophys. J.* 49:231a

63. Verdugo, P., Aitken, M., Langley, L., Villalon, M. J. 1987. Molecular mechanism of product storage and release in mucin secretion. II. The role of extracellular Ca^{++}. *Biorheology* 24:625–33

64. Verdugo, P., Deyrup-Olsen, L. Aitken, M., Villalon, M. J., Johnson, D. 1987. Molecular mechanism of mucin secretion: the role of intragranular charge shielding. *J. Dent. Res.* 66:506–8

65. Verdugo, P., Tam, P. Y., Butler, J. 1983. Conformational structure of respiratory mucus studied by laser correlation spectroscopy. *Biorheology* 20:223–30

66. Widdicombe, J. G. 1989. Airway mucus. *Eur. Respir.* 2:107–15

67. Winet, H. 1987. The role of the periciliary fluid in mucociliary flows: flow velocity profiles in frog palate mucus. *Biorheology* 24:635–42

68. Winkler, H., Westhead, E. 1980. The molecular organization of adrenal chromaffin granules. *Neuroscience.* 5:1803–24

69. Zimmerberg, J., Whitaker, M. 1985. Calcium causes irreversible swelling of secretory granules during exocytosis. *Nature* 315:581–84

70. Kendel, M. V., Warley, A. 1986. Elemental content of mast cell granules measured by x-ray microanalysis if rat thymic sections. *J. Cell Sci.* 83:77–87

71. Villalón, M., Verdugo, P., Fernandez, J. M. 1990. Histamine-induced recondensation of exocytosed mast cell granules. *Biophys. J.* Abstr. In press

Annu. Rev. Physiol. 1990. 52:177–95

IMMUNOGLOBULIN SECRETION IN THE AIRWAYS[1]

R. P. Daniele

Cardiovascular-Pulmonary Division, Department of Medicine, University of Pennsylvania School of Medicine, Philadelphia, Pennsylvania 19104-4283

KEY WORDS: pulmonary immunity, immunoglobulin A, host defense, bronchial secretions, antibody

INTRODUCTION

Besides the gastrointestinal tract, the epithelial surface of the lung constitutes the next largest area that must be protected from invasion by microbes and toxic agents in the environment. Two principal mechanisms have evolved for the surveillance and protection of this epithelial boundary: One is relatively nonspecific and involves the mucociliary apparatus, which mechanically clears particles from the airways. The second is a more adaptive mechanism and involves the secretory immune system, which often operates in concert with the mucociliary escalator.

Well before the recognition of the structure and function of antibodies, it was appreciated that specific neutralizing substances could be found in the secretions of the upper and lower respiratory tract that protected the host from a variety of infectious agents (e.g. influenza virus) (24, 66). Furthermore, these humoral responses to locally applied antigens could occur independently and often in the absence of systemic immunity.

The next major advance was the recognition that the antibody responsible for this specific protection along the mucosal barrier was immunoglobulin A, IgA (61).

---

[1]This review is a revised and updated version of the chapter, "The Secretory Immune System of the Lung," by Ronald P. Daniele, which appeared in the book, *Immunology and Immunologic Diseases of the Lung,* edited by Ronald P. Daniele

0066-4278/90/0315-0177$02.00

SECRETORY IgA—IMMUNOCHEMICAL FEATURES

In man, IgA represents about 5–10% of the total protein recoverable in bronchoalveolar lavage fluid (2) (Table 1). Also, the IgA found in bronchial secretions is not only structurally different from serum IgA but is transported into secretions by a unique cellular mechanism (8, 58). Secretory IgA (SIgA) differs from serum IgA in that it is a dimer (390 kd), whereas serum IgA is a monomer. Secretory IgA is synthesized by the plasma cells located in the lamina propria of the mucosal membranes. The plasma cells polymerize two 7S monomers of IgA using a J-chain glycoprotein (about 15 kd) that is also synthesized within plasma cells. This covalent linkage of the two dimers of IgA occurs within the plasma cell just prior to SIgA secretion. The next step in the secretory sequence is the synthesis of the secretory component of about 80 kd within the epithelial cells (9). The secretory component is then expressed on the epithelial membrane at the basolateral surface and combines by covalent and noncovalent interactions with the dimeric (IgA) or polymeric (IgM) immunoglobulins as secretory immunoglobulins are being transported to the mucosal surface (Figure 1). The secretory component imparts two important functions to secretory IgA. First, it acts as a membrane receptor for dimeric IgA (or polymeric IgM) and facilitates the transport of SIgA and secretory component complexes across the epithelial cell. The complexes are enclosed within cytoplasmic vesicles and transported to the luminal surface

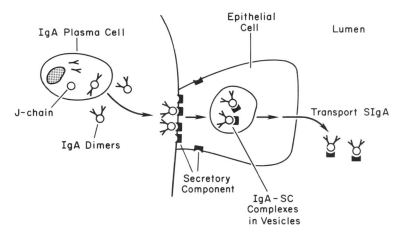

Figure 1 Mechanism of transport of secretory IgA. Dimers of IgA are linked with J-chains within the plasma cell and then secreted into the interstitial space. The dimers then bind to the secretory component expressed on the epithelial cell surface. This provides a transport mechanism via intracellular vesicles for SIgA and secretory component (SC) to be excreted by exocytosis into the bronchial lumen (reproduced from reference 15 with permission).

where they are extruded by exocytosis into bronchial secretions. The transcytosis of complexes of polymeric Ig and the secretory component (SC) receptor represents a unique type of ligand-receptor interaction since the ligand binding domain of the SC receptor is proteolytically cleaved and released into the external secretion in association with the polymeric form of Ig (52). Thus the receptor is used only for one round of transport leading to its designation as a sacrificial receptor (52).

It is unclear whether this is the only way secretory IgA gains entry to mucosal secretions, or whether there are auxiliary mechanisms, as described for the biliary tract, whereby dimeric IgA may be transported directly from serum into biliary secretions (33, 43).

A second function of the secretory component, which may have greater inportance in gastrointestinal secretions, is that it confers resistance to proteolytic degradation of the IgA dimer. Although secretory IgA is resistant to most of the proteolytic enzymes that are normally found in the gut and possibly in the lung, certain bacteria, notably *Streptococcus pneumoniae* and *Haemophilus influenzae,* can produce a protease that cleaves the IgA1 subclass into inactive peptides (30). Bronchial secretions, however, contain the IgA2 subclass that comprises about one-third of the total IgA and is resistant to these bacterial proteases (16). One of the unique structural differences between IgA1 and IgA2 is found in the hinge region of IgA1, which contains a sequence of 13 amino acids that are susceptible to cleavage by bacterial proteases (22, 51).

Functional Characteristics of Secretory IgA

The secretory IgA in bronchial secretions appears to protect the lung in several ways (17, 37). First, it promotes clumping and decreases the adherence of certain bacteria (streptococcus) to mucosal cell surfaces. Second, it inhibits viruses from infecting epithelial cells. For example, secretory anti-

Table 1   Immunoglobulins in bronchoalveolar lavage fluid

	Lavage Fluid[a]
IgA	10.2 ± 1.0[b]
IgG	19.0 ± 1.7
IgM	0.08 ± 0.04
IgD	0 ± 0
IgE	0 ± 0

[a] Healthy volunteers (smokers and nonsmokers).
[b] Values are % of total protein, mean ± SEM (data from Bell et al, reference 2).

bodies confer better protection and neutralization than serum antibodies to a variety of respiratory viruses; equally important, secretory antibodies can abolish the mucosal carrier state for certain viruses. And finally, the combination of lysozyme, SIgA, and perhaps components of complement in bronchial secretions may promote phagocytosis by alveolar macrophages of IgA-coated particles and bacteria (see below).

It is incompletely understood, however, how secretory IgA interacts with the alveolar macrophage. This uncertainty stems from two causes: (a) It remains problematic as to whether alveolar macrophages possess a functional Fc receptor for IgA (47) (see below), and (b) IgA does not fix complement by the classic pathway. Furthermore, bronchial secretions appear to lack certain classic components of complement. Thus, at first glance it appears that the enhanced phagocytosis (and killing) resulting from particles or bacteria that are coated (or opsonized) with antibody and complement might not be operative in the lung. One way out of this dilemma is suggested by the observation that bronchial secretions contain precursors for complement activation by the alternate pathway (49). This is of potential importance because, under certain conditions, IgA may fix complement via the alternate pathway and allow interaction of opsonized particles with the alveolar macrophage C3b receptor.

The debate continues as to whether alveolar macrophages possess a functional Fc receptor for alveolar macrophages, which permits the binding of opsonized bacteria and particles and their subsequent phagocytosis and elimination. A recent report using a cell-bound radiolabeled ligand showed that about 17% of rabbit alveolar macrophages possessed an Fc receptor for IgA (41). Interestingly, the proportion of alveolar macrophages bearing Fc receptors for IgA increased after lung inflammation. The controversy concerning the existence of Fc receptors for IgA on alveolar macrophages may relate to the heterogeneity of this cell population. Resident alveolar macrophages differ with respect to differentiation and maturation (23a). Thus, as alveolar macrophages differentiate and become more mature, they may lose the IgA Fc receptor. The small proportion of lung macrophages exhibiting IgA receptors in some studies may represent newly recruited or immature cells: this is supported by the fact that the proportion of these cells increases with lung inflammation.

A separate but related mechanism by which inflammatory stimuli may cause alveolar macrophages to interact with SIgA involves the secretion of chemotaxins that can recruit polymorphonuclear leukocytes and monocytes from blood into the alveoli to assist in the elimination of particles and microbes (46). Polymorphonuclear leukocytes and blood monocytes do possess functional Fc receptors for IgA and are capable of ingesting and degrading IgA immune complexes (19a, 20).

Thus defense of the distal airways may involve IgA by three mechanisms: (*a*) the opsonization of particles and bacteria by the alveolar macrophage C3b receptor; (*b*) binding and phagocytosis by the IgA receptor of polymorphonuclear leukocytes and blood monocytes; and (*c*) phagocytosis of IgA complexes by early forms of alveolar macrophages recruited during inflammation.

Role of Secretory IgA in Immune Exclusion

Secretory IgA also relates to the theory of immune exclusion. Because of its antiviral properties and capacity to agglutinate and impair the adherence of certain bacteria and antigens to the mucosal surface, IgA is thought to prevent entry of antigens beyond the mucosal barrier by augmenting antigen elimination by phagocytosis and clearance mechanisms (65). This hypothesis is supported by the increased association of allergic disease and circulating antibodies to milk and food proteins in patients with IgA deficiency (14). While such a hypothesis is supported by studies in the gut, evidence involving the lung is lacking.

Other Immunoglobulins in Bronchial Secretions

There are few studies comparing the relative concentrations of specific immunoglobulins in the bronchial tree. In one study (2) it was found that lavage fluid effluents contained predominantly IgG and IgA; little or no IgM, IgD or IgE was found (2) (Table 1). These human studies are in agreement with more detailed studies that were conducted by Kaltreider & Chan in the dog (27). In that study, the concentrations of IgG and IgA were sampled from various levels of the canine respiratory tract, including stimulated salivary secretions, tracheal washes, and bronchoalveolar lavage. Salivary secretions contained mostly IgA, whereas bronchial washes contained predominantly IgG. The contents of IgA and IgG in tracheal washes were intermediate between those of stimulated saliva and bronchial washes. Thus there is a progressive decrease in the concentration of IgA and an increase in the content of IgG, as one proceeds from the upper to the lower respiratory tract.

The measured values of IgA and IgG in the bronchoalveolar lavage are also in reasonable agreement with the immunocyte populations identified in the bronchial mucosa by immunofluorescent staining. Soutar et al (53) reported that at various levels of the bronchial tree IgA cells equaled 56 to 67% and IgG 12 to 16% of the lymphocytes; IgM cells equaled 7 to 11%. There is little agreement on the identification of IgE producing cells in bronchial biopsy specimens.

As mentioned above, under normal conditions little IgM is found in the bronchial secretions. In patients with selective IgA deficiency, however, there may be a compensatory increase in the secretory IgM (11). The incidence of selective IgA deficiency syndrome is approximately 1 in 700 individuals, but few have apparent clinical abnormalities, especially recurrent sinopulmonary infections. The adaptive potential for replacing IgA with IgM may explain this phenomenon. The secretory pathway for multimeric IgM is similar to that of secretory IgA whereby an IgM pentamer is assembled with a J-chain in plasma cells and then secreted into the interstitial fluid. The IgM pentamers also bind the secretory component, thus providing a transport mechanism in vesicles through the epithelial cells; secretory IgM is then released into the airway lumen by exocytosis.

In certain IgA-deficient patients, however, immunoregulatory compensation, instead of leading to the production of IgM antibody, gives rise to a large number of IgD-producing cells in the respiratory mucosa (12, 28). IgD cannot act as a functional secretory antibody, and these patients are prone to have recurrent sinopulmonary infections (12, 28).

IgE was once classified as a secretory immunoglobulin. This notion, however, needs revision in light of the evidence that IgE does not bind to secretory component and is not actively transported by epithelial cells (7). Moreover, earlier estimates of the distribution of IgE immunocytes in the lamina propria of the upper respiratory tract were probably inaccurate. Application of newer immunohistochemical techniques, which distinguish IgE B cells from mast cells, reveals fewer IgE B cells than previously estimated (4, 35).

The concentration of IgE in bronchoalveolar lavage fluid is barely detectable, but may increase with certain allergic inflammatory states. Although the deleterious effects that follow mast cell and basophil sensitization by IgE molecules in the atopic individual have been well studied, the defensive role of IgE in bronchial secretions remains obscure. There is some evidence that IgE possesses antiviral properties and that IgE cooperates with IgA in defending against certain microorganisms. The latter is supported by the clinical observation that patients with a combined deficiency of secretory IgE and IgA but not IgA alone have a greater incidence of sinopulmonary infections (1).

In man, the concentration of IgG in lavage fluid is about 10–20% of the total protein (2) (Table 1). This fact coupled with the evidence of measurable numbers of IgG immunocytes in the bronchial mucosa and IgG-secreting cells in lavage fluid supports the view that IgG plays a major defensive role in the distal airways of the lung.

The way IgG crosses the bronchial mucosa to enter the airways is unsettled. It does not involve a specific epithelial transport mechanism employing secretory component. Instead, IgG, similar to what probably occurs for IgE, is secreted by submucosal plasma cells into the interstitial space. IgG then may cross the mucosa by passive diffusion or by traversing breaks in the epithelial boundary, produced by acute or chronic irritation (4). Even under normal circumstances, the lung is continually exposed to airborne irritants that can alter epithelial permeability and promote the movement of IgG (and IgE) into the airways from the interstitial space.

Regional differences in the class of secreted immunoglobulins have been found along the respiratory tract with IgA predominating in the nasal and upper tracheal secretions, whereas IgG is the major immunoglobulin in the lower respiratory tract. These distinctions are important because the alveolar macrophage, which mainly protects the lower airways, possesses an Fc receptor for IgG. Bacteria are more effectively phagocytized by alveolar macrophages when coated or opsonized with IgG rather than IgA molecules (48).

All four IgG subclasses can be recovered from bronchoalveolar lavage fluid, and their concentrations are similar to those found in serum, with IgG1 and IgG2 being the most abundant (38) (Table 2).

THE GENERATION OF THE LOCAL HUMORAL RESPONSE—GENERAL CONSIDERATIONS

Several distinct phenomena of the lung's secretory immune response need explaining. First, how does antigen cross the epithelial barrier and gain access to organized lymphoid tissue? Antigen must then be processed by accessory cells and presented to responsive lymphocytes, particularly the helper T cell. Second, how is the lung's secretory immune system organized so as to elicit a specific immune response that is often segregated from a systemic immunity? An additional feature of this response is that the secretory antibody is optimally stimulated at the site of antigen application. Finally, despite the relative segregation of the lung's immune response from the systemic immune response, how is the lung's immune response integrated with other sites of mucosal or secretory immunity?

Table 2 IgG subclasses in serum and BAL fluid of normal nonsmokers

	Serum[a]	BAL
IgG1	67 ± 2.4	65 ± 2.4
IgG2	31 ± 0.1	28 ± 0.9
IgG3	0.4 ± 0.01	1.8 ± 0.2
IgG4	1.3 ± 0.02	5.2 ± 0.6

[a] As percent of total IgG, presented as mean ± SEM (adapted from reference 38); n = 15.

Fate of Inhaled Antigens

Current evidence indicates that there may be specialized sites along the tracheobronchial tree where antigen is transported across the bronchial epithelium to submucosal lymphoid tissue (45). As shown in Figure 2, these include areas where a specialized epithelium covers the bronchial-associated lymphoid tissue (BALT) in the proximal airways and less defined lymphoid aggregates in the distal airways. At first it was believed that the sole function of BALT was to provide the precursors of IgA plasma cells to the lamina propria (see below). Newer evidence, however, indicates that the epithelium overlying BALT is capable of pinocytosing and transporting soluble as well as particulate antigens (45). It is noteworthy that BALT is preferentially located at bifurcations in the tracheobronchial tree, thus increasing the likelihood for inertial impaction of inhaled particles at these sites.

In the more distal airways, particularly the respiratory bronchioles, similar epithelial cells cover other collections of lymphoid aggregates. These lymphoid aggregates are also capable of transporting antigens by a pinocytotic mechanism across the mucosal barrier. Morphologically, the epithelial cells covering BALT and lymphoid aggregates share several unique features (3, 6). The cells are flattened and possess irregular microvilli and no cilia; the

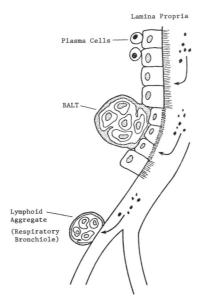

Figure 2 Location in the tracheobronchial tree where epithelial cells may transport antigenic particles across the mucosa: (*a*) The BALT, (*b*) lymphoid aggregates that are near respiratory bronchioles (reproduced from reference 15 with permission).

cytoplasm contains numerous vesicles and vacuoles (Figure 3). This unique type of cell is strikingly similar in morphology to the M cell that covers the epithelium of Peyer's patches. BALT is similar in morphology and structure to the gut-associated lymphoid tissue (GALT), which is associated with Peyer's patches in the gut. Unlike BALT, the lymphoid aggregates in the distal areas are less organized and do not contain true germinal centers.

Thus, similar to what is found in the gut, there appear to be discrete regions of the respiratory tract that act as ports of entry for inhaled antigens. Such transport mechanisms are important in the induction of local humoral responses (see below).

Most of the morphologic studies have considered BALT (or GALT) a relatively static structure. One recent report, however, has investigated the changes occurring in the epithelium covering BALT after stimulation by intratracheal administration of horseradish peroxidase (63). Studies done with morphologic and ultrastructural methods in the rat showed that the epithelium

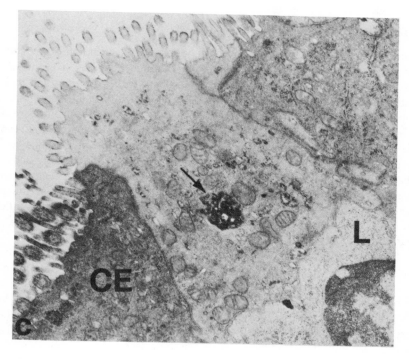

Figure 3   BALT. Lymphoepithelial cell (M cell) containing pinocytosed horseradish peroxidase deposits (arrow) in vacuoles of the lymphoepithelial cell. L = lymphocyte; CE = ciliated epithelial cell, 8900 X (courtesy of Dr. Q. N. Myrvik from reference 45).

was infiltrated with helper T cells, and the BALT epithelial cells expressed membrane Ia antigens and developed microvilli. Also, the number of nonciliated cells in the stimulated BALT increased. Thus BALT appears capable of undergoing changes in both structural and functional capabilities with acute inflammation.

It should be noted that although the existence of Peyer's patches and GALT in the gut is highly reproducible, evidence for BALT in certain species has been questioned. It is possible that the irregular distribution of BALT aggregates is due to a variable degree of antigen stimulation experienced by the animal species under study. Nonetheless, a feature common to the intestinal tract and the bronchi is the existence of a similar lamina propria in which differentiation of individual follicles is possible. Also, the differentiated lympho-epithelium in the lung supports the reality of BALT.

Thus BALT and related lymphoid aggregates have two principal functions: (a) to sample antigen from the bronchial lumen, and (b) to process antigen and generate antigen-reactive B cells that ultimately differentiate into the immunoglobulin-secreting cells.

Generation of IgA-Secreting Cells

Little is known about the identity and topographical distribution of the cells required for the generation of a secretory immune response in bronchial-associated lymphoid tissue. More is known about these cell types and their interactions in Peyer's patches and GALT. Consequently, the description of what most likely occurs in the lung must be drawn, in part, from lessons learned from the gut. Histologically, Peyer's patches, GALT (and BALT) can be divided into three regions (39): (a) the dome that contains lymphocytes, both T and B cells, as well as a significant number of functionally active macrophages; (b) lymphoid follicles that contain several germinal centers that are enriched with B cells committed to IgA. However, unlike germinal centers of lymphoid tissues such as the spleen and lymph nodes, there is little or no B cell differentiation into plasma cells. And finally, (c) there is a parafollicular or T cell-dependent area or zone (39).

Further analysis of the cell types and cell populations has been obtained by enzymatic treatment of isolated mouse Peyer's patches. Almost equal numbers of T and B cells are obtained using monoclonal antibodies to lymphocyte subpopulations (21, 31), with most of the B cells bearing surface IgM (85–92% of total B cells). A significant number of B cells in the B cell zone express surface IgA (12–16%). There are about 35–38% mature T cells in the T cell zone with helper and suppressor cytotoxic T cells comprising about 60 and 20%, respectively, of the total T cells. In the dissociated cell preparations, there are also macrophages (about 5–9%) and dendritic cells (≤ 1%)

in both T and B cell areas; these macrophages also appear to be fully functional in in vitro assays (54).

All the relevant cell types for the induction of the complete immune response appear to be present in Peyer's patches. Furthermore, in dissociated cell preparations of GALT, it was shown in vitro that these cells are capable of developing a full immune response to both T cell-dependent and -independent antigens (18, 31, 32). The situation in vivo is different, however, because the full immune response to antigen does not occur. The development of plasma cells that secrete antibody to specific antigen requires that B cells first leave GALT or BALT and complete terminal differentiation in distant mucosal sites. It is unclear whether this represents a unique structural feature of the mucosal lymphoid tissue because relevant cell types are physically separated into distinct regions, or whether the appropriate terminal inductive stimuli from helper T cells is furnished only at remote mucosal sites.

Soluble and particulate antigens are capable of traversing the specialized epithelial cell (M cell) overlying GALT and BALT. The presence of phagocytic cells, whether airway or interstitial macrophages or dendritic cells, is important because a critical step in the first phase of the immune response is the processing and presentation of antigen in combination with the major histocompatibility determinants (MHC, class II antigens). It is also possible that accessory cell function may be served by epithelial cells per se which, under certain conditions, can express class II antigens (50).

Immune Regulation

Macrophages or accessory cells present foreign antigens to responsive helper T cells. The helper T cells, in turn, provide necessary factor(s) that induce B cell precursors to divide and differentiate. In vitro studies using cloned murine T cells (from Peyer's patches) demonstrate that the helper T cells can switch B cells expressing surface IgM to those bearing IgA (55) (Figure 4). It is proposed that in the upper respiratory tract (BALT) and in tonsillar tissue, B cells are induced to proliferate and switch isotypes sequentially (IgM to IgG to IgA), according to the order of the heavy chain constant (CH) genes (10). This contrasts with the GALT where there is direct switching from IgM to IgA2 (10). These two distinct pathways may explain the preferential IgA2 production in the gut and the IgA1 production in the tonsils and upper respiratory tract. Studies of Peyer's patches and to some extent BALT indicate that there are critical switch T cells that govern the first step in inducing isotypic expression in B cells (19, 29).

It was recently suggested that there are two classes of helper T cells of mucosal lymphoid tissues that can be distinguished on the basis of the lymphokines that they secrete (40). They have been designated T helper 1

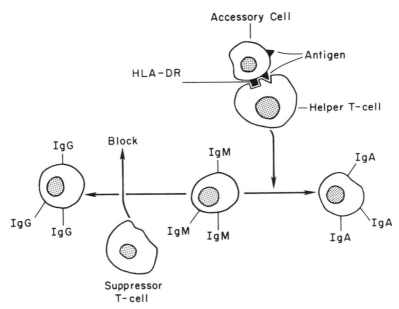

Figure 4 Cell-cell interactions involved in the generation of IgA immunocytes. Antigen is presented by accessory cells to helper T cells in association with HLA-DR determinants. Helper T cells are involved in the switch of IgM to IgA immunocytes. Suppressor cells are involved in preventing the appearance of IgG and IgE immunocytes (reproduced from reference 15 with permission).

(Th1) cells that produce IL-2 and gamma interferon, a T helper 2 (Th2) cell that produces interleukin-4 (previously designated B cell growth factor 1 or B cell stimulatory factor 1), and interleukin-5 (previously called T cell replacing factor). It has been hypothesized that IgA synthesis is principally under the control of the Th2 cell type, whereby interleukin-4 first induces the IgA isotypic switch and then IL-5 assists in the differentiation of committed B cells (those possessing membrane IgA) into IgA-secreting cells (25, 26, 34, 42). Th2 cells are found in Peyer's patches and can be activated at that site, but terminal differentiation involving interleukin-5 takes place mainly in distal mucosal sites. In contrast, the Th1 subset produces gamma interferon, which down-regulates the IL-5 stimulation of IgA secretion. Thus the distribution and relative proportions of these two subsets of helper T cells may explain the preference for IgA production in mucosal lymphoid tissues.

Despite repeated stimulation, precursor B cells for IgA synthesis do not terminally differentiate in Peyer's patches. Instead, precursor cells leave the lymphoid aggregates as large lymphocytes or lymphoblasts and travel by way of the lymphatics to regional lymph nodes (mesenteric or mediastinal) and then to the thoracic duct and the systemic circulation (5, 60) (Figure 5). They may continue to recirculate but ultimately are distributed beneath the mucosa (lamina propria). The relative functional roles of the mediastinal or bronchial lymph nodes are not known, nor is the role of the regions beneath the lamina propria that induce the terminal differentiation of IgA B cells into IgA-secreting (plasma) cells. It is likely that additional T cell help is required for this differentiation step and appropriate T cells are present in the lamina propria (36).

Although less extensively studied, it appears that T lymphoblasts derived from GALT or related lymphoid aggregates follow the same circulation pathway as B cells, with a similar tendency to home to secretory sites (e.g. lamina propria) (5). These considerations raise the possibility that activated

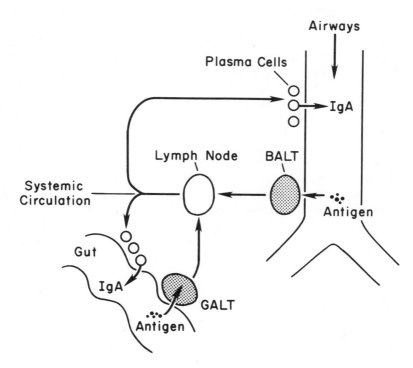

Figure 5 Enteropulmonic pathways of the secretory immune system. BALT and GALT are involved in the generation of IgA precursor cells that leave as lymphoblasts or large lymphocytes by way of the lymphatics to regional lymph nodes (mesenteric and mediastinal or bronchial lymph nodes). IgA precursor cells or differentiated IgA secreting cells then leave lymph nodes to the systemic circulation and populate the lamina propria of the lung or gut (reproduced from reference 15 with permission).

Th2 subsets may also travel with B cells to induce final differentiation with the secretion of interleukin-5.

The deployment of IgA precursor cells along with a population of helper T cells in the bronchial-associated lymphoid tissue and lamina propria might also explain why the secretory (i.e. IgA) responses are somewhat localized to the locus of antigen delivery. When antigen is introduced into a sensitized host at a particular location on the mucosa, it induces T and B cells to proliferate locally and recruits additional circulating lymphoblasts and T cells to that same site.

Thus the generation of IgA-secreting cells involves two steps: first, after antigen stimulation in GALT or BALT, helper T cells induce IgM B cells to switch to IgA precursor cells; second, helper T cells induce the terminal differentiation of these IgA immunocytes into plasma cells either in regional lymph nodes or at their final location beneath the lamina propria or both.

There is no complete explanation as to how IgG-secreting cells populate the lamina propria and what determines their predominant distribution in the distal airways. One explanation may come from the observation that bronchial lymph nodes are a rich source of IgG immunocytes that populate bronchial mucosa (36). Another level of immune regulation that could explain the particular distribution of IgG-producing cells in the bronchial mucosa is the existence of suppressor cells (55, 59). In the gut and possibly upper respiratory tract, they mainly affect IgG, IgM, and IgE immunocytes. Thus the emergence of predominantly IgA immunocytes or lymphoblasts is determined by the balance of specific helper T cells for the IgM-IgA B cell switch and by suppressor cells directed at IgG and IgM immunocytes (Figure 4).

Although based on little experimental evidence, it is also possible that the biological and physicochemical characteristics of the antigen influence the nature of immune regulation of the secretory system. For example, certain types of antigens (e.g. parasites, pollens) may foster the generation of IgE secretory responses. Here, the development of IgE-secreting cells appears to parallel that described for IgA (55). After antigen stimulation in GALT or BALT, there is probably an IgM to IgE B cell switch governed by a specific helper T cell coupled with the absence of suppressor T cells. Further, the terminal differentiation of IgE lymphoblast to plasma cell takes place in lymph node or lamina propria in the presence of a factor produced by T cells that expresses an Fc receptor for IgE (57). It should be emphasized, however, that for most inhaled antigens the balance favors suppression of IgE B cells.

TOLERANCE

A related functional feature of the mucosal immune system comes from the observation that when antigens are given by mouth, they may induce a complete or partial systemic tolerance to the same or related antigens. Suppressor T cells discussed above are probably involved in the regulation of this process (56) (Figure 4). With stimulation, suppressor T cells are activated and are usually class specific because IgM and IgG suppression occurs in the absence of IgA suppression. The question as to whether systemic tolerance occurs after the inhalation of antigen into the respiratory tract has been little studied. Nonetheless, suppressor cells could explain, in part, the selectivity for IgA responses in upper airways and the relative segregation of local pulmonary immune responses from systemic immunity.

COMMON MUCOSAL SYSTEM AND MIGRATORY PATTERNS OF LYMPHOCYTES

The cell-cell interactions of B cells and helper or suppressor T cells in the lamina propria only partly explain the segregation of humoral responses at mucosal sites. For example, studies in experimental animals and in man indicate that when antigen is given by mouth, it may elicit not only a secretory immune response in the gut (without systemic immunity) but the appearance of antibodies to the same antigens in other secretions such as the lung and mammary gland (4, 64). The functional interaction between various mucosal systems is further supported by experiments examining the traffic of cells between these sites (44, 60). When lymphocytes are taken from mesenteric lymph nodes and adoptively transferred to congenic animals, they populate the intestinal lamina propria and other mucosal sites, including the mammary gland and bronchus. Further, IgA-bearing cells from mediastinal lymph nodes selectively populate the bronchus and intestine (Figure 5). Similarly, there is a linkage between BALT and GALT; IgA precursor cells from either location can repopulate the intestinal or bronchial mucosa (60, 67) (Figure 5). Built into this recognition system is an additional level of selectivity whereby lymphocytes derived from the GALT tend to migrate preferentially to the intestines, and cells from BALT tend to home to the lung. Thus the boundaries of the recirculation pathways for IgA precursor cells must be expanded to include other mucosal sites, which together form a common mucosal associated lymphoid (MALT) system. The MALT system includes the gut, lung, salivary, lacrimal, and mammary glands, and the urogenital tract.

The mechanism by which precursor cells recognize or home to specific mucosal locations is unclear and apparently is unrelated to the secretory component. It is known that entry of lymphocytes from the blood to Peyer's patches involves the recognition and binding to specialized endothelial cells lining the high endothelial venules in these lymphoid aggregates. Recent studies (23) have identified a monoclonal antibody that identifies a specific receptor on certain lymphocytes; it appears to be a glycoprotein and mediates the recognition of the high endothelial venule in Peyer's patches. Thus the migratory pathways and ultimate destination of lymphocyte subsets appear to involve membrane recognition units on both lymphocytes and specific endothelial cells (13, 62).

CONCLUDING REMARKS

An elucidation of the structure and function of the lung's secretory immune system is essential for an overall understanding of the lung's host defenses and how specific defects in this system may be remedied. Although much new knowledge has been gained with respect to secretory immunity, there has been relatively little attention directed toward the lung. There appear to be several important areas for future study.

1. Although bronchial associated lymphoid tissue has been well characterized in the rabbit and rat, it is much less conspicuous in humans. In fact, some have questioned whether BALT truly exists in man. It seems important, therefore, to identify more precisely the locations within the tracheobronchial tree that are responsible for antigen sampling and to determine whether these same sites are also involved in antigen processing and the generation of IgA precursor cells. If discrete lymphoid aggregates can be isolated from bronchial mucosa, then it should be possible to better define the identity and function of these cells. Such studies might explain the regional distribution of immunoglobulins in the bronchial secretions (e.g. IgA in the upper airway and IgG in the lower airway).

2. An understanding of the cell-cell interactions and immune regulation that occur after the inhalation of an antigen might clarify why certain antigens selectively induce IgA response, whereas other antigens induce an IgE response. This effort would no doubt shed light on why certain individuals are predisposed to anaphylactic or allergic phenomena in the airways.

3. We are just beginning to understand why lymphocytes originating from the MALT system migrate to the same or different mucosal sites. The continued use of monoclonal antibodies to probe both migrating lymphocytes and recognition determinants on endothelial cells will help to uncover the mechanism underlying the selective targeting of lymphocytes in the mucosal immune system.

4. Finally, the notion of a common mucosal system, particularly an enteropulmonic pathway (Figure 5), has important practical implications for future immunization strategies. For example, it may be possible to immunize or vaccinate against respiratory pathogens or toxins by the ingestion of oral antigens (64).

Literature Cited

1. Ammann, A. J., Cain, W. A., Ishizaka, K., Hong, R., Good, R. A. 1969. Immunoglobulin E deficiency in ataxia-telangiectasia. *New Engl. J. Med.* 281:469–72

2. Bell, D. Y., Haseman, J. A., Spock, A., McLennan, G., Hook, G. E. R. 1981. Plasma proteins of the bronchoalveolar surface of the lung; smokers and nonsmokers. *Am. Rev. Respir. Dis.* 124:72–79

3. Bienenstock, J. 1982. Gut and bronchus associated lymphoid tissue: An overview. In *In Vivo Immunology,* ed. P. Nieuwenhuis, A. A. van den Broek, M. G. Hanna Jr., pp. 471–77. New York: Plenum

4. Bienenstock, J., Befus, A. D. 1980. Mucosal immunology. *Immunology* 41:249–70

5. Bienenstock, J., Befus, A. D., McDermott, M., Mirski, S., Rosenthal, K. 1983. Regulation of lymphoblast traffic and localization in mucosal tissues with emphasis on IgA. *Fed. Proc.* 42:3213–17

6. Bienenstock, J., McDermott, M. R., Befus, A. D. 1982. The significance of bronchus-associated lymphoid tissue. *Bull. Eur. Physiopathol. Respir.* 18:153–77

7. Brandtzaeg, P. 1977. Human secretory component. VI. Immunoglobulin-binding properties. *Immunochemistry* 14:179–88

8. Brandtzaeg, P. 1982. Review and discussion of IgA transport across mucosal membranes. In *Recent Advances in Mucosal Immunity,* ed. W. Strober, L. A. Hanson, K. W. Sell, pp. 267–85. New York: Raven

9. Brandtzaeg, P. 1983. Immunohistochemical characterization of intracellular J chain and binding site for secretory component (SC) in human immunoglobulin (Ig)-producing cells. *Mol. Immunol.* 23:941–66

10. Brandtzaeg, P. 1988. Immunobarriers of the mucosa of the upper respiratory and digestive pathways. *Acta Oto-Laryngol.* 105:172–80

11. Brandtzaeg, P., Fjellanger, I., Gjeruldsen, S. T. 1968. Immunoglobulin M: Local synthesis and selective secretion in patients with immunoglobulin A deficiency. *Science* 160:789–91

12. Brandtzaeg, P., Karlsson, G., Hansson, G., Petruson, B., Bjorkander, J., Hanson, L. A. 1987. Immunohistochemical study of nasal mucosa in patients with selective IgA deficiency. *Int. Arch. Allergy Appl. Immunol.* 82:483–84

13. Chin, Y.-H., Rasmussen, R., Cakiroglu, A. G., Woodruff, J. J. 1984. Lymphocyte recognition of lymph node high endothelium. VI. Evidence of distinct structures mediating binding to high endothelial cells of lymph nodes and Peyer's patches. *J. Immunol.* 133:2961–65

14. Cunningham-Rundles, C., Brandeis, W. E., Good, R. A., Day, N. K. 1978. Milk precipitin, circulating immune complexes and IgA deficiency. *Proc. Natl. Acad. Sci. USA* 75:3387–91

15. Daniele, R. P. 1988. The secretory immune system of the lung. In *Immunology and Immunologic Diseases of the Lung,* ed. R. P. Daniele, pp. 115–26. Boston: Blackwell Scientific. 705 pp.

16. Delacroix, D. L., Dive, C., Rambaud, J. C., Vaerman, J. P. 1982. IgA subclasses in various secretions and in serum. *Immunology* 47:383–85

17. Doe, W. F. 1979. An overview of intestinal immunity and malabsorption. *Am. J. Med.* 67:1077–84

18. Eldridge, J. H., Kiyono, H., Michalek, S. M., McGhee, J. R. 1983. Evidence for a mature B cell subpopulation in Peyer's patches of young adult xid mice. *J. Exp. Med.* 157:789–94

19. Elson, C. O. 1985. Induction and control of the gastrointestinal immune system. *Scand. J. Gastroenterol.* (Suppl.) 114:1–15

19a. Fanger, M. W., Pugh, J., Bernier, G. M. 1981. The specificity of receptors for IgA on human peripheral polymorphonuclear cells and monocytes. *Cell. Immunol.* 60:324–34

20. Fanger, M. W., Shen, L., Pugh, J., Bernier, G. M. 1980. Subpopulations of human peripheral granulocytes and monocytes express receptors for IgA. *Proc. Natl. Acad. Sci. USA* 77:3640–44

21. Frangakis, M. V., Koopman, W. J., Kiyono, H., Michalek, S. M., McGhee, J. R. 1982. An enzymatic method for preparation of dissociated murine Peyer's patch cells enriched for macrophages. *J. Immunol. Methods* 48:33–44

22. Fujiyama, Y., Kobayashi, K., Senda, S., Benno, Y., Bamba, T., Hosoda, S. 1985. A novel IgA protease from *Clostridium sp.* capable of cleaving IgA1 and IgA2 A2m(1) but not IgA2 A2m(2) allotype paraproteins. *J. Immunol.* 134:573–76

23. Gallatin, W. M., Weissman, I. L., Butcher, E. C. 1983. A cell-surface molecule involved in organ-specific homing of lymphocytes. *Nature* 304:30–34

23a. Gil, J., Daniele, R. P. 1988. Morphology of the lung's immune system. In *Immunology and Immunologic Diseases of the Lung*, ed. R. P. Daniele, pp. 21–54. Boston: Blackwell Scientific. 705 pp.

24. Hanson, L. A. 1961. Comparative immunological studies of the immune globulins of human milk and of blood serum. *Int. Arch. Allergy Appl. Immunol.* 18:241–67

25. Harriman, G. R., Kunimoto, D. Y., Elliott, J. F., Paetkau, V., Strober, W. 1988. The role of IL-5 in IgA B cell differentiation. *J. Immunol.* 140:3033–39

26. Harriman, G. R., Strober, W. 1987. Commentary: Interleukin 5, a mucosal lymphokine? *J. Immunol.* 139:3553–55

27. Kaltreider, H. B., Chan, M. K. 1976. The class-specific immunoglobulin composition of fluids obtained from various levels of the canine respiratory tract. *J. Immunol.* 116:423–29

28. Karlsson, G., Brandtzaeg, P., Hansson, G., Petruson, B., Bjorkander, J., Hanson, L. A. 1987. Immunohistochemical study of nasal mucosa in patients with common variable immunodeficiency. *Int. Arch. Allergy Appl. Immunol.* 82:481–82

29. Kawanishi, H., Saltzman, L. E., Strober, W. 1983. Mechanisms regulating IgA class-specific immunoglobulin production in murine gut-associated lymphoid tissues. II. Terminal differentiation of postswitch sIgA-bearing Peyer's patch B cells. *J. Exp. Med.* 158:649–69

30. Kilian, M., Mestecky, J., Kulhavy, R., Tomano, M., Butler, W. T. 1980. IgA1 proteases from *Haemophilus influenzae*, *Streptococcus pneumoniae*, *Neisseria meningitidis* and *Streptococcus sanguis*: Comparative immunochemical studies. *J. Immunol.* 124:2596–2600

31. Kiyono, H., McGhee, J. R., Wannemuehler, M. J., Frangakis, M. V., Spalding, D. M., et al. 1982. In vivo immune response to a T-cell-dependent antigen by cultures of disassociated murine Peyer's patch. *Proc. Natl. Acad. Sci. USA* 79:596–600

32. Kiyono, H., Mosteller, L. M., Eldridge, J. H., Michalek, S. M., McGhee, J. R. 1983. IgA responses in xid mice: Oral antigen primes Peyer's patch cells for in vitro immune responses and secretory antibody production. *J. Immunol.* 131:2616–22

33. Lamitre-Coelho, I., Jackson, G. D. F., Vaerman, J.-P. 1978. High levels of secretory IgA and free secretory component in the serum of rats with bile duct obstruction. *J. Exp. Med.* 147:934–39

34. Lebman, D. A., Coffman, R. L. 1988. The effects of IL-4 and IL-5 on the IgA response by murine Peyer's patch B cell subpopulations. *J. Immunol.* 141:2050–56

35. Mayrhofer, G., Bazin, H., Gowans, J. L. 1976. Nature of cells binding anti-IgE in rats immunized with *Nippostrongylus brasiliensis*: IgE synthesis in regional nodes and concentration in mucosal mast cells. *Eur. J. Immunol.* 6:537–45

36. McDermott, M. R., Bienenstock, J. 1979. Evidence for a common mucosal immunologic system. I. Migration of B immunoblasts into intestinal, respiratory and genital tissues. *J. Immunol.* 122: 1892–98

37. McNabb, P. C., Tomasi, T. B. 1981. Host defense mechanisms at mucosal surfaces. *Annu. Rev. Microbiol.* 35: 477–96

38. Merrill, W. W., Naegel, G. P., Olchowski, J. J., Reynolds, H. Y. 1985. Immunoglobulin G subclass proteins in serum and lavage fluid of normal subjects: Quantitation and comparison with immunoglobulins A and E. *Am. Rev. Respir. Dis.* 131:584–87

39. Mestecky, J., McGhee, J. R. 1987. Immunoglobulin A (IgA): Molecular and cellular interactions involved in IgA biosynthesis and immune response. *Adv. Immunol.* 40:153–275

40. Mosmann, T. R., Coffman, R. L. 1987. Two types of mouse helper T cell clone. Implications for immune regulation. *Immunol. Today* 8:223–27

41. Mota, G., Moraru, I. Jr., Nicolae, M., Moraru, I. 1988. The Fc receptor for IgA expression and affinity on lymphocytes and macrophages. *Mol. Immunol.* 25(2):95–101

42. Murray, P. D., McKenzie, D. T., Swain, S. L., Kagnoff, M. F. 1987. Interleukin 5 and interleukin 4 produced by Peyer's patch T cells selectively enhance immunoglobulin A expression. *J. Immunol.* 139:2669–74

43. Orlans, E., Peppard, J., Reynolds, J., Hall, J. 1978. Rapid active transport of immunoglobulin A from blood to bile. *J. Exp. Med.* 147:588–92

44. Phillips-Quagliata, J. M., Roux, M. E., Arny, M., Kelly-Hatfield, P., McWilliams, M., Lamm, M. E. 1983. Migration and regulation of B cells in the mucosal immune system. *Ann. N.Y. Acad. Sci.* 409:194–203

45. Racz, P., Tenner-Racz, K., Myrvik, Q. N., Fainter, L. K. 1977. Functional

architecture of bronchial associated lymphoid tissue and lymphoepithelium in pulmonary cell-mediated reactions in the rabbit. *J. Reticuloendothel. Soc.* 22:59–83

46. Reynolds, H. Y. 1986. Lung immunology and its contribution to the immunopathogenesis of certain respiratory diseases. *J. Allergy Clin. Immunol.* 78:833–47

47. Reynolds, H. Y., Atkinson, J. P., Newball, H. H., Frank, M. M. 1975. Receptors for immunoglobulin and complement on human alveolar macrophages. *J. Immunol.* 114:1813–19

48. Reynolds, H. Y., Kazmierowski, J. A., Newball, H. H. 1975. Specificity of opsonic antibodies to enhance phagocytosis of *Pseudomonas aeruginosa* by human alveolar macrophages. *J. Clin. Invest.* 56:376–85

49. Robertson, J., Caldwell, J. R., Castle, J. R., Waldman, R. H. 1976. Evidence for the presence of components of the alternate (properdin) pathway of complement activation in respiratory secretions. *J. Immunol.* 117:900–3

50. Scott, H., Solheim, B. G., Brandtzaeg, P., Thorsby, E. 1980. HLA-DR-like antigens in the epithelium of the human small intestine. *Scand. J. Immunol.* 12:77–82

51. Senda, S., Fujiyama, Y., Ushijima, T., Hodohara, K., Bamba, T., et al. 1985. *Clostridium ramosum*, an IgA protease-producing species and its ecology in the human intestinal tract. *Microbiol. Immunol.* 29:1019–28

52. Solari, R., Kraehenbuhl, J.-P. 1985. The biosynthesis of secretory component and its role in the transepithelial transport of IgA dimer. *Immunol. Today* 6:17–20

53. Soutar, C. A. 1976. Distribution of plasma cells and other cells containing immunoglobulin in the respiratory tract of normal man and class of immunoglobulin contained therein. *Thorax* 31:158–66

54. Spalding, D. M., Koopman, W. J., Eldridge, J. H., McGhee, J. R., Steinman, R. M. 1983. Accessory cells in murine Peyer's patch. I. Identification and enrichment of a functional dendritic cell. *J. Exp. Med.* 157:1646–59

55. Strober, W. 1982. The regulation of mucosal immune system. *J. Allergy Clin. Immunol.* 70:225–30

56. Strober, W., Richman, L. K., Elson, C. O. 1981. The regulation of gastrointestinal immune responses. *Immunol. Today* 2:156–62

57. Suemura, M., Yodoi, J., Hirashima, M., Ishizaka, K. 1980. Regulatory role of IgE-binding factors from rat T lymphocytes. I. Mechanism of enhancement of IgE response by IgE-potentiating factor. *J. Immunol.* 125:148–54

58. Tomasi, T. B. Jr. 1976. *The Immune System of Secretions.* Englewood Cliffs, NJ: Prentice-Hall. 161 pp.

59. Tomasi, T. B. Jr. 1983. Mechanisms of immune regulation at mucosal surfaces. *Rev. Infect. Dis.* 5(4):S784–92

60. Tomasi, T. B. Jr., Larson, L., Challacombe, S., McNabb, P. 1980. Mucosal immunity: The origin and migration patterns of cells in the secretory system. *J. Allergy Clin. Immunol.* 65:12–19

61. Tomasi, T. B. Jr., Tan, E. M., Solomon, A., Prendergast, R. A. 1965. Characteristics of an immune system common to certain external secretions. *J. Exp. Med.* 121:101–24

62. van der Brugge-Gamelkoorn, G. J., Kraal, G. 1985. The specificity of the high endothelial venule in bronchus-associated lymphoid tissue (BALT). *J. Immunol.* 134:3746–50

63. van der Brugge-Gamelkoorn, G. J., van de Ende, M., Sminia, T. 1986. Changes occurring in the epithelium covering the bronchus-associated lymphoid tissue of rats after intratracheal challenge with horseradish peroxidase. *Cell Tissue Res.* 245:439–44

64. Waldman, R. H., Stone, J., Lazzell, V., Bergmann, K. C., Khakoo, R., et al. 1983. Oral route as method for immunizing against mucosal pathogens. *Ann. N.Y. Acad. Sci.* 409:510–16

65. Walker, W. A. 1981. Antigen uptake in the gut: Immunologic implications. *Immunol. Today* 2:30–33

66. Walsh, T. E., Cannon, P. R. 1938. Immunization of the respiratory tract. A comparative study of the antibody content of the respiratory and other tissues following active, passive and regional immunization. *J. Immunol.* 35:31–46

67. Weisz-Carrington, P., Grimes, S. R. Jr., Lamm, M. E. 1987. Gut-associated lymphoid tissue as source of an IgA immune response in respiratory tissues after oral immunization and intrabronchial challenge. *Cell. Immunol.* 106:132–38

Annu. Rev. Physiol. 1990. 52:197–213

IONIC CHANNELS AND THEIR REGULATION BY G PROTEIN SUBUNITS

Arthur M. Brown

Department of Molecular Physiology and Biophysics, Baylor College of Medicine, Houston, Texas 77030

Lutz Birnbaumer

Department of Cell Biology and Department of Molecular Physiology and Biophysics, Baylor College of Medicine, Houston, Texas 77030

KEY WORDS: potassium channels, calcium channels, sodium channels, G protein-coupled receptors, G protein-coupled effectors

INTRODUCTION

In the most common forms of signaling, chemical messengers are used to transmit information from one cell to another and, in many cases, guanine nucleotide binding G proteins, coupling receptors to enzyme effectors, play a critical role in the response. Every response seems to include some change in the electrical properties of the cell and of the ionic channels from which these electrical properties are derived. Heretofore such changes were thought to be mediated by cytoplasmic pathways regulated by the G protein effector enzymes, but it is now clear that G proteins also couple membrane receptors to ionic channels by a cytoplasmically independent, membrane-delimited pathway. These two pathways have the respective synonyms indirect and direct (Figure 1). Although a membrane intermediary has not yet been excluded, it is likely that ionic channels will join adenylyl cyclase (AC) and cGMP phosphodiesterase (cGMP PDE) and possibly phospholiphase (PLC) and phospholiphase A_2 (PLA$_2$) as direct targets for G proteins. Furthermore,

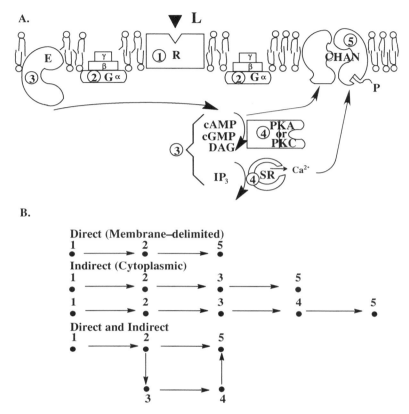

Figure 1 Components of receptor-G protein-ionic channel pathways (*A*) and examples of the pathways (*B*).
1.=R, receptor; 2.=G protein; 3.=Effectors such as adenylyl cyclase, cGMP phosphodiesterase, phospholipase C and phospholipase A_2 and their products such as cAMP, cGMP, DAG, and IP_3; 4.=PKA, protein kinase A, or PKC, protein kinase C, or SR, sarcoplasmic reticulum.

a single G protein may have several membrane targets (63) including more than one type of ionic channel (86, 105), and G proteins may wire these targets into membrane circuits capable of producing complex electrical and metabolic responses. For ionic channel regulation the G proteins may be obligatory for opening, or they may be modulatory with some other stimulus such as membrane potential being obligatory for opening. Examples are muscarinic atrial K^+ channels (direct, obligatory); photoreceptor non-selective cation channels (indirect, obligatory); voltage-gated dihydropyridine (DHP)-sensitive Ca^{2+} channels (direct and indirect, modulatory); and fast TTX-sensitive Na^+ channels (direct and indirect, modulatory).

Regulation of ionic channels by G protein pathways is widespread and its extent may be gauged from the following considerations. G proteins are linked to about 70 different receptors (4), at least eight different K^+ channels, two different Ca^{2+} channels, and TTX-sensitive and amiloride-sensitive Na^+ channels (Table 1). G proteins are $\alpha\beta\gamma$ trimers, and there are presently cDNAs for 12 α-subunits, 2 β-subunits, and 1 γ-subunit. One additional γ is known to exist for a total of 48 possible permutations (4). Ionic transport by membrane carriers may also be under the control of G proteins (88), but this review is restricted to channels and, furthermore, it is restricted to plasmalemmal ionic channels although it is possible that channels in intracellular membranes such as the endoplasmic or sarcoplasmic reticulum may be regulated by G proteins. Mainly we will consider direct G protein pathways since indirect G protein pathways have been considered previously when channel modulation via receptors had been reviewed. At present the direct G protein pathway to the atrial muscarinic K^+ channel has been studied most extensively, and it is instructive to review the historical development of this subject.

DIRECT G PROTEIN GATING OF MUSCARINIC ATRIAL K^+ CHANNELS

One of the earliest measurements in physiology has been the heart rate. Slowing of the heart was tied to the first demonstration of chemical transmission at synapses (58) and to the earliest measurements of intracellular cardiac membrane potentials (38) but, as we shall see, the mechanism by which the

Table 1   Ionic channels directly gated by G proteins

$G\alpha$ Protein	Channel	Receptor	Tissue	References
α_k, α_i-3, $r\alpha_i$-3	K^+, 40pS, IR	M_2, (ACh)	atrium	102, 15, 63, 107
α_k, α_i-3	K^+, 55pS, ?R	M_2, (ACh), SS	GH_3	11, 104
α_o, $r\alpha_o$	K^+, 55pS, NR	unknown	hippocampus	99
	K^+, 38pS, NR	unknown	hippocampus	99
	K^+, 38pS, IR	5 HT-1A	hippocampus	99
	K^+, 13pS, NR	unknown	hippocampus	99
α_i-1, $r\alpha_i$-1	K^+, 40pS, IR	M_2 (ACh)	atrium	107
α_i-2, $r\alpha_i$-2	K^+, 40pS, IR	M_2 (ACh)	atrium	107
α_s	Ca^{2+}, DHP-sensitive, 25pS	β-AR	atrium, ventricle	103, 39
α_s, $r\alpha_s$, splice variants	Ca^{2+}, DHP-sensitive, 10pS	β-AR	skeletal muscle	106
α_s	Na^+, TTX-sensitive	β-AR	atrium, ventricle	86
α_i-3	epithelial Na^+	unknown	kidney	56
α_i-3	K^+_{ATP}		RIN	19
α_o	K^+_{ATP}		skeletal muscle	73
unknown	K^+_{Ca}, 260pS	β-AR	myometrium	77
unknown	Ca^{2+}, T-type	unknown	dorsal root ganglion	61

two phenomena were associated remained elusive until very recently. Loewi (58) established that the "Vagusstoff" responsible for vagal slowing of the heart was acetylcholine. The effect was blocked by atropine, and the receptor was defined as a muscarinic acetylcholine or cholinergic receptor (mAChR). Trautwein & Dudel (95) showed that acetylcholine (ACh) hyperpolarized the atrial membrane by increasing K^+ permeability, and subsequently a latency of 50–150 msec following topical application of ACh or vagal nerve stimulation was established (25, 36, 32, 72, 66, 67). The latency at the neuromuscular junction, where the nicotinic AChR (nAChR) and its channel are one and the same protein, is about 1 msec and an intermediary coupling process between the atrial mAChR and atrial K^+ channel seemed likely.

About twenty years ago biochemical studies showed that guanine nucleotides were important in the linkage between membrane receptors and cellular effectors (79, 80). Binding studies showed that just as for other receptor-ligand interactions, guanine nucleotides modified the affinity with which muscarinic agonists displace the muscarinic antagonist 3-quinuclidinyl benzilate (QNB) from mAChRs (82). Furthermore, pertussis toxin (PTX) substrates, sure evidence of the presence of G proteins, were identified in cardiac tissue (82, 33, 52, 28). Nevertheless a connection between regulation of mAChR and guanine nucleotide binding and the latency of the ACh response recorded electrically was not made at this time, although the alteration in second messenger levels often considered in such processes such as cAMP and cGMP was found to have no effect on atrial membrane potential (96, 67), and the biochemical and electrophysiologic approaches continued along their separate paths. The introduction of methods for dispersing single cardiac cells (76) and studying the isolated cells electrophysiologically with a suction pipette (53, 54) and, ultimately with a patch-pipette (29, 83), led to single-channel studies and the identification of the inwardly rectifying single-channel K^+ currents of atria that were activated by ACh (83). Then, by perfusing the patch-pipette, Soejima & Noma (89) showed that ACh activated this K^+ channel independently of cytoplasmic mediators, but they did not invoke a G protein mechanism. This important observation was followed by reports that demonstrated that PTX blocked the ACh inhibition of atrial pacemaking (20) and atrial hyperpolarization (90); PTX blocked the ACh-activated K^+ current and GTP was required for the ACh effect (74); the ACh-activated K^+ current became irreversible in the presence of the nonhydrolyzable guanosine triphosphate (GTP) analog guanyl-5'-yl imidodiphosphate (GMP-P(NH)P) (7). These experiments established the involvement of G proteins termed G_k (7), but a PTX-insensitive nonselective cation current related to phosphoinositide hydrolysis (94, 90) complicated the whole-cell current measurements, and with awareness of the results of Soejima & Noma (89), the strongest statement on mechanism that could be made was that muscarinic activation was independent of changes in cyclic nucleotides (74).

The possibility of a membrane-delimited or direct pathway between G proteins and the inwardly rectifying K^+ channel activated by ACh finally became clear when another nonhydrolyzable congener, quanosine 5'-0-(3-thiotriphosphate) GTPγS was shown to activate single atrial K^+ channel currents in excised, inside-out membrane patches (49, 50) in a Mg^{2+}-dependent manner (51). The experiments did not identify the G protein involved other than it was a PTX substrate, and the possibility that the G protein was acting indirectly through, for example, a membrane-associated enzyme such as protein kinase C (PKC) had not been specifically excluded although Kurachi et al (49) noted that adenosine triphosphate (ATP) was not required for the GTPγS effect. G proteins purified from human erythrocytes (12, 13, 14) were applied to ACh-sensitive K^+ channels in excised, inside-out, membrane patches from mammalian atrial muscle (102, 15), and an exogenous PTX-sensitive G protein, now identified as G_i-3, preactivated with GTPγS and then denoted as G_k^*, mimicked the mACH effect on K^+[ACh] channels. G_k^* was effective at pM concentrations even in the absence of Mg^{2+}, whereas GTPγS only has effects at 10 nM or greater and requires Mg^{2+} (51). The other principal G protein purified from human red blood cells (RBC), the cholera toxin (CTX)-sensitive G protein G_s, which activates AC when preactivated with GTPγS, had no effect (102, 15), nor did the preactivated G protein transducin (T), prepared from bovine retina. Activated G_o from bovine brain had weak effects that may have been due to contamination with an activated G protein with G_k activity (102), but a direct effect of G_o could not be excluded. The preactivated α-subunit of G_k, α_i^*-3 was equipotent with G_i^*-3, or the mixture of α_i^*-3 plus βγ of G_i-3. The single-channel currents that are identified by their ACh (in this case Carbachol or Carb) responsiveness had a slope conductance of about 40 pS and an average open time at -80 mV of about 1.5 msec. These results were identical for single-channel currents activated by ACh in cell-attached patches, ACh and GTP in the bath solution in excised inside-out patches, GTPγS, G_i^*-3, α_i^*-3, unactivated G_i-3 plus GTP in the presence of ACh, and a recombinant α_i^*-3 expressed in E. coli (63, 8, 107). The G_i^*-3 and α_i^*-3 effects persist even after washes of as long as 30 min, whereas the ACh effects cease after GTP is removed. Opening probability, P_o, in the absence of activation, is nearly zero, and activation is because of an increase in P_o; neither conductance nor open times are affected, and the frequency of simultaneous openings for the customary two to three channels in each atrial patch was fitted from binomial expectations. Considerable efforts were made to rule out activation of the membrane-associated substrate requiring an enzyme such as PKC, and absence of ATP or addition of the nonhydrolyzable congener AMP-PNP, which cannot be used in transphosphorylation, was without effect. Adenosine diphosphate (ADP)-ribosylation with PTX blocked muscarinic activation, and the response was reconstituted by unactivated G_i-3 in the presence of GTP.

Thus endogenous G_k cannot be tightly coupled to the muscarinic receptor since ADP-ribosylation with PTX would, in this case, have led to permanent loss of receptor-G protein-K^+ channel coupling; nor can the endogenous G_k be tightly coupled to the K^+[ACh] channel since exogenous G_i^*-3 or α_i^*-3 activated the channel. While GTP plus the unactivated trimeric G_i-3 stimulated K^+[ACh] channels in the presence of agonist and PTX, GTP plus $\beta\gamma$ could not reconstitute the response, and this finding plus the fact that α_i^*-3 and holo G_i^*-3 were equipotent led us to dispute the conclusion of Logothetis et al (60) and Bourne (5) that $\beta\gamma$-subunits and not α-subunits mediate the G_k effect. It is now agreed that α-subunits are responsible (59, 45, 6), although it has been proposed that $\beta\gamma$-subunits activate phospholipase A_2 (45, 6) and that arachidonic acid (AA) and certain of its metabolities activate these same atrial K^+ channels. The latter follows from the observation (48) that certain eicosanoids activate muscarinic atrial K^+ channels. However this pathway is not operative in muscarinic or purinergic stimulation since eicosanoid pathway blockers are said to have no effect on the agonist-induced responses (45, 48). Furthermore, there are inconsistencies between the observations of Kurachi et al (48) and Kim et al (45) in regards to the postulated mediation of $\beta\gamma$ effects via AA release. The most noteworthy is that the effects of AA and its metabolities observed by Kurachi et al (48) required the presence of GTP, whereas the $\beta\gamma$ effects of Kim et al (45) occur in its absence (60).

The $\beta\gamma$ activator theory has been propelled in part by the idea that the α- and $\beta\gamma$-subunits could each act as effector activators. The idea is interesting, but proof for it is elusive. In most cases where this has been investigated, effects of $\beta\gamma$ have been shown to be inhibitory through a mass action effect on the α-subunit (43, 44), although in the case of retinal PLA_2 a direct stimulatory effect for $\beta\gamma$-subunits has been proposed (40). Evidence for $\beta\gamma$ mediation of the pheromone receptor response in *Saccharomyces cerevisiae* has been summarized in (6). In the retina, the concentrations of $\beta\gamma$ were in the micromolar range, i.e. $\sim 10^6$-fold higher than those needed to obtain an effect with α_i-3 on K^+ channels (15, 11) or on adenylyl cyclase (70). In the atrial K^+ channel experiments nanomolar $\beta\gamma$ was used. The $\beta\gamma$ activator results are doubtful because the zwitterionic detergent CHAPS, used in the experiments of Clapham & collaborators, can by itself activate atrial K^+ channels (47, 10) as well as other ionic channels (47). It is well-known that ionic detergents can act upon Na^+ channels and other membrane proteins including PLA_2 (75).

The idea that $\beta\gamma$-subunits might be stimulatory to atrial K^+ channels has also been challenged by experiments that show that $\beta\gamma$-subunits, including the same ones used by Logothetis et al (60, 59), inhibit these channels. In some of these experiments (71) the detergent Lubrol was used to suspend the $\beta\gamma$-subunits, and care was taken to avoid any direct effects of Lubrol. In others, the hydrophilic $\beta\gamma$ of transducin ($\beta\gamma T$), which does not require detergents, was used with the same result, i.e. inhibition of the muscarinic atrial K^+ channels. Moreover, $\beta\gamma$ was found to be more potent as an inhibitor of channels in the absence of agonist ($EC_{50} \sim$ 10 pM), which suggests that $\beta\gamma$-subunits have the suppression of agonist-independent background noise as one role, thus lending further support to the idea that the inhibitory effect is physiologically relevant.

The experiments to this point dealt mainly with reconstitution of the K^+[ACh] response. To probe further functional aspects, a monoclonal antibody (mAb) that binds to α- but not $\beta\gamma$-subunits was used. mAb 4A binds to α_T and α_i-3 and had been shown to block the light-induced transition of rhodopsin to metarhodopsin II (30, 17). The results showed that mAb 4A blocked the mAChR effect and, furthermore, the block was irreversible only if endogenous G protein was activated. Only two conclusions were possible: (a) that $\beta\gamma$ was liberated at a time when the mACh effect was blocked; or (b) that αGTP$\beta\gamma$ and $\beta\gamma$ were equipotent, which is not the case. Neither result is consistent with a role for $\beta\gamma$ in mAChR activation of K^+[ACh] (105).

While recombinant α_i-3, activated either by GTPγS or A1F^{4-}, does indeed stimulate the atrial muscarinic K^+ channel, thus removing any doubt as to structural identity of the α-subunit of G_k (63, 107), the other recombinant forms of α_i, when tested for effects on atrial K^+ channels, proved to be equipotent (107). This led us to test the native versions that were contaminated by each other at less than 5%. Native GTPγS-activated α_i-1 (α_i^*-1) and α_i-2 (α_i^*-2) were prepared from purified bovine brain G_i-1 and human erythrocyte G_i-2, as described earlier for α_i^*-3, and were tested for effects on atrial K^+ channels. The native type 1 and 2 molecules were active at the same low concentrations as α_i^*-3, and therefore the results from the recombinant forms of the α_i molecules were valid (107). Thus, at least with respect to atrial K^+ channel regulation, types 1, 2, and 3 of the G_is are G_k isoforms.

Little is known about the site of protein-protein interaction at which the α-subunit activates the K^+ channel. Recently Kirsch & Brown (46) have shown that trypsin activates the atrial K^+ channel irreversibly possibly by cleavage at lysine or arginine residues. They suggest that an inhibitory subunit similar to the γ-subunit of cGMP PDE (46) may be present.

DIRECT G PROTEIN PATHWAY TO K^+ CHANNELS IN CLONAL PITUITARY CELLS

An analogous situation to that for muscarinic atrial K^+ channels exists for K^+ channels in GH_3 clonal rat anterior pituitary cells (104, 11). Somatostatin (SST) inhibits secretion, reduces intracellular Ca^{2+} levels (85), and produces cAMP-independent membrane hyperpolarization (101). ACh has the same effects, possibly through the same type of muscarinic receptors as are present in heart. These results implicated K^+ channels, and ACh and SST were found to activate the same subset of GH_3 K^+ channels (11, 104, 102, 15). Just as it did in heart, human RBC G_i^*-3 directly activated single K^+ channel currents but, unlike the conductance of 40 pS for atrial $K^+[G_k]$ currents (102, 15, 47), the conductance of these K^+ channels from this rat anterior pituitary cell line was 55 pS (104). The rectifying properties of $K^+[G_k]$ channel were not fully determined because GH_3 cells, unlike atrial myocytes, have a variety of outward K^+ currents that complicate the recordings. Nevertheless the data indicate that the atrial and clonal pituitary K^+ channels are different. Just as for heart, G_s^* had no effect on this K^+ channel. G_o^* effects were weak and, as for heart, possibly because of contamination with G_k. The GTP-binding α-subunit of G_i-3, not the $\beta\gamma$ complex, was responsible for stimulating GH_3 K^+ channels just as it was responsible for stimulating muscarinic atrial K^+ channels.

DIRECT G PROTEIN GATING OF NEURONAL K^+ CHANNELS

A similar line of experiments to those described for cardiac and pituitary cells led us to suspect that the G protein G_o, the most common G protein in brain for which no known function had been adduced, might activate neuronal K^+ channels directly. Thus acetylcholine M_2, adrenergic α_2, serotonin (5HT-1A), dopamine (D_2), adenosine (A_1), γ-aminobutyric acid ($GABA_B$), and opioid δ and μ SST receptors are coupled to whole-cell neuronal K^+ currents by GTP-dependent, PTX-inhibitable mechanisms (69, 64, 3, 98, 22, 84, 2, 68, 100, 65). The existence of several novel G_o-gated K^+ channels was established in cultured hippocampal neurons (99). Application of purified bovine brain G_o^* to the cytoplasmic aspect of inside-out membrane patches activated four types of single-channel K^+ currents having slope conductances of 13 pS, 38 pS, 38 pS, and 55 pS. One set of 38 pS channels was inwardly rectifying and differed from the other in its burst behavior and in that it was a nonrectifying channel. The 38 pS inwardly rectifying channel was coupled to 5HT-1A receptors, but the receptors to which the other G_o-activated K^+ channels are coupled, if any, are unknown. No such stimulatory effects were observed on these channels with human erythrocyte G_i^*-3 or α_i^*-3. The neuronal results contrasted with earlier observations using the same preparation of G_o^* added to guinea pig atrial membrane patches that showed only marginal effects. The hippocampal K^+ channels are highly sensitive to G_o^*: significant activation was obtained at 1 pM, and half maximal effects were obtained at about 10 pM. In a few cases involving as yet uncharacterized channels it was observed that α_i^*-3 but not α_o^* was an activator.

In order to confirm that the observed channels, on addition of G_o^*, are indeed gated by G_o and not by a contaminant, the G protein specificity of the channel was studied by addition of partially purified recombinant α^* molecules, including α_o^*, α_i-1, α_i-2, and α_i-3, which were obtained by the pT7 expression method discussed below. All of the above mentioned types of K^+ channel were stimulated by recombinant α_o^* under conditions where prior addition of one of the recombinant α_i^* preparations, active on guinea pig atrial muscarinic K^+ channels, had no effect. The G_o-gated channels were stimulated in the absence of Ca^{2+} or ATP, and the presence of AMP-P(NH)P, added routinely to inhibit ATP-sensitive K^+ channels, and EGTA did not interfere with the actions of G_o^* or recombinant α_o^*. Thus in hippocampal pyramidal cells of the rat, G_o is a G_k, and the K^+ channels gated by it are several and differ from those present in atrial cells in various aspects including G protein specificity.

DIRECT G PROTEIN GATING OF Ca^{2+} CHANNELS

K^+ channels are not the only channels proven to be regulated directly by G proteins. G proteins also directly regulate voltage and DHP-sensitive Ca^{2+} channels from rabbit skeletal muscle T-tubules (106) and from guinea pig or bovine cardiac sarcolemma (103, 39). In fact, after the initial studies identifying G_k as the activator of atrial and GH_3 K^+ channels, we turned our attention to Ca^{2+} channels to see how widespread the phenomenon of membrane-delimited direct gating might be because Ca^{2+} channels were the channels par excellence for which cytoplasmic modulatory pathways had been established. Unlike K^+ channels, for which G protein gating is obligatory, in the case of Ca^{2+} channels, G protein gating is modulatory; the G protein is not essential for channel opening, but membrane depolarization is. Suggestions that G proteins might directly regulate Ca^{2+} channels had been in the literature (8). Guanine nucleotides changed the binding of DHPs to their receptors, thought to be Ca^{2+} channels, in cell-free membrane preparations of cardiac muscle (97) and skeletal muscle T-tubules (23). SST-inhibited Ca^{2+} currents in the anterior pituitary AtT-20 cell line by a PTX-sensitive mechanism, and the effect was mimicked by GTPγS (55). GABA$_B$ and α-adrenergic receptor ligands reduced Ca^{2+} currents in avian dorsal root ganglion cells (DRGs), and GDPβS blocked the effects (37). GTPγS inhibited the transient Ca^{2+} current in DRGs and potentiated the inhibition of transient and steady components of Ca^{2+} current caused by the GABA$_B$ agonist baclofen (18). PTX attenuated the effects of baclofen and GDPβS antagonized the effects of GTPγS. Dopamine produces a decrease in Ca^{2+} currents in snail neurons that is mediated by G_o. Opioid peptide agonists reduced Ca^{2+} currents in neuroblastoma x glioma hybrid cells; the effect was PTX-sensitive and was restored by injecting the cells with G_i^* or G_o^* purified from porcine brain, with G_o^* being at least ten times more effective (35). The α_o^* subunit was equipotent with

G_o^*. Direct G protein action might be responsible for these effects, especially since G_o had no known effectors. However Ca^{2+} currents are also reduced by activators of PKC such as 1,2-oleylacetylglycerol (OAG) and phorbol esters (78, 37, 55). Thus although a G protein, possibly G_o, mediates the effects (31), the G protein could be acting indirectly via PKC rather than directly. Perhaps the most convincing evidence comes from neurally-derived dorsal root ganglion cells in which PKC can be down-regulated by phorbol esters while the PTX-sensitive receptor-mediated inhibition persists (21).

To test for direct effects on cardiac Ca^{2+} channels (103, 39), GTPγS and G proteins were applied directly just as for the K^+ channels. However, the predominant DHP-sensitive Ca^{2+} channel, variously referred to as the high threshold, fast deactivating, long-lasting, or L channel, quickly inactivates or runs down following patch excision. Two approaches were used to deal with this problem. In one approach, ventricular Ca^{2+} channels were activated by the β-adrenoreceptor agonist isoproterenol (ISO) or the DHP agonist Bay K 8644 prior to patch excision. ISO phosphorylates Ca^{2+} channels via protein kinase A (PKA) (42, 41), and Bay K 8644 activates the channels directly. Both cause some prolongation of survival time after patch excision, but single-channel currents still ceased quickly. In the other approach, Ca^{2+} channels in vesicles from skeletal muscle T-tubules and cardiac sarcolemma were incorporated into planar phospholipid bilayers. Although both sets of channels are DHP-sensitive, the skeletal muscle channels have smaller conductances (81, 61, 106) and very different kinetics (16, 9). Incorporated skeletal muscle T-tubule single Ca^{2+} channel currents do not run down in the presence of Bay K 8644 (1, 81) and are stable for relatively long periods when the unincorporated material has been removed (106).

In inside-out membrane patches from guinea pig ventricle, GTPγS produced stimulation of ISO-activated (phosphorylated) or Bay K 8644-stimulated Ca^{2+} channels. In both cases, ISO in the patch-pipette was an absolute requirement, presumably to increase the off-rate of GDP from endogenous G protein and to accelerate activation by GTPγS before run down became irreversible. GTP was also effective in these situations. Protocols using combinations of ATP, cAMP, PKA, and forskolin were designed to mimic possible phosphorylating effects of GTPγS, and they failed as did protocols designed to block AC activity (addition of 10 mM ADPβS) or PKA activity (addition of protein kinase inhibitor, PKI). Accessibility to the inside surface of the membrane patch was not a problem because the nucleotide GTPγS and the protein G_s^* had equivalent effects.

Several lines of evidence indicate that the Ca^{2+} channel regulatory protein is none other than G_s, the activator protein of AC. First, GTPγS, to be effective in excised patches, required an agonist-occupied β-adrenergic receptor, and the latter couples to G_s. Second, only activated purified human erythrocyte G_s (G_s^*) and its α-subunit (α_s^*) mimicked the effect of GTPγS. Third, the active G protein is a CTX substrate.

In the reconstitution experiments on skeletal muscle T-tubule Ca^{2+} channels, G_s^* stimulation was more straightforward since the control single Ca^{2+} channel currents were not running down; neither ATP nor Bay K 8644 were required and the addition of exogenous G_s activated either with GTPγS or CTX was effective. Activation of co-incorporated G_s by addition of either GTPγS or GTP plus ISO also increased single Ca^{2+} channel currents. Moreover, activation by GTP plus ISO or G_s^* was asymmetrical. ISO was effective only from the extracellular side, and GTP, GTPγS, and G_s^* were effective only from the intracellular side. GDPβS blocked the stimulation produced by activating co-incorporated G_s with GTPγS. Human erythrocyte G_k^* had no effect and neither activated bovine brain G_{41} nor activated bovine brain G_{39} (G_o) had any clear effect. Single Ca^{2+} channel currents in lipid bilayers were also stimulated by phosphorylation catalyzed by PKA, and such phosphorylated channels were stimulated still further by addition of G_s^* (39). Thus G proteins directly modulate Ca^{2+} channel activity in the case of muscle producing stimulation. In the case of neurons and neurosecretory cells (37, 55, 18, 35, 21), the anticipated direct G protein effect would be inhibitory.

As discussed previously, G_s may not be the only G protein that directly activates Ca^{2+} channels, and DHP-sensitive Ca^{2+} channels may not be the only Ca^{2+} channel targets for direct G protein modulation. Recently it has been shown that brain G_i can reconstitute angiotensin II-activated high threshold, DHP-sensitive Ca^{2+} currents in clonal adrenal glomerulosa cells (34) in a PTX-dependent, cAMP-independent manner, and the low voltage-activated, DHP-insensitive Ca^{2+} channels (T channels) have been altered by GTPγS in excised membrane patches (87).

Both the indirect G_s effect via PKA-mediated phosphorylation and the direct effect are the consequences of occupancy of the β-adrenergic receptor. Hence a single G protein appears to have two effectors, and G proteins may therefore act as integrators in addition to their role as signal transducers. The α_s-subunits are four structures, two pairs differing by a 14/15 amino acid insertion/deletion and members of each pair differing by one serine residue at the carboxy-end of the insertion/deletion (4, 24, 57). The α_s of human erythrocytes is of the short type, and it is not known if both forms are present. To determine if one α_s alone could act on both effectors, the effects of three of the four splice variants, expressed in bacteria, were studied. Each splice variant, when preactivated, stimulated both AC and Ca^{2+} channels thus proving that one α_s can indeed activate two distinct effectors (62).

Recombinant α_s-subunits, when tested for their biological activity in *cyc* reconstitution assays, proved consistently to have low intrinsic activities, ranging between 3 and 5% of that of purified human erythrocyte G_s. Similarly low specific activities were obtained on testing the recombinant forms of α_s acting on Ca^{2+} channels in lipid bilayers and α_i acting on K^+ channels in inside-out membrane patches.

Whatever the reason may be for bacterial α-subunits to have low intrinsic activity, it is not due to the nine extra amino acids at the amino terminal end introduced by the way we had engineered the expression from the pT7 vector (15, 62, 92, 93). When using a bacterial α_s construct with normal amino acid composition and studying its interactions with AC, Graziano et al (26) also needed to use higher concentrations of bacterial α_s to obtain the same degree of AC stimulation as with native α_s. It is relevant that the inverse was found as well, i.e. higher concentrations of AC were required to titrate bacterial α_s than native α_s (27). Other properties of the bacterial α_s were normal, including intrinsic rates of GTP hydrolysis, GTP binding, and GDP release and interaction with $\beta\gamma$ dimers and receptors. It is likely that the lowered affinity of recombinant α_s is because of omission by bacteria of one or more posttranslational modifications that eukaryotic cells can, but bacteria cannot, perform.

The drawback of low potency also occurs for recombinant α_is and α_o and K^+ channels. Thus the GTPγS activated native α_i-3 activates atrial K^+ channels with an EC_{50} of 20 pM while the recombinent activated α_i-3 has an EC_{50} of 500 pM. Since there is such a large shift in potency, if the differences in the specificity of the three α_is depend on differences in affinity, then these specificities could be obscured when recombinant α-subunits are used. Hence it is essential to compare data obtained with recombinant α-subunits with those obtained with the native α-subunits. This has been accomplished for the α_i effects on the atrial K^+ channels (107) and the α_o effects on hippocampal neuron K^+ channels (99). However a careful comparison of potency measurements using the receptor to activate the G protein is essential to develop an understanding of the specificity of G proteins.

Literature Cited

1. Affolter, H., Coronado, R. 1985. Agonists Bay-K8644 and CGP-28392 open calcium channels reconstituted from skeletal muscle transverse tubules. *Biophys. J.* 48:341–47
2. Aghajanian, G. K., Wang, Y.-Y. 1986. Pertussis toxin blocks the outward currents evoked by opiate and α_2-agonists in locus coeruleus neurons. *Brain Res.* 371:390–94
3. Andrade, R., Malenka, R., Nicoll, R. A. 1986. A G protein couples serotonin and GABA_B receptors to the same channels in hippocampus. *Science* 234:1261–65
4. Birnbaumer, L., Codina, J., Mattera, R., Yatani, A., Scherer, N., et al. 1987.

Signal transduction by G proteins. *Kidney Int.* 32:S14–S37
5. Bourne, H. R. 1987. 'Wrong' subunit regulates cardiac potassium channels. *Nature* 325:296–97
6. Bourne, H. R. 1989. G-protein subunits: Who carries what message? *Nature* 337:504–5
7. Breitweiser, G. E., Szabo, G. 1985. Uncoupling of cardiac muscarinic and β-adrenergic receptors from ion channels by a guanine nucleotide analogue. *Nature* 317:538–40
8. Brown, A. M., Yatani, A., Imoto, Y., Kirsch, G. E., Hamm, H., et al. 1988. *Cold Spring Harbor Symp. Quant. Biol.* 53(1):365–73

9. Caffrey, J., Brown, A. M., Schneider, M. D. 1987. Mitogens and oncogenes can block the induction of specific voltage-gated ion channels. *Science* 236: 570–73

10. Cerbai, E., Klöckner, U., Isenberg, G. 1988. The α subunit of the GTP binding protein activates muscarinic potassium channels of the atrium. *Science* 240: 1782–83

11. Codina, J., Grenet, D., Yatani, A., Birnbaumer, L., Brown, A. M. 1987. Hormonal regulation of pituitary GH_3 cell K^+ channels by G_k is mediated by its α-subunit. *FEBS Lett.* 216:104–6

12. Codina, J., Hildebrandt, J. D., Birnbaumer, L., Sekura, R. D. 1984. Effects of guanine nucleotides and Mg on human erythrocyte N_i and N_s, the regulatory components of adenylyl cyclase. *J. Biol. Chem.* 259:11408–18

13. Codina, J., Hildebrandt, J. D., Iyengar, R., Birnbaumer, L., Sekura, R. D., Manclark, C. R. 1983. Pertussis toxin substrate, the putative N_i of adenylyl cyclases, is an $α/β$ heterodimer regulated by guanine nucleotide and magnesium. *Proc. Natl. Acad. Sci. USA* 80: 4276–80

14. Codina, J., Hildebrandt, J. D., Sekura, R. D., Birnbaumer, M., Bryan, J., et al. 1984. N_s and N_i, the stimulatory and inhibitory regulatory components of adenylyl cyclases. Purification of the human erythrocyte proteins without the use of activating regulatory ligands. *J. Biol. Chem.* 259:5871–86

15. Codina, J., Yatani, A., Grenet, D., Brown, A. M., Birnbaumer, L. 1987. The α subunit of G_k opens atrial potassium channels. *Science* 236:442–45

16. Cota, G., Stefani, E. 1986. A fast-activated inward calcium current in twitch muscle fiber of the frog *(Rana montezume)*. *J. Physiol.* 370:151–63

17. Deretic, D., Hamm, H. E. 1987. Topographic analysis of antigenic determinants recognized by monoclonal antibodies to the photoreceptor guanyl nucleotide binding protein, transducin. *J. Biol. Chem.* 262:10839–47

18. Dolphin, A. C., Scott, R. H. 1987. Calcium channel currents and their inhibition by (-)baclofen in rat sensory neurones: modulation by guanine nucleotides. *J. Physiol.* 386:1–17

19. Eddlestone, G. T., Ribalet, B., Ciani, S. 1989. Differences in K channel behavior in glucose-responsive and glucose-unresponsive insulin secreting tumor cell lines. *Biophys. J.* 55:541a

20. Endoh, M., Manyama, M., Tajima, T. 1985. Attenuation of muscarinic cholinergic inhibition by islet-activating protein in the heart. *Am. J. Physiol.* 249:H309–H320

21. Ewald, D. A., Sternweis, P. C., Miller, R. J. 1988. Guanine nucleotide-binding protein G_o-induced coupling of neuropeptide Y receptors to Ca^{2+} channels in sensory neurons. *Proc. Natl. Acad. Sci. USA* 85:3633–37

22. Gähwiler, B. H., Brown, D. A. 1985. $GABA_B$-receptor-activated K^+ current in voltage-clamped CA_3 pyramidal cells in hippocampal cultures. *Proc. Natl. Acad. Sci. USA* 82:1558–62

23. Galizzi, J.-P., Fossett, M., Lazdunski, M. 1984. Properties of receptors for the Ca^{2+} channel blocker verapamil in transverse tubule membranes of skeletal muscle. *Eur. J. Biochem.* 144:211–15

24. Gilman, A. G. 1987. G proteins: transducers of receptor-generated signals. *Annu. Rev. Biochem.* 56:615–49

25. Glitsch, H. G., Pott, L. 1978. Effects of acetylcholine and parasympathetic nerve stimulation on membrane potential in quiescent guinea pig atria. *J. Physiol.* 279:655–68

26. Graziano, M. P., Casey, P. J., Gilman, A. G. 1987. Expression of cDNAs for G proteins in *Escherichia coli*. Two forms of $G_sα$ stimulate adenylate cyclase. *J. Biol. Chem.* 262:11375–87

27. Graziano, M. P., Freissmuth, M., Gilman, A. G. 1989. Expression of $G_sα$ in *Escherichia coli:* purification and properties of two forms of the protein. *J. Biol. Chem.* 264:409–18

28. Halvorsen, S. W., Nathanson, N. M. 1984. Ontogenesis of physiological responsiveness and guanine nucleotide sensitivity of cardiac muscarinic receptors during chick embryonic development. *Biochemistry* 23:5813–21

29. Hamill, O. P., Marty, A., Neher, E., Sakmann, B., Sigworth, F. J. 1981. Improved patch-clamp techniques for high resolution current recording from cells and cell-free membrane patches. *Pflügers Arch.* 391:85–100

30. Hamm, H. E., Deretic, D., Hofmann, K. P., Schleicher, A., Kohl, B. 1988. Mechanism of action of monoclonal antibodies that block the light-activation of the guanyl nucleotide binding protein, transducin. *J. Biol. Chem.* 262:10831–38

31. Harris-Warrick, R. M., Hammond, C., Paupardin-Tritsch, D., Homburger, V., Rouot, B., et al. 1988. An $α_{40}$ subunit of a GTP-binding protein immunologically related to mammalian G_o mediates a dopamine-induced decrease of calcium

current in snail neurons. *Neuron* 1:27–32

32. Hartzell, H. 1980. Distribution of muscarinic acetylcholine receptors and presynaptic nerve terminals in amphibian heart. *J. Cell Biol.* 86:6–20

33. Hazeki, O., Ui, M. 1981. Modification by islet-activating protein of receptor-medicated regulation of cAMP accumulation in isolated rat heart cells. *J. Biol. Chem.* 256:2856–62

34. Hescheler, J., Rosenthal, W., Hinsch, K.-D., Wulfern, M., Trautwein, W., Schultz, G. 1988. Angiotensin II-induced stimulation of voltage-dependent Ca^{2+} currents in an adrenal cortical cell line. *EMBO J.* 7:619–24

35. Hescheler, J., Rosenthal, W., Trautwein, W., Schultz, G. 1987. The GTP-binding protein, G_o, regulates neuronal calcium channels. *Nature* 325:445–47

36. Hill-Smith, I., Purves, R. D. 1978. Synaptic delay in the heart: an ionophoretic study. *J. Physiol.* 279:31–54

37. Holz, G. G. IV, Rane, S. G., Dunlap, K. 1986. GTP-binding proteins mediate transmitter inhibition of voltage-dependent calcium channels. *Nature* 319:670–72

38. Hutter, O. F., Trautwein, W. 1956. Vagal and sympathetic effects on the pacemaker fibers in sinus venosus of the heart. *J. Gen. Physiol.* 39:153–94

39. Imoto, Y., Yatani, A., Reeves, J. P., Codina, J., Birnbaumer, L., Brown, A. M. 1988. The α subunit of G_s directly activates cardiac calcium channels in lipid bilayers. *Am. J. Physiol.* 255:H722–28

40. Jelsema, C. L., Axelrod, J. 1987. Stimulation of phospholipase A_2 activity in bovine rod outer segments by the βγ subunits of transducin and its inhibition by the α subunit. *Proc. Natl. Acad. Sci. USA* 84:3623–27

41. Kameyama, M., Hescheler, J., Hofmann, F., Trautwein, W. 1986. Modulation of Ca current during the phosphorylation cycle in the guinea pig heart. *Pflügers Arch.* 407:123–28

42. Kameyama, M., Hofmann, F., Trautwein, W. 1985. On the mechanism of β-adrenergic regulation of the Ca channel in the guinea pig heart. *Pflügers Arch.* 405:285–93

43. Katada, T., Bokoch, G. M., Northup, J. K., Ui, M., Gilman, A. G. 1984. The inhibitory guanine nucleotide-binding regulatory component of adenylate cyclase. Properties and function of the purified protein. *J. Biol. Chem.* 259:3568–77

44. Katada, T., Bokoch, G. M., Smigel, M.

D., Ui, M., Gilman, A. G. 1984. The inhibitory guanine nucleotide-binding regulatory component of adenylate cyclase. Subunit dissociation and the inhibition of adenylate cyclase in S49 lymphoma cyc- and wild-type membranes. *J. Biol. Chem.* 259:3586–95

45. Kim, D., Lewis, D. L., Graziadei, L., Neer, E. J., Bar-Sagi, D., Clapham, D. E. 1989. G-protein βγ-subunits activate the cardiac muscarinic K^+ channel via phospholipase A_2. *Nature* 337:557–60

46. Kirsch, G. E., Brown, A. M. 1989. Trypsin activation of atrial muscarinic K^+ channels. *Am. J. Physiol.* 257:H334–38

47. Kirsch, G. E., Yatani, A., Codina, J., Birnbaumer, L., Brown, A. M. 1988. α-subunit of G_k activates atrial K^+ channels of chick, rat and guinea pig. *Am. J. Physiol.* 23:H1200–5

48. Kurachi, Y., Ito, H., Sugimoto, T., Shimizu, T., Miki, I., Ui, M. 1989. Arachidonic acid metabolities as intracellular modulators of the G protein-gated cardiac K^+ channel. *Nature* 337:555–57

49. Kurachi, Y., Nakajima, T., Sugimoto, T. 1986. On the mechanism of activation of muscarinic K^+ channels by adenosine in isolated atrial cells: involvement of GTP-binding proteins. *Pflügers Arch.* 407:264–74

50. Kurachi, Y., Nakajima, T., Sugiomto, T. 1986. Acetylcholine activation of K^+ channels in cell-free membrane of atrial cells. *Am. J. Physiol.* 251 (*Heart Circ. Physiol.* 20):H681–84

51. Kurachi, Y., Nakajima, T., Sugimoto, T. 1986. Role of intracellular Mg^{2+} in the activation of muscarinic K^+ channel in cardiac atrial cell membrane. *Pflügers Arch.* 407:572–74

52. Kurose, H., Ui, M. 1983. Functional uncoupling of muscarinic receptors from adenylate cyclase in rat cardiac membranes by the active component of islet-activating protein, pertussis toxin. *J. Cycl. Nucl. Protein Phosphorylation Res.* 9:305–18

53. Lee, K. S., Akaike, N., Brown, A. M. 1978. Properties of internally perfused, voltage-clamped, isolated nerve cell bodies. *J. Gen. Physiol.* 71:489–507

54. Lee, K. S., Weeks, T. A., Kao, R. L., Akaike, N., Brown, A. M. 1979. Sodium current in single heart muscle cells. *Nature* 278:269–71

55. Lewis, D. L., Weight, F. F., Luini, A. 1986. A guanine nucleotide-binding protein mediates the inhibition of voltage-dependent calcium current by somato-

statin in a pituitary cell line. *Proc. Natl. Acad. Sci. USA* 83:9035–39

56. Light, D. B., Ausiello, D., Stanton, B. A. 1989. Guanine nucleotide binding protein, α_i^*-3, directly activates a cation channel in rat renal inner medullary collecting duct cells. *J. Clin. Invest.* 84: 352–56

57. Lochrie, M. A., Simon, M. I. 1988. G protein multiplicity in eukaryotic signal transduction systems. *Biochemistry* 17: 4957–65

58. Loewi, O., Navratil, E. 1926. Über humorale übertragbarkeit der herznervenwirkung. *Pflügers Arch.* 214:678–88

59. Logothetis, D. E., Kim, D., Northup, J. K., Neer, E. J., Clapham, D. E. 1988. Specificity of action of guanine nucleotide-binding regulatory protein subunits on the cardiac muscarinic K^+ channel. *Proc. Natl. Acad. Sci. USA* 85:5814–18

60. Logothetis, D. E., Kurachi, Y., Galper, J., Neer, E. J., Clapham, D. E. 1987. The β subunits of GTP-binding proteins activate the muscarinic K^+ channel in heart. *Nature* 325 (6102):321–26

61. Ma, J., Coronado, R. 1988. Heterogeneity of conductance states in calcium channels of skeletal muscle. *Biophys. J.* 53:387–95

62. Mattera, R., Graziano, M. P., Yatani, A., Zhou, Z., Graf, R., et al. 1989. Splice variants of the α subunit of the G protein G_s activate both adenylyl cyclase and calcium channels. *Science* 243:804–7

63. Mattera, R., Yatani, A., Kirsch, G. E., Graf, R., Olate, J., el al. 1989. Recombinant α_i-3 subunit of G protein activates G_k-gated K^+ channels. *J. Biol. Chem.* 264(1):465–71

64. Mihara, S., North, R. A., Surprenant, A. 1987. Somatostatin increases an inwardly rectifying potassium conductance in guinea-pig submucous plexus neurons. *J. Physiol.* 390:335–55

65. Moore, S. D., Madamba, S. G., Joels, M., Siggins, G. R. 1988. Somatostatin augments the M-current in hippocampal neurons. *Science* 239:278–80

66. Nargeot, J., Lester, H. A., Birdsall, N. J. M., Stockton, J., Wassermann, N. H., Erlanger, B. F. 1982. A photoisomerizable muscarinic antagonist: studies of binding and of conductance relaxations in frog heart. *J. Gen. Physiol.* 79:657–78

67. Nargeot, J., Nerbonne, J. M., Engels, J., Lester, H. A. 1983. Time course of the increase in the myocardial slow inward current after a photochemically generated concentration jump of intracellular cAMP. *Proc. Natl. Acad. Sci. USA* 80:2395–99

68. North, R. A., Williams, J. T. 1985. On the potassium conductance increased by opioids in rat locus coeruleus neurones. *J. Physiol.* 364:265–80

69. North, R. A., Williams, J. T., Surprenant, A., Christie, M. J. 1987. μ and δ receptors belong to a family of receptors that are coupled to potassium channels. *Proc. Natl. Acad. Sci. USA* 84: 5487–91

70. Northup, J. K., Smigel, M. D., Sternweis, P. C., Gilman, A. G. 1983. The subunits of the stimulatory regulatory component of adenylate cyclase. Resolution of the activated 45,000-Dalton (alpha) subunit. *J. Biol. Chem.* 258: 11369–76

71. Okabe, K., Yatani, A., Evans, T., Ho, W.-K., Codina, J., et al. 1989. $\beta\gamma$ subunits of G proteins inhibit muscarinic K^+ channels in heart. *J. Biol. Chem.* Accepted

72. Osterrieder, W., Yang, Q.-F., Trautwein, W. 1981. The time course of the muscarinic response to ionphoretic acetylcholine application to the S-A node of the rabbit heart. *Pflügers Arch.* 389:283–91

73. Parent, L., Coronado, R. 1989. Reconstitution of the ATP-sensitive potassium channel of skeletal muscle. Activation by a G protein-dependent process. *J. Gen. Physiol.* 94(3):445–63

74. Pfaffinger, P. J., Martin, J. M., Hunter, D. D., Nathanson, N. M., Hille, B. 1985. GTP-binding proteins couple cardiac muscarinic receptors to a K channel. *Nature* 317:536–38

75. Pind, S., Kuksis, A. 1988. Solubilization and assay of phospholipase A_2 activity from rat jejunal brush-border membranes. *Biochim. Biophys. Acta* 938:211–21

76. Powell, T., Twist, V. W. 1976. Isoprenaline stimulation of cyclic AMP production by isolated cells from adult rat myocardium. *Biochem. Biophys. Res. Commun. Chem. Pathol. Pharmacol.* 72:1218–25

77. Ramos-Franco, J., Toro, L., Stefani, E. 1989. GTPγS enhances the open probability of K_{Ca} channels from myometrium incorporated into bilayers. *Biophys. J.* 55:536a

78. Rane, S. O., Dunlap, K. 1986. Kinase C activator 1,2-oleylacetylglycerol attenuates voltage-dependent calcium current in sensory neurones. *Proc. Natl. Acad. Sci. USA* 83:184–88

79. Rodbell, M., Krans, H. M. J., Pohl, S. L., Birnbaumer, L. 1971. The glucagon-

sensitive adenyl cyclase system in plasma membranes. IV. Binding of glucagon: Effects of guanyl nucleotides. *J. Biol. Chem.* 246:1872–76

80. Rodbell, M., Birnbaumer, L., Pohl, S. L., Krans, H. M. J. 1971. The glucagon-sensitive adenyl cyclase system in plasma membranes of rat liver. V. An obligatory role guanyl nucleotides in glucagon action. *J. Biol. Chem.* 246:1877–82

81. Rosenberg, R. L., Hess, P., Reeves, J. P., Smilowitz, H., Tsien, R. W. 1986. Calcium channels in planar lipid bilayers: insights into mechanisms of ion permeation and gating. *Science* 231:1564–66

82. Rosenberger, L. B., Roeske, W. R., Yamamura, H. I. 1979. The regulation of muscarinic cholinergic receptors by guanine nucleotides in cardiac tissue. *Eur. J. Pharmacol.* 56:179–80

83. Sakmann, B., Noma, A., Trautwein, W. 1983. Acetylcholine activation of single muscarinic K^+ channels in isolated pacemaker cells of the mammalian heart. *Nature* 303:250–53

84. Sasaki, K., Sato, M. 1987. A single GTP-binding protein regulates K^+-channels coupled with dopamine, histamine and acetylcholine receptors. *Nature* 325:259–62

85. Schlegel, W., Wuarin, F., Zbaren, C., Wolheim, C. B., Zahnd, G. R. 1985. Pertussis toxin selectively abolishes hormone induced lowering of cytosolic calcium in GH_3 cells. *FEBS Lett.* 189:27–32

86. Schubert, B., Van Dongen, A. M. J., Kirsch, G. E., Brown, A. M. 1989. Modulation of cardiac Na channels by β-adrenoreceptors and the G protein, G_s. *Biophys. J.* 55:229a

87. Scott, R. H., Dolphin, A. C., Wooton, J. F. 1986. Photorelease of GTPγS inhibits T-type calcium channel currents in rat dorsal root ganglion neurons. *Biophys. J.* 55:37a

88. Shah, A., Cohen, I. S., Rosen, M. R. 1988. Stimulation of cardiac alpha receptors increases Na/K pump current and decreases g_k via a pertussis toxin-sensitive pathway. *Biophys. J.* 54:219–25

89. Soejima, M., Noma, A. 1984. Mode of regulation of the ACh-sensitive K-channel by the muscarinic receptor in rabbit atrial cells. *Pflügers Arch.* 400:424–31

90. Sorota, S., Tsuji, T., Tajima, T., Pappano, A. J. 1985. Pertussis toxin treatment blocks hyperpolarization by muscarinic agonists in chick atrium. *Circ. Res.* 57:748–58

91. Tabor, S. 1987. Dissection of the bacteriophage T7 DNA replication by the overproduction of its essential genetic elements. PhD thesis. Harvard Univ. Sch. Med. 257 pp.

92. Tabor, S., Huber, H. E., Richardson, C. C. 1987. *Escherichia coli* thioredoxin confers processivity on the DNA polymerase activity of the gene 5 protein of bacteriophage T7. *J. Biol. Chem.* 262:16212–23

93. Tabor, S., Richardson, C. C. 1985. A bacteriophage T7 RNA polymerase/promote system for controlled exclusive expression of specific genes. *Proc. Natl. Acad. Sci. USA* 82:1074–78

94. Tajima, T., Tsuji, Y., Brown, J. H., Pappano, A. J. 1987. Pertussis-insensitive phosphoinositide hydrolysis, membrane depolarization, and positive inotropic effect of carbachol in chick atria. *Circ. Res.* 61:436–45

95. Trautwein, W., Dudel, J. 1958. Zum Mechanismus der Membrane-wirkung des Acetylcholins an der Herzmuskelfaser. *Pflügers Arch.* 266:324–34

96. Trautwein, W., Taniguchi, J., Noma, A. 1982. The effect of intracellular cyclic nucleotides and calcium on the action potential and acetylcholine response of isolated cardiac cells. *Pflügers Arch.* 392:307–14

97. Triggle, D. J., Skattebol, A., Rampe, D., Joclyn, A., Gengo, P. 1986. Chemical pharmacology of Ca^{2+} channel ligands, In *New Insights into Cell and Membrane Transport Processes*, ed. G. Poste, S. T. Crooke, pp. 125–143. New York: Plenum

98. Trussell, L. O., Jackson, M. B. 1987. Dependence of an adenosine-activated potassium current on a GTP-binding protein in mammalian central neurons. *J. Neurosci.* 7:3306–16

99. Van Dongen, A., Codina, J., Olate, J., Mattera, R., Joho, R., et al. 1988. The brain protein, G_o, directly activates K^+ channels in hippocampal pyramidal cells. *Science* 242:1433–37

100. Yakel, J. L., Trussell, L. O., Jackson, M. B. 1988. Three serotonin responses in cultured mouse hippocampal and striatal neurons. *J. Neurosci.* 8(4):1273–85

101. Yamashita, N., Shibuya, N., Ogata, E. 1986. Hyperpolarization of the membrane potential caused by somatostatin in dissociated human pituitary adenoma cells that secrete growth hormone. *Proc. Natl. Acad. Sci. USA* 83:6198–6202

102. Yatani, A., Codina, J., Brown, A. M., Birnbaumer, L. 1987. Direct activation of mammalian atrial muscarinic K channels by a human erythrocyte pertussis toxin-sensitive G protein, G_k. *Science* 235:207–11

103. Yatani, A., Codina, J., Imoto, Y., Reeves, J. P., Birnbaumer, L., Brown, A. M. 1987. Direct regulation of mammalian cardiac calcium channels by a G protein. *Science* 238:1288–92

104. Yatani, A., Codina, J., Sekura, R. D., Birnbaumer, L., Brown, A. M. 1987. Reconstitution of somatostatin and muscarinic receptor mediated stimulation of K^+ channels by isolated G_k protein in clonal rat anterior pituitary cell membranes. *Mol. Endocrinol.* 1:283–89

105. Yatani, A., Hamm, H. E., Codina, J., Mazzoni, M. R., Birnbaumer, L., Brown, A. M. 1988. A monoclonal antibody to the α subunit of G_k blocks muscarinic activation of atrial K^+ channels. *Science* 241:828–31

106. Yatani, A., Imoto, Y., Codina, J., Hamilton, S. L., Brown, A. M., Birnbaumer, L. 1988. The stimulatory G protein of adenylyl cyclase, G_s, also stimulates dihydropyridine-sensitive Ca^{2+} channels: evidence for direct regulation independent of phosphorylation. *J. Biol. Chem.* 263(20):9887–95

107. Yatani, A., Mattera, R., Codina, J., Graf, R., Okabe, K., et al. 1988. The G protein-gated atrial channel is stimulated by three distinct $G_i\alpha$-subunits. *Nature* 336:680–82

ACKNOWLEDGMENT

We are deeply grateful to our collaborators, in particular A. Yatani and J. Codina. Preparation of this manuscript was supported by United States Public Health Service grants HL36930, HL37044, and HL39262 (A. M. B.) and DK19318, HD09581, HL31164, and HL37044 (L. B.)

Annu. Rev. Physiol. 1990. 52:215–42

G-PROTEINS AND POTASSIUM CURRENTS IN NEURONS

David A. Brown

Department of Pharmacology, University College London, Gower Street, London, WC1E 6BT England

KEY WORDS: adenyl cyclase, phospholipase C, phospholipase A, diacylglycerol, inositol trisphosphate

INTRODUCTION

Neurons possess a wide variety of kinetically-distinct K-channels. Many of these can be modified (opened or closed) by neurotransmitters and hormones acting on surface receptors capable of coupling to GTP-binding proteins (G-proteins). This review attempts to summarize some of the experimental evidence available concerning the types of K-channels (or K-currents) controlled by transmitters; the role and identity of the G-proteins involved in coupling the receptors to the channels; and the mechanism whereby the G-proteins exert this control—in particular, whether the G-protein exerts a local (direct) effect on the channel or whether a subsequent enzymatic step leading to the generation of cytoplasmic second messengers is involved. In the latter case, some discussion of the nature of these second messengers is included. For the purpose of this review the term neuron is taken to include both vertebrate and invertebrate nerve cells and also certain excitable endocrine cells and neuron-like cell lines that have proven particularly favorable for experimental study.

Tables 1 and 2 summarize some of the principal experimental work on which this review is based. Some background information about the varieties of neuronal K-channels (72, 140), the general control of ion channels by transmitters, hormones and G-proteins (46, 78, 91, 120, 139), and G-protein function (60, 63, 117, 170) is provided in the additional references indicated.

Table 1 G-protein-mediated activation of neuronal K-channels by transmitters and hormones

Channels	Tissue	γ (pS)	Transmitter/ hormone	G-protein tests				Second messenger	Notes	Refs.
				GTPγS Gpp(NH)p	GDPβS	PTX	G-protein			
I_K(IR)	Hippocampus	38	5-HT	+		+	G_o	None	isolated patches	163
			5-HT (1_A) (GABA(B))	+	+	+			PE−ve, cAMP−ve	5
	Hippocampus		Adenosine	+	+	+			cAMP,	162, 176
	Striatum		5-HT			+			cGMP−ve	155,156
	Hippocampus		GABA(B)	+		+			synaptic ipsp	96
	Thalamus		GABA(B)	+		+				124, 111
			ACh(M)	+					isolated patch	2, 166
	Locus coeruleus	80	Opiates(μ)	+						74
			Opiates (μ/δ)	+		+				37
			NA (α2)							86
			Somatostatin	+		+				73
	Dorsal raphe		GABA(B)			+				
	Substantia nigra		GABA(B)	+		−				
			Dopamine (D2)			+			cAMP−ve	124
			Opiates (μ/δ)	+		+				
	Submucous plexus		Somatostatin	+					cAMP, PE−ve	110
			NA (α2)	+		+			cAMP, PE−ve	153
			ACh	+					cAMP, PE−ve	148
	Sympathetic ganglion GH3	55	Somatostatin	+		+	Gi3		isolated patches G_s−ve	177, 180
			Carbachol							

Current	Cell	γ	Agonist		Effect		Second messenger	Mechanism	References
$I_{K(Ca)}$	NG108-15	40	Bradykinin	[+]	$(+)^{62}$ $-^{71}$	IP_3		GTPase	178, 62, 71, 69, 70
		[3]	ACh (M) (transfected)		−			noise	57, 118
	GH_3	9–14	TRH	[+]	−		IP_3	IP_3/GTPase	45, 88, 137, 95, 151, 173
	Aplysia bag cells	40	Neuropeptides				IP_3		52, 144, 143
	Dorsal raphe		$NA(\alpha_1)$				IP_3	increased $I_{K(Ca)}$	56
$I_{K(IR)}$	Aplysia R15	[7]	5-HT	+	+	G_s	cAMP	noise	161, 90, 44, 14, 94, 64
I_K	Aplysia		Dopamine						142
			Histamine	+	+				
			ACh						
$I_{K(S)}$	Aplysia sensory	55	FRFMamide	+	+		AA metabolites	cAMP−ve	23, 24, 11, 135, 164, 31, 125, 134
			Histamine		−				

Abbreviations: $I_{K(IR)}$ = inwardly-rectifying K-current; $I_{K(Ca)}$ = Ca-activated K-current; I_K = resting K-current; $I_{K(S)}$ = S-current; γ = single channel conductance; PTX = pertussis toxin; NA = noradrenaline; 5-HT = serotonin (5-hydroxytryptamine); ACh(M) = acetylcholine (muscarinic receptors); IP_3 = inositol-1, 4, 5-trisphosphate; PE = phorbol esters; IP_3 = inositol-1, 4, 5-trisphosphate; AA = arachidonic acid; + = positive effect (activation or potentiation), − = no effect; [ ] = indirect evidence.

WHAT K-CHANNELS ARE CONTROLLED BY TRANSMITTERS?

Channels Opened by Transmitters (see Table 1)

$I_{K(IR)}$ This refers to a K-current showing some degree of inward rectification that can be activated in a variety of mammalian central and peripheral neurons by a number of transmitters or hormones, including acetylcholine (ACh), noradrenaline (NA), dopamine, serotonin (5-hydroxytryptamine, 5-HT), γ-aminobutyric acid (GABA), opiates, adenosine, and somatostatin (124). $I_{K(IR)}$ may be analogous to the cardiac K-current activated by ACh (32, 122, 141) and adenosine (13, 85), but much less information is available regarding the nature of the underlying channels in neurons. In isolated patches of hippocampal cell membranes, 5-HT can activate a single channel of 38 pS conductance (in isotonic K) showing marked inward rectification (163). An 80 pS channel (also in isotonic K) activated by the opioid μ-agonist, DAGO, has been reported in cell-attached patch recordings from rat locus coeruleus neurons (111). In GH$_3$ anterior pituitary tumor cells, somatostatin and carbachol activate a 55 pS channel (180), and the macroscopic current induced in the related corticotrophic AtT-20 cell line shows inward rectification (128), but it is not yet known whether the unitary conductance of the pituitary cell channel rectifies. A fast inward rectifier current (I_{fir}) can also be recorded from some neurons in the absence of agonist (39, 140). Although similar in terms of sensitivity to block by external Cs and Ba, the agonist-induced current shows much less pronounced rectification for outward current (58, 171, 172) and may therefore be quite distinct from the endogenous inward rectifier. In contrast, in *Aplysia* R15 neurons, 5-HT does appear to increase the amplitude of an endogenous inward rectifier current (14). The rectification of the 5-HT-induced current shows the same ($V_m - E_K$) relationship as the endogenous rectifier (94) and fluctuation analysis of Cs-blocked currents yielded the same single-channel conductance (7 pS in 40 mM external K) in the absence and presence of 5-HT (64). (It should be noted that the action of 5-HT in *Aplysia* cells is very different from that in mammalian cells, in that enhancement of the R15 current involves cAMP-mediated phosphorylation whereas activation of the inward rectifier channels by 5-HT in hippocampal neurons does not involve a cytoplasmic messenger—see further below.)

$I_{K(Ca)}$ This refers to the various species of Ca-activated K-currents activated by some peptide hormones and transmitters in NG108–15 neuroblastoma hybrid cells (70, 71, 178), GH$_3$ pituitary tumor cells (45, 137), and certain *Aplysia* neurons (52, 144) as a result of transmitter-induced generation of inositol trisphosphate (IP$_3$) and consequent elevation of intracellular Ca (see below). The channels underlying this current belong to the small or medium class of Ca-activated K-channels (64, 70, 88). Those in NG108–15 and GH$_3$ cells are further characterized by their insensitivity to tetraethylammonium (TEA) and sensitivity to block by apamin or tubocurarine (69, 137; cf 34); the *Aplysia* channels show a rather different pharmacology (144). These (or similar) Ca-activated K-currents are common to a variety of mammalian neurons, where they are normally activated by the Ca entering the cell during action potentials, and this naturally-activated current is frequently inhibited by transmitters (see below and Table 2). In spite of the adjuvant presence of comparable biochemical pathways for releasing intracellular Ca, there is no firm evidence that normal mammalian nerve cells are activated in this way by transmitters, though an enhancement by NA of the spike-activated current has been reported in dorsal raphe neurons (56). Also—and in contrast to certain secretory cells (108, 129)—the large-conductance BK channels (107) present in many neurons (16) do not appear susceptible to activation or inhibition by transmitters (partly, perhaps, because of their lower sensitivity to Ca).

$I_{K(s)}$ The S-current is a moderately voltage-sensitive resting K-current carried by 55 pS channels (147) that is present in *Aplysia* sensory neurons (82, 136) and their terminals (12), and in some other molluscan neurons (e.g. 40, 41), which can be enhanced by the peptide FRMFamide (11, 23) or by histamine (134), and inhibited by 5-HT (see Table 2 and below).

I_K This refers to an outward current activated by several transmitters in molluscan neurons (80). Evidence is now strong that a G-protein coupling mechanism is involved in the generation of this current by dopamine, ACh, and histamine in *Aplysia* abdominal neurons (142).

Channels Closed by Transmitters (Table 2)

In vertebrate neurons, transmitters and hormones can inhibit a variety of endogenous K-currents, including resting (voltage-independent) currents ($I_{K(rest)}$), at least two pharmacologically different species of Ca-activated K-currents ($I_{K(Ca)}$), a slow voltage-gated K-current (the M-current, $I_{K(M)}$), and an inwardly rectifying K-current ($I_{K(IR)}$). These effects are responsible for many of the excitatory synaptic phenomena in the nervous system, and therefore have a major signalling function. However there is still relatively little known about the properties of the channels underlying these currents. By analogy with skeletal muscle (136), the channels responsible for the transmitter-sensitive Ca-activated K-current are likely to be of low (10–15 pS) conductance, with high sensitivity to Ca and relative insensitivity to voltage. Appropriate channels of about 15 pS conductance have been detected in excised patches from hippocampal neurons (87). M-channels have not yet

Table 2 G-protein-mediated inhibition of neuronal K-channels by transmitters and hormones

Channels	Tissue	γ (pS)	Transmitter/ hormone	G-protein tests GTPγS Gpp(NH)p	GDPβS	PTX	G-protein	Second messenger	Notes	Refs.
$I_{K(rest)}$	Hippocampus		ACh (M)	+		−		?DAG	PE +ve cAMP −ve	99, 47, 10, 103, 30
$I_{K(M)}$	Frog sympathetic ganglion		ACh (M) LHRH	+	+	−		?DAG ?Ca	PE +ve cAMP −ve IP₃ −ve	130, 76, 93, 131, 25, 132, 18, 159
	Rat sympathetic ganglion	[2]	ACh (M)	+	+	−		?DAG	PE +ve cAMP −ve noise IP₃ −ve	104, 29, 106
	NG108–15	[3]	Bradykinin	+		−		?DAG	PE +ve noise IP₃ −ve	69, 57, 118, 26, 27
	Hippocampus		ACh (M)			−		?IP₃	PE −ve IP₃ +ve	48, 47
$I_{K(IR)}$	Nucleus basalis		Subst. P.	+		−			cAMP −ve	115

	Tissue		Transmitter		G-protein	Messenger	Effect	References
$I_{K(IR)}$	Nucleus basalis		Subst. P.	+	—		cAMP −ve	115
$I_{K(S)}$	Helix		5-HT Dopamine FRMFamide		G_s	cAMP	cAMP +ve	40, 41
	Aplysia sensory neuron	55	5HT Peptides		G_s	cAMP	isolated patches cAMP +ve PKA +ve PKI inhibits	38 147, 33, 165, 146, 12, 1
$I_{K(Ca)}$	Hippocampus	14	NA (β_1) Histamine (H_2)		—	G_s	cAMP	cAMP +ve block- ed by PKA in- hibitor	100, 65, 101, 102, 87
			ACh (M)			?DAG	PE +ve	99, 47, 10, 103
	Frog sympathet- ic ganglion		ACh (M)				PE −ve cAMP −ve	25, 158
	Myenteric and submucous AH-cells		SP 5-HT ACh (M) Bradykinin	− −		?cAMP		174, 61, 119, 126, 145
	Sensory gangl- ion		PGs		G_s	?Ca↓ ?cAMP		145, 113, 123 55, 168, 169

Abbreviations (see also Table 1): $I_{K(rest)}$ = resting (leak) K-current; $I_{K(M)}$ = M-current; DAG = diacylglycerol.

been unequivocally identified in patch recordings, but they are also likely to be of low conductance; noise analysis has yielded estimated conductances of 1–2 pS in sympathetic neurons (106) and 3 pS in neuroblastoma hybrid cells (118). A variety of resting, inwardly rectifying and fast transient and sustained voltage-gated K-channels have also been described in vertebrate neurons (169), but which (if any) of these is closed by transmitters or G-proteins is unknown. Likewise, the K channels expressed from cloned DNA/mRNAs appear to belong to the delayed rectifier/transient variety of voltage-gated channels (152, 157) that are generally insensitive to transmitters, and the effects of G-proteins on these channels have not been reported. (Although inhibition of A-currents has occasionally been reported (45, 116), this does not appear to be a widespread phenomenon.) This paucity of information at the channel/molecular level remains a serious hindrance to the analysis of mechanisms of channel closure.

Equivalent channel closure responses are also widespread in molluscan neurons, the best studied of which is the inhibition by 5-HT of the 55 pS channels responsible for the S-current ($I_{K(S)}$) in *Aplysia* neurons (see above and Table 1).

EVIDENCE FOR G-PROTEIN INVOLVEMENT

Current knowledge of the general structure and modus operandi of the receptors listed in Tables 1 and 2 (e.g. 42) carries a strong implication that any effects they exert on ion channels are very likely to be mediated by G-proteins (170). The aim of this section is, therefore, to examine to what extent this inference is backed by direct experimental evidence when changes in K-channel activity are addressed as the end-point of receptor activation.

The usual test employed in electrophysiologic experiments is based on those pioneered by Levitan et al (14, 161) in *Aplysia* neurons and by Pfaffinger et al (133) and Breitweiser & Szabo (21, 22) in cardiac muscle—namely, to apply analogues of GTP or GDP into the cell (either by microelectrode injection or by inclusion in a whole-cell patch-electrode) in the hope of reducing the rate of reassociation or dissociation respectively of the activated α-subunits. Thus inclusion of stable GTP analogues [GTPγS, Gpp(NH)p] may be expected to augment or prolong agonist-induced effects (and possibly replicate them, if the resting G-protein cycle is sufficiently rapid), while GDPβS might antagonize if present in sufficient amounts to compete with endogenous GTP. Using such approaches, inferences for G-protein involvement in both K-channel opening and closing in a variety of cells can be drawn (Tables 1 and 2). However some limitations to this approach have also become apparent. First, as shown by Breitweiser & Szabo (22), the effectiveness of the GTP analogues (in terms of activation rate) will depend on the endogenous level of GTP [maximal K-current activation rate in cardiac cells in the presence of acetylcholine requiring 5 GTPγS : 1 GTP or 20 Gpp(NH)p : 1 GTP]. The endogenous GTP level is uncertain and likely to vary in microelectrode-impaled cells and may be 25–50 μM (22) in internally dialyzed cells even in the absence of added GTP. Hence, attainment of appropriate concentrations of analogue may not always be easy and negative effects not necessarily conclusive. The same consideration of competition with endogenous GTP applies even more for antagonism by GDPβS, which is not bound irreversibly; as a result, very high concentrations of intracellular GDPβS (100 μM to 1 mM) are necessary for effective antagonism, which confers the risk of complicating side-effect due to (for instance) contaminants (90, 131). A second area of interpretative uncertainty concerns the ability of stable GTP analogues to imitate the effect of receptor activation. This depends on the endogenous turnover rate of the G-protein cycle in the absence of ligand, which in turn depends on the GDP dissociation rate (51). This, coupled with the slow dissociation rate of the GTPγS–α-subunit complex, means that the effect of added GTPγS tends to be slow in onset and slow to reach equilibrium, even when added directly to isolated membrane patches (85) or when applied rapidly by concentration-jump techniques (43). Moreover, the dissociation rate for GDP may differ for different G-proteins, so that effects of GTPγS may be apparently selective even when G-proteins mediate more than one effect. For example, both closure of S-channels by serotonin and opening of S-channels by FRMFamide are mediated by G-proteins (see below), yet only the opening response is normally seen following internal application of GTPγS (24, 164).

An alternative and prospectively useful diagnostic approach might be to apply antibodies that inhibit the GTPase activity or receptor recognition of the G-protein α-subunit. This has been used effectively to inhibit the activation of atrial K-channels in isolated membrane patches by pure G-protein (181). Intracellular injection of anti-G$_o$ antibodies has been found to block the inhibition of Ca currents by dopamine in snail neurons (67, 127) and by noradrenaline in neuroblastoma hybrid cells (28), but has not yet been applied to G-protein controlled K-currents in neurons.

IDENTIFICATION OF G-PROTEIN SPECIES

What G-Proteins Are Present in Nerve Cells?

G-proteins may be classified on the basis of their α-subunits into at least five groups: G$_s$/G$_{olf}$ (adenylate cyclase activating); G$_t$ (transducin, coupling to phosphodiesterase); G$_i$ (cyclase-inhibiting); G$_o$; and G$_p$ (coupling to phospholipase C) (60, 63). There have been a number of studies on their distribution in the nervous system, which use either α-subunit antibody or mRNA localization. G_s and G_o are the most widely abundant. G_o in particular appears to be uniquely associated with the nervous system (6, 20, 35). In striatal cell cultures, G_o comprises up to 0.3% of neuronal protein whereas a 40-kd PTX-ribosylated protein (G_i?) was more prevalent in glial cultures (19). Within the central nervous system quite substantial variations in G-protein distribution have been reported. Brann et al (20) describe mRNA distribution profiles for G_s, G_{i2}, G_{i1}, and G_o in cerebral cortex, hippocampus, caudate putamen, globus pallidus, cerebellum, choroid plexus, liver, heart, and kidney. High concentrations of both G_s and G_{i2} mRNA were present in all regions except the caudate putamen; G_{i1} mRNA was restricted to the brain, but could not be detected in either the caudate putamen or globus pallidus, while G_o mRNA (also restricted to the brain) was absent from the globus pallidus. This differential distribution was confirmed by in situ hybridization. Largent et al (89) also completed an in situ hybridization study on the distribution of mRNAs for $G_{\alpha\text{-}s}$, $G_{\alpha\text{-}o}$, and G_β. $G_{\alpha\text{-}s}$ and G_β were both widely distributed, but $G_{\alpha\text{-}o}$ mRNA showed a more restricted distribution, with high concentrations in the hippocampus (pyramidal cells and dentate gyrus), cerebellar Purkinje cells, habenula, endopiriform nucleus, and claustrum. Using immunohistochemistry, Worley et al (175) reported strong staining for G_o in the molecular layer of the cerebral cortex, the neuropil (but not the pyramidal cell layer) of the hippocampus, the pars reticulata of the substantia nigra, the molecular layer of the cerebellum, the substantia gelatinosa of the spinal cord and the posterior pituitary. Within the peripheral nervous system, dense G_o-immunoreactivity has been reported in the myenteric and submucous plexuses of the intestine, in the superior cervical ganglion (particularly presynaptic terminals), and in the adrenal medulla (but not the adrenal cortex) (154). The presence of G_o, together with two other PTx substrates, in chromaffin cell membranes has also been reported (160). Developmental studies (35) have revealed that G_o in rat brain was low before birth, but increased thereafter reaching a peak at 4 weeks and further that it was associated with nerve cell membranes and synapses, but not the somatic cytoplasm. A close association of G_o with neurons and with the development of neuronal excitability is also indicated by recent studies on neuroblastoma hybrid cells in which immunoreactivity for G_o was present at low levels in undifferentiated (nonexcitable) cells, but increased substantially following their differentiation into excitable neuron-like cells. However G_i immunoreactivity remained at approximately the same level in both differentiated and undifferentiated cells (114).

What G-Proteins Couple to K-Channels?

Given the above information about the species of G-proteins present in nerve cells, how can the species responsible for coupling receptors to K-channels be identified? Three approaches have been used to tackle this question: the use of pertussis toxin (PTx); the application of purified or recombinant G-proteins; and the application of function disrupting antibodies.

PERTUSSIS TOXIN (PTX) SENSITIVITY   The most frequently used first step is to test whether the effect of receptor activation is blocked by PTx, which ADP-ribosylates the α-subunits of G_t, G_o, and the three forms of G_i (60, 63). By this criterion, a rather clear classification emerges in respect to receptor control of K-currents (Tables 1 and 2). Where tested, receptor-mediated activation of the inwardly rectifying current is uniformly blocked by PTx (except 86); whereas activation of the Ca-dependent K-current and inhibition of the various K-currents are not.

RECONSTITUTION   When the resident G-protein can be inactivated by PTx, different G-proteins can be tested for their ability to reconstitute the response to the receptor-ligand. This approach has been used to show that the activation of K-channels in membranes of GH_3 pituitary tumor cells by somatostatin, when blocked by PTx, can be regenerated by direct application of GTPγS-preactivated G_{i3} (G_k), but not by a thousand-fold higher concentration of preactivated G_s (177, 180). These channels can be activated directly by the G-protein (see below) and thus reconstitution tests can be performed in isolated patches—indeed, there is no need to inactivate the native G-protein with PTx as long as agonist is not applied. The same approach can be used for macroscopic currents—witness the preferential reconstitution of Ca-current inhibition by opiates in neuroblastoma hybrid cells (68) and by neuropeptide Y in dorsal root ganglion cells (49) by G_o—but G-protein has not yet been employed to reconstitute macroscopic K-currents. However, reconstitution tests only show which species of G-protein is (or are) potentially capable of mediating the channel response, not which one actually mediates the response in the normal cell. This has become a question of added significance in view of the fact that there appears to be considerable promiscuity both in the ability of a single G-protein to couple to more than one effector (e.g. G_s coupling with equal facility to adenylate cyclase and Ca channels: 109, 179) and in the ability of different homologous G-protein α-subunits to activate the same ion channel (183).

ANTIBODIES   An alternative approach to identification is to use specific antibodies to individual G-proteins that are capable of disrupting the link to the receptor. Appropriate functional antibodies to C-terminal peptide sequences of G_o and G_i have been produced and shown to be capable of discriminating between these two classes of G-protein (98). Intracellular application of these antibodies has shown that noradrenaline and opiate inhibition of Ca-currents in neuroblastoma hybrid cells is probably mediated by G_o rather than G_i (28), as suggested by the reconstitution experiments of Hescheler et al (68). A similar effect of anti-alpha$_o$ antibodies against dopamine-inhibition of Ca-current in mollusc neurons has been reported, though without corresponding tests with antibodies against other G-proteins (67). Clearly there are difficulties to this approach, both in the generation of sufficiently discriminating antibodies and in their technical use in electrophysiologic experiments. However antibody discrimination appears promising and may be helpful in identifying G-proteins coupling to K-channels, since it does not depend on the prior inactivation of the resident G-proteins and can be applied even when the coupling is indirect (see below).

HOW DO G-PROTEINS CONTROL NEURONAL K-CHANNELS?

G-proteins couple receptors to several enzyme systems, so an obvious mechanism for control of K-channels is through the enzymatic generation of soluble second messengers. Experiments on cardiac cell membranes, however, have shown that G-protein subunits can also modify the activity of K- and Ca-channels through a more local effect, without the intermediation of cytoplasmic messengers (85, 97, 179).

One way of distinguishing between these two methods is to record channel activity with a cell-attached patch-electrode and then to discern whether the receptor agonist is more effective when applied outside the patch or in the patch-electrode. By this criterion, the opening of the inwardly rectifying K-channels in neuronal cell membranes by somatostatin (177, 180), serotonin (163), and μ-opiates (111) would appear to be an essentially local phenomenon, since these agonists activated channels when present in the patch-electrode, but not when applied outside the patch. However opening of Ca-dependent K-channels in neuroblastoma cells and pituitary tumor cells by bradykinin and TRH respectively (70, 88) and opening and closing of S-channels in *Aplysia* neurons by FRMFamide and serotonin respectively (111, 147) appear to require more remote control mechanisms, since these agonists were effective when applied to the cell membrane outside the patch. This approach has not yet been applied to other K-channel closure responses, primarily because of the lack of single channel data. (This may not be totally prohibitive since, in principle, local currents might be recorded using a large patch-electrode, 54). However while apparently clear-cut in the instances referred to above, the conclusions drawn from this approach are not always watertight. For instance, there is a notable discrepancy between reported effects of extra-patch applications of noradrenaline on intra-patch Ca-channel activity in chick sensory ganglion cells (3, 54). Moreover, as reported for Ca-channel regulation by G_s (179, 182), K-channels might be subject to both remote and local control through different effects of the same G-protein that are not necessarily exclusive. Nevertheless, the division into local and remote (soluble messenger) effects is a convenient one for further discussion.

Local (direct?) Effects of G-Proteins

As indicated above, there is good evidence that agonists can activate inwardly rectifying channels in neuronal membranes through a local action. The most comprehensively studied of these effects is the response of GH_3 anterior pituitary cells to somatostatin (SST) and carbachol (CCh) (177). Application of 0.5 μM SST or 10 μM CCh via cell-attached patch-pipettes induced the opening of 55 pS channels (in isotonic K) in 30% of trials. No channels were detected with 20 mM TEA or 5 mM Cs in the pipette solution. The channels did not appear to be Ca-activated since they were not blocked by apamin (see 34), and all solutions contained less than 1 nM Ca. It was not established whether the channels rectified positive to E_K since additional outwardly conducting channels appeared at positive potentials. Involvement of a G-protein in channel activation was established by observations after excision that (a) agonist-induced activity disappeared in the absence of GTP in the external (inside-facing) solution and reappeared on adding 100 μM GTP; (b) opening was rapidly inhibited by adding preactivated PTx (10 μg/ml) with NAD; and (c) activity could be induced by 100 μM GTPγS in the absence of agonist. In PTx-treated, agonist-exposed membrane patches or in native membrane patches without added agonist, activity could also be induced by applying 2 pM GTPγS-preactivated erythrocyte G_k (= G_{i3}:36). In contrast, 100-fold higher concentrations of erythrocyte preactivated G_s were needed to produce an equivalent effect. Since these preactivated G-protein preparations contained equimolar free β-γ-subunit concentrations, this differential sensitivity to the two G-proteins was suggested to exclude a major role for the β-γ-subunits (cf 92). Other G-proteins (G_{i1-2}, G_o) were not tested on these channels. Parallel experiments on cardiac cell membranes (183) suggest that the other species of G_i proteins might well exert similar effects, but it would be particularly interesting to know whether G_o was equally effective in view of the effects of G_o on hippocampal cell K-channels described below.

In an interesting extension of this approach, Van Dongen et al (163) have by-passed the receptor-activation step to explore what K-channels in isolated patches of hippocampal cell membranes might be activated by a G-protein. For this they used preactivated G_o prepared from bovine brain and a recombinant G_o. They recorded channel activity in 34/69 patches following application of these G_o preparations; purified G_o was active at 1–10 pM, whereas 15-fold higher concentrations of the recombinant preparation were required. Channels could be divided into three classes in terms of single-channel conductance (55, 38, and 13 pS for inward current in isotonic K). The 38 pS group was further subdivided into two groups with differing mean open times and burst lengths. Some of the 38 pS channels showed strong inward rectification in the single-channel current-voltage curves and appeared to correspond to channels opened by serotonin in the patch-pipette. A fraction of extracted brain protein containing G_i was also tested: this activated the 13 pS channels in 2/5 patches, but was less effective than G_o. Interestingly, GTPγS activated the same three classes of channel. Since GTPγS would be expected to activate any endogenous G-protein, this implies either that these hippocampal cell membrane preparations only contained G_o as the predominant G-protein, or that other G-proteins present were either inactive or activated the same channels. G_o did not affect voltage-gated A-channels or ATP-gated channels present in these membranes: this accords with the usual resistance of A-currents to transmitter modulation (but see reference 116 for an exception).

These experiments answer many questions but raise others.

1. One question concerns the relationship between the ability of agonists such as somatostatin, carbachol, serotonin, and opioids to activate K-channels and their reported ability to inhibit adenylate cyclase. It is clear that a reduction in cytosolic cAMP is not, in itself, the trigger for K-channel opening. This is apparent not only from the above experiments, where channel opening by agonist persisted after patch isolation, but also from other tests in intact cells in which cAMP or forskolin failed to prevent or reverse the K-current induced by these agonists (5, 110, 162; but see also reference 4). Hence these agonists must produce a bifurcating response. In the case of the pituitary cell response, both channel opening and adenylate cyclase inhibition might result from activation of G_i: if so, then one might equally assume that the same agonist receptors are responsible. On the other hand, if the effects of G_o on the hippocampus are representative of other brain neurons (and truly depict the preferred modus operandi of serotonin), then one must assume that cyclase inhibition and K-channel activation involve separate G-proteins, since G_o does not inhibit adenylate cyclase (79, 132). This in turn implies either that the same receptor couples to two G-proteins, or that two distinct receptors are involved. Precisely the same situation arises in respect to the relationship between adenylate cyclase inhibition and Ca-current inhibition by opiates and noradrenaline in neuroblastoma hybrid cells, where cyclase inhibition is clearly mediated by G_i, and Ca-current inhibition is mediated by G_o (28, 68, 97, 98). In this instance, it seems most probable from pharmacological knowledge that two different receptors are involved (97). However there is

also evidence from both G-protein receptor reconstitution studies (60) and expression studies on cloned receptors (7, 150) that a single receptor species is at least potentially capable of coupling with more than one G-protein.

2. Given that activated G-protein α-subunits can induce the opening of single neuronal K-channels within a membrane patch of about 1 μm^2, does this reflect a direct gating of the channel protein or does it involve other adjacent membrane-associated molecules, possibly with the formation of additional local messengers? The plausibility of this latter possibility has been enhanced by the recent report of Kim et al (81) that, even within an isolated patch of cardiac cell membrane, activation of K-channels by solubilized β-γ-subunits from bovine brain can be inhibited by antibodies to PLA_2, or by the lipoxygenase inhibitor, nordihydroguaiaretic acid, which suggests local production and action of arachidonic acid metabolites of membrane lipids (see below). Available kinetic information regarding the activation of K-channels in neuronal membrane patches by pure α-subunits does not rule out such indirect effects, and this question can probably only be answered when recombinant G-protein α-subunits can be applied to recombinant channel proteins in a controlled lipid environment.

Effects Mediated by Soluble Second Messengers

G-proteins can activate or inhibit several enzymes to modify levels of soluble second messengers, which in turn can affect the activity of ion channels. This introduces many divergent potential routes for G-protein mediated control of K-channels. Since these are essentially secondary to the primary action of the G-protein, they might—strictly speaking—be regarded as outside the scope of this review. However some consideration of the most prominent of these second messenger systems seems in order, at least to highlight gaps in knowledge where the nature of the controlling pathway is unclear.

ADENYLATE CYCLASE   A particularly well-studied example of receptor-induced K-channel control mediated through activation of adenylate cyclase is the closure of the voltage-dependent S-channels of *Aplysia* sensory neurons induced by serotonin. In this system it is clear that a soluble messenger is involved, since the individual channels have been recorded with cell-attached patches and their closure recorded following application of serotonin to the membrane outside the patch (147). Involvement of cAMP was initially indicated by the ability of cAMP to replicate the channel closure (147) and subsequently by the demonstration that the catalytic subunit of cAMP-dependent protein kinase (PKA) could induce channel closure in isolated patches (146). Further, the effect of serotonin was substantially reduced by intracellular injection of protein kinase inhibitor protein (33). This implies that activation of adenylate cyclase, rather than direct coupling of G_s to the S-channels (see below), is primarily responsible for S-channel closure. Compatible, though somewhat less complete, evidence has been adduced for the inhibition of the macroscopic S-current by serotonin, dopamine, and FRMFamide in *Helix* neurons (38, 40, 41) and also for the activation of an inwardly rectifying K-current by serotonin in *Aplysia* R15 neurons (14, 44, 64, 90, 94, 161).

In vertebrate neurons, another widely distributed K-current that can be inhibited by activating adenylate cyclase or by adding cAMP (55, 102, 119, 126) is a slow Ca-activated K-current, which is responsible for a long spike after-hyperpolarization in a variety of cell types (AHP-current), and which also contributes to the resting potential in certain enteric neurons. Since this current can also be inhibited by neurotransmitters or hormones capable of activating adenylate cyclase, such as noradrenaline (via beta-receptors), serotonin, histamine, and prostaglandins, one supposes that their effects are mediated through cAMP. In hippocampal pyramidal cells, there is good confirmatory evidence for this in the sense that the inhibitory effect of noradrenaline is reduced by the adenylate cyclase inhibitor SQ 22, 536 (9-tetrahydro-2-furyladenine) (102). However in both hippocampal and myenteric neurons, this type of current can also be inhibited by other transmitters such as ACh, which does not activate adenylate cyclase. In sympathetic ganglion cells the comparable action of ACh is probably secondary to inhibition of the priming Ca-current (105, 112, 167), but this is not true for enteric or hippocampal neurons since (*a*) ACh inhibits the K-current in myenteric cells when applied after the priming Ca-current (59), and (*b*) inhibition of the K-current in hippocampal cells is not accompanied by a clear reduction in the priming Ca-spike (102) nor in the Ca-transient recorded with Fura-2 (83). In the hippocampus the effect of ACh can be replicated by phorbol esters, which suggests a possible role for diacylglycerol (DAG, see below); in myenteric neurons a change in the rate of sequestration of Ca has been suggested (123).

In evaluating the role of adenylate cyclase in the action of putative G_s-coupled transmitter-receptors, cognizance must be given to the recent experiments of Yatani et al (179, 182) in which direct application of purified or recombinant GTPγS-preactivated G_s has been shown to activate Ca-channels in isolated membrane patches or reconstituted into lipid bilayers under conditions where cAMP/PKA-mediated phosphorylation could be excluded; and further, that activation by PKA and by G_s were additive rather than exclusive. Taken in conjunction with the fact that many K-channels are likely to contain amino acid sequences susceptible to PKA-mediated phosphorylation, observations to the effect that the action of a transmitter is replicated by cAMP or by adenylate cyclase activation (or is even potentiated by a phosphodiesterase inhibitor) cannot be regarded as sufficient evidence per se that the effect of a transmitter is mediated through this route rather than through a more direct effect of G_s. It is further necessary to show that the effect of the transmitter is blocked when PKA-mediated phosphorylation or adenylate cyclase activation is prevented. So far such evidence has only been forthcoming for the inhibition of the *Aplysia* S-current by serotonin (33) and the hippocampal AHP-current by noradrenaline (102).

ADENYLATE CYCLASE INHIBITION   A number of the transmitters capable of activating K-currents through a PTx-sensitive G-protein are also able to inhibit adenylate cyclase. However these appear to be quite separate phenomena: in most cases where the question has been addressed, opening of K-channels does not depend on a reduction on cAMP. This is most clearly established in isolated patches (e.g. 176, 180), but has also been inferred from whole-cell recordings in which the activation of the K-current was not modified by prior activation of adenylate cyclase or injection of excess cAMP (5, 110, 124, 148, 153, 176). In only one instance—the hyperpolarization of locus coeruleus neurons by μ-opiates and α_2 adrenoceptor antagonists (4)—was the effect of the agonist apparently reversed by high concentration of cAMP, and subsequent tests (2) suggest that this resulted from activation of an opposing inward current rather than a true reversal of the opiate effect. (Since opiates are capable of activating these channels in membrane patches when present in the patch-electrode, but not outside (111), involvement of a soluble messenger such as cAMP seems unlikely.) Even in *Aplysia* sensory neurons the opposing effect of FRMFamide on the adenylate cyclase mediated inhibition of S-channels by serotonin is not mediated through negative coupling to the adenylate cyclase but through a separate downstream mechanism involving arachidonic acid metabolites (see below). In general, it would seem that there is little evidence that inhibition of adenylate cyclase has any pronounced effect on K-channel function—somewhat surprising, perhaps, in view of the sensitivity of so many K-channels to PKA-mediated phosphorylation.

PHOSPHOLIPASE C (PLC)   A number of the transmitters referred to in Tables 1 and 2 are also capable of activating PLC. This process appears to be dependent on prior activation of a G-protein (50), but the precise identity of the G-protein involved has not been determined, nor is it clear (from studies on pure PLC) whether the G-protein directly couples to PLC or requires an intermediate. Nevertheless, the results of such an activation produces at least two prospective second messengers, inositol 1,4,5 trisphosphate (IP_3) (or derivatives thereof) and diacylglycerol (DAG) (15).

Inositol trisphosphate (IP₃)   The usual effect of this substance is to release Ca from intracellular pools (15), and hence generation of IP_3 might be expected to activate Ca-dependent K-channels. There is strong evidence for such an effect resulting from PLC-linked receptor activation in two neuron-like cell lines: GH_3 cells stimulated by TRH (45, 88, 95, 137, 151, 173) and NG108-15 neuroblastoma/glioma hybrid cells stimulated by bradykinin (62, 69, 70, 71, 178). In the former, the evidence is largely inferential from a correlation of the electrophysiologic effects of TRH with its known bioche-mical effects; in the NG108-15 cells somewhat more compelling evidence is provided by the very close correspondence between the electrophysiologic effects of bradykinin with those of IP_3 and Ca injections (69, 70). In the latter cells, transfection of genes for other receptors (muscarinic m_1 and m_3) capable of activating PLC also endows a bradykinin-like response (57, 118). In nerve cells proper, some evidence for a role of IP_3 in mediating the outward current induced in *Aplysia* bag cells by some neuroactive peptides has been deduced from responses to injected IP_3 (52, 143, 144), and in dorsal raphe neurons the ability of noradrenaline to enhance the Ca-dependent spike after-current can be replicated by IP_3 injections (56). Finally, in hippocampal pyramidal neurons, intracellular infiltration of IP_3 appears capable of inhibiting the voltage-gated M-current, probably by an action which is independent of Ca-release (and which may therefore involve a metabolite) (47). Neverthe-less, in view of the widespread ability of agonists to activate PLC in the nervous system as judged from measurements of inositol phosphate produc-tion or phospholipid turnover, the number of instances where such an effect releases sufficient Ca to produce a demonstrable activation of Ca-dependent K-channels seems surprisingly sparse (53). This pathway appears better suited for, and used more widely as, a process for stimulating secretion rather than for controlling K-channels.

Diacylglycerol (DAG)   The principal effect of DAG is to activate protein kinase C (PKC) (121). The usual method for assessing a prospective role for DAG is to test the effect of exogenous diacylglycerols or other compounds capable of activating PKC such as phorbol esters (PE) (9, 17, 77). By this criterion, DAG might prospectively be involved in the receptor-mediated closure of M-channels in sympathetic ganglion cells and NG108-15 cells (25, 29, 69, 104, 132) and the closure of Ca-activated K-channels in hippocampal cells by ACh (10, 47, 103). However this cannot be regarded as more than suggestive evidence, since the effects of PKC activators show several differ-ences from those of the normal receptor agonist, and tests with a PKC inhibitor have not provided confirmatory evidence (18, 132). Even though there is abundant evidence that agonists that close M-channels are also capable of stimulating PLC, evidence that either product of such stimulation plays a role in M-channel closure is circumstantial at best: although a G-protein linkage is clearly indicated from tests with GTP and GDP analogues, the identity of the G-protein and the subsequent pathway leading to channel closure is still unclear.

PHOSPHOLIPASE A_2 A widely distributed signaling system in a variety of cell types (including nerve cells) involves the formation of arachidonic acid (AA) from membrane phospholipids by phospholipase A_2, with the subsequent formation of a variety of enzymatic products by the cyclo-oxygenase and lipoxygenase pathways (8). In the context of neuronal K-channel control, there is particularly strong biochemical and electrophysiologic evidence that the opening of S-channels in *Aplysia* sensory neurons by FRMFamide is mediated through this pathway, principally by 12-HETE, a product of the lipoxygenase pathway (31, 135). Thus activation of the S-current by FRMFamide is imitated by external AA and blocked by inhibitors of phospholipase (4-bromophenacyl bromide) and lipoxygenase (nordihydroguaiaretic acid), but not by indomethacin, which blocks cyclo-oxygenase (135). Further evidence that AA has to be metabolized is provided by the observation that AA opens channels in cell-attached patches when applied outside the patch (135), but not when applied to the inside face of isolated inside-out patches (31). In the latter configuration, 12-HPETE (20 μM) produced a delayed activation of the channels, whereas the same concentration of 12-HETE (the metabolite of 12-HPETE) produced an immediate increase; this suggests that the latter may be the active product and—since no ATP or GTP was present in the solution—that 12-HETE may gate the channels directly (31). Involvement of a G-protein in coupling the FRMFamide receptors to this cascade is indicated by the ability of GTPγS to activate the S-current (and potentiate the effect of FRMFamide) and of GDPβS to antagonize the effect of the agonist (164). Since GTPγS did not affect the action of AA, the G-protein link appears to be directed at the phospholipase rather than the subsequent steps in the pathway. The precise identity of the G-protein has not yet been established: it is PTx-sensitive, but unlikely to be a member of the G_i-family since FRMFamide does not inhibit adenylate cyclase (125). One possibility is that β-γ-, rather than an α-subunit might be responsible, since PLA_2 can be activated by the β-γ-subunit of transducin (75). Evidence has recently shown that purified β-γ-subunits from bovine brain can activate K-channels in cardiac cell membrane patches through the activation of PLA_2 and local generation of lipoxygenase products (principally leukotrienes) (81, 84).

CONCLUSIONS

It is clear that transmitters and hormones can modify K-channels in neurons through the intervention of G-proteins. However, the great variety of transmitter receptors, cellular transduction systems, and K-channels in neurons, coupled with technical limitations for studying many neurons, means that (with some notable exceptions) analysis of the details of the control mechanisms lags behind that currently existing for certain non-neural tissues, and that it is difficult to formulate any general rules. Nonetheless certain patterns are beginning to emerge, and some general points may be in order.

1. Many transmitters can activate K-channels to generate a K-current which—in macroscopic current terms at least—seems to be rather similar in different nerve cell types and also somewhat similar to that activated in cardiac cells. However preliminary evidence suggests that this may result from activation of more than one type of K-channel, as judged from single-channel conductance levels. Further, in the two cell types so far studied (hippocampal and pituitary tumor cells) there is a clear difference in the G-protein selectivity (G_i vs G_o): this implies that, even where there may be an overall similarity in the macroscopic current or even the single-channel behavior, there must be variations either in the channel structures themselves or in the micro-mechanism for G-protein regulation of the channels.

2. Although some K-channels appear susceptible to a very localized, possibly direct, modification in gating by G-proteins, it is also clear that a number of neuronal K-channels are susceptible to protein kinase-mediated phosphorylation or other forms of second messenger regulated modulation. In some instances (the control of the *Aplysia* S-current, and the activation of Ca-dependent K-currents in certain neural cell lines) such indirect G-protein mediated mechanisms appear to be responsible for transmitter/hormone control of the currents in question. This clearly allows greater flexibility in control, but at the same time imposes greater constraints on the experimental analysis of the mechanisms involved in K-channel regulation. Much more research will be needed to determine which transmitter-operated control mechanisms might involve cytoplasmic messengers and what the details of such messenger systems might be.

3. Since there is evidence from other studies that both the G-protein cycle itself and intracellular phosphorylation/dephosphorylation systems (and possibly other cytosolic messenger systems) can exhibit a slow resting turnover rate in the absence of receptor activation, K-channel function might well be susceptible to tonic G-protein-mediated regulation. At the very least this could be important in determining variations in K-channel behavior in different cells or under different experimental conditions. However, there is as yet little direct information regarding such endogenous control systems for neuronal K-currents from (e.g.) effects of PTx or adenylate cyclase or protein kinase C inhibition.

Literature Cited

1. Abrams, T. W., Castellucci, V., Camardo, S., Kandel, E. R. 1984. Two endogenous neuropeptides modulate the gill and siphon withdrawal reflex in *Aplysia* presynaptic facilitation involving cAMP-dependent closure of a serotonin-sensitive channel. *Proc. Natl. Acad. Sci. USA* 81:7956–60

2. Aghajanian, G. K., Wang, Y.-Y. 1986. Pertussis toxin blocks the outward currents evoked by opiates and α_2 agonists in locus coeruleus neurons. *Brain Res.* 371:390–94

3. Anderson, C. R., Dunlap, K. 1988. Single L-type calcium channels in dorsal root ganglia can be modulated by norepinephrine. *Neurosci. Abstr.* 14:644

4. Andrade, R., Aghajanian, G. K. 1985. Opiate and α_2-adrenoceptor-induced hyperpolarization of locus coeruleus neurons in brain slices: reversal by cyclic adenosine-3'5-monophosphate analogues. *J. Neurosci.* 5:2359–164

5. Andrade, R., Malenka, R. C., Nicoll, R. A. 1986. A G-protein couples serotonin and GABA$_B$ receptors to the same channels in hippocampus. *Science* 234: 1261–65

6. Asano, J., Semba, R., Kamiya, N., Ogasawara, N., Kato, K. 1988. G$_o$, a GTP-binding protein: immunochemical and immunohistochemical localization in the rat. *J. Neurochem.* 50:1164–69

7. Ashkenazi, A., Winslow, J. W., Peralta, E. G., Peterson, G. L., Schimerli, M. I., et al. 1987. An M2 muscarinic receptor subtype coupled to both adenylcyclase and phosphoinositide turnover. *Science* 238:672–67

8. Axelrod, J., Burch, R. M., Jelesma, C. 1988. Receptor-mediated activation of phospholipase A$_2$ via GTP-binding proteins: arachidonic acid and its metabolites as second messengers. *Trends Neurosci.* 11:117–123

9. Baraban, J. M. 1989. Phorbol esters: probes of protein kinase C function in the brain. *Trends Neurosci.* 10:57–59

10. Baraban, J. M., Snyder, S. H., Alger, B. E. 1985. Protein kinase C regulates ionic conductance in hippocampal pyramidal neurons: electrophysiological effects of phorbol esters. *Proc. Natl. Acad. Sci. USA* 82:2538–42

11. Belardetti, F., Kandel, E. R., Siegelbaum, S. 1987. Neuronal inhibition by the peptide FRMFamide involves opening of S K$^+$-channels. *Nature* 325:153–56

12. Belardetti, F., Schacher, S., Kandel, E. R., Siegelbaum, S. A. 1986. The growth cone of *Aplysia* sensory neurons: modulation by serotonin of action potential duration and single potassium channel currents. *J. Neurosci.* 83:7094–98

13. Belardinelli, L., Isenberg, G. 1983. Isolated atrial myocytes: adenosine and acetylcholine increase potassium conductance. *Am. J. Physiol.* 244:H734–37

14. Benson, J. A., Levitan, I. B. 1983. Serotonin increases an anomalously-rectifying K$^+$-current in the *Aplysia* neuron R15. *Proc. Natl. Acad. Sci. USA* 80:3522–25

15. Berridge, M. J. 1987. Inositol trisphosphate and diacylglycerol: two interacting second messengers. *Annu. Rev. Biochem.* 56:159–93

16. Blatz, A. L., Magleby, K. L. 1987. Calcium-activated potassium channels. *Trends Neurosci.* 11:463–67

17. Blumberg, P. M., Jaken, S., Konig, B., Sharkey, N., Leach, K. L., et al. 1984. Mechanism of action of the phorbol ester tumor promoters: specific receptors for lipophilic ligands. *Biochem. Pharmacol.* 33:933–40

18. Bosma, M., Hille, B. 1989. Protein kinase C is not necessary for peptide-induced suppression of M current or for desensitization of the peptide receptor. *Proc. Natl. Acad. Sci. USA* 86:2943–47

19. Brabet, P., Dumuis, A., Sebben, M., Pantaloni, C., Bockaert, J., Homburger, V. 1988. Immunocytochemical localization of the guanine nucleotide-binding protein G$_o$ in primary cultures of neuronal and glial cells. *J. Neurochem.* 8:701–8

20. Brann, M. R., Collins, R. M., Spiegel, A. 1987. Localization of mRNAs encoding the α-subunits of signal-transducing G-proteins within rat brain and among peripheral tissues. *FEBS Lett.* 222:191–98

21. Breitweiser, G., Szabo, G. 1985. Uncoupling of cardiac muscarinic and β-adrenergic receptors from ion channels by a guanine nucleotide analogue. *Nature* 317:538–40

22. Breitweiser, G., Szabo, G. 1988. Mechanism of muscarinic receptor-induced K$^+$ channel activation as revealed by hydrolysis-resistant GTP analogues. *J. Gen. Physiol.* 91:469–93

23. Brezina, V., Eckert, R., Erxleben, C. 1987. Modulation of potassium conductances by an endogenous neuropeptide in neurones of *Aplysia californica*. *J. Physiol.* 382:267–90

24. Brezina, A., Eckert, R., Erxleben, C. 1987. Suppression of calcium current by an endogenous neuropeptide in neurones

of *Aplysia californica. J. Physiol.* 388: 565–95

25. Brown, D. A., Adams, P. R. 1987. Effects of phorbol dibutyrate on M currents and M current inhibition in bullfrog sympathetic neurons. *Cell. Mol. Neurobiol.* 7:255–69

26. Brown, D. A., Higashida, H. 1988. Membrane current responses of NG108–15 mouse neuroblastoma x rat glioma cells to bradykinin. *J. Physiol.* 397:167–84

27. Brown, D. A., Higashida, H. 1988. Inositol 1,4,5-trisphosphate and diacylglycerol mimic bradykinin effects on mouse neuroblastoma x rat glioma hybrid cells. *J. Physiol.* 397:185–207

28. Brown, D. A., McFadzean, I., Milligan, G. R. 1989. Antibodies to the GTP-binding protein G$_o$ attenuate the inhibition of the calcium current by noradrenaline in mouse neuroblastoma x rat glioma (NG108–15) hybrid cells. *J. Physiol.* 415:20P

29. Brown, D. A., Marrion, N. V., Smart, T. G. 1989. On the transduction mechanism for muscarine-induced inhibition of M-current in cultured rat sympathetic neurones. *J. Physiol.* 413:469–88

30. Brown, L. D., Nakajima, S., Nakajima, Y. 1988. Acetylcholine modulates resting K-current through a pertussis toxin-resistant G-protein in hippocampal neurons. *Neurosci. Abstr.* 14:1328

31. Buttner, N., Volterra, A., Siegelbaum, S. A. 1988. Control of S-K$^+$ channel activity by arachidonic acid metabolites in cell-free inside-out patches from *Aplysia* sensory neurons. *Biophys. J.* 55: 197a

32. Carmeliet, E., Mubagwa, K. 1986. Characterization of the acetylcholine-induced potassium current in rabbit cardiac purkinje fibres. *J. Physiol.* 371: 219–37

33. Castellucci, V. F., Nairn, A., Greengard, P., Schwartz, J. H., Kandel, E. R. 1982. Inhibitor of adenosine 3'5'-monophosphate-dependent protein kinase blocks presynaptic facilitation in *Aplysia. J. Neurosci.* 2:1673–81

34. Castle, N. A., Haylett, D. G., Jenkinson, D. H. 1988. Toxins in the characterization of potassium channels. *Trends Neurosci.* 12:59–65

35. Chang, K.-J., Pugh, W., Blanchard, S. G., McDermed, J., Tam, J. P. 1988. Antibody specific to the α-subunit of the guanine-nucleotide-binding regulatory protein G$_o$: developmental appearance and immunohistochemical localization in brain. *Proc. Natl. Acad. Sci. USA* 85:4929–33

36. Codina, J., Olate, J., Abramowitz, J., Mattera, R., Cook, R. G., Birnbaumer, L. 1988. α$_i$-3 cDNA encodes the α subunit of G$_k$, the stimulatory G protein of receptor-regulated K$^+$ channels. *J. Biol. Chem.* 263:6746–50

37. Colmers, W. F., Williams, J. T. 1988. Pertussis toxin discriminates between pre- and postsynaptic actions of baclofen in rat dorsal raphe neurons *in vitro. Neurosci. Lett.* 93:300–6

38. Colombaioni, L., Paupardin-Tritsch, D., Vidal, P. P., Gerschenfeld, H. M. 1985. The neuropeptide FRMFamide decreases both the Ca^{2+} conductance and a cyclic 3'5-adenosine monophosphate-dependent K$^+$ conductance in identified molluscan neurons. *J. Neurosci.* 5:2533–38

39. Constanti, A., Galvan, M. 1983. Fast inward-rectifying current accounts for anomalous rectification in olfactory cortex neurones. *J. Physiol.* 386:153–78

40. Deterre, P., Paupardin-Tritsch, D., Bockaert, J., Gerschenfeld, H. M. 1981. Role of cyclic AMP in a serotonin-evoked slow inward current in snail neurones. *Nature* 290:783–85

41. Deterre, P., Paupardin-Tritsch, D., Bockaert, J., Gerschenfeld, H. M. 1982. cAMP-mediated decrease in K$^+$ conductance evoked by serotonin and dopamine in the same neuron: a biochemical and physiological single-cell study. *Proc. Natl. Acad. Sci. USA* 79: 7934–38

42. Dohlman, H. G., Caron, M. G., Lefkowitz, R. J. 1987. A family of receptors coupled to guanine-nucleotide regulatory proteins. *Biochemistry* 26:2664–68

43. Dolphin, A. C., Wootton, J. F., Scott, R. H., Trentham, D. R. 1988. Photoactivation of intracellular guanosine triphosphate analogues reduces the amplitude and slows the kinetics of voltage-activated calcium channel currents in sensory neurones. *Pflügers Arch.* 411:628–36

44. Drummond, A H., Benson, J. A., Levitan, L. B. 1980. Serotonin-induced hyperpolarization of an identified *Aplysia* neuron is mediated by cyclic AMP. *Proc. Natl. Acad. Sci. USA* 77:5013–17

45. Dubinsky, J. M., Oxford, G. S. 1985. Dual modulation of K-channels by thyrotropin-releasing hormone in clonal pituitary cells. *Proc. Natl. Acad. Sci. USA* 82:4282–86

46. Dunlap, K., Holz, G. G., Rane, S. G. 1987. G-proteins as regulators of ion channel function. *Trends Neurosci.* 10: 241–44

47. Dutar, P., Nicoll, R. A. 1988. Stimula-

tion of phosphatidylinositol (PI) turnover may mediate the muscarinic suppression of the M-current in hippocampal pyramidal cells. *Neurosci. Lett.* 85:89–94

48. Dutar, P., Nicoll, R. A. 1988. Classification of muscarinic responses in hippocampus in terms of receptor subtypes and second-messenger systems: electrophysiological studies *in vitro. J. Neurosci.* 8:4214–24

49. Ewald, D. A., Sternweis, P. C., Miller, R. J. 1988. Guanine nucleotide-binding protein G_o-induced coupling of neuropeptide Y receptors to Ca^{2+} channels in sensory neurons. *Proc. Natl. Acad. Sci. USA* 88:3633–37

50. Fain, J. N., Wallace, M. A., Wojcikiewicz, J. H. 1988. Evidence for involvement of guanine nucleotide-binding regulatory proteins in the activation of phospholipases by hormones. *FASEB J.* 2:2569–74

51. Ferguson, K. M., Higashijima, T., Smigel, M. D., Gilman, A. G. 1986. The influence of bound GDP on the kinetics of guanine nucleotide binding to G proteins. *J. Biol. Chem.* 261:7393–99

52. Fink, L. A., Connor, J. A., Kaczmarek, L. 1988. Inositol trisphosphate releases intracellularly stored calcium and modulates ion channels in molluscan neurons. *J. Neurosci.* 8:2544–55

53. Fink, L. A., Kaczmarek, L. K. 1988. Inositol polyphosphates regulate excitability. *Trends Neurosci.* 11:338–39

54. Forscher, P., Oxford, G. S., Schulz, D. G. 1986. Noradrenaline modulates calcium channels in avian dorsal root ganglion cells through tight receptor-channel coupling. *J. Physiol.* 379:131–44

55. Fowler, J. C., Wonderlin, W. F., Weinreich, D. 1985. Prostaglandins block a Ca^{2+}-dependent slow spike afterhyperpolarization independent of effects of Ca^{2+} influx in visceral afferent neurons. *Brain Res.* 345:345–49

56. Freedman, J. E., Aghajanian, G. K. 1987. Role of phosphoinositide metabolites in the prolongation of afterhyperpolarization by α_1-adrenoceptors in rat dorsal raphe neurons. *J. Neurosci.* 7:3897–3906

57. Fukuda, K., Higashida, H., Kubo, T., Maeda, A., Akiba, I., et al. 1988. Selective coupling with K^+ currents of muscarinic acetylcholine receptor subtypes in NG108-15 cells. *Nature* 335:355–58

58. Gähwiler, B. H., Brown, D. A. 1985. $GABA_B$-receptor-activated K^+ current in voltage-clamped CA_3 pyramidal cells

in hippocampal cultures. *Proc. Natl. Acad. Sci. USA* 82:1558–62

59. Galligan, J. J., North, R. A., Tokimasa, T. 1989. Muscarinic agonists and potassium currents in guinea-pig myenteric neurones. *Br. J. Pharmacol.* 96:193–203

60. Gilman, A. G. 1987. G proteins: Transducers of receptor-generated signals. *Annu. Rev. Biochem.* 56:615–49

61. Grafe, P., Mayer, C. J., Wood, J. D. 1980. Synaptic modulation of calcium-dependent potassium conductance in myenteric neurones in the guinea-pig. *J. Physiol.* 305:235–48

62. Grandt, R., Greiner, C., Zubin, P., Jakobs, K. H. 1986. Bradykinin stimulates GTP hydrolysis in NG108-15 membranes by a high affinity, pertussis toxin-insensitive GTPase. *FEBS Lett.* 196:279–83

63. Graziano, M. P., Gilman, A. G. 1987. Guanine nucleotide-binding regulatory proteins: mediators of transmembrane signalling. *Trends Pharmacol. Sci.* 8:478–81

64. Gunning, R. 1987. Increased numbers of ion channels promoted by an intracellular second messenger. *Science* 235:80–82

65. Haas, H., Konnerth, A. 1983. Histamine and noradrenaline decrease calcium-activated potassium conductance in hippocampal pyramidal cells. *Nature* 302:432–34

66. Haga, T., Uchiyama, H., Haga, T., Ichiyama, A., Kangawa, K., Matsuo, H. 1989. Cerebral muscarinic acetylcholine receptors interact with three kinds of GTP-binding proteins in a reconstitution system of purified components. *Mol. Pharmacol.* 35:286–94

67. Harris-Warwick, R. M., Hammond, C., Paupardin-Tritsch, D., Homburger, V., Rouot, B., et al. 1988. An α_{40} subunit of a GTP-binding protein immunologically related to G_o mediates a dopamine-induced decrease of Ca^{2+} current in snail neurons. *Neuron* 1:27–32

68. Hescheler, J., Rosenthal, W., Trautwein, W., Schultz, G. 1987. The GTP-binding protein, G_o, regulates neuronal calcium channels. *Nature* 325:445–47

69. Higashida, H., Brown, D. A. 1986. Two polyphosphatidylinositol metabolites control two K^+ currents in a neuronal cell. *Nature* 323:333–35

70. Higashida, H., Brown, D. A. 1988. Ca^{2+}-dependent K^+-channels in neuroblastoma hybrid cells activated by intracellular inositol trisphosphate and extracellular bradykinin. *FEBS Lett.* 238:395–400

71. Higashida, H., Streaty, R. A., Klee, W., Nirenberg, M. 1986. Bradykinin-activated transmembrane signals are coupled via N_o or N_i to production of inositol 1,4,5-trisphosphate, a second messenger in NG108-15 neuroblastoma-glioma hybrid cells. *Proc. Natl. Acad. Sci. USA* 83:942–46

72. Hille, B. 1984. *Ion Channels in Excitable Cells*, Sunderland, Mass.: Sinauer

73. Innis, R. B., Aghajanian, G. K. 1987. Pertussis toxin blocks autoreceptor-mediated inhibition of dopaminergic neurons in rat substantia nigra. *Brain Res.* 411:139–43

74. Inoue, M., Nakajima, S., Nakajima, Y. 1988. Somatostatin induces an inward rectification in rat locus coeruleus neurones through a pertussis-toxin sensitive mechanism. *J. Physiol.* 407:177–98

75. Jelesma, C., Axelrod, J. 1987. Stimulation of phospholipase A_2 activity in bovine rod outer segments by the $\beta\gamma$ subunits of transducin and its inhibition by the α subunit. *Proc. Natl. Acad. Sci. USA* 84:3623–27

76. Jones, S. W. 1987. GTP-γ-S inhibits the M-current of dissociated bullfrog sympathetic neurons. *Neurosci. Abstr.* 13:533

77. Kaczmarek, L. 1987. The role of protein kinase C in the regulation of ion channels and neurotransmitter release. *Trends Neurosci.* 10:30–33

78. Kaczmarek, L., Levitan, I. B. 1987. *Neuromodulation. The Biochemical Control of Neuronal Excitability*, Oxford: Oxford Univ. Press. 286 pp.

79. Katada, T., Oinumi, M., Ui, M. 1986. Mechanisms for inhibition of the catalytic activity of adenylate cyclase by the guanine nucleotide-binding proteins serving as the substrate of islet-activating protein, pertussis toxin. *J. Biol. Chem.* 261:5215–21

80. Kehoe, J. S., Marty, A. 1980. Certain slow synaptic responses: their properties and possible underlying mechanisms. *Annu. Rev. Biophys. Bioeng.* 9:437–65

81. Kim, D., Lewis, D., Grziadei, L., Neer, E. J., Bar-Sagi, D., Clapham, D. E. 1989.. G-protein Bγ subunits activate the cardiac muscarinic K^+ channel via phospholipase A_2. *Nature* 337:557–59

82. Klein, M., Camardo, J., Kandel, E. R. 1982. Serotonin modulates a specific potassium current in the sensory neurons that show presynaptic facilitation in *Aplysia*. *Proc. Natl. Acad. Sci. USA* 79:5713–17

83. Knoepfel, T., Brown, D. A. Vranesic, I., Gähwiler, B. H. 1989. Depression of Ca^{2+} activated potassium conductance by muscarine and isoproterenol without alteration of depolarization-induced transient rise in cytosolic free Ca^{2+} in hippocampal CA3 pyramidal cells. *Eur. J. Neurosci. Suppl.* 2:92

84. Kurachi, Y., Ito, H., Sugimoto, T., Shimuzu, T., Miki, I., Ui, M. 1989. Arachidonic acid metabolites as intracellular modulators of the G protein-gated cardiac K^+ channel. *Nature* 337:555–67

85. Kurachi, Y., Nakajima, T., Sugimoto, T. 1986. On the mechanism of activation of muscarinic K^+ channels by adenosine in isolated atrial cells: involvement of GTP-binding proteins. *Pflügers. Arch.* 407:264–74

86. Lacey, M. G., Mercuri, N. B., North, R. A. 1988. On the potassium conductance increase activated by GABA$_B$ and dopamine D_2 receptors in rat substantia nigra neurones. *J. Physiol.* 401:437–53

87. Lancaster, B., Perkel, D. T., Nicoll, R. A. 1987. Small conductance Ca^{2+}-activated K^+ channels in hippocampal neurons. *Neurosci. Abstr.* 13:176

88. Lang, D. G., Ritchie, A. K. 1987. Large and small conductance calcium-activated potassium channels in the GH$_3$ anterior pituitary cell line. *Pflügers Arch.* 410:614–22

89. Largent, B. L., Jones, D. T., Reed, R. R., Pearson, R. C. A., Snyder, S. H. 1988. G protein mRNA mapped in rat brain by *in situ* hybridization. *Proc. Natl. Acad. Sci. USA* 85:2864–68

90. Lemos, J. R., Levitan, I. B. 1984. Intracellular injection of guanyl nucleotide alters the serotonin-induced increase in potassium conductance in *Aplysia* neuron R15. *J. Gen. Physiol.*, 83:269–85

91. Levitan, I. B. 1988. Modulation of ion channels in neurons and other cells. *Annu. Rev. Neurosci.* 11:119–36

92. Logothetis, D. E., Kurachi, Y., Galper, J., Neer, E. J., Clapham, D. E. 1987. The $\beta\gamma$ subunits of GTP-binding proteins activate the muscarinic K^+ channel in heart. *Nature* 325:321–26

93. Lopez, H. S., Brown, D. A., Adams, P. R. 1987. Possible involvement of GTP-binding proteins in coupling of muscarinic receptors to M-current in bullfrog ganglion cells. *Neurosci. Abstr.* 13:532

94. Lotshaw, D. P., Levitan, I. B. 1987. Serotonin and forskolin increase an inwardly rectifying potassium conductance in cultured *Aplysia* neurons. *J. Neurophysiol.* 58:909–21

95. MacPhee, C. H., Drummond, A. H. 1984. Thyrotropin-releasing hormone stimulates rapid breakdown of phosphotidylinositol 4,5-bisphosphate and phosphotidylinositol 4-phosphate in GH$_3$ pituitary tumor cells. *Mol. Pharmacol.* 25:193–200

96. McCormick, D. A. 1988. Interactions and possible second messenger systems involved in neurotransmitter responses in the thalamus. *Neurosci. Abstr.* 14: 913

97. McFadzean, I., Mullaney, I., Brown, D. A., Milligan, G. 1989. Antibodies to the GTP-binding protein, G$_o$, antagonize noradrenaline-induced calcium current inhibition in NG108-15 hybrid cells. *Neuron* 3:177–82

98. McKenzie, F. R., Kelly, E. C. H., Unson, C. G., Spiegel, A. M., Milligan, G. 1988. Antibodies which recognize the C-terminus of the inhibitory guanine-nucleotide-binding protein (G$_i$) demonstrate that opioid peptides and foetal-calf serum stimulate the high-affinity GTPase activity of two separate pertussis-toxin substrates. *Biochem. J.* 249: 653–59

99. Madison, D. V., Lancaster, B., Nicoll, R. A. 1987. Voltage clamp analysis of cholinergic action in the hippocampus. *J. Neurosci.* 7:733–41

100. Madison, D. V., Nicoll, R. A. 1982. Noradrenaline blocks accommodation of pyramidal cell discharge in the hippocampus. *Nature* 299:636–38

101. Madison, D. V., Nicoll, R. A. 1986. Actions of noradrenaline recorded intracellularly in rat hippocampal CA1 pyramidal neurones, *in vitro. J. Physiol.* 372:221–44

102. Madison, D. V., Nicoll, R. A. 1986. Cyclic adenosine 3'5'-monophosphate mediates β-receptor actions of noradrenaline in rat hippocampal pyramidal cells. *J. Physiol.* 372:245–59

103. Malenka, R. C., Madison, D. V., Andrade, R., Nicoll, R. A. 1986. Phorbol esters mimic some cholinergic actions on hippocampal pyramidal cells. *J. Neurosci.* 6:475–80

104. Marrion, N. V. 1987. Probable role of a GTP-binding protein in mediating M-current inhibition by muscarine in rat sympathetic neurones. *J. Physiol.* 396: 87P

105. Marrion, N. V., Smart, T. G., Brown, D. A. 1987. Membrane currents in adult rat superior cervical ganglia in dissociated tissue culture. *Neurosci. Lett.* 77:55–60

106. Marsh, S. J., Owen, D. G. 1989. Fluctuation analysis of M-current in cultured rat sympathetic neurones. *J. Physiol.* 410:31P

107. Marty, A. 1988. Ca-dependent K channels with large unitary conductance in chromaffin cell membranes. *Nature* 291: 497–500

108. Marty, A., Evans, M. G., Tan, Y. P., Trautmann, A. 1986. Muscarinic response in rat lacrimal glands. *J. Exp. Biol.* 124:15–32

109. Mattera, R., Graziano, M. P., Yatani, A., Zhou, Z., Graf, R., et al. 1989. Splice variants of the α subunit of the G protein G$_s$ activate both adenylyl cyclase and calcium channels. *Science* 243:804–7

110. Mihara, S., North, R. A., Surprenant, A. 1987. Somatostatin increases an inwardly rectifying potassium conductance in guinea-pig submucous plexus neurones. *J. Physiol.* 390:335–55

111. Miyaka, M., Christie, M. J., North, R. A. 1988. Single potassium channels opened by opioids in rat central neurons. *Neurosci. Abstr.* 14:401

112. Mochida, S., Kobayashi, K. 1986. Activation of M$_2$ muscarinic receptors causes an alteration of action potentials by modulation of Ca entry in isolated sympathetic neurons of rabbits. *Neurosci. Lett.* 72:199–204

113. Morita, K., North, R. A., Tokimasa, T. 1982. Muscarinic agonists inactivate potassium conductance of guinea-pig myenteric neurones. *J. Physiol.* 333: 125–39

114. Mullaney, I., Milligan, G. R. 1989. Elevated levels of the guanine nucleotide binding protein, G$_o$, are associated with differentiation of neuroblastoma x glioma hybrid cells. *FEBS Lett.* 244: 113–18

115. Nakajima, Y., Nakajima, S., Inoue, M. 1988. Pertussis toxin-insensitive G protein mediates substance P-induced inhibition of potassium channels in brain neurons. *Proc. Natl. Acad. Sci. USA* 85:3643–47

116. Nakajima, Y., Nakajima, S., Leonard, R. J., Yamaguchi, K. 1986. Acetylcholine raises excitability by inhibiting the fast transient potassium current in cultured hippocampal neurons. *Proc. Natl. Acad. Sci. USA* 83:3022–26

117. Neer, E. J., Clapham, D. E. 1988. Roles of G protein subunits in transmembrane signalling. *Nature* 333:129–34

118. Neher, E., Marty, A., Fukuda, K., Kubo, T., Numa, S. 1988. Intracellular calcium release mediated by two muscarinic receptor subtypes. *FEBS Lett.* 240:88–94

119. Nemeth, P. R., Palmer, J. M., Wood, J. D., Zhafirov, D. H. 1986. Effects of forskolin on electrical behaviour of myenteric neurones in guinea-pig small intestine. *J. Physiol.* 376:439–50

120. Nicoll, R. A. 1988. The coupling of neurotransmitter receptors to ion channels in the brain. *Science* 241:545–51

121. Nishizuka, Y. 1984. The role of protein kinase C in cell surface signal transduction and tumour promotion. *Nature* 308: 693–98

122. Noma, A., Trautwein, W. 1978. Relaxation of the ACh-induced potassium current in the rabbit sinoatrial node cell. *Pflügers. Arch.* 377:193–200

123. North, R. A., Tokimasa, T. 1983. Depression of calcium-dependent potassium conductance of guinea-pig myenteric neurones by muscarinic agonists. *J. Physiol.* 342:253–66

124. North, R. A., Williams, J. T., Surprenant, A., Christie, M. J. 1987. μ and δ receptors belong to a family of receptors that are coupled to potassium channels. *Proc. Natl. Acad. Sci. USA* 84: 5487–91

125. Ocorr, K. A., Tabata, M., Byrne, J. H. 1985. Cyclic AMP, a common biochemical locus for the effects of 5-HT and SCP$_B$, but not FRMFamide, in tail sensory neurons of *Aplysia*. *Neurosci. Abstr.* 11:481

126. Palmer, J. M., Wood, J. D., Zafirov, D. H. 1986. Elevation of adenosine 3'5'-phosphate mimics slow synaptic excitation in myenteric neurones of the guinea-pig. *J. Physiol.* 376:451–60

127. Paupardin-Tritsch, D., Hammond, C., Harris-Warwick, R., Gerschenfeld, N. M. 1988. In *Modulation of Synaptic Transmission and Plasticity in Nervous Systems,* ed. G. Hertting, H.-C. Spatz, pp. 271–288. Berlin: Springer-Verlag. 457 pp.

128. Pennefather, P. S., Heisler, S., MacDonald, J. F. 1988. A potassium conductance contributes to the action of somatostatin-14 to suppress ACTH secretion. *Brain Res.* 444:346–50

129. Petersen, O. H., Findlay, I., Suzuki, K., Dunne, M. J. 1986. Messenger-mediated control of potassium channels in secretory cells. *J. Exp. Biol.* 106:33–52

130. Pfaffinger, P. J. 1987. Control of M-current in dialyzed sympathetic ganglion neurons. *Neurosci. Abstr.* 13:152

131. Pfaffinger, P. J. 1988. Muscarine and t-LHRH suppress M-current by activating an IAP-insensitive G-protein. *J. Neurosci.* 8:3343–53

132. Pfaffinger, P. J., Leibowitz, M. D.,

Subers, E. M., Nathanson, N. M., Almers, W., Hille, B. 1988. Agonists that suppress M-current elicit phosphoinositide turnover and Ca^{2+} transients, but these events do not explain M-current suppression. *Neuron* 1:477–84

133. Pfaffinger, P. J., Martin, J. M., Hunter, D. D., Nathanson, N. M., Hille, B. 1985. GTP-binding proteins couple cardiac muscarinic receptors to a K channel. *Nature* 317:536–38

134. Piomelli, D., Shapiro, E., Feinmark, S. J., Schwartz, J. H. 1987. Metabolites of arachidonic acid in the nervous system of *Aplysia:* possible mediators of synaptic modulation. *J. Neurosci.* 7:3675–86

135. Piomelli, D., Volterra, A., Dale, N., Siegelbaum, S. A., Kandel, E. R., et al. 1987. Lipoxygenase metabolites of arachidonic acid as second messengers for presynaptic inhibition of *Aplysia* sensory cells. *Nature* 328:38–43

136. Pollock, J. D., Bernier, L., Camardo, J. S. 1985. Serotonin and cyclic adenosine 3':5'-monophosphate modulate the potassium current in tail sensory neurons in the pleural ganglion of *Aplysia*. *J. Neurosci.* 5:1862–71

137. Ritchie, A. K. 1987. Thyrotropin-releasing hormone stimulates a calcium-activated potassium current in a rat anterior pituitary cell line. *J. Physiol.* 385:611–25

138. Roof, J. D., Applebury, M. L., Sternweis, P. C. 1985. Relationship within the family of GTP-binding proteins isolated from bovine central nervous system. *J. Biol. Chem.* 260:16242–49

139. Rosenthal, W., Schultz, G. 1987. Modulation of voltage-dependent ion channels by extracellular signals. *Trends Pharmacol. Sci.* 8:351–54

140. Rudy, B. 1988. Diversity and ubiquity of K channels. *Neurosci.* 25:729–49

141. Sakmann, B., Noma, A., Trautwein, W. 1983. Acetylcholine activation of single muscarinic K$^+$ channels in isolated pacemaker cells of the mammalian heart. *Nature* 303:250–53

142. Sasaki, K., Sato, M. 1987. A single GTP-binding protein regulates K$^+$ channels coupled with dopamine, histamine and acetylcholine receptors. *Nature* 325: 259–62

143. Sawada, M., Cleary, L. J., Byrne, J. H. 1989. Inositol trisphosphate (IP$_3$) and activators of protein kinase C (PKC) modulate membrane currents in tail motor neurons of *Aplysia*. *J. Neurophysiol.* 61:302–10

144. Sawada, M., Ichinose, M., Maeno, T. 1987. Ionic mechanism of the outward current induced by intracellular injection

of inositol trisphosphate into *Aplysia* neurons. *J. Neurosci.* 7:1470–83

145. Shen, K.-Z., Surprenant, A. 1988. Properties of the potassium conductance decreased by real and putative neurotransmitters in submucous plexus neurones. *Neurosci. Abstr.* 14:280

146. Shuster, M. J., Camardo, J.-S., Siegelbaum, S. A., Kandel, E. R. 1985. Cyclic AMP-dependent protein kinase closes the serotonin-sensitive K⁺-channels of *Aplysia* sensory neurones in cell-free membrane patches. *Nature* 313:392–95

147. Siegelbaum, S. A., Camardo, J. S., Kandel, E. R. 1982. Serotonin and cyclic AMP close single K⁺ channels in *Aplysia* sensory neurones. *Nature* 299: 413–17

148. Smith, P. A., Zidichouski, J. A., Selyanko, A. A. 1988. Transduction mechanisms for muscarine-induced currents in frog sympathetic neurones. *Neurosci. Abstr.* 14:280

149. Stanfeld, P. R., Nakajima, Y., Yamaguchi, K. 1985. Substance P raises neuronal membrane excitability by reducing inward rectification. *Nature* 315:498–501

150. Stein, R., Pinkas-Kramarski, R., Sokolovsky, M. 1988. Cloned M1 muscarinic receptors mediate both adenylate cyclase inhibition and phosphoinositide turnover. *EMBO J.* 7:3031–35

151. Straub, R. E., Gershengorn, M. C. 1986. Thyrotropin-releasing hormone and GTP activate inositol trisphosphate formation in membranes isolated from rat pituitary cells. *J. Biol. Chem.* 261: 2712–17

152. Stühmer, W., Stocker, M., Sakmann, B., Seeburg, P., Baumann, A., et al. 1988. Potassium channels expressed from rat brain cDNA have delayed rectifier properties. *FEBS Lett.* 242:199–206

153. Surprenant, A., North, R. A. 1988. Mechanism of synaptic inhibition by noradrenaline acting at α_2-adrenoceptors. *Proc. R. Soc. Lond.* B234:85–114

154. Terashima, T., Katada, T., Takayama, C., Ui, M., Inoue, Y. 1988. Immunohistochemical detection of GTP-binding regulatory proteins (G_o) in the autonomic nervous system including the enteric system, superior cervical and adrenal medulla. *Brain Res.* 455:353–59

155. Thalmann, R. H. 1987. Pertussis toxin blocks a late inhibitory postsynaptic potential in hippocampal CA_3 neurons. *Neurosci. Lett.* 82:41–46

156. Thalmann, R. H. 1988. Evidence that guanosine triphosphate (GTP)-binding proteins control a synaptic response in brain: effect of pertussis toxin and GTPγS on the late inhibitory postsynaptic potential of hippocampal CA_3 neurons. *J. Neurosci.* 8:4589–4602

157. Timpe, L. C., Schwarz, T. L., Tempel, B. L., Papazian, D. M., Jan, Y. N., Jan, L. Y. 1988. Expression of functional potassium channels from shaker cDNA in *Xenopus* oocytes. *Nature* 331:143–45

158. Tokimasa, T. 1984. Muscarinic agonists depress calcium-dependent g_K in bullfrog sympathetic neurons. *J. Aut. Nerv. Syst.* 10:107–16

159. Tokimasa, T. 1985. Intracellular Ca^{2+} ions inactivate K⁺-current in bullfrog sympathetic neurones. *Brain Res.* 337: 386–91

160. Toutant, M., Aunis, D., Bockaert, J., Homburger, V., Rouot, B. 1987. Presence of three pertussis toxin substrates and $G_o\alpha$ immunoreactivity in both plasma and granule membranes of chromaffin cells. *FEBS Lett.* 215:339–44

161. Treistman, S. N., Levitan, I. B. 1976. Intraneuronal guanylylim/iodiphosphate injection mimics long-term synaptic hyperpolarization in *Aplysia*. *Proc. Natl. Acad. Sci. USA* 73:4689–92

162. Trussell, L. O., Jackson, M. B. 1987. Dependence of an adenosine-activated potassium current on a GTP-binding protein in mammalian central neurons. *J. Neurosci.* 7:3306–16

163. Van Dongen, A. M. J., Codina, J., Olate, J., Mattera, R., Joh, O. R., et al. 1988. Newly identified brain potassium channels gated by the guanine nucleotide binding protein G_o. *Science* 242:1433–37

164. Volterra, A., Siegelbaum, S. 1988. Role of two different guanine nucleotide-binding proteins in the antagonistic modulation of the S-type K⁺ channel by cAMP and arachidonic acid metabolites in *Aplysia* sensory neurons. *Proc. Natl. Acad. Sci. USA* 85:7810–14

165. Walsh, J. P., Byrne, J. H. 1984. Forskolin mimics and blocks a serotonin-sensitive decreased conductance in tail sensory neurons of *Aplysia*. *Neurosci. Lett.* 52:7–11

166. Wang, Y. Y., Aghajanian, G. K. 1987. Intracellular GTPγS restores the ability of morphine to hyperpolarize rat locus coeruleus neurons after blockade by pertussis toxin. *Brain Res.* 436:396–401

167. Wanke, E., Ferroni, A., Malgaroli, A., Ambrosini, A., Pozzan, T., Meldolesi, J. 1987. Activation of a muscarinic receptor selectively inhibits a rapidly inactivating Ca^{2+} current in rat sympa-

thetic neurons. *Proc. Natl. Acad. Sci. USA* 84:4313–17

168. Weinreich, D. 1986. Bradykinin inhibits a slow spike after-hyperpolarization in visceral sensory neurons. *Eur. J. Pharmacol.* 132:61–63

169. Weinreich, D., Wonderlin, W. F. 1987. Inhibition of calcium-dependent spike after-hyperpolarization increases excitability of rabbit visceral sensory neurones. *J. Physiol.* 394:415–27

170. Weiss, E. R., Kelleher, D. J., Woon, C. W., Soparkar, S., Osawa, S., et al. 1988. Receptor activation of G proteins. *FASEB J.* 2:2841–48

171. Williams, J. T., Colmers, W. F., Pan, Z. Z. 1988. Voltage- and ligand-activated inwardly rectifying currents in dorsal raphe neurones *in vitro*. *J. Neurosci.* 8:3499–3506

172. Williams, J. T., North, R. A., Tokimasa, T. 1988. Inward rectification of resting and opiate-activated potassium currents in rat locus coeruleus neurons. *J. Neurosci.* 8:4299–4306

173. Wojikiewicz, R. J. H., Kent, P. A., Fain, J. A. 1986. Evidence that thyrotropin-releasing hormone-induced increases in GTPase activity and phosphoinositide metabolism in GH₃ cells is mediated by a guanine nucleotide-binding protein other than G_i or G_o. *Biochem. Biophys. Res. Comm.* 138:1383–89

174. Wood, J. D., Mayer, C. J. 1979. Serotonergic activation of tonic-type enteric neurons in guinea-pig small intestine. *J. Neurophysiol.* 42:582–93

175. Worley, P. F., Baraban, J. M., Van Dop, C., Neer, E. J., Snyder, S. H. 1986. G_o, a guanine nucleotide-binding protein: Immunohistochemical localization in rat brain resembles distribution of second messenger systems. *Proc. Natl. Acad. Sci. USA* 83:4561–65

176. Yakel, J. L., Trussell, L. O., Jackson, M. B. 1988. Three serotonin responses in cultured mouse hippocampal and striatal neurons. *J. Neurosci.* 8:1273

177. Yamashita, N., Kojima, I., Shibuya, N., Ogata, E. 1987. Pertussis toxin inhibits somatostatin-induced K^+-conductance in human pituitary cells. *Am. J. Physiol.* 253:E28–32

178. Yano, K., Higashida, H., Inoue, R., Nozawa, Y. 1984. Bradykinin-induced rapid breakdown of phosphatidyl inositol 4,5-bisphosphate in neuroblastoma X glioma hybrid NG108–15 cells. A possible link to agonist induced neuronal function. *J. Biol. Chem.* 259:10201–7

179. Yatani, A., Codina, J., Imoto, Y., Reeves, J. P., Birnbaumer, L., Brown, A. M. 1987. A G protein directly regulates mammalian cardiac calcium channels. *Science* 238:1288–92

180. Yatani, A., Codina, J., Sekura, R. D., Birnbaumer, L., Brown, A. M. 1987. Reconstitution of somatostatin and muscarinic receptor mediated stimulation of K^+ channels by isolated G_K protein in clonal rat anterior pituitary cell membranes. *Mol. Endocrinol.* 1:283–89

181. Yatani, A., Hamm, H., Codina, J., Mazzoni, M. R., Birnbaumer, L., Brown, A. M. 1988. A monoclonal antibody to the α subunit of G_K blocks muscarinic activation of atrial K^+ channels. *Science* 241:828–31

182. Yatani, A., Imoto, Y., Codina, J., Hamilton, S. L., Brown, A. M., Birnbaumer, L. 1988. The stimulatory G-protein of adenylyl cyclase, G_s, also stimulates dihydropyridine-sensitive Ca^{2+} channels. *J. Biol. Chem.* 263:9887–95

183. Yatani, A., Mattera, R., Codina, J., Graf, R., Okabe, K., et al. 1988. The G protein-gated atrial K^+ channel is stimulated by three distinct $G_i\alpha$-subunits. *Nature* 336:680–82

Annu. Rev. Physiol. 1990. 52:243–55

G PROTEIN MODULATION OF CALCIUM CURRENTS IN NEURONS

Annette C. Dolphin

Pharmacology Department, St. George's Hospital Medical School, Cranmer Terrace, London SW17 ORE, United Kingdom

KEY WORDS: Calcium channel, guanine nucleotide, second messenger, signal transduction, cyclic nucleotide

IMPORTANCE OF CALCIUM CHANNELS FOR NEURONAL FUNCTION

A neuron represents an extreme example of a specialized cell in which differentiation has generated polarity. Several specialized regions of the cell then perform quite different functions. Voltage-activated calcium (Ca) channels are present throughout nerve cells (43, 61), and appear early in development (50). They are involved in many of the activities of the neuron, including the initial response to neurotransmitters. This response may either involve Ca channels directly or indirectly, since Ca channels will be activated following depolarization of the membrane by other transmitters such as glutamate (15). The activation of Ca channels may lead to the propagation of Ca spikes that are involved in temporal and spatial integration of signals in the dendritic tree (43). These channels also contribute to the propagation of action potentials in the cell body and axon (21), and finally they play an essential role in the release of neurotransmitter, which depends critically on an influx of Ca^{2+} through voltage-gated channels at the presynaptic terminal (3). Neurons also have the property of responding to their degree of activation by exhibiting both short and long term plasticity. It is clear that changes in intracellular Ca^{2+} levels play a role in synaptic plasticity (6), for example by activation of Ca^{2+}-dependent intracellular enzymes and by changes in gene expression.

0066/4278/90/0315-0243$02.00

The different types of Ca channels that have been identified, and probably more that are not yet clearly defined, are certain, from their distinctive properties, to play quite individual roles in these specialized neuronal functions. It is also likely that the different types of Ca channels are localized heterogeneously in differentiated neurons, according to their function (3, 32a). For this reason, the mechanisms for modulation of Ca channels in neurons are likely to be more diverse and to have a greater variety of consequences than in other cell types, such as muscle or secretory cells, which are specialized to perform a more unitary function.

TYPES OF Ca CHANNEL IN NEURONS

The first Ca channel to be investigated was the dihydropyridine-sensitive high voltage activated or L channel, originally described in cardiac myocytes (54). Its existence in several neuronal cell classes has now been well documented. The presence of a low threshold or T channel was subsequently shown in peripheral neurons (12) and heart (48). It was reported to be blocked by octanol, amiloride, and phenytoin (for review see 61), but none of these drugs is specific for the T channel. It is likely that, because of its threshold for activation near the resting potential, this channel takes part in an important homeostatic function of neurons, which is to moderate their own excitability and to regulate the rate of repetitive firing (10, 43). It is suggested that there is another distinct subtype of channel that is present only in neurons (61). This was originally described in dorsal root ganglion neurons and has been termed an N channel (49). It is not thought to be dihydropyridine-sensitive and has a single channel conductance and kinetics of activation and inactivation intermediate between T and L channels (49). It has been suggested that activation of N channels underlies the transient component of the high threshold whole-cell current, with L channels being responsible for the more sustained component (Figure 1a). However it remains unclear whether N current results from activation of a single class of channel, since its properties appear to vary with cell type (61). For this reason all sustained current cannot be attributed to L channels.

New tools are needed to discriminate between the different Ca channel subtypes. The marine snail toxin ω-conotoxin blocks N channels (46) and does not affect L channels in heart and muscle. Initial studies suggested that ω-conotoxin irreversibly blocks all high threshold Ca channels in peripheral neurons (46), but several recent studies indicate that neuronal dihydropyridine-sensitive Ca channels are not affected by ω-conotoxin (1b, 51a). Several newly discovered toxins from *Agenelopsis aperta* may prove to be ligands for high threshold Ca channels in central and peripheral neurons (1, 42a). These toxins are likely to be important tools in future research.

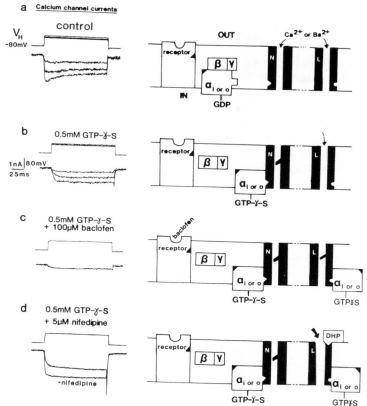

Figure 1   Calcium channel currents recorded from cultured rat dorsal root ganglion neurons.
    (*a*) control Ca channel currents activated at -20, -10 and $+5$ mV;   (*b*) Ca channel currents recorded in the presence of internal GTP-γ-S (500 μM) activated at -20, -10 and 0 mV;   (*c*) the effect of external application of (-)-baclofen (100 μM) on the maximum Ca channel current recorded in (*b*), activated at 0mV;   (*d*) the effect of external application of nifedipine (5 μM) on the maximum Ca channel current recorded at 0 mV in the presence of internal GTP-γ-S.

EVIDENCE THAT MODULATION OF NEURONAL Ca CURRENTS BY NEUROTRANSMITTERS INVOLVES G PROTEINS

Many neurotransmitters and neuromodulators are known to regulate calcium-dependent processes in neurons, and a large number of them require the obligatory activation of a GTP binding protein in the transduction of the neurotransmitter signal. The function of voltage-sensitive Ca channels may be influenced by a variety of means, either directly or involving further second messengers.

Many cells exhibit Ca spikes, or show a substantial calcium-dependent plateau phase of their action potential. In several cell types, neurotransmitters and neuromodulators, including noradrenaline, adenosine, opiates, and GABA, inhibit Ca spikes (21).

Subsequently it has been shown in some cells, including dorsal root ganglion neurons, that Ca currents are inhibited by these agonists (21, 36, 55, 61), although in other cell types it is clear that activation of a potassium conductance is responsible for the observed effect on the action potential. It is noteworthy that a similar subset of receptors is coupled both to activation of K^+ currents and to inhibition of Ca currents. These include $GABA_B$, $5-HT_{1a}$, α_2-adrenergic, muscarinic, somatostatin, neuropeptide Y (NPY), D_2, A_1, μ- and δ-opiate receptors. All these receptor subtypes have, from binding studies, been observed to interact with a GTP binding protein (G protein). Evidence for this includes the ability of GTP to reduce high affinity agonist binding in membrane preparations (27, 34). In several cases the close association with a G protein has been observed to remain in solubilized membranes. Where it has been examined, the G protein has been found to be sensitive to pertussis toxin, and treatment of membranes with this toxin reduces the receptor affinity for agonists by preventing the receptor from interacting with the ADP-ribosylated G protein (27, 37). The most abundant pertussis toxin-sensitive G protein present in neuronal tissue is G_o, but three subtypes of G_i are also present. However in several reconstitution studies several receptors have been observed to associate equally well with exogenously added G_o or G_i (2). Their inhibition of adenylate cyclase occurs largely by interaction of the enzyme with α G_i, also stoichiometrically by free $\beta\gamma$ recombining with α_s (27).

There are several more direct lines of evidence that inhibition of Ca currents by these receptors involves a G protein. The response is pertussis toxin-sensitive and can be mimicked by non-hydrolysable analogues of GTP (Figure 1b) and to a lesser extent by GTP itself (17, 18, for review see 60). In several studies it has been observed that receptor or G protein activation causes a differential inhibition of the transient component of the Ca current (Figure 1b), and in some cases it has been suggested that N current is preferentially inhibited (20, 61). However in several systems agonists also inhibit the slowly inactivating component of the Ca current (Figure 1c) although, as previously discussed, this may not represent L current. GTP analogues cause a marked slowing of the activation kinetics of the whole cell Ca current (Figure 1b). Although this also occurs in response to some neurotransmitters (45), the effect of most neurotransmitters, and GTP itself, on the kinetics of the Ca current is less marked, presumably because of rapid GTP hydrolysis (18).

Like pertussis toxin, GDP analogs oppose the response to neurotransmitters (17, 36). These agents also increase the amplitude of Ca currents in dorsal root ganglion neurons, thus having a particularly marked effect on the transient component (17, 55). This result suggests either that there exists a receptor-independent tonic activation of a pool of G proteins, or that there is a tonic production of an endogenous neuromodulator by the cultured neurons.

More direct evidence for the involvement of G proteins in Ca current inhibition comes from the introduction of purified G proteins into pertussis toxin-treated neuronal cells. Under these circumstances, G_o, and to a lesser extent G_i, restores the ability of an opiate agonist to inhibit Ca currents in NG 108-15 cells (33). Similar experiments have been performed in dorsal root ganglion neurons using NPY (24). However the finding that high concentrations of a particular G protein or its α subunit is effective does not necessarily imply that this is the mediator in vivo. Further evidence comes from the intracellular application of anti-G protein antibodies. These antibodies prevent the response of calcium currents to agonists in snail neurons (32), dorsal root ganglion neurons (24), and neuroblastoma-glioma hybrid cells (9). Although anti-G_o was found to be more effective than antibodies against the G_i species, such experiments are difficult to perform quantitatively because of the different antibody properties. Nevertheless these studies provide evidence that G_o activation can inhibit Ca currents.

There have been fewer studies on the responsiveness of low voltage-activated or T currents to inhibitory modulation by neurotransmitters or G protein activation. Although activation of κ-opiate receptors by dynorphin produced a marked inhibition of the transient component of the high threshold Ca current in rat dorsal root ganglion neurons, it was not observed to inhibit low threshold currents (30). In contrast, dopamine and an adenosine analogue were found to inhibit T currents in chick and rat dorsal root ganglion neurons respectively (25, 56). In addition, photorelease of 10–20 μM GTP-γ-S intracellularly from a photosensitive nitrophenylethyl ester of GTP-γ-S inhibits T currents in rat dorsal root ganglion neurons, whereas a lower concentration of 6 μM GTP-γ-S increases T currents (19).

MECHANISM OF G PROTEIN MODULATION OF Ca CURRENTS

The finding that activation of a G protein is an essential step in the mediation of the response of various components of the whole-cell Ca current to neurotransmitters does not imply a direct interaction between this G protein and the different Ca channels.

Receptor-mediated responses will now be discussed under four sections: (*a*) responses involving activation or inhibition of adenylate cyclase by the mediation of G_s and G_i respectively; (*b*) responses involving activation of phospholipase C by a distinct G protein (G_p); the diacylglycerol arm of this second messenger pathway will be particularly considered; (*c*) responses mediated by a G protein involving other second messenger candidates; (*d*) evidence for responses involving direct interaction with Ca channels.

Responses Involving Cyclic AMP

The first evidence for a neurotransmitter affecting Ca channels was provided by noradrenaline, which increases cardiac Ca currents by β-receptor activation (11). This occurs via G_s, mainly by cAMP-dependent phosphorylation of one of the subunits of the L channel (38), and the effect is on the channel gating kinetics rather than on the single channel conductance or number of channels.

There is less evidence in neurons for a robust response of Ca currents to changes in intracellular cAMP. There are several reports that neuronal Ca currents show little or no sensitivity to cAMP despite the presence of a dihydropyridine-sensitive component of the macroscopic current (47, 59, 63). However we have observed agents that increase cAMP to enhance sustained Ca currents in rat dorsal root ganglion neurons, and conversely agents that inhibit phosphorylation reduce Ca currents (13, 16). There is also evidence that single L channels in hippocampal and sympathetic neurons respond to cAMP (28, 42). It is possible that modulation of Ca currents by cAMP is not obvious in neurons because there is a higher basal adenylate cyclase activity in these cells, and the channels are normally more fully phosphorylated.

The group of agents that inhibit neuronal Ca currents (see previous section) are all capable of being coupled to inhibition of adenylate cyclase. Evidence that Ca current inhibition does not occur by utilizing this route is of two types. Firstly, the inhibitory responses to members of this group of neurotransmitters and neuromodulators cannot be prevented by agents such as forskolin, which will produce a massive increase in intracellular cAMP (16, 47, 59, 63). Secondly, in most cases it has not been found that the response involves a soluble intracellular messenger. This evidence will be discussed in a later section.

Involvement of Phospholipase C

In most tissues, including neurons, the Ca^{2+}-mobilizing class of neurotransmitters and neuromodulators that activate phospholipase C, do so by a pertussis toxin-insensitive mechanism; and the group of neurotransmitters that inhibit Ca currents is not normally considered to belong to this class. There is, nevertheless, a certain amount of indirect evidence that some neurotransmitters may affect at least a component of neuronal Ca currents by production of diacyglycerol and activation of protein kinase C (PKC). Most of this evidence relies on the use of the PKC activators, phorbol esters and synthetic diacylglycerols. These compounds are membrane-permeable, and they have been shown to inhibit Ca currents when applied externally to neurons (52). However in other studies either no effect or an increase in Ca currents has been observed of these agents (16, 47, 63). In addition, they increase single Ca^{2+} channel activity in sympathetic neurons (42), as has been shown previously in cardiac cells (41). Similarly, it has been observed that phorbol esters induce the appearance of new Ca^{2+} channels in *Aplysia* neurons (60).

Most studies have not found inhibitors of PKC to prevent the block of Ca currents by either neurotransmitters or PKC activators (16, 63). However all widely available PKC inhibitors, including H7, polymyxin B, and staurosporine are unsatisfactory, since they show little specificity for PKC, and also inhibit other protein kinases (26). H7 and polymyxin B have also been reported to inhibit neuronal Ca channels, and the latter interacts with ω-conotoxin binding sites (39). Recently a specific peptide inhibitor of PKC has been developed (62), and it has been reported to prevent the effect of PKC activators and the agonists noradrenaline and GABA on dorsal root ganglion Ca currents, when infused in the patch pipette (53). It will be of great interest to examine the effects of this inhibitor in other systems.

Although most transmitters that inhibit neuronal Ca currents are not Ca^{2+} mobilizing, it has been observed that some of these transmitters stimulate diacylglycerol production possibly from non-inositol containing phospholipids, since inositol trisphosphate production is little affected. For example, NPY stimulates diacylglycerol production in dorsal root ganglion neurons, and its effect on Ca currents has been reported to involve PKC (51). This effect is partially prevented when PKC is down-regulated by prolonged exposure of the cells to phorbol esters (22). However PKC activation may also affect receptor sensitivity, as has been observed for the receptors involved in the inhibition of neuronal M currents (7). In one study the Ca mobilizing hormone bradykinin was observed to inhibit Ca currents in sensory neurons, in a pertussis toxin-sensitive manner. It is unusual that the response can be restored by intracellular infusion of two G_i proteins and also by G_o (23), which indicates that in this case several signal transduction mechanisms may be involved. In contrast, in another study bradykinin either had no effect or enhanced Ca channel currents carried by Ba^{2+} in rat sensory neurons (16). A more clear-cut example of the participation of PKC is provided by cholecystokinin, which inhibits Ca currents in neurons of the snail *Helix aspersa*. The effect of this peptide is mimicked by phorbol esters and enhanced by injection of PKC (31).

In conclusion, the evidence for the obligatory mediation of PKC in the inhibition of Ca currents by neurotransmitters remains largely equivocal. However it is likely that most workers would agree that PKC activation is not responsible for neurotransmitter inhibition of the transient component of the whole-cell current.

Responses Involving Other Second Messengers

The S potassium current in *Aplysia* sensory neurons is activated by the peptide transmitter FMRF-amide, which also inhibits Ca currents in these neurons by a G protein dependent mechanism (8). The effect on S channels appears to occur by activation of phospholipase A_2 via a pertussis toxin-sensitive G protein (for review see 4). It is mimicked by external application of arachidonic acid or its lipoxygenase metabolites. Although the mechanism of action of the eicosanoid second messenger on the channel is unknown, it may interact with the cAMP-dependent phosphorylation system activated by serotonin and the small cardioactive peptides, which all decrease the number of functional S channels. It remains to be seen whether the same second-messenger pathway is involved in Ca current inhibition in these neurons, although arachidonic acid does not inhibit Ca currents in dorsal root ganglion neurons (16).

Direct Interaction of G Proteins with Neuronal Ca Channels

To obtain convincing evidence that a G protein-mediated effect on a Ca current does not occur via a second messenger, it must ultimately be shown that the neurotransmitter affects Ca channels under conditions where soluble second messengers cannot be involved, i.e. in a cell-free patch or in a reconstituted system. Such evidence, which has been obtained in the case of neuronal K^+ channels, is more conclusive than studies showing that activators or inhibitors of various second-messenger systems do not mimic, or prevent the responses to the neurotransmitters in question. The examination of neuronal Ca channels in isolated patches has proven difficult in the case of high threshold channels, since their survival in cell-free patches is limited. However low threshold or T channels are more robust, and it has been shown that T channels are inhibited by dopamine in outside-out patches (45) and by GTP analogues in inside-out patches (19). These results clearly suggest a direct interaction involving receptor, G protein, and channel, although they do not rule out the mediation of membrane-bound second messengers whose formation does not require soluble cofactors.

Another experimental approach that has been more fruitful in the examination of high threshold Ca channels is the use of cell-attached patches. The ability of a neurotransmitter to inhibit Ca channels is then compared when it is present in the patch pipette and when it is applied to the cell externally to the patch pipette. This protocol tests whether there is production of a second messenger that can diffuse to the channels under the patch and has proven successful in implicating cAMP as a mediator in S channel inhibition. In the first study of this type, external noradrenaline did not inhibit the Ca channel current recorded from a large cell-attached patch (25). Subsequently, similar results have been observed in the case of noradrenaline on sympathetic neuron Ca channels (42), NPY on myenteric neuron Ca channels (35), and the

GABA$_B$ agonist baclofen on dorsal root ganglion Ca channels (29), although there is a recent report that noradrenaline applied outside the patch inhibits Ca channels in chick dorsal root ganglion neurons (1a). Thus even this technique has not provided unequivocal evidence for a direct interaction between Ca channels and G proteins. Indeed, if the second messenger were diacylglycerol or another membrane-associated compound, it might not be expected to diffuse to the membrane under the patch.

G PROTEIN INTERACTION WITH Ca CHANNEL LIGAND BINDING SITES

We have recently observed an interaction between G protein activation and the Ca channel ligand binding sites, with respect to their effects on Ca channel currents recorded in cultured rat dorsal root ganglion neurons and sympathetic neurons (18, 57). Ca channel antagonists from three different chemical classes showed only agonist properties in the presence of internal guanine nucleotide analogues. The dihydropyridines nifedipine and (-)-202-791, the phenylakylamine D600, and the benzothiazepine diltiazem all inhibit control Ca currents, although in a proportion of neurons an initial transient agonist response was observed, particularly at hyperpolarized holding potentials (18, 57). In contrast, in the presence of internal GTP-γ-S, the agonist response was marked and prolonged for the duration of the application of the drug (18, 57; Figure 1d). These agonist responses, as well as those to the Ca channel agonists Bay K 8644 and (+)-202-791, were prevented by pertussis toxin (58), which suggests that in intact cells G protein activation may be required for Ca channel ligands to act as agonists, or that inactive G proteins prevent the channel from existing in a conformation where the ligands can act as agonists (18). There may be a subset of L channels that responds only to agonists. It seems unlikely that there are different binding sites for the agonist and antagonist isomers of each class of Ca channel ligand, but rather that the Ca channel can exist in several conformations, dependent upon membrane potential and other factors, which interconvert each ligand binding site between the ability to bind agonists or antagonists and produce the corresponding effect. It is clear that in polarized heart cells there is co-operativity between these binding sites (40) and that both homotropic and heterotropic interactions can occur. This novel interaction between Ca channels and pertussis toxin-sensitive G proteins has not yet been shown to involve a direct association, although there is no evidence for the involvement of second messenger (18). An initial binding study on the interaction between G proteins and Ca channel ligands has shown that GTP-γ-S enhanced Bay K 8644 binding (5). It will be interesting to investigate the interaction between G proteins and Ca channel ligand binding and action in polarized cells, and in lipid bilayers. Further experiments are in progress on the physiologic implications of this interaction in terms of the various functions such as transmitter release, in which there is an obligatory role for Ca channel activation.

CONCLUSION

Several different interactions between G proteins and neuronal Ca channels and Ca currents have been described. T channels, which contribute to the modulation of neuronal excitability, can be inhibited by neurotransmitters, as can high threshold channels, particularly N channels, which may be involved in providing Ca^{2+} for transmitter release. However there remains no unequivocal evidence that any of the different classes of neuronal Ca channel are influenced directly by an activated G protein.

ACKNOWLEDGMENT

The author's work is supported by the Medical Research Council (UK) and the Wellcome Trust.

Literature Cited

1. Adams, M. E., Dolphin, A. C., Scott, R. H. 1989. The inhibition of Ca^{2+} channel currents in cultured rat dorsal root ganglion (DRG) neurones by ω-Agatoxin-1A (a funnel-web spider toxin) *J. Physiol.* In press
1a. Anderson, C. S., Dunlap, K. 1988. Single L type calcium channels in dorsal root ganglion neuron can be modulated by norepinephrine. *Soc. Neurosci. Abstr.* 14:644 (Abstr.).
1b. Aosaki, T. Kasai, T. 1989. Characterization of two kinds of high-voltage activated Ca-channel currents in chick sensory neurons: differential sensitivity to dihydropyridines and ω-conotoxin GVIA. *Pflügers Arch.* 414:150–56
2. Asano, T., Ui, M., Ogasawara, N. 1985. Prevention of the agonist binding to γ-aminobutyric acid B receptors by guanine nucleotides and islet activating protein, pertussis toxin in bovine cerebral cortex. *J. Biol. Chem.* 260:12653–58
3. Augustine, G. J., Charlton, M. P., Smith, S. J. 1987. Calcium action in synaptic transmitter release. *Annu. Rev. Neurosci.* 10:633–93
4. Belardetti, F., Siegelbaum, S. 1988. Up- and down- modulation of single K^+ channel function by distinct second messengers. *Trends Neurosci.* 11:232–38
5. Bergamaschi, S., Govoni, S., Com-

inetti, P., Parenti, M., Trabucchi, M. 1988. Direct coupling of a G protein to dihydropyridine binding sites. *Biochem. Biophys. Res. Commun.* 56:1279–86
6. Bliss, T. V. P., Lynch, M. A. 1988. In *Long Term Potentiation: From Biophysics to Behaviour*, ed. P. W. Landfield, S. W. Deadwyler, pp. 3–78. New York: Liss
7. Bosma, M. M., Hille, B. 1989. Protein kinase C is not necessary for desensitization of peptide-induced suppression of M current or for the peptide receptors. *Proc. Natl. Acad. Sci. USA* 86:2943–47
8. Brezina, V., Eckert, R., Erxleben, C. 1987. Suppression of calcium current by an endogenous neuropeptide in neurons of *Aplysia californica*. *J. Physiol.* 388:565–95
9. Brown, D. A., McFadzean, I., Milligan, G. 1989. Antibodies to the GTP binding protein G_o attenuate the inhibition of the calcium current by noradrenaline in mouse neuroblastoma x rat glioma (NG 108-15) hybrid cells. *J. Physiol.* 415:20P
10. Burlhis, T. M., Aghajanian, G. K. 1987. Pacemaker potentials of serotonergic dorsal raphé neurones: Contribution of a low threshold Ca^{2+} conductance. *Synapse* 1:582–88
11. Cachelin, A. B., de Peyer, J. E., Kokubun, S., Reuter, H. 1983. Ca^{2+} channel

modulation by 9-bromocyclic AMP in cultured heart cells. *Nature* 304:462–64

12. Carbone, E., Lux, H. D. 1985. A low voltage-activated, fully inactivating Ca^{2+} channel in vertebrate sensory neurons. *Nature* 310:501–2

13. Chad, J., Eckert, R. 1986. An enzymatic mechanism for calcium current inactivation in dialyzed *Helix* neurons. *J. Physiol.* 378:31–51

14. Deleted in proof

15. Choi, D. W. 1988. Calcium-mediated neurotoxicity: relationship to specific channel types and role in ischaemic damage. *Trends Neurosci.* 11:465–69

16. Dolphin, A. C., McGuirk, S. M., Scott, R. H. 1989. An investigation into the mechanisms of inhibition of calcium channel currents in cultured rat sensory neurons by guanine nucleotide analogues and (-)-baclofen. *Br. J. Pharmacol.* 97:263-73

17. Dolphin, A. C., Scott, R. H. 1987. Calcium-channel currents and their inhibition by (-)-baclofen in rat sensory neurons: modulation by guanine-nucleotides. *J. Physiol.* 386:1–17

18. Dolphin, A. C., Scott, R. H. 1989. Interaction between calcium channel ligands and guanine nucleotides in cultured rat sensory and sympathetic neurons. *J. Physiol.* 413:271–88

19. Dolphin, A. C., Scott, R. H., Wootton, J. F. 1989. Photo-release of GTP-γ-S inhibits a low threshold calcium channel current in cultured rat dorsal root ganglion (DRG) neurons. *J. Physiol.* 410:16P

20. Dolphin, A. C., Wootton, J. F., Scott, R. H., Trentham, D. R. 1988. Photoactivation of intracellular guanosine triphosphate analogues reduces the amplitude and slows the kinetics of voltage-activated calcium channel currents in sensory neurons. *Pflügers Arch.* 411: 628–36

21. Dunlap, K., Fischbach, G. D. 1981. Neurotransmitters decrease the calcium conductance activated by depolarization of embryonic chick sensory neurones. *J. Physiol.* 317:519–35

22. Ewald, D. A., Matthies, H. J. G., Perney, T. M., Walker, M. W., Miller, R. J. 1988. The effect of down regulation of protein kinase C on the inhibitory modulation of DRG Ca^{2+} currents by NPY. *J. Neurosci.* 8:2447–51

23. Ewald, D. A., Miller, R. J., Sternweis, P. C. 1988. G proteins reconstitute inhibition of Ca^{2+} currents by bradykinin in pertussis toxin-treated rat dorsal root ganglion DRG neurons. *Soc. Neurosci. Abstr.* 14:754 (Abstr.)

24. Ewald, D. A., Sternweis, P. C., Miller, R. J. 1988. Guanine nucleotide-binding proteins G_o-induced coupling of neuropeptide Y receptors to Ca^{2+} channels in sensory neurons. *Proc. Natl. Acad. Sci. USA* 85:3633–37

25. Forscher, P., Oxford, G. S., Schultz, D. 1986. Noradrenaline modulates calcium channels in avian dorsal root ganglion cells through tight receptor-channel coupling. *J. Physiol.* 379:131–44

26. Garland, L. G., Bonser, R. W., Thompson, N. T. 1987. Protein kinase C inhibitors are not selective. *Trends Pharmacol. Sci.* 8:334

27. Gilman, A. G. 1987. G proteins: transducers of receptor-generated signals. *Annu. Rev. Biochem.* 56:615–49

28. Gray, R., Johnston, D. 1987. Noradrenaline and β-adrenoceptor agonists increase activity of voltage-dependent calcium channels in hippocampal neurons. *Nature* 327:620–22

29. Green, K. A., Cottrell, G. A. 1988. Actions of baclofen on components of the Ca-current in rat and mouse DRG neurons in culture. *Br. J. Pharmacol.* 94:235–45

30. Gross, R. A., MacDonald, R. L. 1987. Dynorphin A selectively reduces a large transient (N-type) calcium current of mouse dorsal root ganglion neurons in cell culture. *Proc. Natl. Acad. Sci. USA* 84:5469–73

31. Hammond, C., Paupardin-Tritsch, D., Nairn, A. C., Greengard, P., Gerschenfeld, H. M. 1987. Cholecystokinin induces a decrease in Ca^{2+} current in snail neurons that appears to be mediated by protein kinase C. *Nature* 325:809–11

32. Harris-Warwick, R. M., Hammond, C., Paupardin-Tritsch, D., Homburger, V., Rouot, B., et al. 1988. An α_{40} subunit of a GTP binding protein immunologically related to G_o mediates a dopamine-induced decrease of a Ca^{2+} current in snail neurons. *Neuron* 1:27–32

32a. Haydon, P. G., Man-Song-Hing, H. 1988. Low and high voltage-activated calcium currents: their relationship to the site of neurotransmitter release in an identified neuron of Helisoma. *Neuron* 1:919–27

33. Hescheler, J., Rosenthal, W., Trautwein, W., Schultz, G. 1987. The GTP binding protein G_o, regulates neuronal calcium channels. *Nature* 325:445–47

34. Hill, D. R., Bowery, N. G., Hudson, A. L. 1984. Inhibition of $GABA_B$ receptor binding by guanyl nucleotides. *J. Neurochem.* 42:652–57

35. Hirning, L. D., Fox, A. P., Miller, R. J.

1988. Modulation of calcium currents by neuropeptide Y in rat myenteric neuron cultures. *Soc. Neurosci. Abstr.* 14:901 (Abstr.)

36. Holz, G. G. IV, Rane, S. G., Dunlap, K. 1986. GTP binding proteins mediate transmitter inhibition of voltage-dependent calcium channels. *Nature* 319:670–72

37. Hsia, J. A., Moss, J., Hewlett, E. L., Vaughan, M. 1984. Requirement for both choleragen and pertussis toxin to obtain maximal activation of adenylate cyclase in cultured cells. *Biochem. Biophys. Res. Commun.* 119:1068–1074

38. Kameyama, M., Hescheler, J., Hofmann, F., Trautwein, W. 1986. Modulation of Ca current during the phosphorylation cycle in the guinea pig heart. *Pflügers Arch.* 407:123–28

39. Knaus, H.-G., Striessnig, J., Koza, A., Glossmann, H. 1987. Neurotoxic aminoglucoside antibiotics are potent inhibitors of (^{125}I)-omega conotoxin GVIA binding to guinea-pig cerebral cortex membranes. *Naunyn-Schmiedeberg's Arch. Pharmacol.* 336:583–86

40. Kokubun, S., Prod'hom, B., Becker, C., Porzig, H., Reuter, H. 1986. Studies on Ca channels in intact cardiac cells: Voltage dependent effects and cooperative interactions of dihydropyridine enantiomers. *Mol. Pharmacol.* 30:571–84

41. Lacerda, A. E., Rampe, D., Brown, A. M. 1988. Effects of protein kinase C activators on cardiac Ca^{2+} channels. *Nature* 335:249–51

42. Lipscombe, D., Bley, K., Tsien, R. W. 1988. Modulation of neuronal Ca channels by cAMP and phorbol esters. *Soc. Neurosci. Abstr.* 14:153 (Abstr.)

42a. Llinas, R., Sugimori, M., Lin, J.-W., Cherksey, B. 1989. Blocking and isolation of a calcium channel from neurons in mammals and cephalopods utilizing a toxin fraction (FTX) from funnel-web spider poison. *Proc. Natl. Acad. Sci. USA* 86:1689–93

43. Llinas, R., Yarom, Y. 1981. Properties and distribution of ionic conductances generating electroresponsiveness of mammalian inferior olivary neurones in vitro. *J. Physiol.* 315:569–84

44. Deleted in proof

45. Marchetti, C., Carbone, E., Lux, H. D. 1986. Effects of dopamine and noradrenaline on Ca channels of cultured sensory and sympathetic neurons of chick. *Pflügers Arch.* 406:104–11

46. McCleskey, E. W., Fox, A. P., Feldman, D. H., Cruz, L. J., Olivera, B.

M., et al 1987. Direct and persistent blockade of specific types of calcium channels in neurons but not muscle. *Proc. Natl. Acad. Sci. USA* 84:4327–31

47. McFadzean, I., Docherty, R. J. 1989. Noradrenaline and enkephalin-induced inhibition of voltage-sensitive calcium currents in NG108-15 hybrids cells: transduction mechanisms. *Eur. J. Neurosci.* 1:141–47

48. Nilius, B., Hess, P., Lansman, J. B., Tsien, R. W. 1985. A novel type of cardiac calcium channel in ventricular cells. *Nature* 316:443–46

49. Nowycky, M. C., Fox, A. P., Tsien, R. W. 1985. Three types of neuronal calcium channel with different calcium agonist sensitivity. *Nature* 316:440–43

50. O'Dowd, D. K., Ribera, A. B., Spitzer, N. C. 1988. Development of voltage-dependent calcium, sodium and potassium currents in *Xenopus* spinal neurons. *J. Neurosci.* 8:792–805

51. Perney, T. M., Miller, R. J. 1988. Two different G proteins may mediate receptor-stimulated phospholipid breakdown in cultured rat sensory neurons. *Soc. Neurosci. Abstr.* 14:1204 (Abstr.)

51a. Plummer, M. R., Logothetis, D. E., Hess, P. 1989. Elementary properties and pharmacological sensitivities of calcium channels in mammalian peripheral neurons. *Neuron* 2:1453–63

52. Rane, S. G., Dunlap, K. 1986. Kinase-C activator 1,2-oleoylace tyl glycerol attenuates voltage-dependent calcium current in sensory neurons. *Proc. Natl. Acad. Sci USA* 83:184–88

53. Rane, S. G., Walsh, M. P., Dunlap, K. 1987. Norepinephrine inhibition of sensory neuron calcium current is blocked by a specific protein kinase C inhibitor. *Soc. Neurosci. Abstr.* 13:557 (Abstr.)

54. Reuter, H., Stevens, C. F., Tsien, R. W., Yellen, G. 1982. Properties of single calcium channels in cardiac cell culture. *Nature* 297:501–4

55. Scott, R. H., Dolphin, A. C. 1986. Regulation of calcium currents by a GTP analogue: potentiation of (-)-baclofen-mediated inhibition. *Neurosci. Lett.* 69:59–64

56. Scott, R. H., Dolphin, A. C. 1987. In *Topics and Perspectives in Adenosine Research*, eds. E. Gerlach, B. F. Becker, pp. 549–58. Berlin: Springer-Verlag

57. Scott, R. H., Dolphin, A. C. 1987. Activation of a G-protein promotes agonist responses to calcium channel ligands. *Nature* 330:760–62

58. Scott, R. H., Dolphin, A. C. 1988. The agonist effect of Bay K 8644 on neuron-

al calcium channel currents is promoted by G protein activation. *Neurosci. Lett.* 89:170–75

59. Shimahara, T., Icard-Liepkalns, C. 1987. Activation of enkephalin receptors reduces calcium conductance in neuroblastoma cells. *Brain Res.* 415:357–61

60. Strong, J. A., Fox, A. P., Tsien, R. W., Kaczmarek, L. K. 1987. Stimulation of protein kinase C recruits covert calcium channels in *Aplysia* bag cell neurons. *Nature* 325:714–17

61. Tsien, R. W., Lipscombe, D., Madison, D. V., Bley, K. R., Fox, A. P. 1988. Multiple types of neuronal calcium channels and their selective modulation. *Trends Neurosci.* 11:431–37

62. Walsh, M. P., Valentine, K. A., Ngai, P. K., Carruthers, C. A., Hollenberg, M. D. 1984. Ca^{2+}-dependent hydrophobic interaction chromatography. *Biochem. J.* 224:117–27

63. Wanke, E., Ferroni, A., Malgaroli, A., Ambrosini, A., Pozzan, T., Meldolesi, J. 1987. Activation of a muscarinic receptor selectively inhibits a rapidly inactivated Ca^{2+} current in rat sympathetic neurons. *Proc. Natl. Acad. Sci. USA* 84:4313–17

Annu. Rev. Physiol.. 1990. 52:257–74

REGULATION OF CARDIAC L-TYPE CALCIUM CURRENT BY PHOSPHORYLATION AND G PROTEINS

Wolfgang Trautwein and Jürgen Hescheler[1]

II. Physiologisches Institut der Universität des Saarlandes D-6650 Homburg/Saar, West Germany

KEY WORDS: calcium channel control, β-adrenergic stimulation, phosphorylation, signal transduction

INTRODUCTION

Voltage-dependent Ca^{2+} channels play a major role in the electromechanical coupling of cardiac cells. During the plateau phase Ca^{2+} entry induces a Ca^{2+}-dependent Ca^{2+} release from the sarcoplasmic reticulum and consequently the initiation of contraction (for review see 41). Voltage-dependent Ca^{2+} channels are also involved in the spontaneous impulse generation as well as in the duration of the action potentials and hence in refractoriness. Ca^{2+} channels are also the target of various hormones and neurotransmitters. In an *Annual Review of Physiology* that appeared ten years ago, Reuter (112) suggested a hypothetical scheme for the β-adrenergic control of Ca^{2+} channels by cAMP-dependent phosphorylation, but direct experimental evidence for this was still missing (further reviews see 90, 125, 133, 134). In the subsequent decade the concept of regulation via the signal transduction process and phosphorylation became more elaborate by analysis of the

[1]new address: Pharmakologisches Institut der Freien Universität Berlin Thielallee 69–73, D-I000 Berlin 33, West-Germany

0066-4278/90/0315-0257$02.00

biochemical steps involved (17). The progress has been made possible by the availability of purified biochemical compounds and new biophysical techniques, i. e. isolated cells (72, 107) and the patch-clamp technique (53).

β-ADRENERGIC STIMULATION

Whole Cell Current

The best-studied example of an hormonal effect on the calcium channel current (I_{Ca}) is the β-adrenergic stimulation of the L-type Ca^{2+} channel (111, 113, 135; for review see 124, 130, 131). On extracellular application, isoprenaline (ISP) increased I_{Ca} after a latency of a few seconds. The effect could be maintained for up to 30 min without visible desensitization and was reversible after washing out the agonist. The threshold, half-maximal and maximal concentration of ISP was 1, 50, and 100 nM, respectively (Figure 1a; 81, 60). The maximal β-adrenergic increment of I_{Ca} seems to be species-dependent; i.e. in guinea pig ventricular cardiocytes the maximal I_{Ca} increase was three to four-fold (81), while in the frog this was 15-fold (12, 55). The ISP-sensitive I_{Ca} component could be blocked by dihydropyridines or phenylalkylamines, which suggests that L-type Ca^{2+} channels are modulated (12, 101), but T-type channels are not (11, but see 95). In guinea pig preparations, β-adrenergic stimulation did not apparently shift the threshold maximum and reversal potential of the U-shaped I_{Ca} voltage relation, nor alter Ca^{2+} channel selectivity (71, 81, 115). In bullfrog ventricular and rabbit atrial cells, the enhancement of I_{Ca} by β-adrenergic agonists was found to be voltage-dependent; currents elicited by small or moderate depolarizations were increased to a larger degree than currents elicited by strong depolarizations (10, 12). The time course of I_{Ca} inactivation was not altered by β-adrenergic stimulation with physiologic Ca^{2+} concentrations (1.8 mM, 56, 71), but was prolonged under Ba^{2+} (12). Under Ba^{2+} there was also a slowing of I_{Ca} activation (12).

Single Channel Data

The whole cell Ca^{2+} current can be calculated as

$$I_{Ca} = N_T \times p_f \times p_o \times i_{Ca}$$

where N_T is the total number of Ca^{2+} channels, p_f the probability that a channel is available (thus $N_T \times P_f$ = number of functional channels), p_o the probability that the channel will be open, given that it is available, and i_{Ca} the unitary current through the open pore (135).

Adrenaline, ISP, or intracellular cAMP were without effect on i_{Ca} and N_T, but decreased the number of blank traces (p_f) in an ensemble of current traces

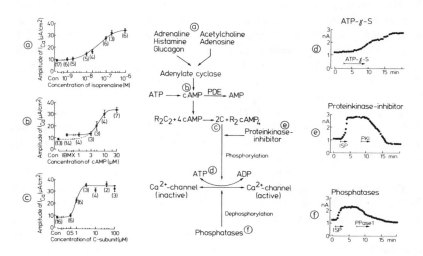

Figure 1 β-adrenergic stimulation of cardiac I_{Ca} via cAMP-dependent phosphorylation. *Middle part:* Scheme of the intracellular cascade. (*a*)–(*f*) refer to the experimental results on the left and right side. *Left side:* Concentration response curves of I_{Ca} densities for ISP (*a*), intracellularly applied cAMP (*b*), or for C-subunit of the cAMP-PK (*c*). The dotted line in (*b*) was estimated for the absence of IBMX. For experimental details see 81. The number of experiments is given in the brackets. *Right side:* Time courses of whole cell I_{Ca} during repetitive voltage clamp pulses from −40 to 0 mV. The following agents were intracellularly applied: ATPγS (5 mM, *d*), PKI (approximately 2 μM, *e*) and PPase 1 (approximately 2 μM, *f*). In (*e*) and (*f*) the ISP concentration amounted to 50 nM (from references 57, 80) (Left side with permission from Springer).

in response to step depolarizations (24, 25, 100, 111, 114, 135). Shorter closed times between bursts and a longer cluster of openings were also observed, which corresponded to the prolonged inactivation of the whole cell current under Ba^{2+} (12). Moreover, a slight increase in open time was reported. A model was proposed, where the Ca^{2+} channel can enter several states; the short-lived states (two closed, one open) being responsible for the voltage-dependent, fast kinetics, whereas the long-lived states (one voltage-dependent one phosphorylation-dependent) being responsible for the number of functional channels (105).

Components of the Signal Transducing Cascade

Biochemically, agonists acting on β-adrenoceptors activate the adenylate cyclase, thus elevating intracellular cAMP (Figure 1; 37, 141). Electrophysiologic measurements suggested a role for this second messenger in the β-adrenergic stimulation of I_{Ca}. (*a*) Direct stimulation of adenylate cyclase by forskolin (122) increased I_{Ca} by the same degree as β-adrenergic stimulation (56, 142). (*b*) Application of the membrane permeable dBcAMP or phosphodiesterase inhibitors (e.g. methylxanthine, IBMX) increased the upstroke velocity of Ca^{2+}-mediated slow action potentials and increased I_{Ca} (113, 124, 133, 134). (*c*) Atrial bullfrog trabeculae loaded with the photolabile cAMP derivative, o-nitrobenzyl cAMP, increased I_{Ca} within 10 to 30 s after light flashes released cAMP (96). (*d*) In guinea pig ventricular cardiocytes, direct intracellular application of cAMP confirmed the cAMP-dependent elevation of the action potential plateau (23, 67, 132) and I_{Ca} increase (see Figure 1b; 43, 44, 67, 81).

Similar to cAMP, intracellular application of the catalytic (C) subunit of the cAMP-dependent protein kinase (cAMP-PK) led to an increase in I_{Ca} (see Figure 1c; 23, 18, 101). All three agonists, ISP, cAMP, as well as C-subunit, modulated I_{Ca} density within the same range, i.e. between 10 and 35 $\mu A/cm^2$ (values for guinea pig ventricular cardiocytes, 81). At maximal concentrations, the effects were not additive, thus supporting the hypothesis that β-adrenergic agonists use a cAMP-dependent phosphorylation as an intracellular signal cascade (see Figure 1). A plot of equipotent concentrations of C-subunit of cAMP-PK vs cAMP is fitted according to a reaction scheme for the dissociation of the holoenzyme cAMP-PK into regulatory (R) and catalytic (C) subunits (32):

$$R_2C_2 + 4\ cAMP \rightarrow R_2cAMP_4 + 2C.$$

The estimated cAMP concentration for half-maximal activation of the cAMP-PK was 5 μM and in good agreement with that measured in vitro (81; for biochemical data see 31, 37, 129, 141).

Blockage of the Cascade

From these results it can be expected that interruption of the cascade should suppress the β-adrenergic stimulation of I_{Ca}. This was clearly observed on intracellular application of the following biochemical tools: (*a*) R_pcAMPS, a cyclic cAMP analogue that binds to the R-subunit preventing dissociation of the cAMP-PK holoenzyme (36, 61); (*b*) purified R-subunit of the cAMP-PK (80, 86, 101); and (*c*) heat stable protein kinase inhibitor (PKI) of the cAMP-PK (6).

On intracellular infusion of 2 μM PKI, enhanced I_{Ca} was fully reversed to a value somewhat below the control amplitude (Figure 1e; see also 80). Similar PKI antagonistic effects were also observed in spontaneously beating cardiocytes (19).

Experiments with ATP and Analogues

Protein phosphorylation requires $Mg^{2+}ATP$ as a phosphate donor. Elevation of intracellular ATP levels from two to nine mM increased I_{Ca} (67) and $[Mg^{2+}]_i$ affected I_{Ca} augmented by cAMP-dependent phosphorylation, but had no effect on basal I_{Ca} (143). The role of phosphorylation in the β-adrenergic stimulation of I_{Ca} was also corroborated using ATP analogues. Infusion of 5'-adenylyl-imidodiphosphate (AMP-PNP), a non-hydrolyzable ATP analogue whose γ-phosphate is not available for protein kinases (146), largely suppressed the β-adrenergic response on I_{Ca} (130). An opposite effect was expected for adenosine-5'-O-(3-thiotriphosphate) (ATPγS), which leads to irreversibly thiophosphorylated substrates resistant to dephosphorylation (146). Intracellular ATPγS resulted in a slow but steady increase of I_{Ca} (Figure 1d), which may reflect basal cAMP-PK activity. This was dramatically augmented if the cardiocyte was additionally superfused with ISP at threshold concentrations (see 80, 81).

Dephosphorylation

The hypothesis of a cAMP-dependent phosphorylation as mediator of the β-adrenergic effect on I_{Ca} became more substantiated by the identification of several protein phosphatases (PPases) that, when applied intracellularly, were able to reverse the increment of I_{Ca}. At least three different PPases were demonstrated to exert such an effect (57, 58; for aplysia bag cell neurones see 27): (a) PPase 1, characterized by its ability to be blocked by the inhibitors 1 and 2, (b) PPase 2A, and (c) PPase 2B, which is identical to the Ca^{2+}-dependent PPase calcineurin (for classification of PPases see 30).

The involvement of more than one PPase in the dephosphorylation of a substrate, closely related or identical to the Ca^{2+} channel, was supported by the observation that all inhibitors that had a relative high specificity for the different PPases only partially elevated I_{Ca}, in contrast to ATPγS, which led to a maximal increase of I_{Ca}. The following inhibitors were available for these studies: (a) inhibitor 1 or 2 for PPase 1, (b) okadaic acid for PPase 2A (59), (c) Ca^{2+} chelator EGTA for PPase 2B.

EXPERIMENTS ON PURIFIED DIHYDROPYRIDINE RECEPTORS

Phosphorylation, Reconstitution, and Primary Structure

Several reports on purified skeletal muscle high affinity dihydropyridine (DHP) receptors, denoted as L-type channels due to pharmacologic and electrical properties (5, 102), revealed a multi-subunit protein with an approximate molecular weight of 400 kd (20, 34, 35, 46, 127; for review see 52).

The protein consisted of several non-covalently associated subunits termed α_1, α_2, β, γ, and δ (8, 26, 89), of which only the α_1-subunit binds the organic Ca^{2+} channel blockers (for review see 63, 64). DHP receptors purified from bovine cardiac tissue have a slightly larger α_1-subunit with homologies, but are not apparently identical (28, 121).

Two techniques have been used to reconstitute functional Ca^{2+} channels from DHP receptors: (a) incorporation of the multi-subunit protein into lipid vesicles (34, 79); Ca^{2+} uptake could then be triggered by K^+ depolarization (i. e. voltage dependency), blocked by addition of DHP, and augmented by C-subunit of the cAMP-PK plus Mg^{2+}ATP (i. e. phosphorylation increasing open probability); (b) incorporation of liposomes containing the purified α, β, γ subunits into planar lipid bilayers (104). This method revealed two types of voltage-dependent Ca^{2+} channels having conductances of 9 and 20 pS with 90 mM Ba^{2+} as charge carrier. The 20 pS channel could be blocked by phenylal-kylamines (L-type like) and respond to phosphorylation by the cAMP-PK C-subunit with an increased open probability (46).

The model shown in Figure 2 is deduced from the primary structure of the DHP receptor α_1-subunit from rabbit skeletal muscle (128; for review see 26). The cloned DHP receptor contains seven potential phosphorylation sites (six serine, one threonine), one between repeat II and III, and six between repeat IV and the carboxy terminal. Phosphorylation by cAMP-dependent protein kinase incorporated within 10 min up to 1.6 mol phosphate/mol protein into the α-subunit from rabbit skeletal muscle and 1 mol/mol into the β-subunit (46, 97). The serine 687 (i. e. the phosphorylation site between repeat II and III) was determined as a rapidly phosphorylated site, possibly responsible for the increase in open probability. A second site, presumably serine 1617

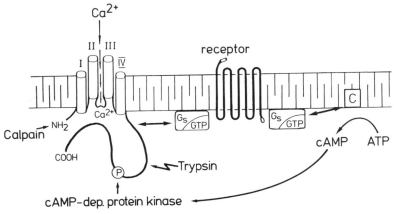

Figure 2 Model of the Ca^{2+} channel protein and its regulation by various mechanisms. C=catalytic subunit of the adenylate cyclase. For further explanation see text.

(located at the carboxy terminus), was phosphorylated at a slower rate (117, 118).

Other kinases can also phosphorylate the α_1- or β-subunit of the Ca^{2+} channel protein. Casein kinase II phosphorylated the α_1- and the β-subunit at similar rates, while cGMP-dependent protein kinase, protein kinase C, and calmodulin kinase II preferentially phosphorylated the β-subunit. The latter was phosphorylated ten times faster by cGMP-dependent protein kinase and protein kinase C than by cAMP-PK (73). The physiologic role of β-subunit phosphorylation is not clear.

MODIFICATION BY PROTEASES

It is generally assumed that the regulatory parts of the Ca^{2+} channel, especially the phosphorylation site(s), are facing the cytoplasm (Figure 2). Proteolytic enzymes, intracellularly applied, might therefore first affect the regulation of the channels. The endoproteases, trypsin and chymotrypsin, as well as exocarboxypeptidase increased the amplitude of I_{Ca} by a factor of three to four without affecting the voltage dependency or the sensitivity towards DHPs or phenylalkylamines. Exoaminopeptidase did not increase the amplitude, but accelerated the run-down of I_{Ca} (see below, 62). The increase in I_{Ca} induced by proteolysis or by ISP were of similar magnitude and not additive at maximal concentrations. Since intracellular application of R_pcAMPS or AMP-PNP did not abolish the trypsin effect, it was assumed that the cAMP-PK cascade may not be involved but rather that the protease directly modifies a regulating site of the channel (62).

The results obtained with proteases suggest that the carboxy terminal containing the cAMP-PK phosphorylation site may work as a biochemical inactivation gate (see Figure 2). Phosphorylation or proteolytic cleavage may remove this gate, thus resulting in a higher availability to pass current on depolarization. Alternatively, proteolytic modification may induce a global change in channel protein affecting serine 687 (in vitro phosphorylation site, see above).

The dependence of I_{Ca} on pH_1 has also been explained by an interaction of H^+ ions with the channel protein. The relationship between open-state probability and pH_1 was fitted by the Hill equation with pK of 6.6 (68, 138), which suggests that protons interact with histidin residues (78).

COUPLING OF HORMONAL RECEPTORS TO THE CASCADE: ROLE OF G PROTEINS

Hormones Acting on the Adenylate Cyclase

As depicted in Table 1, histamine and glucagon are adenylate cyclase stimulating factors. Acetylcholine (ACh), adenosine, and atrial natriuretic factor (ANF) were reported to lower the cytosolic cAMP level. Hence these agents are thought to affect I_{Ca} via the same intracellular cascade as proposed for the β-adrenergic stimulation. In cardiac preparations, histamine (0.1 to 10 μM) enhanced the upstroke velocity of slow action potentials, elevated the plateau (39), and increased I_{Ca} (61). The effect of histamine on I_{Ca} (maximal concentrations) was not additive to that of β-adrenergic agonists and was abolished by R_pcAMPS (61).

In mammalian ventricular preparations, ACh (0.1 to 10 μM) and adenosine (1 to 200 μM) lowered I_{Ca} only when enhanced by stimulation of the adenylate cyclase (13, 44, 56, 77, 99, 142), but not by intracellular applica-

Table 1   Effects of various hormones on cardiac action potential and I_{Ca}

Hormone transmitter	Plateau level up-stroke slow ap	I_{Ca} amplitude	Possible mechanism	Ref.
Nor/adrenaline (β-adrenoceptor)	↑	↑	cAMP ↑	81, 113, 115, 129, 137
Nor/adrenaline (α-adrenoceptor)	0	0	IP$_3$ ↑	2, 60, 106
Histamine (H$_2$-receptor)	↑	↑	cAMP ↑	39, 60, 90, 93
Glucagon	↑	nd	cAMP ↑	42, 108
Acetylcholine (muscarine receptor)	↓ after β-adrenergic stimulation	↓ after β-adrenergic stimulation	cAMP ↓ cGMP ↑ IP$_3$ ↑	9, 44, 48, 56, 75, 77, 109
Adenosine (A1 receptor)	↓ after β-adrenergic stimulation	↓ after β-adrenergic stimulation	cAMP	69, 72, 142
Angiotensin II	↑	↑	cAMP 0 IP$_1$/IP$_2$ ↑ PKC ↑	1, 38, 47, 84
Opiate	↓	nd	nd	120
Hyperthyroidism 8 days Thyroxin	↓	↑	nd	16
Atrial natriuretic factor (ANF)	nd	↓ β-adrenergic stimulation ↓ cAMP stimulation	cAMP ↓ cGMP ↑	3, 51

Abbreviations and symbols represent ↑ = stimulation; nd = not done; ↓ = inhibition; PKC = protein kinase C; 0 = no effect; slow ap = slow action potential.

cAMP or cAMP-PK C-subunit. This suggested that muscarinic receptors affect I_{Ca} at the adenylate cyclase level (44, 56, 75, 92).

How Can Different Receptors Operate on the Same Intracellular Signaling System?

This is accomplished by a class of GTP-binding transducer proteins (G proteins), that link different receptors to the cellular (mostly membranous) effectors (29, 50; for review see 17, 119). In the case of the fore-mentioned hormones, the effector involved seems to be the adenylate cyclase, which controls Ca^{2+} channel activity indirectly via cAMP.

Stimulatory effects are transduced by a G_s protein, inhibitory effects by G_i. This concept was confirmed by several electrophysiologic studies.

GDP/GTP ANALOGUES   G protein activation releases GDP from α-subunits which allows GTP to bind and activate them (17, 29, 50); this release can be prevented by guanosine-5'-O-(2-thiodiphosphate) (GDPβS, 74). Intracellularly infused GDPβS almost completely prevented the increase of I_{Ca} evoked by histamine or by β-adrenergic agonists (61). 5'-Guanylyl-imido-diphosphate (GMP-PNP) cannot be hydrolyzed by the active α-subunit, thus resulting in permanent activation of G proteins because of inhibition of GTPase activity (123). When infused into a cardiocyte, this compound only slightly increased I_{Ca}, presumably because both G_s and G_i were fully activated. Under this condition, hormonal responses of ISP and ACh on I_{Ca} were absent (21, 56; for slow action potentials see 125). Similarly, guanosine-5'-O-(3'-thiotriphosphate) (GTPγS) inhibits the intrinsic GTPase activity of the G protein α-subunit (76, 123) but evokes a more pronounced increment of I_{Ca}, perhaps due to the larger affinity of GTPγS for G_s over G_i. As with GMP-PNP, GTPγS also inhibited hormonal modulations of I_{Ca} (61). The larger effect of GTPγS may also be due to direct activation of the Ca^{2+} channel by a G_s (see below).

BACTERIOTOXINS   Cholera toxin activates G_s irreversibly by ADP-ribosylation, stimulates adenylate cyclase (49, 103), and elevates the plateau of slow action potentials (91). Pertussis toxin inhibits by ADP-ribosylation the ability of G_i, but not of G_s, to be activated by hormone receptors (136). Cardiocytes exposed to pertussis toxin exhibited a larger amplitude of I_{Ca} than control cells (because of a block of the basal inhibitory influence of G_i on the adenylate cyclase), and ACh failed to depress I_{Ca} stimulated by β-adrenergic agonists (56). Results with adenosine in guinea pig atrial cells were similar (70).

DIRECT EFFECTS OF G PROTEINS ON Ca^{2+} CHANNELS

Blockage of the cAMP-dependent cascade by R-subunit of the cAMP-PK, heat stable PKI, R_pcAMPS, AMP-PNP, and PPase 1 and 2 reduced the amplitude of basal I_{Ca} by only approximately 20% (80). It seems, therefore, that phosphorylation only modulates the Ca^{2+} channel activity, but is not a requirement for basal availability, especially since unphosphorylated DHP receptors in lipid bilayers formed functional Ca^{2+} channels. However, in dialysed cells and inside-out patches, I_{Ca} declined in the course of the experiment. This run-down could not be prevented or restored by cAMP-PK (15, 88; for neuronal cells see 4, 85), which suggests that another cytosolic factor was necessary to control I_{Ca}.

In regard to the mechanisms that maintain basal I_{Ca} activity, direct stimulation of Ca^{2+} channels by G_s has been suggested (22, 66, 144). In inside-out patches, GTPγS caused a slowing of the run-down of Ca channel activity (see Birnbaumer & Brown, this volume; but note 82), and the preactivated α-subunit of G_s, but not of G_i, G_o or $\beta\gamma$, maintained channel activity (144). Furthermore, GTPγS and preactivated G_s applied to bovine cardiac sarcolemmal vesicles incorporated into planar lipid bilayers increased the single channel activity (66). Whether this direct G_s effect on Ca^{2+} channels also plays a role in the β-adrenergic stimulation of I_{Ca} remains unclear. The contribution is expected to be small since β-adrenergic agonists were almost ineffective in increasing I_{Ca} when the cAMP-dependent cascade was blocked. Recently, however, concentration jumps of ISP reveal that the rise of I_{Ca} could be fitted with two time constants; with $\tau=200$ ms attributed to a direct G_s effect, and $\tau=30$ s for the cAMP-dependent phosphorylation. On concentration jumps of forskolin, the fast time constant was absent (145).

OTHER PATHWAYS CONTROLLING Ca^{2+} CHANNELS

Possible Mediators for the Action of the Atrial Natriuretic Factor (ANF)

Superfusion of frog cardiocytes with ANF (3 to 300 nM) produced negligible effects on basal I_{Ca}, but markedly reduced I_{Ca} when enhanced by ISP (51). The observation that the reduction was less on I_{Ca} stimulated by infusion of cAMP indicates a mechanism similar to that reported for ACh; i.e. G_i-mediated inhibition of adenylate cyclase (in line with biochemical data; 3). The remaining partial inhibition of cAMP-stimulated I_{Ca} may be caused by a different mechanism. Possibly cGMP is involved, since ANF is known to be a potent activator of the guanylate cyclase (65; for cardiocytes see 33). There is no evidence for the involvement of G proteins in the regulation of the guanylate cyclase, unlike the case of ACh, where it is suggested that the ANF receptor is inherent to the guanylate cyclase protein (140).

Role of cGMP in the Regulation of I_{Ca}

In guinea pig papillary muscles 8-bromo-cGMP depressed slow action potentials (139), and pressure injection of dBcGMP into guinea pig cardiocytes shortened the action potential (132). In cultured chick embryonic heart cells intracellular application of cGMP (liposome method) slowed the rise of the action potential upstroke (18). The underlying mechanism of these observations and the possible involvement of I_{Ca} remained unclear until the studies of Flitney & Singh (45). Superfusion of frog myocardium with 8-bromo-cGMP led to a lowering of the endogenous cAMP concentration via a cGMP-stimulated cyclic nucleotide phosphodiesterase (40, 54). This hypothesis was supported by the finding that in frog ventricular cardiocytes, 3'5'cGMP (but not 2'3'cGMP) reduced the amplitude of I_{Ca} enhanced by β-adrenergic stimulation and that this effect was blocked by the phosphodiesterase inhibitor IBMX or M and B 22948 (43, 55). An effect on the cGMP-dependent protein kinase was excluded since 8-bromo-cGMP, a very potent activator of this kinase (40), had no effect on I_{Ca} (43).

Possible Mediators for Angiotensin II (AII) Action

AII (10 nM to μM) increased the spontaneous rate of action potentials in neonatal rat heart preparations (47) and I_{Ca} in Purkinje fibers (84). The increase in I_{Ca} by AII occurred without an effect on the control of ISP-stimulated adenylate cyclase activity, but was accompanied by an increased level of inositol monophosphate and inositol biphosphate (but not inositol triphosphate; 1). The modulation of I_{Ca} by AII was apparently receptor mediated since the EC_{50} was nearly identical to the K_D for the high affinity binding site in these cells (7, 116). Since phorbol esters increased I_{Ca} in cultured neonatal rat hearts similar to AII, it was assumed that the AII effects may be mediated by protein kinase C (1, 38). In the same preparation, superfusion with 12-O-tetradekanoyl-phorbol 13 acetate initially increased and then depressed whole cell I_{Ca} and single channel activity (87). However, 12 myristate-phorbol 13 acetate had only a small depressing effect on I_{Ca} in guinea pig ventricular cardiocytes (J. Hescheler, W. Trautwein, unpublished observation); and intracellular application of protein kinase C was ineffective on I_{Ca} (M. Kameyama, personal communication).

POSSIBLE MECHANISMS INVOLVED IN THE LONG-TERM REGULATION OF Ca^{2+} CHANNELS

The run-down of Ca^{2+} channel activity in isolated patches could be much delayed on application of cytosolic fluid to the intracellular membrane face

(82, 83; for whole cell I_{Ca} see 15). Using HPCL chromatography, an active cytosolic compound has been isolated ($\sim$ mol wt 200 kd, 83). Interestingly, the molecular weight is similar to that of calpastatin, the endogenous inhibitor of the Ca^{2+}-dependent proteases calpain I and II, found in heart muscle in relatively high concentrations (94, 126). An involvement of such a protease had already been suggested since the run-down of whole cell I_{Ca} was found to be faster at raised $[Ca^{2+}]_i$ (15, 88). Indeed, intracellular application of purified calpain I and II greatly accelerated the run-down of I_{Ca}, while the inhibitor calpastatin delayed it (14). The results suggest that the calpain/calpastatin system plays a role in the degradation, or turnover, of Ca^{2+} channel protein (see Figure 2). Proteins that have a high turnover share a specific recognition sequence, the so-called PEST sequence (110), and such sequences occur at least in three domains of the Ca^{2+} channel α_1-subunit (M. Rechsteiner, J. Hescheler, unpublished result). At present no data are available on the turnover of Ca^{2+} channels. It may be rewarding to study the role of hormones, phosphorylation, and G proteins on this turnover.

CONCLUSIONS

Recent literature has proposed several mechanisms concerning the chemical gating of voltage-dependent L-type Ca^{2+} channels in cardiocytes. The best established mechanism is the cAMP-dependent phosphorylation cascade where G proteins play an indirect role by signal transduction from the receptor to the adenylate cyclase. Evidence has also emerged for direct coupling of G_s protein to the Ca^{2+} channel. Other mechanisms proposed for hormones like ANF and AII may add different possible pathways to this complex regulation. In the long-term regulation of cardiac Ca^{2+} channels, Ca^{2+} dependent proteases, and their inhibitors may also be of importance.

ACKNOWLEDGMENTS

We wish to thank Dr. T. J. Allen for reading the manuscript and Mrs. H. Leser for unfailing secretarial help. This work was supported by the Deutsche Forschungsgemeinschaft, SFB 246

Literature Cited

1. Allen, I. S., Cohen, N. M., Dhallan, R. S., Gaa, S. T., Lederer, W. J., Rogers, T. B. 1988. Angiotensin II increases spontaneous contractile frequency and stimulates calcium current in cultured neonatal rat heart myocytes: Insights into the underlying biochemical mechanisms. *Circ. Res.* 62:524–34

2. Alvarez, J. L., Mongo, K. G., Vassort, G. 1987. Effects of alpha$_1$-adrenergic stimulation on Ca current in single ventricular frog cells. *J. Physiol.* 390:66P

3. Anand-Srivastava, M. B., Cantin, M. 1986. Atrial natriuretic factors are negatively coupled to adenylate cyclase in cultured atrial and ventricular cardiocytes. *Biochem. Biophys. Commun.* 138:427–36

4. Armstrong, D., Eckert, R. 1987. Voltage-activated calcium channels that

must be phosphorylated to respond to membrane depolarization. *Proc. Natl. Acad. Sci. USA* 84:2518–22

5. Arreola, J., Calvo, J., Garcia, M. C., Sánchez, J. A. 1987. Modulation of calcium channels of twitch skeletal muscle fibers of the frog by adrenaline and cyclic adenosine monophosphate. *J. Physiol.* 393:307–30

6. Ashby, C. D., Walsh, D. A. 1972. Characterization of the interaction of a protein inhibitor with adenosine 3',5'monophosphate-dependent protein kinase. *J. Biol. Chem.* 247:6637–41

7. Baker, K. M., Campanile, C. P., Trachte, G. J., Peach, M. J. 1984. Identification and characterization of the rabbit angiotensin II myocardial receptor. *Circ. Res.* 54:286–93

8. Barhanin, J., Coppola, T., Schmid, A., Borsotto, M., Lazdunski, M. 1987. The calcium channel antagonist receptor from rabbit muscle. Reconstitution after purification and subunit characterization. *Eur. J. Biochem.* 164:525–31

9. Bailey, J. C., Watanabe, A. M., Besch, H. R., Lathrop, D. A. 1979. Acetylcholine antagonism of the electrophysiological effects of isoproterenol on canine cardiac Purkinje fibers. *Circ. Res.* 44: 378–83

10. Bean, B. P. 1989. Multiple types of calcium channels in heart muscle and neurons: Modulation by drugs and neurotransmitters. In *Calcium Channels, Structure and Function*, ed. D. W. Wray, R. I. Norman, P. Hess, *Ann. N.Y. Acad. Sci.* 560:334–45

11. Bean, B. P. 1985. Two kinds of calcium channels in canine atrial cells. Differences in kinetics, selectivity, and pharmacology. *J. Gen. Physiol.* 86:1–30

12. Bean, B. P., Nowycky, M. C., Tsien, R. W. 1984. β-adrenergic modulation of calcium channels in frog ventricular heart cells. *Nature* 307:371–75

13. Belardinelli, L., Isenberg, G. 1983. Actions of adenosine and isoproterenol on isolated mammalian ventricular myocytes. *Circ. Res.* 53:287–97

14. Belles, B., Hescheler, J., Trautwein, W., Blomgren, K., Karlsson, J. O. 1988. A possible physiological role of the Ca-dependent protease calpain and its inhibitor calpastatin on the Ca current in guinea pig myocytes. *Pflügers Arch.* 412:554–56

15. Belles, B., Malécot, C. O., Hescheler, J., Trautwein, W. 1988. "Run-down" of the Ca current during long whole-cell recordings in guinea pig heart cells: role of phosphorylation and intracellular calcium. *Pflügers Arch.* 411:353–60

16. Binah, O., Rubinstein, I., Gilat, E. 1987. Effects of thyroid hormone on the action potential and membrane currents of guinea pig ventricular myocytes. *Pflügers Arch.* 409:214–16

17. Birnbaumer, L., Codina, J., Mattera, R., Cerione, R. A., Hildebrandt, J. D., et al. 1985. Regulation of hormone receptors and adenyl cyclases by guanine nucleotide binding N proteins. *Rec. Prog. Hormone. Res.* 41:41–97

18. Bkaily, G., Sperelakis, N. 1985. Injection of guanosine 5'-cyclic monophosphate into heart cells blocks calcium slow channels. *Am. J. Physiol.* 248: H745–49

19. Bkaily, G., Sperelakis, N. 1984. Injection of protein kinase inhibitor into cultured heart cells blocks slow calcium channels. *Am. J. Physiol.* 246: H630–34

20. Borsotto, M., Barhanin, J., Fosset, M., Lazdunski, M. 1985. The 1,4-dihydropyridine receptor associated with the skeletal muscle voltage-dependent Ca^{2+} channel. Purification and subunit composition. *J. Biol. Chem.* 260:14255–263

21. Breitwieser, G. E., Szabo, G. 1985. Uncoupling of cardiac muscarinic and β-adrenergic receptors from ion channels by a guanine nucleotide analogue. *Nature* 317:538–40

22. Brown, A. M., Birnbaumer, L. 1988. Direct G protein gating of ion channels. *Am. J. Physiol.* 254:H401–10

23. Brum, G., Flockerzi, V., Hofmann, F., Osterrieder, W., Trautwein, W. 1983. Injection of catalytic subunit of cAMP-dependent protein kinase into isolated cardiac myocytes. *Pflügers Arch.* 398: 147–54

24. Brum, G., Osterrieder, W., Trautwein, W. 1984. β-adrenergic increase in the calcium conductance of cardiac myocytes studied with the patch clamp. *Pflügers Arch.* 401:111–18

25. Cachelin, A. B., de Peyer, J. E., Kokubun, S., Reuter, H. 1983. Ca^{2+} channel modulation by 8-bromocyclic AMP in cultured heart cells. *Nature* 304:462–64

26. Catterall, W. A. 1988. Structure and function of voltage-sensitive ion channels. *Science* 242:50–61

27. Chad, J. E., Eckert, R. 1986. An enzymatic mechanism for calcium current inactivation in dialyzed Helix neurones. *J. Physiol.* 378:31–51

28. Chang, F. C., Hosey, M. M. 1988. Dihydropyridine and phenylalkylamine receptors associated with cardiac and skeletal muscle calcium channels are structurally different. *J. Biol. Chem.* 263:18929–37

29. Codina, J., Hildebrandt, J., Sunyer, T., Sekura, R., Manclark, C., et al. 1984. Mechanism in vectorial receptor-adenylate cyclase signal transduction. *Adv. Cyclic Nucleotide Res.* 17:111–25

30. Cohen, P. 1982. The role of protein phosphorylation in neural and hormonal control of cellular activity. *Nature* 296:613–20

31. Corbin, J. D., Keely, S. L. 1977. Characterization and regulation of heart adenosine 3',5'-monophosphate-dependent protein kinase isozymes. *J. Biol. Chem.* 252:910–18

32. Corbin, J. D., Sugden, P. H., West, L., Flockhart, D. A., Lincoln, T. M. 1978. Studies on the properties and mode of action of the purified regulatory subunit of bovine heart adenosine 3',5'-monophosphate-dependent protein kinase. *J. Biol. Chem.* 253:3997–4003

33. Cramb, G., Banks, R., Rugg, E. L., Aiton, J. F. 1987. Actions of atrial natriuretic peptide (ANF) on cyclic nucleotide concentrations and phosphatidylinositol turnover in ventricular myocytes. *Biophys. Biochem. Res. Comm.* 148:962–70

34. Curtis, B. M., Catterall, W. A. 1986. Reconstitution of the voltage-sensitive calcium channel purified from skeletal muscle transverse tubules. *Biochemistry* 25:3077–83

35. Curtis, B. M., Catterall, W. A. 1984. Purification of the calcium antagonist receptor of the voltage-sensitive calcium channel from skeletal muscle transverse tubules. *Biochemistry* 23:2113–18

36. DeWit, R., Hekstra, D., Jastorff, B., Stec, W., Baraniak, J., et al. 1984. Inhibitory action of certain cyclophosphate derivatives of cAMP on cAMP-dependent protein kinase type I. *Eur. J. Biochem.* 142:255–60

37. Dobson, J. G., Ross, J., Mayer, S. E. 1976. The role of cyclic adenosine 3',5'-monophosphate and calcium in the regulation of contractility and glycogen phosphorylase activity in guinea pig papillary muscle. *Circ. Res.* 39:388–95

38. Dösemeci, A., Dhallan, R. S., Cohen, N. M., Lederer, W. J., Rogers, T. B. 1988. Phorbol ester increases calcium current and simulates the effects of angiotensin II on cultured neonatal rat heart myocytes. *Circ. Res.* 62:347–57

39. Eckel, L., Gristwood, R. W., Nawrath, H., Owen, D. A. A., Satter, P. 1982. Inotropic and electrophysiological effects of histamine on human ventricular heart muscle. *J. Physiol.* 330:111–23

40. Erneux, C., Couchie, D., Dumont, J. E., Baraniak, J., Stec, W. J., et al. 1981. Specificity of cyclic GMP activation of a multi-substrate cyclic nucleotide phosphodiesterase from rat liver. *Eur. J. Biochem.* 115:503–10

41. Fabiato, A., Fabiato, F. 1979. Calcium and cardiac excitation-contraction coupling. *Annu. Rev. Physiol.* 41:473–84

42. Farah, A. E. 1983. Glucagon and the heart. In: *Handbook of Experimental Pharmacology, Glucagon II*, ed. P. J. Lefèbvre, 66/2:553–609. Berlin/Heidelberg/New York: Springer-Verlag

43. Fischmeister, R., Hartzell, H. C. 1987. Cyclic guanosine 3'-5'-monophosphate regulates the calcium current in single cells from frog ventricle. *J. Physiol.* 387:453–72

44. Fischmeister, R., Hartzell, H. C. 1986. Mechanism of action of acetylcholine on calcium current in single cells from frog ventricle. *J. Physiol.* 376:183–202

45. Flitney, F. W., Singh, J. 1981. Evidence that cyclic GMP may regulate cyclic AMP metabolism in the isolated frog ventricle. *J. Mol. Cell. Cardiol.* 13:963–79

46. Flockerzi, V., Oeken, H. J., Hofmann, F., Pelzer, D., Cavalié, A., Trautwein, W. 1986. Purified dihydropyridine-binding site from skeletal muscle t-tubules is a functional calcium channel. *Nature* 323:66–68

47. Freer, R. T., Pappano, A. J., Peach, M. J., Bing, K. T., McLean, M. J., et al. 1976. Mechanism for the positive inotropic effect of angiotensin II on isolated cardiac muscle. *Circ. Res.* 39:178–83

48. Giles, W., Noble, S. J. 1976. Changes in membrane currents in bull-frog atrium produced by acetylcholine. *J. Physiol.* 261:103–23

49. Gill, D. M., Meren, R. 1978. ADP-ribosylation of membrane proteins catalyzed by cholera toxin: Basis of the activation of adenylate cyclase. *Proc. Natl. Acad. Sci. USA* 75:3050–54

50. Gilman, A. 1984. G proteins and dual control of adenylate cyclase. *Cell* 36:577–79

51. Gisbert, M.-P., Fischmeister, R. 1988. Atrial natriuretic factor regulates the calcium current in frog isolated cardiac cells. *Circ. Res.* 62:660–67

52. Glossmann, H., Striessnig, J. 1988. Calcium channels. In *Vitamins and Hormones*, ed. D. B. McCormick, 44:155–328 San Diego: Academic

53. Hamill, O. P., Marty, A., Neher, E., Sakmann, B., Sigworth, F. J. 1981. Improved patch-clamp techniques for high resolution current recording from cells

and cell-free membrane patches. *Pflügers Arch* 391:85–100

54. Harrison, S. A., Reifsnyder, D. H., Gallis, B., Cadd, G. G., Beavo, J. A. 1986. Isolation and characterization of bovine cardiac muscle cGMP-inhibited phosphodiesterase: A receptor for new cardiotonic drugs. *Mol. Pharmacol.* 29:506–14

55. Hartzell, H. C., Fischmeister, R. 1986. Opposite effects of cyclic GMP and cyclic AMP on Ca current in single heart cells. *Nature* 323:273–75

56. Hescheler, J., Kameyama, M., Trautwein, W. 1986. On the mechanism of muscarinic inhibition of the cardiac Ca current. *Pflügers Arch.* 407:182–89

57. Hescheler, J., Kameyama, M., Trautwein, W., Mieskes, G., Soeling, H. D. 1987. Regulation of the cardiac calcium channel by protein phosphatases. *Eur. J. Biochem.* 165:261–66

58. Hescheler, J., Kameyama, M., Trautwein, W., Mieskes, G., Hofmann, F. 1987. Regulation of the Ca-channel by phosphorylation-dephosphorylation. In *Signal Transduction and Protein Phosphorylation,* ed. L. M. G. Heilmeyer, pp. 177–81, New York: Plenum

59. Hescheler, J., Mieskes, G., Rüegg, J. C., Takai, A., Trautwein, W. 1988. Effects of a protein phosphatase inhibitor, okadaic acid, on membrane currents of isolated guinea-pig cardiac myocytes. *Pflügers Arch.* 412:248–52

60. Hescheler, J., Nawrath, H., Tang, M., Trautwein, W. 1988. Adrenoceptor-mediated changes of excitation and contraction in ventricular heart muscle from guinea-pigs and rabbits. *J. Physiol.* 397:657–70

61. Hescheler, J., Tang, M., Jastorff, B., Trautwein, W. 1987. On the mechanism of histamine induced enhancement of the cardiac Ca^{2+} current. *Pflügers Arch.* 410:23–29

62. Hescheler, J., Trautwein, W. 1988. Modification of L-type calcium current by intracellularly applied trypsin in guinea pig ventricular myocytes. *J. Physiol.* 404:259–74

63. Hofmann, F., Nastainczyk, W., Röhrkasten, A., Schneider, T., Sieber, M. 1987. Regulation of the L-type calcium channel. *Trends Pharmacol. Sci.* 8:393–98

64. Hosey, M. M., Lazdunski, M. 1988. Calcium channels: Molecular pharmacology, structure and regulation. *J. Membr. Biol.* 104:81–105

65. Huang, C.-L., Ives, H. E., Cogan, M. G. 1986. In vivo evidence that cGMP is the second messenger for atrial natriuretic factor. *Proc. Natl. Acad. Sci. USA* 83:8015–18

66. Imoto, Y., Yatani, A., Reeves, J. P., Codina, J., Birnbaumer, L., Brown, A. M. 1988. α-subunit of G_s directly activates cardiac calcium channels in lipid bilayers. *Am. J. Physiol.* 255:H722–28

67. Irisawa, H., Kokubun, S. 1983. Modulation by intracellular ATP and cyclic AMP of the slow inward current in isolated single ventricular cells of the guinea pig. *J. Physiol.* 338:321–37

68. Irisawa, H., Sato, R. 1986. Intra- and extracellular actions of proton on the calcium current of isolated guinea pig ventricular cells. *Circ. Res.* 59:348–55

69. Isenberg, G., Belardinelli, L. 1984. Ionic basis for the antagonism between adenosine and isoproterenol on isolated mammalian ventricular myocytes. *Circ. Res.* 55:309–25

70. Isenberg, G., Cerbai, E., Klöckner, U. 1987. Ionic channels and adenosine in isolated heart cells. In: *Topics and Perspectives in Adenosine Research,* ed. E. Gerlach, B. F. Becker, pp. 323–35. Berlin: Springer-Verlag

71. Isenberg, G., Klöckner, U. 1982. Calcium currents of isolated bovine ventricular myocytes are fast and of large amplitude. *Pflügers Arch.* 395:30–41

72. Isenberg, G., Klöckner, U. 1982. Calcium tolerant ventricular myocytes prepared by preincubation in "KB medium." *Pflügers Arch.* 395:6–18

73. Jahn, H., Nastainczyk, W., Röhrkasten, A., Schneider, T., Hofmann, F. 1988. Site-specific phosphorylation of the purified receptor for calcium-channel blockers by cAMP- and cGMP-dependent protein kinases, protein kinases C, calmodulin-dependent protein kinase II and casein kinase II. *Eur. J. Biochem.* 178:535–42

74. Jakobs, K. H. 1983. Determination of the turn-off reaction for the epinephrine-inhibited human platelet adenylate cyclase. *Eur. J. Biochem.* 132:125–30

75. Jakobs, K. H., Aktories, K., Schultz, G. 1979. GTP-dependent inhibition of cardiac adenylate cyclase by muscarinic cholinergic agonists. *Naunyn Schmiedeberg's Arch. Pharmacol.* 310:113–19

76. Jakobs, K. H., Gehring, U., Gaugler, B., Pfeuffer, T., Schultz, G. 1983. Occurrence of an inhibitory guanine nucleotide-binding regulatory component of the adenylate cyclase system in cyc-variants of S49 lymphoma cells. *Eur. J. Biochem.* 130:605–11

77. Josephson, I., Sperelakis, N. 1982. On the ionic mechanism underlying

adrenergic-cholinergic antagonism in ventricular muscle. *J. Gen. Physiol.* 79: 69–86

78. Kaibara, M., Kameyama, M. 1988. Inhibition of the calcium channel by intracellular protons in single ventricular myocytes of the guinea pig. *J. Physiol.* 403:621–40

79. Kameyama, A., Nakayama, T. 1988. Calcium efflux through cardiac calcium channels reconstituted into liposomes—flux measurement with fura-2. *Biochem. Biophys. Res. Commun.* 154:1067–74

80. Kameyama, M., Hescheler, J., Hofmann, F., Trautwein, W. 1986. Modulation of Ca current during the phosphorylation cycle in the guinea pig heart. *Pflügers Arch.* 407:123–28

81. Kameyama, M., Hofmann, F., Trautwein, W. 1985. On the mechanism of β-adrenergic regulation of the Ca channel in the guinea pig heart. *Pflügers Arch.* 405:285–93

82. Kameyama, M., Kameyama, A., Kaibara, M., Nakayama, T. 1987. Involvement of intracellular factor(s) in "run down" of the cardiac L-type Ca channel. *J. Physiol. Soc. Jpn.* 49:501

83. Kameyama, M., Kameyama, A., Nakayama, T., Kaibara, M. 1988. Tissue extract recovers cardiac calcium channels from "run-down". *Pflügers Arch.* 412:328–30

84. Kass, R. S., Blair, M. L. 1981. Effects of angiotensin II on membrane current in cardiac Purkinje fibers. *J. Mol. Cell. Cardiol.* 13:797–809

85. Kostyuck, P. G. 1984. Intracellular perfusion of nerve cells and its effects on membrane currents. *Physiol. Rev.* 64: 435–54

86. Krebs, E. G., Beavo, J. A. 1979. Phosphorylation-dephosphorylation of enzymes. *Annu. Rev. Biochem.* 48:923–59

87. Lacerda, A. E., Rampe, D., Brown, A. 1988. Effects of protein kinase C activators on cardiac Ca^{2+} channels. *Nature* 335:249–51

88. Lee, K. S., Tsien, R. W. 1984. High selecitity of calcium channels in single dialysed heart cells of the guinea pig. *J. Physiol.* 354:253–72

89. Leung, A. T., Imagawa, T., Campbell, K. P. 1987. Structural characterization of the 1,4-dihydropyridine receptor of the voltage-dependent Ca^{2+} channel from rabbit skeletal muscle. Evidence for two distinct high molecular weight subunits. *J. Biol. Chem.* 262:7943–46

90. Levi, R., Owen, D. A. A., Trzeciakoswki, J. 1982. Actions of histamine on the heart and vasculature. In *Pharmacology of Histamine Receptors,* ed. C. R. Gnellin, M. E. Parson, Bristol: *Wright & Sons,* 236 pp.

91. Li, T., Sperelakis, N. 1983. Stimulation of slow action potentials in guinea pig papillary muscle cells by intracellular injection of cAMP, Gpp(NH)p, and cholera toxin. *Circ. Res.* 52:111–17

92. Linden, J., Hollen, C., Patel, A. 1985. The mechanism by which adenosine and cholinergic agents reduce contractility in rat myocardium. Correlation with cyclic AMP and receptor densities. *Circ. Res.* 56:728–35

93. McNeill, J. 1984. Histamine and the heart. *Can. J. Physiol. Pharmacol.* 62: 720–26

94. Mellgren, R. 1987. Calcium-dependent proteases: an enzyme system active at the cellular membranes? *FASEB J.* 1:110–15

95. Mitra, R., Morad, M. 1986. Two types of calcium channels in guinea pig ventricular myocytes. *Proc. Natl. Acad. Sci. USA* 83:5340–44

96. Nargeot, J., Nerbonne, J. M., Engels, J., Lester, H. A. 1983. The time course of the increase in the myocardial slow inward current after a photochemically generated concentration jump of intracellular cAMP. *Proc. Natl. Acad. Sci. USA* 80:2395–99

97. Nastainczyk, W., Röhrkasten, A., Sieber, M., Rudolph, C., Schächtele, C., et al. 1987. Phosphorylation of the purified receptor for calcium channel blockers by cAMP kinase and protein kinase C. *Eur. J. Biochem.* 169:137–42

98. Niedergerke, R., Page, S. 1977. Analysis of catecholamine effects in single atrial trabeculae of the frog heart. *Proc. R. Soc. Lond. B* 197:333–62

99. Ochi, R. 1981. Decrease in calcium conductance by acetylcholine in mammalian ventricular muscle. In *The Mechanism of Gated Calcium Transport across Biological Membranes,* ed. T. Ohnishi, M. Endo, pp. 79–86. New York: Academic

100. Ochi, R., Hino, N., Okuyama, H. 1986. β-adrenergic modulation of the slow gating process of cardiac calcium channels. *Jpn. Heart J.* 27 (Suppl):51–55

101. Osterrieder, W., Brum, G., Hescheler, J., Trautwein, W., Flockerzi, V., Hofmann, F. 1982. Injection of subunits of cyclic AMP-dependent protein kinase into cardiac myocytes modulates Ca^{2+} current. *Nature* 298:576–78

102. Palade, P. T., Almers, W. 1985. Slow calcium and potassium currents in frog skeletal muscle: their relationship and pharmacologic properties. *Pflügers Arch.* 405:91–101

103. Pappano, A. J., Hartigan, P. M., Coutu, M. D. 1982. Acetylcholine inhibits the positive inotropic effect of cholera toxin in ventricular muscle. *Am. J. Physiol.* 243:H434–41

104. Pelzer, D., Cavalié, A., Flockerzi, V., Hofmann, F., Trautwein, W. 1988. Reconstitution of solubilized and purified dihydropyridine receptor from skeletal muscle microsomes as two single calcium channel conductances with different functional properties. In *The Calcium Channel: Structure, Function and Implications*, ed. M. Morad, W. Nayler, S. Kazda, M. Schramm. pp. 217–30. Berlin/Heidelberg: Springer-Verlag

105. Pelzer, D., Cavalié, A., Trautwein, W., 1986. Activation and inactivation of single calcium channels in cardiac cells. In *Calcium Electrogenesis and Neuronal Functioning, Exp. Brain Res., Series 14*, ed. U. Heinemann, M. Klee, E. Neher, W. Singer, pp. 17–34. Berlin: Springer-Verlag

106. Poggioli, J., Sulpice, J. C., Vassort, G. 1986. Inositol phosphate production following alpha$_1$-adrenergic, muscarinic or electrical stimulation in isolated rat heart. *FEBS Lett.* 206:292–98

107. Powell, T., Terrar, D. A., Twist, V. W. 1980. Electrical properties of individual cells isolated from adult rat ventricular myocardium. *J. Physiol.* 302:131–53

108. Prasad, K. 1975. Glucagon-induced changes in the action potential, contraction, and ATPase of cardiac muscle. *Cardiovasc. Res.* 9:335–65

109. Rardon, D. P., Pappano, A. T. 1986. Carbachol inhibits electrophysiological effects of cyclic AMP in ventricular myocytes. *Am. J. Physiol.* 251:H601–11

110. Rechsteiner, M., Rogers, S., Rote, K. 1987. Protein structure and intracellular stability. *Trends Biol. Sci.* 12:390–94

111. Reuter, H. 1983. Calcium channel modulation by neurotransmitters, enzymes and drugs. *Nature* 301:569–74

112. Reuter, H. 1979. Properties of two inward membrane currents in the heart. *Annu. Rev. Physiol.* 41:413–24

113. Reuter, H. 1974. Localization of β-adrenergic receptors and effects of noradrenaline and cyclic nucleotides on action potentials, ionic currents and tension in mammalian cardiac muscle. *J. Physiol.* 242:429–51

114. Reuter, H., Kokubun, S., Prod'hom, B. 1986. Properties and modulation of cardiac calcium channels. *J. Exp. Biol.* 124:191–201

115. Reuter, H., Scholz, H. 1977. The regu-lation of the calcium conductance of cardiac muscle by adrenaline. *J. Physiol.* 264:49–62

116. Rogers, T. B., Gaa, S. T., Allen, I. S. 1986. Identification and characterization of functional angiotensin II receptors on cultured heart myocytes. *J. Pharmacol. Exp. Ther.* 236:438–44

117. Röhrkasten, A., Meyer, H. E., Nastainczyk, W., Sieber, M., Hofmann, F. 1988. cAMP-dependent protein kinase rapidly phosphorylates Serine-687 of the skeletal muscle receptor for calcium channel blockers. *J. Biol. Chem.* 263:15325–29

118. Röhrkasten, A., Meyer, H. E., Schneider, T., Nastainczyk, W., Sieber, M., et al. 1988. Site-specific phosphorylation of the skeletal muscle receptor for calcium-channel blockers by cAMP-dependent protein kinase. In *The Calcium Channel: Structure, Function and Implications*, ed. M. Morad, W. Nayler, S. Kazda, M. Schramm, pp. 193–99. Berlin/Heidelberg: Springer-Verlag

119. Rosenthal, W., Schultz, G. 1987. Modulations of voltage-dependent ion channels by extracellular signals. *Trends Pharmacol. Sci.* 8:351–54

120. Saxon, M. E., Ivanitsky, G. R., Beloyartsev, F. F., Safronova, V. G. K., Kokoz, Y. M., Freydin, A. A. 1982. Myocardial opiate receptors. *Gen. Physiol. Biophys.* 1:447–52

121. Schneider, T., Hofmann, F. 1988. The bovine cardiac receptor for calcium channel blockers is a 195-kDa protein. *Eur. J. Biochem.* 174:369–75

122. Seamon, K., Wetzel, B. 1984. Interaction of forskolin with dually regulated adenylate cyclase. *Adv. Cyclic Nucleotide Res.* 17:91–99

123. Selinger, Z., Cassel, D. 1981. Role of guanine nucleotides in hormonal activation of adenylate cyclase. *Adv. Cyclic Nucleotide Res.* 14:15–22

124. Sperelakis, N. 1988. Regulation of calcium slow channels of cardiac muscle by cyclic nucleotides and phosphorylation. *J. Mol. Cell. Cardiol.* 20:75–105 (Suppl. II)

125. Sperelakis, N. 1985. Phosphorylation hypothesis of the myocardial slow channels and control of Ca^{2+} influx. In *Cardiac Electrophysiology and Arrhythmias*, ed. D. P. Zipes, J. Jalife, pp. 123–35. Orlando: Grune & Stratton

126. Suzuki, K., Kawashima, K., Imahori, K. 1984. In *Calcium Regulation in Biological Systems*, ed. S. Ebashi et al., pp. 213–26. New York: Academic

127. Talvenheimo, J. A., Worley, J. F. III, Nelson, M. T. 1987. Heterogenity of

calcium channels from a purified dihydropyridine receptor preparation. *Biophys. J.* 52:891–99

128. Tanabe, T., Takeshima, H., Mikami, A., Flockerzi, V., Takahashi, H., et al. 1987. Primary structure of the receptor for calcium channel blockers from skeletal muscle. *Nature* 328:313–18

129. Terasaki, W. L., Brooker, G. 1977. Cardiac adenosine 3',5'-monophosphate. *J. Biol. Chem.* 252:1041–50

130. Trautwein, W., Kameyama, M., Hescheler, J., Hofmann, F. 1986. Cardiac calcium channels and their transmitter modulation. In *Membrane Control of Cellular Activity, Progress in Zoology, Vol. 33*, ed. H. Ch. Lüttgau, pp. 163–82. Stuttgart: Fischer-Verlag

131. Trautwein, W., Osterrieder, W. 1986. Mechanisms of β-adrenergic and cholinergic control of Ca and K currents in the heart. In *Cardiac Muscle: The Regulation of Excitation and Contraction*, ed. R. D. Nathan, pp. 87–127. Orlando: Academic

132. Trautwein, W., Taniguchi, J., Noma, A. 1982. The effect of intracellular cyclic nucleotides and calcium on the action potential and acetylcholine response of isolated cardiac cells. *Pflügers Arch.* 392:307–14

133. Tsien, R. W. 1983. Calcium channels in excitable cell membranes. *Annu. Rev. Physiol.* 45:341–58

134. Tsien, R. W. 1977. Cyclic AMP and contractile activity in heart. *Adv. Cyclic Nucleotide Res.* 8:363–420

135. Tsien, R. W., Bean, B. P., Hess, P., Lansman, J. B., Nilius, B., Nowycky, M. C. 1986. Mechanisms of calcium channel modulation by β-adrenergic agents and dihydropyridine calcium agonists. *J. Mol. Cell. Cardiol.* 18:691–710

136. Ui, M. 1984. Islet-activating protein, pertussis toxin: a probe for functions of the inhibitory guanin nucleotide regulatory component of adenylate cyclase. *Trends Pharmacol. Sci.* 5:277–79

137. Vassort, G., Rougier, O., Garnier, D., Sauviat, M. P., Coraboeuf, E., Gargouil, Y. M. 1969. Effects of adrenaline on membrane inward currents during the cardiac action potential. *Pflügers Arch.* 309:70–81

138. Vogel, S., Sperelakis, N. 1977. Blockade of myocardial slow inward current at low pH. *Am. J. Physiol.* 233:C99–103

139. Wahler, G. M., Sperelakis, N. 1985. Intracellular injection of cGMP depresses cardiac slow action potentials. *J. Cyclic Nucleotide Protein Phosphoryl. Res.* 10:83–95

140. Waldman, S. A., Murad, F. 1987. Cyclic GMP synthesis and function. *Pharmacol. Rev.* 39:163–96

141. Watanabe, A. M., Besch, H. R. Jr. 1975. Interaction between cyclic adenosine monophosphate and cyclic guanosine monophosphate in guinea pig ventricular myocardium. *Circ. Res.* 37:309–17

142. West, G. A., Isenberg, G., Belardinelli, L. 1986. Antagonism of forskolin effects by adenosine in isolated hearts and ventricular myocytes. *Am. J. Physiol.* 250:H769–77

143. White, R. E., Hartzell, H. C. 1988. Effects of intracellular free magnesium on calcium current in isolated cardiac myocytes. *Science* 239:778–80

144. Yatani, A., Codina, J., Imoto, Y., Reeves, J. P., Birnbaumer, L., Brown, A. M. 1987. A G protein directly regulates mammalian cardiac calcium channels. *Science* 238:1288–92

145. Yatani, A., Okabe, K., Brown, A. M. 1989. Time course of cardiac Ca^{2+} current after a concentration jump of isoproterenol. *Biophys. J.* 55:36a

146. Yount, R. G. 1975. ATP analogs. *Adv. Enzymol.* 34:1–56

Annu. Rev. Physiol. 1990. 52:275–92

ROLE OF G PROTEINS IN CALCIUM CHANNEL MODULATION

G. Schultz, W. Rosenthal, and J. Hescheler

Institut für Pharmakologie, Freie Universität Berlin, Thielallee 69/73, D-1000 Berlin 33, West Germany

W. Trautwein

Physiologisches Institut, Universität des Saarlandes, D-6650 Homburg/Saar, West Germany

KEY WORDS: signal transduction, Ca^{2+} influx, ion channels, pertussis toxin, guanine nucleotides

INTRODUCTION

Modulation of Ca^{2+}-permeable ion channels by hormones and neurotransmitters is accomplished by reversibly interacting signal transduction components of the plasma membrane and the cytosol. The first component of the signal transduction chain is a transmembranous receptor that binds extracellular signal molecules with high specificity. Typically, the receptors are glycosylated monomers with an amino acid sequence predictive for seven membrane spanning regions (57). Following the binding of an agonist, receptors interact with and thereby activate heterotrimeric ($\alpha\beta\gamma$) guanine nucleotide-binding proteins (G proteins) attached to the inner face of the plasma membrane (Brown & Birnbaumer, this volume). Activation of G proteins leads to an exchange of GDP for GTP bound to their α-subunit. GTP-liganded α-subunits affect the activity of effectors that generate intracellular signals. In the case of the ubiquitous cAMP-generating enzyme, the adenylate cyclase, and the retinal light-sensitive cGMP-phosphodiesterase activity changes result from direct interactions with G protein α-subunits, as was shown in reconstitution experiments with purified components (17, 28).

A direct interaction of G protein subunits with ion channels has not been demonstrated. However evidence is increasing that receptor-activated G proteins can affect the activity of ion channels by membrane-confined mechanisms.

The best studied example for a close control of ion channels by G proteins is cardiac K^+ channels. In excised membrane patches of guinea pig atrial cells, activated G protein α-subunits of the G_i family, (G_{i1-3}), purified from human erythrocytes or bovine brain are sufficient to stimulate K^+ channels if applied to the cytoplasmic face of the patch at subpicomolar concentrations (101); recombinant G_i α-subunits are also active. Surprisingly, G protein $\beta\gamma$-complexes have also been reported to activate atrial K^+ channels in membrane patches; the stimulatory effect is observed at relatively high (nM) concentrations and apparently requires metabolites of arachidonic acid (52; see also Szabo this volume).

In addition, the α-subunit of the G protein, G_k (representing a mixture of G_{i2} and G_{i3}) stimulates K^+ channels in isolated membrane patches of a pituitary cell line, GH_3, if applied at subpicomolar concentrations (11). Moreover the G protein, G_o, isolated from bovine brain activates a variety of otherwise quiescent K^+ channels in cell-free membrane patches of neuronal cells if employed at a concentration of 1 pM (92); the ability is retained in a recombinant G_o α-subunit.

A close control by G-proteins also appears to apply to voltage-dependent Ca^{2+} channels. The main purpose of this contribution is to review data suggesting that G proteins exert both a membrane-confined stimulatory and a membrane-confined inhibitory control of voltage-dependent Ca^{2+} channels. We also discuss other G protein involving mechanisms by which receptor agonists modulate Ca^{2+} influx through ion channels.

CLOSE CONTROL OF VOLTAGE-DEPENDENT Ca^{2+} CHANNELS BY G PROTEINS

Inhibition of Voltage-Dependent Ca^{2+} Channels in Neuronal and Endocrine Cells

INVOLVED RECEPTOR AGONIST AND CELL TYPES   In neuronal cells of vertebrates the inhibition of voltage-dependent Ca^{2+} channels by receptor agonists provides a molecular mechanism for the inhibition of neurosecretion via presynaptic receptors. In endocrine cells the inhibition of Ca^{2+} currents by receptor agonists may represent a molecular mechanism for the inhibition of secretion. In most studies investigators used the patch-clamp technique (whole-cell recording; 37) to study the inhibitory modulation of Ca^{2+} currents.

In dorsal root ganglion cells of chick, Ca^{2+} currents are inhibited by noradrenaline (via α_2-adrenoceptors), γ-aminobutyric acid (GABA, via GABA$_B$-receptors), serotonin and dopamine (via D$_2$-receptors) (14, 22, 31[1], 43, 63). In dorsal root ganglion neurons of rat, 2-chloroadenosine (via A$_1$-receptors), baclofen (via GABA$_B$-receptors), neuropeptide Y and opioid peptides (via μ-receptors) reduce Ca^{2+} currents (18, 20, 26, 34, 82, 83), and in dorsal root ganglion neurons of mouse, baclofen and opioid peptides (via κ-receptors) decrease Ca^{2+} currents (35[2]). In sympathetic ganglion neurons of chick, noradrenaline and dopamine inhibit Ca^{2+} currents (63); in the same cell type of rat, acetylcholine (via muscarinic receptors) induces Ca^{2+} current inhibition (97). Acetylcholine also inhibits voltage-dependent Ca^{2+} currents in hippocampal neurons of rat (89). Finally, in mouse/rat neuroblastoma x glioma hybrid cells (108CC15), opioid peptides (via δ-receptors) and soma-tostatin reduce Ca^{2+} currents (40, 91). The extent of Ca^{2+} current inhibition at maximally effective concentrations of neurotransmitters ranges from 30% (mouse dorsal root ganglion neurons, 35; rat sympathetic ganglion neurons, 97), 40% (rat hippocampal neurons, 89), 60% (rat dorsal root ganglion neurons, 18) to 70% (neuroblastoma x glioma hybrid cells, 40, 91).

In pituitary cell lines from mouse (AtT-20) and rat (GH$_3$), somatostatin, a secretion-inhibiting hormone, inhibits voltage-dependent Ca^{2+} channels by about 34 and 50%, respectively (58, 80).

In both neuronal and pituitary cells the inhibitory modulation of Ca^{2+} currents occurs fast (within seconds) and is rapidly reversed by removal of the receptor agonist (35, 40, 43, 58, 80, 83, 89, 91, 97).

EFFECTS OF GUANINE NUCLEOTIDES   The agonists mentioned above are known to activate transmembranous receptors coupled to G proteins. The involvement of G proteins in the inhibitory Ca^{2+} current modulation is evident from the effects of intracellularly applied analogs of guanine nucleo-tides. Intracellular application of high concentrations (100 to 500 μM) of the GTP analog, guanosine-5'-0-(3-thiotriphosphate) (GTPγS), an activator of G proteins, reduces Ca^{2+} currents in neuronal (40, 43, 83, 89, 97) and pituitary cells (58). GTPγS applied intracellularly at a low concentration (1 μM) has no effect on Ca^{2+} currents of neuroblastoma x glioma hybrid cells in the absence of a receptor agonist, but renders irreversible the inhibition caused by a δ-receptor agonist (41). Similarly, somatostatin causes an irreversible in-hibition of Ca^{2+} currents in AtT-20 cells infused with a GTPγS-containing solution (58). Using caged GTPγS, which is released by light, Dolphin & coworkers showed that the maximum of Ca^{2+} current inhibition induced by

---

[1] In this study currents through single channels of a cell-attached membrane patch were measured.

[2] Currents were measured by the use of microelectrodes instead of patch-pipettes.

moderate concentrations of GTPγS (20 μM) is reached within 5 to 10 min (21). This rather slow time course of GTPγS action on Ca^{2+} currents, also described for AtT-20 cells (58), corresponds well to the slow activation of G proteins by GTP analogs in the absence of receptor agonists (Brown & Birnbaumer, this volume).

Intracellular application of the GDP analog, guanosine-5'-0-(2-thiodiphos-phate) (GDPβS), which prevents receptor-induced activation of G proteins, also prevents the inhibition of Ca^{2+} currents by receptor agonists (40, 41, 43, 83, 97).

Activation of G proteins specifically requires GTP. However in almost all studies mentioned above, patch-pipettes were filled with solutions containing ATP but not GTP. Only in few studies (89, 97) pipette solutions contained both ATP and GTP. The apparent ability of ATP to substitute for GTP may be explained by the action of hormone-sensitive, G protein-associated nucleoside diphosphokinases that convert ATP to GTP, thus providing the nucleotide required for G protein activation (53, 75, 84). There is no easy explanation for the fact that some investigators observe receptor-mediated Ca^{2+} channel inhibition when infusing nucleotide-free solutions into cells (63, 91). Since under these experimental conditions reversible inhibition of Ca^{2+} currents is observed up to 20-30 min after achievement of the whole-cell configuration (63), one has to assume that a sufficient concentration of GTP is maintained at the inner face of the plasma membrane, either by permanent synthesis of nucleotides, tight binding of nucleotides to the plasma membrane, or by the existence of compartments that are not easily accessible to the pipette solution.

SENSITIVITY TOWARDS PERTUSSIS TOXIN   The main exotoxin of *Bordetella pertussis,* pertussis toxin, prevents coupling of activated receptors to some G proteins (e.g. members of the G_i family and G_o) by ADP-ribosylation of G protein α-subunits (Brown & Birnbaumer, this volume). Treatment with pertussis toxin for several hours prevented the agonist-induced inhibition of Ca^{2+} currents in dorsal root ganglion neurons (86), AtT-20 cells (58), neuroblastoma x glioma hybrid cells (40), GH_3 cells (80), and hippocampal neurons (89). Analogous to data obtained with regard to inhibition of adenylate cyclase, GTPγS-induced inhibition of Ca^{2+} currents in neuroblastoma x glioma hybrid cells was not abolished by pertussis toxin (41).

POSSIBLE ROLE OF INTRACELLULAR SIGNAL MOLECULES OR PROTEIN KINASES   Agonists that inhibit Ca^{2+} currents also inhibit adenylate cyclase thereby reducing cytosolic cAMP levels (e.g. adrenaline via α_2-adrenoceptors, GABA via $GABA_B$-receptors, dopamine via D_2-receptors, opioids via δ-, μ- and κ-receptors, adenosine via A_1-receptors) (49). Inhibition of both Ca^{2+} channels and adenylate cyclase are mediated by pertussis toxin-sensitive G proteins. However in contrast to the hormonal modulation of cardiac Ca^{2+} channels (Trautwein & Hescheler this volume), cAMP or cAMP-dependent protein kinase are not involved in the receptor-mediated inhibition of Ca^{2+} currents in neuronal and pituitary cells for several reasons. (a) Intracellular infusion of cAMP in the absence of a hormonal agonist does not affect Ca^{2+} channel activity (40, 80, 97). (b) Agonists inhibit Ca^{2+} currents in cells loaded with cAMP (43, 58, 97). (c) Extracellular application of the adenylate cyclase-stimulating diterpene, forskolin, does not modify Ca^{2+} currents in neuroblastoma x glioma hybrid cells (41), or GH$_3$ cells (80), nor does it prevent the inhibition of Ca^{2+} currents by a GABA$_B$ receptor agonist in rat dorsal root ganglion neurons (19). For effects of cAMP on neuronal L-type Ca^{2+} currents see chapter by Dolphin, this volume.

Based on data obtained with modulators of protein kinase C, both a stimulatory and an inhibitory control of neuronal and pituitary Ca^{2+} currents by protein kinase C have been suggested (Dolphin, this volume; 62, 86[3]). The inhibitory effects led to the hypothesis that protein kinase C is involved in the receptor-mediated inhibition of Ca^{2+} currents (78). This assumption, however, appears to be unlikely for several reasons. (a) The main activator of protein kinase C, diacylglycerol, is formed by phosphoinositide hydrolysis catalyzed by a phospholipase C (6). However most receptor agonists that inhibit Ca^{2+} currents in neuronal and pituitary cells do not stimulate phosphoinositide hydrolysis; consequently, they do not activate protein kinase C via this pathway. (b) In contrast to Ca^{2+} current inhibition, the receptor-mediated phosphoinositide hydrolysis in pituitary cells is not blocked by pertussis toxin (64, 69, for review see Reference 27). (c) Activators and inhibitors of protein kinase C do not affect the agonist-induced inhibition of Ca^{2+} currents in rat sympathetic ganglion neurons (97) and in chick dorsal root ganglion neurons (51). (d) Bradykinin, which stimulates phospholipase C in both cell types, does not inhibit voltage-dependent Ca^{2+} channels in neuroblastoma x glioma hybrid cells (G. Schultz et al, unpublished), or in rat dorsal root ganglion cells (19). In addition, there is convincing evidence that in neuroblastoma x glioma hybrid neurons, bradykinin-induced phosphoinositide hydrolysis is insensitive to pertussis toxin (33, 74), although there is a contradictory report (42). Also opposed to the findings described above is a report by Ewald et al (25); according to this group, bradykinin inhibits voltage-dependent Ca^{2+} currents of rat dorsal root ganglion neurons in a pertussis toxin-sensitive manner; however in this study the possible involvement of protein kinase C has not been examined.

Fatty acids, in particular arachidonic acid, also activate protein kinase C (85). Arachidonic acid is formed following the activation of phospholipase A$_2$

---

[3]Ca^{2+} influx was determined by the use of the fluorescent Ca^{2+} chelator, fura-2.

or—subsequent to phosphoinositide hydrolysis—by a diacylglycerol lipase. At least in some cell types, receptor-mediated stimulation of a phospholipase A_2 is sensitive to pertussis toxin (for review see Reference 27). However arachidonic acid or an inhibitor of phospholipases does not affect Ca^{2+} currents in chick (51) or rat dorsal root ganglion neurons (19).

Arachidonic acid may also affect Ca^{2+} channel activity by stimulation of a cGMP-generating enzyme, i.e. soluble guanylate cyclase, and subsequent activation of cGMP-dependent protein kinase (32). In contrast to snail neurons (76), this pathway is apparently not involved in the inhibition of Ca^{2+} currents in neuronal cells of vertebrates, since cGMP, applied intracellularly, does not affect Ca^{2+} currents in neuroblastoma x glioma hybrid cells (G. Schultz et al, unpublished observation), nor does nitroprusside, a potent stimulator of soluble guanylate cyclase, affect Ca^{2+} currents in chick dorsal root ganglion neurons (51). Thus a role of a phospholipase A_2 in the inhibitory modulation of neuronal Ca^{2+} channels appears unlikely. In pituitary cells a possible involvement of phospholipase A_2 in the receptor-induced Ca^{2+} channel inhibition has not yet been investigated.

In conclusion, intracellular signal molecules or protein kinases stimulated by intracellular signal molecules are apparently not involved in the pertussis toxin-sensitive inhibitory Ca^{2+} current modulation. A membrane-confined mechanism is also supported by experiments in which currents through single Ca^{2+} channels of a cell-attached patch (37) were recorded. In this configuration, the membrane under the tip of the pipette is not accessible for agonists applied to the bath solution. In chick and mouse dorsal root ganglion cells (31, 34), application of inhibitory agonists to the bath solution does not induce an inhibition of Ca^{2+} channels in the patch, which suggests that readily diffusible intracellular signal molecules are not involved in the inhibitory modulation of Ca^{2+} currents (see also Dolphin, this volume).

IDENTITY OF THE G PROTEINS INVOLVED IN THE INHIBITORY Ca^{2+} CHANNEL MODULATION   The G protein that physiologically mediates pertussis toxin-sensitive inhibition of voltage-dependent Ca^{2+} channels in neuronal and endocrine cells has not been identified with certainty. There is, however, some experimental evidence suggesting that the G protein, G_o, may be involved. (*a*) G_o is an abundant G protein in cell types that exhibit pertussis toxin-sensitive inhibition of Ca^{2+} currents, i.e. neuronal cells (2), neuroblastoma x glioma hybrid cells (67), rat pituitary cells (2), and GH_3 cells (80). (*b*) Following the treatment of cells with pertussis toxin, intracellular application of G_o or its α-subunit efficiently restores the ability of agonists to inhibit Ca^{2+} currents in neuroblastoma x glioma hybrid cells (40), rat dorsal root ganglion neurons (26), snail neurons (38), and rat hippocampal neurons (60). (*c*) Antibodies against the G_o α-subunit attenuate the inhibitory modulation of

Ca^{2+} currents in snail neurons (38) and in neuroblastoma x glioma hybrid cells (8). (*d*) The expression of the G_o α-subunit in rat pituitary tumor cells correlates with the ability of dopamine to inhibit prolactin secretion (13). (*e*) Inhibitory agonists efficiently stimulate guanine nucleotide-binding to a 39-kd membrane protein presumably representing N, the G_o α-subunit in neuroblastoma x glioma hybrid cells and GH_3 cells (S. Offermanns, G. Schultz, & W. Rosenthal, unpublished).

According to Attali & coworkers (3), G_{i1} is involved in the inhibition of Ca^{2+} currents induced by κ-receptor agonists. They found that chronic exposure of rat spinal cord-dorsal root ganglion cocultures to κ-receptor agonists attenuates the receptor-mediated inhibition of $^{45}Ca^{2+}$ uptake and down regulates the G_{i1} α-subunit, but not the G_o α-subunit.

TYPES OF Ca^{2+} CHANNELS INHIBITED BY G PROTEINS   Based on electrophysiological and pharmacological properties, neuronal voltage-dependent Ca^{2+} channels have been classified as L-, N-, and T-type channels (90). Inhibitory neurotransmitters acting via pertussis toxin-sensitive G proteins mainly appear to affect Ca^{2+} channels of the N- and the T-type (Dolphin this volume). Since N-type channels play a dominant role in neurosecretion (90), the inhibition of N-type channels by neurotransmitters may be relevant for the inhibition of neurosecretion via presynaptic receptors.

Isolated and clonal cells from the anterior pituitary possess fast and slowly inactivating Ca^{2+} currents that apparently correspond to Ca^{2+} fluxes through L- and T-type channels (e.g. 15, 62, 80). GH_3 cells may, in addition, possess slowly inactivating N-type Ca^{2+} channels (88). In GH_3 cells, somatostatin exclusively inhibits slowly inactivating Ca^{2+} currents (80). Whether these currents represent currents through L- or N-type channels is not known. Evidence for a control of neuronal and pituitary L-type Ca^{2+} channels by pertussis toxin-sensitive G proteins is based on experiments with Ca^{2+} channel-blocking and -activating ligands (Dolphin, this volume, 81).

Stimulation of Voltage-Dependent Ca^{2+} Channels in Endocrine Cells and in Myocytes of the Heart and Skeletal Muscle

ENDOCRINE CELLS   Data reviewed here were obtained by applying the patch-clamp technique in the whole-cell configuration (37). In bovine adrenal glomerulosa cells (12), as well as in the adrenocortical cell line, Y1 (39), angiotensin II, the major stimulator of aldosterone secretion, stimulates voltage-dependent Ca^{2+} currents up to about 1.7-fold. According to preliminary data, angiotensin II is also active in isolated porcine (39) and in pituitary GH_3 cells (80). In Y1 cells, stimulation is observed a few seconds after addition of the hormone and is rapidly reversed by its removal from the bath (39).

Similarly to angiotensin II, the secretion-stimulating hormone, luteinizing hormone-releasing hormone (gonadotropin-releasing hormone, GnRH, LHRH), stimulates voltage-dependent Ca^{2+} currents of GH_3 cells about 1.5-fold in a rapid and reversible fashion (80). Thus in this cell type, receptor agonists exert a dual control of voltage-dependent Ca^{2+} currents (see above).

Effects of pertussis toxin   Stimulation of Ca^{2+} currents in Y1 cells is abolished by treatment of cells with pertussis toxin (39). This observation confirms a previous finding that pertussis toxin abolishes the stimulation of $^{45}Ca^{2+}$ influx by angiotensin II (54).

In pituitary GH_3 cells, pertussis toxin not only abolishes the inhibitory but also the stimulatory Ca^{2+} current modulation (80). Consistent with this observation is the finding that both stimulatory and inhibitory hormones stimulate high-affinity GTPases in membranes from GH_3 cells (representing the enzymatic activity of G proteins) and that this effect is sensitive to pertussis toxin (72). Thus in GH_3 cells both stimulatory and inhibitory hormones apparently modulate Ca^{2+} channels via pertussis toxin-sensitive G proteins.

Independency of cAMP   While Ca^{2+} currents in cardiac and skeletal myocytes are stimulated by cAMP-dependent phosphorylation (Trautwein & Hescheler, this volume), the stimulatory modulation of Ca^{2+} currents in adrenocortical and pituitary cells appears to be independent of cAMP for several reasons. (*a*) Intracellularly applied cAMP or extracellularly applied forskolin does not stimulate Ca^{2+} currents in Y1 or GH_3 cells (39, 80). (*b*) In membranes of adrenocortical and pituitary cells, angiotensin II does not stimulate but rather inhibits adenylate cyclase (23, 80, 98). (*c*) LHRH does not affect adenylate cyclase activity in membranes of GH_3 cells (80). (*d*) The sensitivity of the stimulatory Ca^{2+} current modulation towards pertussis toxin further indicates that elevation of cAMP is not an intermediate step since stimulation of adenylate cyclase is mediated by G_s, a G protein that is a substrate for cholera toxin but not for pertussis toxin (Brown & Birnbaumer, this volume).

Possible involvement of phospholipases   In adrenocortical (24, 54) and pituitary cells (64, 69), angiotensin II, LHRH, and thyrotropin-releasing hormone (TRH) stimulate a phospholipase C and, thereby, phosphoinositide hydrolysis via pertussis toxin-insensitive mechanisms. It is, therefore, unlikely that activation of protein kinase C or mobilization of intracellularly stored Ca^{2+} via this pathway is involved in the Ca^{2+} current stimulation by angiotensin II and LHRH.

Another possible mechanism underlying the agonist-induced Ca^{2+} current stimulation is the liberation of arachidonic acid by receptor-mediated, pertussis toxin-sensitive activation of a phospholipase A_2 (see above). In Y1 cells, a protein kinase C-activating phorbol ester did not affect Ca^{2+} currents nor did cGMP affect the Ca^{2+} current stimulation by angiotensin II (39). It remains to be determined whether or not either of these pathways activated by arachidonic acid provides a mechanism for the stimulatory control of Ca^{2+} currents in pituitary cells. In both adrenocortical and pituitary cells the direct effect of arachidonic acid or its metabolites on Ca^{2+} channel activity has not been examined.

While the data reviewed above are consistent with a membrane-confined mechanism, other investigators suggest that cytosolic components are required for the stimulatory Ca^{2+} current modulation in pituitary cells. Taking advantage of the cell-attached variation of the patch-clamp technique, Mason & Waring (65) found that cation channels permeable to Ca^{2+} are stimulated by LHRH applied to the bath solution, which therefore suggested the involvement of a cytosolic messenger.It is however, not clear, whether the cation channels activated by LHRH represent classical voltage-dependent Ca^{2+} channels. Measuring cytosolic Ca^{2+} with a fluorescent Ca^{2+} chelator, Shangold & colleagues (86) showed that a protein kinase C-activating phorbol ester promotes the portion of the LHRH-induced increase in cytosolic Ca^{2+}, which apparently depends on nitrendipine-sensitive Ca^{2+} influx. Pertussis toxin was not applied in either of these studies.

Identity of the G protein involved in the pertussis toxin-sensitive stimulatory Ca^{2+} channel modulation   Data from reconstitution experiments with purified G proteins are still missing. Since only two groups of pertussis toxin-sensitive G proteins are known in nonretinal tissues (i.e. G_i and G_o), and since G_o apparently mediates inhibition of Ca^{2+} currents, it appears plausible that a G_i-type G protein is involved in the pertussis toxin-sensitive stimulation of voltage-dependent Ca^{2+} channels. This hypothesis is supported by the finding that membranes of Y1 cells contain G proteins of the G_i-type, but are devoid of G_o (39). The hypothesis is also consistent with the finding that membranes of GH_3 cells possess—besides large amounts of G_o—at least two G_i-type G proteins (80).

CARDIAC AND SKELETAL MYOCYTES   The cholera toxin-sensitive G protein, G_s, confers hormonal activation to adenylate cyclase. This leads to stimulation of cAMP-dependent protein kinase, which, in turn, activates cardiac Ca^{2+} channels (Trautwein & Hescheler, this volume). Similarly, cAMP-dependent protein kinase phosphorylates and, thereby, activates the L-type Ca^{2+} channel purified from T tubules of skeletal muscle (30). Recent evidence suggests that G_s also activates Ca^{2+} channels independently of a cAMP-dependent step. In isolated inside-out patches of cardiac myocytes and in cardiac sarcolemma or T tubule membranes incorporated into phospholipid bilayers, various forms of the G_s α-subunit activate Ca^{2+} channels if applied to the cytoplasmic side (45, 66, 100). Thus G_s controls Ca^{2+} channels by a cAMP-independent, membrane-confined mechanism and by a cAMP-dependent mechanism requiring cytosolic components. While the former mechanism appears to be fast (observable within tens of milliseconds), the latter mechanism appears to be slow (observable within tens of seconds) (99).

TYPES OF Ca^{2+} CHANNELS STIMULATED BY G PROTEINS   In Y1 and GH_3 cells, hormone-sensitive currents inactivate slowly, exhibit a high threshold potential, and are in a large portion sensitive to Ca^{2+} channel agonists and antagonists of the dihydropyridine type, which suggests that fluxes through L-type Ca^{2+} channels mainly contribute to these currents; low threshold, fast inactivating currents (probably representing currents through T-type channels) are not sensitive to hormones (39, 80). Also consistent with a modulation of L-type Ca^{2+} channels by G proteins is the observation that pertussis toxin and guanine nucleotides affect the responses of L-type Ca^{2+} channels to organic Ca^{2+} channel agonists and antagonists (Dolphin, this volume). On the other hand, angiotensin II-sensitive Ca^{2+} currents in bovine glomerulosa cells represent currents through T-type channels (12). In cardiac and skeletal muscle, the G protein-controlled channels apparently represent dihydropyridine-sensitive L-type channels (45, 66, 100).

G PROTEIN-INVOLVING MECHANISMS BY WHICH HORMONAL FACTORS MODULATE Ca^{2+} INFLUX THROUGH ION CHANNELS

Voltage-Dependent Ca^{2+} Channels

Membrane-confined interactions of G proteins with voltage-dependent Ca^{2+} channels appear to provide a rapid mechanism by which receptor agonists affect ion channel activity (see above; Table 1). In contrast to the close control of voltage-dependent Ca^{2+} channels by G proteins, G proteins also exert a distant control of Ca^{2+} channel activity by modulating enzymatic effectors that generate intracellular signals (e.g. cAMP, cGMP, diacylglycerol, inositol-1,4,5-trisphosphate). In most instances these signal molecules activate protein kinases that stimulate or inhibit Ca^{2+} channels by phosphorylation of either a regulatory component or of the channel protein itself (50, 79). In skeletal muscle, inositol 1,4,5-trisphosphate may affect dihydropyridine-sensitive Ca^{2+} channels directly (93). Whether stimulatory hormonal effects

Table 1 Direct and indirect regulations of voltage-dependent Ca^{2+} channels via receptors and G proteins

Cell/tissue	Effect	Agonist (example)	Sensitive to toxin	G protein	Intracellular signal, PK	Method	References
Neuronal, endocrine	↓	SST, opiate	PT	G_o	—	whole-cell	See text
Endocrine	↑	A II, LHRH	PT	G_i	—	whole-cell	See text
Cardiac, skeletal muscle	↑	β-adrenergic	CT	G_s	—	inside-out patch, lipid bilayer	See text
Cardiac, skeletal muscle	↑	β-adrenergic	CT ?	G_s	cAMP-PK	whole-cell, cell-attached patch, lipid bilayer	Trautwein & Hescheler (this volume)
Endocrine, neuronal, intestinal smooth muscle	↑	β-adrenergic	CT ?	G_s	cAMP-PK	whole-cell, cell-attached patch, inside-out patch	1, 50, 73
Neuronal	↑	Serotonin	nk	nk	cGMP-PK	whole-cell	76
Cardiac, neuronal, endocrine	↓↑		nk		PKC	whole-cell, cell-attached patch	56, 78, 62
Cardiac, neuronal, endocrine	↑	LHRH	nk		PKC	whole-cell, cell-attached patch, fura-2	16, 56, 86
Stomach smooth muscle	↑	Acetylcholine	nk	nk	PKC	whole-cell	94
Skeletal muscle	↑	—	nk	nk	IP_3	lipid bilayer	93
Vascular smooth muscle	↑	Noradrenaline, A II	nk	nk	nk	whole-cell, cell-attached patch	4, 7, 70
Tracheal smooth muscle	↑	Carbachol	nk	nk	nk	fura-2	29

Abbreviations: PK = protein kinase; SST = somatostatin; A II = angiotensin II; LHRH = luteinizing hormone-releasing hormone; fMLP = N-formyl-L-methionyl-L-leucyl-L-phenylalanine; CT = cholera toxin; PT = pertussis toxin; cAMP-PK = cAMP-dependent protein kinase; cGMP-PK = cGMP-dependent protein kinase; PKC = protein kinase C; IP_3 = inositol 1,4,5-trisphosphate; IP_4 = inositol 1,3,4,5-tetrakisphosphate; nk = not known.

on voltage-dependent Ca^{2+} channels in vascular and tracheal smooth muscle involve intracellular signal molecules and/or protein kinase C has not yet been clarified.

Voltage-Dependent and Independent Ca^{2+}-Permeable Cation Channels

In contrast to highly selective voltage-dependent Ca^{2+} channels, Ca^{2+}-permeable cation channels show no or little selectivity for Ca^{2+} and are insensitive to organic Ca^{2+} channel ligands; many of them may also lack a voltage-dependent gating mechanism. As suggested by electrophysiological and biochemical experiments, cation channels, which exist in many cells, are controlled by agonists acting on G protein-coupled receptors (Table 2).

G proteins may control cation-channel activity by a membrane-confined mechanism, although at present the experimental evidence for such a mechanism is less conclusive than that for voltage-dependent Ca^{2+} channels. Benham & Tsien (5) reported that in isolated outside-out patches (37) cation channels of vascular smooth muscle cells are activated by ATP applied to the bath solution. Although the stimulatory modulation apparently does not require exogenous GTP added to the cytoplasmic face of membrane patches (see above), it is plausible that G proteins are involved, since purinergic receptors are known to act via G proteins. Recently a membrane-confined control of renal epithelial cation channels by G proteins was proposed by Light & coworkers (59), who found that the G_{i3} α-subunit directly activates cation channels in isolated inside-out patches.

In most instances, however, the control of cation channels by G proteins is indirect. Here, an intracellular signal, generated by a G protein-regulated enzymatic effector, modulates cation channels either by direct interaction or via an enzymatic step. The latter pathway may apply to cation channels of platelets. These channels are active in membrane vesicles incorporated into planar phospholipid bilayers provided the intact cells have been exposed to thrombin (102). This suggests that a covalent modification, possibly phosphorylation by thrombin-activated protein kinase C, may cause activation of these cation channels. In various cell types, inositol 1,4,5-trisphosphate (10, 55, 77, 87) or inositol 1,4,5-trisphosphate in combination with inositol 1,3,4,5-tetrakisphosphate (48, 68) have been postulated to stimulate Ca^{2+} entry through ion channels. A cation channel stimulated by cytosolic Ca^{2+} may play a significant role in the sustained activation of neutrophils (95). Finally, many receptor agonists, all of which stimulate phosphoinositide hydrolysis, stimulate Ca^{2+} influx by unknown mechanisms (9, 36, 44, 46, 47, 61, 71, 96); in some instances (44, 46, 47) a pertussis toxin-sensitive G protein appears to be involved.

Table 2 Direct and indirect regulations of Ca^{2+}-permeable cation channels via receptors and G proteins

Cell/tissue	Effect	Agonist (example)	Sensitive to toxin	G protein	Intracellular signal, PK	Method	References
Vascular smooth muscle	↑	ATP	nk	nk	—	outside-out patch	5
Renal epithelium	↑		nk	G_{i3}	—	inside-out patch	59
Platelets	↑	Thrombin	nk	nk	PKC?	lipid bilayer	102
Mast cells	↑		nk	nk	IP_3	whole cell	77
T-lymphocytes	↑	Mitogens	nk	nk	IP_3	cell-attached patch, inside-out patch	55
Epithelial cells (A 431)	↑		nk	nk	IP_3	cell-attached patch, inside-out patch	10
Xenopus laevis oocytes	↑	Acetylcholine	nk	nk	IP_3	whole-cell, Cl^- current	87
Xenopus laevis oocytes	↑		nk	nk	$IP_3 + IP_4$	maturation	48
Lacrimal acinar cells	↑		nk	nk	$IP_3 + IP_4$	whole-cell, K^+ current	68
Neutrophils	↑	fMLP	PT	nk	Ca^{2+}	inside-out patch	95
Ileum smooth muscle	↑	Acetylcholine	nk	nk	nk[4]	whole-cell	47
J774 macrophages	↑	ATP	nk	nk	nk[4]	whole-cell	9
Hepatocytes	↑	Vasopressin	PT	nk	nk[4]	^{45}Ca	44
PC-12 pheochromocytoma	↑	Muscarinic	PT	nk		^{45}Ca	46
Vascular smooth muscle	↑	Vasopressin	nk	nk	nk[4]	^{45}Ca	96
Jurkat T-lymphatic cells	↑	Immunoglobulins	nk	nk		^{45}Ca	71
B-lymphocytes	↑	Immunoglobulins	nk	nk		indo-1	61
Endothelium	↑	Thrombin, histamine	nk	nk	nk[4]	fura-2	36

See Table 1 footnote for abbreviations.

[4]Since the respective receptor agonists stimulate phosphoinositide hydrolysis, IP_3, Ca^{2+}, or PKC may be involved.

CONCLUSIONS

There is increasing evidence that G proteins exert a close membrane-confined control of ion channels permeable for Ca^{2+}. Proof for a direct interaction of G proteins and ion channels—analogous to the interaction of G proteins with enzymatic effectors (17, 28)—is missing. The determination of signal transduction components essential for the receptor-mediated modulation of Ca^{2+} permeable ion channels awaits reconstitution of agonist-responsive systems with purified or recombinant components.

ACKNOWLEDGMENT

Work of the authors reported herein was supported by the Deutsche Forschungsgemeinschaft, Sonderforschungsbereich 246 and the Fonds der Chemischen Industrie.

Literature Cited

1. Armstrong, D., Eckert, R. 1987. Voltage-activated calcium channels that must be phosphorylated to respond to membrane depolarization. *Proc. Natl. Acad. Sci. USA* 84:2518–22
2. Asano, T., Semba, R., Kamiya, N., Ogasawara, N., Kato, K. 1988. G_o, a GTP- binding protein: immunohistochemical localization in the rat. *J. Neurochem.* 50:1164–69
3. Attali, B., Saya, D., Nah, S., Vogel, Z. 1989. Chronic kappa opiate agonist treatment induces down-regulation of G_i proteins in rat spinal cord-dorsal root ganglion cocultures. *Pflügers Arch.* 413:R55 (Suppl.)
4. Benham, C. D., Tsien, R. W. 1988. Noradrenaline modulation of calcium channels in single smooth muscle cells from rabbit ear artery. *J. Physiol.* 404:767–84
5. Benham, C. D., Tsien, R. W. 1987. A novel receptor-operated Ca^{2+}-permeable channel activated by ATP in smooth-muscle. *Nature* 328:275–78
6. Berridge, M. J. 1987. Inositol trisphosphate and diacylglycerol: Two interacting second messengers. *Annu. Rev. Biochem.* 56:159–93
7. Bkaily, G., Peyrow, M., Sculptoreanu, A., Jacques, D., Chahine, M., et al. 1988. Angiotensin II increases I_{si} and blocks I_k in single aortic cell of rabbit. *Pflügers Arch.* 412:448–50
8. Brown, D. A., McFadzean, I., Milligan, G. 1989. Antibodies to the GTP binding protein G_o attenuate the inhibition of the calcium current by noradrena-

line in mouse neuroblastoma x rat glioma (NG 108-15) hybrid cells. *J. Physiol.* 415:20P (Suppl.)
9. Buisman, H., Steinberg, T., Fischbarg, J., Silverstein, S., Vogelzang, S., et al. 1988. Extracellular ATP induces a large nonselective conductance in macrophage plasma membranes. *Proc. Natl. Acad. Sci. USA* 85:7988–92
10. Chapron, Y., Cochet, C., Crouzy, S., Jullien, T., Keramidas, M., Verdetti, J. 1989. Tyrosine protein kinase activity of the EGF receptor is required to induce activation of receptor-operated calcium channels. *Biochem. Biophys. Res. Commun.* 158:527–33
11. Codina, J., Grenet, D., Yatani, A., Birnbaumer, L., Brown, A. M. 1987. Hormonal regulation of pituitary GH$_3$ cell K^+ channels by G_k is mediated by its α-subunit. *FEBS Lett.* 216:104–6
12. Cohen, C., McCarthy, R., Barrett, P., Rasmussen, H. 1988. Ca channels in adrenal glomerulosa cells: K^+ and angiotensin II increase T-type Ca channel current. *Proc. Natl. Acad. Sci. USA* 85:2412–16
13. Collu, R., Bouvier, C., Lagacé, G., Unson, C., Milligan, G., et al. 1988. Selective deficiency of guanine nucleotide-binding protein G_o in two dopamine-resistant pituitary tumors. *Endocrinology* 122:1176–78
14. Deisz, R. A., Lux, H. D. 1985. γ-Aminobutyric acid-induced depression of calcium currents of chick sensory neurons. *Neurosci. Lett.* 56:205–10
15. DeRiemer, S. A., Sakmann, B. 1985.

Two calcium currents in normal rat anterior pituitary cells identified by a plaque technique. *Exp. Brain Res.* 14:139–54

16. DeRiemer, S. A., Strong, J. A., Albert, K. A., Greengard, P., Kaczmarek, L. K. 1985. Enhancement of calcium current in Aplysia neurones by phorbol ester and protein kinase C. *Nature* 313:313–16

17. Deterre, P., Bigay, J., Forquet, F., Robert, M., Chabre, M. 1988. cGMP phosphodiesterase of retinal rods is regulated by two inhibitory subunits. *Proc. Natl. Acad. Sci. USA* 85:2424–28

18. Dolphin, A. C., Forda, S. R., Scott, R. H. 1986. Calcium-dependent currents in cultured rat dorsal root ganglion neurones are inhibited by an adenosine analogue. *J. Physiol.* 373:47–61

19. Dolphin, A. C., McGuirk, S. M., Scott, R. H. 1989. An investigation into the mechanisms of inhibition of calcium channel currents in rat cultured sensory neurones by guanine nucleotide analogues and (-)- baclofen. *Br. J. Pharmacol.* 97:263–73

20. Dolphin, A. C., Scott, R. H. 1987. Calcium-channel currents and their inhibition by (-)-baclofen in rat sensory neurons: modulation by guanine-nucleotides. *J. Physiol.* 386:1–17

21. Dolphin, A. C., Wootton, J. F., Scott, R. H., Trentham, D. R. 1988. Photoactivation of intracellular guanosine triphosphate analogues reduces the amplitude and slows the kinetics of voltage-activated calcium channel currents in sensory neurons. *Pflügers Arch.* 411:628–36

22. Dunlap, K., Fischbach, G. D. 1981. Neurotransmitters decrease the calcium conductance activated by depolarization of embryonic chick sensory neurones. *J. Physiol.* 317:519–35

23. Enjalbert, A., Sladeczek, F., Guillon, G., Bertrand, P., Shu, C., et al. 1986. Angiotensin II and dopamine modulate both cAMP and inositol phosphate production in anterior pituitary cells. *J. Biol. Chem.* 261:4071–75

24. Enyedi, P., Mucsi, I., Hunyady, L., Catt, K. J., Spät, A. 1986. The role of guanyl nucleotide binding-proteins in the formation of inositol phosphates in adrenal glomerulosa cells. *Biochem. Biophys. Res. Commun.* 140:941–47

25. Ewald, D. A., Miller, R. J., Sternweis, P. C. 1988. G proteins reconstitute inhibition of Ca^{2+} currents by bradykinin (BK) in pertussis toxin-treated rat dorsal root ganglion (DRG) neurons. *Soc. Neurochem. Abstr.* 14:754

26. Ewald, D. A., Sternweis, P. C., Miller, R. J. 1988. Guanine nucleotide-binding protein G$_o$-induced coupling of neuropeptide Y receptors to Ca^{2+} channels in sensory neurons. *Proc. Natl. Acad. Sci. USA* 85:3633–37

27. Fain, J. N., Wallace, M. A., Wojcikiewicz, R. J. H. 1988. Evidence for involvement of guanine nucelotide-binding regulatory proteins in the activation of phospholipases by hormones. *FASEB J.* 2:2569–74

28. Feder, D., Im, M. J., Klein, K. W., Hekman, M., Holzhöfer, A., et al. 1986. Reconstitution of β$_1$-adrenoceptor dependent adenylate cyclase from purified components. *EMBO J.* 5:1509–14

29. Felbel, J., Trockur, B., Ecker, T., Landgraf, W., Hofmann, F. 1988. Regulation of cytosolic calcium by cAMP and cGMP in freshly isolated smooth muscle cells from bovine trachea. *J. Biol. Chem.* 263:16764–71

30. Flockerzi, V., Oeken, H. J., Hofmann, F., Pelzer, D., Cavalié, A., Trautwein, W. 1986. Purified dihydropyridine-binding site from skeletal muscle t-tubules is a functional calcium channel. *Nature* 323:66–68

31. Forscher, P., Oxford, G. S., Schulz, D. 1986. Noradrenaline modulates calcium channels in avian dorsal root ganglion cells through tight receptor-channel coupling. *J. Physiol.* 379:131–44

32. Gerzer, R., Brash, A., Hardman, J. 1986. Activation of soluble guanylate cyclase by arachidonic acid and 15-lipoxygenase products. *Biochem. Biophys. Acta* 886:383–89

33. Grandt, A., Greiner, C., Zubin, P., Jakobs, K. H. 1986. Bradykinin stimulates GTP hydrolysis in NG108–15 membranes by a high-affinity, pertussis toxin-insensitive GTPase. *FEBS Lett.* 196:279–84

34. Green, K. A., Cottrell, G. A. 1988. Actions of baclofen on components of the Ca-current in rat and mouse DRG neurones in culture. *Br. J. Pharmacol.* 94:235–45

35. Gross, R. A., MacDonald, R. L. 1987. Dynorphin-A selectively reduces a large transient (N-type) calcium current of mouse dorsal-root ganglion neurons in cell culture. *Proc. Natl. Acad. Sci. USA* 84:5469–73

36. Hallam, T., Jacob, R., Merritt, J. 1988. Evidence that agonists stimulate bivalent-cation influx into human endothelial cells. *Biochem. J.* 255:179–84

37. Hamill, O. P., Marty, A., Neher, E., Sakmann, B., Sigworth, F. J. 1981. Improved patch clamp techniques for high-

resolution current recording from cells and cell-free membrane patches. *Plügers Arch.* 391:85–100

38. Harris-Warrick, R. M., Hammond, C., Paupardin-Tritsch, D., Homburger, V., Rouot, B., et al. 1988. An α_{40} subunit of a GTP-binding protein immunologically related to G_o mediates a dopamine-induced decrease of Ca^{2+} current in snail neurons. *Neuron* 1:27–32

39. Hescheler, J., Rosenthal, W., Hinsch, K., Wulfern, M. Trautwein, W., Schultz, G. 1988. Angiotensin II-induced stimulation of voltage-dependent Ca^{2+} currents in an adreno-cortical cell line. *EMBO J.* 7:619–24

40. Hescheler, J., Rosenthal, W., Trautwein, W., Schultz, G. 1987. The GTP-binding protein, G_o, regulates neuronal calcium channels. *Nature* 325:445–47

41. Hescheler, J., Rosenthal, W., Wulfern, M., Tang, M., Yajima, M., Trautwein, W., Schultz, G. 1988. Involvement of the guanine nucleotide-binding protein, N_o, in the inhibitory regulation of neuronal calcium channels. *Adv. 2nd Messenger Phosphoprotein Res.* 21:165–74

42. Higashida, H., Streaty, R. A., Klee, W., Nirenberg, M. 1986. Bradykinin-activated transmembrane signals are coupled via N_o or N_i to production of inositol 1,4,5-trisphosphate, a second messenger in NG108-15 neuroblastoma-glioma hybrid cells. *Proc. Natl. Acad. Sci. USA* 83:942–46

43. Holz, G. G. IV, Rane, S. G., Dunlap, K. 1986. GTP-binding proteins mediate transmitter inhibition of voltage-dependent calcium channels. *Nature* 319:670–72

44. Hughes, B. P., Crofts, J. N., Auld, A. M., Read, L. C., Barritt, G. 1987. Evidence that a pertussis toxin-sensitive substrate is involved in the stimulation by epidermal growth factor and vasopressin of plasma-membrane Ca^{2+} inflow in hepatocytes. *Biochem. J.* 248:911–18

45. Imoto, Y., Yatani, A., Reeves, J. P., Codina, J., Birnbaumer, L., Brown, A. M. 1988. α-subunit of G_s directly activates cardiac calcium channels in lipid bilayers. *Am. J. Physiol.* 255:H722–28

46. Inoue, K., Kenimer, J. 1988. Muscarinic stimulation of calcium influx and norepinephrine release in PC12 cells. *J. Biol. Chem.* 263:8157–61

47. Inoue, R., Isenberg, G. 1989. Receptor-operated currents in ileal smooth muscle cells: G-proteins involved in transduction for muscarinic acetylcholine recep-

tors to non-specific cation channels. *J. Physiol.* In press

48. Irvine, R. F., Moor, R. M. 1987. Inositol (1,3,4,5) tetrakisphosphate-induced activation of sea urchin eggs requires the presence of inositol trisphosphate. *Biochem. Biophys. Res. Commun.* 146:284–90

49. Jakobs, K. H., Aktories, K., Minuth, M., Schultz, G. 1985. Inhibition of adenylate cyclase. *Adv. Cycl. Nucleotide Protein Phosphorylation Res.* 19:137–50

50. Kaczmarek, L. K. 1988. The regulation of neuronal calcium and phosphorylation. *Adv. 2nd Messenger Phosphoprotein Res.* 22:113–38

51. Kasai, H., Aosaki, T. 1989. Modulation of Ca-channel current by an adenosine analog mediated by a GTP-binding protein in chick sensory neurons. *Pflügers Arch.* 414:145–49

52. Kim, D., Lewis, D., Graziadei, L., Neer, E. J., Bar-Sagi, D., Clapham, D. E. 1989. G-protein $\beta\gamma$-subunits activate the cardiac muscarinic K^+ channels via a phospholipase A_2. *Nature* 337:557–60

53. Kimura, N., Shimada, N. 1988. Direct interaction between membrane-associated nucleoside diphosphate kinase and GTP-binding proteins (G_s), and its regulation by hormones and guanine nucleotides. *Biochem. Biophys. Res. Commun.* 151:248–56

54. Kojima, I., Shibata, H., Ogata, E. 1986. Pertussis toxin blocks angiotensin II-induced calcium influx but not inositol trisphosphate production in adrenal glomerulosa cell. *FEBS Lett.* 204:347–51

55. Kuno, M., Gardner, P. 1987. Ion channels activated by inositol 1,4,5-trisphosphate in plasma membrane of human T-lymphocytes. *Nature* 326:301–4

56. Lacerda, A. E., Rampe, D., Brown, A. M. 1988. Effects of protein kinase C activators on cardiac Ca^{2+} channels. *Nature* 335:249–51

57. Lefkowitz, R. J., Caron, M. C. 1988. Adrenergic receptors. *J. Biol. Chem.* 263:4993–96

58. Lewis, D. L., Weight, F. F., Luini, A. 1986. A guanine nucleotide-binding protein mediates the inhibition of voltage-dependent calcium current by somatostatin in a pituitary cell line. *Proc. Natl. Acad. Sci. USA* 83:9035–39

59. Light, D., Ausiello, D., Stanton, B. 1989. G-protein regulation of a cation channel in renal epithelial cells. *J. Clin. Invest.* 84:352–56

60. Lux, H., Toselli, M., Tokutomi, N.

1989. Transmitter-modulation of neuronal Ca channels. *Pflügers Arch.* 413: R48 (Suppl.)

61. MacDougall, S. L., Grinstein, S., Gelfand, E. W. 1988. Detection of ligand-activated conductive Ca^{2+} channels in human B lymphocytes. *Cell* 54:229–34

62. Marchetti, C., Brown, A. M. 1988. Protein kinase activator 1-oleyl-2-acetyl-sn-glycerol inhibits two types of calcium currents in GH$_3$ cells. *Am. J. Physiol.* 254:C206–10

63. Marchetti, C., Carbone, E., Lux, H. D. 1986. Effects of dopamine and noradrenaline on Ca channels of cultured sensory and sympathetic neurons of chick. *Pflügers Arch.* 406:104–11

64. Martin, T. F. J., Bajjalieh, S. M., Lucas, D. O., Kowalchyk, J. A. 1986. Thyrotropin-releasing hormone stimulation of polyphosphoinositide hydrolysis in GH$_3$ cell membranes is GTP dependent but insensitive to cholera or pertussis toxin. *J. Biol. Chem.* 261:10141–43

65. Mason, W., Waring, D. 1986. Patch clamp recordings of single ion channel activation by gonadotropin-releasing hormone in ovine pituitary gonadotrophs. *Neuroendocrinology* 43:205–19

66. Mattera, R., Graziano, M. P., Yatani, A., Zhou, Z., et al. 1989. Splice variants of the G protein G$_s$ activate both adenylyl cyclase and calcium channels. *Science* 243:804–7

67. Milligan, G., Gierschik, P., Spiegel, A. M., Klee, W. A. 1986. The GTP-binding regulatory proteins of neuroblastoma x glioma, NG108-15, and glioma C6, cells. *FEBS Lett.* 195:225–30

68. Morris, A. P., Gallacher, D. V., Irvine, R. F., Petersen, O. H. 1987. Synergism of inositol trisphosphate and tetrakisphosphate in activating Ca^{2+}-dependent K$^+$ channels. *Nature* 330:635–55

69. Naor, Z., Azrad, A., Limor, R., Zakut, H., Lotan, M. 1986. Gonadotropin-releasing hormone activates a rapid Ca^{2+}-independent phosphodiester hydrolysis of polyphosphoinositides in pituitary gonadotrophs. *J. Biol. Chem.* 261:12506–12

70. Nelson, M. T., Standen, N. B., Brayden, J. E., Worley, J. F. III. 1988. Noradrenaline contracts arteries by activating voltage-dependent calcium channels. *Nature* 336:382–85

71. Ng, J., Fredholm, B. B., Jondal, M., Andersson, T. 1988. Regulation of receptor-mediated calcium influx across the plasma membrane in a human leukemic T-cell line: evidence of its dependence on an initial calcium mobilization from intracellular stores. *Biochim. Biophys. Acta* 971:207–14

72. Offermanns, S., Schultz, G., Rosenthal, W. 1989. Secretion-stimulating and secretion-inhibiting hormones stimulate high-affinity pertussis-toxin-sensitive GTPases in membranes of a pituitary cell line. *Eur. J. Biochem.* 180:283–87

73. Okya, Y., Kitamura, K., Kuriyama, H. 1987. Modulation of ionic currents in smooth muscle walls of the rabbit intestine by intracellularly perfused ATP and cyclic AMP. *Pflügers Arch.* 408:465–73

74. Osugi, T., Imaizumi, T., Mizushima, A., Uchida, S., Yoshida, H. 1987. Role of a protein regulating guanine-nucleotide binding in phosphoinositide breakdown and calcium mobilization by bradykinin in neuroblastoma x glioma hybrid NG108-15 cells: Effects of pertussis toxin and cholera toxin on receptor-mediated signal transduction. *Eur. J. Pharmacol.* 137:207–18

75. Otero, A. S., Breitwieser, G. E., Szabo, G. 1988. Activation of muscarinic potassium currents by ATP-γS in atrial cells. *Science* 242:443–45

76. Paupardin-Tritsch, D., Hammond, C., Gerschenfeld, H. M., Nairn, A. C., Greengard, P. 1986. cGMP-dependent protein kinase enhances Ca$^+$ current and potentiates the serotonin-induced Ca^{2+} current increase in snail neurons. *Nature* 323:812–14

77. Penner, R., Matthews, G., Neher, E. 1988. Regulation of calcium influx by second messengers in rat mast cells. *Nature* 334:499–504

78. Rane, S. G., Dunlap, K. 1986. Kinase C activator 1,2-oleoylacetylglycerol attenuates voltage-dependent calcium current in sensory neurons. *Proc. Natl. Acad. Sci. USA* 83:184–88

79. Reuter, H. 1983. Calcium channel modulation by neurotransmitters, enzymes and drugs. *Nature* 301:569–74

80. Rosenthal, W., Hescheler, J., Hinsch, K.-D., Spicher, K., Trautwein, W., Schultz, G. 1988. Cyclic AMP-independent, dual regulation of voltage-dependent Ca^{2+} currents by LHRH and somatostatin in a pituitary cell line. *EMBO J.* 7:1627–33

81. Schettini, G., Meucci, O., Florio, T., Grimaldi, M., Landolfi, E., Magri, G., Yasumoto, T. 1988. Pertussis toxin pretreatment abolishes dihydropyridine inhibition of calcium flux in the 235-1 pituitary cell line. *Biochem. Biophys. Res. Commun.* 151:361–69

82. Schroeder, J. E., Fischbach, P. S., Mamo, M., McClesky, E. W. 1989. Mu opioids inhibit calcium channels. *Biophys. J.* 55:38a

83. Scott, R. H., Dolphin, A. C. 1986. Regulation of calcium currents by a GTP analogue: potentiation of (-)-baclofen-mediated inhibition. *Neurosci. Lett.* 69:59–64

84. Seifert, R., Rosenthal, W., Schultz, G., Wieland, T., Gierschik, P., Jakobs, K. H. 1988. The role of nucleoside-diphosphate kinase reactions in G protein activation of NADPH oxidase by guanine and adenine nucleotides. *Eur. J. Biochem.* 175:51–55

85. Seifert, R., Schächtele, C., Rosenthal, W., Schultz, G. 1988. Activation of protein kinase C by *cis-* and *trans-*fatty acids and its potentiation by diacylglycerol. *Biochem. Biophys. Res. Commun.* 154:20–26

86. Shangold, G., Murphy, S., Miller, R. 1988. Gonadotropin-releasing hormone-induced Ca^{2+} transients in single identified gonadotropes require both intracellular Ca^{2+} mobilization and Ca^{2+} influx. *Proc. Natl. Acad. Sci. USA* 85:6566–70

87. Snyder, P. M., Krause, K.-H., Welsh, M. J. 1988. Inositol trisphosphate isomers, but not inositol 1,3,4,5,-tetrakisphosphate, induce calcium influx in *Xenopus laevis* oocytes. *J. Biol. Chem.* 263:11048–51

88. Suzuki, N., Yoshioka, T. 1987. Differential blocking action of synthetic ω-conotoxin on components of Ca^{2+} channel current in clonal GH$_3$ cells. *Neurosci. Lett.* 75:235–39

89. Toselli, M., Lux, H. D. 1989. GTP-binding proteins mediate acetylcholine inhibition of voltage-dependent calcium channels in hippocampal neurons. *Pflügers Arch.* 413:319–21

90. Tsien, R. W., Lipscombe, D., Madison, D. V., Bley, K. R., Fox, A. P. 1988. Multiple types of neuronal calcium channels and their selective modulation. *Trends Neurosci.* 11:431–37

91. Tsunoo, A., Yoshii, M., Narahashi, T. 1986. Block of calcium channels by enkephalin and somatostatin in neuroblastoma-glioma hybrid NG108-15 cells. *Proc. Natl. Acad. Sci. USA* 83:9832–36

92. VanDongen, A. M. J., Codina, J., Olate, J., Mattera, R., Joho, R., et al. 1988. Newly identified brain potassium channels gated by the guanine nucleotide binding protein G$_o$. *Science* 242:1433–37

93. Vilven, J., Coronado, R. 1988. Opening of dihydropyridine calcium channels in skeletal muscle membranes by inositol trisphosphate. *Nature* 336:587–89

94. Vivaudou, M. B., Clapp, L. H., Walsh, J. V. Jr., Singer, J. J. 1988. Regulation of one type of Ca^{2+} current in smooth muscle cells by diacylglycerol and acetylcholine. *FASEB J.* 2:2497–504

95. von Tscharner, V., Prod'hom, B., Baggiolini, M., Reuter, H. 1986. Ion channels in human neutrophils activated by a rise in free cytosolic calcium concentration. *Nature* 324:369–72

96. Wallnöfer, A., Cauvin, C. Rüegg, U. 1987. Vasopressin increases ^{45}Ca^{2+} influx in rat aortic smooth muscle cells. *Biochem. Biophys. Res. Commun.* 148:273–78

97. Wanke, E., Ferroni, A., Malgaroli, A., Ambrosini, A., Pozzan, T., Meldolesi, J. 1987. Activation of a muscarinic receptor selectively inhibits a rapidly inactivated Ca^{2+} current in rat symphathetic neurons. *Proc. Natl. Acad. Sci. USA* 84:4313–17

98. Woodcook E., McLeod, J. 1986. Adenylate cyclase inhibition is not involved in the adrenal steroidogenic response to angiotensin II. *Endocrinology* 119:1697–702

99. Yatani, A., Brown, A. M. 1989. Time course of Ca^{2+} current after a concentration jump of isoproterenol. *Science* 245:71–74

100. Yatani, A., Codina, J., Imoto, Y., Reeves, J. P., Birnbaumer, L., Brown, A. M. 1987. A G protein directly regulates mammalian cardiac calcium channels. *Science* 238:1288–92

101. Yatani, A., Mattera, R., Codina, J., Graf, R., Okabe, K., et al. 1988. The G protein-gated K$^+$ channel is stimulated by three distinct G$_i$α-subunits. *Nature* 336:680–82

102. Zschauer, A., van Breemen, C., Bühler, F. R., Nelson, M. T. 1988. Calcium channels in thrombin-activated human platelet membrane. *Nature* 334:703–5

Annu. Rev. Physiol. 1990. 52:293–305

G PROTEIN MEDIATED REGULATION OF K⁺ CHANNELS IN HEART

Gabor Szabo and Angela S. Otero

Department of Physiology and Biophysics, University ot Texas Medical Branch, Galveston, Texas 77550-2781

KEY WORDS: muscarinic receptors, guanine nucleotides, potassium conductance, activation kinetics, neurotransmitters

INTRODUCTION

Neuroendocrine control of cardiac function involves extensive regulation of potassium (K^+) currents via specific receptors in various anatomical regions of the heart (22, 53, 54, 60). Recent evidence, to be considered here, indicates that these regulatory processes involve a relatively complex cascade in which receptor activation is coupled to channel opening by guanine nucleotide binding proteins (G proteins). Of the various K^+ channels in the heart (see, for example 60), the inwardly rectifying K^+ current $I_{K_{(ACh)}}$ activated by muscarinic agonists or adenosine, the delayed rectifier I_K, and the background K^+ conductance g_K are thought to be regulated via G proteins either directly or indirectly. The regulation of $I_{K_{(ACh)}}$ is of particular interest, not only because it has been the most thoroughly studied, but also because it represents a novel mechanism involving the direct activation of a channel by a receptor-linked G protein. Moreover, $I_{K_{(ACh)}}$ serves as a rapid, sensitive and specific indicator of G protein function that may be used to explore with unprecedented time resolution the receptor-G protein interactions that underlie a large number of neuroendocrine responses.

0066-4278/90/0315-0293$02.00

THE MUSCARINIC POTASSIUM CHANNEL K$_{(Ach)}$: PROTOTYPE OF A G PROTEIN GATED CHANNEL

Acetylcholine (ACh) and other muscarinic agonists induce an inwardly rectifying K$^+$ current I$_{K_{(ACh)}}$ in most myocardial tissues except mammalian ventricle (11, 24, 48, 54, 61, 65, 68). Agonists elicit I$_{K_{(ACh)}}$ after a considerable delay, the duration of which is highly dependent on temperature (23; see 54 for review). The discovery of this behavior, reminiscent of slow synaptic responses, prompted early suggestions that multiple biochemical events were interposed between receptor activation and channel opening and might involve a receptor-induced formation of intracellular second messengers (50). However, as demonstrated later by Soejima & Noma (68), muscarinic activation of I$_{K_{(ACh)}}$ does not involve diffusible cytoplasmic factors. Using the cell-attached mode of the patch-clamp technique, these authors observed that channel activity in a patch of membrane isolated by the recording pipette was increased by the addition of a muscarinic agonist to the pipette solution, but not to the bath. This elegant experiment clearly indicated that coupling between channel and receptor is achieved at the level of the membrane; it also implied that if any second messengers are involved, they are not free to diffuse laterally in the bilayer, either as a result of some intrinsic property of the system or as a consequence of the barrier created by the patch-pipette.

Subsequently, the existence of a membrane bound G protein that couples muscarinic receptors to K$^+$ channels in atrial myocytes was revealed by the following observations: (*a*) intracellular perfusion with hydrolysis-resistant GTP analogues produces persistently activated I$_{K_{(ACh)}}$ currents in a receptor-dependent manner (5); (*b*) intracellular GTP is required for channel activation (61), and (*c*) pertussis toxin, which inactivates a number of G proteins by ADP-ribosylation, abolishes receptor-dependent activation of I$_{K_{(ACh)}}$ (18, 47, 61, 69). Thus activated muscarinic receptors do not interact directly with K$_{(ACh)}$ channels; instead, binding of the agonist triggers channel openings via a pertussis toxin-sensitive, inhibitory (G$_i$) type G protein, designated G$_k$ by Breitwieser & Szabo (5). The conclusions of these initial observations were corroborated and extended by further evidence considered below.

Note that the action of adenosine on cardiac tissues closely resembles that of ACh (1, 2, 23, 43). Specifically, adenosine and ACh activate the same population of K$^+$ channels in atrial myocytes. Moreover, channel activation by adenosine requires GTP, and it is abolished by pertussis toxin, which suggests that adenosine receptors activate I$_{K_{(ACh)}}$ also via a G protein (41, 43). Thus while the adenosine response is not well characterized, the analysis of the muscarinic activation of K$^+$ channels is likely to apply to adenosine elicited K$^+$ currents as well.

Quantitative Aspects of Muscarinic $K_{(ACh)}$ Activation in Cardiac Myocytes

KINETIC STEPS OF G PROTEIN MEDIATED CHANNEL OPENING   The mechanism by which G_K couples receptor activation to channel opening was studied in vivo with the aid of hydrolysis-resistant GTP analogues (GppNHp, guanylyl-imidodiphosphate; GTPγS, guanosine-5'-0-(3-thiotriphosphate); and GppCHp, guanylyl (β,γ-methylene)-diphosphate), collectively designated here as GXP. These compounds are easily introduced into cardiac myocytes using the broken-patch, whole-cell gigaseal technique (5,6). Even in the absence of an extracellular agonist, intracellular application of GTP analogues elicits the progressive development of an ionic conductance identical to $I_{K_{(ACh)}}$ (6, 40, 43). This receptor-independent current and that produced by muscarinic agonists are not additive; in particular, a fully developed receptor-independent current completely eliminates the response to agonists (6, 43). Moreover, the GXP-induced current is insensitive to muscarinic antagonists such as atropine. Uncoupling of $K_{(ACh)}$ channels from receptor implies that channel opening is not a direct effect of channel-receptor interactions, but rather it is produced by interaction of channels with G proteins that become persistently activated in the presence of GXP and Mg^{2+}.

When cells are dialyzed with solutions containing known concentrations of both GTP and GXP, the rate of receptor-independent, GXP-induced activation of $I_{K_{(ACh)}}$ depends only upon the GXP/GTP ratio and not on the absolute concentration of the nucleotides (6). The activation process shows a certain degree of specificity, since each GTP analogue activates G_k at different GXP/GTP ratios, with an order of relative effectiveness GTPγS>GTP>GppNHp>GppCHp (6). The rates of $I_{K_{(ACh)}}$ activation by all three analogues increase as a function of the GXP/GTP ratio and saturate at the same value, near 0.3/min, which suggests the existence of a rate limiting step that precedes nucleotide binding. This step is likely to be the basal, receptor-independent release of GDP from the inactive, GDP-bound G protein. The activated receptor is expected to act on the G protein by increasing the rate of GDP release, thereby facilitating GDP-GTP exchange and promoting the appearance of an active, GTP-bound G protein (12, 21, 70). Indeed, even nanomolar concentrations of ACh catalyze the rate of appearance of $I_{K_{(ACh)}}$ for all three analogues without affecting the relative affinity of G_k for GTP or its analogues (6). Thus activated receptors simply accelerate GDP-GXP exchange regardless of the analogue structure. The rate of activation of $K_{(ACh)}$ currents depends linearly on ACh concentration and, for bullfrog atrial myocytes, is given by the following expression:

$$k_{ACh} = 8.4 \times 10^8 \text{ min}^{-1} \text{ M}^{-1} \text{ [ACh]} + 0.44 \text{ min}^{-1}$$

the first term of which reflects the receptor-catalyzed rate of GDP release from $G_k \cdot$ GDP, while the second term corresponds to the basal rate of GDP release in the absence of an agonist (6).

Note that since all the nucleotide analogues should diffuse to the nucleotide binding site at approximately the same rate, the specificity of GXP binding cannot be explained by a diffusion-limited on-rate for the nucleotide-G_k reaction. This suggests that immediately after the release of GDP the binding site in the G protein is transiently open, and the interaction with GTP or its analogues is freely reversible; a conformational change then locks the nucleotide in the binding site (6). Direct evidence of occlusion of a transiently accessible guanine nucleotide binding site in vivo has been obtained recently. Moreover, results from these experiments suggest that the subsequent occlusion process is relatively slow (G. Szabo, A. Otero, unpublished results).

MECHANISM OF CHANNEL DEACTIVATION   Deactivation of $K_{(ACh)}$ channels upon removal of an agonist is thought to result from GTP hydrolysis, as indicated by the results obtained with hydrolysis-resistant GTP analogues. This view is supported by a large body of biochemical studies (21, 44, 70). In frog atrial myocytes the rate of deactivation of the muscarinic response could be estimated from the rate of decay of $I_{K_{(ACh)}}$ following agonist washout and also from extrapolation of the activation rate of the muscarinic response to the half-maximal concentration of $K_{(ACh)}$ activation by ACh. Both of these methods yield similar values for the rates of deactivation, near 150 min^{-1} (6). These and other estimates of deactivation rates in vivo (56) are much higher than those measured in vitro (near 2 min^{-1}; 12, 21). Since there are reports that persistently activated G proteins may release tightly bound GTP analogues in the presence of activated receptors (reviewed in 44), this discrepancy could conceivably arise from a deactivation step involving not hydrolysis, but the release of intact GTP. However, even though brief application of an agonist does remove persistent activation produced by low GXP/GTP ratios (G. Szabo, A. Otero, unpublished results), this process shows an absolute requirement for GTP. This observation suggests that release of GXP has to be followed by GTP binding and hydrolysis if deactivation is to occur. Therefore, in physiologic circumstances deactivation results from GTP hydrolysis and not from GTP/GDP exchange. The higher rates of deactivation seen in vivo imply an enhanced GTPase activity either by interaction with the effector (e.g. the ion channel) or some as yet unidentified regulatory component. The observation that at least in the adenylate cyclase system the effector actually decreases GTPase activity (14) may favor the second alternative.

Properties of $K_{(ACh)}$ at the Single-Channel Level

The G protein link between muscarinic receptors and K^+ channels in cardiac myocytes has also been examined at the single-channel level. K^+ channels activated by muscarinic agonists in intact cells are characterized by short mean open times (1–5 ms) and single-channel conductances of the order of 40 pS for $[K^+_o] \simeq 150$ mM (41, 54, 65). The single-channel conductance shows inward rectification when Mg^{2+} is present at the inner surface of the membrane (29, 30). In excised, inside-out patches, extracellular muscarinic agonists do not elicit $K_{(ACh)}$ channels unless GTP (or a GTP analogue) and Mg^{2+} are present at the cytoplasmic aspect (39, 41, 42). In the absence of an agonist, $K_{(ACh)}$ channels are slowly activated by application of hydrolysis-resistant GTP analogues to the inner surface of the membrane (39, 41, 46). Treatment of inside-out patches with the A protomer of pertussis toxin and nicotinamide adenine dinucleotide (NAD) prevents receptor-dependent channel activation in the presence of GTP (39, 41, 42), but it does not inhibit GTPγS-induced channel opening (46). Therefore, ADP-ribosylation of G_k prevents the interaction of G_k with receptor but not with effector, and does not affect the channel itself.

Taken together, these data support the hypothesis that receptors G_k and $K_{(ACh)}$ are separate, membrane-bound molecular entities, and that it is the coupling protein G_k, not the receptor, that activates the $K_{(ACh)}$ channel. This interpretation was tested directly through external application of purified G proteins or their resolved subunits to the intracellular surface of excised atrial cell membrane patches and proven to be correct.

Role of the G Protein Subunits in Channel Opening

The structural and biochemical properties of G proteins involved in transmembrane signaling have been recently reviewed (7, 12, 21, 51, 63, 70). These membrane-bound coupling proteins are characterized by a heterotrimeric structure, with α, β, and γ subunits. The α-subunits bind and hydrolyze GTP, can be ADP-ribosylated by bacterial toxins, and interact with both receptors and effectors. $\beta\gamma$ dimers anchor α-subunits to the membrane and are essential for the coupling between α-subunits and receptors (19, 21), but their ability to interact directly with effectors is controversial (12, 51). In the resting state the three subunits are associated, and the α-subunit contains tightly bound GDP. Activation of the G protein by receptors is thought to promote exchange of bound GDP for GTP; loading of the holoprotein with GTP results in its dissociation into active, GTP-liganded α-subunits, and $\beta\gamma$ dimers (21, 62, 70). The α-subunit is deactivated by its intrinsic GTPase activity, and α-GDP reassociates with $\beta\gamma$.

Activation of cyclic nucleotide phosphodiesterase by transducin in the visual system and enhancement of adenylate cyclase activity via G_s appears to result from interaction between the GTP-bound α-subunit with the effector (7, 21). By analogy, the expectation is that $K_{(ACh)}$ channels should be activated by GTP-bound α-subunits. This generalization seems to be valid. After initial conflicting reports (46, 75), a consensus has now emerged to the effect that under physiologic conditions muscarinic opening of potassium channels results from the interaction between channel and activated α-subunits. Evidence for this conclusion comes from studies in which purified G proteins or their resolved α-subunits, stably activated by GTPγS and Mg^{2+}, were applied to the cytosolic aspect of excised patches of sarcolemma (13, 15, 36, 75). Initial results demonstrated that a G_i-like protein (G_{i-3}), could activate $K_{(ACh)}$-like channels in excised patches through its α-subunit, while G_s was ineffective. A monoclonal antibody that reacted with the activated holoprotein or with the resolved α-subunit of G_{i-3} blocked agonist-induced channel opening, thereby suggesting that the α-subunit is the physiologic activator of the channel (76). Unexpectedly, the GTPγS-bound forms of $G_{i\alpha-1}$ and $G_{i\alpha-2}$ are also found to open $K_{(ACh)}$ channels (77). This lack of specificity is not a result of cross contamination, since the recombinant forms of these α-subunits activate $K_{(ACh)}$ channels in a manner that is not additive with stimulation by an agonist plus GTP or by GTPγS (77). Injection of activated α-subunits from G proteins of the G_i subgroup into intact atrial cells elicits K^+ selective currents with a similar lack of specificity (71). Unlike $I_{K_{(ACh)}}$ (6, 67), these currents are not characterized by voltage-dependent relaxations or by an inwardly rectifying steady-state current-voltage relationship. It is likely that in addition to $K_{(ACh)}$, other ionic channels are activated under these circumstances.

Contrary to expectation, application of $\beta\gamma$-subunits to the intracellular surface of excised cardiac cell membranes has also been reported to activate $K_{(ACh)}$-like channels at subnanomolar concentrations (13, 35, 37, 45, 46). Since $\beta\gamma$-subunits obtained from the brain and heart are highly hydrophobic, detergents are required to maintain the purified complex in solution. Unfortunately, some detergents also specifically influence $K_{(ACh)}$ activation (13, 36), so the interpretation of the results of these experiments must be made with care. A number of control experiments addressing this question indicate that artifacts cannot account for the observed stimulatory effects of $\beta\gamma$ dimers on muscarinic K^+ channels (37, 45). Recently it was suggested that stimulation of phospholipase A_2 (PLA$_2$) may underlie the action of $\beta\gamma$ on $K_{(ACh)}$ channels, since an antibody raised against PLA$_2$ blocks the effects of exogenous $\beta\gamma$ (35). This hypothesis is supported by the observation of receptor-independent activation of $K_{(ACh)}$ channels by arachidonic acid (AA), a product of the reaction catalyzed by PLA$_2$, as well as some of its metabolites generated by lipoxygenases (35, 38). These effects are not blocked by treatment with pertussis toxin. Some of the AA derivatives are effective in atrial membranes from neonatal rat, but do not activate the channel in guinea pig atrial membranes; the reason for this discrepancy is not clear. It is unlikely, however, that this mechanism contributes significantly to the physiologic activation of $K_{(ACh)}$ channels, since antibodies to PLA_2 do not prevent $K_{(ACh)}$ activation by GTPγS and, more importantly, blocking of either the PLA_2 or the lypoxygenase pathway does not hinder agonist-induced channel activation.

Kurachi & co-workers report (38) that $K_{(ACh)}$-like channels induced by ACh, AA, or leukotriene C_4 during cell-attached recording disappear rapidly upon excision from the cell but can be restored by cytoplasmic GTP. Interestingly, this effect of GTP is observed in the absence of a purinergic or muscarinic agonist. Application of GTPγS also revives the channels in AA-treated patches (38), but without the delay that characterizes receptor-independent activation of G proteins by GTP analogues in membrane patches or intact cells (6, 40, 41, 75). Based on these observations it was suggested (38) that AA or its metabolites may act by stimulating GDP/GTP exchange in G_k. Because GTP does not alter channel activation by AA in inside-out patches from rat atrial cells (35), such a mechanism may not be widespread.

The foregoing results strongly suggest that under physiologic circumstances, the α-subunit mediates K^+ channel opening. One should recognize, however, that the presently available data do not rule out a possible involvement of the $\beta\gamma$-subunit or other unidentified membrane-bound components in the process of channel opening, since these would be intrinsic to native systems such as atrial cell membranes.

INDIRECT REGULATION OF K^+ CHANNELS BY G PROTEINS

Delayed Rectifier

Activation of receptors that stimulate or inhibit hormone sensitive adenylate cyclase markedly affects ion transport across the plasma membrane of cardiac myocytes. In this paradigm of second messenger-mediated response, receptors that are coupled to adenylate cyclase by stimulatory (G_s) or inhibitory (G_i) G proteins are able to affect the rate of cAMP synthesis. The ensuing changes in the cellular level of cAMP alter the activity of cAMP-dependent protein kinase and thus modify the phosphorylation state of cellular proteins involved in channel function.

Although the modulation of L-type calcium channels by β-adrenergic agonists is the classic example of channel control via the adenylate cyclase-G_s-G_i system in heart, it is by no means unique. Currents that appear to be regulated by an analogous mechanism include the hyperpolarization-activated current, I_f (16), the transient outward current, I_{to} (49), as well as the delayed outward current carried by potassium ions, I_K, considered here.

Tsien & coworkers (72) first demonstrated that β-adrenergic agonists increased I_K in calf Purkinje fibers, and that this response could be elicited independently of β-receptors by perfusion with cyclic nucleotide phosphodiesterase inhibitors, cAMP, or with a lipid soluble cAMP analogue. These results were confirmed and expanded in subsequent work with these as well as other multicellular preparations (3, 8, 34, 52, 55).

Further support for the hypothesis that cAMP mediates the effects of various agonists on I_K was obtained from experiments performed in isolated cardiac myocytes. In ventricular cells the basal I_K is increased in response to β agonists (4, 33, 73, 74) and to elevation in the intracellular concentration of cAMP brought about by perfusion of cells with forskolin (73) or membrane permeable cAMP analogues (74). Intracellular application of the catalytic subunit of cAMP-dependent protein kinase also stimulates I_K in the absence of β-adrenergic agonists (9, 33, 57, 74), while dialysis with either the regulatory subunit or the specific protein inhibitor of this enzyme counteracts β-receptor dependent rises in I_K (31). β-agonist stimulation of I_K is potentiated by the phosphatase inhibitor okadaic acid, and it is not observed in cells perfused with protein phosphatases (26, 27, 32). These results strongly suggest that β-adrenergic stimulation of I_K occurs by phosphorylation of an intracellular protein and can be reversed by phosphatase-catalyzed dephosphorylation. An interesting feature of the response of delayed rectifier (but not Ca^{2+}) channels to agents that promote this phosphorylation event is its steep temperature dependence (73, 74).

A model of regulation through receptor-dependent changes in adenylate cyclase activity predicts that the target will respond in a similar way to stimulatory agonists that activate G_s, and that inhibitory agonists should oppose these effects by activating G_i. Indeed, activation of histamine receptors also enhances I_K by a mechanism that depends on cAMP, since R_p-cAMPS, an inhibitor of cAMP-dependent protein kinase prevents the histamine effect (28). Conversely, muscarinic cholinergic agonists antagonize β-adrenergic stimulation of I_K currents in ventricular myocytes (25), thus supporting the notion that receptors linked to adenylate cyclase by G_i are also involved in I_K modulation.

Although I_K and I_{Ca} are similarly affected by most manipulations, the control of I_K by different agonists is not likely to be secondary to changes in the rate of Ca^{2+} entry into cells via calcium channels. Modulation of the two currents by cAMP-related phosphorylation differs in terms of temperature sensitivity (74), cAMP concentration dependence, and kinetics (52). More importantly, β-agonists and cAMP-dependent protein kinase are able to stimulate I_K in the presence of calcium channel blockers (3, 4, 34, 73, 74).

Because some of the results summarized here originate from studies that chiefly addressed the regulation of I_{Ca}, the description of the mechanism of receptor regulation of I_K is far from complete. In particular, the involvement of G_s and G_i in the responses of delayed rectifier currents to activated receptors has not been rigorously demonstrated. Nevertheless the evidence for a role of adenylate cyclase (and therefore G_s and G_i) in the modulation of I_K is compelling. Furthermore, as pointed out by Hescheler & colleagues (28), the general observation of parallel changes in I_K and in I_{Ca} supports the conclusion that both currents are controlled through similar processes.

Background K^+ Channels

In Purkinje fibers, stimulation of α_1-adrenergic receptors by submicromolar concentrations of phenylephrine leads to a decrease in automaticity. Recently it was shown that this effect arises through receptor-mediated activation of the Na/K pump and inhibition of the background potassium conductance, g_K (66). The response to phenylephrine is rendered partially irreversible in the presence of internal GppNHp and is blocked in cells treated with pertussis toxin (66). These results suggest that a G protein couples α_1-adrenergic receptors to the decrease in g_K and the increase in pump currents. The nature of the g_K component affected by phenylephrine is uncertain, although Shah et al (66) indicate that it may be the inward rectifier current, I_{K1}. The identity of the effector system that interacts with the activated G protein is also unknown. Since the negative chronotropic effect of phenylephrine in Purkinje fibers and in ventricular tissue was shown to be associated with the presence of a pertussis toxin substrate of $M_r \simeq 41$ kd (64), the G protein involved in the inhibition of g_K presumably belongs to the G_i subgroup.

CONCLUSIONS

The discovery that, in addition to membrane potential and cytoplasmic second messengers, ion channels can be also gated by membrane-bound coupling factors, of which G proteins may be but one example, has imparted a new dimension to the array of cellular regulatory processes controlled by neuroendocrine signals. This is particularly significant for cardiac, neuronal, and other excitable cells in which ion channels are the fundamental units that provide physiologically relevant cellular responses.

Much remains to be learned about the detailed role of G proteins in channel gating. The number of channels found to be regulated by G proteins is increasing and may well encompass all membrane channels. For example, G proteins were recently implicated in the regulation of ATP-sensitive K^+ channels in pancreatic β-cells (17, 20) and skeletal muscle (59); similar channels present in cardiac cells may also be regulated likewise. It is presently difficult to understand the physiologic specificity of G protein-mediated responses in light of the apparent similarity of a given class of purified G proteins with respect to their interactions with different receptors and effectors. A better understanding of the role of G protein subunits and the spatial arrangement of these relative to receptor and effector is required to clarify this issue. The direct gating of channels by activated G protein subunits has been demonstrated only in native cell membranes, which may contain unidentified coupling factors. Unambiguous demonstration of direct gating of channels by G protein subunits will require a system in which purified subunit and channel protein are brought together in a well-defined lipid environment. Moreover, there is a possibility that other factors, for example nucleoside diphosphokinases (58) or cytoskeletal components, are necessary for a physiologically functional system. The muscarinic $K_{(ACh)}$ response is characterized by both short and long term desensitization (43) and prominent voltage-dependent relaxations (67). The origin of these phenomena is not understood and is the object of current research. The major challenge, however, is to understand how G proteins achieve the integration of extracellular signals into physiologically appropriate cellular responses.

Literature Cited

1. Belardinelli, L., Giles, W. R., West, A. 1988. Ionic mechanism of adenosine actions in pacemaker cells from rabbit heart. *J. Physiol.* 405:615–33
2. Belardinelli, L., Isenberg, G. 1983. Isolated atrial myocytes: adenosine and acetylcholine increase potassium conductance. *Am. J. Physiol.* 224:H734–37
3. Bennett, P., Mckinney, L., Begenisich, T., Kass, R. S. 1986. Adrenergic modulation of the delayed rectifier potassium channel in calf cardiac Purkinje fibers. *Biophys. J.* 49(4):839–48
4. Bennett, P. B., Begenisich, T. B. 1987. Catecholamines modulate the delayed rectifying potassium current (Ik) in guinea pig ventricular myocytes. *Pflügers Arch.* 410:217–19
5. Breitwieser, G. E., Szabo, G. 1985. Uncoupling of cardiac muscarinic and β-adrenergic receptors from ion channels by a guanine nucleotide analogue. *Nature* 317:538–40
6. Breitwieser, G. E., Szabo, G. 1988. Mechanism of muscarinic receptor-induced K channel activation as revealed by hydrolysis resistant GTP analogues. *J. Gen. Physiol.* 91:469–93
7. Brown, A. M., Birnbaumer, L. 1988. Direct G protein gating of ion channels. *Am. J. Physiol.* 254(23):H401–10

8. Brown, H., Noble, S. J. 1974. Effects of adrenaline on membrane currents underlying pacemaker activity in frog atrial muscle. *J. Physiol.* 238, 51P–53P
9. Brum, G., Flockerzi, V., Hofmann, F., Osterrieder, W., Trautwein, W. 1983. Injection of catalytic subunit of cAMP-dependent protein kinase into isolated cardiac myocytes. *Pflügers Arch.* 398: 147–54
10. Carmeliet, E., Mubagwa, K. 1986. Changes by acetylcholine of membrane currents in rabbit cardiac Purkinje fibers. *J. Physiol.* 371:201–17
11. Carmeliet, E., Mubagwa, K. 1986. Characterization of the acetylcholine-induced potassium current in rabbit Purkinje fibres. *J. Physiol.* 371:219–37
12. Casey, P. J., Gilman, A. G. 1988. G Protein involvement in receptor-effector coupling. *J. Biol. Chem.* 263:2577–80
13. Cerbai, E., Klockner, U., Isenberg, G. 1988. The α subunit of the GTP binding protein activates muscarinic potassium channels of the atrium. *Science* 240: 1782–83
14. Cerione, R. A., Sibley, D. R., Codina, J., Benovic, J., Winslow, J., et al. 1984. Reconstitution of a hormone-sensitive adenylate cyclase system. The pure β-adrenergic receptor and guanine

nucleotide regulatory protein confer hormone responsiveness on the resolved catalytic unit. *J. Biol. Chem.* 259:9979–82

15. Codina, J., Yatani, A., Grenet, D., Brown, A. M., Birnbaumer, L. 1987. The α subunit of the GTP binding protein G_K opens atrial potassium channels. *Science* 236:442–44

16. DiFrancesco, D., Tromba, C. 1988. Muscarinic control of the hyperpolarization-activated current (i_f) in rabbit sinoatrial node myocytes. *J. Physiol.* 405: 493–510

17. Dunne, M. J., Bullett, M. J., Guodong, L., Wollheim, C. B., Peterson, O. H. 1989. Galanin activates nucleotide-dependent K^+ channels in insulin secreting cells via a pertussis toxin-sensitive G-protein. *EMBO J.* 8:413–20

18. Endoh, M., Maruyama, M., Iijima, T. 1985. Attenuation of muscarinic cholinergic inhibition by islet-activating protein in the heart. *Am. J. Physiol.* 249:H309–20

19. Florio, V. A., Sternweis, P. C. 1989. Mechanisms of muscarinic receptor action on G_o in reconstituted phospholipid vesicles. *J. Biol. Chem.* 264:3909–15

20. Fosset, M., Schmid-Antomarchi, H., de Weille, J. R., Lazdunski, M. 1988. Somatostatin activates glibenclamide-sensitive ATP-regulated K^+ channels in insulinoma cells via a G-protein. *FEBS Lett.* 242:94–96

21. Gilman, A. G. 1987. G Proteins: Transducers of Receptor-Generated Signals. *Annu. Rev. Biochem.* 56:615–49

22. Gintant, G. A., Cohen, I. S. 1988. Advances in cardiac cellular electrophysiology: implications for automaticity and therapeutics. *Annu. Rev. Pharmacol. Toxicol.* 28:61–81

23. Hartzell, H. C. 1979. Adenosine receptors in frog sinus venosus: slow inhibitory potentials produced by adenosine compounds and acetylcholine. *J. Physiol.* 293:23–49

24. Hartzell, H. C., Simmons, M. A. 1987. Comparison of the effects of acetylcholine on calcium and potassium currents in frog atrium and ventricle. *J. Physiol.* 389:411–22

25. Hescheler, J., Kameyama, M., Trautwein, W. 1986. On the mechanism of muscarinic inhibition of the cardiac Ca current. *Pflügers Arch.* 407:182–89

26. Hescheler, J., Kameyama, M., Trautwein, W., Mieskes, G., Soling, H.-D. 1987. Regulation of the cardiac calcium channel by protein phosphatases. *Eur. J. Biochem.* 165:261–66

27. Hescheler, J., Mieskes, G., Takai, A.,

Trautwein, W. 1988. Effects of a protein phosphatase inhibitor, okadaic acid, on membrane currents of isolated guinea-pig cardiac myocytes. *Pflügers Arch.* 412:248–52

28. Hescheler, J., Tang, M., Jastorff, B., Trautwein, W. 1987. On the mechanism of histamine induced enhancement of the cardiac Ca^{2+} current. *Pflügers Arch.* 410:23–29

29. Horie, M., Irisawa, H. 1987. Rectification of muscarinic K current by magnesium ion in guinea pig atrial cells. *Am. J. Physiol.* 253:H210–14

30. Horie, M., Irisawa, H. 1989. Dual effects of intracellular magnesium on muscarinic potassium channel current in single guinea-pig atrial cells. *J. Physiol.* 408:313–332

31. Kameyama, M., Hescheler, J., Hofmann, F., Trautwein, W. 1986. Modulation of Ca current during the phosphorylation cycle in the guinea pig heart. *Pflügers Arch.* 407:123–28

32. Kameyama, M., Hescheler, J., Mieskes, G., Trautwein, W. 1986. The protein-specific phosphatase 1 antagonizes the β-adrenergic increase of the cardiac Ca current. *Pflügers Arch.* 407:461–63

33. Kameyama, M., Hofmann, F., Trautwein, W. 1985. On the mechanism of β-adrenergic regulation of the Ca channel in the guinea-pig heart. *Pflügers Arch.* 405:285–93

34. Kass, R. S., Wiegers, S. E. 1982. The ionic basis of concentration-related effects of noradrenaline on the action potential of calf cardiac Purkinje fibers. *J. Physiol.* 322:541–58

35. Kim, D., Lewis, D. L., Graziadei, L., Neer, E. J., Bar-Sagi, D., et al. 1989. G-protein $\beta\gamma$-subunits activate the cardiac muscarinic K^+-channel via phospholipase A_2. *Nature* 337:557–60

36. Kirsch, G. E., Yatani, A., Codina, J., Birnbaumer, L., Brown, A. M. 1988. α-Subunit of G_K activates atrial K^+ channels of chick, rat, and guinea pig. *Am. J. Physiol.* 254:1200–5

37. Kurachi, Y., Ito, H., Katada, T., Ui, M. 1989. Activation of atrial muscarinic K^+ channels by low concentrations of $\beta\gamma$ subunits of rat brain G protein. *Pflügers Arch.* 413:325–27

38. Kurachi, Y., Ito, H., Sugimoto, T., Shimizu, T., Miki, I., et al. 1989. Arachidonic acid metabolites as intracellular modulators of the G protein cardiac K^+ channel. *Nature* 337:555–57

39. Kurachi, Y., Nakajima, T., Sugimoto, T. 1986. Acetylcholine activation of K^+

channels in cell-free membrane of atrial cells. *Am. J. Physiol.* 251:H681–84

40. Kurachi, Y., Nakajima, T., Sugimoto, T. 1987. Quinidine inhibition of the muscarinic receptor-activated K^+ channel current in atrial cells of the guinea pig. *Naunyn-Schmiedeberg's Arch. Pharmacol.* 335:216–18

41. Kurachi, Y., Nakajima, T., Sugimoto, T. 1986. On the mechanism of activation of muscarinic K^+ channels by adenosine in isolated atrial cells: involvement of GTP-binding proteins. *Pflügers Arch.* 407:264–74

42. Kurachi, Y., Nakajima, T., Sugimoto, T. 1986. Role of intracellular Mg^{2+} in the activation of muscarinic K channel in cardiac atrial cell membrane. *Pflügers Arch.* 407:572–74

43. Kurachi, Y., Nakajima, T., Sugimoto, T. 1987. Short-term desensitization of muscarinic K^+ channel current in isolated atrial myocytes and possible role of GTP-binding proteins. *Pflügers Arch.* 410:227–33

44. Levitzki, A. 1987. Regulation of adenylate-cyclase by hormones and G-proteins. *FEBS Lett.* 211:113–18

45. Logothetis, D. E., Kim, D., Northup, J. K., Neer, E. J., Clapham, D. E. 1988. Specificity of action of guanine nucleotide-binding regulatory protein subunits on the cardiac muscarinic K^+ channel. *Proc. Natl. Acad. Sci. USA* 85:5814–18

46. Logothetis, D. E., Kurachi, Y., Galper, J., Clapham, D. E., Neer, E. J. 1987. The $\beta\gamma$ subunits of GTP-binding proteins activate the muscarinic K^+ channel in heart. *Nature* 325:321–26

47. Martin, J. M., Hunter, D. D., Nathanson, N. M. 1985. Islet activating protein inhibits physiological responses evoked by cardiac muscarinic acetylcholine receptors. Role of guanosine triphosphate binding proteins in regulation of potassium permeability. *Biochemistry* 24:7521–25

48. Momose, Y., Giles, W., Szabo, G. 1984. Acetylcholine-induced K^+ current in amphibian atrial cells. *Biophys. J.* 45:20–22

49. Nakayama, T., Fozzard, H. A. 1988. Adrenergic modulation of the transient outward current in isolated canine Purkinje cells. *Circ. Res.* 62:162–72

50. Nargeot, J., Lester, H. A., Birdsall, N. J. M., Stockton, J., Wassermann, N. H., et al. 1982. A photoisomerizable muscarinic antagonist: studies of binding and of conductance relaxations in frog heart. *J. Gen. Physiol.* 79:657–78

51. Neer, E. J., Clapham, D. E. 1988.

Roles of G protein subunits in transmembrane signalling. *Nature* 333:129–34

52. Nerbonne, J. M., Richard, S., Nargeot, J., Lester, H. A. 1984. New photoactivatable cyclic nucleotides produce intracellular jumps in cyclic AMP and cyclic GMP concentrations. *Nature* 310:74–76

53. Noble, D. 1984. The surprising heart: a review of recent progress in cardiac electrophysiology. *J. Physiol.* 353:1–50

54. Noma, A. Chemical-receptor dependent potassium channels in cardiac muscle 1987. In *Electrophysiology of Single Cardiac Cells*, eds. D. Noble, T. Powell, pp. 223–246. Orlando: Academic

55. Noma, A., Kotake, H., Irisawa, H. 1980. Slow inward current and its role in mediating the chronotropic effect of epinephrine in the rabbit sinoatrial node. *Pflügers Arch.* 388:1–9

56. Okabe, K., Yatani, A., Brown, A. M. 1989. Coupling between the G Protein G_k and atrial K^+ channels studied by a concentration jump method. *Biophys. J.* 55:586a

57. Osterrieder, W., Brum, G., Hescheler, J., Trautwein, W., Flockerzi, V., et al. 1982. Injection of subunits of cyclic AMP-dependent protein kinase into cardiac myocytes modulates Ca^{2+} current. *Nature* 298:576–78

58. Otero, A. S., Breitwieser, G. E., Szabo, G. 1988. Activation of muscarinic potassium currents by ATPγS in atrial cells. *Science* 242:443–45

59. Parent, L., Coronado, R. 1989. Reconstitution of the ATP-sensitive potassium channel of skeletal muscle. Activation by a G-protein dependent process. *Biophys. J.* 55:587a

60. Pennefather, P., Cohen, I. S. 1989. Molecular mechanisms of cardiac potassium channel regulation. In: *Cardiac Electrophysiology and Arrhythmias from Cell to Bedside*, eds. D. P. Zipes, J. Jalife, Philadelphia: Saunders

61. Pfaffinger, P. J., Martin, J. M., Hunter, D. D., Nathanson, N. M., Hille, B. 1985. GTP-binding proteins couple cardiac muscarinic receptors to a K channel. *Nature* 317:536–38

62. Ransnäs, L. A., Insel, P. A. 1988. Subunit dissociation is the mechanism for hormonal activation of the G protein in native membranes. *J. Biol. Chem.* 263:17239–42

63. Robishaw, J. D., Foster, K. A. 1989. Role of G proteins in the regulation of the cardiovascular system. *Annu. Rev. Physiol.* 51:229–44

64. Rosen, M. R., Steinberg, S. F., Chow, Y.-K., Bilezikian, J. P., Danilo, P. Jr. 1988. Role of a pertussis toxin-sensitive protein in the modulation of canine Purkinje fiber automaticity. *Circ. Res.* 62: 315–23

65. Sakmann, B., Noma, A., Trautwein, W. 1983. Acetylcholine activation of single muscarinic K^+ channels in isolated pacemaker cells of the mammalian heart. *Nature* 303:250–53

66. Shah, A., Cohen, I. S., Rosen, M. R. 1988. Stimulation of cardiac alpha receptors increases Na/K pump current and decreases g_k via a pertussis toxin-sensitive pathway. *Biophys. J.* 54:219–25

67. Simmons, M. A., Hartzell, H. C. 1987. A quantitative analysis of the acetylcholine-activated potassium current in single cells from frog atrium. *Pflügers Arch.* 409:454–61

68. Soejima, M., Noma, A. 1984. Mode of regulation of the ACh-sensitive K-channel by the muscarinic receptor in rabbit atrial cells. *Pflügers Arch.* 400: 424–31

69. Sorota, S., Tsuji, Y., Tajiima, T., Pappano, A. J. 1985. Pertussis toxin treatment blocks hyperpolarization by muscarinic agonists in chick atrium. *Circ. Res.* 57:748–58

70. Stryer, L., Bourne, H. R. 1986. G proteins: a family of signal transducers. *Annu. Rev. Cell Biol.* 2:391–419

71. Szabo, G., Pang, I. H., Sternweis, P. C. 1988. Activation of a K^+ current by exogenous G proteins in atrial myocytes. *Biophys. J.* 53:424a.

72. Tsien, R. W., Giles, W., Greengard, P. 1972. Cyclic AMP mediates the effects of adrenaline on cardiac Purkinje fibers. *Nature New Biol.* 240:181–83

73. Walsh, K. B., Begenisich, T. B., Kass, R. S. 1988. β-Adrenergic modulation in the heart. *Pflügers Arch.* 411:232–34

74. Walsh, K. B., Kass, R. S. 1988. Regulation of a heart potassium channel by protein kinase A and C. *Science* 242:67–69

75. Yatani, A., Codina, J., Brown, A. M., Birnbaumer, L. 1987. Direct activation of mammalian atrial potassium channels by GTP regulatory protein G_k. *Science* 235:207–11

76. Yatani, A., Hamm, H., Codina, J., Mazzoni, M. R., Birnbaumer, L., et al. 1988. A monoclonal antibody to the α subunit of G_k blocks muscarinic activation of atrial K^+ Channels. *Science* 241:828–31

77. Yatani, A., Mattera, R., Codina, J., Graf, R., Okabe, K., et al. 1988. The G protein-gated atrial K^+ channel is stimulated by three distinct G_i α-subunits. *Nature* 336:680–682

Annu. Rev. Physiol. 1990. 52:307–319

ELECTROPHYSIOLOGY OF THE PARIETAL CELL

Jeffery R. Demarest

Department of Zoology, University of Arkansas, Fayetteville, Arkansas 72701

Donald D. F. Loo

Department of Physiology, University of California, School of Medicine, Los Angeles, California 90024-1751

KEY WORDS: epithelium, acid secretion, membrane fusion, ion channels, patch-clamp

INTRODUCTION

Recently the application of new biophysical methods, such as patch-clamping and intracellular ion-sensitive fluorescent probes, has resulted in substantial gains in understanding the mechanisms that underlie HCl secretion by the gastric mucosa. The stimulation of acid secretion by the parietal or oxyntic cells of the gastric mucosa involves membrane fusion that results in the insertion of proton pumps (the H,K-ATPase) and the activation of ion transport pathways in the membranes of the cells. Although the process of gastric acid secretion has been the focus of research by several generations of electrophysiologists, direct identification of the cell types responsible for transepithelial ion transport, measurement of the intracellular electrical properties of oxyntic cells, and identification of the ion channels contributing to them have only been achieved within the last five years. The present review is concerned with these recent advances in the electrophysiology of oxyntic cells, particularly those obtained using patch-clamp techniques. Other methodologies and much previous work on gastric secretion and its regulation will be summarized briefly in this review. The interested reader is referred to other cited recent reviews for further details. In this review we will proceed from a brief overview of the function of the intact epithelium and changes in

0066-4278/90/0315-0307$02.00

307

cellular morphology associated with the stimulation of HCl secretion to the membrane and molecular mechanisms that underlie secretion.

Epithelial and Cellular Morphology of Acid Secretion

The multicellular exocrine glands of the gastric epithelium of mammals contain acid-secreting parietal cells and enzyme-secreting chief cells. In nonmammalian vertebrates a single cell type, the oxyntic cell, performs both functions. In humans, each of the cell types contributes to the one to three liters of gastric juice secreted by the glands each day (8). This gastric juice is an approximately isosmotic solution of HCl that has a K^+ concentration higher than that of plasma. Organic constituents, primarily mucoproteins and the acid-activated proenzyme, pepsinogen, account for only about 10 mOsm/liter.

Membrane fusion, which results in a large increase in secretory membrane surface, is an important process for the activation of HCl and fluid secretion by oxyntic cells (18). The apical cytoplasm of a resting oxyntic cell that is not secreting acid is packed with vesicles formed of membrane containing H,K-ATPase (the proton pump that exchanges cytosolic protons for luminal K^+), but has no other specific ion permeabilities (46). Lack of permeability for K^+ maintains the ATPase in an arrested state in the resting cell by depriving it of intravesicular K^+ ions to exchange for cytosolic protons (47). Stimulation of the cell by a variety of secretagogues (e.g. histamine, cholinergic agonists, gastrin, cAMP) results in the fusion of these so-called tubulovesicles with the apical membrane of the cell. This process takes from 10 to 30 min and by morphometric measurement results in at least a tenfold increase in the apical membrane area (18, 27). Electrical capacitance measurements suggest that the actual membrane area increase may be more than 100-fold (5). Concurrently with these fusion events, permeability pathways for Cl^- and K^+ are thought to be activated in the apical membrane. In mammalian parietal cells a deep invagination of the apical membrane called the secretory canaliculus is formed in continuity with the lumen of the gastric gland (18). In the amphibian oxyntic cell no canaliculus is formed, but there is an increase in the number of folds and density of microvillae on the apical membrane (27). In addition, since the amphibian oxyntic cell also secretes pepsinogen, some of the increase in apical membrane in these cells is because of the addition of zymogen granule membrane when protein secretion is stimulated. In both parietal and oxyntic cells the membranes added during stimulation are retrieved when the stimulus is removed and recycled for subsequent bouts of secretion (19).

Ion Transport

Each of the membranes of the polarized oxyntic cell performs a specific function with respect to acid secretion. The basolateral membrane acts as a pathway for Cl^- entry into the cell and for the extrusion of bicarbonate produced by the reaction catalyzed by carbonic anhydrase during the intracellular generation of protons for secretion. This membrane also contains the ubiquitous Na,K-ATPase and exhibits a dominant conductance for K^+ (14, 24). The apical membrane acts as a pathway for Cl^- and H^+ exit from the cell in to the lumen of the gastric gland. Protons are actively secreted from the cell by the H,K-ATPase located in the apical membrane. The presence of active exchange pumps in the basolateral and apical membranes, which are dependent on extracellular K^+, indicates that K^+ must be recycled across both membranes. For the basolateral membrane, K^+ leaving the cell through the basolateral conductance is recycled in exchange for Na^+ by the Na,K-ATPase, as is the case in most epithelial cells. K^+ must also be recycled across the apical membrane, however, in order to replenish lumen K^+ depleted by the H,K-ATPase. The distribution of some of these ion pathways in an oxyntic cell is illustrated in Figure 1.

ELECTRICAL PROPERTIES AND CONDUCTANCE PATHWAYS

Parietal cells are not accessible for microelectrode impalement in intact mammalian gastric mucosa. Attempts to make microelectrode measurements from mammalian parietal cells in isolated gastric glands have encountered technical difficulties such as low resting potentials and thus have not proven satisfactory (see 15). Further, there has been only limited success with electrical measurements from parietal cells in culture where functional polarity of the cells is lost (34). Consequently, most intracellular electrical measurements have been made using amphibian tissues.

Amphibian Oxyntic Cell

The first intracellular electrical measurements from oxyntic cells obtained from isolated *Necturus* cells indicated that the intracellular potential was

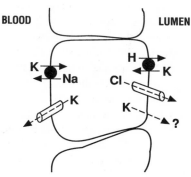

Figure 1 Ion transport pathways in oxyntic cells. Filled circles refer to ATP-driven pumps (Na,K and H,K-ATPases). Cylinders refer to conductance channels (K and Cl). The nature of the luminal membrane pathway for K^+ is uncertain (see text).

about -44 mV (2). In these isolated cells, however, the contribution of the apical and basolateral membranes to the membrane potential could not be determined.

A methodological advance was made by Demarest & Machen (14) who developed an intact preparation of *Necturus* gastric epithelium mounted seros-al side up in an Ussing chamber with the basolateral membrane of the oxyntic cells exposed by dissection of the submucosal connective tissue. The upward-facing basolateral membrane could then be impaled by a microelectrode. Measurements from oxyntic cells in this intact preparation indicated a baso-lateral membrane potential of about -45 mV under resting conditions (i.e. in the presence of the histamine type II receptor blocker cimetidine), which increased to about -60 mV following stimulation with histamine (14). Apical cell membrane potential with respect to the mucosal bathing solution was -20 mV at rest and is hyperpolarized to -25 mV after stimulation. The potential profile across this layer of cells has the shape of a well, similar to that found in the majority of other epithelial cells. The transepithelial electrical potential of the serosal with respect to the mucosal surface was about 25 mV at rest and 30 mV in acid-secreting epithelia. In both resting and stimulated cells, suddenly increasing the serosal K^+ concentration from 5 mM/liter to 50 mM/liter by substituting K^+ for Na^+ rapidly depolarized the basolateral membrane poten-tial and markedly reduced the resistance of the basolateral membrane (14). Replacing an equivalent amount of Na^+ with n-methyl-D-glucamine$^+$ or lowering the Cl^- concentration by tenfold had no significant effect on the cellular electrical properties (14, 13). Thus the dominant conductance in the basolateral membrane of *Necturus* oxyntic cells is K^+ conductance with little or no conductance for Na^+ or Cl^- in both the resting and stimulated states. Similar techniques have been applied to frog oxyntic cells, thus confirming the dominance of the basolateral K^+ conductance, absence of a basolateral Cl^- conductance, and hyperpolarizations of V_{mc} and V_{cs} upon stimulation with histamine (40a). Evidence for an electrogenic Na/HCO_3 cotransporter has also been reported for frog oxyntic cells (7).

Accurate assessment of apical membrane conductance properties using rapid ion substitution experiments in the intact mucosa is problematic because of potential inaccessibility of the apical membranes, presumably because of restricted diffusion within the glandular lumen. It is clear, however, that the apical membrane must contain a significant conductance for Cl^-, since localized transepithelial ionic current measured using a vibrating probe in-dicates that oxyntic cells alone are responsible for the electrogenic secretion of Cl^- by the mucosa (16). The following observations in isolated frog gastric mucosa suggest that the apical K^+ conductance must be small compared to that for Cl^-: (*a*) transepithelial potential changes in response to tenfold changes in mucosal K^+ concentration are only about 4 mV; (*b*) Ba^{2+}, a potent blocker of K^+ conductances at concentrations up to 20 mM in the mucosal solution, has no affect on acid secretion or the short circuit current due to Cl^- transport (23, 31, 41). In addition, only a Cl^--dependent noise component could be detected in the short-circuit current across frog gastric mucosa under control conditions; a K^+-dependent component could only be demonstrated in Cl^--free solutions (49).

In *Necturus* oxyntic cells the ratio of the resistance of the apical to basolateral membrane is close to unity at rest and is unchanged upon stimulation (14). Since oxyntic cells are the major conductive pathway across the *Necturus* mucosa, even at rest, and the reduction in the transepithelial resistance that accompanies stimulation can be attributed to changes in oxyntic cell conductance alone, the constancy of the relative resistances of the apical and basolateral membranes indicates that the conductance of both membranes increases by the same amount as the result of stimulation (14). This observation is another example of the well-documented cellular homeostatic feedback mechanisms found in the cells of other transporting epithelia (9, 12, 17, 43). These mechanisms coordinate the activities of the apical and basolateral components of transepithelial transport in order to preserve the ionic and volume balance of the cell. For example, intracellular pH is remarkably stable during the course of maximal stimulation of parietal cells, while transepithelial H^+ flux is increasing from zero to very high levels (29, 34a).

Mammalian Parietal Cell

As a result of the complex morphology of the mammalian gastric epithelium, much of the current understanding of the ion permeability pathways in parietal cells has been obtained from studies of isolated rabbit gastric glands, purified parietal cells, and membrane vesicles (1, 21, 38). The high density of glands in the mammalian mucosa provides an abundant source of material for these studies as well as for biochemical investigations. Fluorescence and isotopic tracer flux techniques reveal an array of co- and counter-transport activities and ionic conductances in the membranes of parietal cells. These mechanisms may participate directly in the acid secretory process or have an indirect role by contributing to cellular ionic and volume homeostasis (21, 29). Biochemical studies have focused on the mechanism of the H,K-ATPase, which has been determined to be a neutral one-for-one exchange mechanism (38). Current knowledge of the cellular regulation of acid secretion by parietal cells has recently been reviewed by Chew (3). We will only summarize briefly results from these studies relevent to the conductive pathways and active ion pumps directly involved in acid secretion.

The conductance pathways in the mammalian parietal cell identified from biochemical, fluorescent, and isotopic flux studies are different from those derived from electrophysiologic studies on amphibian material in several significant respects. Investigations using isolated gastric glands, apical membrane vesicle fractions, and isolated parietal cells infer that the H,K-ATPase containing membranes of the resting cell have little or no conductance for Cl^- (6, 48). Evidence for a significant Cl^- conductance is found in stimulation-associated vesicles derived from the expanded canalicular membrane that results, following stimulation, from the fusion of intracellular vesicles. In vesicle studies the presence of a K^+ conductance in the resting membranes is disputed, as is its activation upon stimulation (6, 48). Studies of acid accumulation in digitonin-permeabilized gastric glands suggest the presence of a Cl^- conductance in both resting and stimulated apical membranes, but do not indicate a K^+ conductance in either condition (36).

Work with isolated parietal cells and basolateral membrane vesicles indicates the presence of a large basolateral K^+ conductance, but no Cl^- conductance (32).

PATCH-CLAMP STUDIES OF OXYNTIC AND PARIETAL CELLS

The patch-clamp technique is based on the isolation of very small areas of membrane ($\leq$ 1–10 μm^2) at the tip of a fire-polished glass pipette (39). Interaction of a clean pipette tip with the cell membrane results in the formation of a seal with an electrical resistance on the order of 10^{10} Ω, which isolates the membrane patch electrically as well as physically, and permits the measurement of specific membrane currents of less than 10^{-12} A. This technique allows the observation of either the activity of single molecules (tight seal or single-channel recording) or the ensemble behavior of all of the channels in a cell (whole-cell recording). Since the membranes of interest must be accessible to patch pipettes, most investigations of glandular and tubular epithelia have been performed on cells or groups of cells isolated by enzymatic digestion. Gastric ion channels have been studied using parietal cells in primary culture, partially dispersed gastric glands, and isolated oyntic cells, all of which retain apical-to-basolateral membrane polarity (for exceptions, see below) and allow access to one or both of these membranes that are otherwise inaccessible in the intact mucosa.

Polarity of Gastric Secretory Cells

The only membrane that can be studied directly in isolated parietal cells is the basolateral membrane because of the formation of the secretory canaliculus. Although several studies employing cultured parietal cells have claimed that the basolateral membrane orients downward during attachment of the cells to the culturing support matrix and that the apical membrane faces upwards and is exposed (4, 10, 34, 42), the retention of polarity by parietal cells in culture has not been established.

In contrast, the apical and basolateral membranes of isolated amphibian oyntic cells are exposed in the resting cell, and no intracellular canaliculus is formed upon stimulation. Instead stimulation-induced membrane fusion increases the exposed apical membrane area (16, 27). The polarity between these two membranes could be lost, however, because of lateral diffusion and mixing of membrane constituents during the isolation procedure. Two methods have been used to distinguish the basolateral and apical membranes in patch-clamp studies. (*a*) Small clusters of cells or partially dispersed gastric glands can be isolated from *Necturus* mucosa (45). In this preparation of partially dispersed glands, the lumina of the glands are visible with a light microscope, and the basolateral membrane of the oxyntic cells, which is distant from the lumen, is exposed, thus allowing the approach by a patch pipette. (*b*) Oxyntic cells isolated from the resting gastric mucosa of *Necturus* by enzymatic digestion with pronase and collagenase in the presence of 10^{-4} M cimetidine have been found to retain the distinct polarity between the apical and basolateral membranes (13). In addition, these cells respond to stimulation (10^{-4} M isobutylmethylxanthine and 10^{-3} M cAMP) with a marked increase in their apical membrane area following a time course similar to that observed in the intact epithelium (13, 27). This preparation has made the apical membrane readily accessible to patch pipettes for the first time.

Ion Channels in Oxyntic Cells

BASOLATERAL MEMBRANE Potassium conductance dominates the basolateral membrane conductance of resting and stimulated oxyntic cells (14). Single-channel recordings from basolateral membranes of *Necturus* oxyntic cells reveal that there are at least two types of channels that are highly selective for K^+ (45). These two types of channels can be distinguished on the basis of conductance, voltage dependence, and activation by intracellular cAMP or Ca^{2+} (Table 1). The cAMP-activated K^+ channel has a conductance of 33 pS and is relatively voltage-independent. The channel activated by Ca^{2+} has a larger conductance, 67 pS, and is activated by depolarization of the membrane. This class of channel shows several of the characteristics of maxi K^+ channels, such as the large single-channel conductance and the high selectivity for K^+ over Na^+ (Table 1; 26). Ca^{2+} had no effect on the AMP-activated K^+ channel, similarly the activity of the Ca^{2+}-activated K^+ channel was unaffected by cAMP. Ca^{2+} and cAMP increase the open probability of their respective channels without affecting single-channel conductance, rather than causing the recruitment of new channels into the patch. Both carbachol, presumably acting to elevate intracellular Ca^{2+}, and exogenous cAMP activate oxyntic cell basolateral K^+ channels in cell-attached patches when added to the medium bathing the cells (45). Therefore, these K^+ channels may account for at least part of the increase in basolateral conductance and hyperpolarization measured with microelectrodes in oxyntic cells in the intact epithelium (13). In addition, increased turnover of the Na,K-ATPase because of increased basolateral-coupled Na^+ entry probably contributes to the stimulation-induced hyperpolarization. What is not clear is the contribution of each class of K^+ channels to the resting conductance, and whether these K^+ channels alone can account for the resting basolateral K^+ conductance.

APICAL MEMBRANE   Single-channel recording methods have also been applied to determine the ion channels in the apical membrane of resting and stimulated oxyntic cells (13). Cell-attached patches formed on resting apical membranes contained a single class of Cl^- channels with a conductance of 12 pS at the resting membrane potential. As the membrane potential is hyperpolarized from 20 to 100 mV from the resting potential, the channels showed approximately a fivefold increase in single-channel conductance and approximately a 2,000-fold increase in channel open probability (P_o) (13). Stimulation of oxyntic cells with cAMP and isobutylmethylxanthine resulted in an expansion of the apical membrane area and a concurrent increase in P_o. Both changes were gradual. Starting approximately 10 min after stimulation, P_o increased progressively for 20 min to a steady-state value up to 30-fold greater than resting levels. In patches with channel activity, stimulation resulted in an increase in open probability of the channels. In other experiments, stimulation resulted in the appearance of ion channels in patches formed on resting cells that had exhibited no channel openings. In oxyntic cells in the isolated intact epithelium, stimulation of acid secretion is accompanied by a hyperpolarization of the apical membrane (14). Such a hyperpolarization would cause both an increase in the conductance of this Cl^- channel and an increase in its open probability. These effects would be consistent with the increase in apical membrane conductance and electrogenic Cl^- secretion that accompanies the stimulation of acid secretion by oxyntic cells (14, 16). These Cl^- channels may be related to the fluid and enzyme secretory functions of these cells (13).

K^+ channels were absent from the apical membrane (13). Thus apical and basolateral membranes of oxyntic cells showed a segregation of ion channels.

Table 1 Properties of oxyntic cell ion channels

Channel	K^+	K^+	Cl^-
Location	Basolateral	Basolateral	Apical
Conductance (pS)	67	33	12[a]
Voltage dependence	Depolarization activated	Voltage independent	Hyperpolarization activated
Selectivity	$P_K/P_{Na} > 10$	$P_K/P_{Na} > 10$	Anion
Ca^{2+} sensitivity	yes	no	—
cAMP sensitivity	no	yes	yes
Reference	45	45	13

[a] Rectifying I/V relationship. The value is for pipette potentials between 20 and 50 mV.

K^+ channels are found only in the basolateral membrane while Cl^- channels are located exclusively in the apical membrane.

Ion Channels in Parietal Cells

Patch-clamp methods have also been applied to freshly dissociated parietal cells from rabbit and dog (28, 30), to cultured explants from fetal rat mucosa (10, 44), and to rabbit parietal cells in culture (42). The following brief account of the conflicting results is based on preliminary reports that have appeared only in abstract form. Basolateral K^+ channels have been identified in freshly dissociated parietal cells isolated from the rabbit and dog mucosa (28, 30, 38a). A peculiar observation is that the density of these K^+ channels is extremely low, one channel per fifteen patches with acceptable seal resistance, which suggests that the cells have a very low resting conductance (28). This low rate may be related to the finding that membrane potentials of parietal cells in isolated gastric glands is very low, from -9 to -26 mV (25, 40; J. R. Demarest, unpublished observations). Sakai et al (38a) have reported the rare occurence of a 230 pS inward rectifying K^+ channel and a 22 pS nonselective cation channel in cell attached patches of the basolateral membrane of isolated rabbit parietal cells. Both channels were observed in only one percent of the patches. In cultured explants from rat fetal stomach, nonselective channels with conductances of 21 pS have been described (10), and K^+ and Cl^- channels activated by intracellular Ca^{2+} have also been described (44). Parietal cells in these cultured explants respond to stimulation with carbachol with a decrease in input resistance as measured with microelectrodes and a hyperpolarization of their membrane potential (34).

In cultured rabbit parietal cells, a K^+ channel with a conductance of 65 pS that is sensitive to voltage, intracellular Ca^{2+} level, and pH has been described (42). Although these channels were attributed to the secretory membrane, the membrane location of the channels described remains in doubt because of the uncertainly of the origin of the membrane being studied (see the section on polarity of gastric secretory cells).

ION TRANSPORT PATHWAYS IN GASTRIC AND OTHER SECRETORY EPITHELIA

Active electrogenic Cl^- transport appears to follow similar patterns in a variety of epithelia (22, 37). Chloride is accumulated within the cell above its equilibrium distribution across the basolateral membrane by a secondarily active sodium-dependent process, such as Na/K/2Cl cotransport or linked Na/H and Cl/HCO_3 exchange. This latter mode of basolateral chloride entry has been demonstrated in parietal cells (35). In these cells the basolateral Cl/HCO_3 exchanger has a important dual role. It provides Cl^- for secretion and eliminates the large quantities of base generated intracellularly by active proton secretion, thus contributing to the regulation of intracellular pH in concert with the basolateral Na/H exchanger (29). It has been assumed that Cl^- leaves the cells passively down its electrochemical gradient through an apical channel. Although this model has been applied generally to exocrine cells (37), little direct evidence for an apical Cl^- channel has been available. Evidence for both K^+ and Cl^- channels in zymogen granule membranes isolated from pancreatic and other acinar cells (11) suggests that stimulation of protein secretion could also result in the insertion of these types of channels in the apical membrane of amphibian oxyntic cells.

K^+ enters the cell on the basolateral Na,K-ATPase and is recycled to the interstitum via basolateral K^+ channels, or in the case of the oxyntic cell, it may leave the cell across the apical membrane by an unidentified mechanism (see below) to be recycled by the apical H,K-ATPase.

The existence of an apical K^+ permeability in oxyntic cells has been most controversial. Studies of isolated membrane vesicles have yielded conflicting results. The earliest studies of vesicles isolated from stimulated rabbit mucosa indicated that K^+ and Cl^- were nonconductively cotransported (47). Later investigations, however, indicated that there was a lone Cl^- conductance (6), or that Cl^- and K^+ conductances were present in parallel (48). Recent studies of the acid transporting compartment in permeabilized gastric glands support the presence of a Cl^- conductance (36). The direct demonstration of a single class of apical Cl^- channel by Demarest et al (13), using patch-clamp techniques, is in agreement with this study. In addition, neither of these studies produced evidence for the presence of an apical K^+ channel. Lack of an apical K^+ conductance is consistent with the repeated reports in the transepithelial literature (see above) that addition of the well-known K^+ channel blocker Ba^{2+} to the mucosal solution has no effect on the transepithelial potential, resistance, and acid secretory rate of isolated amphibian and mammalian gastric mucosa (31, 41). The absence of a K^+ conductance in the apical membrane suggests that K^+ exit occurs via a nonchannel mechanism (13).

The currently accepted model of the transport processes in the apical membrane of the parietal cell, based on vesicle studies, proposes parallel K^+ and Cl^- conductances that are activated upon stimulation. An alternative model based on electrophysiologic studies, shown in Figure 1, has a Cl^- conductance alone. During stimulation, fusion of tubulovesicles with the apical membrane results in an expansion of the apical membrane area and exposure of the H,K-ATPase to the gland lumen. K^+ is supplied to the luminal surface of the H,K-ATPase by a nonchannel mechanism. Although alternatives to a true exchange mechanism for this ATPase have been proposed (20), the enzyme is generally considered to be an electrically neutral counter-transport mechanism (38). During stimulation, activation of the baso-lateral K^+ conductance and faster turnover of the Na,K-ATPase result in hyperpolarization of the cell, thus providing an increased driving force for Cl^- secretion across the apical membrane. Apical membrane Cl^- conductance is increased because of the insertion or activation of additional Cl^- channels, increased channel open probability, and single-channel conductance. Thus, the overall decrease in the electrical resistance of both the basolateral and apical membranes upon stimulation results from the activation of basolateral K^+ and apical Cl^- channels.

FUTURE DIRECTIONS

We will summarize here only a few broad areas of particular interest that require further study. Although there is a growing literature on the regulation of intracellular pH in parietal cells, there is very little information concerning other intracellular ion concentrations of oxyntic and parietal cells. The technology is developing rapidly in this area, however, and preliminary studies using the Na^+ - sensitive fluorescent indicator, SBFI, promise to help elucidate the role of the Na,K-ATPase in acid secretion (33). Further study is needed on the regulation of ion channels by intracellular mediators as well as by membrane fusion. The technical challenge presented by the mammalian parietal cell will no doubt require that its ion channels be isolated and incorporated into lipid bilayers for sucessful study. Finally, as for an increasing number of membrane transport studies, molecular biological techniques will allow selective modifications of proteins involved in the mechanisms and control of acid secretion.

Acknowledgments

The authors wish to thank Duncan W. Martin and Terry Machen for their helpful comments on the manuscript. This work was supported by grants DK38664 and DK40615 from the National Institutes of Health.

Literature Cited

1. Berglindh, T. 1984. The mammalian gastric parietal cell in vitro. *Annu. Rev. Physiol.* 46:377–92
2. Blum, A. L., Shah, G. T., Wiebelhaus, V. D., Brennan, F. T., Helander, H. F., et al. 1971. Pronase method for isolation of viable cells from Necturus gastric mucosa. *Gastroenterology* 61:189–200
3. Chew, C. S. 1989. Intracellular activation events for parietal cell HCl secretion. In *Handbook of Physiology. Salivary, Gastric, Pancreatic and Hepato-*
biliary Secretion, ed. S. G. Schultz, 3:229–53. Washington D.C: Am. Physiol. Soc.
4. Chew, C. S., Ljungstrom, M., Smolka, A., Brown, M. R. 1989. Primary culture of secretagogue-responsive parietal cells from rabbit gastric mucosa. *Am. J. Physiol.* 256:G254–63
5. Clausen, C., Machen, T. E., Diamond, J. M. 1982. Changes in the cell membranes of the bullfrog gastric mucosa with acid secretion. *Science* 217:448–59

6. Cuppoletti, J., Sachs, G. 1984. Regulation of gastric acid secretion via modulation of a chloride conductance. *J. Biol. Chem.* 259:14952–59

7. Curci, S., Debellis, L., Fromter, E. 1987. Evidence for rheogenic sodium bicarbonate cotransport in the basolateral membrane of oxyntic cells of frog gastric fundus. *Pflügers Archiv.* 408:497–504

8. Davenport, H. W. 1971. *Physiology of the Digestive Tract* 3rd Edition, Chicago: Year Book Medical Pub. pp. 229

9. Davis, C. W., Finn, A. L. 1985. Cell volume regulation in frog urinary bladder. *Fed. Proc.* 44:2520–25

10. Debellis, L., Krasus, P., Christine, C. W., Gitter, A. H., Fromter, E. 1987. Non-selective ion channels in the apical membrane of parietal cells from cultured gastric mucosa. *Pflügers Archiv.* 408:R48 (Abstr.)

11. DeLisle, R. C., Hopfer, U. 1986. Electrolyte permeabilities of pancreatic zymogen granules: implications for pancreatic secretion. *Am J. Physiol.* 250:G489–96

12. Demarest, J. R., Finn, A. L. 1987. Interaction between the basolateral K^+ and apical Na^+ conductances in Necturus urinary bladder. *J. Gen. Physiol.* 89:563–80

13. Demarest, J. R., Loo, D. D. F., Sachs, G. 1989. Activation of apical chloride channels in the gastric oxyntic cell. *Science* 245:402–4

14. Demarest, J. R., Machen, T. E. 1985. Microelectrode measurements from oxyntic cells in intact Necturus gastric mucosa. *Am. J. Physiol.* 249:C535–40

15. Demarest, J. R., Machen, T. E. 1989. Electrophysiology of the gastric mucosa. See Ref. 3, pp. 185–205

16. Demarest, J. R., Scheffey, C., Machen, T. E. 1986. Segregation of gastric Na and Cl transport: a vibrating probe and microelectrode study. *Am. J. Physiol.* 251:C643–48

17. Diamond, J. 1982. Transcellular cross-talk between epithelial cell membranes. *Nature* 300:683–5

18. Forte, J. G., Forte, T. M., Black, J. A., Okamoto, C., Wolosin, J. M. 1981. Ultrastructural changes related to functional activity in gastric oxyntic cells. *Am. J. Physiol.* 241:G349–58

19. Forte, T. M., Machen, T. E., Forte, J. G. 1977. Ultrastructural changes in oxyntic cells associated with secretory function: A membrane recycling hypothesis. *Gastroenterology* 73:941–55

20. Forte, J. G., Machen, T. E., Obrink, K. J. 1980. Mechanisms of gastric H^+ and

Cl^- transport. *Annu. Rev. Physiol.* 42:111–26

21. Forte, J. G., Wolosin, J. M. 1987. HCl secretion by the gastric oxyntic cell. In *Physiology of the Gastrointestinal Tract,* ed L. R. Johnson, pp. 853–63. New York: Raven

22. Frizzell, R. A., Field, M., Schultz, S. G. 1978. Sodium-coupled chloride transport in epithelial tissues. *Am. J. Physiol.* 236:F1–8

23. Harris, J. B., Edelman, I. S. 1964. Chemical concentration gradients and electrical properties of gastric mucosa. *Am. J. Physiol.* 206:769–82

24. Helander, H. F., Durbin, R. P. 1982. Localization of ouabain binding sites in frog gastric mucosa. *Am. J. Physiol.* 243:G297–303

25. Kafoglis, K., Hersey, S. J., White, J. F. 1984. Microelectrode measurements of K^+ and pH in rabbit gastric glands: effect of histamine. *Am. J. Physiol.* 246:G433–44

26. Latorre, R., Miller, C. 1983. Conduction and selectivity in potassium channels. *J. Membr. Biol.* 71:11–30

27. Logsdon, C. D., Machen, T. E. 1982. Ultrastructural changes during stimulation of amphibian oxyntic cells viewed by scanning and transmission electron microscopy. *Anat. Rec.* 202:73–83

28. Loo, D. D. F., Mendlein, J. D., Berglindh, T., Soll, A. H., Sachs, G., Wright, E. M. 1985. Single channel and whole cell currents in unstimulated isolated parietal cells. *Fed. Proc.* 44:643 (Abstr.)

29. Machen, T. E., Paradiso, A. M. 1987. Regulation of intracellular pH in the stomach. *Annu. Rev. Physiol.* 49:19–33

30. Mendlein, J. D., Loo, D. D. F., Berglindh, T., Wright, E. M., Sachs, G. 1985. Patch clamp studies of parietal cells using a rapid method cell isolation. *Gastroenterology* 88:1717 (Abstr.)

31. McLennan, W. L., Machen, T. E., Zeuthen, T. 1980. Ba^{2+} inhibition of electrogenic Cl^- secretion in vitro piglet and bullfrog gastric mucosa. *Am. J. Physiol.* 239:G151–60

32. Muallem, S., Burnham, C., Blissard, D. T., Berglindh, T., Sachs, G. 1985. Electrolyte transport across the basolateral membrane of the parietal cells. *J. Biol. Chem.* 260:6641–49

33. Negulescu, P. A., Minta, A., Tsien, R. Y., Machen, T. E. 1989. Intracellular Na dependence of the parietal cell Na/K ATPase assessed with a fluorescent sodium indicator. *FASEB J.* 3:A564 (Abstr.)

34. Okada, Y., Ueda, S. 1984. Electrical

membrane responses to secretagogues in parietal cells of the rat gastric mucosa in culture. *J. Physiol.* 354:109–19

34a. Paradiso, A., Townsley, M., Wenzl, E., Machen, T. 1989. Regulation of intracellular pH in resting and in stimulated parietal cells. *Am. J. Physiol.* 257:C554–61

35. Paradiso, A. M., Tsien, R. Y., Demarest, J. R., Machen, T. E. 1988. Na/H and Cl/HCO₃ exchange in rabbit oxyntic cells using fluorescence microscopy. *Am. J. Physiol.* 253:C30–36

36. Perez, A., D. Blisard, D., Sachs, G., Hersey, S. J., 1989. Evidence for a chloride conductance in the secretory membrane of the parietal cell. *Am. J. Physiol.* 256:G299–305

37. Petersen, O. H. 1986. Calcium-activated potassium channels and fluid secretion by exocrine glands. *Am. J. Physiol.* 251:G1–13

38. Sachs, G. 1987. The gastric proton pump: the H⁺, K⁺-ATPase. See Ref. 21, pp. 865–81

38a. Sakai, H., Okada, Y., Morii, M., Takeguchi, N. 1989. Anion and cation channels in the basolateral membrane of rabbit parietal cells. *Pflügers Archiv.* 414:185–92

39. Sakmann, B., Neher, E. 1983. *Single Channel Recording,* New York: Plenum pp. 503

40. Schettino, T., M. Kohler, M., Fromter, E. 1985. Membrane potentials of individual cells of isolated gastric glands of rabbit. *Pflügers Arch.* 405:58–65

40a. Schettino, T., Trischitta, F. 1989. Transport properties of the basolateral membrane of the oxyntic cells in the frog fundic gastric mucosa. *Pflügers Archiv.* 414:469–76

41. Schwartz, M., Pacifico, A. D., Mack-

rell, T. N., Jacobson, A., Rehm, W. S. 1968. Effects of barium on the in vitro frog gastric mucosa. *Proc. Soc. Exp. Biol. Med.* 127:223–25

42. Shoemaker, R. L., Veldkamp, P. J., Saccomani, G. 1988. Potassium channels in the apical membrane of isolated parietal cells. *Biophys. J.* 53:525 (Abstr.)

43. Schultz, S. G. 1981. Homocellular regulatory mechanisms in sodium-transporting epithelia: avoidance of extinction by "flush-through". *Am. J. Physiol.* 241:F579–90

44. Ueda, S., Kotera, T., Okada, Y. 1987. Operation of K⁺ and Cl⁻ channels in cultured rat parietal cells upon the stimulation with acid secretagogues. *Comp. Biochem. Physiol.* 90:836 (Abstr.)

45. Ueda, S., Loo, D. D. F., Sachs, G. 1987. Regulation of K channels in the basolateral membrane of Necturus oxyntic cells. *J. Membr. Biol.* 97:31–41

46. Wolosin, J. M., Forte, J. G. 1981. Functional differences between K⁺-ATPase membranes isolated from resting or stimulated rabbit fundic mucosa. *FEBS Lett.* 125:208–12

47. Wolosin, J. M., Forte, J. G. 1983. Kinetic properties of the KCl transport at the secreting apical membrane of the oxyntic cell. *J. Membr. Biol.* 71:195–207

48. Wolosin, J. M., Forte, J. G. 1984. Stimulation of oxyntic cell triggers K⁺ and Cl⁻ conductances in apical (H⁺-K⁺)-ATPase membrane. *Am. J. Physiol.* 246:C537–45

49. Zeiske, W., Machen, T. E., Van Driessche, W. 1983. Cl⁻ - and K⁺ - related fluctuations of ionic current through oxyntic cells in frog gastric mucosa. *Am. J. Physiol.* 245:G797–807

Annu. Rev. Physiol. 1990. 52:321–44

THE MECHANISM AND STRUCTURE OF THE GASTRIC H,K-ATPase[1]

Edd C. Rabon and Michael A. Reuben

Center for Ulcer Research and Education, Veterans Administration Center, Wadsworth Division Los Angeles, California 90073 and the Department of Medicine, University of California at Los Angeles, School of Medicine, Los Angeles, California 90024

KEY WORDS: stomach, proton pump, potassium, conformation, phosphoenzyme

INTRODUCTION

The H,K-ATPase (E.C. 3.6.1.3) is a H transporting ATPase distinct from the mitochondrial F_1F_o and other H-ATPases found in intracellular organelles such as lysosomes and secretory and chromaffin granules. The H,K-ATPase belongs to a family of eukaryotic transport ATPases that includes the Na,K-ATPase and the Ca-ATPase. These transport ATPases use a characteristic acid-stable phosphorylated intermediate in the cycle of substrate catalysis and ion transport. The H,K-ATPase is located on secretory membrane structures within the mammalian gastric parietal cell and produces the H component of HCl secretion within the gastric lumen. Other topics of interest that have been reviewed include the physiologic role of the H,K-ATPase in acid secretion (19, 20, 79, 81), the gastric ATPase as a therapeutic target (83), the localization and function of the H,K-ATPase preparations derived from gastric mucosa (80, 85, 116), the preparation of membrane-bound H,K-ATPases (67), and the catalytic sequence and general transport properties of the H,K-ATPase in membrane vesicles (9, 80, 85, 86, 120).

Recently, attention has focused on emerging relationships between structure and function of the gastric H,K-ATPase. Topics of interest include the electrogenicity of H and K transport, the binding and catalytic selectivity of ion transport sites of the H,K-ATPase, the regulation of the H,K-ATPase by the stimulus-dependent appearance of K and Cl pathways in parallel to the ATPase, and the molecular composition of the functional unit of the H,K-ATPase. A further impetus for exploration of structure-function relationships has been the elucidation of the primary sequence of the rat and hog H,K-ATPases and the discovery of acid-activated or pH gradient-dependent pump inhibitors that may label the luminal or hydrophobic sectors of the membrane embedded pump. This article reviews recent investigations of enzyme function and structure to provide a current picture of ion transport within the H,K-ATPase, mechanisms of regulation of the activity of this enzyme, and the composition and structure of the functional pump complex.

STRUCTURE OF THE H,K-ATPase

Molecular Organization of the Functional H,K-ATPase

The membrane-bound particles of the H,K-ATPase preparation aggregate into coherent arrays in medium containing KC1, vanadate, and DMSO. A two-dimensional crystalline lattice has been reconstructed from the light diffraction pattern (63). The unit crystal, exhibiting P-2 symmetry was resolved to 27 Å. The crystalline unit was composed of two centers of mass with molecular dimensions of 56×110 Å.

Presently, several lines of information suggest that the functional unit of the H,K-ATPase is not a monomer of the catalytic peptide. Using radiation inactivation analysis, studies of the frozen H,K-ATPase have shown that the functional catalytic unit of the H,K-ATPase is an oligomeric structure ranging in size from 200 to 275 kd (66, 77). A larger target size was reported in lyophylized samples, but it is possible that the removal of water from the sample has introduced unaccounted variations into this measurement (89). Rabon et al measured a smaller target size range (92–146 kd) for the destruction of the catalytic protein and the phosphoenzyme that would be limited to a single monomer of the catalytic peptide and possibly a second, significantly smaller peptide (66).

A cross-linking analysis of the $C_{12}E_8$ solubilized H,K-ATPase indicated that protein associations were a prominent feature of active solutions (65). In a $C_{12}E_8$-solubilized preparation exhibiting about twice the activity of membrane-bound controls, approximately 75% of the original protein migrating at $M_r = 94$ kd was rapidly cross-linked by glutaraldehyde. The catalytic monomer was converted into a larger particle of unknown composition migrating at approximately $M_r = 168$ kd. The most likely candidates would be a dimer of similar sized proteins within the $M_r = 94$ kd band or a complex of the $M_r = 94$ kd catalytic protein and a protein within the poorly stained region between $M_r = 60$ and 80 kd.

Recently, a second glycoprotein recognized by wheat germ agglutinin has been identified in H,K-ATPase preparations. Endoglycosidase F treatment of a heavily glycosylated band migrating on SDS gels between $M_r = 60$ and 80 kd produced a core protein of $M_r = 34$ kd (7, 25, 55). Munson et al have obtained evidence that the radioactive Schering derivative mDAZIP labeled a second tryptic fragment in H,K-ATPase preparations that was distinct from the catalytic protein (53). There is no evidence of identity between this peptide and the core protein obtained by Endoglycosidase F treatment, but the identification of a second peptide sequence labeled with a putative probe of the K site and the discovery of a heavily glycosylated region between $M_r = 60$ and 80 kd fuels speculation that the catalytic subunit of the H,K-ATPase may be associated with a glycoprotein. A glycoprotein, putatively associated with the H,K-ATPase, is included in the structure shown in Figure 1.

Primary Sequence of the Catalytic Subunit

The primary amino acid sequence of the H,K-ATPase has recently been deduced from the cDNA sequence of rat and hog (50, 93). A molecular mass of about 114 kd is obtained from each sequence. The predicted sequence

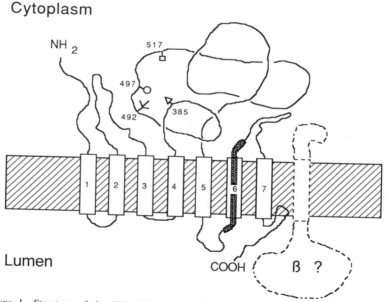

Figure 1 Structure of the HK-ATPase. The H,K-ATPase is modeled with 7 membrane-spanning domains that define 4 luminal and 5 cytoplasmic loops. Several specific labels of the nucleotide binding region and a segment labeled by a K competitive inhibitor are placed within these designated regions. A putative β subunit is included in the molecular organization, although evidence is preliminary. The following symbols represent identified features of these molecules; carbohydrates ⋎ , the phosphorylation site (Asp 385) ⚶ , the pyridoxal phosphate binding site (Lys 497) ♀ , the FITC binding site (Lys 517) ⌇ , the mDAZIP fragment (Leu 854 to Lys 921) ▨ .

homology between these two species is 97%, showing virtual identity. The greatest difference between the two proteins is at the amino terminus, where there are 9 amino acid changes in the first 75 residues, and in the hog sequence, where an alanine residue is inserted at position 4. Comparisons of sequence homology show that the H,K-ATPase is more closely related to the Na,K-ATPases (63% homology) (94) and the Ca-ATPases (24% homology) (49) than the H transporting ATPases of *Neurospora crassa* (14% homology) (1) and yeast (17%) (92). This has led to the suggestion by Jorgensen that the family of phosphoenzyme-forming ATPases is derived from an ancestral ATPase that diverged at an early stage of evolution from the more primative H-ATPases (34).

Amino acid sequence has been obtained from several regions of the H,K-ATPase, some of which are included in Figure 1. The predicted amino acid sequence from hog cDNA matched that of the N-terminal 17 amino acid sequence identified by Lane et al (39). The N termini of even the related ATPases are poorly conserved. An ATP binding region, defined as the phosphorylation site (109), the ATP-protectable fluorescein-5-isothiocyanate (FITC) (16, 33), and pyridoxal phosphate sites (51, 107), include asp 385, lys 517, and lys 496, respectively (rat H,K-ATPase sequence). These amino acid residues comprising the ATP-binding regions of closely related ATPases are highly conserved. Moreover, H4, the most conserved of the hydrophobic domains, has 72% homology with Na,K-ATPase (94) and 52% homology with Ca-ATPase (49). Shull has suggested that H4 may serve to transmit conformational changes between the luminal and cytoplasmic domains (94).

The first sequence labeled by an inhibitor displaying competitive inhibition kinetics with the K site was recently obtained by Munson et al from an enzyme fragment labeled by a radioactive photoaffinity analogue, [^{3}H]-8-[(4-azidophenyl)methoxy]1,2,3-trimethylimidazo[1,2-a] pyridinium iodide (mDAZIP), derived from the Schering 28080 inhibitor (53). The Schering derivative labeled a 44 amino acid sequence beginning at leu 854 and terminating at arg 897. This amino acid sequence is partially conserved with the Na,K-ATPase, although the inhibitor blocks K transport by the H,K-ATPase (111) with much greater affinity than the Na,K-ATPase (S. J. D. Karlish, personal communication).

The H,K-ATPase exhibits three potential glycosylation sites at asn 224, asn 492, and asn 729. These sites are conserved within the Na,K-ATPases, although the latter enzyme has two additional potential sites (94). In both rat and hog H,K-ATPase preparations, tryptic fragments labeled by both con A and FITC have been obtained (24, 103). In the hog preparations, the sequence obtained from the N terminal and CnBr cleavage fragments suggested the N-linked glycosylation of asn 492 (493 in hog) (24, 25).

Secondary Structure

Despite many regions of poor amino acid identity between the ATPases, they retain a striking similarity of secondary structure that is most easily visualized by their hydropathy plots. The model of Figure 1 contains seven membrane-spanning domains, though up to nine potential transmembrane domains have been deduced from hydropathy plots of amino acid sequence and comparisons to the previously cloned Na,K-ATPases and Ca-ATPases (49, 94). The four major hydrophobic domains (H1–H4) in the N-terminal region match those of the Na,K-ATPase, Ca-ATPase, and H-ATPase (92). The C-terminal organ-ization is less certain, thus assignment of hydrophobic, luminal, and cytoplasmic domains is more speculative. Within this region, H5 is suf-ficiently long to cross the membrane twice. The degree of hydropathy of H6 falls short of the criteria outlined by Kyte & Doolittle, although the analogous H6 region in the Na,K-ATPases and Ca-ATPases is more strongly hydrophobic and is thought to be transmembrane. Two or three segments form predicted transmembrane domains in the final portion of the C terminal (50, 93).

Assignment of the cytoplasmic loop containing the ATP-binding region can be made with some certainty because each of the amino acids within the nucleotide site must be oriented toward the cytoplasmic face. These amino acids are contained within the cytoplasmic loop C3 that connects the hydrophobic segments, H4/H5.

Luminal assignment of the N-linked carbohydrate at asn 492 would in-troduce two unsuspected hydrophobic segments between the hydrophobic segments H4/H5 (24). This assignment could be controversial because partial identification of the ATP binding region with FITC and pyridoxal phosphate labeling at lys 497 and lys 517 would not appear to leave sufficient room for a membrane-spanning segment. Alternatively, the faint intensity of the Con A label of this protein may indicate that a restricted population of molecules is glycosylated (25).

Assignment of a peptide region involved in cation binding is tentative since the region is identified exclusively by inhibitor binding. Because of inhibition by SCH 28080, (see inhibitors below), it is likely that the derivatized se-quence would be luminally or hydrophobically placed. The labeled tryptic fragment that begins at leu 854 is modeled as part of the third luminal loop, L3, defined by hydrophobic segments H5/H6; the sequence extends through H6 and into the fourth cytoplasmic domain.

The assignment of additional hydrophobic segments as well as the place-ment of the C-terminal position is controversial. The Kyte-Doolittle plots predict four C-terminal hydrophobic segments ending in a cytoplasmically placed C terminal (93). Immunological studies of the Na,K-ATPase suggest that an epitope near the C-terminal portion of this enzyme is luminal (56, 57).

There is also a putative phorphorylation site for a cAMP-dependent protein kinase at amino acid residues 949–953 (93). As a functional regulatory site, it would be located on the cytoplasmic face of the membrane. This placement would eliminate a hydrophobic segment suggested by Kyte-Doolittle plots but would preserve the C-terminal position so that the molecule could end in a luminal domain in agreement with Ovchinnikov's antibody data for the Na,K-ATPase (57).

Conformational Structure

Conformational transitions within the nucleotide domain have been identified by ligand-induced fluorescence responses of FITC and eosin (26, 33). Jackson et al has shown that the H,K-ATPase, but not its associated pNPPase activity, was inhibited by FITC binding. The low fluorescence state, produced by saturation of a K site or vanadate binding in the presence of Mg, was defined as the E_2 conformational state (33). Recently, it was demonstrated that the K-induced fluorescence quench was reversed by Na binding and that a similar high fluorescence state was induced by Na addition to the K-free enzyme (64). The low and high fluorescence states provided a tool to investigate the E_2 and E_1 conformational species, respectively. Analysis of the conformational equilibrium using the Na- and K-dependent fluorescence species suggests that about 70% of the unliganded H,K-ATPase resides in the E_1 conformation. The proton concentration was a weak promoter of the conformational equilibrium and decreased the affinity of cation binding at more acidic pH. The Na-dependent induction of the high fluorescence species exhibited a K_m of approximately 48 mM at pH 6.4 and 10 mM at pH 8.0.

Eosin fluorescence provided a fluorescent marker for the high affinity ATP site, competing with ATP in the ATPase reaction with a $K_i = 1.2$ μM (26). A fluorescence quench was produced by saturation of a K site or displacement of noncovalently bound eosin by ATP. At acidic pH, the enzyme exhibited a high affinity ATP site and a low affinity K site characteristic of the E_1 conformation, whereas at alkaline pH the enzyme displayed a lower affinity ATP site and a higher affinity K site characteristic of the E_2 conformation (E. C. Rabon, unpublished data). These results were consistent with information from FITC fluorescence, which showed that the biochemical specificity of ligand binding was related to its effect on the conformational equilibrium.

Limited trypsin digestion has provided direct information on conformational structures of the E_1E_2 enzyme family because the site of primary cleavage is conformationally dependent (34, 35). Distinct fragmentation patterns have been obtained from the H,K-ATPase with limited trypsin digestion in either ATP or KCl (29). Peptide fragments of $M_r = 42$ and 56 kd were produced by proteolytic digestion in the K-dependent E_2 conformation, while fragments of $M_r = 35$ and 67 kd were produced by digestion in the ATP-dependent E_1 conformation. The phosphorylated residue asp 386 was obtained on the 42 kd fragment of the E_2 conformation and the 67 kd fragment of the E_1 conformation. The characterization of the two conformationally dependent tryptic patterns does not eliminate the possibility of other ligand-induced conformations. A less characterized pattern, unlike K or ATP, was obtained with proteolysis in 30 mM Mg. The specific cleavage points in the H,K-ATPase are not known but Jorgensen suggests that homologies with the Na,K-ATPase can provide probable assignments (34). Additional studies are needed to determine the effects of specific bond cleavage on the conformational equilibrium and on the conformationally dependent transport and catalytic reactions.

It is clear that conformational changes are an integral part of the catalytic cycle and that numerous amino acid residues are involved in these transitions. It is not certain that these changes require gross structural changes in alpha helical or beta sheet content. Mitchell et al using fourier transform infrared spectroscopic studies probed K-induced changes in secondary structure and concluded that a lack of effect on the amide I band precluded a gross change in the protein secondary structure (52). In their view, conformational changes were restricted to local changes not detectable by this method. These observations are in contrast to those presented by Sachs et al, whose measurements of circular dichroism indicated that the alpha helical structure of the H,K-ATPase was increased by addition of ATP to enzyme solutions containing Mg and K (76, 82).

CATALYTIC AND TRANSPORT FUNCTION

Summary of the Basic Reaction Scheme

The H,K-ATPase catalyzes an equal exchange of H for K (21, 41, 79) that is coupled to the formation and hydrolysis of a covalently linked β-aspartyl phosphate intermediate (70, 78, 102). Several variations of a basic scheme have been proposed to account for the coupling of this intermediate to ion transport and ATP hydrolysis (6, 80, 81, 86).

The scheme presented in Figure 2 is intended to provide a useful framework for understanding the various reactions of this enzyme, but it should only be considered a working model destined for further refinement. The basic tenet of this scheme is that the sidedness of ion binding is dependent upon an equilibrium between two basic conformations, designated E_1 and E_2. The E_1 conformation exposes ion binding sites at the cytoplasmic enzyme face, while the E_2 conformation exposes ion binding sites at the extracellular enzyme face. The cycle is simplified by combining the H/cation displacement steps at each enzyme face and by omitting the formalization of a K/K exchange occurring in the absence of MgATP. The transport cycle accounts for the binding of 2 H molecules at the cytoplasmic face of the H,K-ATPase, their transport to the luminal enzyme face, and their equivalent exchange for 2 K molecules in the opposite direction.

In this scheme, substrate catalysis and transport kinetics reflect a conformational equilibrium influenced by various ligands. K binding to the enzyme promotes the E_2 enzyme conformation (26, 29, 33) characterized by luminal-facing ion sites and a low ATP affinity. An occluded K intermediate, thought to occur during K transport through the membrane, is included in the scheme of Figure 2 even though its isolation has been problematic. ATP saturation of a low affinity nucleotide site (115) promotes a conformational change of the E_2K enzyme to the E_1K form. The E_1 conformation presents cytoplasmic-facing ion sites and exhibits a high affinity ATP site. 2H ions displace 2K ions in this conformation (68, 96). MgATP phosphorylates the E_1H enzyme, which is thought to change sequentially from a high energy, ADP-sensitive E_1H phosphoenzyme intermediate to a low energy, K-sensitive E_2H phosphoenzyme intermediate (27, 62). Events that may occur with the conformational change include the transport of 2H and their release at the luminal enzyme face. The displacement of 2H ions at the luminal face and the subsequent binding of 2K then catalyzes the rapid dephosphorylation of the E_2 phosphoenzyme to complete the transport cycle.

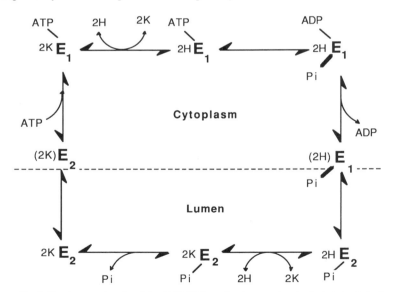

Figure 2   Active transport cycle of the H,K-ATPase. Ion transport and substrate hydrolysis are coupled to the cyclical conversion of two basic enzyme-conformations, E_1 and E_2. The model provides that a high energy β-aspartyl phosphate bond is utilized in the conversion of a high affinity, cytoplasmically placed H binding site to a low affinity luminally placed H binding site. The rationale for components of this scheme is presented in the text.

Distinct enzyme conformations within the transport cycle were deduced from several types of experiments, including the kinetics of phosphoenzyme formation and degradation (6, 102, 114, 115), the sidedness of the K and H requirements for H transport and ATP hydrolysis (79, 86), proteolytic fragmentation patterns obtained with limited trypsin digestion (29), and analysis of conformational probes at or near the nucleotide site (26, 33). Although the evidence suggests that the transport cycle involves at least two basic enzyme conformations, it does not exclude a greater diversity of conformational forms. The influence of Mg on tryptic fragmentation patterns and the kinetics of the ADP-sensitive phosphoenzyme and ATP/ADP exchange suggest that Mg may promote a third conformation, although at present this conformation is not well characterized (27, 29, 62). Several features of this scheme, including the H/ATP stoichiometry under physiologic conditions, the nature of the substrate binding site(s), and the electrogenicity of the individual H and K transport steps, are controversial and are considered in greater detail.

Partial Reactions of the Phosphoenzyme Intermediate

The general properties of H,K-ATPase-mediated substrate catalysis and ion transport have been reviewed, so this subject is not presented in detail (80, 86). More recently, several investigations of enzyme functions have provided some mechanistic insights and are discussed below.

SUBSTRATE HYDROLYSIS   A prominent feature of ATP-dependent hydrolysis and phosphoenzyme formation is the non-hyperbolic ATP dependence (73, 115). The explanation for these kinetics is controversial. Reenstra et al (73) proposed that ATP binds to an active site on a phosphoenzyme form to increase the rate of a putative limiting step, i.e. the conversion of an additional phosphoenzyme form. This formulation was developed to account for the researchers' measurements of the ATP dependence of ATP hydrolysis and steady-state phosphoenzyme and the inhibitory effects of inorganic phosphate. The authors argue that a ternary complex of ATP-Enz-Pi would account for their measurements of partial ATPase inhibition at low ATP concentrations and noncompetitive inhibition at high ATP concentrations. The slow phase of biphasic K-dependent dephosphorylation kinetics, originally demonstrated by Wallmark & Mardh (114), would result from a rapid reequilibration of the two phosphoenzyme forms followed by a slower rate of inorganic phosphate loss from the ternary phosphoenzyme complex. The binding of ATP to the phosphoenzyme might explain the demonstration of Helmich-de Jong et al (28) that ATP saturation of a low affinity site inhibits dephosphorylation of the phosphoenzyme and may account for reported differences in stoichiometry between ATP analogues or inhibitors and the phosphoenzyme. The molar ratio of the transition state inhibitor, vanadate, to phosphoenzyme in the H,K-ATPase, unlike the Na,K-ATPase, is reportedly 2

(13, 15). Similar ratios have been reported for the ATP analogues (2'(3')trinitrophenyladenosine-5-triphosphate-ATP (TNP-ATP) (87) and adenylyl imido diphosphate (AMPPNP) (108). An alternative explanation presented for the non-hyperbolic ATP dependence of substrate hydrolysis is that the affinity of the ATP site in the E_1 and E_2 enzyme conformations differ (6, 43). The consequence of this model is that the affinity of ATP to the E_1 conformation is 1000 times greater than the affinity of ATP to E_2 conformation, that the slow phase of biphasic K-dependent dephosphorylation kinetics is unlikely to be associated with the normal catalytic cycle, and there is a near equivalence of several rate constants within the reaction scheme, each of which can become rate-limiting under appropriate conditions.

THE ADP-SENSITIVE PHOSPHOENZYME   Several partial reactions are described within the overall transport cycle. One of these reactions, the ATP/ADP substrate exchange, is obtained by the synthesis of ATP from ADP (62). This exchange, catalyzed by nucleotide binding at a low affinity site, is regulated in a complex manner by K, Mg, and pH and was the first indirect evidence of an ADP-sensitive phosphoenzyme intermediate. The high energy, ADP-sensitive phosphoenzyme was demonstrated directly in enzyme preparations modified by 5,5'-dithiobis(2) dinitrobenzoic acid (DTNB) in low Mg medium (62). Recently, the ADP-sensitive phosphoenzyme has been demonstrated in an unmodified enzyme in medium containing low Mg (27).

THE LOW ENERGY PHOSPHOENZYME   The presence of a low energy phosphoenzyme intermediate has been inferred from studies of the catalysis of ^{18}O exchange occurring between inorganic phosphate and H_2O (14). The rate of exchange was faster than overall ATPase activity and sensitive to vanadate. Vanadate inhibition of exchange was compatible with competitive binding between vanadate and inorganic phosphate. The ^{18}O exchange was stimulated by K to approximately the rate of K-dependent dephosphorylation, although the K-stimulated exchange did not alter the kinetic pattern of ^{18}O distribution. Faller has suggested that this isotope exchange, in the presence and absence of K, occurs within the same enzyme form and that K acts to increase the amount of this conformer (15).

Current Concepts

H/ATP STOICHIOMETRY   The stoichiometry of H transport determines the maximal electrochemical gradient that can be formed by an ion-translocating ATPase. The gastric H,K-ATPase produces a pH gradient for gastric HCl secretion of about 6 pH units. Since H transport utilizes the free energy of hydrolysis available in ATP, physiologically attained pH gradients are expected from a pump stoichiometry of one H molecule transported per ATP molecule hydrolyzed.

Several investigators have compared the stoichiometry of H transport to that of K-stimulated ATP hydrolysis in gastric vesicle preparations obtained from dog and hog stomach. The stoichiometric ratios reported are considerably closer to 2 than to 1 (68, 96–98). Some reports of a H/ATP stoichiometry approaching 1 have utilized total ATP hydrolysis rather than the K-stimulated component (74, 98). These measurements do not account for a contaminating Mg-ATPase or K-stimulated ATPase occurring in broken vesicles. If, as the authors believe, these components are not negligible, this would lead to an underestimation of the vesicular H/ATP stoichiometry.

A H/ATP stoichiometry of 2, while compatible with the limited pH gradient obtained in gastric vesicles (60), would not be obtained in vivo with pH gradients of 6 pH units. Possibly, the H,K-ATPase stoichiometry is not a fixed molecular stoichiometry. Until recently, the stoichiometry of the phosphoenzyme-forming pumps was considered to be fixed at 2 Ca per ATP and 3Na/2K per ATP hydrolyzed for the Ca-ATPase and the Na,K-ATPase, respectively. This view of a constant stoichiometry has recently been challenged by Goldshlegger et al who observed that at low Na concentrations the Na,K-ATPase functioned in an apparently electroneutral manner (22). Their suggestion that the Na pump transports less than three Na ions under some circumstances introduces a possible mechanism for achieving variable coupling ratios. Experiments are needed to determine if this phenomena is a general principle applicable to the H,K-ATPase.

Na/K SELECTIVITY   Kinetic effects of Na on the H,K-ATPase have been observed in the catalytic reactions involving the phosphoenzyme, paranitrophenyl phosphate (pNPP) and ATP hydrolysis (44, 71, 114, 115). Na inhibition of the H,K-ATPase has been reported at alkaline pH. This inhibition is thought to result from the competition between Na and H at the E_1 enzyme face because of the alkaline pH dependence of the enzyme (44, 72) and because it has been shown that it is the formation of the phosphoenzyme, and not its dephosphorylation, that is affected by Na at this concentration (44, 114).

Evidence suggests that Na transport occurs passively from either face of the H,K-ATPase. Na binding and transport from the E_2 to the E_1 enzyme face was demonstrated with the measurement of $^{86}Rb_{in}/Na_{out}$ exchange in NaCl-loaded proteoliposomes containing the reconstituted H,K-ATPase (61). ATP-dependent H transport, requiring internal K, was obtained after dilution of the NaCl-loaded proteoliposomes into KCl, but not NaCl, medium. This suggests that luminal K was obtained through the K/Na exchange mechanism prior to the addition of MgATP.

Na binding and transport from the E_1 to E_2 enzyme face was demonstrated in $^{86}RbCl$-loaded gastric vesicles by the fivefold stimulation of ^{86}Rb efflux with cytoplasmic Na (88). Cytoplasmic Na has been shown to inhibit H transport in KCl loaded gastric microsomes (44, 102). This inhibition could result from KCl depletion of essential intravesicular K by the Na_{in}/K_{out} exchange prior to the addition of MgATP or from a Na-dependent shift in the conformational equilibrium towards the E_1 conformation (see Na effects on conformational equilibrium below).

The active transport of Na from either enzyme face has also been shown. Polvani et al recently demonstrated a slow, ATP-dependent Na uptake from the E_1 enzyme face of gastric vesicles at alkaline pH (58, 59). Active Na transport from the E_2 face must be inferred from indirect observations. A slow, MgATP-dependent H transport has been demonstrated in gastric vesicles containing 500 mM NaCl after dilution into Na-free transport medium (10).

These types of experiments suggest that under limited circumstances Na can be transported actively or passively from either the E_1 or the E_2 face of the H,K-ATPase. Na binding appears to compete with H at the E_1 face, which suggests competition between Na and H at a common site on the cytoplasmic face of the membrane, and with K at the E_2 face. The action of Na in the catalytic and transport cycles is complex and may result from both ion binding and biochemical selectivity. Possibly, the selectivity is based on size. Na, with only one water at hydration, is a poor surrogate in comparison to K and Rb, larger ions containing a second water molecule. Further work is needed to define the relationship between the selectivity of cation binding and the biochemical specificity resulting from that binding.

THE ELECTROGENICITY OF ION TRANSPORT   A characteristic property of ion pumps is the electrogenicity of ion translocation. The H,K-ATPase functions as an effectively electroneutral pump with H transport inward equal to K transport outward. For a review of the transport characteristics leading to this conclusion see references (9, 86). Recently, however, evidence indicates that ATP-dependent activation of the proton pump incorporated into membrane bilayers produces a transient capacitive current (17). This observation and recent reports that the rates of active H transport and ATPase activity are potential-sensitive (17, 47) suggests that specific reaction steps involving either H or K transport carry charge and that in the H,K-ATPase both arms may carry an equal and opposite charge.

The initial evidence that functional electroneutrality may result from the separate contributions of two electrogenic processes was presented by Fendler & Bamberg's demonstration that the release of ATP from an inactive, photolabile derivative produced a transient capacitive current in black lipid membranes reconstituted with the H,K-ATPase (17). This transient current was eliminated by K addition to the medium before release of the caged ATP. The ATP-dependent transient current and its inhibition by K suggests that K induced the E_2K conformation or that both H and K transport are charge carrying steps that balance each other in the active transport cycle.

Lorentzon et al demonstrated that ATPase activity was sensitive to membrane potentials produced in gastric vesicles (47, 48). The authors compared K-stimulated ATPase activity in intact vesicles as a function of increasing medium KCl. Maximal K-stimulated ATPase activity, obtained in the presence of the K/H exchange ionophore nigericin, was progressively inhibited at KCl concentrations above 10 mM KCl. The saturation of the inhibitory K site was decreased by an inward positive potential produced by addition of the electrogenic K ionophore valinomycin. They suggested that the experiment reversed the E_2K to E_1 transition, a potential-sensitive, rate limiting step produced by saturation of the low affinity cytoplasmic K site.

Implicit within these experiments is the belief that effects of voltage would only be observed if the rate constant was limiting or the ion-binding site not saturated under the experimental conditions. Recent theoretical analysis points out that charge movements include not only the transported ion but also groups on the protein to which the ions bind, as well as charge movements or dipole displacements on the protein that are not directly related to transport. (40, 75). Future experiments with the H,K-ATPase must explore potential effects on ion-binding constants as well as conformational parameters to obtain a more detailed characterization of charge effects related to the catalytic and transport cycle.

Solubilization and Reconstitution of the H,K-ATPase

Several detergents including cholate, n-octylglucoside, emulgen, and $C_{12}E_8$ have been used to solubilize the H,K-ATPase. Soumarmon et al first reported the disassociation of the H,K-ATPase into large, partially active molecular aggregates by a mild extraction with n-octyglucoside (100). Determination of particle mass by sedimentation through a glycerol gradient suggested that the solubilized enzyme was distributed into several aggregates ranging in size from 220 to 440 kd (101). Depolymerization of these particles with stronger treatment of n-oxtylglucoside or cholate inactivated the enzyme. The inactivation at high n-octylglucoside concentrations was prevented by protection of the enzyme with Mg,ATP, and acidic pH (61). Takaya et al solubilized the unprotected H,K-ATPase with emulgen and purified the soluble protein by polyethylene glycol fractionation and sepharose chromatography steps (104). The protein was purified to a single band on SDS gels but was apparently inactivated during purification. The instability of the soluble protein limited conclusions as to the final purity of the catalytic subunit and precluded experiments addressing the state of association of the molecular species within the functional ATPase complex. Recently, a fully competent soluble preparation was obtained with the nonionic detergent, $C_{12}E_8$. The catalytic properties and inhibitor sensitivities of this preparation appear almost identical to the native enzyme; thus it is a promising candidate for studies including final purification of the catalytic subunit and the identification of molecular associations of the active enzyme.

Some information about enzyme mechanism has been obtained from reconstituted proteoliposomes containing the H,K-ATPase. Ion transport has been reconstituted into proteoliposomes using either cholate or n-octyglucoside solubilized preparations (61, 95, 97). The enzyme was incorporated into proteoliposomes oriented with the cytoplasmic face (70%) outward in contrast to 90% in native gastric vesicles (61). Both active H/K transport and passive K/K exchange activities appeared similar to those occurring in the native vesicles. Because of the extended initial rates of transport observed in reconstituted proteoliposomes, it was demonstrated that the rates of active Rb efflux and passive Rb/Rb exchange were similar (61). This suggested that K occlusion within the H,K-ATPase, unlike the Na,K-ATPase, was not a prominent feature limiting K transport in the absence of ATP. Skrabanja et al have suggested that a passive H/K operates via the H,K-ATPase at about 5% of the rate of active transport. The authors claim that a K gradient-dependent, vanadate-sensitive H movement can be generated in proteoliposomes containing the H,K-ATPase (95). The authors have also identified an amiloride-sensitive Na/H transporter in this preparation; thus a more detailed analysis of the properties of the passive transporters is needed. The H/ATP stoichiometry of proteoliposomes containing the H,K-ATPase has been determined and, like native gastric vesicles, was two (97). Finally, some purification of the H,K-ATPase was also obtained by sedimentation of proteoliposomes through glycerol gradients. The peak specific ATPase activity was enriched about twofold above that found in native vesicle preparations; by SDS PAGE it was singularly enriched in the 94 kd band containing the catalytic subunit (61). The activity peak was not homogeneous, however, and several peptides including a poorly stained region migrating at approximately 68 kd were also present.

Regulation of the H,K-ATPase

The obligatory coupling of H for K constrains models of physiologic H,K-ATPase activity to include K and Cl pathways to provide luminal K. This pathway is missing from vesicles derived from hog because the H,K-ATPase is fully competent, but it is largely inactive without lengthy preequilibration in K-containing medium (21, 84). Several lines of evidence suggest that the membrane environment of the H,K-ATPase changes with the onset of acid secretion and that as a consequence K and Cl pathways support H,K-ATPase-mediated H transport. Some aspects of the secretory cycle of the parietal cell, including its morphological transformation and the characterization of ion pathways present in heterogeneous vesicle preparations derived from secreting tissue, have been reviewed (20, 116). The exact nature of these ancillary ion pathways and whether or not they are proteins distinct from the H,K-ATPase is not known. This section will summarize the evidence, largely derived from transport studies, of this controversial topic.

Wolosin & Forte first demonstrated that membrane fractions derived from stimulated or resting rabbit gastric mucosa show significant differences in H transport function (117, 118). The H,K-ATPase-dependent H pump, in a heterogeneous class of dense vesicles derived from the stimulated stomach, functioned independently of lengthy equilibration of KCl-containing medium. The mechanism for KCl movement was first attributed to a KCl cotransporter from observations that H transport in these vesicles was insensitive to the protonophore carbonylcyanide-m-chlorophenyl hydrazone (CCCP) and that the rate of H transport was a saturable function of medium K and Cl (18, 119, 120). More recently, the authors have found that the protonophore, tetrachlorosalicylanilide (TCS), rapidly dissipated the H pump-generated pH gradients in Cl-free, K medium and inhibited dissipation of the pH gradient in K-free, Cl medium (121). Because both K and Cl effects were absent in H,K-ATPase preparations of gastric microsomes, the authors suggested that the dissipation resulted from separate K and Cl conductances introduced into the H,K-ATPase environment with the onset of acid secretion (121, 122).

Gunther et al compared Rb transport pathways in the dense vesicle fraction derived from the stimulated stomach and gastric microsomes. They attributed cation transport in gastric microsomes exclusively to the vanadate-sensitive cation exchange mechanism of the H,K-ATPase. In contrast, cation transport in the dense vesicles was attributed to two distinct mechanisms, one the vanadate-sensitive exchange of the H,K-ATPase and the other a potential-sensitive K conductance (23).

The conclusion that both K and Cl conductance pathways are absent in gastric microsomes or that these pathways are an intrinsic property of the H,K-ATPase is controversial. Cuppoletti & co-workers used the cationic potential probe, 3,3'-dipropylthiadicarbocyanine iodide [diSC$_3$(5)] to obtain measurements of K and Cl conductances in gastric vesicles. They reported a furosemide-sensitive Cl conductance in vesicles derived from stimulated stomach, but in contrast to Gunther et al, they reported measurements of a vanadate-sensitive, K-dependent potential in preparations from both stimulated and resting rabbit membrane fractions (8). They suggested that the vanadate-sensitive K exchanger observed in hog microsomal vesicles may resemble the K conductance observed in their experiments with rabbit vesicles. These diverse conclusions are difficult to reconcile, and it may be that these studies reflect preparational differences of isolated ion transport systems. The conclusions derived by Wolosin were based on the H leak characteristics of pH gradients generated by the H,K-ATPase and may be particularly relevant (121, 122).

Takeguchi et al have shown that the treatment of gastric vesicles with the S-S cross-linking reagent Cu^{2+}-o-phenanthroline can increase net KCl permeability and that these changes are influenced by pretreatment with SH reagents (3, 105, 106). Their measurements of light scatter (presumably a measure of net KCl influx) indicated that KCl entry was increased by pretreatment of hog gastric microsomes with Cu^{2+}-o-phenanthroline (105). The authors suggested that the increased flux involved S-S modification of the H,K-ATPase, since protection was afforded by ATP, the H,K-ATPase inhibitor SCH 28080, and an inhibitory IgG monoclonal antibody raised to the H,K-ATPase (3, 105). The increased KCl flux was attributed to a specific modification affecting Cl permeability because Cl efflux (exchange) rather than Rb efflux (exchange) was increased by cross-linking (106). The authors have claimed that these changes represent the opening or closing within the H,K-ATPase of a native physiologic Cl channel that would function together with an intrinsic K conductance to control the flux of K and Cl across the gastric secretory membrane.

In contrast to the view that the H,K-ATPase provides functional channels for the flux of K and Cl, Im et al have identified a KCl permeable vesicle population from resting rat gastric microsomes that they believe is distinct from the vesicle population containing the H,K-ATPase (30). The authors suggest that during the stimulation of secretion this vesicle class is fused to other vesicles containing the H,K-ATPase and is incorporated into the denser, canalicular membrane. The authors have also presented evidence for an electrogenic ATPase, distinct from the H,K-ATPase, that is present in membrane vesicles thought to contain the K transport pathway (31). The electrogenic ATPase was identified by vanadate and ATP affinities distinct from the H,K-ATPase. RbCl uptake was inhibited by both vanadate and low concentrations of MgATP, but the vanadate inhibition was reversed by the K ionophore valinomycin. Presumably, the electrically mediated valinomycin response provided a Rb uptake pathway, coupled to a H conductance present in the membranes, and failed to restore the MgATP-dependent inhibition because the positive inside potential produced by the electrogenic H pump maintained $Rb_{out} > Rb_{in}$. In their view, the electrogenic H pump might produce an electrochemical gradient functioning to regulate K influx in vesicles containing the H,K-ATPase and the K pathways.

Ray reported that a soluble protein obtained from hog gastric mucosal preparations functioned directly as an activator of the H,K-ATPase (69). This protein is reportedly a 40-kd protein functioning as an 80-kd dimer (4, 5). Titration of the purified activator with the H,K-ATPase displayed a complex behavior with sigmoidal activation at low H,K-ATPase-to-activator ratios and inhibition at higher ratios (4). Reports of the extent of stimulation of the H,K-ATPase and its associated pNPPase activity have been variable, and the activation phenomena does not increase phosphoenzyme levels or appear to significantly affect H transport coupled to ATP hydrolysis (5, 71). The protein is reported to be heat labile and sensitive to endogenous protease inhibition; thus a more detailed characterization of its own phosphatase activity and of the mechanism of its interaction with the H,K-ATPase have not been obtained (5).

Inhibitors of the H,K-ATPase

Many ligands and group-specific reagents have been shown to interact with the H,K-ATPase. The enzyme modification by some of these compounds has been reviewed (9).

The H,K-ATPase is inhibited by vanadate, a potent inhibitor of the phosphoenzyme-forming ATPases (12). Inhibition is characterized by the saturation of high and low affinity sites at the cytosolic enzyme face. At 100% inhibition, 3 nmol of vanadate are reportedly bound per 1.5 nmol of phosphoenzyme. The reason for the discrepancy between the stoichiometry of vanadate binding and phosphoenzyme levels is not understood though Faller et al have suggested that the inhibitor binds competitively with the substrate at two distinct catalytic sites (13, 15).

The substituted benzimidazoles represent a new class of antisecretory compounds that are H,K-ATPase inhibitors. This class of inhibitor is typified by the compound omeprazole {5-methoxy-2-[((4-methoxy-3,5-dimethyl-2-pyridinyl)methyl)sulfinyl]-1H-benzimidazole}. Omeprazole, a weak base (pK $\approx$ 4), undergoes acid catalyzed conversion into an impermeant cation. The active intermediate is labile ($t_{1/2} = 3$ min), and the reversal of its inhibition by mercaptans such as B-mercaptoethanol (45, 110, 112) suggests that SH groups are most likely involved in its reaction with the H,K-ATPase. The chemistry leading to the acid activation of omeprazole has been investigated (2, 32, 42), and its use as an inhibitor of gastric acid secretion and as a selective inhibitor of the gastric H,K-ATPase has been recently reviewed (80, 83). Lorentzon et al proposed that the primary inhibitory complex was a disulfide linkage between the inhibitor and the enzyme (45).

The potency of omerprazole is dependent on the conditions used. Keeling et al showed a pH dependency for inhibition by the compound with an $IC_{50} = 36$ μM at pH 7.4 and an $IC_{50} = 5.2$ μM at pH 6.1 (36). Incorporation of (^{14}C) omeprazole at 100% H,K-ATPase inactivation required 10 to 20 nmol of omeprazole per phosphorylation site (37, 45). Under these relatively nonspecific conditions, omeprazole also inhibited the Na,K-ATPase, albeit with a lower potency ($IC_{50} = 186$ μM at pH 7.4 vs $IC_{50} = 19$ μM at pH 6.1) (36). The specificity of omeprazole for the H,K-ATPase is related to the unique acid environment produced in the lumen of gastric vesicles by the H,K-ATPase. Lorentzon & Wallmark demonstrated that omeprazole was an ineffectual inhibitor of the H,K-ATPase in hog gastric vesicles in the absence of a pH gradient (46). When the H pump was stimulated, however, omeprazole inhibited the H,K-ATPase of the transport-competent vesicles. This inhibition was directly related to incorporation of (^{14}C) omeprazole. At 100% inhibition, 1 to 2 mol of omeprazole were incorporated per mol of phosphoenzyme (37, 46). Omeprazole treatment inactivates the H,K-ATPase and its associated K-phosphatase and phosphoenzyme intermediate (45, 46, 113).

Protonatable amines provide a second class of reversible H,K-ATPase inhibitors. One in particular, {2-methyl-8-[phenyl methoxy] imidazo-(1-2-a) pyrine-3-acetonitrile}, SCH 28080, was shown to have potent antisecretory activity in man (11) and in isolated parietal cell fundic mucosa (91). Scott & Sundell first suggested that the antisecretory activity was due to direct inhibition of the H,K-ATPase (90). This suggestion was confirmed in gastric membrane preparations where the drug was shown to be a competitive inhibitor of the H,K-ATPase with a K_i ranging from 0.024 to 0.12 μM (38, 91, 111). This inhibition was fully reversible and was unaffected by reduction of sulfhydryl groups with DTT or B-mercaptoethanol (91). It is though that SCH 28080 is a luminally acting inhibitor, since as a weak base (pK = 5.5) it would be accumulated into acidic spaces. A less permeable n-methylated derivative was also shown to be a poorer inhibitor of the H,K-ATPase and its associated K phosphatase in intact vesicles compared with lyophilized preparations (38). Wallmark et al have shown that SCH 28080 inhibited passive K/K exchange and produced the low fluorescence state of the FITC-labeled enzyme that was suggestive of the E_2 enzyme form (111). It seems likely that SCH 28080 can react with either the dephosphoenzyme or the phosphoenzyme. The existence of an E-I inhibitor complex was suggested by the inhibition of Rb exchange and MgATP-dependent phosphorylation (111), while the E-P-I complex was inferred from SCH 28080 inhibition of K-stimulated dephosphorylation (38). Recently, a light-sensitive derivative 2,3-dimethyl-8-[(4-azidophenyl)methoxy]imidazo(1,2a) pyridine (DAZIP) has been shown to be a K competitive inhibitor of the H,K-ATPase in the dark. Irradiation of DAZIP produced an irreversible loss of activity, a component of which was protected by K (54). The development of compounds exhibiting light-dependent covalent insertion into the H,K-ATPase may provide powerful probes of the luminal cation sites.

CONCLUSIONS

Since its discovery in 1973, many studies of the H,K-ATPase have focused on refinement of the operations of the catalytic and transport pathways. Much of this information has been incorporated into the reaction scheme of Figure 2. Some fundamental questions remain: Is variable coupling possible in the ion transport process, what are the functional consequences of ion binding and catalytic selectivity, and are individual transport steps are electrogenic? It is likely that the exploration of these phenomena will proceed at both mechanistic and structural levels. An early model of H,K-ATPase structure is provided in Figure 1. Sequence comparisons of related enzymes may provide clues of essential structural features so that improved models of structural features may be obtained. The pharmacology of the ATPase inhibitors, developed because of their physiologic relevance in the treatment of ulcer disease, may provide the specificity needed to obtain the first clues of luminal ion-binding domains. In the near future, the functional consequences of site-directed mutations to single amino acid residues may contribute to unraveling the intricate relationship between structural features and their functional correlates. The refinement of enzyme structure by high resolution crystallographic techniques remains elusive because of the difficulty of crystallizing membrane bound proteins, and even the molecular composition of the fundamental unit of activity is not established. Expression of the active unit from its cDNAs may be the most convincing way of establishing the basic catalytic complex.

ACKNOWLEDGMENTS

We would like to thank S. J. D. Karlish, G. Sachs, K. Hall, and K. B. Munson for their interest and numerous discussions of topics related to this review. This work was supported by National Institutes of Health Grant ROI AM 34286, DK17328 and VAMC Research Funds.

Literature Cited

1. Addison, R. 1986. Primary structure of the Neurospora plasma membrane H-ATPase deduced from the gene sequence. *J. Biol. Chem.* 261:14896–14901
2. Adelstein, G. W., Yen, C. H., Haack, R. A., et al. 1988. Substituted 2 - ((2 - Benzimidazoleylsulfinyl)methyl) anilines as potential inhibitors of H, K-ATPase. *J. Med. Chem.* 31:1215–20
3. Asano, S., Inoie, M., Takeguchi, N. 1987. The Cl channel in hog gastric vesicles is part of the function of the H,K-ATPase. *J. Biol. Chem.* 262: 13263–68
4. Bandopadhyay, S., Das, P. K., Wright, M. V., Nandi, J., Bhattacharyyay, D., Ray, T. K. 1987. Characteristics of a pure endogenous activator of the gastric H,K-ATPase system. Evaluation of the role as a possible intracellular regulator. *J. Biol. Chem.* 262:5664–70
5. Bandopadhyay, S., Ray, T. K. 1986. Purification and characterization of a cytosolic activator protein for the gastric H,K-ATPase system from dog fundic mucosa. *Prep. Biochem.* 16:21–32
6. Brzezinski, P., Malmstrom, B. G., Lorentzon, P., Wallmark, B. 1988. The catalytic mechanism of gastric H/K-ATPase: simulations of pre- steady-state and steady-state kinetic results. *Biochim. Biophys. Acta* 942:215–19
7. Chow, D., Okamoto, C., Forte, J. 1989. Immunological characterization of a 60–80 kDa glycoprotein associated with the gastric microsomal H,K-ATPase. *FASEB J.* 3:A873 (Abstr.)
8. Cuppoletti, J., Sachs, G. 1984. Regula-

tion of gastric acid secretion via modulation of a chloride conductance. *J. Biol. Chem.* 259:14952–59

9. De Pont, J. J. H. H. M., Bonting, S. L. 1981, Anion-sensitive ATPase and K,H-ATPase. In *Membrane Transport,* ed. S. L. Bonting, J. J. H. H. M. De Pont, pp. 209–234. New York/Holland: Elsevier/ North-Holland Biomedical

10. Ditmars, M., Mendlein, J., Sachs, G. 1989. The selectivity of monovalent cations for the H,K-ATPase. *FASEB J.* 3:A873 (Abstr.)

11. Ene, M. D., Daneshmend, K., Roberts, C. J. C. 1982. A study of the inhibitory effects of SCH 28080 on gastric secretion in man. *Br. J. Pharmacol.* 76:389–391

12. Faller, L., Jackson, R., Malinowska, D., Mukidjam, E., Rabon, E., et al. 1982. Mechanistic aspects of gastrict (H + K)-ATPase. *Ann. NY Acad. Sci.* 402:146–63

13. Faller, L., Smolka, A., Sachs, G. 1985. The gastric H,K-ATPase. In *The Enzymes of Biological Membranes, Vol. 3,* ed. A. N. Martonosi, 3:431–48. New York/London: Plenum,

14. Faller, L. D., Elgavish, G. A. 1984. Catalysis of oxygen-18 exchange between inorganic phosphate and water by the gastric H,K-ATPase. *Biochemistry.* 23:6584–90

15. Faller, L. D., Rabon, E., Sachs, G. 1983. Vanadate binding to the gastric H,K-ATPase and inhibition of the enzyme's catalytic and transport activities. *Biochemistry.* 22:4676–85

16. Farley, R. A., Faller, L. D. 1985. The amino acid sequence of an active site peptide from the H,K-ATPase of gastric mucosa. *J. Biol. Chem.* 260:3899–3901

17. Fendler, K., van der Hijden, H., Nagel, G., de Pont, J. J. H. H. M., Bamberg, E. 1988. Pump currents generated by renal Na,K-ATPase and gastric H,K-ATPase on black lipid membranes. *Prog. Clin. Biol. Res.* 268:501–10

18. Forte, J. G., Forte, T. M., Black, J. A., Okamoto, C., Wolosin, J. M. 1983. Correlation of parietal cell structure and function. *J. Clin. Gastroenterol.* 5:17–27

19. Forte, J. G., Lee, H. C. 1977. Gastric adenosine triphosphatases: a review of their possible role in HCl secretion. *Gastroenterology* 73:921–26

20. Forte, J. G., Machen, T. E., Obrink, K. J. 1980. Mechanisms of gastric H and Cl transport. *Annu. Rev. Physiol.* 42:111–26

21. Ganser, A. L., Forte, J. G. 1973. K-stimulted ATPase in purified micro-

somes of bullfrog oxyntic cells. *Biochim. Biophys. Acta* 307:169–180

22. Goldshlegger, R., Shahak, Y., Karlish, S. J. D. 1989. Electrogenic and electroneutral transport modes of renal Na,K-ATPase reconstituted into phospholipid vesicles. *J. Memb. Biol.* In press

23. Gunther, R. D., Bassilian, S., Rabon, E. C. 1987. Cation transport in vesicles from secreting rabbit stomach. *J. Biol. Chem.* 262:13966–72

24. Hall, K., Perez, G., Anderson, D., Sachs, G., Hersey, S., Kaplan, J. 1989. An unsuspected membrane spanning peptide in gastric H,K-ATPase. *FASEB J.* 3:A873 (Abstr.)

25. Hall, K., Perez, G., Gutierrez, C., et al. 1989. Location of the carbohydrates present in the H,K-ATPase vesicles isolated from hog gastric mucosa. *Biochemistry* In press

26. Helmich-de Jong, M. L., van Duynhoven, J. P. M., Schuurmans Stekhoven, F. M. A. H., De Pont, J. J. H. H. M. 1986. Eosin, a fluorescent marker for the high-affinity ATP site of (K + H)-ATPase. *Biochim. Biophys. Acta* 858:254–62

27. Helmich-de Jong, M. L., van Emst-de Vries, S. E., De Pont, J. J. H. H. M., Schuurmans Stekhoven, F. M. A. H., Bonting, S. L. 1985. Direct evidence for an ADP-sensitive phosphointermediate of (K + H)-ATPase. *Biochim. Biophys. Acta* 821:377–83

28. Helmich-de Jong, M. L., van Emst-de Vries, S. E., Swarts, H. G. P., Schuurmans Stekhoven, F. M. A. H., De Pont, J. J. H. H. M. 1986. Presence of a low affinity nucleotide binding site on the K,H-ATPase phosphoenzyme. *Biochim. Biophys. Acta* 860:641–49

29. Helmich-de Jong, M. L., van Emst-de Vries, S. E., and De Pont, J. J. H. H. M. 1987. Conformational states of (K + H)-ATPase studied using tryptic digestion as a tool. *Biochim. Biophys. Acta* 905:358–70

30. Im, W. B., Blakeman, D. P., Davis, J. P. 1985. Studies on K permeability of rat gastric microsomes. *J. Biol. Chem.* 260:9452–60

31. Im, W. B., Blakeman, D. P., Davis, J. P. 1986. Finding of a KCl-independent, electrogenic, and ATP-driven H-pumping activity in rat light gastric membranes and its effect on the membrane K transport activity. *J. Biol. Chem.* 261:11686–92

32. Im, W. B., Sih, J. C., Blakeman, D. P., McGrath, J. P. 1985. Omeprazole, a specific inhibitor of gastric (H-K)-

ATPase, is a H-activated oxidizing agent of sulfhydryl groups. *J. Biol. Chem.* 260:4591–97

33. Jackson, R. J., Mendlein, J., Sachs, G. 1983. Interaction of fluorescein isothiocyanate with the H,K-ATPase. *Biochim. Biophys. Acta* 731:9–15

34. Jorgensen, P. L., Andersen, J. P. 1988. Structural basis for E1–E2 conformational transitions in Na,K-ATPase and Ca-pump proteins. *J. Membr. Biol.* 103:95–120

35. Jorgensen, P. L., Farley, R. A. 1988. Proteolytic cleavage as a tool for studying structure and conformation of pure membrane-bound Na,K-ATPase. *Methods Enzymol.* 156:291–301

36. Keeling, D. J., Fallowfield, C., Milliner, K. J., Tingley, S. K., Ife, R. J., Underwood, A. H. 1985. Studies on the mechanism of action of omeprazole. *Biochem. Pharmacol.* 34:2967–73

37. Keeling, D. J., Fallowfield, C., Underwood, A. H. 1987. The specificity of omeprazole as an (H + K)-ATPase inhibitor depends upon the means of its activation. *Biochem. Pharmacol.* 36:339–44

38. Keeling, D. J., Laing, S. M., Seen-Bilfinger, J. 1988. SCH 28080 is a lumenally acting, K-site inhibitor of the gastric (H + K)-ATPase. *Biochem. Pharmacol.* 37:2231–36

39. Lane, L. K., Kirley, T. L., Ball, W. J. 1986. Structural studies on H,K-ATPase: Determination of the NH_2-terminal amino acid sequence and immunological cross-reactivity with Na,K-ATPase. *Biochem. Biophys. Res. Commun.* 138:185–92

40. Lauger, P., Appell, H. J. 1986. A microscopic model for the current-voltage behavior of the Na,K pump. *Eur. Biophy. J.* 13:309–21

41. Lee, J. G., Simpson, G., Scholes, P. 1974. An ATPase from dog gastric mucosa; changes in outer pH in suspensions of membrane vesicles accompanying ATP hydrolysis. *Biochem. Biophys. Res. Commun.* 60:825–32

42. Lindberg, P., Nordberg, P., Alminger, T., Brandstrom, A. 1986. The mechanism of action of the gastric acid secretion inhibitor omeprazole. *J. Med. Chem.* 29:1327–29

43. Ljungstrom, M., Mardh, S. 1985. Kinetics of the acid pump in the stomach. Proton transport and hydrolysis of ATP and p-nitrophenyl phosphate by the gastric H,K-ATPase. *J. Biol. Chem.* 260:5440–44

44. Ljungstrom, M., Vega, F. V., Mardh, S. 1984. Effects of pH on the interaction of ligands with the (H + K)-ATPase purified from pig gastric mucosa. *Biochim. Biophys. Acta* 769:220–30

45. Lorentzon, P., Eklundh, B., Brandstrom, A., Wallmark, B. 1985. The mechanism for inhibition of gastric (H + K)-ATPase by omeprazole. *Biochim. Biophys. Acta* 817:25–32

46. Lorentzon, P., Jackson, R., Wallmark, B., Sachs, G. 1987. Inhibition of (H + K)-ATPase by omeprazole in isolated gastric vesicles requires proton transport. *Biochim. Biophys. Acta* 897:41–51

47. Lorentzon, P., Sachs, G., Wallmark, B. 1988. Inhibitory effects of cations on the gastric H,K-ATPase. A potential-sensitive step in the K^+ limb of the pump cycle. *J. Biol. Chem.* 263:10705–10

48. Lorentzon, P., Scott, D., Hersey, S., Wallmark, B., Rabon, E., Sachs, G. 1988. The gastric H,K-ATPase. *Prog. Clin. Biol. Res.* 273:247–54

49. MacLennan, D. H., Brandl, C. J., Korczak, B., Green, N. M. 1985. Amino acid sequence of a Ca-Mg-dependent ATPase from rabbit muscle sarcoplasmic reticulum, deduced from its complementary DNA sequence. *Nature* 316:696–700

50. Maeda, M., Ishizaki, J., Futai, M. 1988. cDNA cloning and sequence determination of pig gastric H,K-ATPase. *Biochem. Biophys. Res. Commun.* 157:203–9

51. Maeda, M., Tagaya, M., Futai, M. 1988. Modification of gastric (H + K)-ATPase with pyridoxal 5'-phosphate. *J. Biol. Chem.* 263:3652–56

52. Mitchell, R. C., Haris, P. I., Fallowfield, C., Keeling, D. J., Chapman, D. 1988. Fourier transform infrared spectroscopic studies on gastric H/K-ATPase. *Biochim. Biophys. Acta* 941:31–38

53. Munson, K. B., Gutierrez, C., Hall, K., Sachs, G. 1989. Labeling of the H,K-ATPase with a K-competitive photoaffinity inhibitor, discovery of a β subunit. *Prot. Soc.* S138 (Abstr.)

54. Munson, K. B., Sachs, G. 1988. Inactivation of H,K-ATPase by a K-competitive photoaffinity inhibitor. *Biochemistry* 27:3932–38

55. Okamoto, C., Reenstra, W. W., Li, W., Forte, J. G. 1989. Partial characterization of a 60–80 kDa glycoprotein associated with the hog gastric microsomal

H,K-ATPase. *J. Cell Biol.* 107(6, Pt.3):125a (Abstr.)

56. Ovchinnikov, Y. A. 1987. Probing the folding of membrane proteins. *Trends Biochem. Sci.* 12:434–38

57. Ovchinnikov, Y. A., Luneva, N. M., Arystarkhova, E. A., Gevondyan, N. M., Arzamazova, N. M., et al. 1988. Topology of Na,K-ATPase. *FEBS. Lett.* 227:230–34

58. Polvani, C., Sachs, G., Blostein, R. 1989. Sodium transport by the gastric H,K-ATPase. *Biochem. J.* 55:337a (Abstr.)

59. Polvani, C., Sachs, G., Blostein, R. 1989. Sodium transport by the gastric H,K-ATPase. *J. Biochem. Chem.* In press

60. Rabon, E., Chang, H., Sachs, G. 1978. Quantitation of hydrogen ion and potential gradients in gastric plasma membrane vesicles. *Biochemistry.* 17:3345–53

61. Rabon, E., Gunther, R. D., Soumarmon, A., Bassilian, S., Lewin, M., Sachs, G. 1985. Solubilization and reconstitution of the gastric H,K-ATPase. *J. Biol. Chem.* 260:10200–7

62. Rabon, E., Sachs, G., Mardh, S., Wallmark, B. 1982. ATP/ADP exchange activity of gastric (H + K)-ATPase. *Biochim. Biophys. Acta* 688:515–24

63. Rabon, E., Wilke, M., Sachs, G., Zampighi, G. 1986. Crystallization of the gastric H,K-ATPase. *J. Biol. Chem.* 261:1434–39

64. Rabon, E. C., Bassilian, S., Faller, L., Sachs, G., Karlish, S. 1989. Conformational transitions of the H,K-ATPase studied with sodium ions as surrogates for protons. In preparation

65. Rabon, E. C., Bassilian, S. 1988. Solubilization of the hog gastric H,K-ATPase. *FASEBJ.* 2:2451 (Abstr.)

66. Rabon, E. C., Gunther, R. D., Bassilian, S., Kempner, E. S. 1988. Radiation inactivation analysis of oligomeric structure of the H,K-ATPase. *J. Biol. Chem.* 263:16189–94

67. Rabon, E. C., Im, W. B., Sachs, G. 1988. Preparation of gastric H,K-ATPase. *Methods Enzymol.* 157:649–54

68. Rabon, E. C., McFall, T. L., Sachs, G. 1982. The gastric (H,K)-ATPase: H/ATP stoichiometry. *J. Biol. Chem.* 257:6296–99

69. Ray, T. K. 1978. Gastric K$^+$-stimulated adenosine-triphosphatase demonstration of an endogenous activator. *FEBS. Lett.* 92:49–52

70. Ray, T. K., Forte, J. G. 1976. Studies on the phosphorylated intermediates of a K-stimulated ATPase from rabbit gastric mucosa. *Biochim Biophys. Acta* 443:451–67

71. Ray, T. K., Nandi, J. 1983. Regulation of the gastric microsomal (H + K)-transporting ATPase system by the endogenous activator. Effect of phospholipase A2 treatment. *Biochem. J.* 212:887–90

72. Ray, T. K., Nandi, J. 1985. Modulation of gastric H,K-transporting ATPase function by sodium. *FEBS. Lett.* 185:24–28

73. Reenstra, W. W., Bettencourt, J. D., Forte, J. G. 1988. Kinetic studies of the gastric H,K-ATPase. *J. Biol. Chem.* 263:19618–25

74. Reenstra, W. W., Forte, J. G. 1981. H/ATP stoichiometry for the gastric (K + H)-ATPase. *J. Membr. Biol.* 61:55–60

75. Reynolds, J. A., Johnson, E. A., Tanford. C. 1985. Incorporation of membrane potential into theoretical analysis of electrogenic ion pumps. *Proc. Natl. Acad. Sci. USA* 82:6869–73

76. Saccomani, G., Chang, H. H., Spisni, A., Helander, H. G., Spitzer, H. F., Sachs, G. 1979. Effect of phospholipase A2 on purified gastric vesicles. *J. Supramol. Struct.* 11:429–44

77. Saccomani, G., Sachs, G., Cuppoletti, J., Jung, C. Y. 1981. Target molecular weight of the gastric (H + K)-ATPase functional and structural molecular size. *J. Biol. Chem.* 256:7727–29

78. Saccomani, G., Shah, G., Spenney, J. G., Sachs, G. 1975. Characterization of gastric mucosal membranes. *J. Biol. Chem.* 250:4802–9

79. Sachs, G. 1977. H transport by a non-electrogenic gastric ATPase as a model for acid secretion. *Rev. Physiol. Biochem. Pharmacol.* 79:133–62

80. Sachs, G. 1987. The gastric proton pump: The H,K-ATPase. In *Physiology of the Gastrointestinal Tract,* ed. L. R. Johnson, pp. 865–81. New York: Raven

81. Sachs, G., Berglindh, T. 1981. Physiology of the parietal cell. See Ref. 80, pp. 567–602

82. Sachs, G., Berglindh, T., Rabon, E., Stewart, H. B., Barcellona, M. L. et al. 1980. Aspects of parietal cell biology: cells and vesicles. *Ann. NY Acad. Sci.* 341:312–34

83. Sachs, G., Carlsson, E., Lindberg, P., Wallmark, B. 1988. Gastric H,K-ATPase as therapeutic target. *Annu. Rev. Pharmacol. Toxicol.* 28:269–84

84. Sachs, G., Chang, H. H., Rabon, E., Schackmann, R., Lewin, M., Saccoma-

ni, G. 1976. A nonelectrogenic H pump in plasma membranes of hog stomach. *J. Biol. Chem.* 251:7690–98

85. Sachs, G., Spenney, J. G., Lewin, M. 1978. H transport: regulation and mechanism in gastric mucosa and membrane vesicles. *Physiol. Rev.* 58:106–73

86. Sachs, G., Wallmark, B., Saccomani, G., Rabon, E., Stewart, B. et al. 1982. The ATP-dependent component of gastric acid secretion. *Curr. Top. Membr. Transp.* 16:135–59

87. Sartor, G., Mukidjam, E., Faller, L., Saccomani, G., Sachs, G. 1982. Nucleotide probes of gastric ATPase. *Biophys. J.* 37:375a (Abstr.)

88. Schackmann, R., Schwartz, A., Saccomani, G., Sachs, G. 1977. Cation transport by gastric H,K-ATPase. *J. Memb. Biol.* 32:361–81

89. Schrijen, J. J., Van Groningen-Luyben, W. A. H. M., Nauta, H ., De Pont, J. J. H. H. M., Bonting, S. L. 1983. Studies on (K + H)-ATPase. VI. Determination on the molecular size by radiation inactivation analysis. *Biochim. Biophys. Acta* 731:329–37

90. Scott, C. K., Sundell, E. 1985. Inhibition of H,K-ATPase by SCH 28080 and SCH 32651. *Eur. J. Pharmacol.* 112:268–70

91. Scott, C. K., Sundell, E., Castrovilly, L. 1987. Studies on the mechanism of action of the gastric microsomal (H + K)-ATPase inhibitors SCH 32651 and SCH 28080. *Biochem. Pharmacol.* 36:97–104

92. Serrano, R., Kielland-Brandt, M. C., Fink, G. R. 1986. Yeast plasma membrane ATPase is essential for growth and has homology with Na-K, K and Ca-ATPases. *Nature* 319:689–93

93. Shull, G. E., Lingrel, J. B. 1986. Molecular cloning of the rat stomach (H + K)-ATPase. *J. Biol. Chem.* 261: 16788–91

94. Shull, G. E., Schwartz, A., Lingrel, J. B. 1985. Amino acid sequence of the catalytic subunit of the Na-K ATPase deduced from a complementary DNA. *Nature* 316:691–95

95. Skrabanja, A. T. P., Asty, P., Soumarmon, A., De Pont, J. J. H. H. M., Lewin, M. J. M. 1986. H transport by reconstituted H,K-ATPase. *Biochim. Biophys. Acta* 860:131–36

96. Skrabanja, A. T. P., De Pont, J. J. H. H. M., Bonting, S. L. 1984. The H/ATP transport ratio of the (K + H)-ATPase of pig gastric membrane vesicles. *Biochim. Biophys. Acta* 774:91–95

97. Skrabanja, A. T. P., van der Hijden, H., De Pont, J. J. H. H. M. 1987.

Transport ratios of reconstituted (H + K)-ATPase. *Biochim. Biophys. Acta* 903:434–40

98. Smith, G. S., Scholes, P. B. 1982. The H+/ATP stoichiometry of the (H + K)-ATPase of dog gastric microsomes. *Biochim. Biophys. Acta* 688:803–7

99. Smolka, A., Helander, H. F., Sachs, G. 1983. Monoclonal antibodies against gastric (H + K)-ATPase. *Am. J. Physiol.* 245:G589–96

100. Soumarmon, A., Grelac, F., Lewin, M. J. 1983. Solubilization of active (H + K)-ATPase from gastric membrane. *Biochim. Biophys. Acta* 732:579–85

101. Soumarmon, A., Robert, J. C., Lewin, M. J. 1986. Depolymerization of solubilized gastric (H + K)-ATPase by n-octylglucoside or cholate. *Biochim. Biophys. Acta* 860:109–17

102. Stewart, B., Wallmark, B., Sachs, G. 1981. The interaction of H^+ and K^+ with the partial reactions of gastric (H + K)-ATPase. *J. Biol. Chem.* 256:2682–90

103. Tai, M. M., Im, W. B., Davis, J. P., Blakeman, D. P., Zurcher-Neely, H. A., Heinrikson, R. L. 1989. Evidence for the presence of a carbohydrate moiety in FITC-labelled fragments of rat gastric H,K-ATPase. *J. Biol. Chem.* 28:3183–87

104. Takaya, J., Omori, K., Taketani, S., Kobayashi, Y., Tashiro, Y. 1987. Solubilization, purification, and characterization of (H,K)-ATPase from hog gastric microsomes. *J. Biochem. (Tokyo)* 102:903–11

105. Takeguchi, N., Joshima, R., Inoue, Y., Kashiwagura, T., Morii, M. 1983. Effects of Cu^{2+}-o-phenanthroline on gastric (H + K)-ATPase Evidence for opening of a closed anion conductance by S-S cross-linkings. *J. Biol. Chem.* 258:3094–98

106. Takeguchi, N., Yamazaki, Y. 1986. Disulfide cross-linking of H,K-ATPase opens Cl conductance, triggering proton uptake in gastric vesicles. Studies with specific inhibitors. *J. Biol. Chem.* 261:2560–66

107. Tamura, S., Tagaya, M., Maeda, M., Futai, M. 1989. Pig gastric H,K-ATPase. Lys 497 conserved in cation transporting ATPases is modified with pyridoxal 5-phosphate *J. Biol. Chem.* 264:8580–84

108. van de Ven, F. J. M., Schrijen, J. J., De Pont, J. J. H. H. M., Bonting, S. L. 1981. Studies on (K + H)-ATPase III. Binding of adenylyl imidodiphosphate. *Biochim. Biophys. Acta* 640:487–99

109. Waldenhaug, M. O., Post, R. L., Sac-

comani, G., Leonard, R. T., Briskin, D. P. 1985. Structural relatedness of three ion-transport adenosine triphosphatases around their active sites of phosphorylation. *J. Biol. Chem.* 260:3852–59

110. Wallmark, B., Brandstrom, A., Larsson, H. 1984. Evidence for acid-induced transformation of omeprazole into an active inhibitor of (H + K)-ATPase within the parietal cell. *Biochim. Biophys. Acta* 778:549–58

111. Wallmark, B., Briving, C., Fryklund, J., Munson, K., Jackson, R. et al. 1987. Inhibition of gastric H,K-ATPase and acid secretion by SCH 28080, a substituted pyridyl(1,2a)imidazole. *J. Biol. Chem.* 262:2077–84

112. Wallmark, B., Jaresten, B. M., Larsson, H., Ryberg, B., Brandstrom, A., Fellenius, E. 1983. Differentiation among inhibitory actions of omeprazole, cimetidine, and SCN- on gastric acid secretion. *Am. J. Physiol.* 245:G64–71

113. Wallmark, B., Lorentzon, P., Larsson, H. 1985. The mechanism of action of omeprazole—a survey of its inhibitory actions in vitro. *Scand. J. Gastroenterol.* 20(Suppl. 108):37–51

114. Wallmark, B., Mardh, S. 1979. Phosphorylation and dephosphorylation kinetics of potassium stimulated ATP phosphohydrolase from hog gastric mucosa. *J. Biol. Chem.* 254:11899–11902

115. Wallmark, B., Stewart, H. B., Rabon, E., Saccomani, G., Sachs, G. 1980. The catalytic cycle of gastric (H + K)-ATPase. *J. Biol. Chem.* 255:5313–19

116. Wolosin, J. M. 1985. Ion transport studies with H,K-ATPase-rich vesicles: implications for HCl secretion and parietal cell physiology. *Am. J. Physiol.* 248:G595–607

117. Wolosin, J. M., Forte, J. G. 1981. Functional differences between K-ATPase rich membranes isolated from resting or stimulated rabbit fundic mucosa. *FEBS. Lett.* 125:208–12

118. Wolosin, J. M., Forte, J. G. 1981. Changes in the membrane environment of the (K + H)-ATPase following stimulation of the gastric oxyntic cell. *J. Biol. Chem.* 256:3149–52

119. Wolosin, J. M., Forte, J. G. 1981. Isolation of the secreting oxyntic cell apical membrane-identification of an elecroneutral KCl symport. In *Membrane Biophysics: Structure and Function in Epithelia* pp. 189–204. New York: Liss

120. Wolosin, J. M. and Forte, J. G. 1983. Kinetic properties of the KCl transport at the secreting apical membrane of the oxyntic cell. *J. Membr. Biol.* 71:195–207

121. Wolosin, J. M., Forte, J. G. 1984. Stimulation of oxyntic cell triggers K+ and Cl− conductances in apical (H,K)-ATPase membrane. *Am. J. Physiol.* 246:C537–45

122. Wolosin, J. M., Forte, J. G. 1985. K and Cl conductances in the apical membrane from secreting oxyntic cells are concurrently inhibited by divalent cations. *J. Membr. Biol.* 83:261–72

Annu. Rev. Physiol. 1990. 52:345–61

PERMEABLE CELL MODELS IN STIMULUS-SECRETION COUPLING

S. J. Hersey and A. Perez

Department of Physiology, Emory University, Atlanta, Georgia 30233

KEY WORDS: digitonin, electropermeability, liver, pancreas, stomach

INTRODUCTION

Stimulus-secretion coupling has come to be a generic term indicating a complex set of intracellular reactions initiated by an external stimulus, and resulting in the elaboration of a secretory product. Substantial interest has focused on identifying the individual reactions. From an investigative point of view, the complex set of reactions may be grouped into three phases: receptor-associated events, including second messenger production; reactions mediated by the second messengers; and activation of the secretory mechanism itself. Attempts to define and monitor stimulus-secretion events in intact cells have met with limited success. A major obstacle with intact cells is the presence of a plasma membrane that restricts measurements of intracellular events and prevents control of the cytosolic environment. Three general approaches have been utilized to overcome the limitations imposed by the plasma membrane. The most frequent approach is to examine selected aspects of stimulus-secretion coupling in isolated subcellular components. This approach has yielded substantial information, but suffers from an inability to correlate events with the actual secretory process. A second approach has been to employ intracellular probes, e.g. microelectrodes, optical probes, and so on, to monitor changes of intracellular components. This approach is limited by the specificity of the available probes. A third approach to this problem is through selective removal of the plasma membrane diffusion barrier. This approach originated with mechanical techniques for skinning

345

muscle fibers (65) and evolved to the use of physical forces or chemical agents to permeabilize the plasma membrane without disrupting intracellular organelles. Permeabilization of the plasma membrane results in a loss of soluble components of the cell while allowing for control of cytosolic composition and direct measurement of residual biochemical reactions. Thus permeabilized cells represent a compromise preparation that is intermediate between the intact cell and the isolated subcellular components. The permeabilization techniques have been applied to many cell types, including those of the gastrointestinal tract.

Various intracellular events have been studied in permeabilized cells. In terms of stimulus-secretion coupling, these preparations have proven particularly useful for investigation of the role of second messengers and the involvement of organelles in the secretory process.

Here we present a summary of the permeabilization techniques with emphasis on studies of stimulus-secretion coupling events in gastrointestinal cells. Selected information on other cell types and other areas of investigation is included to indicate the versatility of permeabilized cell preparations.

METHODS FOR PERMEABILIZING CELLS

The process of plasma membrane permeabilization denotes any procedure that results in a nonselective increase in permeability. This definition excludes solute-select agents, e.g. ionophores and membrane-permeant chemical species. In addition, an effective permeabilization procedure should preserve normal ultrastructural relationships and enzyme activities and should be selective for the plasma membrane relative to organelle membranes. Among the various procedures employed, some appear to be generally applicable while others are cell-type specific. Therefore, it is necessary to test several procedures with the cell-type of interest before identifying an appropriate method.

Detergents: Digitonin, Saponin, and Lysolecithin

The saponins, including digitonin, are steroid or triterpene glycosides that specifically react with cholesterol and other β-hydroxysterols thus resulting in the formation of an insoluble equimolar complex (1, 69). This interaction results in the creation of permanent pores in the plasma membrane (18). The molar ratio cholesterol/phospholipid of the plasma membrane differs considerably from the one for the intracellular membranes (45, 94). The cholesterol/phospholipid ratio for the plasma membrane of hepatocytes is 0.76, for the outer mitochondrial membrane and microsomes is 0.12, and for the rough endoplasmic reticulum is 0.06 (58). Thus treatment with digitonin or saponin brings about a selective increase in the permeability of the plasma membrane and spares the membranes of the intracellular organelles. The pores in the surface membrane of saponin-treated cells are seen by scanning electron microscopy to range in size from 100 nm to 1 μm (12). Analysis of different types of digitonin-treated cells (pancreatic islet cells, isolated gastric glands, and isolated hepatocytes) by electron microscopy shows no significant ultrastructural differences when compared with nontreated cells (7, 16, 49). Mooney & McDonald (54) reported that digitonin-permeabilized adipocytes are more fragile and prone to breakage during pipetting than intact cells. It is important to determine the optimum concentration of digitonin relative to tissue concentration for each system. The extent of tissue permeabilization as well as cell fragility appears to depend on this ratio (26, 61). The permeabilization induced by saponin-like detergents is stable and does not reverse upon removing the detergent.

Lysolecithin (L-α-lysophosphatidyl choline) is an ionic detergent that has been used to permeabilize many monolayer and suspension cultured cells (53). At low lysolecithin concentrations, cells become permeable to small molecules (Trypan Blue) and maintain viability as evidenced by continued growth after returning to culture medium; at higher concentrations, cells do not retain viability. The size of the molecules that can be incorporated into lysolecithin-treated cells depends on the concentration of lysolecithin used. The permeability change is reversed in about 15–20 min upon replacing the lysolecithin solution with growth medium (53).

Electropermeabilization

The exposure of cells to high voltage discharge renders them permeable by causing dielectric breakdown of the membrane (41, 44). The dielectric breakdown is due to mechanical compression of the membrane by the electric field. At a critical voltage, there is a rapid, localized membrane breakdown or formation of pores at two oppositely positioned sites on the cell. With successive voltage discharges, more pores (two at a time) will be created as long as the electrical field is interrupted by an intact membrane (the field is at 90° with respect to the sites of breakdown). Thus successive discharges initially increase the permeability of the cells by increasing the number of pores. As the fraction of membrane containing pores increases, however, the effectiveness of successive discharges declines (41, 44). The intensity of the externally applied field required to produce dielectric breakdown is inversely proportional to the diameter of a sphere; thus by applying a field of proper intensity, it is possible to produce localized dielectric breakdown of the plasma membrane without affecting the membrane of the intracellular organelles (3, 41, 43, 44, 63). Furthermore, it is possible, in a heterogeneous cell population, to permeabilize only larger cells while leaving smaller cells intact (44). This could also represent a disadvantage of the technique since, if the goal is to permeabilize all cells in a heterogeneous population, the applied field must be of sufficient intensity to affect the small cells and this may result in damage to the larger cells. If the electropermeabilized cells have not suffered extensive damage, the cells will reseal. The length of time required for the cells to reseal depends on the parameters used in the shocking procedure as well as on the electromechanical properties of the plasma membrane of each cell type (67). Erythrocytes are able to reseal and form ghosts when incubated at 37°C (67). Ileal brush-border vesicles remain permeable for about 15 min (17), pancreatic islet cells reseal after 30 min (63), and bovine adrenal medullary cells remain freely accessible up to an hr (3, 5, 41). Knight & Baker (3, 41, 44) determined that electropermeabilization of bovine adrenal medullary cells results in the creation of pores with an effective radius of about 1–4 nm. The size range of molecules reported to permeate plasma membranes after electropermeabilization is quite broad. Knight & Baker (41) reported that bovine adrenal medullary cells can be rendered leaky to molecules up to M_r 1000. Zimmerman et al (67, 95) showed that hemoglobin (M_r 64,500) can be released from red blood cells after electropermeabilization, and radioactively labeled albumin (M_r 60,000) can be incorporated and retained after cells reseal. Donowitz et al (17) reported the incorporation of dextran (M_r 70,000) into ileal brush-border membrane vesicles after high voltage discharge. Merritt et al (52) showed that exposure of pancreatic acinar cells to low field strength made them permeable to $^{86}Rb^+$, but not to inositol phosphates or Trypan Blue (M_r 960). When the intensity of the field was increased, the cells became permeable to Trypan Blue.

Electron micrographs of electropermeabilized ileal brush-border vesicles (17), insulin-secreting cells (RINm5F) (91), pancreatic islet cells (63), bovine adrenal medullary cells (41), and parathyroid cells (62) showed no major ultrastructural differences in comparison with the controls. In contrast, electron microscopy of isolated rabbit gastric glands that were electropermeabilized showed massive mitochondria damage, indicated by swelling and vacuolation (49). The electropermeabilization technique can be applied not only to cell suspensions but also to immobilized cells (87). But immobilization may restrict the ability to make multiple plasma membrane lesions as a consequence of repeated exposures to the applied electrical field.

Toluene

Toluene has been used to render bacteria and yeast (32, 73), hepatocytes (29, 30), and mitochondria (47, 50, 81, 82) permeable. The mechanism by which toluene achieves this is not known. Matlib et al (50) proposed that for mitochondrial membranes toleuene causes a small loss of cholesterol and phospholipids from the membranes and makes them less rigid. This is thought to allow the aggregation of membrane proteins so that channels are formed through which nucleotides and coenzymes can penetrate the mitochondrial membrane. Electron microscopy of toluene-permeabilized mitochondria showed that there was relatively little damage caused to the mitochondrial structure; the outer mitochondrial membrane was discontinuous, but the inner mitochondrial membrane was intact (50). In order to obtain a stable mitochondrial preparation and prevent release of matrix enzymes, Matlib et al (50) had to included 8.5% polyethylene glycol (M_r 6000–7500) in their medium.

Sendai Virus

Among the different types of virus, only two have been shown to produce permeability changes in plasma membranes, the *Sendai* virus and the *Newcastle-disease* virus (66). The permeability changes induced by these viruses have little cell specificity (22). This is probably because the attachment site for these viruses, a sialic acid group present either as a glycoprotein (2) or as a glycolipid (25), is present at the surface of most, if not all, animal cells. The permeability changes seem to be due to a cluster of viral glycoproteins that when fused with the cells form a hydrophilic channel similar to the one formed by polypeptide ionophores (93). Wyke et al (93) have shown that the presence of the F glycoprotein in the envelope of the paramyxovirus is a necessary factor for virally mediated changes to occur. One advantage of the virus-mediated permeabilization is that the extent and duration of the permeability change can be effectively controlled by calcium. Calcium temporarily restores the permeability barrier. Thus when calcium is withdrawn by chelation with EGTA or by washing the cells, the permeability change is restored (24, 33). A permanent recovery of the permeability barrier can be achieved by incubating the cells at 37°C. This process requires 2–4 hr for HeLa cells (66). One disadvantage of this method is that it tends to produce a significant amount of cell lysis. Wyke et al (93) estimated the size of virally mediated pores at about 1 nm in diameter.

Ca^{2+} Free Solutions

Streb & Schulz (78) reported that pancreatic acinar cells became permeable to Ca^{2+} and ATP when they were incubated in solutions containing a very low calcium concentation. The leakiness of the cells was assessed by Trypan Blue uptake (varying from 60–100%) and by release of the cytosolic enzyme lactate dehydrogenase (LDH); more than 80% of total LDH was released (71, 72, 78). The increase in cell permeability was not reversed upon readdition of calcium. The leaky pancreatic acinar cells retained the ability to react to secretagogues (carbamylcholine and cholecystokinin), even though they were permeable to high molecular weight molecules (77, 78).

Velasco et al (86) reported that they could generate permeable enterocytes by including EDTA in the isolation procedure. The enterocytes became permeable to calcium and other ions and did not accumulate α-methyl glucoside, which indicates a dissipation of the Na^+ gradient (86). The enterocytes accumulated calcium in both mitochondrial and nonmitochondrial compartments. Inositol trisphosphate released calcium selectively from the nonmitochondrial compartment (86).

Filipin

Filipin is a polyene antibiotic that increases the plasma membrane permeability by interacting with the cholesterol present in natural and artificial membranes (23). Filipin has been used to permeabilize isolated hepatocytes (23, 36, 75). The requirements for selective permeabilization seem to be strict. Gankema et al (23) reported that a dose of 50 μM with an incubation time of 1 min gave the best results, as indicated by leakage of glycerol 3-phosphate and retention of lactate dehydrogenase. Higher concentrations of filipin produce disintegration of the plasma membrane as indicated by extensive leakage of lactate dehydrogenase from the cells. The goal of Gankema & colleagues was to create a cell system permeable to low molecular weight compounds, e.g. glycerol 3-phosphate, but still able to retain cytosolic enzymes. This was achieved by using a low concentration of filipin with a short incubation time and the addition of ATP and reduced glutathione (23).

Dextran Sulfate

Dextran sulfate 500 is a polyanion that has been used to increase the permeability of Ehrlich ascites tumor cells (15, 39, 51). The exact mechanism by which dextran sulfate produces this permeability increase is unknown. Dextran sulfate 500 is known to cause the sorbitol space (impermeable space) to increase so that it becomes almost equal to the $[^3H]$ H_2O space (39). In Ehrlich ascites tumor cells, the permeability increase is nonspecific for small molecules, e.g. sorbitol, erythrosin B, orotate (OA), AMP, and ATP. Cells still maintain a permeability barrier to macromolecules such as inulin and OA phosphoribosyltransferase (15, 39, 51), however. In order to stabilize the dextran sulfate-treated cells, 7.5% (wt/vol) polyethylene glycol (PEG) was included in the medium and the incubation temperature lowered to room temperature (15). Kasahara (39) showed that ascites fluid or calcium ions plus glucose are able to restore active transport and to repair the permeability barrier in dextran sulfate-treated Ehrlich ascites tumor cells (39).

Hypertonicity

Castellot et al (13) reported the permeabilization of BHK cells by exposure to hypertonic solutions. The cells became permeable to nucleotides while they retained most macromolecules. The cells either remained permeable, or they could be resealed by returning them to a complete medium. The time required for $\geq$ 95% of the cells to take up Trypan Blue varied from 40 to 50 min. Electron micrographs of permeable and intact BHK cells indicated little structural damage. After permeabilization, cells remained viable and when supplied with appropriate substrates and cofactors, the cells were able to synthesize DNA, RNA, and protein (13).

APPLICATION TO GASTROINTESTINAL CELLS

The availability of methods for selective permeabilization of the plasma membrane allows for some unique approaches to study stimulus-secretion coupling events. In particular, use of these techniques has led to an improved understanding of the role of cellular organelles and the action mechanism of putative second messengers. In this section we review some of the applications of cell permeabilization to understand stimulus-secretion coupling in tissues from the gastrointestinal tract.

Liver

The use of permeabilized hepatocytes has contributed significantly to the understanding of the role of inositol trisphosphate [INS(1,4,5)P$_3$] in intracellular calcium mobilization. It is known that the glycogenolytic action of α_1-adrenergic agonists and vasoactive peptide hormones in the liver are mediated by an increase in the cytosolic-free calcium concentration, which leads to an allosteric activation of phosphorylase b kinase. The calcium appears to derive from intracellular organelles and not by entry through the plasma membrane (9, 19, 38, 88). Joseph et al (37), using saponin-treated hepatocytes, demonstrated that INS(1,4,5)P$_3$ was responsible for the calcium mobilization and that the calcium originated from a nonmitochondrial compartment. In addition, they showed that calcium reaccumulation was associated with dephosphorylation of INS(1,4,5)P$_3$. The mechanism by which INS(1,4,5)P$_3$ activates calcium channels in intracellular membranes is not well understood. Recently Worley et al (92) demonstrated the presence of high affinity binding sites for ^{3}H-INS(1,4,5)P$_3$ in rat cerebellum. The binding of ^{3}H-INS(1,4,5)P$_3$ to these sites was inhibited by heparin (92). Hill et al (31) were able to show heparin inhibition of INS(1,4,5)P$_3$ induced calcium release in electropermeabilized hepatocytes. In these studies, heparin did not affect the passive calcium release nor the calcium sequestration into intracellular storage sites; it was concluded that heparin was interacting with the INS(1,4,5)P$_3$ receptor binding site (31).

The use of saponin-treated hepatocytes has led to the confirmation that endotoxicosis and sepsis produced by Gram-negative bacterial endotoxins alter the Ca^{2+}-associated information flow, not only at the level of the plasma membrane but also at intracellular sites. Spitzer & Deaciuc (74) showed that endotoxicosis and sepsis affect the interaction of INS(1,4,5)P$_3$ with endoplasmic reticulum. They suggested that it is not so much the bacteria as it is the mediators produced as a consequence of the bacteria present in the medium that induce such alterations (74).

By combining the results obtained from using intact and digitonin-treated hepatocytes, Murphy et al (57) were able to follow the effects of the α-adrenergic agents norepinephrine and phenylephrine on the intracellular distribution of calcium as well as on the kinetics and dose-response relationship of changes in the cytosolic free Ca^{2+} concentration. From their experiments, it was concluded that there is a cause and effect relationship between binding of phenylephrine to the α-receptor, the increase of cytosolic-free calcium, and the activation of phosphorylase. The α-receptor antagonist, phentolamine, inhibited the increase in cytosolic-free calcium and the phosphorylase activity, while the β-receptor antagonist, propranolol, did not affect either parameter (57).

By using digitonin-treated hepatocytes, Rubin et al (68) were able to show that the activation of phospholipase C by ethanol and other membrane-disordering agents may depend on the presence of an intact receptor G protein complex in the plasma membrane.

Gastric Mucosa

Permeabilized gastric chief cells have been used to investigate the intracellular mechanisms associated with stimulation of pepsinogen secretion. Norris & Hersey (61) demonstrated that digitonin-permeabilized isolated gastric glands retained the capacity to secrete pepsinogen in response to a variety of agents. Thus the chief cells appear to retain sufficient regulatory components after permeabilization to carry out stimulus-secretion coupling. The permeabilized glands responded to the secretagogues, cholecystokinin octapeptide (CCK-OP), forskolin, and 8-bromo-adenosine 3',5'-cyclic monophosphate (8BrcAMP) as well as to calcium and vanadate, which suggest that both calcium and cAMP-mediated pathways are retained (61). Tsunoda et al (83, 84) investigated the mechanism by which intracellular calcium is released by INS(1,4,5)P$_3$ in chief cells. The saponin-permeabilized cells released calcium in response to INS(1,4,5)P$_3$, Ca^{2+} ionophores, and CCK-OP. From these experiments, Tsunoda et al concluded that the permeable cells respond to CCK-OP by releasing Ca^{2+} from the same INS-(1,4,5)P$_3$-sensitive pool. For intact chief cells, CCK-OP produces a biphasic response of pepsinogen secretion. The initial but transient response is associated with a rapid rise of cytoplasmic calcium that is independent of extracellular Ca^{2+} and probably is mediated by INS(1,4,5)P$_3$-induced Ca^{2+} release from intracellular stores. The sustained phase of secretion depends on extracellular Ca^{2+} and appears to be mediated by receptor-regulated Ca^{2+} entry from the extracellular space. The influx of Ca^{2+} from the extracellular medium may be mediated by diacylglycerol (84). In addition, it was found that cholchicine or cytochalasin D (cytoskeletal disrupting agents) inhibited the Ca^{2+} release elicited by INS(1,4,5)P$_3$, CCK-OP, or Ca^{2+} ionophores, and the CCK-OP-induced initial pepsinogen release (83). These results suggest that release of Ca^{2+} from the INS(1,4,5)P$_3$-sensitive pool requires an appropriate organization of the cytoskeletal system; thus the cytoskeleton is involved in the regulation of intracellular calcium metabolism (83).

Permeabilized gastric glands and parietal cells have been used to study the mechanisms underlying stimulation of acid secretion. Investigation of acid secretion in permeabilized parietal cells may provide a unique model system. This secretory process involves transmembrane ion transport rather than release of specific molecules into the bathing solution. Thus these studies require measurement of transmembrane ion gradients. Since the ion gradients of interest occur across a plasma membrane, the permeabilization procedures should, in theory, prevent ion gradient formation. Fortuitously, the secretory membrane of the parietal cell appears to be relatively unusual because permeabilization procedures do not alter this membrane, but selectively permeabilize the basolateral membrane. Although other ion transporting cells have not been studied in detail, it may be that the parietal cell represents a truly unique system for studying intracellular regulation of ion transport.

Permeabilized gastric glands retain the ability to generate proton gradients upon addition of ATP (16, 27, 49). The proton transport occurs in two phases, a spontaneous phase and a phase that requires the addition of valinomycin, a K^+-ionophore (27, 64). Addition of intracellular second messengers to the permeabilized cells does not alter proton transport. Pretreatment of the cells to establish secreting or resting states prior to permeabilization, however, results in retention of the transport characteristics following permeabilization (26, 28, 64). The secreting state has been correlated with spontaneous proton transport, while the resting state is associated with valinomycin-dependent transport (26, 64). These results supported the hypothesis that stimulation of the parietal cell leads, in part, to the activation of a KCl permeability in the secretory membrane. Further studies using the permeabilized cells demonstrated the existence of a Cl^- conductance in the acidifying membrane, but failed to show the existence of a significant K^+ conductance, which suggests that the KCl permeability consists of a neutral cotransport pathway in parallel with a Cl^- conductance (64). The permeabilized parietal cell system also is used to measure activity of the proton transporting ATPase, H,K-ATPase, in situ. Hersey et al (28) showed that a major effect of stimulating the parietal cell is an increase in the activity of the H,K-ATPase primarily because of an increase in the number of active enzyme molecules. The increase in number of active H,K-ATPase molecules is thought to result from recruitment of enzyme from a reserve pool of inactive H,K-ATPase. Thus stimulation of the parietal cell involves at least two major events, recruitment of H,K-ATPase molecules into the secretory membrane and activation of a KCl permeability.

Pancreas

Permeabilized acinar cells have been used to investigate the action of putative second messengers in stimulating enzyme secretion by the exocrine pancreas. Acinar cells permeabilized by digitonin or exposure to calcium-free solutions secrete amylase in response to Ca^{+2}, cAMP and analogues, and phorbol esters (40, 56). It is thought that the permeabilized cells retain stimulus-secretion coupling systems for both Ca^{+2} and cAMP-mediated pathways. Moreover, the findings support the concept that both protein kinase A and protein kinase C are involved in the stimulation of enzyme secretion (40). Stimulation of intact acinar cells by cholinergic agents and CCK-OP involves an increase in intracellular free Ca^{+2} associated with formation of INS-$(1,4,5)P_3$ (56). Studies using permeabilized cells indicate that $INS(1,4,5)P_3$ acts by releasing Ca^{+2} from a nonmitochondrial pool (77), which is thought to be the endoplasmic reticulum (76). It is suggested that both products of phosphatidylinositol breakdown, e.g. diacylglycerol and $INS(1,4,5)P_3$, are involved in the stimulation of enzyme secretion by acetylcholine and CCK (40). Although both acetylcholine and CCK appear to activate phospholipase C, Schnefel et al (70), using permeabilized acinar cells, presented evidence indicating that these stimuli are coupled to the enzyme through distinct GTP-binding proteins. The relationship between phosphoinositides and calcium appears to be interactive, since addition of calcium to permeabilized cells stimulates the formation of $INS(1,4,5)P_3$ (8, 80). At present it is not clear whether Ca^{+2} activation of phospholipase C represents a physiologically relevant component of receptor-initiated $INS(1,4,5)P_3$ production (80).

Permabilization techniques also have been used to investigate the endocrine pancreas, in particular to elucidate insulin secretion. Glucose-induced insulin secretion is thought to be mediated by an increase in intracellular calcium (90). Wolf et al (89) and Best (78) have shown that $INS(1,4,5)P_3$ can mediate the release of calcium from digitonin-treated pancreatic islets. Nilsson et al (59) suggested that Ca^{2+} released by $INS(1,4,5)P_3$ is taken up by a part of the endoplasmic reticulum that is not sensitive to $INS(1,4,5)P_3$. Upon metabolism of $INS(1,4,5)P_3$, Ca^{2+} recycles to the $INS(1,4,5)P_3$-sensitive pool. As in hepatocytes, heparin inhibits $INS(1,4,5)P_3$-induced Ca^{2+} release in electropermeabilized pancreatic β-cells in a dose-dependent manner. This effect is not due to inhibition of Ca^{2+} uptake into the $INS(1,4,5)P_3$-sensitive pool (60). Evidence indicates that insulin release can be modulated independent of changes in intracellular Ca^{2+} concentration. Tamagawa et al

(79) showed that forskolin and 12-O-tetradecanoylphorbol-13-acetate (TPA) are able to evoke insulin release without a rise in intracellular calcium concentration. Their findings suggest that activation of both protein kinase A and protein kinase C can modulate insulin release without a concomitant increase in cytosolic free Ca^{2+}. Jones et al (34) also reported that in electrically permeabilized islets cAMP-induced insulin secretion was not dependent on changes in cytosolic Ca^{2+}. Kimura et al (40), on the other hand, suggest that both pathways are Ca^{2+}-dependent and interact with each other. These contradictory results might be explained by the finding that phorbol esters are capable of activating protein kinase C in the absence of Ca^{2+}, although to a reduced extent (85). Also, Jones & Howell (35) found that TPA shifts the Ca^{2+}-activation curve to the left, thus inducing exocytosis at lower levels of intracellular Ca^{2+}. They suggested the possibility that the physiologic activation of protein kinase C by 1,2 diacylglycerol could stimulate insulin secretion without the need for elevation in cytosolic Ca^{2+}. Wolheim et al (91) reported that a Ca^{2+}-independent guanine nucleotide-sensitive site is involved in the control of exocytosis at a late or distal step in the chain of events leading to insulin secretion. Based on studies of the exocrine pancreas (52, 70), it appears that the G protein that couples Ca^{2+}-mobilizing receptors to phospholipase C is distinct from the G proteins that couple receptors to adenylate cyclase. This concept suggests a striking parallel with receptor regulation of adenylate cyclase, yet allows independent control of each of these signaling pathways.

ADDITIONAL APPLICATION OF THE PERMEABILIZATION TECHNIQUE

Permeabilization techniques have been employed to study various cellular properties in tissues other than those of the gastrointestinal tract. We include some of these findings primarily to illustrate the general application of this technique.

Secretory Processes

Considerable knowledge about Ca^{2+}-dependent catecholamine release has been gained by the use of permeabilized adrenal chromaffin cells. Indeed, the initial development of the electropermeabilization technique was performed with this preparation (4,5). In a series of studies, Baker & Knight (3,4,5,41) showed that catecholamine release from adrenal medullary cells is activated by micromolar concentrations of Ca^{2+}, requires MgATP, and can be inhibited by Mg, detergents, trifluoperazine, high osmotic pressure, and chaotropic anions. The Ca^{2+}-dependent catecholamine release is unaffected by Ca-channel blockers such as D600, which indicates a direct access to the activating site. Phorbol esters, as for pancreatic islets cells (35), increase the apparent affinity of exocytosis for calcium (42), which indicates a role for protein kinase C in the exocytosis process. Lelkes et al (46), using digitonin-treated chromaffin cells, suggested that microfilaments may play a role in the secretory process. Accordingly, F-actin destabilizing agents, such as cytochalasin D or DNase 1, promoted Ca^{2+}-stimulated (as well as basal) secretion, while stabilizers like phalloidin produced the opposite effect.

Mooney & McDonald (54) demonstrated that digitonin-permeabilized adipocytes retain adenylate cyclase activity, which is activated by β-adrenergic agonists and inhibited by adenosine analogues. The same preparation was used also to provide the first direct evidence that insulin does not need to affect adenylate cyclase activity in order to elicit an antilipolitic effect (55).

The parathyroid cell is unusual for its inverse relationship between the extracellular and cytosolic Ca^{2+} concentrations and parathyroid hormone (PTH) release. High Ca^{2+} concentrations inhibit rather than stimulate PTH release in the parathyroid cell. Oetting et al (62), using electropermeabilized parathyroid cells, provided evidence that PTH release is mediated by a guanine-nucleotide regulatory protein. Nonhydrolysable analogues of GTP, e.g. GppNHp, produce a dose-dependent stimulation of PTH release while GDPβS, a nonhydrolysable GDP analogue, completely abolishes GppNHp-stimulated hormone release. PTH release was maximal at free $[Ca^{2+}]$ less than 200 nM and progressively decreased as the free $[Ca^{2+}]$ increased from 300 nM to 100 μM; this is similar to the Ca^{2+}-induced suppression of PTH secretion in nonpermeabilized cells. These findings indicate that the inhibitory effects of Ca^{2+} on PTH release may result from a Ca^{2+}-induced reduction in guanine-nucleotide-stimulated PTH secretion either via inhibition of a stimulatory G protein (62), or activation of an inhibitory G protein as suggested by Fitzpatrick & Aurbach (21).

Bradford & Rubin (11), using saponin-treated rabbit neutrophils, showed that the activity of phospholipase C in neutrophils is regulated by a G protein. This regulatory protein appears to sensitize phospholipase C to physiologically relevant Ca^{2+} concentrations and thus could result in activation of the enzyme in the absence of any increase in the calcium concentration (11). This mechanism appears to be analogous to the role of diacylglycerol in pancreatic islets (35) and adrenal medullary cells (42), i.e. to sensitize protein kinase C to low $[Ca^{2+}]$ (11). Barrowman et al (6) suggest that GTP analogues can activate secretory processes in virus-permeabilized neutrophils, not only at the level of the receptors, but also by exerting a direct effect on the exocytotic process.

Saponin-treated and virus-treated mast cells were used by Chakravarty (14) and Gomperts et al (24) to show Ca^{2+}-dependent histamine secretion. The histamine secretion showed characteristics of a normal secretory exocytotic mechanism as regards Ca^{2+} concentration dependence and a requirement for metabolic energy.

Measurement of Enzyme Activity

In addition to permitting access of exogenous substances to the cytosol, selective permeabilization of the plasma membrane releases soluble components into the bathing medium. This allows measurement of soluble metabolites, e.g. ATP and ADP (96), without requiring homogenization or the use of protein denaturing agents. Soluble enzymes that are released by permeabilization can be isolated from particulate material easily and assayed directly (48, 97). Moreover, for enzymes that distribute between soluble and membrane-associated compartments, e.g. protein kinase C, it is possible to assay the redistribution with rapid separation of the two compartments.

The permeabilization techniques also permit the measurement of membrane-associated enzymes in situ. Selective permeabilization of the plasma membrane allows ready access of normally impermeable substrates to enzymes associated with organelles. This approach has been used to study the properties of several enzymes including H,K-ATPase in gastric parietal cells (28); carnitine palmitoyltransferase in hepatocytes (10, 75); and adenylate cyclase in adipocytes (54). The development of procedures to make mitochondria permeable to normally nonpenetrating substrates and cofactors by treatment with toluene allows measurement of mitochondrial enzymes in situ (47, 50, 81, 82). The use of permeabilization techniques to assay enzymes in situ is very likely to be extended to other cell types and other enzyme activities.

SUMMARY

A number of mechanical and chemical methods have been developed to achieve selective permeabilization of the plasma membrane. These methods have been applied to many cell types and have proven to be highly useful for studying stimulus-secretion coupling mechanisms. Thus far, this approach has contributed significantly to our understanding of phosphoinositide metabolism and the regulation of intracellular calcium. The permeabilization techniques also have contributed important information regarding cAMP-dependent pathways. In addition to studies of stimulus-secretion coupling, permeabilized cell preparations can be employed for investigations of enzyme activity in situ and the properties of intracellular organelles in general. Since cell permeabilization, particularly with chemical agents, is surprisingly easy, these techniques should find wide application for future studies.

Literature Cited

1. Akiyama, T., Takagi, S., Sankawa, U., Inari, S., Saitô, H. 1980. Saponin-cholesterol interaction in the multibilayers of egg yolk lecithin as studied by deuterium nuclear magnetic resonance: digitonin and its analogues. *Biochemistry* 19:1904–11

2. Bächi, T., Deas, J. E., Howe, C. 1977. Virus-erythrocyte membrane interactions. *Cell Surf. Rev.* 2:83–127

3. Baker, P. F., Knight, D. E. 1981. Calcium control of exocytosis and endocytosis in bovine adrenal medullary cells. *Phil. Trans. R. Soc. London Ser. B* 296:83–103

4. Baker, P. F., Knight, D. E. 1978. Calcium-dependent exocytosis in bovine adrenal medullary cells with leaky plasma membranes. *Nature* 276:620–22

5. Baker, P. F., Knight, D. E. 1980. Gaining access to the site of exocytosis in bovine adrenal medullary cells. *J. Physiol. (Paris)* 76:497–504

6. Barrowman, M. M., Cockcroft, S., Gomperts, B. D. 1986. Two roles for guanine nucleotides in the stimulus-secretion sequence of neutrophils. *Nature* 319:504–7

7. Benedetti, A., Fulceri, R., Romani, A., Comporti, M. 1987. Stimulatory effect of glucose 6-phosphate on the non-mitochondrial Ca^{2+} uptake in permeabilized hepatocytes and Ca^{2+} release by inositol trisphosphate. *Biochim. Biophys. Acta* 928:282–86

8. Best, L. 1986. A role for calcium in the breakdown of inositol phospholipids in intact and digitonin-permeabilized pancreatic islets. *Biochem. J.* 238:773–79

9. Blackmore, P. F., Hughes, B. P., Shuman, E. A., Exton, J. H. 1982. alpha-Adrenergic activation of phosphorylase in liver cells involves mobilization of intracellular calcium without influx of extracellular calcium. *J. Biol. Chem.* 257(1):190–97

10. Boon, M. R., Zammit, V. A. 1988. Use of a selectively permeabilized isolated rat hepatocyte preparation to study changes in the properties of overt carnitine palmitoyltransferase activity in situ. *Biochem. J.* 249:645–52

11. Bradford, P. G., Rubin, R. P. 1986. Guanine nucleotide regulation of phospholipase C activity in permeabilized rabbit neutrophils. *Biochem. J.* 239:97–102

12. Brooks, J. C., Carmichael, S. W. 1983. Scanning electron microscopy of chemically skinned bovine adrenal medullary chromaffin cells. *Mikroskopie* 40(11–12):347–56

13. Castellot, J. J. Jr., Miller, M. R., Pardee, A. B. 1978. Animal cells reversibly permeable to small molecules. *Proc. Natl. Acad. Sci. USA* 75(1):351–55

14. Chakravarty, N. 1986. Histamine secretion from permeabilized mast cells by calcium. *Life Sci.* 39:1549–54

15. Chen, J. J., Jones, M. E. 1979. Effect of 5-phosphoribosyl-1-pyrophosphate on de novo pyrimidine biosynthesis in cultured Ehrlich ascites cells made permeable with dextran sulfate 500. *J. Biol. Chem.* 254(8):2697–2704

16. Colca, J. R., Wolf, B. A., Comens, P. G., McDaniel, M. L. 1985. Protein phosphorylation in permeabilized pancreatic islet cells. *Biochem. J.* 228:529–36

17. Donowitz, M., Emmer, E., McCullen, J., Reinlib, L., Cohen, M. E., et al. 1987. Freeze-thaw and high voltage discharge allow macromolecule uptake into ileal brush-border vesicles. *Am. J. Physiol.* 252 (*Gastrointest. Liver Physiol.* 15):G723–35

18. Dunn, L. A., Holz, R. W. 1983. Catecholamine secretion from digitonin-treated adrenal medullary chromaffin cells. *J. Biol. Chem.* 258(8):4989–93

19. Exton, J. H. 1981. Molecular mechanisms involved in alpha-adrenergic responses. *Mol. Cell Endocr.* 23(3):233–64

20. Fiskum, G., Craig, S. W., Decker, G. L., Lehninger, A. L. 1980. The cytoskeleton of digitonin-treated rat hepatocytes. *Proc. Natl. Acad. Sci. USA* 77(6):3430–34

21. Fitzpatrick, L. A., Aurbach, G. D. 1986. Calcium inhibition of parathyroid hormone secretion is mediated via a guanine nucleotide regulatory protein. *J. Bone Miner. Res.* 1(1):140 (Abstr. 320)

22. Foster, K. A., Gill, K., Micklem, K. J., Pasternak, C. A. 1980. Survey of virally mediated permeability changes. *Biochem. J.* 190:639–46

23. Gankema, H. S., Laanen, E., Groen, A. K., Tager, J. M. 1981. Characterization of isolated rat-liver cells made permeable with filipin. *Eur. J. Biochem.* 119:409–14

24. Gomperts, B. D., Baldwin, J. M., Micklem, K. J. 1983. Rat mast cells permeabilized with *Sendai* virus secrete histamine in response to Ca^{2+} buffered in the micromolar range. *Biochem. J.* 210:737–45

25. Haywood, A. M. 1974. Characteristics of *Sendai* virus receptors in a model membrane. *J. Mol. Biol.* 83:427–36

26. Hersey, S. J., Steiner, L. 1985. Acid formation by permeable gastric glands: enhancement by prestimulation. *Am. J. Physiol.* 248 (*Gastrointest. Liver Physiol.* 11):G561–68

27. Hersey, S. J., Steiner, L. 1988. Stimulation of acid formation in permeable gastric glands by valinomycin. *Am. J. Physiol.* 255 (*Gastrointest. Liver Physiol.* 18):G313–18

28. Hersey, S. J., Steiner, L., Matheravidathu, S., Sachs, G. 1988. Gastric H^+-K^+-ATPase in situ: relation to secretory state. *Am. J. Physiol.* 254 (*Gastrointest. Liver Physiol.* 17):G856–63

29. Hilderman, R. H., Deutscher, M. P. 1974. Aminoayl transfer ribonucleic acid synthesis in toluene-treated liver cells. *J. Biol. Chem.* 249:5346–48

30. Hilderman, R. H., Goldblatt, P. J., Deutscher, M. P. 1975. Preparation and characterization of liver cells made permeable to macromolecules by treatment with toluene. *J. Biol. Chem.* 250:4796–4801

31. Hill, T. D., Berggren, P.-O., Boynton, A. L. 1987. Heparin inhibits inositol trisphosphate-induced calcium release from permeabilized rat liver cells. *Biochem. Biophys. Res. Commun.* 149(3):897–901

32. Hower, S. H., Walker, L. L. 1972. Synthesis of DNA in toluene-treated *Chlamydomonas reinhardi* (DNA replication-chloroplast DNA-cell cycle-electron microscopy). *Proc. Nat. Acad. Sci. USA* 69:490–94

33. Impraim, C. C., Foster, K. A., Mickelem, K. J., Pasternak, C. A. 1980. Nature of virally mediated changes in membrane permeability to small molecules. *Biochem. J.* 186:847–60

34. Jones, P. M., Fyles, J. M., Howell, S. L. 1986. Regulation of insulin secretion by cAMP in rat islets of Langerhans permeabilized by high-voltage discharge. *FEBS Lett.* 205(2):205–9

35. Jones, P. M., Howell, S. L. 1986. Insulin secretion studied in islets permeabilized by high voltage discharge. *Adv. Exp. Med. Biol.* 211:279–91

36. Jorgenson, R. A., Nordlie, R. C. 1980. Multifunctional glucose-6-phosphatase studied in permeable isolated hepatocytes. *J. Biol. Chem.* 255(12):5907–15

37. Joseph, S. K., Thomas, A. P., Williams, R. J., Irvine, R. F., Williamson, J. R. 1984. myo-Inositol 1,4,5-trisphosphate. A second messenger for the hormonal mobilization of in-

tracellular Ca^{2+} in liver. *J. Biol. Chem.* 259(5):3077–81

38. Joseph, S. K., Williamson, J. R. 1983. The origin, quantitation, and kinetics of intracellular calcium mobilization by vasopressin and phenylephrine in hepatocytes. *J. Biol. Chem.* 258 (17):10425–32

39. Kasahara, M. 1977. A permeability change in Ehrlich ascites tumor cells caused by dextran sulfate and its repair by ascites fluid or Ca^{2+} ions. *Arch. Biochem. Biophys.* 184:400–7

40. Kimura, T., Imamura, K., Eckhardt, L., Schultz, I. 1986. Ca^{2+}-, phorbol ester-, and cAMP-stimulated enzyme secretion from permeabilized rat pancreatic acini. *Am. J. Physiol.* 250 (*Gastrointest. Liver Physiol.* 13):G698–708

41. Knight, D. E., Baker, P. F. 1982. Calcium-dependence of catecholamine release from bovine adrenal medullary cells after exposure to intense electric fields. *J. Membr. Biol.* 68:107–40

42. Knight, D. E., Baker, P. F. 1983. The phorbol ester TPA increases the affinity of exocytosis for calcium in "leaky" adrenal medullary cells. *FEBS Lett.* 160(1,2):98–100

43. Knight, D. E., Koh, E., 1984. Ca^{2+} and cyclic nucleotide dependence of amylase release from isolated rat pancreatic acinar cells rendered permeable by intense electric fields. *Cell Calcium* 5:401–18

44. Knight, D. E., Scrutton, M. C. 1986. Gaining access to the cytosol: the technique and some applications of electropermeabilization. *Biochem. J.* 234:497–506

45. Lange, Y., Ramos, B. V. 1983. Analysis of the distribution of cholesterol in the intact cell. *J. Biol. Chem.* 258 (24):15130–34

46. Lelkes, P. I., Friedman, J. E., Rosenheck, K., Oplatka, A. 1986. Destabilization of actin filaments as a requirement for the secretion of catecholamines from permeabilized chromaffin cells. *FEBS Lett.* 208(2):357–63

47. Lof, C., Cohen, M., Vermeulen, L. P., Van Roermund, C. W. T., Wanders, R. J. A., Meijer, A. J. 1983. Properties of carbamoyl-phosphate synthetase (ammonia) in rat-liver mitochondria made permeable with toluene. *Eur. J. Biochem.* 135(2):251–58

48. Mackall, J., Meredith, M., Lane, M. D. 1979. A mild procedure for the rapid release of cytoplasmic enzymes from cultured animal cells. *Anal. Biochem.* 95:270–74

49. Malinowska, D. H., Koelz, H. R., Hersey, S. J., Sachs, G. 1981. Proper-

ties of the gastric proton pump in unstimulated permeable gastric glands. *Proc. Natl. Acad. Sci. USA* 78(9):5908–12

50. Matlib, M. A., Shannon, W. A. Jr., Srere, P. A. 1977. Measurement of matrix enzyme activity in isolated mitochondria made permeable with toluene. *Arch. Biochem. Biophys.* 178:396–407

51. McCoy, G. D., Resch, R. C., Racker, E. 1976. Characterization of dextran sulfate-treated ascites tumor cells and their repair by ascites fluid. *Cancer Res.* 36:3339–45

52. Merrit, J. E., Taylor, C. W., Rubin, R. P., Putney, W. Jr. 1986. Evidence suggesting that a novel guanine nucleotide regulatory protein couples receptors to phospholipase C in exocrine pancreas. *Biochem J.* 236:337–43

53. Miller, M. R., Castellot, J. J. Jr., Pardee, A. B. 1979. A general method for permeabilizing monolayer and suspension cultured animal cells. *Exp. Cell Res.* 120:421–25

54. Mooney, R. A., McDonald, J. M. 1986. In situ analysis of adenylate cyclase activity in permeabilized rat adipocytes: sensitivity to GTP, isoproterenol, and N^6-(phenylisopropyl)adenosine. *J. Biochem.* 18(8):713–18

55. Mooney, R. A., Swicegood, C. L., Marx, R. B. 1986 Coupling of adenylate cyclase to lipolisis in permeabilized adipocytes: direct evidence that an antilipolytic effect of insulin is independent of adenylate cyclase. *Endocrinology* 119:2240–48

56. Muallem, S., Pandol, S. J., Beeker, T. G. 1989. Hormone-evoked calcium release from intracellular stores is a quantal process. *J. Biol. Chem.* 264(1):205–12

57. Murphy, E., Coll, K., Rich, T. L., Williamson, J. R. 1980. Hormonal effects on calcium homeostasis in isolated hepatocytes. *J. Biol. Chem.* 255(14):6600–8

58. Nachbaur, A. C., Vignais, P. M. 1971. Enzymic characterization and lipid composition of rat liver subcellular membranes. *Biochim. Biophys. Acta* 249:462–92

59. Nilsson, T., Arkhammar, P., Hallberg, A., Hellman, B., Berggren, P.-O. 1987. Characterization of the inositol 1,4,5-trisphosphate-induced Ca^{2+} release in pancreatic β-cells. *Biochem. J.* 248:329–36

60. Nilsson, T., Zwiller, J., Boynton, A. L., Berggren, P.-O. 1988. Heparin inhibits IP_3-induced Ca^{2+} release in permeabilized pancreatic β-cells. *FEB Lett.* 229(1):211–14

61. Norris, S. H., Hersey, S. J. 1985. Stimulation of pepsinogen secretion in permeable isolated gastric glands. *Am. J. Physiol.* 249 (*Gastrointest. Liver Physiol.* 12):G408–15

62. Oetting, M., LeBoff, M., Swiston, L., Preston, J., Brown, E. 1986. Guanine nucleotides are potent secretagogues in permeabilized parathyroid cells. *FEBS Lett.* 208(1):99–104

63. Pace, C. S., Tarvin, J. T., Neighbors, A. S., Pirkle, J. A., Greider, M. H. 1980. Use of a high voltage technique to determine the molecular requirements for exocytosis in islet cells. *Diabetes* 29:911–18

64. Perez, A., Blissard, D., Sachs, G., Hersey, S. J. 1989. Evidence for a chloride conductance in secretory membrane of parietal cells. *Am. J. Physiol.* 256 (*Gastrointest. Liver Physiol.* 19):G299–305

65. Podolsky, R. J., Costantin, L. L. 1964. Regulation by calcium of the contractions and relaxation of muscle fibers. *Fed. Proc.* 23:933–39

66. Poste, G., Pasternack, C. A. 1978. Virus-induced cell fusion. *Cell Surf. Rev.* 5:306–49

67. Riemann, F., Zimmermann, U., Pilwat, G. 1975. Release and uptake of haemoglobin and ions in red blood cells induced by dielectric breakdown. *Biochim. Biophys. Acta* 394:449–62

68. Rubin, R., Thomas, A. P., Hoek, J. B. 1987. Ethanol does not stimulate guanine nucleotide-induced activation of phospholipase C in permeabilized hepatocytes. *Arch. Biochem. Biophys.* 256(1):29–38

69. Scallen, T. J., Dietert, A. E. 1969. The quantitative retention of cholesterol in mouse liver prepared for electron microscopy by fixation in a digitonin-containing aldehyde solution. *J. Cell Biol.* 40:802–13

70. Schnefel, S., Banfic, H., Eckhardt, L., Schultz, G., Schulz, I. 1988. Acetylcholine and cholecystokinin receptors functionally couple by different G-proteins to phospholipase C in pancreatic acinar cells. *FEBS Lett.* 230(1,2)125:130

71. Schulz, I., Streb, H., Bayerdörffer, E., Imamura, K. 1986. Intracellular messengers in stimulus-secretion coupling of pancreatic acinar cells. *J. Cardiovasc. Pharmacol.* (Suppl. 8):S91–96

72. Schulz, I., Streb, H., Bayerdörffer, E., Thévenod, F. 1985. Stimulus-secretion coupling in exocrine glands: the role of inositol-1,4,5-trisphosphate, calcium and cAMP. *Curr. Eye Res.* 4(4):467–73

73. Serrano, R., Gancedo, J. M., Gancedo, C. 1973. Assay of yeast enzymes in situ.

A potential tool in regulation studies *Eur. J. Biochem.* 34:479–82

74. Spitzer, J. A., Deaciuc, I. V. 1987. IP_3-dependent Ca^{2+} release in permeabilized hepatocytes of endotoxemic and septic rats. *Am. J. Physiol.* 253 (*Endocrinol. Metab.* 16):E130–34

75. Stephens, T. W., Harris, R. A. 1987. Effect of starvation and diabetes on the sensitivity of carnitine palmitoyltransferase I to inhibition by 4-hydroxyphenylglyoxylate. *Biochem. J.* 243:405–12

76. Streb, H., Bayerdörffer, E., Haase, W., Irvine, R. F., Schulz, I. 1984. Effect of inositol-1,4,5-trisphosphate on isolated subcellular fractions of rat pancreas. *J. Membr. Biol.* 81:241–53

77. Streb, H., Irvine, R. F., Berridge, M. J., Schulz, I. 1983. Release of Ca^{2+} from a nonmitochondrial intracellular store in pancreatic acinar cells by inositol-1,4,5-trisphosphate. *Nature* 306:67–68

78. Streb, H., Schulz, I. 1983. Regulation of cytosolic free Ca^{2+} concentration in acinar cells of rat pancreas. *Am. J. Physiol.* 245 (*Gastrointest. Liver Physiol.* 8):G347–57

79. Tamagawa, T., Niki, H., Niki, A. 1985. Insulin release independent of a rise in cytosolic free Ca^{2+} by forskolin and phorbol ester. *FEBS Lett.* 183(2):430–32

80. Taylor, C. W., Merritt, J. E., Putney, J. W. Jr., Rubin, R. P. 1986. Effects of Ca^{2+} on phosphoinositide breakdown in exocrine pancreas. *Biochem. J.* 238:765–72

81. Thomas, A. P., Denton, R. M. 1986. Use of permeabilized mitochondria in the study of insulin-induced pyruvate dehydrogenase activation. *Biochem. Soc. Trans.* 14:314–15

82. Thomas, A. P., Denton, R. M. 1986. Use of toluene-permeabilized mitochondria to study the regulation of adipose tissue pyruvate dehydrogenase in situ. *Biochem. J.* 238:93–101

83. Tsunoda, Y. 1987. The cholecystokinin-induced Ca^{2+} shuttle from the inositol trisphosphate-sensitive and ATP-dependent pool, and initial pepsinogen release connected with cytoskeleton of the chief cell. *Biochim. Biophys. Acta* 901:35–51

84. Tsunoda, Y., Takeda, H., Otaki, T., Asaka, M., Nakagaki, I., Sasaki, S. 1988. A role for Ca^{2+} in mediating hormone-induced biphasic pepsinogen secretion from the chief cell determined by luminescent and fluorescent probes

and X-ray microprobe. *Biochim. Biophys. Acta* 941:83–101

85. Vandenbark, G. R., Kuhn, L. J., Niedel, J. E. 1984. Possible mechanism of phorbol diester-induced maturation of human promyelocytic leukemia cells. *J. Clin. Invest.* 73(2):448–57

86. Velasco, G., Shears, S. B., Michell, R. H., Lazo, P. S. 1986. Calcium uptake by intracellular compartments in permeabilized enterocytes. Effect of inositol 1,4,5 trisphosphate. *Biochem. Biophys. Res. Commun.* 139(2):612–18

87. Whitaker, M. J. 1985. Polyphosphoinositide hydrolysis is associated with exocytosis in adrenal medullary cells. *FEBS Lett.* 189(1):137–40

88. Williamson, J. R., Cooper, R. H., Hoek, J. B. 1981. Role of calcium in the hormonal regulation of liver metabolism. *Biochim. Biophys. Acta* 639(3, 4):243–95

89. Wolf, B. A., Comens, P. G., Ackermann, K. E., Sherman, W. R., McDaniel, M. L. 1985. The digitonin-permeabilized pancreatic islet model. Effect of myo-inositol 1,4,5-trisphosphate on Ca^{2+} mobilization. *Biochem. J.* 227:965–69

90. Wollheim, C. B., Sharp, G. W. G. 1981. Regulation of insulin release by calcium. *Physiol. Rev.* 61(4):914–73

91. Wollheim, C. B., Ullrich, S., Meda, P., Vallar, L. 1987. Regulation of exocytosis in electrically permeabilized insulin-secreting cells. Evidence for Ca^{2+} dependent and independent secretion. *Biosci. Rep.* 7(5):443–54

92. Worley, P. F., Baraban, J. M., Supattapone, S., Wilson, V. S., Synder, S. H. 1987. Characterization of inositol trisphosphate receptor binding in brain. Regulation by pH and calcium. *J. Biol. Chem.* 262(25):12132–36

93. Wyke, A. M., Impraim, C. C., Knutton, S., Pasternak, C. A. 1980. Components involved in virally mediated membrane fusion and permeability changes. *Biochem. J.* 190:625–38

94. Yeagle, P. L. 1985. Cholesterol and the cell membrane. *Biochim. Biophys. Acta* 822:267–87

95. Zimmermann, U., Pilwat, G., Riemann, F. 1975. Preparation of erythrocyte ghosts by dielectric breakdown of the cell membrane. *Biochim. Biophys. Acta* 375:209–19

96. Zuurendonk, P. F., Tager, J. M. 1974. Rapid separation of particulate components and soluble cytoplasm of isolated rat-liver cells. *Biochim. Biophys. Acta* 333:393–99

SPECIAL TOPIC: ION MOVEMENTS IN LEUKOCYTES

Louis Simchowitz, Section Editor

Departments of Medicine, Cell Biology, and Physiology, V.A. Medical Center and Washington University School of Medicine, St. Louis, Missouri 63110

INTRODUCTION

Spurred by recent advances in our understanding of the physiology of excitable tissues and epithelia, there has been a tremendous renaissance of interest in the study of small, nonpolarized cells. While erythrocytes have always enjoyed a loyal and devoted following, it has only been in the last decade or so that other blood cells, in particular lymphocytes, neutrophils, monocytes, platelets, and their mast cell cousins, have stirred the curiosity of those versed in cellular physiology. Even a cursory glance at the index pages of most biological journals will convey some sense of the intense activity accorded this area of inquiry today. For a comprehensive treatment of this subject, readers are referred to the proceedings of a recent symposium on "Cell Physiology of Blood" that was organized by Drs. Robert Gunn and John Parker at the 1987 annual meeting of the Society of General Physiologists in Woods Hole (1).

The next five reviews deal mainly with neutrophils, lymphocytes, and platelets. As will be outlined in these chapters, the functional attributes of these cells are as diverse as their morphology. Nonetheless, a recurring theme will emerge in terms of the basic membrane properties and pathways of ion movement in resting as well as stimulated cells. This is especially true of the cascade of physiologic and biochemical events characterizing the transition from quiescent phase to the activated state, a process generally known as stimulus-response coupling. In this context, changes in intracellular pH, membrane potential, and cytosolic Ca^{2+}, all directly linked to the transport of various ions, are thought to play central roles in the locomotor and secretory responses so vital to the normal function of these cells. It is the dynamic interplay of these ion fluxes, either as fundamental intracellular messengers or

363

as permissive, regulatory factors, plus a host of intermediary metabolic steps that underlie the signal transduction apparatus.

The section opens with a chapter by Dr. Ramadan Sha'afi who was among the first to apply a physiologic approach to the study of the ionic basis of neutrophil function. His review details recent developments in the scheme of cell activation in neutrophils with emphasis on the roles of intracellular pH, G-proteins, protein kinase C, and cytosolic calcium transients. In the second chapter, Dr. James Bibb and I summarize information on the modes of anion transport, especially the physiologic role of Cl^-/HCO_3^- exchange in intracellular pH regulation, in neutrophils and HL-60 cells. The third article, by Drs. Sergio Grinstein and Kevin Foskett, focuses on the various ionic mechanisms of cell volume regulation after osmotic shock. This is followed by a discussion by Drs. Michael Cahalan and Richard Lewis on the electrophysiology of lymphocytes and the role of K^+ channels in mitogenesis. In the final chapter, Drs. Timothy Rink and S. Sage outline concepts regarding calcium homeostasis and cytoplasmic free calcium as a potential second messenger of signal activation in platelets.

While limitations on space unfortunately do not permit an exhaustive recounting of all of the accomplishments in this burgeoning field, I sincerely hope that the efforts of the contributors to this section may be rewarded by enticing others to enter this arena of research.

Literature Cited

1. Gunn, R. B., Parker, J. C., eds. 1988. *Cell Physiology of Blood. Soc. Gen. Physiol. Ser.,* Vol. 43. New York: Rockefeller Univ. Press. 402 pp.

Annu. Rev. Physiol. 1990. 52:365–79

ROLE OF ION MOVEMENTS IN NEUTROPHIL ACTIVATION

Ramadan I. Sha'afi and Thaddeus F. P. Molski

Department of Physiology, University of Connecticut Health Center, Farmington Connecticut, 06032

KEY WORDS: motility, degranulation, oxidative burst, GM-CSF, calcium

INTRODUCTION

The neutrophils represent the first line of defense against foreign pathogens. They are highly specialized for the performance of this primary function, the phagocytosis and destruction of microorganisms. The microbial invasion elicits several neutrophil responses. They include: chemotaxis, phagocytosis, oxidative burst, digestion, extracellular release, and aggregation. In this chapter we will restrict our discussion to the possible role of ion (Na^+, K^+, Ca^{2+}) movements in these cell responses. Discussion of the methods for measuring ion movements will not be presented since this subject has been reviewed recently (27). Other aspects of the excitation-response coupling of neutrophil activation will not be dealt with since this subject has been discussed extensively (7, 8, 12, 29, 32–35, 42, 43, 46).

SODIUM AND POTASSIUM IONS

The intracellular concentration of K^+ in neutrophils, like that in other mammalian cells, is much higher than the corresponding value in the extracellular fluid, whereas the reverse is true for Na^+. The plasma membrane of the neutrophil is permeable to these ions. Depending on the species studied, the value of the unidirectional flux for Na^+ is 1–5 meq/liter cell water/min; the corresponding value for K^+ is 1–7 meq/liter cell water/min.

0066-4278/90/0315-0365$02.00

These values are at least 50 times faster than those obtained with mammalian red cells. The experimentally determined values for the intracellular concentrations of Na^+ and K^+ vary considerably among different investigators and most likely reflect the experimental differences (temperature, pH) under which these values were determined. The physiologic values should be in the range of 20 mM for Na^+ and 120 mM for K^+.

These concentration gradients are maintained by the Na^+, K^+ pump, which is driven by metabolic energy derived from the hydrolysis of ATP by membrane-associated $(Mg^{2+} + Na^+ + K^+)$ activated adenosine triphosphatase (ATPase). This view is based on the following observations: (a) ouabain inhibits the rates of K^+ influx and Na^+ efflux; (b) the rate of Na^+ efflux is significantly reduced when extracellular K^+ is removed, and (c) a Na^+, K^+ activated, ouabain-inhibited ATPase activity is present in the plasma membrane of neutrophils (6, 10, 28, 33, 35, 38–41).

Sodium ions should be able to enter the cell by at least one or more of three known distinct pathways (Figure 1). They include the Na^+/H^+ antiport, the Na^+/Ca^{2+} exchange, and the Na^+ channel. The plasma membrane of the neutrophil contains a 1:1 tightly coupled antiport that exchanges extracellular Na^+ for internal H^+, and it has an affinity for Li^+ and NH^+_4 in addition to Na^+ (17, 34). The interaction of external Na^+ with the antiport follows Michaelis-Menten kinetics and suggests a single binding site. This component of Na^+ inward movement is inhibited by amiloride and its analogues and is stimulated by, among other things, protein kinase C activation. A second mechanism by which Na^+ can enter the cell is through the Na^+/Ca^{2+} exchange system. This low affinity high capacity transport system for regulating the free concentration of intracellular calcium in which Na-influx is coupled to Ca-efflux is quite common in muscle and probably non-muscle cells. Although such a system most likely is found in the plasma membrane of the neutrophil, its presence has been difficult to demonstrate experimentally (44). Unlike the Na^+/H^+ antiport, there are no known specific inhibitors for the Na^+/Ca^{2+} exchange system. A third possible mechanism for Na^+ entry is through channels. Again, because of the lack of specific inhibitors, the presence of such a transport mechanism is difficult to demonstrate experimentally.

The main mechanism for Na^+-efflux is through the well-known Na^+, K^+ pump that exchanges $3Na^+$ for $2K^+$, and it is driven by metabolic energy derived from the hydrolysis of ATP (28, 35, 41). This transport system is inhibited by ouabain and requires the presence of K^+ in the bathing medium. A second pathway for Na^+-efflux has been demonstrated recently in human neutrophils (40). This system transports $3Na^+$ out of the cell in exchange for $1Ca^{2+}$. This counter exchange system is noncompetitively inhibited by benzamil and by some other amiloride analogues bearing a substituent on the terminal nitrogen atom of the guanidine group (40).

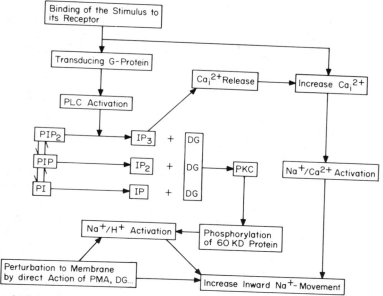

Figure 1   Schematic representation of the various pathways for Na^+-influx. The symbols are as follows: PLC, phospholipase C; PIP_2 phosphatidylinositol 4,5-bis-phosphate; PIP, phosphatidylinositol 4-phosphate; PI, phosphatidylinositol; DG, diacylglycerol; IP_2 inositol 1,4-bisphosphate; IP, inositol 1-phosphate; IP_3, inositol 1,4,5-trisphosphate.

Potassium can enter the cell by at least two transport mechanisms. The first transport system involves the above mentioned ouabain inhibited Na^+, K^+ pump (28, 41). A second mechanism for K^+ entry is through K^+ channels. The presence of K^+ channels and their specificity is difficult to demonstrate experimentally because of the lack of suitable inhibitors. There are several channels through which K^+ can leave the cells: those that are present when the cells are under resting conditions and those that are normally quiescent and become evident following cell activation. The most widely known system is the calcium-activated potassium channel. This system, which can be inhibited by oligomycin, furosemide, quinine, and quinidine, was first described in red cells, and it is known as the Gardos effect (21). The rise in Ca^{2+} also activates other non-selective cation channels as measured by the patch-clamp method (45).

Na^+-influx is enhanced by agonists that are known to activate the neutrophils. These agonists include fMet-Leu-Phe, leukotriene B_4, platelet-activating factor, arachidonic acid, phorbol 12-myristate, 13-acetate (but not inactive phorbol esters), and others (25, 28, 40, 41; for review see 34, 35). These stimuli activate one or more of the pathways through which Na^+ can enter the cell (Figure 1). This enhancement of Na^+-influx can be inhibited by amiloride and its analogues but not by the protein kinase C inhibitor 1-(5-isoquinolinesulphonyl)-2-methylpiperazine dihydrochloride (H-7) or by the calmodulin inhibitor trifluoperazine (TFP) (25, R. Sha'afi, unpublished data).

Among the various agonists, the effect of the chemotactic factor fMet-Leu-Phe on cation transport has been the most studied. The chemotactic factor produces a rapid and concentration-dependent increase in Na^+-influx. Smaller enhancements of K^+-influx and Na^+-efflux are also produced by fMet-Leu-Phe. The chemotactic factor-sensitive increase in K^+-influx and Na^+-efflux are inhibited by ouabain. In addition, the observed increase in Na^+-efflux is abolished in the absence of extracellular K^+. Unlike Na^+-efflux the efflux of K^+ is not stimulated by fMet-Leu-Phe.

In considering the role of Na^+ and K^+ in neutrophil responses elicited by soluble and particulate agents, we would like to distinguish between the two ways in which they may be involved. First, they may modulate cell responses indirectly by affecting one or more steps in the main sequence of events in the excitation response mechanism (receptor binding, guanine nucleotide binding protein, or phospholinase C activity), or they may modify the biochemical or biophysical changes (pH, actin polymerization, levels of cyclic nucleotides) that are elicited by agonists. Such a role implies that Na^+ and K^+ are not necessary to elicit the response by the stimulus, but they could be necessary for optimal stimulation. Second, Na^+ and/or K^+ may play a direct role in some or all of the neutrophil responses elicited by various stimuli. Such a role implies that Na^+ and/or K^+ are either necessary and sufficient, necessary but not sufficient, or sufficient but not necessary to elicit the response. The role of univalent cations in the physiologic responses of neutrophils has been thoroughly investigated using various experimental manipulations (3, 4, 18, 20, 25, 30, 31, 33, 35–37, 46–48). These studies can be conveniently divided into substitution experiments in which one or more ionic species is removed and/or replaced by another and investigations into the effects of ionophores. It is noteworthy that a change in the concentration of any one of the ions in the bathing medium results in rapid and significant changes in the concentrations of other intracellular ionic species. This is true because the permeability of the plasma membrane of the neutrophils to Na^+ and K^+ is relatively high, and the movements of the various cations are coupled. Rarely can the effects of the removal of one ionic species from the extracellular fluid be pinpointed precisely. Therefore the results from substitution experiments, though informative, must be interpreted with caution.

The basic assumption in the use of ionophores to investigate the role of a given ion in a specific event is that the basal permeability of the plasma membrane of the cell under study is very low and that the addition of the ionophore significantly increases the membrane permeability to this specific ion. This assumption holds true in many but not necessarily all cases. Studies in which ionophores specific to K^+ or Na^+ are used in neutrophils must be viewed with reservation and interpreted cautiously unless the ionophoretic ability is directly demonstrated.

Modulatory influences of extracellular Na^+ and K^+ on chemotaxis have been studied, and it has been found that physiologically balanced salt solutions are necessary for optimal cell locomotion. If the concentration of Na^+ or K^+ is varied quite widely, a locomotor response can still be obtained though the strength of the response is significantly diminished (3, 35, 46, for recent review see reference 11). For example, removal of K^+ from the bathing medium and/or the addition of ouabain depress the chemotactic responsiveness of neutrophils by about 50%, i.e. the concentration of the chemotactic factor required to elicit a specific level of responsiveness is doubled in the presence of ouabain. Under these conditions chemotaxis is not abolished. The dose-response curve is simply displaced to the right. In addition, increasing the concentration of K^+ can overcome the ouabain inhibition of chemotaxis. Furthermore, increasing the extracellular K^+ concentration causes a polarizing response in neutrophils similar to the response produced by fMet-Leu-Phe, and this response is not inhibited by ouabain (18). It is worth noting that the K^+ channel blocker tetraethylammonium chloride does not inhibit cell polarization produced by fMet-Leu-Phe.

The effects of the known K^+ ionophores valinomycin and nigericin on chemotaxis in neutrophils have been thoroughly studied. Valinomycin at low concentrations ($10^{-7}M$) slightly enhances chemotaxis in the presence of extracellular K^+ but has no effect in its absence. Nigericin at the same concentration has no effect on chemotaxis in the presence of K^+ and slightly inhibits chemotaxis in its absence. The differential effects of these two K^+ ionophores suggest that the potentiating action of valinomycin on chemotaxis may not be mediated by its K^+ transporting ability.

Brief removal of extracellular sodium leads to an increase in spontaneous (i.e. in the absence of the chemotactic factor) motility (3, 18, 35, 36). This enhancement in spontaneous activity is dependent on the presence of extracellular Ca^{2+} and may result from the inhibition of a Na^+ influx, Ca^{2+} efflux exchange mechanism. On the other hand, replacing sodium by choline significantly inhibits cell polarization induced by fMet-Leu-Phe (18). The number of polarized cells decreases with decreasing Na^+ concentration in the extracellular solution. One likely interpretation of these results is that the stimulated influx of sodium produced by fMet-Leu-Phe is required for cell polarization and subsequent locomotion. The observed increase in spontaneous activity in the absence of Na^+ may account for this decrease in cell polarization. Since the increased spontaneous activity is dependent on the presence of Ca^{2+}, it will be interesting to examine the effect of this ion on the observed decrease in cell polarization produced by the removal of Na^+.

The roles of extracellular Na^+ and K^+ in degranulation induced by various stimuli have been examined (4, 20, 33, 35). The effect of extracellular K^+ on degranulation by cytochalasin B-treated neutrophils stimulated by fMet-Leu-Phe is essentially similar to that observed for chemotaxis. Removal of K^+ from the bathing medium shifts the dose-response curve to the right, and ouabain is essentially without any effect. The two ionophores tested, valinomycin and nigericin, have no effect on chemotactic factor-induced degranulation from cytochalasin B-treated cells. However, valinomycin at concentrations greater than 10^{-7} M causes rabbit neutrophils to degranulate to a small but significant extent. Its secretory action requires the presence of extracellular Ca^{2+} and is enhanced by cytochalasin B. The most likely explanation for this finding is that valinomycin may act as a weak Ca^+ ionophore.

Replacing extracellular sodium with choline inhibits the release of lysozyme and β-glucuronidase in human neutrophils stimulated with immune complexes fMet-Leu-Phe or the calcium ionophore A23187 (20, 35). These results suggest that a Na^+-influx may be necessary for degranulation. On the other hand, amiloride, which inhibits most of the stimulated Na^+-influx, has little, if any, inhibitory action on the release of lysozyme or β-glucuronidase in neutrophils stimulated with several agonists (4). These agonists include fMet-Leu-Phe, PMA, and A23187. This argues against a necessary role for Na^+-influx in degranulation. Moreover the Na^+ ionophore monensin, which has been shown to increase Na^+-influx, does not elicit β-glucuronidase release (20). These data strongly suggest that Na^+-influx is not sufficient to stimulate degranulation.

Replacement of extracellular Na^+ by other univalent cations such as choline significantly inhibits ($>50\%$) superoxide generation stimulated with various agonists including fMet-Leu-Phe (20, 33, 38). Furthermore, prolonged incubation of human neutrophils with amiloride (10^{-3}M) greatly reduces superoxide generation produced by fMet-Leu-Phe, but it does not affect the corresponding increase produced by the protein kinase activator PMA (4). On the other hand, monensin does not elicit superoxide generation (20), and protein kinase C inhibitors, though they block PMA-induced superoxide production, do not alter the stimulation of Na^+-influx generated by PMA. These data strongly suggest that the presence of Na^+ and/or Na^+-influx are necessary for fMet-Leu-Phe but not PMA-produced stimulation of the oxidative burst, and that Na^+-influx is not sufficient for this response.

It has been suggested that the apparent requirement for Na^+ for a stimulated oxidative burst in neutrophils is due to exposing the cells to an erythrocyte lysis medium that contains NH^+_4 (30). We tested this point by examining the effect of replacing sodium chloride with choline chloride on superoxide production in rabbit peritoneal neutrophils stimulated with fMet-Leu-Phe and

PMA. We found that at the lower concentration of the stimulus, removal of Na^+ has no effect on the magnitude of superoxide production. At the higher concentration of the stimulus, however, removal of Na^+ significantly depresses ($>25\%$) superoxide production by the two stimuli.

The role, if any, of the univalent cations Na^+ and K^+ in stimulated neutrophil responses appears to be modulatory in nature, and these cations are not an essential part of the basic sequence of the excitation-response coupling. Having the proper intracellular concentration of Na^+ and K^+ is important for the optimum responsiveness of the cells. The main points concerning the role of Na^+ and K^+ in neutrophil response are summarized in Table 1.

CALCIUM MOVEMENT

The regulation of the intracellular concentration of free calcium, Ca_i^{2+}, in the neutrophils is achieved by pump-leak systems at the plasma membrane and by binding of Ca^{2+} by cytoplasmic constituents and plasma membrane (35). There are probably two separate channels by which Ca^{2+} could leak into the cells. The first channel is independent of membrane potential, whereas the second channel could be controlled by the membrane potential. In addition, there are at least two different energy-dependent mechanisms for the control of Ca^{2+} efflux: a specific calcium pump driven by the hydrolysis of ATP by a Mg^{2+}, Ca^{2+}-activated ATPase, the presence of which has been demonstrated in the plasma membrane of neutrophils, and a Na^+ influx, Ca^{2+} efflux

Table 1 The effects of changing Na^+ and K^+ movements by several experimental manipulations on the neutrophil responses produced by the chemotatic factor fMet-Leu-Phe

1. Removal of extracellular Na^+ inhibits cell polarization, reduces chemotaxis, and significantly inhibits ($>50\%$) degranulation and superoxide production. The effect on chemotaxis and degranulation is to shift the dose-response curve to the right.

2. Amiloride ($10^{-3}M$), which inhibits Na^+-influx, slightly inhibits ($<25\%$) degranulation and greatly ($>50\%$) reduces superoxide generation. The PMA-induced superoxide production is not inhibited by amiloride.

3. Ouabain, which inhibits the Na^+, K^+ pump, reduces chemotaxis but has no effect on either degranulation or the oxidative burst.

4. The Na^+ ionophore monensin, which stimulates Na^+-influx in neutrophils, does not by itself elicit superoxide generation or significant degranulation (β-glucuronidase).

5. The potassium ionophores valinomycin and nigericin do not significantly enhance chemotaxis, and they do not by themselves produce significant degranulation.

exchange system. This component depends on maintaining the Na^+ gradient across the cell membrane by the classic Na^+, K^+ pump.

In addition to these membrane events, control of cytosol Ca^{2+} is also dependent on binding to the membrane, buffering by cytosol constituents such as soluble proteins and others, and accumulating into intracellular organelles such as mitochondria, endoplasmic reticulum, granules, and others.

With the exception of PMA, all agonists that have been tested that stimulate neutrophils cause an increase in the intracellular concentration of free calcium, Ca_i^{2+} (7, 8, 9, 12, 19, 24, 26, 29, 32, 33). This rise in Ca_i^{2+} is brought about by a net influx from the outside because of an increase in plasma membrane permeability to calcium and a release of bound calcium from internal stores. Evidence that supports an increase in the plasma membrane permeability to calcium includes (7–9, 12, 29, 32, 33): (a) an increase in Ca^{2+} influx, and in the presence of extracellular Ca^{2+}, an increase in steady-state levels of Ca^{2+}; (b) chemotactic factors increase the specific activity of neutrophil Ca^{2+} and increase the pool of exchangeable Ca_i^{2+}; (c) the cytoplasmic Ca^{2+} signals monitored by quin2 and other calcium-sensitive dyes that are produced by fMet-Leu-Phe are reduced in the presence of EGTA; and (d) a rise in the Ca_i^{2+} seems to open nonspecific ion channels as measured by patch-clamp methods. The main evidence supporting a release of calcium from intracellular compartments following stimulation of neutrophils include (7–9, 12, 29, 32, 33): (a) chemotactic factors cause an efflux of Ca^{2+} from preloaded neutrophils, and in the absence of extracellular Ca^{2+} cause a transient decrease in steady-state levels of cell-associated Ca^{2+}; (b) these agents cause an early transient decrease in Ca^{2+} specific activity in the neutrophil; and (c) chemotactic factors cause a transient decrease in the fluorescence of chlorotetracycline-treated neutrophils, and an increase in quin2 and other calcium-sensitive dye signals. The intracellular messenger responsible for calcium release is inositol 1,4,5-trisphosphate, IP_3 (1, 5). The increase in membrane permeability to calcium is probably initiated by the depletion of calcium from the IP_3-sensitive pool.

In discussing the role of Ca^{2+} in various cell responses, one must distinguish between the basal level of Ca^{2+} and the stimulus-induced rise in Ca^{2+}. In some responses a rise in Ca_i^{2+} may be necessary while in others the basal level of Ca_i^{2+} may be sufficient. While it is easier to determine if a rise in Ca_i^{2+} is necessary for a given cell response, it is extremely difficult to determine if calcium per se is required (it is experimentally difficult to reduce Ca_i^{2+} to zero). The role of calcium in locomotion, degranulation, oxidative burst, and other cell responses will be discussed with this point in mind.

The migration of the neutrophil into inflamed tissue is important in fulfilling its vital function. Neutrophil locomotion, whether random or directed, depends on the displacement of the cell. Such displacement requires the conversion of chemical energy to mechanical energy, and the motile apparatus, with actin and myosin as the major components, must be involved in the locomotive activities of the cell. Regardless of whether the motility of the neutrophil is actin-based or actin-myosin based, it is most likely that calcium is closely related to this activity. For example, calcium and gelsolin may regulate the length of the actin filaments and/or activate the actin-myosin ATPase. Although there is no one single experiment that establishes unequivocally a role for calcium in cell motility, it is generally thought that Ca^{2+} is important for motility (3, 11, 35, 42, 46, 47).

The available experimental data concerning calcium and cell motility can be summarized in several points. (a) In spite of early observations, extracellular calcium is not necessary for fMet-Leu-Phe-induced chemotaxis as assayed by migration through micropore filters and by time-lapse videomicroscopy (48). (b) Increasing Ca_i^{2+} excessively (this is normally achieved by incubating the cells with a calcium ionophore in the presence of calcium) inhibits locomotion of neutrophils stimulated with fMet-Leu-Phe (23, 48). (c) Binding of intracellular free calcium by quin2 or chlorotetracycline or inhibiting the release of calcium by TMB-8 inhibits chemotaxis toward fMet-Leu-Phe (13, 22; see original citation 34). The effects of these agents are probably not due to their actions on Ca^{2+} alone, since they are likely to have other effects as well. Consistent with this conclusion is the observation that reducing Ca_i^{2+} by incubating the cells with the calcium ionophore A23187 and EGTA has no effect on fMet-Leu-Phe-induced chemotaxis (48). (d) Inhibitors of calmodulin reduce chemotaxis toward fMet-Leu-Phe (22). Since calmodulin is known to mediate certain calcium-dependent enzymatic activities, it appears that Ca^{2+} is necessary for chemotaxis. Again the inhibitory effect of these compounds is probably not due solely to their action on calcium. A reasonable conclusion, based on the available experimental data, is that a very low concentration of Ca^{2+} is sufficient, if Ca^{2+} is indeed necessary, for chemotaxis.

The addition of chemotactic factors and other soluble and insoluble agonists to neutrophils cause, under the appropriate conditions, the release of both the azurophil and specific granule contents. Since secretion requires the fusion of intracellular granules with the plasma membrane, it is reasonable to hypothesize that chemotactic factor-induced degranulation in neutrophils involves Ca^{2+} and that the level of Ca^{2+}_i necessary for degranulation is most likely higher than that needed for locomotion. Different requirements are needed for the release from the azurophil and specific granules (2). With certain stimuli such as PMA, a rise in cellular Ca^{2+} does not seem to be necessary for the small, slow lysosomal enzyme release. But even in this case, a role for calcium cannot be completely ruled out. It is expected that a reduction in the basal level of Ca_i^{2+} will inhibit PMA-induced lysosomal enzyme release.

The available data in the neutrophil system strongly suggest that the calcium ion is required for degranulation and that in most cases a rise in Ca_i^{2+} is also necessary. This conclusion is supported by several experimental findings (7, 8, 12, 29, 33). (*a*) The calcium ionophore A23187 stimulates degranulation, and the addition of EGTA significantly reduces lysozyme release and abolishes β-glucuronidase release. Removal of extracellular calcium diminishes, but does not totally abolish, degranulation produced by chemotactic factors such as C_{5a}. The pattern of granule fusion as visualized in freeze-fracture replicas is influenced by calcium in the suspending medium during stimulation by fMet-Leu-Phe or C_{5a}. It has been found that the directed pattern of fusion is initiated by release of intracellular calcium or a calcium-independent pathway, and the nondirected convoluted pattern of fusion is initiated by entry of extracellular calcium. (*b*) Incubation of neutrophils for 20 min or longer in calcium-free medium reduces lysosomal enzyme release produced by fMet-Leu-Phe, and this inhibition can be restored by the addition of calcium. The addition of EGTA totally inhibits N-acetyl-β-glucosaminidase release induced by platelet-activating factor. (*c*) Calcium causes degranulation in permeabilized cells. Calmodulin inhibitors and the intracellular calcium release antagonist TMB-8 reduce degranulation produced by various stimuli. However, the effects of these inhibitors may be unrelated to their actions on calcium or calcium-calmodulin. (*d*) The extent of exocytosis from specific granules (vitamin B_{12} binding protein), azurophil granules (β-glucuronidase), and secretory vesicles (gelatinase) is a function of the intracellular concentration of free calcium. Although the minimum concentration of Ca^{2+} that causes significant release from the three granule populations is similar, the EC_{50} values are significantly different for the three compartments. The rank order of increasing EC_{50} values is specific as follows: < secretory < azurophil (33). Rabbit neutrophils maintained, washed, and reacted in the absence of extracellular Ca^{2+} give a dose-response curve that is shifted to the right and in which the maximal level of release is significantly decreased. Depletion of intracellular calcium by exposure to the calcium ionophore blocks the ability of fMet-Leu-Phe to stimulate enzyme release.

A number of soluble and particulate agents stimulate the oxidative metabolism in the neutrophil, and this activation increases the production of superoxide radicals (O_2^-). Although a rise in intracellular concentration of free calcium is likely to be necessary for optimal stimulation of the oxidative burst, it is not absolutely required. Moreover, a rise in Ca_i^{2+} alone is not sufficient since several soluble and insoluble stimuli can produce a rise in Ca_i^{2+}, but do not stimulate superoxide generation. Based on the available data, it is most likely that, although a rise in intracellular calcium may not be absolutely necessary, a rise in Ca_i^{2+} is closely involved in this response to certain stimuli. This hypothesis is supported by numerous studies (7, 8, 12, 16, 29, 32, 33, 43). (a) The calcium ionophore A23187 stimulates superoxide release, and this release is abolished in the presence of EGTA. The action of A23187 may be mediated through the generation of one or more lipid mediators. These mediators are produced by activation of phospholipase A_2, which is critically dependent on Ca^{2+}. (b) There is a good correlation between the rise in Ca_i^{2+} and O_2^- generation produced by fMet-Leu-Phe. (c) The addition of EGTA reduces superoxide generation by most stimuli tested. (d) Although outside calcium may not be required for O_2^- generation, cells depleted of calcium show no release of O_2^- on stimulation with fMet-Leu-Phe when calcium is absent in the outside medium, and this inhibition can be overcome by the addition of calcium. It must be pointed out, however, that under calcium depletion conditions, the level of Ca_i^{2+} may be too low to sustain phospholipase C activation by fMet-Leu-Phe. This depressed state will interfere with the hydrolysis of PIP_2 and the generation of diacylglycerol, which is important for O_2^- production.

The role of Ca^{2+} in the stimulated oxidative burst can be best summarized as follows: First, with some but not all stimuli, a rise in Ca_i^{2+} is neither necessary nor sufficient. Second, although a rise in Ca_i^{2+} is not necessary, some calcium ion is most likely required. The basal, or somewhat lower, concentration of Ca_i^{2+} is probably sufficient to fulfill this requirement. Third, the involvement of calcium is most likely in the translocation and/or activation of protein kinase C to the membrane.

HYDROGEN ION MOVEMENT

The presence in the plasma membrane of the neutrophil of an antiport that exchanges outside sodium for intracellular hydrogen has been demonstrated (17, 34). The exchanger is a ubiquitous transport system with a tightly coupled 1:1 stoichiometry, and it has affinity for Li^+ and NH_4^+ in addition to Na^+ and H^+. The energy required for this exchange is derived from the inwardly directed Na^+ concentration gradient, which is generated by the ouabain sensitive Na^+, K^+ pump. In neutrophils this Na^+/H^+ exchange system is largely quiescent near the physiologic pH.

It is found that the addition of the chemotactic factor fMet-Leu-Phe to neturophils causes rapid and biphasic changes in intracellular pH. Initially there is a rapid drop followed by a slower and larger increase. The importance of the Na^+/H^+ antiport in relation to maintaining ionic and pH equilibrium during normal cell metabolism is obvious. The importance of changes in

Table 2 Effect of GM-CSF on the basal and stimulated level of intracellular concentration of free calcium in human neutrophils

Stimulus	Intracellular concentrations of free calcium, nM	
	Control cells	GM-CSF-treated cells[1]
No addition	100	110
fMet-Leu-Phe	276	700
Platelet activating factor (5 nM)	318	430

[1] The cells were incubated with GM-CSF (200 pM) for 30 min (Similar results were first reported in reference 26).

intracellular pH in cell function or as a signal in the activation and/or regulation of cell activation has been reviewed recently (34).

EFFECT OF GRANULOCYTE-MACROPHAGE COLONY STIMULATING FACTOR ON ION MOVEMENTS IN HUMAN NEUTROPHILS

The human hormone granulocyte-macrophage colony stimulating factor (GM-CSF), which is released by several activated cells such as T lymphocytes, is an important stimulus for the proliferation of erythroid and myelomonocytic stem cells in vitro (14). Although the addition of GM-CSF to mature human neutrophils does not activate cells responses, it primes these cells to subsequent stimulation by the chemotactic factor fMet-Leu-Phe. Thus GM-CSF plays an important role in the host defense. In spite of its importance, the mechanism of GM-CSF action is totally unknown.

The effects of GM-CSF on the basal and stimulated ion (Na^+, Ca^{2+}, pH, $PO^=_4$) movements in human neutrophils stimulated wth fMet-Leu-Phe have been studied, and the results are summarized in Tables 2 and 3 (15). Several

Table 3 GM-CSF-induced stimulation of ion movements in control and pertussis toxin-treated human neutrophils

Ion	GM-CSF-induced change (relative to control)	
	− pertussis toxin	+ pertussis toxin[2]
PAF-induced		
$[Ca_i^{2+}]$ rise	1.35	1.20
$^{22}Na^+$-influx	2.3	1.60
PO_4 uptake	1.90	1.50

[2] Cells were incubated with 0.5 μg/ml pertussis toxin for 45 min before the addition of GM-CSF (200pM). The remaining conditions are the same as those for Table 2.

points can be made from these results. Both the basal and fMet-Leu-Phe stimulated Na^+-influx are increased in GM-CSF-treated neutrophils. GM-CSF causes a rise in the intracellular pH (3). The changes in Na^+ and H^+ movements produced by GM-CSF are rapid, and they can be abolished by amiloride, protein kinase C inhibitors, and they are significantly reduced by pertussis toxin. The stimulation of the Na^+/H^+ antiport by GM-CSF deactivates this system to further activation by PMA or fMet-Leu-Phe. While the basal concentration of Ca_i^{2+} is not affected, the rise in Ca_i^{2+} produced by fMet-Leu-Phe or platelet activating factor (PAF) is greatly increased in GM-CSF treated cells. GM-CSF stimulates the uptake of radioactive phosphate. Unlike Na^+-influx, the action of GM-CSF on phosphate uptake is much slower. The GM-CSF-induced increase in cell-associated radioactive phosphate reflects several biochemical changes such as increased ATP generation, phosphorylation of proteins by tyrosine and other kinases, and other cellular modifications (R. Sha'afi, unpublished data). The observed stimulation of phosphate uptake is inhibited by pertussis toxin, but not by cholera toxin or botulinum D toxin.

ACKNOWLEDGMENTS

This work was supported in part by National Institutes of Health grants AI-24937 and GM-37694.

Literature Cited

1. Abdel-Latif, A. A. 1986. Calcium-mobilizing receptors, polyphosphoinositides, and the generation of second messengers. *Pharmacol. Rev.* 38:227–72

2. Barrowman, M. M., Cockcroft, S., Gomperts, B. D. 1987. Differential control of azurophilic and specific granule exocytosis in *Sendaivirus*-permeabilized rabbit neutrophils. *J. Physiol.* 383:115–24

3. Becker, E. L. 1980. Chemotaxis. *J. Allergy Clin. Immunol.* 66:97–105

4. Berkow, R. L., Dodson, R. W., Kraft, A. S. 1987. Dissociation of human neutrophil activation events by prolonged treatment with amiloride. *J. Lab. Clin. Med.* 110:97–105

5. Berridge, M. J. 1987. Inositol trisphosphate and diacylglycerol: Two interacting second messengers. *Annu. Rev. Biochem.* 56:159–94

6. Block, J. B., Bonting, S. L. 1964. Sodium-potassium activated adenosinetriphosphatase and cation transport in normal and leukemic human leukocytes. *Enzymol. Biol. Clin.* 4:183–98

7. Boxer, G. J., Curnutte, J. T., Boxer, L. A. 1985. Polymorphonuclear leukocyte function. *Hosp. Pract.* 20:69–90

8. Boxer, L. A., Smolen, J. E. 1988. Neutrophil granule constituents and their release in health and disease. In *Hematology/Oncology Clinics of North America;* ed. J. T. Curnutte, 2:101–34. Philadelphia: Saunders

9. Chandler, D. E., Kazilek, C. J. 1987. Calcium signals in neutrophils can be divided into three distinct phases. *Biochim. Biophys. Acta* 931:175–79

10. Cividalli, G., Nathan, D. G. 1974. Sodium and potassium transmembrane fluxes in leukocytes. *Blood* 43:861–869

11. Devreotes, P. N., Zigmond, S. H. 1988. Chemotaxis in eukaryotic cells: A focus on leukocytes and Dictyostelium. *Annu. Rev. Cell Biol.* 4:649–86

12. Dillon, S. B., Verghese, M. W., Snyderman, R. 1988. Signal transduction in cells following binding of chemoattractants to membrane receptors. *Virchaus Archiv.* B 55:65–80

13. Elferink, J. G. R., Deierkauf, M. 1985.

Involvement of intracellular Ca^{2+} in chemotaxis and metabolic burst by neutrophils. The use of antagonists of intracellular Ca^{2+}. *Res. Commun. Chem. Pathol. Pharmacol.* 50:67–81

14. Golde, D. W., Gasson, J. C. 1988. Hormones that stimulate the growth of blood cells. *Sci. Am.* 259:62–70

15. Gomez-Cambronero, J., Yamazaki, M., Metwally, F., Molski, T. F. P., Bonak, V. A., et al. 1989. Granulocyte-macrophage colony-stimulating factor and human neutrophils: Role of guanine-nucleotide regulatory proteins. *Proc. Natl. Acad. Sci. USA* 86:3569–73

16. Grinstein, S., Furuya, W. 1988. Receptor-mediated activation of electropermeabilized neutrophils. *J. Biol. Chem.* 263:1779–83

17. Grinstein, S., Rothstein, A. 1986. Mechanisms of regulation of the Na^+/H^+ exchanger. *J. Membr. Biol.* 90:1–12

18. Haston, W. S., Shields, J. M. 1986. Signal transduction in human neutrophil leukocytes: Effects of external Na^+ and Ca^{2+} on cell polarity. *J. Cell Sci.* 82:249–61

19. Korchak, H. M., Vosshall, L. B., Zagon, G., Ljubich, P., Rich, A. M., Weissman, G. 1988. Activation of the neutrophil by calcium-mobilizing ligands. *J. Biol. Chem.* 263:11090–97

20. Korchak, H. M., Weissmann, G. 1980. Stimulus-response coupling in the human neutrophil: transmembrane potential and the role of extracellular Na^+. *Biochim. Biophys. Acta* 601:180–94

21. Lew, V. L., Ferreira, H. G. 1977. The effect of Ca on the K permeability of red cells. In *Membrane Transport in Red Cells*, ed. J. C. Ellory, V. L. Lew pp. 93–100. New York: Academic

22. Lohr, K. M., Felix, J. B., Kurth, C. 1984. Chlorpromazine inhibits neutrophil chemotaxis beyond the chemotactic receptor-ligand interaction. *J. Infect. Dis.* 150:643–52

23. Marasco, W. A., Becker, E. L., Oliver, J. M. 1980. The ionic basis of chemotaxis: separate cation requirements for neutrophil orientation and locomotion in a gradient. *Am. J. Pathol.* 98:749

24. Meshulam, T., Diamond, R. D., Lyman, C. A., Wysong, D. R., Melnick, D. A. 1988. Temporal association of calcium mobilization, inositol trisphosphate generation, and superoxide anion release by human neutrophils activated by serum opsonized and nonopsonized particulate stimuli. *Biochem. Biophys. Res. Commun.* 150:532–39

25. Molski, T. F. P., Ford, C., Weisman, S. J., Sha'afi, R. I., 1986. Cell alkaliniza-

tion is not necessary and increased sodium influx is not sufficient for stimulated superoxide production. *FEBS. Lett.* 203:267–72

26. Naccache, P. H., Faucher, N., Borgeat, P., Gasson, J. C., Dipersio, J. F. 1988. Granulocyte-macrophage colony-stimulating factor modulates the excitation-response coupling sequence in human neutrophils. *J. Immunol.* 140:3541–46

27. Naccache, P. H., Sha'afi, R. I. 1988. Measurements of ionic events relevant to neutrophil activation. *Methods Enzymol.* 162:283–98

28. Naccache, P. H., Showell, H. J., Becker, E. L., Sha'afi, R. I. 1977. Transport of sodium, potassium and calcium across rabbit polymorphonuclear leukocyte membranes: Effect of chemotactic factor. *J. Cell Biol.* 73:428–44

29. Omann, G. M., Allen, R. A., Bokoch, G. M., Painter, R. G., Traynor, A. E., Sklar, L. A. 1987. Signal transduction and cytoskeletal activation in the neutrophil. *Physiol. Rev.* 67:285–322

30. Pfefferkorn, L. C. 1984. Transmembrane signaling: An ion flux-independent model for signal transduction by complexed F_c receptors. *J. Cell Biol.* 99:2231–40

31. Roberts, R. L., Mounessa, N. L., Gallin, J. I. 1984. Increasing extra-cellular potassium causes calcium-dependent shape change and facilitates concanavalin-A capping in human neutrophils. *J. Immun.* 132:2000–5

32. Rossi, F. 1986. The O_2^--forming NADPH oxidase of the phagocytes: nature, mechanisms of activation and function. *Biochim. Biophys. Acta* 853:65–89

33. Sha'afi, R. I., Molski, T. F. P. 1988. Activation of the neutrophil. *Prog. Allergy* 42:1–64

34. Sha'afi, R. I., Molski, T. F. P. 1988. Effects of neutrophils and platelet activators. In Na^+/H^+ *Exchange*, ed. S. Grinstein pp. 271–283. Boca Raton: CRC Press

35. Sha'afi, R. I., Naccache, P. H. 1981. Ionic events in neutrophil chemotaxis and secretion. *Adv. Inflamm. Res.* 2:115–48

36. Showell, H. J., Becker, E. L. 1976. The effects of external K^+ and Na^+ on the chemotaxis of rabbit peritoneal neutrophils. *J. Immunol.* 116:99–105

37. Showell, H. J., Naccache, P. H., Sha'afi, R. I., Becker, E. L. The effects of extracellular K^+, Na^+ and Ca^{2+} on lysosomal enzyme secretion from polymorphonuclear leukocytes. *J. Immunol.* 119:804–811

38. Simchowitz, L., Spilberg, I. 1979. Chemotactic factor-induced generation of superoxide radicals by human neutrophils: Evidence for the role of sodium. *J. Immunol.* 123:2428–35

39. Simchowitz, L. 1985. Chemotactic factor-induced activation of Na^+/H^+ exchange in human neutrophils. I. sodium fluxes. *J. Biol. Chem.* 260:13237–47

40. Simchowitz, L., Cragoe, E. J. Jr. 1988. Na^+-Ca^{2+} exchange in human neutrophils. *Am. J. Physiol.* (Cell Physiol.) 23:C150–64

41. Simchowitz, L., Spilberg, I., De Weer, P. 1982. Sodium and potassium fluxes and membrane potential of human neutrophils. Evidence for an electrogenic sodium pump. *J. Gen. Physiol.* 79:453–79

42. Snyderman, R., Goetzl, E. J. 1981. Molecular and cellular mechanisms of leukocyte chemotaxis. *Science* 21:830–37

43. Tauber, A. I. 1987. Protein kinase C and the activation of the human neutrophil NADPH-oxidase. *Blood* 69:711–20

44. Volpi, M., Naccache, P. H., Sha'afi, R. I. 1983. Calcium transport in inside-out membrane vesicles prepared from rabbit neutrophils. *J. Biol. Chem.* 258:4153–58

45. Von Tscharner, V., Prod'hom, B., Baggiolini, M., Reuter, H. 1986. Ion channels in human neutrophils activated by a rise in free cytosolic calcium concentration. *Nature* 324:369–72

46. Wilkinson, P. C. 1982. In *Chemotaxis and Inflammation,* ed. P. C. Wilkinson, pp. 61. 2nd ed. Edinburgh: Churchill Livingstone

47. Zigmond, S. H. 1978. Chemotaxis by polymorphonuclear leukocytes. *J. Cell Biol.* 77:269–87

48. Zigmond, S. H., Slonczewski, J. L., Wilde, M. W., Carson, M. 1988. Polymorphonuclear leukocyte locomotion is insensitive to lowered cytoplasmic calcium levels. *Cell Motil. Cytoskel.* 9:184–89

Annu. Rev. Physiol. 1990. 52:381–97

FUNCTIONAL ANALYSIS OF THE MODES OF ANION TRANSPORT IN NEUTROPHILS AND HL-60 CELLS

Louis Simchowitz and James A. Bibb

Department of Medicine, the John Cochran Veterans Administration Medical Center, and Departments of Medicine, Cell Biology, and Physiology, Washington University School of Medicine, St. Louis, Missouri 63110

KEY WORDS: Cl^-/HCO_3^- exchange, Cl^- fluxes, leukocytes

INTRODUCTION

As the title implies, the subject of this review is anion transport, with particular emphasis on anion exchange in neutrophils and their close relatives, HL-60 cells. Neutrophils are bone marrow-derived white blood cells of the myeloid series. Also known as granulocytes or polymorphonuclear leukocytes, they represent one of the body's major cellular defense mechanisms against invading microbes, and they also contribute to the pathophysiology of tissue injury in a number of diseases. Following appropriate stimulation, neutrophils display a number of well-known responses that are vital to their normal function. These include chemotaxis, phagocytosis, free radical generation, and degranulation. Ultimately, these biological expressions of cell activation can be traced to, or at least regulated by, the movement of various ions across the plasma membrane, which results in changes in intracellular pH, membrane potential, and cytosolic free Ca^{2+} levels, to name a few.

Neutrophils are related to another cell type, also phagocytic, referred to as monocytes when circulating in the blood and as macrophages when present in the extravascular tissues. The close relationship between neutrophils and monocytes, both developmentally and functionally, is graphically illustrated

0066-4278/90/0315-0381$02.00

by HL-60 cells, a stable precursor cell line of granulocyte lineage derived from a patient with promyelocytic leukemia (6, 19). Exposure of HL-60 cells to a variety of agents induces them to undergo terminal differentiation along either of two distinct pathways (6, 20): one that bears many of the surface properties and functional characteristics of mature neutrophils (following exposure to dimethylsulfoxide, dibutyryl cAMP, or retinoic acid) and the other that resembles monocytes/macrophages (following addition of phorbol diesters).

Compared to the wealth of information on anion exchange in red blood cells that has accumulated over the past three decades, knowledge of anion transport in neutrophils and HL-60 cells is relatively limited and recent. In this review, our principal aim has been to highlight articles that provide important background material for future endeavors and that shed light on what may eventually be significant differences between these two leukocytic cell forms and the classical band 3 protein of erythrocytes.

Steady-State Cl^- Movements

It has been known for almost a century that anions readily cross the plasma membrane of mixed leukocytes. In 1902, Hamburger & van der Schroeff (25) first reported reversible exchanges of HCO_3^- for Cl^- or NO_3^- with concomitant acidity changes in horse leukocytes. Using a similar model, Fleischmann (18) in 1930 demonstrated permeability to I^-, SCN^-, and salicylate ions. Later, Wilson & Manery (72) showed that rabbit peritoneal leukocytes gain or lose Cl^- depending on the Cl^- concentration of the bathing medium. The study of Cl^- transport in isolated neutrophils in the modern era dates only to the present decade.

When bathed in a normal Cl^- medium ($[Cl^-]_o \geq 100$ mM) similar to that of the body's extracellular fluid and blood, neutrophils and HL-60 cells transfer $^{36}Cl^-$ between the cytosol and their environment at rates of ~ 1.5 and ~ 20–40 meq/liter of cell water·min, respectively (12, 52, 64, 65). Electrically silent anion exchange accounts for the vast majority of the total one-way steady-state $^{36}Cl^-$ influx and efflux of both cells. By way of comparison, these transport rates are 3–4 orders of magnitude lower than that of human red blood cells under comparable conditions (28, 33, 42, 49).

It is of considerable interest that in neither cell is Cl^- distributed passively. Rather, Cl^- is accumulated intracellularly to levels appreciably greater than that dictated by thermodynamic considerations: ~ 80 meq/liter of cell water for neutrophils [$V_m \sim -60$ mV (58, 64, 67)] and ~ 35 meq/liter of cell water for HL-60 cells [$V_m \sim -80$ mV (52)]. In an earlier study using HL-60 cells, Dissing et al (12) first reported an intracellular Cl^- concentration of 84 meq/liter of cell water. The disparity between this and the value of ~ 35 meq/liter reported by Restrepo et al (52) may relate in part to the presence of physiologic concentrations (25 mM) of HCO_3^- in the medium in the latter studies. This interpretation is given credence by the finding by Restrepo et al (53) that the internal Cl^- level rises to ~53 meq/liter of cell water under HCO_3^--free conditions.

Nonetheless, the high internal Cl^- content (~4- and ~10-fold above electrochemical equilibrium in neutrophils and HL-60 cells, respectively) seems to be maintained by an active Cl^- transport system whose properties have yet to be precisely identified and characterized. In neither cell does the uptake appear to be Na^+-dependent. In neutrophils, however, the uphill transport of Cl^- is dependent on metabolic energy (it is absent in cells depleted of ATP by exposure to 2-deoxy-D-glucose) and is sensitive to the loop diuretics, furosemide and ethacrynic acid, and to α-cyano-4-hydroxycinnamate, which also blocks anion exchange (64). In HL-60 cells, the process is reportedly resistant to furosemide, bumetanide, and H_2DIDS (52). The existence of a primary ATP-driven Cl^- pump remains speculative. For both preparations, Cl^- permeability is rather low (52, 64, 67); electro-diffusive Cl^- fluxes are small and account for only a minor fraction of the total. Likewise, Na^+ movements through conductance pathways are low and K^+ permeability determines the membrane potential, the cells behaving nearly as K^+-selective electrodes for most practical purposes.

Dissing et al (12) compared $^{36}Cl^-$ fluxes in undifferentiated HL-60 cells and in DMSO-induced cells that possess phenotypic features characteristic of mature neutrophils. They observed a 2.5-fold reduction in steady-state exchange in differentiated cells. The rates were still roughly one order of magnitude greater than in normal neutrophils under resting conditions. As the activities of other transport systems are reportedly reduced in concert (7, 20), this reduction may be part of a generalized process that accompanies differentiation and functional maturation in these cells. At this point, the role of anion exchange in development is unclear.

Inhibitors

As compared to erythrocytes, the anion exchanger of human neutrophils, which functions physiologically as a Cl^-/HCO_3^- exchanger in intracellular pH regulation (66), exhibits several notable features in its sensitivity to drugs. The most profound difference involves the disulfonic stilbenes, the classical inhibitors of the band 3 protein of red cells (28, 33, 42, 49). For example, DIDS (4,4'-diisothiocyanostilbene-2,2'-disulfonate) and H_2DIDS are essentially inert towards anion exchange in neutrophils and SITS (4-acetamido-4'-isothiocyanostilbene-2,2'-disulfonate) has only modest activity at concentrations $\geq$ 1 mM (61, 64), whereas these compounds are effective in erythrocytes at concentrations in the micromolar range. In neutrophils, however, anion exchange can be competitively inhibited by a number of cinnamic (phenylpropenoic) acid derivatives (61, 65). These agents, originally synthesized as inhibitors of monocarboxylate transport in mitochondria (23, 24), also behave as mixed inhibitors of anion exchange in the red cell (11). The parent compound, α-cyano-4-hydroxycinnimate (CHC), is a weak inhibitor of anion exchange in neutrophils with an apparent K_i of $\sim$9 mM (65). The most potent analogue thus far identified in this series is α-cyano-β-(1-phenylindol-3-yl)acrylate (UK-5099) which is $\sim$300-fold more active (61). To date, these compounds have not been evaluated in HL-60 cells as far as we are aware.

In neutrophils, anion exchange is also sensitive to MK-473 (an indanyloxyacetate derivative), flufenamate, and niflumate (61). All of these compounds, including CHC and UK-5099, are weak organic acids by virtue of their carboxyl groups and compete with Cl^-, presumably by sharing the same binding site on the exchange carrier. In addition, a variety of compounds including NAP-taurine and eosin-5-isothiocyanate, which dramatically suppress red cell anion exchange, are either completely inert or only marginally effective in the millimolar concentration range (61). These properties serve to emphasize that major differences exist between human neutrophils and human erythrocytes in their sensitivity to various drugs.

Present literature indicates that HL-60 cells bear a much closer resemblance to red cells, at least in regard to the profile of inhibitors. The pattern is similar: HL-60 cells are very sensitive to the disulfonic stilbenes DIDS and H_2DIDS, which exhibit apparent K_i values of $\sim$10 and $\sim$100 μM, respectively (12, 52). Moreover, the loop diuretics furosemide (apparent K_i $\sim$500 μM) and ethacrynic acid (apparent K_i $\sim$200 μM) block the exchange in HL-60 cells (51, D. Restrepo, unpublished data), whereas these compounds seem to be rather ineffective in neutrophils (64). From the work of Restrepo & colleagues (51, D. Restrepo, unpublished data), the anion exchanger of HL-60 cells may also be blocked by pentachlorophenol, 3,5-diiodosalicylate, and 2,3,5-trinitrobenzoate with apparent K_i values of $\sim$15, $\sim$30, and $\sim$200 μM. These compounds also display substantial activity in neutrophils (L. Simchowitz, unpublished observations).

It should be stressed that all of these agents exhibit considerably less activity in HL-60 cells than in red cells, the inhibition constants being higher by 2–3 orders of magnitude. Similar results have been obtained in K-562 cells, an erythroleukemic cell line (12, 41). Thus it would appear that each of these forms of nonerythroid anion exchange is inherently less sensitive to a variety of classical inhibitors of erythrocyte band 3. Viewed in this perspective, the relative resistance of the exchange carrier of neutrophils to the disulfonic stilbenes may merely signify a quantitative change reflecting an alteration in the affinity of drug binding sites rather than a fundamental difference between the two proteins.

Substrate Selectivity

Cl^-/HCO_3^- EXCHANGE   The anion exchanger of human neutrophils exhibits broad specificity for a variety of inorganic as well as organic anions (60, 61, 63, 65). Its natural substrates, Cl^- and HCO_3^-, bind with high affinity. In addition, a variety of other monovalent anions are bound and transported in exchange for Cl^-. The rank order of decreasing affinities is as follows, the values given in parentheses represent the apparent half-saturation constants (in mM) for transport: HCO_3^- (2.5), Cl^- (5), NO_3^- (8), Br^- (9), formate$^-$ (13), F^- (23), I^- (44), p-aminohippurate$^-$ (50), SCN^- (56). Glucuronate and gluconate appear devoid of affinity. This selectivity sequence is remarkably similar to that reported by Aickin & Brading (1) for the Cl^-/HCO_3^- exchanger of smooth muscle cells of guinea pig vas deferens. When directly measured there is an equality between the magnitude of the influx of radiolabeled Cl^-, Br^-, I^-, or p-aminohippurate$^-$ and the corresponding counter-efflux of $^{36}Cl^-$, the usual intracellular exchange partner, which indicates that the kinetics are those of an obligate one-for-one counter-transport (60, 65). This 1:1 stoichiometry implies an electroneutral process and is in keeping with the observation that anion exchange is not appreciably affected by large changes in membrane voltage (64). This, too, is the case for HL-60 cells (12).

Of note is the fact that the principal anion (Cl^-/HCO_3^-) exchanger of neutrophils lacks affinity for SO_4^{2-} and other divalent anions such as oxalate and phosphate (60, 61). This finding is in contrast with that in red blood cells where Cl^- and SO_4^{2-} bind with comparably high affinity, although the maximal transport rate for Cl^- is 3–4 orders of magnitude greater than for SO_4^{2-} (33, 45, 56); oxalate is also handled by the erythrocyte carrier albeit slowly transported.

SO_4^{2-}/Cl^- EXCHANGE   Several years ago, Korchak et al (37, 38) reported that $^{35}SO_4^{2-}$ fluxes in human neutrophils could be blocked by SITS and DIDS. In view of the insensitivity of Cl^- transport to these inhibitors, this finding suggests that SO_4^{2-} and Cl^- must, for the most part, cross the plasma membrane via different routes. Recently, Simchowitz & Davis (62) described a separate mechanism for SO_4^{2-} transport that is distinct from Cl^-/HCO_3^- exchange. This system, which accounts for essentially all of the steady-state $^{35}SO_4^{2-}$ fluxes (~17 μmol/liter·min) across the membranes of these cells, consists of an electroneutral SO_4^{2-}/Cl^- counter-transport that displays many features reminiscent of classical anion exchange in erythrocytes. As will be summarized briefly below, the SO_4^{2-}/Cl^- exchange carrier of neutrophils also shares many general properties with other Na^+-independent SO_4^{2-}-transporting exchangers in epithelia and isolated cells (for reviews, see 26, 46). These include its marked sensitivity to SITS and ethacrynic acid (apparent K_i values of ~ 50 and ~ 7 μM). Unlike the Cl^-/HCO_3^- exchanger of neutrophils, the carrier is also inhibited by probenecid and furosemide; both are blocked by CHC.

The SO_4^{2-} carrier binds SO_4^{2-} and Cl^- with K_m values of ~ 14 and ~ 25 mM (62) as well as other divalent anions such as tungstate, oxalate, molybdate, and selenate (K_m values of ~ 1, 6, 45, and 60 mM, respectively). In addition, monovalent anions such as NO_3^-, Br^-, I^-, and formate$^-$ can also be handled, though with considerably lower affinity than was the case for the Cl^-/HCO_3^- exchanger. In fact, HCO_3^- appears to be inert. These findings leave little doubt that there are two distinct transport functions. To dramatize the similarity to red cells even further, the SO_4^{2-} carrier of human neutrophils exhibits a characteristic pH-dependence (62): extracellular acidification enhances the transport rate, while alkalinization reduces it. The relationship to pH relates to the fact that protons are substrates for the reaction, the carrier mediating an $H^+ + SO_4^{2-}$ cotransport in exchange for Cl^-. For details on this well-studied system in red cells, readers are referred to the original articles by Jennings (27) and by Milanick & Gunn (44, 45) as well as to recent reviews (28, 33).

The substrate selectivity of anion exchange in HL-60 cells has not been well studied. To date, the apparent K_m value for external Cl^- of ~ 5 mM measured at high intracellular Cl^- and the apparent K_m value for internal Cl^- of ~ 28 mM measured at saturating extracellular Cl^- (53) are similar to those parameters (~ 5 and ~ 35 mM, respectively) determined for neutrophils (65). Also, gluconate seems to be an inert spectator anion (52), but data on the affinities for other ions are currently unavailable. When comparing and contrasting the erythrocyte, neutrophil, and HL-60 cell exchangers, it is interesting to speculate as to whether or not Cl^- and SO_4^{2-} share the same transport system in HL-60 cells.

Effect of pH; Temperature-Dependence

The rate of anion exchange in both neutrophils and HL-60 cells is very sensitive to changes in pH within the physiologic range (51, 61). The relationship to extracellular pH (pH$_o$) echoes that in erythrocytes and is the reverse of that seen for SO_4^{2-} transport alluded to above. Extracellular alkalinization leads to a dramatic enhancement of the maximal velocity of $^{36}Cl^-$ exchange, while lowering the pH$_o$ of the medium has the opposite effect. These attributes seem to be common among anion exchangers throughout the animal kingdom since essentially identical findings have been observed in monkey renal epithelial cells (Vero line) and sheep cardiac Purkinje fibers, as well as in L, HeLa, and Hep-2 cells (47, 68, 69, 70). The biochemical basis underlying this alteration in transport rate and the nature of putative pH-regulatory sites of carrier activity are currently unknown. These observations have important implications for modulating the functional activity of Cl^-/HCO_3^- exchange during intracellular pH and cell volume regulation.

In the only study to address the issue of temperature-dependence, Dissing et al (12) reported an apparent activation energy of 32 kcal/mol for Cl^-/Cl^- exchange in HL-60 cells. Comparably high values have been observed for anion exchange in erythrocytes (33, 42).

Kinetics; Asymmetry

In erythrocytes, there is an obligatory one-for-one anion exchange that follows so-called ping-pong kinetics. The characteristics of such a tightly coupled system and the predictions of this model have been dealt with in great detail in several recent reviews (17, 28, 33) and will not be outlined here. Operationally, the mechanism involves the ordered, sequential binding of anions to both the internal and external translocation sites followed by a local conformational change allowing the ions to gain access to the other side, the two taking turns crossing the membrane. In red blood cells, the binding sites change orientation only when anions are bound; the empty, unloaded carrier cannot cross the permeability barrier. The current concept is that of a single site that alternately faces either the cytoplasm or the exterior (28, 30). At present, no systematic experimental data exist that address the issue of whether anion exchange in neutrophils conforms to a similar reaction scheme. It has generally been assumed that all forms of nonerythroid anion exchangers are likely to share in this basic principle.

Recently, Restrepo et al (53), working with HL-60 cells, have presented compelling evidence that this expectation may not necessarily be valid. By carefully correlating the dependence of the rate of Cl^-/Cl^- exchange on the intracellular and extracellular Cl^- concentrations, they found that anion exchange in resting, undifferentiated HL-60 cells seems to follow simultaneous kinetics. According to the simple reaction cycle proposed by the authors, the internal and external translocation sites are occupied by Cl^- in random order after which the two anions are simultaneously transported across the plasma membrane barrier. This is different from the ping-pong model where the translocation events take place sequentially. This finding raises the intriguing question as to whether one is dealing with a transport system that is fundamentally different from that of red cells, a point to which we shall return in discussing the molecular biology of these proteins.

On a related issue, evidence compatible with asymmetry of the neutrophil exchange carrier has been observed (63): binding constants for Cl^- and HCO_3^- ($\sim$22 and $\sim$10 mM, respectively) were $\sim$4-fold higher at the internal translocation site of the exchanger than for the external site ($\sim$5 and $\sim$2.5 mM). Data consistent with a similar $\sim$5-fold asymmetry (the carrier preferring to bind external Cl^-) in HL-60 cells have also been noted on the basis of a detailed kinetic analysis as reported by Restrepo et al (53). This property has been recognized for many years in red cells where a $\sim$15-fold asymmetry exists (and in the same direction) between inward- and outward-facing conformational states (17, 33, 49).

Function

In analogy to other cell types, a major physiologic role for Cl^-/HCO_3^- exchange has been postulated in intracellular pH (pH_i) regulation (54); recent consensus holds that a variety of neutrophil functional responses are regulated by pH_i (32, 57). In addition, pH_i may be an important factor in controlling the growth and development of HL-60 cells (39). For instance, cellular differentiation may depend on the anion exchanger for maintenance of the proper pH_i. By way of precedent, the v-erbA oncogene blocks differentiation of avian erythrocytes by specifically suppressing transcription of the band 3 gene (73). Furthermore, Cl^-/HCO_3^- exchange plays a crucial part in the uptake of solutes during cell volume regulation while SO_4^{2-}/Cl^- exchange seems to be involved in SO_4^{2-} transport into the cell.

INTRACELLULAR pH RECOVERY FROM ALKALINIZATION   Compared with the wealth of information regarding cellular mechanisms of acid extrusion (54), the processes underlying recovery from intracellular alkalinization have received relatively little attention. Passive ion fluxes and metabolic acid production have been invoked as possible mechanisms in the past. Only recently have more specialized membrane transport systems been recognized as a result of the original work of Vaughan-Jones (69, 70), who first clearly identified a SITS-sensitive Cl^-/HCO_3^- exchange as being chiefly responsible for pH_i recovery from alkalinization in sheep cardiac Purkinje fibers. In neutrophils, Simchowitz & Roos (66) documented an important contribution of Cl^-/HCO_3^- exchange in pH_i recovery after imposition of an alkaline load. Restoration of pH_i to its normal resting value ($\sim$7.25 at pH_o 7.40) was dependent on external Cl^-, enhanced by HCO_3^-, and blocked by inhibitors of anion exchange in these cells. The ion selectivity sequence and sensitivity of this alkalinization-induced anion exchange to various drugs were identical to those for Cl^-/Cl^- self-exchange in resting cells (63), which strongly implies that the same transport system is involved. It appears that the Cl^-/HCO_3^- exchanger in HL-60 cells subserves a similar role in the regulation of pH_i after alkalinization (52). An analogous mechanism occurs in monkey kidney cells (47, 68).

INTRACELLULAR pH RECOVERY FROM ACIDIFICATION   In other preparations, a Cl^-/HCO_3^- exchange seems to promote recovery from acidification by acting in concert with a separate Na^+/H^+ exchange. This is the case in mouse skeletal muscle, monkey kidney cells, and human epidermoid carcinoma cells (2, 43, 47, 55). In human neutrophils and HL-60 cells that possess both transport systems, however, Na^+/H^+ exchange constitutes the dominant, if not exclusive, mechanism for recovery from acid loads (7, 21, 50, 66), at least following marked acidification. A similar dichotomy of function between the two exchanges has also been reported in sheep cardiac Purkinje fibers (9, 69).

The situation may be somewhat more complex in HL-60 cells wherein Ladoux et al (39) suggested a minor contribution to pH_i recovery from acidosis by a Na^+-dependent mechanism other than Na^+/H^+ exchange. This activity could only be uncovered in the presence of a potent amiloride analogue. The requirements for extracellular Na^+ and HCO_3^- led the authors to speculate that this second pH-regulatory device might be a $Na^+ + HCO_3^-$ cotransport. Conceivably this could represent a Na^+-dependent Cl^-/HCO_3^- exchange as has been found in other cells (5, 40, 43, 55). Clearly, more work is required in defining the biochemical properties of this putative mechanism.

STEADY-STATE pH_i In common with a variety of other nucleated cells (54), intracellular pH in neutrophils and HL-60 cells is maintained at levels considerably more alkaline than predicted for electrochemical equilibrium (7, 21, 52, 59, 66). As measured by weak acid distribution methods and by fluorescent probes, steady-state pH_i is ~7.25 and ~7.00, respectively, at an extracellular pH of 7.40. These values far exceed (by 0.7–0.9 pH units) those expected on thermodynamic grounds for passive H^+ distribution. It is also clear that factors other than Na^+/H^+ exchange are likely to play a major part in governing the resting pH_i: (a) Na^+/H^+ exchange seems to be quiescent in both cells under resting conditions (21, 50, 59); and (b) suppression of Na^+/H^+ exchange using potent amiloride analogues or alteration of the chemical driving forces for the exchange by removal of extracellular Na^+ has only a negligible effect on pH_i (21, 50, 52, 66).

In HL-60 cells, Restrepo et al (52) postulated a dominant role for Cl^-/HCO_3^- exchange in setting the intracellular pH. Reversing the Cl^- gradient (by complete removal of extracellular Cl^-) led to a marked intracellular alkalinization that was dependent on HCO_3^- and blocked by H_2DIDS. Moreover, in the normal Cl^- medium, application of H_2DIDS or pentachlorophenol, at concentrations sufficient to virtually abolish Cl^-/HCO_3^- exchange, caused a decline in pH_i of up to 0.4 pH units. These findings suggest that under resting conditions the anion exchange carrier mediates net HCO_3^- influx and Cl^- efflux.

As pointed out by Restrepo et al (52), the equilibrium pH_i for Cl^-/HCO_3^- exchange based on the Cl^- gradient is ~6.9, very close to the value of 7.00 measured experimentally in steady-state HL-60 cells. The authors further hypothesized that the chemical gradient for Cl^- ultimately provides the energy required to actively pump H^+-equivalents out of the cell. This enticing notion is plausible on theoretical grounds since internal $[Cl^-]$ is itself well above electrochemical equilibrium (12, 52). In principle, it is equally possible for H^+ to be regulating intracellular Cl^- via Cl^-/HCO_3^- exchange as it is for Cl^- to be setting pH_i. In practice, however, Restrepo et al (52) demonstrated that changes in the magnitude of the Cl^- gradient over a wide range are independent of the pH gradient. These results largely exclude the possibility that the H^+ gradient is supplying the energy to move Cl^- thermodynamically uphill.

On the other hand, it may be argued that since, as in most cells under steady-state conditions, the inward Cl^- gradient is greater than that for HCO_3^-, an electroneutral Cl^-/HCO_3^- exchanger is likely to facilitate net Cl^- influx in return for HCO_3^- efflux (5). Thus this transport system would impose an additional acid load on the cells instead of serving to extrude H^+ equivalents as in the model proposed by Restrepo et al (52). More work is therefore necessary to decide between these two alternatives.

In neutrophils, where the equilibrium pH_i (~7.10) for Cl^-/HCO_3^- exchange is also remarkably close to the steady-state value (~7.25), a substantial decline in pH_i is seen in association with inhibition of anion exchange by the cinnamate derivatives CHC and UK-5099 (63, 66). However, at least a portion of this acidification is most likely because of a concomitant block of lactic acid secretion, a known property of these compounds (23, 24), with secondary accumulation of lactic and perhaps other organic acids inside the cell. Whether the same considerations apply to those agents used with HL-60 cells remains to be seen.

Incidentally, Restrepo et al (52) found no changes in the pH_i of DMSO-induced HL-60 cells nor could they detect any qualitative changes in pH_i regulation upon differentiation. This point is somewhat controversial in that Ladoux et al (39) previously reported that induction of terminal differentiation along the granulocyte pathway by retinoic acid elicited a rise in pH_i from 7.03 to 7.37. This disparity may be due to the fact that HCO_3^- was present in the former, but not in the latter studies. Of note, Costa-Casnellie et al (7) also failed to detect any changes in resting pH_i even though their studies were conducted in the absence of HCO_3^-.

CELL VOLUME REGULATION Cl^-/HCO_3^- exchange also plays a major part in cell volume regulation after osmotic shock, specifically in the recovery of cell size (volume regulatory increase) following the initial shrinkage in hypertonic media (16). In neutrophils, Grinstein et al (22) have shown that the restoration to a normal cell size, a process that ultimately depends on the net uptake of salt from the bathing solution, is impaired when Na^+ is removed from the medium or when amiloride is applied to block Na^+/H^+ exchange. It would appear that recovery involves the coordinated movements of Na^+ and Cl^- through the dual operation of two independent exchanges: Na^+ uptake via Na^+/H^+ exchange and Cl^- uptake in parallel via Cl^-/HCO_3^- exchange. This thesis is supported by other experimental evidence. Restrepo et al (50) have shown that when undifferentiated HL-60 cells are subjected to hypertonic shock, little change in pH_i occurs. Treatment of cells with H_2DIDS to block Cl^-/HCO_3^- exchange, however, unmasked a cytoplasmic alkalinization mediated by Na^+/H^+ exchange. This is as expected since the net HCO_3^- efflux through the Cl^-/HCO_3^- exchanger would otherwise serve to blunt the alkalinizing transient.

SULFATE UPTAKE   As is the case with Cl^-, SO_4^{2-} distribution in steady-state human neutrophils is not at thermodynamic equilibrium (37, 62). Instead, SO_4^{2-} is concentrated intracellularly at ~25-fold above the passive distribution level ($[SO_4^{2-}]_i \sim 1$ mM for $[SO_4^{2-}]_o = 2$ mM). Simchowitz & Davis (62) have presented evidence that the energy derived from the Cl^- gradient may provide the driving force for net SO_4^{2-} uptake via the SO_4^{2-}/Cl^- exchanger. Thus from the standpoint of SO_4^{2-}, this represents a form of secondary (or tertiary) active transport. As significant alternate pathways for SO_4^{2-} influx could not be identified, it seems reasonable to conclude that this system functions to promote the entry of SO_4^{2-} and perhaps other divalent anions into the cell. The SO_4^{2-} ion is particularly important during granulocyte differentiation and maturation as a precursor in the biosynthesis of sulfated proteoglycans (48). These macromolecules facilitate the storage and packaging of lysosomal enzymes and other constituents during granule development.

Molecular Aspects

In red cells, anion transport is mediated chiefly through the band 3 protein, an integral membrane glycoprotein with a molecular weight of ~97 kd (33, 49). Functional domains and topology of the protein, as it exists in the membrane, have been studied using a variety of chemical modifying agents and proteolytic enzymes (28, 30, 49). The erythrocyte band 3 protein contains two distinct structural domains. The N-terminal ~400 amino acid residues constitute a very hydrophilic region that functions in the anchoring of cytoskeletal proteins as well as in the binding of hemoglobin and intracellular enzymes. Anion exchange is mediated by the ~500 amino acids of the C-terminus, which contains several highly conserved hydrophobic membrane-spanning regions (for reviews, see 28, 49).

Antisera raised against purified band 3 protein usually bind to epitopes within the cytoplasmic domain, namely, antigenic sites restricted to the 23-kd amino terminal section (15). Polyclonal antibodies directed against the band 3 protein of senescent red blood cells have been found to cross-react with membrane proteins of human neutrophils, as well as mouth squamous epithelial cells, mouse neuroblastoma, and rat hepatocytes (14, 31). These antibodies also recognize surface polypeptides in human fibroblasts, monocytes, umbilical cord vascular smooth muscle tissue, and mesenchymal cells. Such a commonality of membrane localization in diverse cell types is consistent with the ubiquitous nature of anion exchange mechanisms among mammalian species.

The neutrophil membrane protein that is immunologically related to the erythroid band 3 exhibits a capping phenomenon involving cytoskeletal processes (14, 31). Comparable studies conducted in rat kidney (13) have shown that a similar protein colocalizes with ankyrin and spectrin at the basolateral membrane of intercalated cells. This suggests that the ankyrin binding domain is probably conserved and that the same basic features of erythrocyte membrane architecture, which include cytoskeletal anchoring, may be used in different types of cells.

Monoclonal antibodies have also been generated that react with another antigenic determinant on the human erythrocyte band 3 molecule. The epitope is within 7 kd of the C-terminus and therefore represents a portion of the anion exchanging domain that is exposed to the cytoplasmic side of the plasma membrane (29). This antibody immunoprecipitates two distinct membrane proteins in human neutrophils with molecular weights of 125 and 97 kd (71), which suggests that multiple forms of the same polypeptide are likely being expressed in the same cell. It is tempting to postulate that these proteins could conceivably correspond to the two anion exchange activities, Cl^-/HCO_3^- and SO_4^{2-}/Cl^-, that have thus far been identified in human neutrophils on the basis of physiologic studies (62, 64).

Band 3 cDNA probes detect mRNA transcripts of related genes in pancreas, colon, lung, testis, and liver tissue (4). With regard to leukocytes, a cDNA probe derived from a chronic myelogenous leukemia cell line (K-562) hybridized to HL-60 cell RNA as well as to RNA from Jurkat (T cell lymphoma), U-937 (monocytic lymphoma), BL-2 (Burkitt lymphoma), and GM-1056 (lymphoblastoid) cells (10).

The nucleotide sequences of the cDNAs coding for band 3-related proteins in mouse red (36), human K-562 (10), and mouse kidney (3) cells have been elucidated. This information has made possible a model of the primary structure and transmembrane orientation of this family of proteins. The proteins being expressed share a high degree of sequence homology in the membrane-traversing anion transporting domain. Despite the strong similarities in primary sequence, it is readily apparent that the properties of several forms of nonerythroid anion transport, including neutrophils and HL-60 cells, are very different from those catalyzed by band 3. Nonetheless, the weight of evidence strongly suggests that the mechanism of exchange is intrinsically similar to red cells and differs only quantitatively in relative affinities for substrates and inhibitors, rather than being a fundamentally distinct mode of transport.

Thus diverse membrane proteins that have clearly been shown to be related either antigenically or by coding nucleotide sequence homology are found in a wide variety of species. It remains to be conclusively demonstrated, however, that anion exchanging activity is expressed in every instance. Assuming that all anion exchangers carry the band 3 epitope, how might this have evolved? It could potentially be the result of an extended gene family, wherein multiple copies of the band 3 gene are present. However, Southern blot analysis indicates that only a single copy of the anion exchanger gene exists in the erythroid (34) and kidney (3) cell genomes. Alternatively, the observed differences in transport kinetics, inhibitor binding, substrate selectivity, and molecular weight among neutrophils, HL-60 cells, and erythrocytes suggest that cell type-specific expression is probably occurring. This could be regulated at the point of transcriptional initiation (via alternate promoter elements) or post-translational processing and splicing. In fact, there is precedent for both (8, 35). Hopefully, the answers to these questions will soon be resolved in neutrophils and HL-60 cells as data on the molecular biology and structural correlates of anion exchange activity are forthcoming.

FUTURE DIRECTIONS

The various roles that the anion exchanger plays in leukocyte function are just beginning to be addressed at the physiologic, biochemical, and molecular levels. Besides the need to broaden our knowledge of the more descriptive aspects of the cellular physiology of anion transport in neutrophils and HL-60 cells, strategies for the future include the application of modern molecular biological techniques. The construction of oligonucleotide and cDNA probes as well as the production of monoclonal antibodies specifically directed against these anion exchangers will allow one to screen appropriate cDNA libraries and eventually clone the relevant genes. In addition, the use of selection pressures to create mutant clones of cultured cells that are either defective, or over-express anion exchange activity, will no doubt lead to rapid advances in the field. Together, these approaches will provide powerful new research tools for the study of membrane transport in these cells.

It may be suspected that some cellular dysfunctions could be the result of defective anion exchange. Currently, it is still much too early to come to any firm conclusion as to the role of anion exchange in neutrophil function. Early reports indicate that the disulfonic stilbenes block certain stimulated responses

(37), but the significance of this observation needs to be explored more fully. Further research along these lines should provide valuable clues as to the pathophysiology of the many clinical syndromes associated with disorders of neutrophil function.

ACKNOWLEDGMENTS

The authors acknowledge the secretarial skills of Ms. Annette Irving. We also wish to express our sincere gratitude to Drs. Diego Restrepo and Philip Knauf for supplying preprints, manuscripts, and unpublished data on HL-60 cells. This work was supported by funds provided by the Veterans Administration and by National Institutes of Health grant GM38094.

Literature Cited

1. Aickin, C. C., Brading, A. F. 1985. The effects of bicarbonate and foreign anions on chloride transport in smooth muscle of the guinea-pig vas deferens. *J. Physiol.* 366:267–80
2. Aickin, C. C., Thomas, R. C. 1977. An investigation of the ionic mechanism of intracellular pH regulation in mouse soleus muscle fibres. *J. Physiol.* 273: 295–316
3. Alper, S. L., Kopito, R. R., Libresco, S. M., Lodish, H. F. 1988. Cloning and characterization of the murine band 3-related cDNA from kidney and from a lymphoid cell line. *J. Biol. Chem.* 263:17092–99
4. Alper, S. L., Kopito, R. R., Lodish, H. F. 1987. A molecular biological approach to the study of anion transport. *Kidney Int.* 32(Suppl. 23):S117–28
5. Boron, W. F. 1983. Transport of H^+ and of ionic weak acids and bases. *J. Membr. Biol.* 72:1–16
6. Collins, S., Ruscetti, F. W., Gallagher, R. E., Gallo, R. C. 1978. Terminal differentiation of promyelocytic leukemia cells induced by dimethyl sulfoxide and other polar compounds. *Proc. Natl. Acad. Sci. USA* 75:2458–62
7. Costa-Casnellie, M. R., Segel, G. B., Cragoe, E. J. Jr., Lichtman, M. A. 1987. Characterization of the Na^+/H^+ exchanger during maturation of HL-60 cells induced by dimethyl sulfoxide. *J. Biol. Chem.* 262:9093–97
8. Cox, J. V., Lazarides, E. 1988. Alternative primary structures in the transmembrane domain of the chicken erythroid anion transporter. *Mol. Cell. Biol.* 8:1327–35
9. Deitmer, J. W., Ellis, D. 1980. Interactions between the regulation of the intracellular pH and sodium activity of sheep cardiac Purkinje fibres. *J. Physiol.* 304:471–88
10. Demuth, D. R., Showe, L. C., Ballantine, M., Palumbo, A., Fraser, P. J., et al. 1986. Cloning and structural characterization of a human non-erythroid band 3-like protein. *EMBO J.* 5:1205–14
11. Deuticke, B. 1982. Monocarboxylate transport in erythrocytes. *J. Membr. Biol.* 70:89–103
12. Dissing, S., Hoffman, R., Murnane, M. J., Hoffman, J. F. 1984. Chloride transport properties of human leukemic cell lines K562 and HL60. *Am. J. Physiol.* 247:C53–60
13. Drenckhahn, D., Schluter, K., Allen, D. P., Bennett, V. 1985. Colocalization of band 3 with ankyrin and spectrin at the basal membrane of intercalated cells in the rat kidney. *Science* 230:1287–89
14. Drenckhahn, D., Zinke, K., Schauer, U., Appell, K. C., Low, P. S. 1984. Identification of immunoreactive forms of human erythrocyte band 3 in nonerythroid cells. *Eur. J. Cell Biol.* 34:144–50
15. England, B. G., Gunn, R. B., Steck, T. L. 1982. An immunological study of band 3, the anion transport protein of the human red blood cell membrane. *Biochim. Biophys. Acta* 623:171–82
16. Eveloff, J. L., Warnock, D. G. 1987. Activation of ion transport systems during cell volume regulation. *Am. J. Physiol.* 252:F1–10
17. Fröhlich, O., Gunn, R. B. 1986. Erythrocyte anion transport: the kinetics of a single-site obligatory exchange system. *Biochim. Biophys. Acta* 864:169–94

18. Fleischmann, W. 1930. Ueber die Permeabilität der Leukocyten für Ionen. *Pflügers Arch.* 223:47–55

19. Gallagher, R., Collins, S., Trujillo, J., McCredie, K., Ahearn, M., et al. 1979. Characterization of the continuous differentiating myeloid cell line (HL-60) from a patient with acute promyelocytic leukemia. *Blood* 54:713–33

20. Gargus, J. J., Adelberg, E. A., Slayman, C. W. 1985. Coordinated changes in potassium fluxes as early events in the differentiation of the human promyelocyte line HL-60. In *Regulation and Development of Membrane Transport Processes*, ed. J. S. Graves, pp. 179–91. New York: Wiley

21. Grinstein, S., Furuya, W. 1986. Characterization of the amiloride-sensitive Na-H antiport of human neutrophils. *Am. J. Physiol.* 250:C283–91

22. Grinstein, S., Furuya, W., Cragoe, E. J. Jr. 1986. Volume changes in activated human neutrophils: the role of Na^+/H^+ exchange. *J. Cell. Physiol.* 128:33–40

23. Halestrap, A. P. 1976. Transport of pyruvate and lactate into human erythrocytes. Evidence for the involvement of the chloride carrier and a chloride-independent carrier. *Biochem. J.* 156:193–207

24. Halestrap, A. P., Denton, R. M. 1975. The specificity and metabolic implications of the inhibition of pyruvate transport in isolated mitochondria and intact tissue preparations by α-cyano-4-hydroxycinnamate and related compounds. *Biochem. J.* 148:97–106

25. Hamburger, H. J., van der Schroeff, J. J. 1902. Die Permeabilität von Leukocyten und Lymphdrüsenzellen für die Anionen von Natriumsalzen. *Arch. Physiol.* 26:119–165 (Suppl.)

26. Hoffmann, E. K. 1986. Anion transport systems in the plasma membrane of vertebrate cells. *Biochim. Biophys. Acta* 864:1–31

27. Jennings, M. L. 1976. Proton fluxes associated with erythrocyte membrane anion exchange. *J. Membr. Biol.* 28:187–205

28. Jennings, M. L. 1985. Kinetics and mechanism of anion transport in red blood cells. *Annu. Rev. Physiol.* 47:519–33

29. Jennings, M. L., Anderson, M. P., Monaghan, R. 1986. Monoclonal antibodies against human erythrocyte band 3 protein. *J. Biol. Chem.* 261:9002–10

30. Jennings, M. L., Al-Rhaiyel, S. 1988. Modification of a carboxyl group that appears to cross the permeability barrier in the red blood cell anion transporter. *J. Gen. Physiol.* 92:161–78

31. Kay, M. M. B., Tracey, C. M., Goodman, J. R., Cone, J. C., Bassel, P. S. 1983. Polypeptides immunologically related to band 3 are present in nucleated somatic cells. *Proc. Natl. Acad. Sci. USA* 80:6882–86

32. Klempner, M. S., Styrt, B. 1983. Alkalinizing the intralysosomal pH inhibits degranulation of human neutrophils. *J. Clin. Invest.* 72:1793–1800

33. Knauf, P. A. 1979. Erythrocyte anion exchange and the band 3 protein: Transport kinetics and molecular structure. *Curr. Top. Membr. Transp.* 12:249–363

34. Kopito, R. R., Andersson, M., Lodish, H. F. 1987. Structure and organization of the murine band 3 gene. *J. Biol. Chem.* 262:8035–40

35. Kopito, R. R., Andersson, M. A., Lodish, H. F. 1987. Multiple tissue-specific sites of transcriptional initiation of the mouse anion antiport gene in erythroid and renal cells. *Proc. Natl. Acad. Sci. USA* 84:7149–53

36. Kopito, R. R., Lodish, H. F. 1985. Primary structure and transmembrane orientation of the murine anion exchange protein. *Nature* 316:234–38

37. Korchak, H. M., Eisenstat, B. A., Hoffstein, S. T., Dunham, P. B., Weissmann, G. 1980. Anion channel blockers inhibit lysosomal enzyme secretion from human neutrophils without affecting generation of superoxide anion. *Proc. Natl. Acad. Sci. USA* 77:2721–25

38. Korchak, H. M., Eisenstat, B. A., Smolen, J. E., Rutherford, L. E., Dunham, P. B., Weissmann, G. 1982. Stimulus-response coupling in the human neutrophil: the role of anion fluxes in degranulation. *J. Biol. Chem.* 257:6916–22

39. Ladoux, A., Cragoe, E. J. Jr., Geny, B., Abita, J. P., Frelin, C. 1987. Differentiation of human promyelocytic HL60 cells by retinoic acid is accompanied by an increase in the intracellular pH. The role of the Na^+/H^+ exchange system. *J. Biol. Chem.* 262:811–16

40. L'Allemain, G., Paris, S., Pouysségur, J. 1985. Role of a Na^+-dependent Cl^-/HCO_3^- exchange in regulation of intracellular pH in fibroblasts. *J. Biol. Chem.* 260:4877–83

41. Law, F.-Y., Steinfeld, R., Knauf, P. A. 1983. K562 cell anion exchange differs markedly from that of mature red blood cells. *Am. J. Physiol.* 244:C68–74

42. Lowe, A. G., Lambert, A. 1983. Chloride-bicarbonate exchange and related

transport processes. *Biochim. Biophys. Acta* 694:353–74

43. Madshus, I. H., Olsnes, S. 1987. Selective inhibition of sodium-linked and sodium-independent bicarbonate/chloride antiport in vero cells. *J. Biol. Chem.* 262:7486–91

44. Milanick, M. A., Gunn, R. B. 1982. Proton-sulfate cotransport: mechanism of H^+ and sulfate addition to the chloride transporter of human red blood cells. *J. Gen. Physiol.* 79:87–114

45. Milanick, M. A., Gunn, R. B. 1984. Proton-sulfate cotransport: external proton activation of sulfate influx into human red blood cells. *Am. J. Physiol.* 247:C247–59

46. Murer, H., Burckhardt, G. 1983. Membrane transport of anions across epithelia of mammalian small intestine and kidney proximal tubule. *Rev. Physiol. Biochem. Pharmacol.* 96:1–51

47. Olsnes, S., Tonnessen, T. I., Sandvig, K. 1986. pH-regulated anion transport in nucleated mammalian cells. *J. Cell Biol.* 102:967–71

48. Parmley, R. T., Doran, T., Boyd, R. L., Gilbert, C. 1986. Unmasking and redistribution of lysosomal sulfated glycoconjugates in phagocytic polymorphonuclear leukocytes. *J. Hist. Cytochem.* 34:1701–7

49. Passow, H. 1986. Molecular aspects of band 3 protein-mediated anion transport across the red blood cell membrane. *Rev. Physiol. Biochem. Pharmacol.* 103:61–203

50. Restrepo, D., Kozody, D. J., Knauf, P. A. 1987. Changes in Na^+-H^+ exchange regulation upon granulocytic differentiation of HL60 cells. *Am. J. Physiol.* 253:C619–24

51. Restrepo, D., Kozody, D. J., Knauf, P. A. 1988. Initial characterization of anion exchange in promyelocytic HL60 cells. *Biophys. J.* 53:331a.

52. Restrepo, D., Kozody, D. J., Spinelli, L. J., Knauf, P. A. 1988. pH homeostasis in promyelocytic leukemic HL60 cells. *J. Gen. Physiol.* 92:489–507

53. Restrepo, D., Kozody, D. J., Spinelli, L. J., Knauf, P. A. 1989. Cl/Cl exchange in promyelocytic HL60 cells follows simultaneous kinetics. *Am. J. Physiol.* 26:C520–27

54. Roos, A., Boron, W. F. 1981. Intracellular pH. *Physiol. Rev.* 61:296–433

55. Rothenberg, P., Glaser, L., Schlesinger, P., Cassel, D. 1983. Activation of Na^+/H^+ exchange by epidermal growth factor elevates intracellular pH in A431 cells. *J. Biol. Chem.* 258:12644–53

56. Schnell, K. F., Gerhardt, S., Schöppe-Fredenburg, A. 1977. Kinetic characteristics of the sulfate self-exchange in human red blood cells and red blood cell ghosts. *J. Membr. Biol.* 30:319–50

57. Segal, A. W., Geisow, M., Garcia, R., Harper, A., Miller, R. 1981. The respiratory burst of phagocytic cells is associated with a rise in vacuolar pH. *Nature* 290:406–9

58. Seligmann, B. E., Gallin, J. I. 1980. Use of lipophilic probes of membrane potential to assess human neutrophil activation. Abnormality in chronic granulomatous disease. *J. Clin. Invest.* 66:493–503

59. Sha'afi, R. I., Naccache, P. H., Molski, T. F. P., Volpi, M. 1982. Chemotactic stimuli-induced changes in the pH of rabbit neutrophils. In *Intracellular pH: Its Measurement, Regulation and Utilization in Cellular Functions,* ed. R. Nuccitelli, D. W. Deamer, pp. 513–25. New York: Liss

60. Simchowitz, L. 1988. Interactions of bromide, iodide, and fluoride with the pathways of chloride transport and diffusion in human neutrophils. *J. Gen. Physiol.* 91:835–60

61. Simchowitz, L. 1988. Properties of the principal anion exchange mechanism in human neutrophils. In *Cell Physiology of Blood. Soc. Gen. Physiol. Ser.* 43: ed. R. B. Gunn, J. C. Parker, 43:193–208. New York: Rockefeller Univ. Press

62. Simchowitz, L., Davis, A. O. 1989. Sulfate transport in human neutrophils. *J. Gen. Physiol.* 94:95–124

63. Simchowitz, L., Davis, A. O. 1989. Intracellular pH recovery from alkalinization: characterization of chloride and bicarbonate transport by the anion exchange system of human neutrophils. Submitted

64. Simchowitz, L., De Weer, P. 1986. Chloride movements in human neutrophils: exchange, diffusion, and active transport. *J. Gen. Physiol.* 88:167–94

65. Simchowitz, L., Ratzlaff, R., De Weer, P. 1986. Anion/anion exchange in human neutrophils. *J. Gen. Physiol.* 88:195–217

66. Simchowitz, L., Roos, A. 1985. Regulation of intracellular pH in human neutrophils. *J. Gen. Physiol.* 85:443–70

67. Simchowitz, L., Spilberg, I., De Weer, P. 1982. Sodium and potassium fluxes and membrane potential of human neutrophils. Evidence for an electrogenic sodium pump. *J. Gen. Physiol.* 79:453–79

68. Tonnessen, T. I., Ludt, J., Sandvig, K.,

Olsnes, S. 1987. Bicarbonate/chloride antiport in vero cells: I. Evidence for both sodium-linked and sodium-independent exchange. *J. Cell. Physiol.* 132:183–91

69. Vaughan-Jones, R. D. 1982. Chloride-bicarbonate exchange in the sheep cardiac Purkinje fibre. See Ref. 59. pp. 239–52

70. Vaughan-Jones, R. D. 1982. Chloride activity and its control in skeletal and cardiac muscle. *Phil. Trans. R. Soc. Lond. Ser. B: Biol. Sci.* 299:537–48

71. Veach, L. A., Nauseef, W. M., Jen-nings, M. L., Clark, R. A. 1987. Band 3-like molecules in human neutrophils. *Clin. Res.* 35:618A

72. Wilson, D. L., Manery, J. F. 1949. The permeability of rabbit leucocytes to sodium, potassium and chloride. *J. Cell. Comp. Physiol.* 34:493–519

73. Zenke, M., Kahn, P., Disela, C., Vennström, B., Leutz, A., et al. 1988. V-erbA specifically suppresses transcription of the avian erythrocyte anion transporter (band 3) gene. *Cell* 52:107–19

Annu. Rev. Physiol. 1990. 52:399–414

IONIC MECHANISMS OF CELL VOLUME REGULATION IN LEUKOCYTES

Sergio Grinstein and J. Kevin Foskett

Division of Cell Biology, The Hospital for Sick Children, 555 University Avenue, Toronto, Ontario, M5G 1X8 Canada

KEY WORDS: lymphocytes, antiport, intracellular pH, cytosolic calcium, patch-clamp

INTRODUCTION

Mammalian cells, including leukocytes, tend to gain volume passively because of the presence of intracellular charged macromolecules, which are impermeant. This tendency of the cells to swell is counteracted by the active extrusion of monovalent ions, which results in the maintenance of cellular volume. In fact, many cell types preserve an approximately constant cell size in the face of variations in the osmolarity of the medium. The precise coupling between the inward ion leak and the active outward pumping under both isotonic and anisotonic conditions is unlikely to be fortuitous. Instead, the preservation of near-normal size under such a variety of conditions suggests that the cells are able to sense their volume and to compensate for departure from an optimal, physiologic state. This implies the existence of volume-sensitive ion transport pathways that mediate the net loss of solutes when enlarged cells are required to shrink and vice versa. Under physiologic conditions, such transport pathways are likely activated by minute departures from the normal volume. Though subtle and effective, such responses are obviously difficult to study. Instead, several groups have resorted to a more convenient experimental paradigm to investigate the regulation of cellular volume. In this approach, substantial volume changes are imposed by abruptly varying the tonicity of the medium, in the expectation that the responses

0066-4278/90/0315-0399$02.00

will be proportionately magnified, facilitating their detection. The findings obtained using this approach with leukocytes are the subject of this review, with emphasis on advances made in recent years. For details of previous work, the reader is referred to earlier reviews dealing specifically with volume control in white blood cells (17, 32), or in nucleated cells in general (9, 20, 51).

Regulatory Volume Decrease

When leukocytes are suddenly exposed to a dilution of the bathing medium, they swell during the initial 0.5–2 min to levels predicted from osmotic theory. Following the intial swelling phase, the volume of the cells is quickly (5–15 min) restored to near control levels. This regulatory volume decrease (RVD) is associated with enhanced solute efflux, which osmotically withdraws water from the cell. The mechanisms responsible for enhanced solute permeabilities during RVD have been extensively studied and reviewed elsewhere (17, 32). This section will emphasize recent information, most notably patch-clamp electrophysiologic characterization of ion channels in lymphocytes, which has helped define the molecular mechanisms underlying ion efflux during RVD and has provided new insights into the regulation of these pathways.

CATION PERMEABILITY   In leukocytes, as in other cell types that display RVD, K^+ efflux is a critical component of the response. RVD is associated with a diminished cellular K^+ content (5, 12, 18, 27), which is accompanied by the appearance of K^+ in the medium (18). The magnitude of the K^+ loss, if associated with an equivalent anion flux, is sufficient to account for RVD (32). The loss of K^+ is attributable to an increased permeability to this ion, a conclusion based on tracer measurements using ^{86}Rb as a K^+ analogue. Hypotonic shock causes a > ten-fold increase of ^{86}Rb efflux, which temporally parallels RVD (5, 12, 21, 27, 46). Thus the cumulative evidence indicates that a swelling-induced activation of K^+ permeability underlies the cationic basis of RVD.

In contrast to the role of internal K^+, ion substitution experiments demonstrate that external cations are not essential for RVD. High external K^+ inhibits RVD, however, which suggests that an outward K^+ gradient is required (3, 5, 12, 18, 27). The rate of RVD is inversely proportional to the concentration of external K^+ (12), and at $[K^+]_o > 60$ mM, the net flux is reversed, and cells undergo a secondary swelling phase following the initial osmotic volume gain, because of the entry of K^+, accompanying anions and water.

ANION PERMEABILITY   Since Cl^- is the major freely diffusible anion in leukocytes, it is likely that Cl^- efflux, together with K^+ efflux, occurs during

RVD. Although fewer studies have examined the anionic component of RVD in leukocytes, the evidence strongly supports this hypothesis. In mouse lymphoblasts, Cl^- content decreases in parallel with K^+ during RVD (46). Moreover, isotopic flux measurements indicate that swelling activates Cl^- permeability. Efflux of ^{36}Cl from human peripheral blood lymphocytes (PBL) is markedly increased in cells subjected to hypotonicity. The increase is observed despite the fact that swelling dilutes intracellular Cl^- and causes membrane depolarization (21), which reduces the driving force for Cl^- efflux. The selectivity of the anion pathway, determined by examining the effects of anion substitution on the rate of secondary swelling observed in high K^+ media (discussed above), is as follows: $SCN^- = I^- > NO_3^- > Br^- \geq Cl^- >$ acetate$^- > SO_4^= =$ gluconate$^-$ (21).

COUPLING BETWEEN K^+ AND Cl^- FLUXES   A number of different KCl transport pathways appear to be involved in RVD in different cell types, including parallel K^+/H^+ and Cl^-/HCO_3^- exchanges, KCl cotransport, and independent K^+ and Cl^- conductances. The data summarized below indicate that the latter mechanism underlies RVD in lymphocytes.

A variety of evidence indicates that the fluxes of K^+ and Cl^- activated by hypotonic cell swelling proceed through independent pathways. Replacement of bath Cl^- by $SO_4^=$ blocks secondary cell swelling following the initial osmotic response to hypotonicity in high K^+ medium. The volume-induced increase in ^{86}Rb flux persists under these conditions however (21). Conversely, ^{36}Cl efflux is similarly stimulated by hypotonicity in control cells and in cells that have been depleted of intracellular K^+. Moreover, whereas addition of the conductive cation ionophore, gramicidin, to cells in isotonic Na^+-rich medium causes only a very slight change in cell volume, subsequent hypotonic stress induces a Cl^--dependent secondary swelling. The latter is due to NaCl influx driven by the inward Cl^- gradient. In the presence of gramicidin, net Cl^- uptake is observed despite the net outward K^+ movement, thus suggesting independent fluxes (21).

Further evidence for the independence of the volume-induced cation and anion permeation paths was obtained from studies of RVD in lymphocytes of different lineages. Purified T cells regulate volume at a rate comparable to unfractionated PBL (which are composed of >75% lymphocytes). In contrast, B cells display only a significantly reduced RVD (13). The differences in the capacity to regulate volume are attributed to the relative inability of B cells to increase their K^+ permeability in response to hypotonicity (13). Nevertheless, hypotonicity increases the rate of ^{36}Cl efflux comparably in B and T cells, in spite of the poor K^+ response of the former (22, 32).

Experiments using gramicidin not only point to the independence of the fluxes, but also suggest that K^+ and Cl^- migrate through conductive pathways during RVD. In Na^+-rich medium, the channel-forming antibiotic reverses the direction of the volume change by enabling Na^+ to enter the cells. In Na^+-free (e.g. choline$^+$) media, gramicidin accelerates RVD and can also by-pass the K^+ transport deficiency inherent to B cells (32), or that induced in T cells by treatment with K^+ channel inhibitors (47). In all cases, the movement of cations mediated by gramicidin is conductive and must be accompanied by a conductive anion flux to produce a volume change. Therefore, these experiments imply that a volume-activated Cl^- conductance underlies RVD and that the rate of normal RVD is limited by the magnitude of the volume-activated K^+ conductance (21, 49).

The activation of a Cl^- conductance during RVD has been confirmed by measurements of membrane potential. Whereas resting (isotonic) plasma membrane conductance is low and dominated by the K^+ permeability (21, 22), RVD is associated with an increase in permeability, which is relatively greater for anions, causing the membrane potential (E_m) to depolarize and approach the Cl^- equilibrium potential E_{Cl} (21). This increases the driving force for K^+ loss, which is electrically coupled to the exit of Cl^-.

SWELLING-INDUCED K^+ CONDUCTANCE   The nature of the conductive pathways involved in RVD was first probed pharmacologically. The inhibitory effects of quinine, cetiedil, and two phenothiazines, trifluoperazine and chlorpromazine, on RVD suggested that Ca^{2+} might play a role in the activation or regulation of the volume-induced K^+ permeability. Quinine and cetiedil had been previously demonstrated to block Ca^{2+}-activated K^+ permeability in red blood cells and, although phenothiazines are known to be rather nonspecific, the data were consistent with an effect on calmodulin (27, 47, 48). In addition, depletion of intracellular Ca^{2+} by prolonged exposure to Ca^{2+}-free media with EGTA blocked RVD by inhibiting the volume-activated K^+ permeability (27, 48). Thus the observations suggested that Ca^{2+}-activated K^+ conductance is the cationic basis of RVD. Further support for this idea came from studies using Ca^{2+} ionophores on cells in isotonic media. In the presence of extracellular Ca^{2+}, the ionophores cause a hyperpolarization, an increase in K^+ fluxes, and a relatively small volume decrease (27, 33, 48). As for RVD, these effects can be blocked by quinine and trifluoperazine. The accumulated evidence led to the hypothesis that osmotic swelling elevates the intracellular level of Ca^{2+}, which in turn activates the Ca^{2+}-sensitive K^+ channels.

However, this hypothesis was not supported by measurements of intracellular Ca^{2+} using the fluorescent Ca^{2+}-indicator dyes quin-2 (45) and, more recently, indo-1 (33). No significant increase in $[Ca^{2+}]_i$ was detectable in PBL treated hypotonically. Furthermore, patch-clamp studies failed to demonstrate the presence of Ca^{2+}-activated K^+ channels in PBL. Instead, studies of human T cells, on which most of the volume regulatory studies have been conducted, revealed the presence of a voltage-activated K^+ channel with properties similar to the delayed rectifier of muscle and nerve (6, 14, 40). This so-called type n channel has a unitary conductance of 12–18 pS, becomes activated at voltages more positive than ≈ -50 mV, and deactivates during sustained depolarization (6, 14, 16, 38, 40). There are several features of type n K^+ channels that suggest their involvement in RVD. First, the voltage-activation properties of the channel indicate that the depolarization, which occurs during osmotic swelling, could trigger their opening (see below). Second, the density of type n channels correlates with the ability of lymphocytes to regulate volume. Thus in a mouse T cell line (L2), volume regulation following osmotic swelling is deficient in quiescent cells because of insufficient K^+ permeability. Activation with interleukin-2 causes a four-fold enhancement in K^+ conductance and the development of a limited RVD in these cells (37). Similarly, though K^+ currents like those observed in T cells are also found in B cells, the current in the latter cells is 70–80% lower (16), which correlates with the differential ability of T and B lymphocytes to undergo RVD (13).

In light of these correlations, it is necessary to re-evaluate the pharmacology of RVD within the context of the pharmacology of the type n channel. While quinine-sensitivity of RVD was originally perceived as evidence for involvement of Ca^{2+}-activated K^+ channels (32), the type n channel has also been found to be inhibited by quinine (14, 40). Additionally, the type n channel is blocked by cetiedil, tetraethylammonium (TEA; $K_i \approx 10$ mM), 4-aminopyridine, Ni^{2+}, Cd^{2+}, Co^{2+}, La^{3+}, organic calcium channel antagonists, including verapamil, nifedipine, and diltiazem, and by charybdotoxin (CTX; $K_i \approx 0.5$ nM) (4, 7, 10, 14, 15, 37, 38). Of these agents, cetiedil, TEA, verapamil, and CTX have been demonstrated to inhibit RVD at least partially (12, 33, 37, 47). Therefore, available pharmacological data are consistent with activation of n type K^+ channels during RVD.

While CTX effectively inhibits type n channels, it was initially described as a selective inhibitor of Ca^{2+}-activated K^+ channels (41). In fact, the toxin has been used to demonstrate that Ca^{2+}-activated K^+ channels do exist in lymphocytes (33), notwithstanding the inability of patch-clamp studies to detect them. Yet despite the presence of CTX-sensitive Ca^{2+}-activated K^+ channels in lymphocytes, inhibition of RVD by the toxin does not appear to be because of blockade of such channels. This conclusion is based on the following observations. First, osmotic swelling is not associated with elevated $[Ca^{2+}]_i$ (33, 45). Second, buffering of intracellular Ca^{2+} with sufficient chelator to largely abolish ionomycin-induced $[Ca^{2+}]_i$ transients has no effect on RVD. Third, substantial RVD is observed under conditions where intracellular Ca^{2+} stores are depleted by preincubation in Ca^{2+}-free medium with ionomycin (33). Finally, rat thymocytes also display a Ca^{2+}-induced and K^+-gradient dependent hyperpolarization, which is sensitive to CTX, yet RVD in these cells is insensitive to the toxin (33). Thus the accumulated evidence argues against a role of Ca^{2+}-activated K^+ channels in the RVD response, which suggests instead involvement of type n or similar voltage-sensitive channels. CTX-sensitive n channels cannot account for the volume activated K^+ conductance in all cases, however, since the toxin blocks RVD in human PBL only partially and has no effect in rat thymocytes. Therefore, other types of K^+ channels involved in RVD remain to be identified.

SWELLING-INDUCED Cl^- CONDUCTANCE   The Cl^- conductance of resting lymphocytes is quite low, as demonstrated by the small transference number estimated measuring E_m, and by the failure of gramicidin to induce appreciable changes of cell volume under isotonic conditions (21). Upon swelling, however, Cl^- conductance increases markedly, exceeding the conductance to cations. Unlike the volume-induced K^+ permeability, which displays a graded response proportional to the degree of swelling, the Cl^- conductance rises more abruptly (49), which requires cell size to increase by 10–15% before it becomes activated.

Recent patch-clamp studies have identified three different Cl^- channels in the plasma membranes of lymphoid cells. A large conductance (≈ 400 pS) voltage-dependent Cl^- channel is present in both T and B lymphocytes (7). In T cells patch-clamped in the whole-cell mode, this channel is normally shut, but can be induced to open by prolonged (2–3 min) depolarizations (to +20 to +40 mV) (7). A similar channel is present in macrophages where it can be induced to open with Ca^{2+} ionophores in whole cells, but not in excised patches (50). A second type of Cl^- channel, which resembles the epithelial anion channel that is defective in cystic fibrosis, has been recently detected in human B and T cell lines (11). This channel is outwardly rectifying with a conductance at 0 mV of ≈ 40 pS and is activated by cAMP-dependent protein kinase and by sustained large depolarizations. Because $[Ca^{2+}]_i$ remains constant during RVD, and since a role for cAMP in this process has been ruled out (49), there is no evidence implicating these channels in volume regulation.

Cahalan & Lewis (7) described a so-called mini Cl^- channel that is present in human and murine T cells and in a human T cell line. The properties of this channel, in particular its mode of activation, suggest its involvement in RVD. The channel is outwardly rectifying, anion selective, and is not voltage-gated. Its unitary conductance in whole-cell patch-clamp mode at -80 mV is 2.6 pS. In spite of the small single-channel conductance, the anion selectivity is weak with the following permeability sequence: $NO_3^- > Br^-$, Cl^-, $F^- >$ methanesulfonate$^- >$ ascorbate$^- >$ aspartate$^-$. This selectivity is consistent with the anion selectivity of RVD (21). A most interesting property of the Cl^-

current through this channel is that, in the whole-cell configuration, it is activated when the solution in the patch-pipette is hypertonic to the medium (7), which suggests that the current is triggered by cell swelling. Accordingly, the activation is sensitive to osmotic manipulation of the bath; it can be terminated by exposing the cell to a hypertonic solution. Conversely, if following channel activation the bathing medium is made hypotonic, the Cl^- current activates further. Suction on the pipette reversibly inhibits activation of the osmotic gradient-induced Cl^- conductance, thus implying that cell swelling per se activates the channel and that return to normal size turns it off. During peak stimulation of the Cl^- current, ≈ 1000 Cl^- channels are activated. The calculated current flowing through this number of channels is sufficient to account for the Cl^- flux observed during RVD (7). Taken together, these observations strongly suggest that the mini Cl^- channel underlies the increased anion conductance recorded in leukocytes during RVD.

MECHANISM OF ACTIVATION OF RVD   It has been suggested (7, 16, 37) that Cl^- channel activation is the primary event associated with RVD. The osmotic/suction sensitivity of the mini Cl^- channel is consistent with this hypothesis. In this scheme, Cl^- permeability becomes predominant in swollen cells and, as a result, membrane potential depolarizes approaching E_{Cl}. The depolarization in turn activates the voltage-sensitive K^+ channels and provides a pathway for counter-ion transport, which results in salt efflux and volume loss. However attractive, this explanation cannot fully account for the increase in K^+ permeability, since swelling increases ^{86}Rb fluxes in cells already depolarized by high K^+ media and in cells in which the Cl^- flux has been eliminated (21, 32, 33). Thus, depolarization-independent processes must also exist to activate the K^+ channel(s). In summary, while stretch-induced opening of mini Cl^- channels can account for the observed anion permeability changes during RVD, the mechanisms of activation of the K^+ conductance(s) are as yet incompletely understood.

Regulatory Volume Increase

The ability of cells to reswell following osmotically imposed shrinkage has been termed regulatory volume increase (RVI). Unlike other cell types, which restore their original volume following hyperosmotic stress, lymphocytes and neutrophils display only a modest volume recovery under these conditions (23, 28, 34, 46). However, a phenomenon resembling RVI is observed when leukocytes are returned to medium of normal osmolarity after undergoing RVD in hypotonic solutions. Such cells, which have regained their original volume in the hypotonic environment, shrink upon resuspension in the more concentrated normotonic medium. This is followed by a significant regulatory volume gain, attributed to increased solute uptake accompanied by osmotically coupled water. The mechanisms underlying this process have been studied extensively in lymphoid cells, while relatively little is known about RVI in myeloid cells.

CATION TRANSPORT PATHWAYS IN RVI   In leukocytes, extracellular Na^+ is required for RVI. The volume gain is associated with a net increase in the cellular content of Na^+ and also of K^+, which results primarily from enhanced influx rates (23, 46). The stimulated uptake of K^+ is largely eliminated by ouabain, which indicates translocation via the Na^+/K^+ pump (23). Even though ouabain inhibits the accumulation of K^+, RVI is unaffected by the glycoside. Under these conditions, the volume gain persists and is attributed to intake of Na^+, accompanying anions and water. These findings indicate that Na^+ influx is the primary phenomenon in RVI and that exchange of Na^+ for K^+ through the pump is a secondary event.

Comparatively high concentrations of quinine and furosemide produce partial inhibition of RVI in lymphocytes (23). In contrast, nearly complete inhibition is attained using amiloride (23, 28) and related pyrazine derivatives (S. Grinstein, J. D. Smith, unpublished observations) in both lymphocytes and neutrophils. The latter agents also preclude the uptake of Na^+ associated with the volume gain. This pharmacological profile, together with the Na^+ dependence of RVI, suggested the involvement of Na^+/H^+ exchange in this process. Such a mechanism had been postulated earlier to underlie volume regulation in *Amphiuma* erythrocytes (8). Several lines of evidence support the notion that Na^+/H^+ exchange is activated during RVI in white blood cells (23, 31): (a) In nominally bicarbonate-free media, cell shrinking is accompanied by a 0.2 to 0.3 pH unit alkalinization of the cytoplasm; (b) In lightly buffered media, the intracellular alkalosis is paralleled by an extracellular acidification, indicative of transmembrane flux of H^+ equivalents. Both the intra- and extracellular pH changes are dependent on the availability of external Na^+ and are precluded by amiloride and its analogues; (c) No marked changes in membrane potential were recorded during RVI, despite the magnitude of the associated ion fluxes. These observations are consistent with uptake of Na^+ via an electroneutral Na^+/H^+ exchanger.

The mechanism whereby Na^+/H^+ exchange is activated during volume regulation has been studied in some detail. The number of transporters, estimated using the radiolabeled ligand, [^{3}H]-(N-methyl-N-isobutyl)amiloride, was not noticeably different before and after osmotic challenge (19). While it is not possible to ascertain that all the binding sites represent functional exchangers, the available data do not support changes in the number of transport sites as the mechanism responsible for the stimulation of Na^+/H^+ exchange. Similarly, a change in the affinity of the exchanger for extracellular Na^+ cannot account for the activation, as the apparent K_m of the antiport for external Na^+ (≈ 51 mM) was unaffected by shrinking the cells (31). The affinity for extracellular H^+ ions, which are inhibitory to forward (Na^+_o/H^+_i) exchange, was also found to be indistinguishable in normal and shrunken cells (31).

Under physiologic conditions, pH_i is the primary determinant of the rate of Na^+/H^+ exchange (1, 26). This pronounced sensitivity to pH_i has been attributed to the existence of an allosteric modifier site that controls the rate of countertransport (2). When protonated, the allosteric site activates exchange, thereby protecting the cytosol against excessive acidification. At higher pH_i, deprotonation of the modifier curtails the activity of the antiport and prevents alkalinization of the cytosol beyond the physiologic level. Protonation of the modifier could also explain the activation of transport during RVI. This may result from acidification of the cytosol or from an alteration in the pH_i sensitivity of the allosteric site. Direct measurements revealed that pH_i does not drop following osmotic shrinking of lymphocytes or neutrophils (23, 28, 31). In fact, as discussed above, RVI is accompanied by a sizable alkalinization of the cytosol. As shown in Figure 1, this results from an osmotically induced alkaline shift in the pH_i dependence of the antiport. Inasmuch as the allosteric modifier largely determines the pH_i sensitivity of the antiport, the alkaline shift probably reflects an alteration in the behavior of this site.

Na^+/H^+ exchange is also activated in white blood cells by mitogens, tumor promoters, and chemotactic factors (25, 35, 42). As in the case of RVI, stimulation by these agents is associated with cytosolic alkalinization, due to an upward displacement of the pH_i sensitivity of the modifier site. The analogy between the receptor-mediated and osmotically induced effects on the antiport also extends to their pharmacological properties (24). Such similarities, and the finding that the effects induced osmotically and through receptors are not additive, suggested a common mechanism of activation. Because protein phosphorylation is central to the conveyance of signals by receptors, and since phorbol esters effectively stimulate Na^+/H^+ exchange, activation of protein kinase C was postulated to mediate the osmotic activation of the antiport (24). In support of this hypothesis, ATP was found to be required for the activation of Na^+/H^+ exchange not only by phorbol esters, but also by shrinking (24). The occurrence of protein phosphorylation during RVI was analyzed directly, incorporating [^{32}P]phosphate into the nucleotide pool of intact cells. Analysis of membranes by polyacrylamide gel electrophoresis revealed a marked increase in the phosphorylation of a 60-kd polypeptide and smaller changes in the 50–55 kd region (29). Notably, these polypeptides were also phosphorylated in cells treated with phorbol ester. Moreover, phosphoamino acid analysis of the 60-kd band showed increased formation of phosphoserine, as expected from stimulation of protein kinase C.

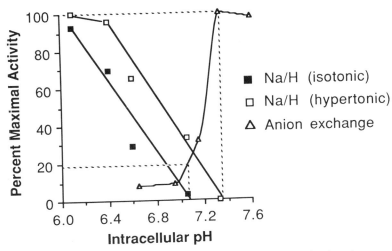

Figure 1 Comparison of the intracellular pH (pH_i) dependence of Na^+/H^+ exchange and of anion exchange in lymphocytes. The pH_i dependence of Na^+/H^+ exchange in cells suspended in isotonic medium (285 mosM; *solid squares*) and in cells shrunken in hypertonic medium (550 mosM; *open squares*) are replotted from (31). The pH_i dependence of anion exchange *(triangles)*, measured as the uptake of ^{36}Cl, is replotted from (39). The anion and cation transport rates were normalized to facilitate comparison. The dotted lines were included to estimate the relative rate of anion exchange at the pH_i where Na^+/H^+ exchange attains quiescence under isotonic or hypertonic conditions. In hypertonic bicarbonate containing media, pH_i equilibrates at an intermediate level, where both Na^+/H^+ exchange and Cl^-/HCO_3^- exchange are active.

Despite the accumulated circumstantial evidence, there is no direct indication that protein kinase C is, in fact, activated during volume regulation. In other systems the kinase is stimulated by diacylglycerol, generated from the hydrolysis of phosphoinositides by phospholipase C (43). In osmotically shrunken cells, however, no decrease in phosphatidylinositol 4,5-bisphosphate levels was observed. Moreover, the concentrations of inositol phosphates, including inositol trisphosphate, were not altered under these conditions (29). It is conceivable that diacylglycerol or other stimulants of protein kinase C such as fatty acids were released from lipids other than phosphoinositides. This possibility appears unlikely, however, since migration of kinase C from the cytosol to the membrane, an index of activation of the enzyme (36), was not detected. In addition, observations made in cells depleted of cellular protein kinase C by down-regulation argue strongly against the involvement of protein kinase C in RVI (30). In these cells, the Na^+/H^+ antiport is no longer responsive to the addition of phorbol esters, which provides functional confirmation that down-regulation of the kinase took place. Nevertheless, when treated hypertonically, such kinase C-depleted cells respond with a Na^+-dependent and amiloride-sensitive alkalinization, diagnostic of activated Na^+/H^+ exchange (30). The conclusion is therefore that at least two distinct mechanisms can activate the antiport in leukocytes: phosphorylation by protein kinase C and an unidentified process triggered by osmotic shrinking, which neither stimulates phospholipase C nor requires the presence of functional protein kinase C. The two pathways must share the final activation step, inasmuch as the responses to hypertonicity and to phorbol esters are not additive.

ANION TRANSPORT PATHWAYS IN RVI   The presence of extracellular Cl^- is an absolute requirement for RVI in lymphocytes. The volume gain is also inhibited, albeit only partially, by the nominal omission of HCO_3^- (23). In accordance with the model put forward by Cala (8), these observations suggest that volume gain results from the coupling of Na^+/H^+ exchange with a parallel, presumably independent, exchange of Cl^- for HCO_3^-. The existence of electroneutral anion exchange in both neutrophils (52, 53) and lymphocytes (39) has been established comparing measurements of net and unidirectional Cl^- flux and measuring pH_i to estimate the transport of HCO_3^-. Evidence for the existence of tightly coupled anion (Cl^-/HCO_3^-) exchange in white blood cells can be summarized as follows: (a) a substantial fraction of the Cl^- flux is electroneutral, insensitive to changes in transmembrane potential, and strictly dependent on the availability of a transported anion (e.g. Cl^- or HCO_3^-) on the *trans* side of the membrane. The flux is inhibited by disulfonic stilbenes in lymphocytes and by hydroxycinnamic acid derivatives in neutrophils; (b) in HCO_3^--containing media, removal of extracellular Cl^- leads to an intracellular alkalosis that can be reversed by reintroducing Cl^-. The pH_i increase likely reflects uptake of extracellular HCO_3^- in exchange for exiting Cl^-; (c) in Cl^- free media, the efflux of intracellular Cl^- is promoted by the availability of extracellular HCO_3^-.

In its simplest form, Cala's model (8) assumes that the primary event during RVI is the activation of Na^+/H^+ exchange. Coupling between cation and anion exchange is thought to be secondary and indirect, through changes in the concentration of intracellular HCO_3^-, which result from the elevation of pH_i generated by H^+ extrusion through the antiport. Recent data suggest that, in addition, a more direct interaction may exist between Na^+/H^+ and anion exchange. Olsnes & collaborators (44) demonstrated that the anion exchangers of some nucleated mammalian cells are exquisitely sensitive to pH_i changes in the physiologic range, their activity being greatly stimulated when the cytosol becomes alkaline. Therefore, by increasing pH_i, activation of the Na^+/H^+ antiport could conceivably stimulate anion exchange directly, independently of changes in $[HCO_3^-]_i$. The validity of this model was recently assessed in rat thymic lymphocytes (39). Three lines of evidence demonstrate the pronounced pH_i dependence of anion exchange in these cells. First, when pH_i was varied over the 6.95 to 7.35 range by means of ionophores, the rate of ^{36}Cl uptake measured in media nominally devoid of HCO_3^- increased more than tenfold. Second, the rate of the alkalinization induced by suspending cells in Cl^--free, HCO_3^--containing solutions was much greater in neutral than in acid-loaded cells, despite the reduced intracellular buffering power and the larger inwardly directed HCO_3^- gradient in the latter. Thirdly, the time course of the alkalinization recorded in Cl^--free media with HCO_3^- was generally sigmoidal, which indicated lower rates of anion exchange at more acidic pH_i.

Does the alkalinization generated by Na^+/H^+ countertransport suffice to activate the anion exchanger during RVI? Osmotic shrinking of cells suspended in media with HCO_3^- induces an alkalinization that, though smaller than in HCO_3^--free media, is nevertheless substantial (39). In thymocytes this ΔpH_i suffices to stimulate anion exchange since the rate of ^{36}Cl uptake was elevated in hypertonically shrunken cells, compared to their isotonic counterparts. Stilbene disulfonates prevented this stimulation, as did N-ethyl-N-(1-methylethyl)amino amiloride, a potent inhibitor of the cation antiport. These findings imply that ^{36}Cl uptake proceeded through anion exchange and, more importantly, that the stimulation required a functional Na^+/H^+ exchanger and the associated alkalinization. Together, these findings indicate that in leukocytes $(Cl^-)_o/(HCO_3^-)_i$ exchange is activated during RVI by two independent mechanisms: a rise in the concentration of the intracellular substrate (i.e. HCO_3^-) and an increase in the turnover number of the exchanger, due to deprotonation of a regulatory pH-sensitive site.

MECHANISM OF VOLUME GAIN DURING RVI   Figure 1 compares the pH_i dependence of Na^+/H^+ and anion exchange in lymphocytes. The behavior of the cation antiport in isotonic and hypertonic conditions is also compared. Note that at ≈ 7.1, the pH_i prevailing under physiologic (isoosmotic) conditions, both Na^+/H^+ exchange and Cl^-/HCO_3^- exchange are relatively inactive, minimizing the inward leak of NaCl, yet are poised to defend pH_i against either acid or alkaline challenge. Na^+/H^+ exchange becomes activated by and counteracts cytosolic acidification, while Cl^-/HCO_3^- exchange is stimulated by and antagonizes alkalinization. In shrunken cells, the set point of Na^+/H^+ exchange is shifted upward and cation exchange remains active at more alkaline levels. As a result, there exists a pH_i range where both Na^+/H^+ and Cl^-/HCO_3^- exchange operate in parallel at substantial rates. This joint operation produces a net gain of NaCl, which, together with the uptake of osmotically obliged water, tends to restore the original cell volume with minimal disturbance of pH_i homeostasis.

It is noteworthy that some degree of volume recovery could be obtained even in the absence of Cl^-/HCO_3^- exchange. Though Na^+/H^+ exchange is, in principle, an osmotically neutral event, the extruded H^+ are readily replaced from the intracellular buffers (≥25 mmole/liter cells.pH), which causes a net osmotic gain. Yet, the presence of HCO_3^- not only increases the physicochemical buffering capacity of the cytoplasm, but promotes Cl^-/HCO_3^- exchange. Exchange of external Cl^- for cellular HCO_3^- counteracts the alkalosis induced by Na^+/H^+ exchange and effectively increases the dynamic buffering power and magnifies the osmotic gain. As discussed elsewhere (31), the combined effects of Na^+/H^+ and Cl^-/HCO_3^- exchange are required to account for the volume gain recorded during RVI in lymphoid cells.

Significance of Volume Regulation in Leukocytes

The changes in ion transport observed when leukocytes are suspended in anisotonic media are consistent with a role in cell volume regulation. The responses are graded, proportional to the degree of volume distortion. Moreover, the transport changes cease when the cells regain their normal (isotonic) size, as expected for a volume-stat. Yet, mammalian white blood cells are rarely exposed to media of abnormal tonicity, as the renal system maintains the osmolarity of serum within very narrow boundaries. Thus the function of RVD and RVI may be restricted to the occurrence of anisosmolar syndromes such as potomania and dehydration, respectively. Alternatively, the transport systems involved in anisoosmotic volume regulation may have as their primary function the maintenance of cell volume under isotonic conditions. Volume maintenance is generally acknowledged to result from a balance between ion pumps and leaks (51, 54). Efficient volume control requires that one or both of these pathways be sensitive and responsive to changes in cellular volume. To the best of our knowledge, the Na^+/K^+ pump has not been demonstrated to perceive or react to alterations in cell size. In contrast, as discussed in detail above, K^+ and Cl^- conductances are known to increase in swollen cells, while Na^+/H^+ exchange and Cl^-/HCO_3^- exchange are stimulated upon shrinking. While these effects have been documented in cells subjected to anisotonic conditions, the permeability changes seem to arise in response to alterations of cell volume and not of medium tonicity or ionic strength. Thus if responsive to smaller departures from the normal volume, the same pathways could constitute the volume-sensitive component of the leak responsible for the maintenance of cell size in isotonic media. It is tempting to speculate that modifications in the behavior of these pathways could also underlie cell growth. In this regard, it is relevant that the set point of the Na^+/H^+ antiport is reset upwards when cells are stimulated by mitogens and tumor promoters. In the presence of HCO_3^- this is expected to induce an amiloride-sensitive volume gain, as has indeed been demonstrated for cells treated with phorbol esters (25). An increase in salt and water content may be a necessary prelude to the synthesis of macromolecules that follows mitogenic stimulation.

ACKNOWLEDGMENTS

Original work from the authors' laboratories included in this review was supported by the Medical Research Council of Canada and the National Cancer Institute. S. G. is a Medical Research Council Scientist. J. K. F. is a Canadian Cystic Fibrosis Foundation Scholar.

Literature Cited

1. Aronson, P. S. 1985. Kinetic properties of the plasma membrane Na^+/H^+ exchanger. *Annu. Rev. Physiol.* 47:545–60
2. Aronson, P. S., Nee, J., Suhm, M. A. 1982. Modifier role of internal H in activating the Na/H exchanger in renal microvillar membrane vesicles. *Nature* 299:161–63
3. Ben-Sasson, S., Shaviv, R., Bentwich, Z., Slavin, S., Doljanski, F. (1975). Osmotic behavior of normal and leukemic lymphocytes. *Blood* 46:891–99
4. Bregestovski, P., Redkozubov, A., Alexeev, A. 1986. Elevation of intracellular calcium reduces voltage-dependent potassium conductance in human T cells. *Nature* 319:776–78
5. Bui, A. H., Wiley, J. S. 1981. Cation fluxes and volume regulation by human lymphocytes. *J. Cell Physiol.* 108:47–54
6. Cahalan, M. D., Chandy, K. G., DeCoursey, T. E., Gupta, S. 1985. A voltage-gated potassium channel in human T lymphocytes. *J. Physiol.* 358:197–237
7. Cahalan, M. D., Lewis, R. S. 1988. Role of potassium and chloride channels in volume regulation by T lymphocytes. In *Cell Physiology of Blood*, eds. R. B. Gunn, J. C. Parker, pp. 281–301. New York: Rockefeller Univ. Press, 402 pp.
8. Cala, P. M. 1980. Volume regulation by *Amphiuma* red cells. The membrane potential and its implications regarding the nature of the ion flux pathways. *J. Gen. Physiol.* 76:683–708
9. Chamberlin, M. E., Strange, K. 1989. Anisosmotic cell volume regulation: A comparative view. *Am. J. Physiol.* 257:C159–73
10. Chandy, K. G., DeCoursey, T. E., Cahalan, M. D., McLaughlin, C., Gupta, S. 1984. Voltage-gated potassium channels are required for human T lymphocyte activation. *J. Exp. Med.* 160:369–385
11. Chen, J. H., Schulman, H., Gardner, P. 1989. A cAMP-regulated chloride channel in lymphocytes that is affected in cystic fibrosis. *Science* 243:657–60
12. Cheung, R. K., Grinstein, S., Dosch, H.-M., Gelfand, E. W. 1982. Volume regulation by human lymphocytes: characterization of the ionic basis for regulatory volume decrease. *J. Cell. Physiol.* 12:189–96
13. Cheung, R. K., Grinstein, S., Gelfand, E. W. 1982. Volume regulation by human lymphocytes. Identification of differences between the two major lymphocyte subpopulations. *J. Clin. Invest.* 70:632–38
14. DeCoursey, T. E., Chandy, K. G., Gupta, S., Cahalan, M. D. 1984. Voltage-gated K^+ channels in human T lymphocytes: a role in mitogenesis? *Nature* 307:465–68
15. DeCoursey, T. E., Chandy, K. G., Gupta, S., Cahalan, M. D. 1987. Two types of potassium channels in murine T lymphocytes. *J. Gen. Physiol.* 89:379–404
16. Deutsch, C., Krause, D., Lee, S. C. 1986. Voltage-gated potassium conductance in human T lymphocytes stimulated with phorbol ester. *J. Physiol.* 372:405–23
17. Deutsch, C., Lee, S. C. 1988. Cell volume regulation in lymphocytes. *Renal Physiol. Biochem.* 35:260–76
18. Deutsch, C., Slater, L., Goldstein, P. 1982. Volume regulation of human peripheral blood lymphocytes and stimulated proliferation of volume-adapted cells. *Biochim. Biophys. Acta* 721:262–67
19. Dixon, S. J., Cohen, S., Cragoe, E. J. Jr., Grinstein, S. 1987. Estimation of the number and turnover rate of Na^+/H^+ exchangers in lymphocytes. Effect of

phorbol ester and osmotic shrinking. *J. Biol. Chem.* 262:3626–32

20. Eveloff, J. L., Warnock, D. G. 1987. Activation of ion transport systems during cell volume regulation. *Am. J. Physiol.* 252:F1–10

21. Grinstein, S., Clarke, C. A., DuPre, A., Rothstein, A. 1982. Volume-induced increase of anion permeability in human lymphocytes. *J. Gen. Physiol.* 80:801–23

22. Grinstein, S., Clarke, C. A., Rothstein, A. 1982. Increased anion permeability during volume regulation in human lymphocytes. *Phil. Trans. R. Soc. London Ser. B.* 299:509–18

23. Grinstein, S., Clarke, C. A., Rothstein, A. 1983. Activation of Na^+/H^+ exchange in lymphocytes by osmotically induced volume changes and by cytoplasmic acidification. *J. Gen. Physiol.* 82:619–38

24. Grinstein, S., Cohen, S., Goetz, J. D., Rothstein, A. 1985. Osmotic and phorbol ester-induced activation of Na^+/H^+ exchange: possible role of protein phosphorylation in lymphocyte volume regulation. *J. Cell. Biol.* 101:269–76

25. Grinstein, S., Cohen, S., Goetz, J. D., Rothstein, A., Gelfand, E. W. 1985. Characterization of the activation of Na^+/H^+ exchange in lymphocytes by phorbol esters: change in cytoplasmic pH dependence of the antiport. *Proc. Nat. Acad. Sci. USA* 82:1429–33

26. Grinstein, S., Cohen, S., Rothstein, A. 1984. Cytoplasmic pH regulation in thymic lymphocytes by an amiloride-sensitive Na^+/H^+ antiport. *J. Gen. Physiol.* 83:341–69

27. Grinstein, S., DuPre, A., Rothstein, A. 1982. Volume regulation of human lymphocytes. Role of Ca^{++}. *J. Gen. Physiol.* 79:849–68

28. Grinstein, S., Furuya, W., Cragoe, E. J. Jr. 1986. Volume changes in activated human neutrophils: The role of Na^+/H^+ exchange. *J. Cell. Physiol.* 128:33–40

29. Grinstein, S., Goetz-Smith, J. D., Stewart, D., Beresford, B. J., Mellors, A. 1986. Protein phosphorylation during activation of Na^+/H^+ exchange by phorbol esters and by osmotic shrinking. *J. Biol. Chem.* 261:8009–16

30. Grinstein, S., Mack, E., Mills, G. B. 1986. Osmotic activation of the Na^+/H^+ antiport in protein kinase C-depleted lymphocytes. *Biochem. Biophys. Res. Commun.* 134:8–13

31. Grinstein, S., Rothstein, A., Cohen, S. 1985. Mechanism of osmotic activation of Na^+/H^+ exchange in rat thymic lymphocytes. *J. Gen. Physiol.* 85:765–87

32. Grinstein, S., Rothstein, A., Sarkadi, R., Gelfand, E. W. 1984. Responses of lymphocytes to aniosmotic media: volume-regulating behavior. *Am. J. Physiol.* 246:C204–15

33. Grinstein, S., Smith, J. D. 1989. Calcium-independent cell volume regulation in human lymphocytes. Inhibition by charybdotoxin. *J. Gen. Physiol.* In press

34. Hempling, H. G., Thompson, S., DuPre, A. 1977. Osmotic properties of human lymphocyte. *J. Cell. Physiol.* 93:293–302

35. Hesketh, T. R., Moore, J. P., Morris, J. D. H., Taylor, M. V., Rogers, J., et al. 1985. A common sequence of calcium and pH signals in the mitogenic stimulation of eukaryotic cells. *Nature* 313:481–84

36. Kraft, A. S., Anderson, W. B. 1983. Phorbol esters increase the amount of Ca, phospholipid-dependent protein kinase associated with plasma membrane. *Nature* 301:621–24

37. Lee, S. C., Price, M., Prystowsky, M. B., Deutsch, C. 1988. Volume response of quiescent and interleukin 2-stimulated T-lymphocytes to hypotonicity. *Am. J. Physiol.* 254:C286–96

38. Lewis, R. S., Cahalan, M. D. 1988. Subset-specific expression of potassium channels in developing murine T lymphocytes. *Science* 239:771–75

39. Mason, M. J., Smith, J. D., Garcia-Soto, J. J., Grinstein, S. 1989. Internal pH-sensitive site couples Cl^--HCO_3^- exchange to Na^+/H^+ antiport in lymphocytes. *Am. J. Physiol.* 256:C428–33

40. Matteson, D. R., Deutsch, C. 1984. K channels in T lymphocytes: a patch clamp study using monoclonal antibody adhesion. *Nature* 307:468–71

41. Miller, C., Moczydlowski, E., Latorre, R., Phillips, M. 1985. Charybdotoxin, a protein inhibitor of single Ca^{2+}-activated K^+ channels from mammalian skeletal muscle. *Nature* 313:316–18

42. Molski, T. F. P., Naccache, P. H., Volpi, M., Wolpert, L. M., Sha'afi, R. I. 1980. Specific modulation of the intracellular pH of rabbit neutrophils by chemotactic factors. *Biochem. Biophys. Res. Commun.* 94:508–14

43. Nishizuka, Y. 1986. Studies and perspectives of protein kinase C. *Science* 233:305–12

44. Olsnes, S., Tonnessen, T. I., Ludt, J., Sandvig, K. 1987. Effect of intracellular pH on the rate of chloride transport in different mammalian cell lines. *Biochemistry* 26:2778–85

45. Rink, T. J., Sanchez, A., Grinstein, S.,

Rothstein, A. 1983. Volume restoration in osmotically swollen lymphocytes does not involve changes in cytoplasmic pH or free Ca^{2+} concentration. *Biochim. Biophys. Acta* 762:593–96

46. Roti-Roti, L. W., Rothstein, A. 1973. Adaptation of mouse leukemic cells (L5178Y) to anisotonic media. *Exp. Cell Res.* 79:295–310

47. Sarkadi, B., Cheung, R, Mack, E., Grinstein, S., Gelfand, E. W., Rothstein, A. 1985. Cation and anion transport pathways in volume regulatory response of human lymphocytes to hypotonic media. *Am. J. Physiol.* 248:C480–87

48. Sarkadi, B., Mack, E., Rothstein, A. 1984. Ionic events during the volume response of human peripheral blood lymphocytes to hypotonic media. I. Distinctions between the volume-activated Cl^- and K^+ conductance pathways. *J. Gen. Physiol.* 83:497–512

49. Sarkadi, B., Mack, E., Rothstein, A. 1984. Ionic events during the volume response of human peripheral blood lymphocytes to hypotonic media. II. Volume- and time-dependent activation and inactivation of ion transport pathways. *J. Gen. Physiol.* 83:513–27

50. Schwarze, W., Kolb, H. A. 1984. Voltage-dependent kinetics of an ion channel of large conductance in macrophages and myotube membranes. *Pflügers Arch* 402:281–91

51. Siebens, A. W. 1985. Cellular volume control. In *The Kidney: Physiology and Pathophysiology.* ed. D. W. Seldin, G. Giebisch, New York: Raven. 91 pp.

52. Simchowitz, L., De Weer, P. 1986. Chloride movements in human neutrophils. Diffusion, exchange and active transport. *J. Gen. Physiol.* 88:167–94

53. Simchowitz, L., Ratzlaff, R., De Weer, P. 1986. Anion/anion exchange in human neutrophils. *J. Gen. Physiol.* 88:195–217

54. Tosteson, D. C., Hoffman, J. F. 1960. Regulation of cell volume by active cation transport in high and low potassium sheep red cells. *J. Gen. Physiol.* 4:169–94

Annu. Rev. Physiol. 1990. 52:415–30

ION CHANNELS AND SIGNAL TRANSDUCTION IN LYMPHOCYTES

Richard S. Lewis and Michael D. Cahalan

Department of Physiology and Biophysics, California College of Medicine, University of California, Irvine, California 92717

KEY WORDS: cell activation, volume regulation, ion transport, patch-clamp, calcium signaling

INTRODUCTION

T and B lymphocytes play fundamental and diverse roles in the immune response, which include recognition of antigens, secretion of lymphokines and antibodies, and killing of foreign or virus-infected cells. Ionic fluxes associated with lymphocyte activation, mitogenesis, and volume regulation have been studied extensively in cell suspensions (for reviews, see 67, 103, 124, Grinstein & Foskett, this volume). More recently, the advent of patch-clamp recording techniques (55) and video imaging of fluorescent ion-sensitive dyes (53, 131) has placed a new emphasis on the responses of individual cells in the immune system. In this review we address recent advances in the exploration of ion-channel functions in T and B lymphocytes at the single-cell level, with particular emphasis on three lymphocyte behaviors: cell activation and mitogenesis, cytotoxicity, and volume regulation.

LYMPHOCYTE BEHAVIORS AND TRANSMEMBRANE ION FLUXES

Lymphocytes are activated in vivo by the binding of specific antigens to the T-cell receptor complex (for T cells) or surface immunoglobulin molecules (for B cells). Monoclonal antibodies that cross-link selected cell surface glycoproteins, as well as several lectins, are commonly used together with

415

0066-4278/90/0315-0415$02.00

phorbol esters to initiate cell activation in vitro. The ensuing activation response encompasses a coordinated series of lineage-dependent and -independent differentiation events, culminating in DNA synthesis and cell division (reviewed in 14, 81). Some of the earliest events, commencing within minutes of exposure to mitogens, include transmembrane ion movements, efflux of K^+ (41, 121) and H^+ (57, 108), and influx of Na^+ (30, 101, 121) and Ca^{2+} (61, 132, 137, reviewed in 134). During the same time period membrane phosphatidylinositol 4,5-bisphosphate is hydrolyzed, yielding inositol 1,4,5-trisphosphate (IP$_3$), which mobilizes Ca^{2+} from intracellular stores, and diacylglycerol, which activates protein kinase C (14, 134). Commitment of lymphocytes to the activation pathway is incompletely understood, but it is generally thought to involve both a sustained rise of intracellular free Ca^{2+} concentration ($[Ca^{2+}]_i$) and activation of protein kinase C, based on several lines of evidence. First, many Ca^{2+}-mobilizing stimuli, when combined with phorbol esters, activate T cells (134), while preventing the sustained $[Ca^{2+}]_i$ rise prevents cell activation (42, 56, 93, 135, 136). In addition, elevation of intracellular $[Ca^{2+}]$ with ionophores, in the presence of phorbol esters, bypasses the involvement of cell-surface receptors and activates lymphocytes (86, 89, 130, 133), leading to expression of early activation genes, such as c-*fos,* c-*myc,* and the T-cell-specific interleukin-2 (IL-2) gene (22, 94, 105, 134). Ca^{2+}-independent pathways may also exist, however, as a variant T-cell hybridoma can be activated by surface-receptor crosslinking to secrete IL-2 in the absence of a detectable $[Ca^{2+}]_i$ rise (125).

The process by which cytotoxic T cells and natural killer cells destroy foreign or virus-infected cells is thought to occur in three phases, referred to as binding, programming-for-lysis, and lethal hit. Although binding of the effector cell to its target is Ca^{2+}-independent, programming and delivery of the lethal hit require extracellular Ca^{2+} (84). K^+ efflux (109) and Ca^{2+} influx (100) in the effector cells both accompany and are required for the cell-killing reaction.

When exposed to a hypotonic environment, T cells swell passively, then spontaneously shrink over a period of minutes to approximately their normal volume. This regulatory volume decrease (RVD) is characteristic of a variety of cell types and is reviewed in detail by Grinstein & Foskett in this volume. RVD is mediated through the efflux of K^+ and Cl^- from the cell, which drives out osmotically obligated water and causes the cell to shrink (18, 45, 112–114).

The patch-clamp technique (55) has enabled characterization of a variety of ion channels in cells of the immune system, several of which appear to underlie the ion fluxes described above (for reviews, see 12, 24, 36). The high membrane resistance (10–100 G Ω) and low surface area (1–2 × 10^{-6} cm^2) and volume (2–3 × 10^{-10} cm^3) of lymphocytes make it possible for small numbers of ion channels to have a powerful influence on both membrane potential and intracellular $[Ca^{2+}]$. For these reasons, the patch-clamp technique, offering both high sensitivity and the ability to introduce specific second messengers into the cytoplasm (95), is ideally suited to the detailed study of channel function and regulation in lymphocytes. The following sections review the present knowledge of lymphocyte K^+, Cl^-, and Ca^{2+} channels as derived from patch-clamp experiments.

VOLTAGE-GATED POTASSIUM CHANNELS

Properties

Three distinct types of voltage-gated K^+ channels have been identified in lymphoid cells based on their voltage dependence, tendency to inactivate, opening and closing kinetics, and pharmacologic profiles (for review, see 76). The most commonly observed K^+ channel, named type n for its prevalence in normal human T cells (11, 23, 28, 87), opens at potentials positive to -50 mV, a voltage dependence that enables the cell to maintain a negative membrane potential. Type n K^+ channels are activated by depolarization per se, not by intracellular Ca^{2+}; instead, raising $[Ca^{2+}]_i$ accelerates inactivation (10, 21, 50). These channels have a unitary conductance of 12–16 pS and are sensitive to a variety of classical K^+ channel blockers, such as tetraethylammonium (TEA) and 4-aminopyridine (4-AP) (23, 51). Interestingly, type n channels are also blocked by drugs thought at one time to be specific inhibitors of Ca^{2+}-activated K^+ channels, including quinine (23, 87, 116) and charybdotoxin (CTX) (111); by classical Ca^{2+}-channel blockers, such as verapamil, diltiazem, dihydropyridines, Ni^{2+}, Cd^{2+}, and Co^{2+} (15, 24, 87); and by the calmodulin antagonists chlorpromazine and trifluoperazine (24).

Two additional varieties of K^+ channels have been characterized in murine T cells and thymocytes. Compared with type n K^+ channels, n' channels do not accumulate inactivation during repetitive depolarizing pulses, and are $\approx$10-fold less sensitive to block by TEA, although they display a similar sensitivity to CTX and similar unitary conductance (75). Type l K^+ channels, named for their larger conductance (21–27 pS) and prevalence in autoimmune mice bearing the lpr mutation, are even more distinct, showing a lack of cumulative inactivation, a more positive voltage threshold for activation, faster closing kinetics, and a 10-fold higher sensitivity to block by TEA compared to n or n' channels (16, 25, 75). Type l channels are not blocked by CTX (111).

Expression

Subtypes of K^+ channels are distributed in a characteristic pattern among functional and developmental subsets of T cells. Type n channels are the most common and are found in human peripheral blood T cells (23, 87), thymocytes (117), and leukemic cell lines (24), and in most subsets of murine thymocytes (immature $CD4^-CD8^-$ and $CD4^+CD8^+$ cells, and helper-phenotype $CD4^+CD8^-$ cells; 75, 90), peripheral T cells, and clonal cell lines (24, 25, 34, 74). Type n channels have also been detected in B lymphocytes (127), macrophages (38, 102, 141), platelets (85), and type II alveolar epithelial cells (27). In contrast, expression of type n' and l channels is restricted to murine thymocytes and peripheral T cells of the cytotoxic/suppressor phenotype ($CD4^-CD8^+$) (52, 75), while abundant expression of type l channels marks functionally aberrant $CD4^-CD8^-$ T cells from mice with autoimmune disease (16, 52). Thus far, type n' or l channels have not been observed in human T or B cells, although l channels are present in a human B-cell lymphoma line (122).

Functions

Several lines of evidence point to a requirement for functional n-type K^+ channels in the activation of T and B lymphocytes by mitogens. First, expression of type n K^+ channels is correlated with the degree of cell proliferation. In the thymus, actively cycling cell subsets express 10- to 20-fold the K^+-channel density of quiescent cells (75, 90), and K^+ channel expression in resting peripheral T and B cells is boosted by a similar amount following mitogenic stimulation (26, 74, 126, 127). In addition, mitogenic lectins have been reported to affect the voltage dependence of K^+ channel gating (11, 23, 24, 117) and maximum K^+ conductance (117) of thymocytes and T cells, but the mechanism of these acute effects and their physiologic significance remain to be determined. The most compelling evidence for a role of K^+ channels in lymphocyte activation is the dose-dependent inhibition of mitogenesis by K^+ channel blocking agents. A variety of structurally distinct compounds, including TEA, 4-AP, quinine, cetiedil, verapamil, nifedipine, and diltiazem, inhibit mitogenesis of T and B cells and antibody secretion by B cells at levels required to block type n channels (15, 16, 23, 24, 28, 110, 115, 126, 127). K^+ channels appear to be necessary for some, but not all, cell activation events (15, 110); for example, while protein and DNA synthesis and IL-2 production are inhibited by the blockers, expression of IL-2 receptors is unaffected. K^+ channel blockers also inhibit the cytotoxic activity of human natural killer cells, apparently by interfering with the programming phase of the reaction (116, 123). Similar effects have been observed using human cytotoxic T cells and a murine natural killer cell line (K. G. Chandy, et al, unpublished observations).

The important question remains, how do K^+ channels exert their influence on lymphocyte activation? The sensitivity of mitogenesis to K^+ channel blockade declines after several hours of mitogen stimulation, which suggests a role during early stages of cell-cycle progression (15, 110). One hypothesis, that K^+ channels conduct Ca^{2+} into the cell (11), now appears unlikely, as full K^+ channel activation by voltage-clamp depolarization does not alter $[Ca^{2+}]_i$ measured in single T cells with fura-2 (78). K^+ channel blockers depolarize T cells (138), and depolarization by high $[K^+]_o$ inhibits Ca^{2+} signaling (40, 43, 97), thereby supporting the notion that K^+ channels indirectly facilitate Ca^{2+} influx through mitogen-stimulated Ca^{2+} channels by maintaining a negative membrane potential (11). However, K^+ channel blockers, such as TEA and 4-AP, only reduce the early $[Ca^{2+}]_i$ rise evoked by phytohemagglutinin (PHA) in T cells by 10–25% (41). This issue may be resolved when the blockers are tested for longer-term effects on $[Ca^{2+}]_i$. Functional K^+ channels may be required for normal transport of essential metabolites, since TEA and 4-AP have been found to inhibit uptake of thymidine and phenylalanine by cloned T cells (115). These inhibitory effects are most likely the result of K^+ channel block rather than of nonspecific action of the blockers themselves, since these agents do not inhibit growth of a lymphoid cell line known to lack K^+ channels (15).

Two types of experimental evidence suggest that type n K^+ channels are involved in the RVD response of T lymphocytes. First, the abundance of n channels directly parallels the ability of T and B cells to volume regulate (19, 28, 73, 127). Second, drugs known to block type n channels in T cells, such as TEA, quinine, cetiedil, verapamil, trifluoperazine, chlorpromazine, and CTX, inhibit RVD at comparable concentrations (13, 18, 24, 47, 48, 73, 113). RVD and type n K^+ channels also exhibit similar sensitivities to intracellular pH (28a). It has been proposed that Cl^- channels activated by osmotic swelling depolarize the membrane to open n-type K^+ channels during RVD (13).

CALCIUM-ACTIVATED POTASSIUM CHANNELS

At least two major classes of Ca^{2+}-activated K^+ channels have been found in the nervous system: a high-conductance (≈ 200 pS) maxi-K^+ channel that is opened by depolarization and intracellular Ca^{2+} and is highly sensitive to block by the scorpion toxin component, CTX (2, 3, 92); and a lower-conductance, voltage-insensitive, Ca^{2+}-activated channel that is blocked by the bee venom peptide, apamin (8, 60). Indirect evidence supporting the existence of Ca^{2+}-activated K^+ channels in lymphocytes includes membrane hyperpolarization and $^{86}Rb^+$ flux induced by raising $[Ca^{2+}]_i$ with ionophores or mitogens (29, 46, 47, 82, 128, 132, 138). The early work on this subject has been reviewed (106).

Two recent patch-clamp studies have identified Ca^{2+}-activated K^+ channels in rat thymocytes and human B cells (83a) and in Jurkat leukemic T cells (49). In cell-attached patches exposed to 140 mM K^+, K^+-selective channels with conductances of 8 and 25 pS are activated upon elevation of $[Ca^{2+}]_i$ (83a). The channels show little voltage dependence and in excised patches exhibit a threshold of several hundred nanomolar Ca^{2+} for activation. Gallin (37) has described a similar 36-pS K^+ channel activated in human macrophages by the Ca^{2+} ionophore, ionomycin. The time course of Ca^{2+}-activated K^+ current in single Jurkat T cells follows the transient elevation of $[Ca^{2+}]_i$ induced by ionomycin or PHA (49; R. S. Lewis & M. D. Cahalan, unpublished observations), and the current is blocked by apamin (S. Grissmer & M.D. Cahalan, unpublished observations).

Ca^{2+}-activated K^+ channels are likely to be involved in generating the membrane hyperpolarization observed in mitogen-treated B and T cells, since the time-course of the hyperpolarization closely parallels that of the $[Ca^{2+}]_i$ increase (82, 132). By maintaining a negative resting potential these channels may enhance the driving force for Ca^{2+} influx. Until recently, no ligand specific for the Ca^{2+}-activated K^+ channel in lymphocytes was known (quinine and CTX block voltage-gated K^+ channels in lymphocytes). The ability to selectively block Ca^{2+}-activated K^+ channels with apamin should allow tests of their involvement in T- and B-cell activation.

The possibility that Ca^{2+}-activated K^+ channels constitute the K^+ efflux pathway of RVD was proposed originally by Grinstein & colleagues based on observations that RVD is inhibited by quinine, calmodulin antagonists, or prolonged incubation in Ca^{2+}-free medium, and that calcium ionophores can induce cell shrinkage (46, 47). Such a role is questionable, however, as a $[Ca^{2+}]_i$ rise is undetectable during RVD of human T cells (107), and the pharmacologic sensitivity of K^+ efflux during RVD closely parallels that of voltage-gated, type n K^+ channels (discussed above).

CHLORIDE CHANNELS

Several varieties of Cl^- channels have been found in lymphocytes, which cover a spectrum of unitary conductances: a 1–2-pS mini channel (13), a 40-pS channel (17), and a 300–400-pS maxi-Cl^- channel (12, 120). Because the normal lymphocyte resting potential of -60 mV lies below the estimated Cl^- equilibrium potential of ≈ -35 mV, activation of Cl^- channels causes Cl^- efflux and membrane depolarization (45).

Mini-Cl^- channels have been found in human and murine T cells and related lines and in both immature and mature thymocyte subsets in mice (13; R. S. Lewis & M. D. Cahalan, unpublished observations). Single channels are too small to be clearly evident in whole-cell recording; the unitary conductance is estimated from fluctuation analysis to be 1–2 pS. Cl^- channel activation is triggered during whole-cell recording by hypoosmotic extracellular or hyperosmotic intracellular solutions and requires the presence of intracellular ATP. Suction applied to the whole-cell recording pipette retards or reverses the activation of the current induced by hypotonic media, thus suggesting that these channels are activated by membrane stretch produced by cell swelling. The acute modulation of mini-Cl^- channels by changes in extracellular tonicity suggests that they underlie the anion transport limb of the RVD pathway. This conclusion is supported by the parallel anion selectivity of the Cl^- conductance ($NO_3^- > Br^- \geq Cl^-$) and of RVD (13, 45). Identification of blocking compounds for the mini-Cl^- channels will facilitate further tests of their role in RVD.

A second type of Cl^- channel has been described recently in human leukemic T cells and transformed B lymphoblasts (17). Its unitary conductance of 40 pS and its activation by prolonged membrane depolarization or by intracellular cAMP and cAMP-dependent protein kinase suggest a close resemblance to the Cl^- channels of secretory cells in airway epithelia (80, 119). The role of the 40-pS Cl^- channel in lymphocyte functions is not known. Regulation of the channels by cAMP-dependent protein kinase, however, appears to be defective in lymphoblasts derived from patients with cystic fibrosis (CF) (17). A similar defect is known to affect Cl^- channels in airway epithelia from CF patients and underlies the pathogenesis of the disease (80, 119). The finding that lymphocytes, a highly accessible biological material, may express the same channel-regulation defect suggests their use as a model preparation for both diagnosis and research on the molecular basis of defective Cl^- transport in cystic fibrosis.

Large conductance maxi-Cl^- channels have been found in murine thymocytes, T cells, and in a B-cell hybridoma (9, 12, 13, 120), as well as in a variety of other cell types (7, 44, 54, 69). The channels are easily recognized by their 300–400-pS conductance, multiple subconductance states, and voltage dependence. Activation is complex; the channels can be opened by several min of membrane depolarization to potentials of >0 mV, by treatment of the cell with ionomycin, or by patch excision. Once induced, the channel is maximally active at 0 mV, closing at both positive and negative potentials. The activation by ionomycin may involve Ca^{2+}-dependent intracellular biochemical events, since following patch excision the channel's activity is unaffected by changes in $[Ca^{2+}]$ bathing the intracellular face (120). A clear function for the maxi-Cl^- channel has not yet been demonstrated. In a recent report showing a similar channel in sarcoplasmic reticulum (SR) from skeletal muscle, Hals et al (54) propose that the channel may indirectly regulate Ca^{2+} release from the SR. If the maxi-Cl^- channels also exist in the endoplasmic reticulum membranes of lymphocytes, one could envision an analogous role in regulating intracellular Ca^{2+} release during lymphocyte activation.

MITOGEN-ACTIVATED CALCIUM CHANNELS

The existence of mitogen-regulated Ca^{2+} channels in T and B lymphocytes was initially inferred from indirect measurements, beginning with observations of $^{45}Ca^{2+}$ uptake induced by polyclonal mitogens (32, 136, 137). Although Ca^{2+} influx is electrogenic (83), voltage-gated Ca^{2+} channels do not appear to be involved, since depolarization of cells with high $[K^+]_o$ before or after exposure to mitogens does not elicit a rise in $[Ca^{2+}]_i$ (40, 77, 97). Likewise, voltage-clamp depolarization fails to evoke inward Ca^{2+} current in T or B cells (11, 34, 126), although voltage-gated Ca^{2+} channels are detectable in murine myeloma and B-cell hybridomas (33, 35). A recent report suggesting the presence of voltage-sensitive Ca^{2+} channels in Jurkat leukemic T cells (28b) must be regarded with skepticism until the ability of Ca^{2+} to carry the current is established. Inhibition of $^{45}Ca^{2+}$ uptake and mitogenesis by Ca^{2+}-channel blockers such as verapamil and dihydropyridines has been taken as evidence for mitogen-gated Ca^{2+} channels in T cells (6), although this interpretation is complicated by the fact that these compounds block type n K^+ channels (15, 24).

Three groups have reported direct measurements of mitogen-stimulated Ca^{2+} or Ba^{2+} currents in T cells or T-cell membranes, but no common consensus has been reached on their characteristics. Gardner & colleagues have described single-channel and whole-cell currents evoked in human T cells by PHA and antibodies to CD2 or CD3 (39, 70, 71). In cell-attached patches exposed to isotonic external $BaCl_2$, the channels have a conductance of ≈ 7 pS and show some selectivity for Ba^{2+}. Channel openings are brief (0.4–0.5 msec), occur in short bursts, and are not measurably voltage-dependent. The ability of bath-applied PHA to elicit channel activity in cell-attached patches indicates that the underlying activation mechanism involves a diffusible intracellular second messenger. A possible role for 1,4,5-IP_3 in this regard is consistent with its ability to activate the channel in excised inside-out patches (70). Micromolar levels of intracellular Ca^{2+} block the channel reversibly, suggesting a means of auto-regulation during the mitogenic response. Whole-cell currents induced by mitogens were large (up to -130 pA at -50 mV) and showed poor selectivity for Ba^{2+} over monovalent cations (39, 71).

A different type of antibody triggered channel activity has been described in bilayers formed from plasma membranes of a human T-cell line (98). Antibodies to CD3 or T-cell receptor epitopes unique to these cells elicit single-channel currents having a small conductance (2–6 pS in symmetrical 100 mM $CaCl_2$, 7–8 pS in symmetrical 50 mM $BaCl_2$). These channels are distinct from those described by Gardner & coworkers in several ways. First, channel opening persists in the presence of millimolar levels of intracellular

Ca^{2+}. Second, the openings are long-lived, in some instances lasting more than 50 sec. Finally, the frequency of openings decreases with depolarization. In addition, channel activation occurs in the bilayer presumably by direct interaction of the antibodies with the channel or an associated protein; in the experiments of Kuno et al (39, 70, 71), second messengers appear to be involved, although additional activation by direct interaction cannot be ruled out.

Recently, a mitogen-activated Ca^{2+} current in T cells has been described using a combination of whole-cell or perforated-patch recording (58) and single-cell Ca^{2+} measurement using fura-2 (77, 79). The advantage of this combined approach is that it allows the correlation of particular components of membrane current with the $[Ca^{2+}]_i$ rise in an individual cell. This advantage is an important one because, given the cell volume of lymphocytes, an extremely small Ca^{2+}-selective inward current in principle could suffice to elevate $[Ca^{2+}]_i$ to micromolar levels. PHA treatment of Jurkat cells induces a small inward Ca^{2+} current (< 1 to ≈ 10 pA) after a delay of 100–300 sec, closely followed by a rise in $[Ca^{2+}]_i$. The conductance is not voltage-dependent and appears to be inhibited by intracellular Ca^{2+} (77). In some cases the current undergoes periodic slow fluctuations that closely parallel $[Ca^{2+}]_i$ oscillations (see below), which is consistent with a role in the oscillation mechanism. The high selectivity of the current for Ca^{2+} distinguishes it from the mitogen-gated, whole-cell currents reported previously (71). Its precise relationship to the single-channel events reported by Gardner & colleagues (39, 70, 71) is at present unclear. The absence of readily detectable current fluctuations during its induction suggests that, if the current is conducted by channels, they must have an extremely small conductance or exceedingly brief openings (R. S. Lewis & M. D. Cahalan, unpublished observations). A similarly smooth Ca^{2+} current has been reported in mast cells following stimulation by substance P or compound 48/80 and is believed to represent the major Ca^{2+} influx pathway activated by those agents (88, 99).

Transmembrane Ca^{2+} flux can be evoked in T and B lymphocytes by a variety of stimuli. For T cells, Ca^{2+} signals have been elicited by antigenic recognition, mitogenic lectins, and cross-linking antibodies directed against the cell-surface glycoproteins CD2 through CD8, CD28, thy-1, and the T cell receptor (1, 31, 59, 62, 63, 65, 66, 68, 72, 96, 129, 133). For B cells, the most effective stimulus is anti-Ig antibodies (5, 83, 104, 139). For at least several of these stimuli, the Ca^{2+} rise occurs via release of Ca^{2+} from intracellular pools, with influx being necessary to sustain the response (1, 5, 57, 61, 62, 65, 77, 79, 104). Several kinds of indirect evidence, reviewed above, suggest that a sustained $[Ca^{2+}]_i$ rise is an important triggering signal for lymphocyte activation. The identification of blocking drugs specific for the mitogen-regulated Ca^{2+} channel should greatly facilitate future studies of its role in transducing extracellular stimuli into cytosolic Ca^{2+} signals for lymphocyte activation and other behaviors such as cytotoxicity.

An unsuspected degree of complexity in the pattern of mitogen-stimulated Ca^{2+} signaling in single cells has been revealed recently by dynamic measurements of $[Ca^{2+}]_i$ using fura-2. These experiments show that the sustained phase of the $[Ca^{2+}]_i$ rise in T and B cells results largely from repetitive, asynchronous $[Ca^{2+}]_i$ oscillations occurring at the level of individual cells (77, 79, 131, 139). Oscillations of $[Ca^{2+}]_i$ are a common consequence of cell activation in a number of systems (4, 64, 131, 140). There is currently great interest in identifying the molecular basis of the oscillation mechanism, and several models have been proposed that involve repetitive release from intracellular stores (4, 4a, 91) or oscillatory Ca^{2+} influx across the plasma membrane (77).

CONCLUSIONS AND FUTURE DIRECTIONS

Patch-clamp techniques have enabled the characterization of a diverse set of ion channels in lymphocytes with diverse functional roles. One theme guiding future work in this area is the control of ion-channel activity by intracellular messengers. Regulated patterns of electrical activity in lymphocytes, including the activation and deactivation of Cl^- channels during the volume regulation response and the periodic activity of Ca^{2+} channels underlying mitogen-triggered $[Ca^{2+}]_i$ oscillations, most likely arise from biochemical or mechanical rather than electrical feedback because the underlying channels are voltage-insensitive. Evidence exists for biochemical modulation of voltage-dependent n-type K^+ channels by cAMP and serotonin in B cells (20, 21), which suggests that neurotransmitters may influence immune function through their effects on ion channels.

The single-cell approach to studying membrane properties is a powerful one. In addition to providing high-resolution detection of ion channels down to the level of single-channel molecules in the cell, advantages include the ability to characterize properties of identified subpopulations of cells (as in thymocytes), to reveal dynamic aspects of cell behavior that are obscured in cell suspensions (e.g. $[Ca^{2+}]_i$ oscillations), and to temporally correlate ion channel activity with ionic signals. An increasingly effective and sophisticated array of experimental approaches is being developed to study ionic signaling and modulation at the single -cell level that includes perforated-patch recording, photoreleasable messengers, and imaging with ion-sensitive dyes. As imaging techniques evolve to provide for real-time detection of enzyme activity and gene transcription, the entire signal transduction pathway from membrane to nucleus may ultimately be visualized in single cells.

ACKNOWLEDGMENTS

The authors' work was supported by National Institutes of Health grants GM41514 and NS14609, and the Office of Naval Research.

Literature Cited

1. Alcover, A., Weiss, M. J., Daley, J. F., Reinherz, E. L. 1986. The T11 glycoprotein is functionally linked to a calcium channel in precursor and mature T-lineage cells. *Proc. Natl. Acad. Sci. USA* 83:2614–18

2. Anderson, C. S., MacKinnon, R., Smith, C., Miller, C. 1988. Charybdotoxin block of single Ca^{2+}-activated K^+ channels. Effects of channel gating, voltage, and ionic strength. *J. Gen. Physiol.* 91:317–33

3. Barrett, J. N., Magleby, K. L., Pallotta, B. S. 1980. Properties of single calcium-activated potassium channels in cultured rat muscle. *J. Physiol.* 331:211–30

4. Berridge, M. J., Cobbold, P. H., Cuthbertson, K. S. R. 1988. Spatial and temporal aspects of cell signalling. *Phil. Trans. R. Soc. Lond. Ser. B* 320:325–43

4a. Berridge, M. J., Galione, A. 1988. Cytosolic calcium oscillators. *FASEB J.* 2:3074–82

5. Bijsterbosch, M. K., Rigley, K. P., Klaus, G. G. B. 1986. Cross-linking of surface immunoglobulin on B lymphocytes induces both intracellular Ca^{2+} release and Ca^{2+} influx: analysis with indo-1. *Biochem. Biophys. Res. Comm.* 137:500–6

6. Birx, D. L., Berger, M., Fleisher, T. A. 1984. The interference of T cell activation by calcium channel blocking agents. *J. Immunol.* 133:2904–9

7. Blatz, A. L., Magleby, K. L. 1983. Single voltage-dependent chloride-selective channels of large conductance in cultured rat muscle. *Biophys. J.* 43:237–41

8. Blatz, A. L., Magleby, K. L. 1986. Single apamin-blocked Ca-activated K^+ channels of small conductance in cultured rat skeletal muscle. *Nature* 323:718–20

9. Bosma, M. M. 1986. Chloride channels in neoplastic B lymphocytes. *Biophys. J.* 49:413a (Abstr.)

10. Bregestovski, P., Redkozubov, A., Alexeev, A. 1986. Elevation of intracellular calcium reduces voltage-dependent potassium conductance in human T cells. *Nature* 319:776–78

11. Cahalan, M. D., Chandy, K. G., DeCoursey, T. E., Gupta, S. 1985. A voltage-gated potassium channel in human T lymphocytes. *J. Physiol.* 358:197–237

12. Cahalan, M. D., Chandy, K. G., DeCoursey, T. E., Gupta, S., Lewis, R. S., et al. 1987. Ion channels in T lymphocytes. In *Mechanisms of Lymphocyte Activation and Immune Regulation*, pp. 85–101, ed. S. Gupta, W. E. Paul, A. S. Fauci. New York: Plenum

13. Cahalan, M. D., Lewis, R. S. 1988. Role of potassium and chloride channels in volume regulation by T lymphocytes. In *Cell Physiology of Blood*, pp. 281–301, ed. R. B. Gunn, J. C. Parker. New York: Rockefeller Univ. Press

14. Cambier, J. C., Ransom, J. T. 1987. Molecular mechanisms of transmembrane signaling in B lymphocytes. *Annu. Rev. Immunol.* 5:175–99

15. Chandy, K. G., DeCoursey, T. E., Cahalan, M. D., McLaughlin, D., Gupta, S. 1984. Voltage-gated potassium channels are required for human T lymphocyte activation. *J. Exp. Med.* 160:369–85

16. Chandy, K. G., DeCoursey, T. E., Fischbach, M., Talal, N., Cahalan, M. D., et al. 1986. Altered K^+ channel expression in abnormal T lymphocytes from mice with the *lpr* gene mutation. *Science* 233:1197–1200

17. Chen, J. H., Schulman, H., Gardner, P. 1989. A cAMP-regulated chloride channel in lymphocytes that is affected in cystic fibrosis. *Science* 243:657–60

18. Cheung, R. K., Grinstein, S., Dosch, H.-M., Gelfand, E. W. 1980. Volume regulation by human lymphocytes: characterization of the ionic basis for regulatory volume decrease. *J. Cell. Physiol.* 112:189–96

19. Cheung, R. K., Grinstein, S., Gelfand, E. W. 1980. Volume regulation by human lymphocytes: identification of differences between the two major lymphocyte subpopulations. *J. Clin. Invest.* 70:632–38

20. Choquet, D., Korn, H. 1988. Dual effects of serotonin on a voltage-gated conductance in lymphocytes. *Proc. Natl. Acad. Sci. USA* 85:4557–61

21. Choquet, D., Sarthou, P., Primi, D., Cazenave, P.-A., Korn, H. 1987. Cyclic AMP-modulated potassium channels in

murine B cells and their precursors. *Science* 235:1211–14

22. Crabtree, G. R. 1989. Contingent genetic regulatory events in T lymphocyte activation. *Science* 243:355–61

23. DeCoursey, T. E., Chandy, K. G., Gupta, S., Cahalan, M. D. 1984. Voltage-gated K$^+$ channels in human T lymphocytes: a role in mitogenesis? *Nature* 307:465–68

24. DeCoursey, T. E., Chandy, K. G., Gupta, S., Cahalan, M. D. 1985. Voltage-dependent ion channels in T-lymphocytes. *J. Neuroimmunol.* 10:71–95

25. DeCoursey, T. E., Chandy, K. G., Gupta, S., Cahalan, M. D. 1987. Two types of potassium channels in murine T lymphocytes. *J. Gen. Physiol.* 89:379–404

26. DeCoursey, T. E., Chandy, K. G., Gupta, S., Cahalan, M. D. 1987. Mitogen induction of ion channels in murine T lymphocytes. *J. Gen. Physiol.* 89:405–20

27. DeCoursey, T. E., Jacobs, E. R., Silver, M. R. 1988. Potassium currents in rat type II alveolar epithelial cells. *J. Physiol.* 395:487–505

28. Deutsch, C., Krause, D., Lee, S. C. 1986. Voltage-gated potassium conductance in human T lymphocytes stimulated with phorbol ester. *J. Physiol.* 372:405–23

28a. Deutsch, C., Lee, S. C. 1989. Modulation of K$^+$ currents in human lymphocytes by pH. *J. Physiol.* 413:399–413

28b. Dupuis, G., Héroux, J., Payet, M. D. 1989. Characterization of Ca^{2+} and K$^+$ currents in the human Jurkat T cell line: effects of phytohaemagglutinin. *J. Physiol.* 412:135–54

29. Felber, S. M., Brand, M. D. 1983. Early plasma-membrane-potential changes during stimulation of lymphocytes by concanavalin A. *Biochem. J.* 210:885–91

30. Felber, S. M., Brand, M. D. 1983. Concanavalin A causes an increase in sodium permeability and intracellular sodium content of pig lymphocytes. *Biochem. J.* 210:893–97

31. Finkel, T. H., McDuffie, M., Kappler, J. W., Marrack, P., Cambier, J. C. 1987. Both immature and mature T cells mobilize Ca^{2+} in response to antigen receptor crosslinking. *Nature* 330:179–81

32. Freedman, M. H., Raff, M. C., Gomperts, B. 1975. Induction of increased calcium uptake in mouse T lymphocytes by concanavalin A and its modulation by cyclic nucleotides. *Nature* 255:378–80

33. Fukushima, Y., Hagiwara, S. 1983. Voltage-gated Ca^{2+} channel in mouse myeloma cells. *Proc. Natl. Acad. Sci. USA* 80:2240–42

34. Fukushima, Y., Hagiwara, S., Henkart, M. 1984. Potassium current in clonal cytotoxic T lymphocytes from the mouse. *J. Physiol.* 351:645–56

35. Fukushima, Y., Hagiwara, S., Saxton, R. E. 1984. Variation of calcium current during the cell growth cycle in mouse hybridoma lines secreting immunoglobulins. *J. Physiol.* 355:313–21

36. Gallin, E. K. 1986. Ionic channels in leukocytes. *J. Leukocyte Biol.* 39:241–54

37. Gallin, E. K. 1988. The effects of Ba, quinine, and TEA on ionomycin-induced K channel activity in human macrophages. *J. Gen. Physiol.* 92:40a (Abstr.)

38. Gallin, E. K., Sheehy, P. A. 1985. Differential expression of inward and outward potassium currents in the macrophage-like cell line J774.1. *J. Physiol.* 369:475–99

39. Gardner, P., Alcover, A., Kuno, M., Moingeon, P., Weyand, C. M., et al. 1989. Triggering of T-lymphocytes via either T3-Ti or T11 surface structures opens a voltage-insensitive plasma membrane calcium-permeable channel: requirement for interleukin-2 gene function. *J. Biol. Chem.* 264:1068–76

40. Gelfand, E. W., Cheung, R. K., Grinstein, S. 1984. Role of membrane potential in the regulation of lectin-induced calcium uptake. *J. Cell. Physiol.* 121:533–39

41. Gelfand, E. W., Cheung, R. K., Grinstein, S. 1986. Mitogen-induced changes in Ca^{2+} permeability are not mediated by voltage-gated K$^+$ channels. *J. Biol. Chem.* 261:11520–23

42. Goldsmith, M. A., Weiss, A. 1988. Early signal transduction by the antigen receptor without commitment to T cell activation. *Science* 240:1029–31

43. Gray, L. S., Gnarra, J. R., Russell, J. H., Engelhard, V. H. 1987. The role of K$^+$ in the regulation of the increase of intracellular Ca^{2+} mediated by the T lymphocyte antigen receptor. *Cell* 50:119–27

44. Gray, P. T. A., Bevan, S., Ritchie, J. M. 1984. High conductance anion-selective channels in rat cultured Schwann cells. *Proc. R. Soc. Lond. Ser. B* 221:395–409

45. Grinstein, S., Clarke, C. A., Dupre, A., Rothstein, A. 1980. Volume-induced increase of anion permeability in human lymphocytes. *J. Gen. Physiol.* 80:801–23

46. Grinstein, S., Cohen, S., Sarkadi, B., Rothstein, A. 1983. Induction of ^{86}Rb fluxes by Ca^{2+} and volume changes in thymocytes and their isolated membranes. *J. Cell. Physiol.* 116:352–62

47. Grinstein, S., Dupre, A., Rothstein, A. 1982. Volume regulation by human lymphocytes: role of calcium. *J. Gen. Physiol.* 79:849–68

48. Grinstein, S., Smith, J. D., Miller, C. 1988. Charybdotoxin inhibits regulatory volume decrease and mitogen- or Ca^{2+} ionophore-induced hyperpolarization in lymphocytes. *Biophys. J.* 53:148a (Abstr.)

49. Grissmer, S., Cahalan, M. 1989. Ionomycin activates a potassium-selective conductance in human T lymphocytes. *Biophys. J.* 55:245a (Abstr.)

50. Grissmer, S., Cahalan, M. D. 1989. Divalent ion trapping inside potassium channels of human T lymphocytes. *J. Gen. Physiol.* 93:609–30

51. Grissmer, S., Cahalan, M. D. 1989. TEA prevents inactivation while blocking open K^+ channels in human T lymphocytes. *Biophys. J.* 55:203–6

52. Grissmer, S., Cahalan, M. D., Chandy, K. G. 1988. Abundant expression of type *l* K^+ channels. A marker for lymphoproliferative diseases? *J. Immunol.* 141:1137–42

53. Grynkiewicz, G., Poenie, M., Tsien, R. Y. 1985. A new generation of Ca^{2+} indicators with greatly improved fluorescence properties. *J. Biol. Chem.* 260:3440–50

54. Hals, G. D., Stein, P. G., Palade, P. T. 1989. Single channel characteristics of a high conductance anion channel in "sarcoballs." *J. Gen. Physiol.* 93:385–410

55. Hamill, O. P., Marty, A., Neher, E., Sakmann, B., Sigworth, F. J. 1981. Improved patch-clamp techniques for high-resolution current recording from cells and cell-free membrane patches. *Pflügers Arch.* 391:85–100

56. Hesketh, T. R., Bavetta, S., Smith, G. A., Metcalfe, J. C. 1983. Duration of the calcium signal in the mitogenic stimulation of thymocytes. *Biochem. J.* 214:575–79

57. Hesketh, T. R., Moore, J. P., Morris, J. D. H., Taylor, M. V., Rogers, J., et al. 1985. A common sequence of calcium and pH signals in the mitogenic stimulation of eukaryotic cells. *Nature* 313:481–84

58. Horn, R., Marty, A. 1988. Muscarinic activation of ionic currents measured by a new whole-cell recording method. *J. Gen. Physiol.* 92:145–59

59. Huenig, T., Tiefenthaler, G., zum Bues-
chenfelde, K.-H. M., Meuer, S. C. 1987. Alternative pathway activation of T cells by binding of CD2 to its cell-surface ligand. *Nature* 326:298–301

60. Hugues, M., Romey, G., Duval, D., Vincent, J. P., Lazdunski, M. 1982. Apamin as a selective blocker of the calcium-dependent potassium channel in neuroblastoma cells: Voltage-clamp and biochemical characterization of the toxin receptor. *Proc. Natl. Acad. Sci. USA* 79:1308–12

61. Imboden, J. B., Stobo, J. D. 1985. Transmembrane signalling by the T cell antigen receptor. *J. Exp. Med.* 161:446–56

62. Imboden, J. B., Weiss, A. 1987. The T-cell antigen receptor regulates sustained increases in cytoplasmic free Ca^{2+} through extracellular Ca^{2+} influx and ongoing intracellular Ca^{2+} mobilization. *Biochem. J.* 247:695–700

63. Imboden, J. B., Weiss, A., Stobo, J. D. 1985. The antigen receptor on a human T cell line initiates activation by increasing cytoplasmic free calcium. *J. Immunol.* 134:663–65

64. Jacob, R., Merritt, J. E., Hallam, T. J., Rink, T. J. 1988. Repetitive spikes in cytoplasmic calcium evoked by histamine in human endothelial cells. *Nature* 335:40–45

65. June, C. H., Ledbetter, J. A., Rabinovitch, P. S., Martin, P. J., Beatty, P. G., et al. 1986. Distinct patterns of transmembrane calcium flux and intracellular calcium mobilization after differentiation antigen cluster 2 (E rosette receptor) or 3 (T3) stimulation of human lymphocytes. *J. Clin. Invest.* 77:1224–32

66. June, C. H., Rabinovitch, P. S., Ledbetter, J. A. 1987. CD5 antibodies increase intracellular ionized calcium concentration in T cells. *J. Immunol.* 138:2782–92

67. Kaplan, J. G. 1978. Membrane cation transport and the control of proliferation of mammalian cells. *Annu. Rev. Physiol.* 40:19–41

68. Kroczek, R. A., Gunter, K. C., Germain, R. N., Shevach, E. M. 1986. Thy-1 functions as a signal transduction molecule in T lymphocytes and transfected B lymphocytes. *Nature* 322:181–84

69. Krouse, M. E., Schneider, G. T., Gage, P. W. 1986. A large anion-selective channel has seven conductance levels. *Nature* 319:58–60

70. Kuno, M., Gardner, P. 1987. Ion channels activated by inositol 1,4,5-trisphosphate in plasma membrane of

human T-lymphocytes. *Nature* 326:301–4

71. Kuno, M., Goronzy, J., Weyand, C. M., Gardner, P. 1986. Single-channel and whole-cell recordings of mitogen-regulated inward currents in human cloned helper T lymphocytes. *Nature* 323:269–73

72. Ledbetter, J. A., June, C. H., Grosmaire, L. S., Rabinovitch, P. S. 1987. Crosslinking of surface antigens causes mobilization of intracellular ionized calcium in T lymphocytes. *Proc. Natl. Acad. Sci. USA* 84:1384–88

73. Lee, S. C., Price, M., Prystowsky, M. B., Deutsch, C. 1988. Volume response of quiescent and interleukin 2-stimulated T-lymphocytes to hypotonicity. *Am. J. Physiol.* 254:C286–96

74. Lee, S. C., Sabath, D. E., Deutsch, C., Prystowsky, M. B. 1986. Increased voltage-gated potassium conductance during interleukin 2-stimulated proliferation of a mouse helper T lymphocyte clone. *J. Cell Biol.* 102:1200–8

75. Lewis, R. S., Cahalan, M. D. 1988. Subset-specific expression of potassium channels in developing murine T lymphocytes. *Science* 239:771–75

76. Lewis, R. S., Cahalan, M. D. 1988. The plasticity of ion channels: parallels between the nervous and immune systems. *Trends Neurosci.* 11:214–18

77. Lewis, R. S., Cahalan, M. D. 1989. Mitogen-induced oscillations of cytosolic Ca^{2+} and transmembrane Ca^{2+} current in human leukemic T cells. *Cell Regul.* In press

78. Lewis, R. S., Cahalan, M. D. 1988. Voltage-dependent calcium signalling in single T lymphocytes. *Soc. Neurosci. Abstr.* 14:298 (Abstr.)

79. Lewis, R. S., Cahalan, M. D. 1989. Ion channels and calcium signaling in single mitogen-stimulated T lymphocytes. In *Immunogenicity, UCLA Symp. Molec. Cell. Biol., New Series.* Vol. 113, ed. C. Janeway, J. Sprent, E. Sercarz. New York: Liss. In press

80. Li, M., McCann, J. D., Liedtke, C. M., Nairn, A. C., Greengard, P., et al. 1988. Cyclic AMP-dependent protein kinase opens chloride channels in normal but not cystic fibrosis airway epithelium. *Nature* 331:358–60

81. MacDonald, H. R., Nabholz, M. 1986. T-cell activation. *Annu. Rev. Cell Biol.* 2:231–253

82. MacDougall, S. L., Grinstein, S., Gelfand, E. W. 1988. Activation of Ca^{2+}-dependent K^+ channels in human B lymphocytes by anti-immunoglobulin. *J. Clin. Invest.* 81:449–54

83. MacDougall, S. L., Grinstein, S., Gelfand, E. W. 1988. Detection of ligand-activated conductive Ca^{2+} channels in human B lymphocytes. *Cell* 54:229–34

83a. Mahaut-Smith, M. P., Schlichter, L. C. 1989. Ca^{2+}-activated K^+ channels in human B lymphocytes and rat thymocytes. *J. Physiol.* 415:69–83

84. Martz, E. 1977. Mechanism of specific tumor-cell lysis by alloimmune T lymphocytes: resolution and characterization of discrete steps in the cellular interaction. *Contemp. Top. Immunobiol.* 7:301–61

85. Maruyama, Y. 1987. A patch-clamp study of mammalian platelets and their voltage-gated potassium current. *J. Physiol.* 391:467–85

86. Mastro, A. M., Smith, M. C. 1983. Calcium-dependent activation of lymphocytes by ionophore, A23187, and a phorbol ester tumor promoter. *J. Cell. Physiol.* 116:51–56

87. Matteson, D. R., Deutsch, C. 1984. K channels in T lymphocytes: a patch clamp study using monoclonal antibody adhesion. *Nature* 307:468–71

88. Matthews, G., Neher, E., Penner, R. 1989. Second messenger-activated calcium influx in rat peritoneal mast cells. *J. Physiol.* In press

89. McCrady, C. W., Ely, C. M., Westin, E., Carchman, R. A. 1988. Coordination and reversibility of signals for proliferative activation and interleukin-2 mRNA production in resting human T lymphocytes by phorbol ester and calcium ionophore. *J. Biol. Chem.* 263:18537–44

90. McKinnon, D., Ceredig, R. 1986. Changes in the expression of potassium channels during mouse T cell development. *J. Exp. Med.* 164:1846–1861

91. Meyer, T., Stryer, L. 1988. Molecular model for receptor-stimulated calcium spiking. *Proc. Natl. Acad. Sci. USA* 85:5051–55

92. Miller, C., Moczydlowski, E., Latorre, R., Phillips, M. 1985. Charybdotoxin, a protein inhibitor of single Ca^{2+}-activated K^+ channels from mammalian skeletal muscle. *Nature* 313:316–18

93. Mills, G. B., Cheung, R. K., Grinstein, S., Gelfand, E. W. 1985. Increase in cytosolic free calcium concentration is an intracellular messenger for the production of interleukin 2 but not for expression of the interleukin 2 receptor. *J. Immunol.* 134:1640–43

94. Moore, J. P., Todd, J. A., Hesketh, T. R., Metcalfe, J. C. 1986. c-*fos* and c-*myc* gene activation, ionic signals, and

DNA synthesis in thymocytes. *J. Biol. Chem.* 261:8158–62

95. Neher, E. 1988. The use of the patch clamp technique to study second messenger-mediated cellular events. *Neuroscience* 26:727–34

96. Nisbet-Brown, E., Cheung, R. K., Lee, J. W. W., Gelfand, E. W. 1985. Antigen-dependent increase in cytosolic free calcium in specific human T-lymphocyte clones. *Nature* 316:545–47

97. Oettgen, H. C., Terhorst, C., Cantley, L. C., Rosoff, P. M. 1985. Stimulation of the T3-T cell receptor complex induces a membrane-potential-sensitive calcium influx. *Cell* 40:583–90

98. Pecht, I., Corcia, A., Liuzzi, M. P. T., Alcover, A., Reinherz, E. L. 1987. Ion channels activated by specific Ti or T3 antibodies in plasma membranes of human T cells. *EMBO J.* 6:1935–39

99. Penner, R., Matthews, G., Neher, E. 1988. Regulation of calcium influx by second messengers in rat mast cells. *Nature* 334:499–504

100. Poenie, M., Tsien, R. Y., Schmitt-Verhulst, A.-M. 1987. Sequential activation and lethal hit measured by $[Ca^{2+}]_i$ in individual cytolytic T cells and targets. *EMBO J.* 6:2223–32

101. Prasad, K. V. S., Severini, A., Kaplan, J. G. 1987. Sodium ion influx in proliferating lymphocytes: An early component of the mitogenic signal. *Arch. Biochem. Biophys.* 252:515–25

102. Randriamampita, C., Trautmann, A. 1987. Ionic channels in murine macrophages. *J. Cell Biol.* 105:761–69

103. Ransom, J. T., Cambier, J. C. 1988. Membrane events during lymphocyte activation. In *Handbook of Experimental Pharmacology*, ed. M. A. Bray, J. Morley, 85:53–82. New York: Springer-Verlag

104. Ransom, J. T., Chen, M., Sandoval, V. M., Pasternak, J. A., Digiusto, D., Cambier, J. C. 1988. Increased plasma membrane permeability to Ca^{2+} in anti-Ig-stimulated B lymphocytes is dependent on activation of phosphoinositide hydrolysis. *J. Immunol.* 140:3150–55

105. Reed, J. C., Nowell, P. C., Hoover, R. G. 1985. Regulation of c-*myc* mRNA levels in normal human lymphocytes by modulators of cell proliferation. *Proc. Natl. Acad. Sci. USA* 82:4221–24

106. Rink, T. J., Deutsch, C. 1983. Calcium-activated potassium channels in lymphocytes. *Cell Calcium* 4:463–73

107. Rink, T. J., Sanchez, A., Grinstein, S., Rothstein, A. 1983. Volume restoration in osmotically swollen lymphocytes does not involve changes in free Ca^{2+} concentration. *Biochim. Biophys. Acta* 762:593–96

108. Rosoff, P. M., Cantley, L. C. 1985. Stimulation of the T3-T cell receptor-associated Ca^{2+} influx enhances activity of the Na^+/H^+ exchanger in a leukemic human T cell line. *J. Biol. Chem.* 260:14053–59

109. Russell, J. H., Dobos, C. B. 1983. Accelerated $^{86}Rb^+$ (K^+) release from the cytotoxic T lymphocyte is a physiologic event associated with delivery of the lethal hit. *J. Immunol.* 131:1138–41

110. Sabath, D. E., Monos, D. S., Lee, S. C., Deutsch, C., Prystowsky, M. B. 1986. Cloned T-cell proliferation and synthesis of specific proteins are inhibited by quinine. *Proc. Natl. Acad. Sci. USA* 83:4739–43

111. Sands, S. B., Lewis, R. S., Cahalan, M. D. 1989. Charybdotoxin blocks voltage-gated K^+ channels in human and murine T lymphocytes. *J. Gen. Physiol.* 93:1061–74

112. Sarkadi, B., Cheung, R., Mack, E., Grinstein, S., Gelfand, E. W., et al. 1985. Cation and anion transport pathways in volume regulatory response of human lymphocytes to hyposmotic media. *Am. J. Physiol.* 248:C480–87

113. Sarkadi, B., Mack, E., Rothstein, A. 1984. Ionic events during the volume response of human peripheral blood lymphocytes to hypotonic media. I. Distinctions between volume-activated Cl^- and K^+ conductance pathways. *J. Gen. Physiol.* 83:497–512

114. Sarkadi, B., Mack, E., Rothstein, A. 1984. Ionic events during the volume response of human peripheral blood lymphocytes to hypotonic media. II. Volume- and time-dependent activation and inactivation of ion transport pathways. *J. Gen. Physiol.* 83:513–27

115. Schell, S. R., Nelson, D. J., Fozzard, H. A., Fitch, F. W. 1987. The inhibitory effects of K^+ channel-blocking agents on T lymphocyte proliferation and lymphokine production are "nonspecific." *J. Immunol.* 139:3224–30

116. Schlichter, L., Sidell, N., Hagiwara, S. 1986. Potassium channels mediate killing by human natural killer cells. *Proc. Natl. Acad. Sci. USA* 83:451–55

117. Schlichter, L., Sidell, N., Hagiwara, S. 1986. K channels are expressed early in human T-cell development. *Proc. Natl. Acad. Sci. USA* 83:5625–29

118. Deleted in proof

119. Schoumacher, R. A., Shoemaker, R. L., Halm, D. R., Tallant, E. A., Wallace, R. W., et al. 1987. Phosphorylation fails to activate chloride channels from cystic fibrosis airway cells. *Nature* 330:752–54

120. Schwarze, W., Kolb, H.-A. 1984. Voltage-dependent kinetics of an anionic channel of large unit conductance in macrophages and myotube membranes. *Pflügers Arch.* 402:281–91

121. Segel, G. B., Simon, W., Lichtman, M. A. 1979. Regulation of sodium and potassium transport in phytohemagglutinin-stimulated human blood lymphocytes. *J. Clin. Invest.* 64:834–41

122. Shapiro, M. S., DeCoursey, T. E. 1988. Two types of potassium channels in a lymphoma cell line. *Biophys. J.* 53:550a (Abstr.)

123. Sidell, N., Schlichter, L. C., Wright, S. C., Hagiwara, S., Golub, S. H. 1986. Potassium channels in human NK cells are involved in discrete stages of the killing process. *J. Immunol.* 137:1650–58

124. Soltoff, S. P., Cantley, L. C. 1988. Mitogens and ion fluxes. *Annu. Rev. Physiol.* 50:207–23

125. Sussman, J. J., Merćep, J., Saito, T., Germain, R. N., Bonvini, E., et al. 1988. Dissociation of phosphoinositide hydrolysis and Ca^{2+} fluxes from the biological responses of a T-cell hybridoma. *Nature* 334:625–28

126. Sutro, J. B., Vayuvegula, B. S., Gupta, S., Cahalan, M. D. 1988. Up-regulation of voltage-sensitive K^+ channels in mitogen-stimulated B lymphocytes. *Biophys. J.* 53:460a (Abstr.)

127. Sutro, J. B., Vayuvegula, B. S., Gupta, S., Cahalan, M. D. 1989. Voltage-sensitive ion channels in human B lymphocytes. In *Mechanisms of Lymphocyte Activation and Immune Regulation,* ed. S. Gupta, W. E. Paul, A. S. Fauci. New York: Plenum In press

128. Tatham, P. E. R., O'Flynn, K., Linch, D. C. 1986. The relationship between mitogen-induced membrane potential changes and intracellular free calcium in human T-lymphocytes. *Biochim. Biophys. Acta* 856:202–11

129. Treves, S., Di Virgilio, F., Cerundolo, V., Zanovello, P., Collavo, D., et al. 1987. Calcium and inositolphosphates in the activation of T cell-mediated cytotoxicity. *J. Exp. Med.* 166:33–42

130. Truneh, A., Albert, F., Golstein, P., Schmitt-Verhulst, A.-M. 1985. Early steps of lymphocyte activation bypassed by synergy between calcium ionophores and phorbol ester. *Nature* 313:318–20

131. Tsien, R. Y., Poenie, M. 1986. Fluorescence ratio imaging: a new window into intracellular ionic signaling. *Trends Biochem. Sci.* 11:450–55

132. Tsien, R. Y., Pozzan, T., Rink, T. J. 1982. T-cell mitogens cause early changes in cytoplasmic free Ca^{2+} and membrane potential in lymphocytes. *Nature* 295:68–71

133. Weiss, A., Imboden, J., Shoback, D., Stobo, J. 1984. Role of T3 surface molecules in human T-cell activation: T3-dependent activation results in an increase in cytoplasmic free calcium. *Proc. Natl. Acad. Sci. USA* 81:4169–73

134. Weiss, A., Imboden, J. B. 1987. Cell surface molecules and early events involved in human T lymphocyte activation. *Adv. Immunol.* 41:1–38

135. Weiss, M. J., Daley, J. F., Hodgdon, J. C., Reinherz, E. L. 1984. Calcium dependency of antigen-specific (T3-Ti) and alternative (T11) pathways of human T-cell activation. *Proc. Natl. Acad. Sci. USA* 81:6836–40

136. Whitney, R. B., Sutherland, R. M. 1972. Requirement for calcium ions in lymphocyte transformation stimulated by phytohemagglutinin. *J. Cell. Physiol.* 80:329–38

137. Whitney, R. B., Sutherland, R. M. 1973. Characteristics of calcium accumulation by lymphocytes and alterations in the process induced by phytohemagglutinin. *J. Cell. Physiol.* 82:9–20

138. Wilson, H. A., Chused, T. M. 1985. Lymphocyte membrane potential and Ca^{2+}-sensitive potassium channels described by oxonol dye fluorescence measurements. *J. Cell. Physiol.* 125:72–81

139. Wilson, H. A., Greenblatt, D., Poenie, M., Finkelman, F. D., Tsien, R. Y. 1987. Crosslinkage of B lymphocyte surface immunoglobulin by anti-Ig or antigen induces prolonged oscillations of intracellular ionized calcium. *J. Exp. Med.* 166:601–6

140. Woods, N. M., Cuthbertson, K. S. R., Cobbold, P. H. 1986. Repetitive transient rises in cytoplasmic free calcium in hormone-stimulated hepatocytes. *Nature* 319:600–2

141. Ypey, D. L., Clapham, D. E. 1984. Development of a delayed outward-rectifying K^+ conductance in cultured mouse peritoneal macrophages. *Proc. Natl. Acad. Sci. USA* 81:3083–87

Annu. Rev. Physiol. 1990. 52:431–49
Copyright © 1990 by Annual Reviews Inc. All rights reserved

CALCIUM SIGNALING IN HUMAN PLATELETS

T. J. Rink

Smith Kline & French Research Limited, The Frythe, Welwyn, Herts, AL6 9AR, United Kingdom

S. O. Sage

Physiological Laboratory, Downing Street, Cambridge, CB2 3EG, United Kingdom

KEY WORDS: receptor, channel, fluorescent indicator, second messenger, Mn^{2+}

INTRODUCTION

In this chapter we outline our current understanding of the processes by which external Ca^{2+} and internal Ca^{2+} stores are mobilized to generate cytosolic free Ca^{2+} ($[Ca^{2+}]_i$) signals in human platelets, and note briefly what is known of how resting $[Ca^{2+}]_i$ is restored and maintained. Due to limitations of space we will not cover the downstream events of calcium interaction with intracellular targets that evoke functional and structural changes: see Reference 71 for a recent, comprehensive review of platelet activation.

A central role for Ca^{2+} in platelet activation was deduced initially by analogy with other secretory and contractile cells where Ca^{2+} had been established as a key mediator of stimulus-secretion and excitation-contraction coupling. A variety of approaches then supported this notion for platelets. Several groups showed that calcium ionophores could evoke platelet responses similar to those seen with natural ligands acting at surface receptors:[45]Ca uptake was found to be increased on stimulation; measurement of chlortetracycline fluorescence (81) was consistent with stimulus-evoked discharge of an internal Ca store; and secretion from electro-permeabilized platelets was stimulated by Ca^{2+} in the range of 0.1 to $10\mu M$ (e.g. 21, 52,

0066-4278/90/0315-0431$02.00

53). The first analyses of agonist-evoked $[Ca^{2+}]_i$ signals awaited the development, in the early 80s, of the fluorescent indicator, quin2, which could be introduced into populations of small cells by cytosolic esterase hydrolysis of the membrane-permeant acetoxymethyl ester (59). This "first-generation" indicator provided considerable insights, which have been summarized in earlier reviews (21, 53). Since 1986 most workers have turned to the "second-generation" dye fura-2. Its greater fluorescence signal permits lower intracellular concentrations of indicator, and hence less cytosolic buffering, and has the advantage of a significant shift of excitation spectrum on calcium binding that allows dual or multiple wavelength ratio techniques e.g. (9). Also, a few groups have made measurements with the photo-protein aequorin (e.g. 26, 84), loaded by reversible cell permeabilization induced by ATP^{4-}, and there have been some further significant data from $^{45}Ca^{2+}$ flux measurements (4, 55). This account will refer mainly to work published between January 1986 and March 1989, but key findings from early work are also referenced. We have focused on studies of human platelets, judged by us to provide important new data and/or insights; we offer the usual apologies for the inevitable omission of some good and significant work.

It is worth noting that the ability to measure and manipulate $[Ca^{2+}]_i$ also allows clearer understanding of the role of other cellular messengers. For instance, it soon became apparent that some functional responses, including secretory exocytosis, shape-change, and myosin phosphorylation, could occur with little or no measured rise in $[Ca^{2+}]_i$ (18, 58, 59). The "Ca-independent" secretory response is probably mediated via protein kinase C (58), which in turn is activated at basal $[Ca^{2+}]_i$ by increased formation of diacylglycerol formed by receptor-mediator activation of phospholipases acting on inositol lipids or on phosphatidylcholine. Ca^{2+}-independent shape-change and myosin phosphorylation seem not to reflect activity of protein kinase C (18, 21) and point to the existence of another excitatory signaling pathway, so far unidentified. Experiments with agents that elevate cAMP and inhibit responses to almost all agonists have shown that cAMP, acting presumably via A-kinase, inhibits both the generation and the actions of intracellular messengers, including elevated $[Ca^{2+}]_i$ (e.g. 1, 39, 41, 57, 64).

IONIC GRADIENTS AND MEMBRANE POTENTIAL

Platelets are in a sense cell fragments, which bud off from megakaryocytes in the bone marrow; they are very small, approximately discoidal, 1 by 3 μm. They lack nuclei and any significant components of protein synthesis, but otherwise appear to have the major components common to larger cell types. The available evidence indicates that platelets share with other cells the usual gradients of Na^+ and K^+, established and maintained by an ouabain-sensitive Na-K ATPase, and have a plasma membrane selectively permeable to K^+ (23, 31, 43, 69). Mass measurements indicate $[K^+]_i$ to be about 135 mM and $[Na^+]_i$ about 20 mM. There are no measurements of intracellular activities for those ions. Resting pH_i is around 7.0 at 37°C, depending somewhat on the experimental conditions (e.g. 72, 73, 74). We recently found that in the usual bicarbonate-free suspending medium pH_i was 7.02, whereas in the presence of 25 mM HCO_3^- with 5% CO_2, pH_i was 7.15 (25). There is clear evidence for the presence of $Na^+:H^+$ exchange in platelets (72, 89), though it is not clear to what extent this is responsible for the maintainance of pH_i. A recent paper has put free Mg^{2+} in the range of 0.1 to 0.3 mM (85), which is markedly lower than that reported for lymphocytes, and many other cell types. This finding needs independent confirmation.

Resting $[Ca^{2+}]_i$ measured by fluorescence indicators is typically close to 0.1 μM. In more recent work with quin2 or fura-2, values for basal $[Ca^{2+}]_i$ tend to be in the range 70–80 nM. These lower values may reflect closer attention to leaked indicator and perhaps better preparation of the cells. Basal $[Ca^{2+}]_i$ is remarkably insensitive to large changes in external $[Ca^{2+}]$. Estimates of basal $[Ca^{2+}]_i$ in aequorin-loaded platelets have been much higher than measurements with quin2 or fura-2 (26, 84). The reason is not known, although the main proponents of the technique have recently proposed that lower than expected free Mg^{2+} in platelets compared with, for example, lymphocytes (60) may account for part of the discrepancy since the calibration of aequorin signals is markedly influenced by $[Mg^{2+}]$ (85). Other aspects of this aequorin technique are discussed in a previous review (9).

Estimates with fluorescent potential-sensitive dyes, or the distribution of radio-labeled lipophilic cations, indicate a platelet resting potential of −60 to −70 mV (e.g. 31, 43). This potential is dominated by the K^+ gradient and substitution of Na^+ or Cl^- with large organic ions has little detectable effect. Recently, whole cell patch-clamp recordings have been made on rabbit, rat, and human platelets (32, 33). The initial zero-current potential was about −52 mV, and the only detectable conductance was a voltage-dependent K^+ conductance. It is possible that sporadic opening of these channels provides the resting K^+ permeability that supports the resting potential. As in many cells, none of the main cations is at electrochemical equilibrium. Therefore there must be primary (ATP-fueled) or secondary active transporters for them. Clearly one is the Na^+/K^+ ATPase which generates the Na^+ gradient, which in turn can provide the potential energy for secondary active transport e.g. of H^+ by $Na^+:H^+$ exchange.

There is controversy in the literature as to whether $Na^+:Ca^{2+}$ exchange or a Ca^{2+}-ATPase in the plasma membrane provides the Ca^{2+} extrusion needed for maintainence of, and recovery to, the resting state (e.g. 5, 14, 16, 35, 50, 55, 56, 70). We judge the evidence to favor a more important role for a Ca^{2+}-ATPase.

Features of $Na^+ : Ca^{2+}$ exchange are clearly seen in microsomal fractions enriched in plasma membrane (50). Some authors have not found Ca^{2+}-ATPase in plasma membrane fractions, but others have reported two classes of Ca^{2+}-ATPase in platelet membranes and proposed that one, analogous to the real cell Ca-ATPase, serves as a Ca^{2+} pump in the platelet plasma membrane (14, 16). Brass observed a reduced ^{45}Ca efflux and increased uptake into human platelets when N-methyl-D-glucamine replaced external Na^+ (5). However, he observed no measurable change in $[Ca^{2+}]_i$ measured by quin2, a result reflected in other reports. More significant, perhaps, was the limited effect of Na^+ substitution in the recovery of $[Ca^{2+}]_i$ or the efflux of $^{45}Ca^{2+}$ following elevation of $[Ca^{2+}]_i$ by thrombin or ionomycin (55, 56). In a very recent paper it is reported that addition of Na^+ but not K^+, to platelets, gel-filtered, treated with ouabain, and suspended in sucrose solution, promoted a decline in $[Ca^{2+}]_i$ (70). This result is consistent with $Na^+ : Ca^{2+}$ exchange, but there were no flux measurements to confirm an efflux rather than sequestration of Ca^{2+}.

INTERNAL CALCIUM RELEASE

The persistence of functional responses, attributed to elevated $[Ca^{2+}]_i$, in the absence of external Ca^{2+} provided indirect evidence for agonist-evoked discharge of intracellular Ca^{2+} stores. This analysis neglected the possibility that non-Ca^{2+} pathways might mediate such responses (as we now believe can happen); but the ability of Ca^{2+} ionophores to activate platelets in the absence of external calcium was more convincing evidence for a pool of Ca^{2+} sequestered in intracellular organelles. The existence of a microsome fraction capable of ATP-dependent accumulation of Ca^{2+}, analogous to sarcoplasmic reticulum (SR) fractions of muscle, was also consistent with this concept (e.g. 7, 39, 40). The demonstration of rapid agonist-evoked elevation of $[Ca^{2+}]_i$ in quin2-loaded platelets suspended in Ca-free medium (59) confirmed the existence of receptor-mediated internal discharge. Subsequent investigation has shown that many platelet receptors including those for platelet activating factor (PAF), vasopressin, thromboxane A_2, 5-hydroxytryptamine, and ADP can mediate internal Ca^{2+} release (13, 21, 53, 81). By contrast, adrenaline and collagen, which are capable of stimulating human platelets to aggregate and secrete, do not appear directly to elevate $[Ca^{2+}]_i$ (at least as measured by quin2 or fura-2) via their own receptors (13, 21, 53). Rather the involvement of Ca^{2+} is indirect: these agents promote aggregation and the liberation of arachidonic acid, probably from phosphatidylcholine, via Ca^{2+}-independent pathways (46). The arachidonic acid is then converted to thromboxane A_2, which acts on its receptors to cause a delayed $[Ca^{2+}]_i$ response. Activators of protein kinase C, such as oleoylacetylglycerol or phorbol myristate acetate, do not increase platelet $[Ca^{2+}]_i$ (in the presence or absence of external Ca^{2+}) as measured by quin2 (26, 58) or fura-2 (47, 85). These agents do produce a modest increase in light emission from aequorin-loaded platelets, but the implication of such signals in terms of Ca^{2+} mobilization and cell signaling remains unclear (84).

The amount of Ca^{2+} discharged from internal stores can be estimated from the size of the $[Ca^{2+}]_i$ transient in quin2-loaded platelets and the intracellular quin2 concentration (59). Such calculations give values of 2–300 μmol Ca^{2+} per liter cell water. This is a plausible value for Ca^{2+} sequestered in organelles, presumably in the dense tubular system, which occupy a few percent of the cytoplasmic volume. The total Ca^{2+} content in such organelles would then be in the range of 10–20 mM, and the expectation is that much of this Ca^{2+} would be reversibly bound to a calsequestrin-like molecule so that the free $[Ca^{2+}]$ in these organelles might be several hundred μM. This arrangement would be analogous to the sacroplasmic reticulum in muscle and to the specialized calcium-sequestering and discharging organelles, "calciosomes", proposed for nonmuscle cells (34).

The amount of internal Ca^{2+} discharged by thrombin is virtually the same as that discharged by Ca^{2+} ionophores (59), which suggests that all the readily mobilized intracellular Ca^{2+} is accessible to receptor-mediated pathways. The minimal Ca^{2+} release evoked by mitochondrial uncouplers indicates that, as in most other cells, mitochondria are not a significant source of releasable Ca^{2+}. Mass measurements of Ca^{2+} and analysis of the amine-storage dense granules show that the total content of Ca^{2+} in platelets is much higher than the dischargeable store, about 10–20 mmol per liter of cell water. Most of this Ca^{2+} forms an insoluble matrix with biogenic amines and ATP within the secretory granules, thereby permitting a content of secretable product far in excess of that possible if the granule contents were in solution, and thus at osmotic balance with the cytosol.

Experiments with fura-2, loaded at low cell content, have shown that agonist-evoked internal release can increase $[Ca^{2+}]_i$ to at least 1 μM (47) and thus well into the range of $[Ca^{2+}]$, which is expected to influence target proteins. Use of stopped-flow equipment has allowed us to examine the subsecond kinetics of Ca^{2+} mobilization (62, 66, 67). In Ca^{2+}-free solution, thrombin, PAF, vasopressin, U46619 (a thromboxane mimetic), and ADP can elicit a $[Ca^{2+}]_i$ rise after a minimum delay of only some 200 msec, with a peak being reached within one sec. These results show that surface ligands can elicit a greater than tenfold elevation of $[Ca^{2+}]_i$ within a few hundred msecs, just by internal release. The delay and the time to peak response lengthen as agonist concentration is reduced from the optimal level, or when the cells are treated with forskolin to increase cAMP levels (56, 67).

Inositol Phosphates

The role of inositol 1,4,5-trisphosphate, IP_3, as a link between receptor occupation and Ca^{2+} discharge is as well established for platelets as for many other cell types. Several agonists elicit a prompt formation of IP_3 and diacylglycerol from PIP_2 hydrolysis (10, 13, 17, 71, 80), though it has yet to be shown that IP_3 is formed quickly enough to account for the rapid $[Ca^{2+}]_i$ responses described above. IP_3 can cause Ca^{2+} release from platelet microsomes and from saponin-permeabilized platelets (e.g. 2, 6, 7, 11, 15, 40). The concentration range over which IP_3 is effective, 1–10 μM, is similar to that required in many other preparations and is compatible with the amount of PIP_2 breakdown and with mass measurement of the stimulated formation of inositol phosphates (80). At this point there is no reason to believe that the IP_3 receptor, or the calcium channel it is coupled to, differ from those in other cell types. As in many other systems, IP_3 is subject to a complex array of metabolic conversions starting with dephosphorylation to the 1,4-bisphosphate, or phosphorylation to form the 1,3,4,5-tetrakisphosphate (71). Thus within 10–20 secs much of the trisphosphate is actually in the form of the 1,3,4 isomer (80). Also, a small proportion of 1,2-cyclic 4,5-trisphosphate is formed. The available evidence suggests that the 1,4,5-tris isomer has the major, perhaps exclusive, role in Ca^{2+} release by the inositol lipid pathway; it appears that formation of cyclic IP_3 is too little and too late to be physiologically important (80). The possible role of inositol phosphates in gating Ca^{2+} entry is considered briefly below.

We have not assumed that IP_3 is the only pathway in nonexcitable cells for discharge of internal Ca^{2+} stores (53, 54, 56, 67). In human platelets ADP is effective in generating $[Ca^{2+}]_i$ signals in the absence of external Ca^{2+} (20). However ADP directly causes little (11) or no (13, 17) PIP_2 hydrolysis and IP_3 formation. These findings could indicate alternative pathways for internal Ca^{2+} discharge.

cAMP and cGMP

The role of cAMP in modulating Ca^{2+} sequestration and IP_3-evoked release remains unclear. Early and more recent reports indicate that cAMP-dependent kinase may act via a 23 kd protein (possibly related to phospholamban) to enhance Ca^{2+}-ATPase and Ca^{2+} uptake by platelet microsomes (1, 39, 71). This has been proposed as a major mechanism for cAMP inhibition of platelet function. However some workers have proposed that cAMP-dependent kinase is facilitatory for IP_3-induced release and reported that "PKI", a peptide inhibitor of cAMP-dependent kinase catalytic subunit, inhibited IP$_3$-evoked Ca^{2+} release from a vesicle fraction (15), while another group found PKI to suppress Ca^{2+} uptake (1). O'Rourke et al (39) have re-examined this point and find first, no effect of protein phosphorylation by the catalytic subunit on Ca^{2+} uptake or IP$_3$-evoked release, and second, no effect of a highly purified PKI on either process. They suggest that previous work may have been confounded by impurities in commercially produced PKI. Our present view is that the main way that cAMP interacts with the inositol phosphate/Ca^{2+} discharge pathway is by inhibiting PIP$_2$ hydrolysis, but other effects are clearly not excluded (41, 57). A recent paper reports that cAMP-dependent kinase can stimulate Ca^{2+} uptake in a microsome fraction from neurons and also reduce the potency of IP$_3$ in promoting Ca^{2+} release (76); these findings indicate that interactions between cAMP and IP$_3$-dischargeable Ca^{2+} pools may be widespread.

Agents such as nitroprusside, which elevate cGMP, also cause inhibition of platelet responses to different agonists, as do permeant forms of cGMP such as dibutyrylcGMP (e.g. 13, 21, 36, 79). Nitroprusside was less effective in reducing responses to Ca^{2+} ionophores or phorbol ester, which suggests that the main site of inhibitory action is in the generation of second messengers (36). Interestingly, cGMP was more effective in inhibiting Ca^{2+} entry evoked by ADP than inhibiting internal release (36), whereas no such differential inhibition is seen with PAF or thrombin stimulation. Because cGMP can increase cAMP, for instance, by effects on cyclic nucleotide phosphodiesterases, it is important to measure both cyclic nucleotides. Morgan & Newby (36) showed that nitroprusside elevated cGMP up to tenfold with no significant effect on cAMP.

C-Kinase

Another important kinase, protein kinase C, can also reduce agonist-evoked PIP$_2$ hydroylsis (e.g. 90) and internal Ca^{2+} release (13, 30, 45, 90). In a broken cell system diacylglycerol was found to release sequestered Ca^{2+} (7), but we have never seen any elevation of [Ca^{2+}]$_i$ evoked by diacylglycerol or phorbol ester in intact platelets (46, 58). Another report has suggested that phorbol esters can stimulate Ca^{2+} sequestration in permeabilized platelets (87). Thus again we have apparently conflicting mechanisms deduced from broken cell systems and no clear relation to what is observed in intact platelets.

pH$_i$ and Na$^+$/H$^+$ Exchange

The role of pH$_i$ and Na$^+$/H$^+$ exchange in Ca^{2+} mobilization in platelets has been controversial (25, 51, 68, 72, 73, 89). It is found that thrombin activates Na$^+$/H$^+$ exchange and can promote, over many seconds, a 0.1 to 0.2 unit increase in pH_i (23, 25, 72, 73, 74, 89). Some workers have seen an inhibition in the thrombin-evoked rise in $[Ca^{2+}]_i$ in Ca^{2+}-free medium when Na^+ is replaced by large cations, or in the presence of amiloride or its analogues that inhibit Na^+/H^+ exchange (72, 73). Moreover, IP_3-evoked Ca^{2+} release from permeabilized platelets was found to be enhanced by modest elevations in pH (6). It seems therefore that pH_i can modulate internal Ca^{2+} discharge, at least in some circumstances. For a complex train of biological processes, comprising many polyvalent-charged solutes and macromolecules, this is not too surprising. It has been implied, and even explicitly stated, that elevation of pH_i is a prerequisite of Ca^{2+} mobilization (72). However the available evidence indicates that pH_i elevation is neither sufficient nor necessary for Ca^{2+} mobilization (25, 51, 68, 74, 88). For instance, complete replacement of external Na^+ by N-methyl-D-glucamine or K^+ did not measurably reduce Ca^{2+} release evoked by thrombin, at near maximal effective concentrations, or by PAF (65). [The literature discrepancies in the effects of Na^+ substitution or amiloride and its analogues may partly reflect the different concentrations of agonist as these experimental manipulations seem to shift the thrombin dose-effect curve to the right (72, 77, 78)]. Changes of pH_i imposed by addition of CO_2, nigericin, or NH_4Cl did not alter resting $[Ca^{2+}]_i$ in fura-2-loaded platelets (74). Incidentally, large changes in $[Ca^{2+}]_i$ evoked by ionomycin did not alter pH_i (74). PAF and ADP produced little or no alkalinization under conditions where they produce a substantial discharge of internal Ca^{2+} (25). A particularly critical point is the temporal relation of the observed changes in pH_i and $[Ca^{2+}]_i$, since for alkalinization to play a significant role in Ca^{2+} mobilization, the increase in pH_i must come first (51, 74). In the published experimental records this does not appear to be the case: $[Ca^{2+}]_i$ peaks well ahead of pH_i and typically before measurable increases in pH_i (e.g. 72, 74). We have confirmed these kinetic patterns with stopped-flow measurements (25). Siffert et al have proposed that this may be because shape-changes optically interfere with pH_i records and generate an artifactual fall in pH_i immediately after activation (73). We doubt this interpretation (25) on the basis of our own data wth HCO_3^--containing medium. We find that shape-change is similar to that under HCO_3^--free conditions, but the dip in pH_i is smaller as expected due to the extra buffering of HCO_3^-. A particularly telling result is shown in Figure 4 of Siffert et al (73) in previously shape-changed cells; the thrombin-evoked $[Ca^{2+}]_i$ transient in Ca^{2+}-free medium is clearly much faster than the pH_i rise.

Other Factors

Membrane potential does not appear to influence internal Ca^{2+} discharge in platelets. Depolarization imposed by high K^+ or gramicidin does not elicit Ca^{2+} release, and thrombin, PAF, and ADP evoke their usual $[Ca^{2+}]_i$ rise in K^+-rich Ca^{2+}-free medium (65). In our hands, caffeine, dantroline, and ryanodine are without obvious effect on basal $[Ca^{2+}]_i$ or on agonist-evoked Ca^{2+} mobilization in human platelets (T. Rink, S. Sage unpublished data), and caffeine was unable to release Ca^{2+} from human platelet internal membrane vesicles (11). Thus agents that have a marked effect on calcium discharge from sarcoplasmic reticulum in striated and smooth muscle appear to have little effect on this process in human platelets. A recent interesting result has been the identification of a monoclonal antibody that binds to platelet membrane vesicles and rather specifically inhibits IP_3-evoked Ca^{2+} release (39). This reagent should prove a valuable tool in elucidating these processes in platelets and most likely in other cell types as well.

Refilling Internal Stores

Following stimulation, the dischargeable store can be refilled. Probably a significant resequestration occurs because the elevation $[Ca^{2+}]_i$ causes enhanced Ca^{2+} pumping into the dense tubular system. However it is also likely that a significant part of the discharged Ca^{2+} is pumped out across the plasma membrane (55, 56). Indeed, in Ca^{2+}-free medium, stimulation by thrombin promotes a loss of approximately half of the ^{45}Ca taken up over a previous 30 min loading period (55). In normal Ca^{2+}-containing medium, the dense tubular system could regain lost Ca^{2+} in two ways. A receptor-mediated Ca^{2+} entry into the cytosol could provide extra Ca^{2+} for subsequent pumping by the Ca-ATPase, or the depletion of Ca^{2+} from the store might induce filling directly from the external medium, as has been suggested for other cell types (see e.g. 22, 54). The available evidence, as discussed below and in Reference 62, does not preclude this second class of mechanism in human platelets.

CALCIUM INFLUX

Four main types of evidence indicate the presence of a significant Ca^{2+} entry into stimulated platelets (3): (a) increased uptake of ^{45}Ca (29, 52); (b) a much larger $[Ca^{2+}]_i$ response in quin2-loaded platelets in the presence than in the absence of external Ca^{2+} (59); (c) stimulated entry of Mn^{2+} detected by the ability of this ion to quench quin2 or fura-2 fluorescence (19, 62); (d) stopped-flow fluorescence measurements showing an earlier agonist-evoked $[Ca^{2+}]_i$ signal in the presence rather than in the absence of external Ca^{2+} (65, 66, 67). As mentioned above, if one loads platelets with low concentrations of fura-2 to minimize cytosolic Ca^{2+} buffering, the peak $[Ca^{2+}]_i$ evoked by thrombin is little reduced in Ca^{2+}-free medium (46), but the declining phase of the response is prolonged in the presence of external Ca^{2+}, as in many other cell types. With stimulation by ADP, we also find, as detailed below, a very fast early phase of Ca^{2+} entry (66, 67). Thus Ca^{2+} entry can provide a faster and more prolonged signal than that provided by internal release only.

Lack of Voltage-Gated Ca^{2+} Channels

Voltage-operated Ca^{2+} channels do not appear to mediate agonist-evoked Ca^{2+} entry in platelets (12, 52, 56, 65). Although a number of agonists have been demonstrated to evoke Na^+-dependent depolarization of the platelet membrane (23, 31, 43), these are only 5–10 mV in magnitude, less than typically required to promote voltage-gated Ca^{2+} entry. Replacement of external Na^+ with impermeant organic cations such as choline or N-methyl-D-glucamine converts the small depolarization into a small hyperpolarization (43), but it does not reduce the elevations in $[Ca^{2+}]_i$ evoked by thrombin or PAF (65). Imposed depolarization using high K^+ does not elevate $[Ca^{2+}]_i$ (65), although agonist-evoked Ca^{2+} influx is substantially reduced in high K^+ (56, 65). A similar reduction in Ca^{2+} influx in high K^+ has been reported in other nonexcitable cells. This effect may be attributed to a reduced driving force for Ca^{2+} entry following depolarization, an idea supported by the finding that depolarization of the platelet membrane using gramicidin also reduces agonist-evoked Ca^{2+} entry. (S. Sage & T. Rink unpublished observations). Organic Ca^{2+} antagonists are relatively ineffective in blocking the agonist-evoked rise in $[Ca^{2+}]_i$ in platelets at concentrations that are effective in excitable cells, although these compounds are reported to have inhibitory effects at high concentrations (e.g. 3, 20). Also, there are no detectable binding sites for verapamil and nitrendipine on human platelets (38), while such sites are readily found on cells such as smooth or cardiac muscle with well documented voltage-dependent Ca^{2+} channels. Interestingly, the platelet plasma membrane has voltage-gated K^+ channels (33). The threshold for activation of these channels lies close to the resting membrane potential, such that they would oppose membrane depolarization during cation entry and maintain the gradient for influx.

Receptor-Mediated Calcium Entry

Receptor-mediated calcium entry may be divided into at least three classes (22): (a) receptor-operated calcium channels, which open as a direct consequence of agonist-receptor binding; (b) Ca^{2+} entry coupled to activated receptors via G-proteins; and (c) second messenger-operated calcium channels, which are opened by a messenger produced in response to agonist-receptor interaction.

Receptor-Operated Channels

Analysis of the subsecond kinetics of rises in $[Ca^{2+}]_i$ in fura-2-loaded platelets by stopped-flow fluorimetry has revealed that, in the presence of extracellular Ca^{2+}, optimal concentrations of ADP evoke a response without measurable delay, i.e. within 10 to 20 msec (66, 67). This early event is due to Ca^{2+} influx. ADP evokes Mn^{2+} entry with similar kinetics (61, 62), and, in the absence of external Ca^{2+}, the onset of the rise in $[Ca^{2+}]_i$ due to discharge of the intracellular stores is delayed by at least 200 msec (66). Rapid ADP-evoked responses have also been observed in indo-1-loaded cells using a continuous flow system (27), although temporal resolution was not at the 10 msec level achieved in our stopped-flow system. The rapidity of ADP-evoked influx suggests close coupling between receptor occupation and the Ca^{2+} channel. A delay of less than 20 msec may point to direct ligand gating, but the finding that there is a delay in ADP-evoked influx at sub-optimal ligand concentrations might be more easily explained by coupling of the receptor to channel opening by a G-protein, (56, 67).

Recently, we obtained direct electrophysiologic evidence from cell-attached patch recordings that ADP can stimulate the opening of channels that carry inward current in intact human platelets (32). Single channel inward currents are observed in physiologic saline solutions containing 1 mM Ca^{2+}. The currents are very similar when Cl^- is replaced with gluconate, which indicates cation entry rather than Cl^- efflux. The slope conductance of the channel in physiologic saline is approximately 11pS at a pipette potential of 0mV (the resting potential), and the open probability is not obviously dependent on potential (32). Similar channels, approximately 10 pS, are evoked when the pipette contains 110 mM $BaCl_2$, thus indicating that divalent cations can permeate. Therefore it appears that ADP opens channels in the plasma membrane through which Ca^{2+} could enter. We suspect that these channels provide the pathway for the early Ca^{2+} entry, but need further data to support this idea.

Channels selective for Ba^{2+} over Na^+ have been demonstrated by the incorporation of platelet membrane vesicles into artificial bilayers (91). Channel activity was present only in membranes from thrombin-stimulated platelets, but not from resting platelets. The channel gating was not influenced by the potential across the bilayer and the activity was blocked by Ni^{2+}, which is known to block thrombin-stimulated Ca^{2+} and Mn^{2+} entry in intact platelets (19, 67). The rather surprising finding that the thrombin-evoked channels survive the cell-fractionation procedure (91) suggests that there may be some covalent modification of the channel, for example by phosphorylation. The prolonged survival of this channel is consistent with the finding that thrombin responses, unlike those evoked by other agonists, do not rapidly desensitize (e.g. 62). Although these reconstitution studies provide direct evidence for a thrombin-evoked calcium channel, it is at present unclear whether the origin of the channel was the plasma membrane or contaminating membrane from intracellular organelles and how it may be coupled to the receptor. From its Ba^{2+}/Na^+ selectivity, this channel seems to be different from the one we have detected in ADP-stimulated intact platelets.

Second Messenger-Operated Channels

Stopped-flow kinetic studies indicate that, of the agonists we have tested, only ADP evokes Ca^{2+} influx without measurable delay. Responses evoked by other agonists, including thrombin, PAF, vasopressin, and U46619, show an irreducible delay of at least 200 msec (56, 67). These results suggest that, with the exception of the ADP response, one or more biochemical steps lie between receptor occupation and the generation of Ca^{2+} influx, which could therefore be explained by the action of a diffusible second messenger.

Possible intermediaries in channel gating include Ca^{2+} and inositol phosphates (8, 22, 28, 83). Calcium-sensitive Ca^{2+} channels in the plasma membrane, which would be opened following the elevation of $[Ca^{2+}]_i$ by discharge of the intracellular store, have been proposed to mediate Ca^{2+} influx in neutrophils (83). Stopped-flow studies suggest that a similar pathway does not operate in platelets (62, 67). The onset of $[Ca^{2+}]_i$ rise in the presence of external Ca^{2+} precedes that observed in the absence of external Ca^{2+} or when Ca^{2+} influx is blocked using Ni^{2+}, which indicates that Ca^{2+} influx precedes the discharge of the intracellular stores.

There is currently little evidence concerning the possible role of inositol phosphates in mediating calcium influx directly across the platelet plasma membrane (as opposed to entry via the intracellular store, discussed below). A model in which $Ins(1,4,5)P_3$ opened Ca^{2+} channels in both the plasma and intracellular store membranes would be compatible with the observed temporal separation of Ca^{2+} influx and store discharge: since the messenger is generated at the plasma membrane, it might be expected to take longer to reach the receptors of the store (67). The only evidence supporting a direct role for $Ins(1,4,5)P_3$ in the generation of Ca^{2+} influx in platelets at present is the finding that this ligand released Ca^{2+} from membrane vesicles enriched in plasma membrane (49). Inward currents evoked by $Ins(1,4,5)P_3$ has been reported in human T-lymphocytes (28) and in rat mast cells (42). There has yet to be a similar direct electrophysiologic investigation of this point in platelets. Agonist-evoked phosphatidyl-$Ins(4,5)P_2$ breakdown in many cells results in the accumulation of $Ins(1,3,4)P_3$ formed from the initial hydrolysis product, $Ins(1,4,5)P_3$. This conversion is particularly rapid in platelets (80). There has been considerable speculation over the possible signaling roles of $Ins(1,3,4,5)P_4$, the intermediate in the conversion of $Ins(1,4,5)P_3$ to $Ins-(1,3,4)_3$. In particular, the possible role of $Ins(1,3,4,5)P_3$ in the generation of Ca^{2+} influx has been considered (24, 37). Evidence that $Ins(1,3,4,5)P_4$, acting in concert with $Ins(1,4,5)P_3$, may be involved in mediating Ca^{2+} influx has been obtained in lacrimal gland cells (8).

Store-Regulated Calcium Influx

In recent years evidence has been presented in a number of cell types suggestive of a pathway by which Ca^{2+} enters the cytosol via some fraction of the intracellular Ca^{2+} store (see e.g. 22, 54). The evidence from refilling experiments, where the stores are discharged in the absence of extracellular Ca^{2+} and are then shown to be recharged after brief exposure to Ca^{2+}, indicates some kind of private pathway between the extracellular space and the store, since $[Ca^{2+}]_i$ is not elevated during the refilling. The simplest explanation of these phenomena is that some form of channel, perhaps like a gap junction, links the lumen of intracellular store to the extracellular space and that the opening of this channel is controlled by the $[Ca^{2+}]$ inside the store. It has been considered that Ca^{2+} entering the store by such a route might gain entry into the cytosol only after passage into an $Ins(1,4,5)P_3$-sensitive fraction of the store, which might require another messenger such as $Ins(1,3,4,5,)P_4$ (8). Recently results consistent with a store-regulated Ca^{2+} influx have been seen in platelets (62, 63). ADP evokes a biphasic rise in $[Ca^{2+}]$, which is poorly resolved at 37°C, but is clearly separated into two events at 17°C. At this temperature an initial rise in $[Ca^{2+}]_i$ occurs without measurable delay and is followed by a further elevation approximately 700 msec later. When the cells are stimulated in the presence of both Ca^{2+} and Mn^{2+}, the second phase of $[Ca^{2+}]_i$ rise coincides wth Mn^{2+} entry. In the absence of external Ca^{2+} there is a single ADP-evoked rise in $[Ca^{2+}]_i$ delayed in onset by approximately 1400 msec. When the cells are stimulated in the presence of Mn^{2+} alone, an early Mn^{2+} entry occurs without measurable delay, followed by a second phase of entry, also delayed by approximately 1400 msec. Hence the second phase of divalent-cation entry coincides with discharge of the intracellular Ca^{2+} stores, which could reflect regulation of influx by the Ca^{2+} in the store. These experiments also indicate that the timing of the second ADP-evoked event is modulated by the presence of external Ca^{2+}, since the second phase of Mn^{2+} entry occurs at a markedly earlier time if both ions are present in the external medium, perhaps because the key event in eliciting an earlier second phase of entry is the elevation of $[Ca^{2+}]_i$ during the initial phase. One can only speculate on the way in which $[Ca^{2+}]_i$ modulates store discharge. For example, it could be that Ca^{2+} stimulation of phospholipase C results in an earlier generation of Ins-$(1,4,5)P_3$.

Modulation of Calcium Entry

Activation of platelet protein kinase C inhibits Ca^{2+} influx (82). This may in part reflect the inhibition of PIP_2 hydrolysis (90) with consequently reduced Ca^{2+} entry through second messenger-operated Ca^{2+} channels and by the store-dependent pathway, since intracellular release is also diminished. Inhibition by protein kinase C may involve a change in receptor affinity, but there also appears to be inhibition at the level of the G-protein, which stimulates the phosphoinositidase, or at a subsequent stage of transduction, since fluoride-stimulated Ca^{2+} entry is reduced (44). The channels responsible for gating Ca^{2+} influx may also be modulated, but as yet there has been no direct electrophysiologic test. Influx, assessed by Mn^{2+} entry, does not appear to be as sensitive to protein kinase C-mediated inhibition as is intracellular release (82), although influx is slower to recover from prolonged exposure to diacylglycerol (DAG).

Cyclic AMP also inhibits Ca^{2+} influx (e.g. 41, 57). As with protein kinase C, the cAMP-dependent kinase probably has several sites of action. Inositol lipid hydrolysis is inhibited (see 71), which could reduce Ca^{2+} influx through putative inositol phosphate-operated channels as well as through the putative store-dependent pathway. There may also be phosphorylation of the Ca^{2+} channels that conduct the influx, although the early phase of ADP-evoked entry is surprisingly insensitive; elevation of cAMP using forskolin can completely inhibit ADP-evoked release of the intracellular stores while Ca^{2+} influx continues to be evoked without measurable delay (67). Resolution of the ADP-evoked influx into its constituent phases at low temperature shows that the second phase of Ca^{2+} or Mn^{2+} entry can be completely abolished while the initial phase, generated without measurable delay, persists (63). In contrast, influx and intracellular release evoked by thrombin or PAF shows similar sensitivity to inhibition by cAMP (64, 67).

Agents that elevate cGMP also inhibit Ca^{2+} influx in platelets (21, 36, 56). As with cAMP, the mechanism probably involves, at least in part, a reduction in PIP_2 hydrolysis (79). But recent results (36) show that Ca^{2+} or Mn^{2+} entry evoked by ADP are preferentially inhibited by nitroprusside. This contrasts with the effect of forskolin mentioned above, which indicates that cAMP preferentially spares the rapid phase of ADP-evoked Ca^{2+} or Mn^{2+} entry.

There is little evidence that pH_i mediates agonist-evoked influx. Abolition of Na^+-dependent alkalinization by ionic substitution has no effect on the magnitude of agonist-evoked rises in $[Ca^{2+}]_i$ (65), while kinetic studies indicate that peak $[Ca^{2+}]_i$ is attained before pH_i rises above basal levels (25).

At present little is known of the structural elements in the plasma membrane that conduct the entry of Ca^{2+} into the cell. The IIb.IIIa membrane glycoprotein complex may be involved in Ca^{2+} transport across the plasma membrane in resting (4) and stimulated cells (48, 86). Monoclonal antibodies or smaller peptide fragments, which bind to the IIb.IIIa complex, reduce agonist-evoked influx (48, but see also 20), although at present it is not clear if these proteins are associated with any of the putative pathways for Ca^{2+} entry.

SUMMARY

The past three years have seen significant advances in our knowledge and understanding of Ca^{2+} mobilization in platelets. Some of the data has shown that systems demonstrated in other cell types operate in platelets, while in certain respects platelet studies have provided the lead with new insights and approaches. An increasing body of evidence supports a key role for Ins1,4,5-trisphosphate in mediating internal release, but it has yet to be experimentally demonstrated that this messenger is formed fast enough to account for the observed kinetics of internal release that can reach its maximum rate within 250 msec. There also remains a question as to the presence of an alternative or additional pathway linking at least ADP receptors to internal Ca^{2+} release. The controversy over the role of pH_i in Ca^{2+} mobilization appears to be resolved; changes in pH_i are neither sufficient nor necessary but can modulate the process in some instances. Elevated cAMP and protein kinase C inhibit Ca mobilization, but the sites and mechanisms of action are not worked out. Analysis of receptor-mediated Ca^{2+} entry by stopped-flow fluorescence has increasingly revealed a complex array of mechanisms, but there is no evidence for voltage-gated Ca^{2+} entry. There are indications of at least three pathways: a fast entry closely coupled to the ADP receptor; a process that may be generated by a diffusible second messenger, possibly an inositol phosphate; and an entry regulated by the state of filling of the discharged Ca^{2+} store. A recent advance has been the successful application of the patch-clamp to these tiny cells, with evidence for voltage-gated K^+ channels and ADP-stimulated single channels that could be the pathway for the fast phase of ADP-evoked $[Ca^{2+}]_i$ elevation.

Acknowledgments

We thank M. Bowden, B. Leigh, and S. Luker for help in preparing the manuscript, Dr. M. Mahaut-Smith for permission to cite unpublished work, and many workers for providing preprints.

Literature Cited

1. Adunyah, S. E., Dean, W. L. 1987. Regulation of human platelets membrane Ca^{2+} transport by cAMP and calmodulin-dependent phosphorylation. *Biochim. Biophys. Acta* 930:401–9
2. Authi, K. S., Crawford, N. 1985. Inositol 1,4,5-trisphosphate release of sequestered Ca^{2+} from highly purified human platelet intracellular membranes. *Biochem. J.* 230:247–53
3. Avodin, P. V., Menshikor, M. Y., Svitina-Ulitana, I. V., Tkachuk, V. A. 1988. Blocking of the receptor-stimulated calcium entry into human platelets by verapamil and nicardipine *Thromb. Res.* 52:587–97
4. Brass, L. F. 1985. Ca^{2+} Transport across the platelet plasma membrane. A

role for membrane glycoproteins IIB & IIIA. *J. Biol. Chem.* 260:2231–6
5. Brass, L. F. (1984). The effect of Na^+ on Ca^+ homeostasis in unstimulated platelets. *J. Biol. Chem.* 259:12571–5
6. Brass, L. F., Joseph, S. K. 1985. A role for inositol trisphosphate in intracellular Ca^{2+} mobilization and granule secretion in platelets. *J. Biol. Chem.* 260:15172–79
7. Grass, L. F., Laporta, M. 1987. Diacylglycerol causes Ca release from the platelet dense tubular system: comparison with Ca release caused by inositol tris 1,4,5-trisphosphate. *Biochem. Biophys. Res. Commun.* 142:7–14
8. Changya, L., Gallacher, D. V., Irvine, R. F., Potter, B. V. L., Peterson, O. H.

1989. Inositol 1,3,4,5 tetratasphosphate is essential for substained activation of the Ca^{2+}-dependent K^+ current in single internally perfused mouse lacrimal acinar cells. *J. Membrane. Biol.* 109:85–93

9. Cobbold, P. J., Rink, T. J. 1987. Fluorescent and bioluminescent measurement of cytosolic free calcium. *Biochem. J.* 248:1–16

10. Daniel, J. L., Dangelmaier, C. A., Selak, M., Smith, J. B. 1986. ADP stimulates IP_3 formation in human platelets. *FEBS Letts.* 206:299–303

11. Dean, W. C., Adunyah, S. E. 1986. Effects of sulfhydryl reagents and other inhibitors on Ca^{2+} transport and inositol trisphosphate-induced Ca^{2+} release from human platelet membranes. *J. Biol. Chem.* 261:13071–75

12. Doyle, V. M., Ruegg, U. T. 1985. Lack of evidence for voltage dependent calcium channels on platelets. *Biochem. Biophys. Res. Comm.* 127:161–67

13. Drummond, A. H., MacIntyre, D. E. 1987. Inositol lipid metabolism and calcium flux. *In Platelets in Biology and Pathology III*, eds. D. E. MacIntyre, J. L. Gordon, pp. 373–431. Amsterdam: Elsevier. 589 pp.

14. Enouf, J., Bredeux, R., Bourdean, N., Levy-Toledano, S. 1987. Two different Ca^{2+} transport systems are associated with plasma and intracellular human platelet membranes. *J. Biol. Chem.* 262:9293–97

15. Enouf, J., Girand, F., Bredoux, R., Bourdean, N., Levy-Toledano, S. 1987. Possible role of a cAMP-dependent phosphorylation in the calcium release mediated by inositol 1,4,5-trisphosphate in human platelet membrane vesicles. *Biochim. Biophys. Acta* 928:76–82

16. Enyedi, A., Sakardi, B., Folder-Papp, Z., Monostory, J., Gardos, G. 1986. Demonstration of two distinct calcium pumps in human platelet membrane vesicles. *J. Biol. Chem.* 261:9558–563

17. Fisher, G. J., Bakshian, S., Baldassare, J. J. 1985. Activation of human platelets by ADP causes a rapid rise in cytosolic free Ca^{2+} without hydrolysis of phosphatidylinositol-4,5-bisphosphate. *Biochem. Biophys. Res. Commun.* 129:958–64

18. Hallam, T. J., Daniel, J. L., Kendrick-Jones, J., Rink, T. J. 1985. Relationship between cytoplasmic free calcium and myosin light chain phosphorylation in intact platelets. *Biochem. J.* 232:373–77

19. Hallam, T. J., Rink, T. J. 1985. Agonists stimulate divalent cation channels in the plasma membrane of human platelets. *FEBS Lett.* 186:175–79

20. Hallam, T. J., Rink, T. J. 1985. Responses to adenosine diphosphate in human platelets loaded with the fluorescent calcium indicator quin2. *J. Physiol.* 368: 131–46

21. Hallam, T. J., Rink, T. J. 1987. Insights into platelet function gained with fluorescent Ca^{2+} indicators. In: *Platelets in Biology and Pathology III*. eds. D. F. MacIntyre, J. L. Gordon, pp. 353–372. Amsterdam:Elsevier. 589 pp.

22. Hallam, T. J., Rink, T. J. 1989. Receptor-mediated Ca^{2+} entry: diversity of mechanism and function. *Trends Pharm. Sci.* 10:8–10

23. Horne, W. C., Norman, N. E., Schwartz, D. B., Simons, E. R. 1981. Changes in cytoplasmic pH and in membrane potential in thrombin-stimulated human platelets. *Eur. J. Biochem.* 120: 295–302

24. Irvine, R. F., Moor, R. M. 1986. Micro-injection of inositol 1,3,4,5-tetrakisphosphate activates sea urchin eggs by a mechanism dependent on external Ca^{2+}. *Biochem. J.* 240:917–20

25. Jobson, T. M., Rink, T. J., Sage, S. O. 1990. Agonist-evoked changes in cytosolic pH and calcium concentration in human platelets: Studies in physiological bicarbonate. *J. Physiol.* In press

26. Johnson, P. C., Ware, J. A., Cliveden, P. B., Smith, M., Dvorak, A. M., Salazman, E. W. 1985. Measurement of ionized calcium in blood platelets with the photoprotein aequorin. *J. Biol. Chem.* 260(4):2069–76

27. Jones, G. D., Gear, A. R. L. 1988. Subsecond calcium dynamics in ADP- and thrombin-stimulated platelets: A continuous-flow approach using Indo-1. *Blood* 71:1539–43

28. Kuno, M., Gardner, P. 1987. Ion channels activated by inositol 1,4,5-trisphosphate in plasma membrane of human T-lymphocytes. *Nature* 326:301–4

29. Lee, T., Malone, B., Blank, M. L., Synder, F. 1981. PAF stimulates Ca influx into rabbit platelets. *Biochem. Biophys. Res. Commun.* 102:1262

30. MacIntyre, D. E., McNicol, A., Drummond, A. H. 1985. Tumor-promoting phorbol esters inhibit agonist-induced phosphate formation and CA^{2+} flux in human platelets. *FEBS Lett.* 180:160–64

31. MacIntyre, D. E., Rink, T. J. 1982. The role of platelet membrane potential in the initiation of platelet aggregation. *Thromb. Haemost.* 47:22–26

32. Mahaut-Smith, M. P., Rink, T. J., Sage, S. O. 1989. Single channels in

human platelets activated by ADP. *J. Physiol.* 415:24P

33. Maruyama, Y. 1987. A patch-clamp study of mammalian platelets and their voltage-gated potassium current. *J. Physiol.* 391:467–85

34. Meldolesi, J., Volpe, P., Pozzan, T. 1988. The intracellular distribution of calcium. *Trends Neurosci.* 11:449–52

35. Menashi, S., Authi, K. S., Carey, F., Crawford, N., 1984. Characterization of the calcium-sequestering process associated with human platelet intracellular membranes isolated by free-flow electrophoresis. *Biochem. J.* 222:413–17

36. Morgan, R. O., Newby, A. C. 1989. Nitroprusside differentially inhibits ADP-stimulated calcium influx and mobilization in human platelets. *Biochem. J.* 258:447–54

37. Morris, A. P., Gallacher, D. V., Irvine, R. F., Petersen, O. H. 1987. Synergism of inositol trisphosphate and tetrakisphosphate in activating Ca^{2+}-dependent K^+ channels. *Nature* 330:653–56

38. Motulsky, H. J., Snavely, M. D., Hughes, P. J., Insel, P. A., 1983. Interaction of verapamil and other calcium channel blockers with α- and β-adrenergic receptors. *Cir. Res.* 52:226–31

39. O'Rourke, F., Zavoico, G. B., Feinstein, M. B. 1989. Release of Ca^{2+} by inositol 1,4,5-trisphosphate in platelet membrane vesicles is not dependent on cyclic AMP-dependent protein kinase. *Biochem. J.* 257: In press

40. O'Rourke, F., Zavoico, G. B., Smith, L. H., Feinstein, M. B. 1987. Stimulus response-coupling in a cell-free platelet membrane system. *FEBS Lett.* 214:176–80

41. Pannocchia, A., Hardisty, R. M. 1985. Cyclic AMP inhibits platelet activation independently of its effect on cytosolic free calcium. *Biochem. Biophysical. Res. Commun.* 127:339–45

42. Penner, R., Matthew, G., Neher, E. 1988. Regulation of calcium influx by second messengers in rat mast cell. *Nature* 334:499–504

43. Pipili, E. 1985. Platelet membrane potential: Simultaneous measurements of dis-C₃-(5) fluorescence and optical density. *Thromb. Haemost.* 54:645–49

44. Poll, C., Kryle, P., Westwick, J. 1986. Activation of protein kinase-C inhibits sodium fluoride-induced elevation of human platelet cytosolic free calcium and thromboxane B_2 generation. *Biochem. Biophys. Res. Commun.* 136:381–89

45. Poll, C., Westwick, J. 1987. Phorbol esters modulate thrombin-operated calcium mobilization and dense granule release in human platelets. *Biochim. Biophys. Acta* 886:434–40

46. Pollock, W. K., Rink, T. J. 1986. Thrombin and ionomycin can raise platelet cytosolic Ca^{2+} to micromolar levels by discharge of internal Ca^{2+} stores: studies using fura-2. *Biochem. Biophys. Res. Commun.*

47. Pollock, W. K., Rink, T. J., Irvine, R. F. 1986. Liberation of [³H] arachidonic acid and changes in cytosolic free calcium in fura-2-loaded human platelets stimulated by ionomycin and collagen. *Biochem. J.* 235:869–77

48. Powling, M. J., Hardisty, R. M. 1985. Glycoprotein IIb-IIIa complex and Ca^{2+} influx in stimulated platelets. *Blood* 66:731–33

49. Rengasamy, A., Feinberg, H. 1988. Inositol 1,4,5-trisphosphate-induced calcium release from platelet plasma membrane vesicles. *Biochem. Biophys. Res. Commun.* 150:1021–26

50. Rengasamy, A., Soura, S., Feinberg H., 1987. Platelet Ca^{2+} hemostasis: Na^+-Ca^{2+} exchange in plasma membrane vesicles. *Thromb. Haemost.* 57:337–40

51. Rink, T. J. 1987. Intracellular pH and cytoplasmic free Ca^{2+}. *Nature* 327:375–76

52. Rink, T. J. 1988. Cytosolic calcium in platelet activation. *Experientia* 44:97–100

53. Rink, T. J., Hallam, T. J. 1984. What turns platelets on? *Trends Biochem. Sci.* 9:215–19

54. Rink, T. J., Hallam, T. J. 1989. Calcium signaling in non-excitable cells: Notes on oscillations and store refilling. *Cell Calcium* In press

55. Rink, T. J., Sage, S. O. 1987. Stimulated calcium efflux from fura-2-loaded human platelets. *J. Physiol.* 393:513–24

56. Rink, T. J., Sage, S. O. 1988. Initiation and termination of Ca^{2+} signals. Studies in human platelets. In *Cell Physiology of Blood.* eds. R. B. Gunn, J. C. Parker. *Soc. Gen. Physiol. 41st Symp.* pp. 381–394. New York: Rockefeller Univ. Press. 402 pp.

57. Rink, T. J., Sanchez, A. 1984. Effects of prostaglandin I_2 and forskolin on the secretion from platelets evoked at basal concentrations of cytoplasmic free calcium by thrombin, collagen, phorbol ester, and exogenous diacylglycerol. *Biochem. J.* 222:833–36

58. Rink, T. J., Sanchez, A., Hallam, T. J. 1983. Diacylglycerol and phorbol ester stimulate secretion without raising cytoplasmic free calcium in human platelets. *Nature* 305:317–19

59. Rink, T. J., Smith, S. W., Tsien, R. 1982. Cytoplasmic free Ca^{2+} in human platelets: Ca^{2+} thresholds and Ca-independent activation for shape change and secretion. *FEBS. Lett.* 148:21–26

60. Rink, T. J., Tsien, R. Y., Pozzan, T. 1982. Cytoplasmic pH and free Mg^{2+} in lymphocytes. *J. Cell. Biol.* 95:189–96

61. Sage, S. O. 1987. Kinetics of ADP-evoked and thrombin-evoked rises in cytosolic calcium in human platelets studies with manganese and nickel. *J. Physiol.* 396:43P

62. Sage, S. O., Merritt, J. E., Hallam, T. J., Rink, T. J. 1989. Receptor-mediated calcium entry in fura-2-loaded human platelets stimulated with ADP and thrombin: Dual wavelength studies with Mn^+. *Biochem. J.* 258:923–26

63. Sage, S. O., Reast, R., Rink, T. J. 1989. ADP evokes a biphasic Ca^{2+} influx in human platelets: Evidence for store-dependent Ca^{2+} entry. *Biochem. J.* In press

64. Sage, S. O., Rink, T. J. 1985. Inhibition by forskolin of cytosolic calcium rise, shape change and aggregation in quin2-loaded human platelets. *FEBS Lett.* 188:135–40

65. Sage, S. O., Rink, T. J. 1986. Effects of ionic substitution on $[Ca^{2+}]_i$ rises evoked by thrombin and PAF in human platelets. *Eur. J. Pharm.* 128:99–107

66. Sage, S. O., Rink, T. J. 1986. Kinetic differences between thrombin-induced and ADP-induced calcium influx and release from internal stores in fura-2-loaded human platelets. *Biochem. Biophys. Res. Commun.* 136:1124–29

67. Sage, S. O., Rink, T. J. 1987. The kinetics of changes in intracellular calcium concentrations in fura-2-loaded human platelets. *J. Biol. Chem* 262:16364–69

68. Sanchez, A., Alouso, M. T., Collazos, J. M. 1988. Thrombin-induced changes of intracellular $[Ca^{2+}]$ and pH_i in human platelets. *Biochim. Biophys. Acta* 938:497–500

69. Sandler, W. C., Le Breton, G. C., Feinberg H. 1980. Movement of sodium into human platelets. *Biochim. Biophys. Acta* 600:448–55

70. Schaeffer, J., Blaustein, M. P. 1989. Platelet free calcium concentrations measured with fura-2 are influenced by the transmembrane sodium gradient. *Cell Calcium* 10:101–13

71. Siess, W. 1989. Molecular mechanisms of platelet activation. *Physiol. Rev.* 69:58–178

72. Siffert, W., Akkerman, J. W. N. 1987. Activation of sodium-proton exchange is a prerequisite for Ca^{2+} mobilization in human platelets. *Nature* 325:456–58

73. Siffert, W., Siffert, G., Scheid, P., Akkerman, J. W. N. 1989. Activation of Na^+/H^+ exchange and Ca^{2+} mobilization start simultaneously in thrombin-stimulated platelets. Evidence that platelet shape change disturbs early rises of BCECF fluorescence which causes an underestimation of actual cytosolic alkalinization. *Biochem. J.* 258:521–27

74. Simpson, A. W. M., Rink, T. J. 1987. Elevation of pH_i is not an essential step in calcium mobilization in fura-2-loaded human platelets. *FEBS Lett.* 22:144–48

75. Sinigaglia, F., Bisio, A., Torti, M., Balduini, C.-L., Balduini, C. 1988. Effects of GPIIb-IIIa complex ligands on calcium ion movement and cytoskeleton organization in activated platelets. *Biochem. Biophys. Res. Commun.* 154:258–64

76. Supattapone, S., Danoff, S. K., Theibert, A., Joseph, S. K., Sieiner, J., Snyder, S. H. 1988. Cyclic AMP-dependent phosphorylation of a brain inositol trisphosphate receptor decreases its release of calcium. *Proc. Natl. Acad. Sci. USA* 85:8747–50

77. Sweatt, J. D., Blair, I. A., Cragoe, E. J., Limbird, L. E. 1986. Inhibitors of Na^+/H^+ exchange block epinephrine- and ADP-induced stimulation of human platelets phospholipase C by blockade of arachidonic acid release at a prior step. *J. Biol. Chem.*261:8660–66

78. Sweatt, J. D., Connolly, T. M., Cragoe, E. J., Limbird, L. E. 1986. Evidence that Na^+/H^+ exchange regulates receptor-mediated phospholipase A_2 activation in human platelets. *J. Biol. Chem.*261:8667–73

79. Takai, Y., Kaibuchi, K., Samo, K., Nishizuta, Y. 1982. Counteraction of calcium activated phospholipid-dependent protein kinase activation by adenosine 3'5' monophosphate and guanosine 3',5'-monophosphate in platelets. *J. Biochem.* 91:403–6

80. Tarver, A. P., King, W. G., Rittenhouse, S. E. 1987. Inositol 1,4,5-trisphosphate and inositol 1,2-cyclic 4,5-trisphosphate are minor components of total mass of inositol trisphosphate in thrombin-stimulated platelets. *J. Biol. Chem.* 262:17268–71

81. Thompson, N. T., Scrutton, M. C. 1985. Intracellular calcium fluxes in human platelets. *Eur. J. Biochem.* 147(2):421–27

82. Valone, F. H., Johnson, B. 1987. Mod-

ulation of platelet-activating-factor-induced calcium influx and intracellular calcium release in platelets by phorbol esters. *Biochem. J.* 247:669–74

83. von Tscharner, V., Prod'hom, B., Baggiolini, M., Reuter, H. 1986. Ion channels in human neutrophils activated by a rise in free cytosolic calcium concentration. *Nature* 324:369–72

84. Ware, J. A., Saitah, M., Smith, M., Johnson, P. C., Slazman, E. W. 1989. Response of aequorin-loaded platelets to activators of protein kinase-C. *Am. J. Physiol.* 256:C35-C43

85. Ware, J. A., Smith, M., Fossel, E. T., Slazman, E. W. 1988. Cytoplasmic Mg^{2+} concentration in platelets: implications for determination of Ca^{2+} with aequorin. *Am. J. Physiol.* 255:H855–59

86. Yamaguchi, A., Yamamoto, N., Kitagawa, H., Tamone, K., Yamazaki, H. 1987. Ca^{2+} influx mediated through the GPIIb/IIIa complex during platelet activation. *FEBS Lett.* 225:228–32

87. Yoshida, K., Nachmias, V. T. 1987. Phorbol ester stimulates calcium sequestration in saponinized human platelets. *J. Biol. Chem.* 262:16048–54

88. Zavoico, G. B., Cragoe, E. J. 1988. Ca^{2+} mobilization can occur independently of acceleration of Na^+/H^+ exchange in thrombin-stimulated human platelets. *J. Biol. Chem.* 263:9635–39

89. Zavoico, G. B., Cragoe, E. J., Feinstein, M. B. 1986. Regulation of intracellular pH in human platelets. Effects of thrombin, A23187, and ionomycin and evidence for activation of Na^+/H^+ exchange and its inhibition by amiloride analogs. *J. Biol. Chem.* 261:13160–67

90. Zavoico, G. B., Halenda, S. P., Sha'afi, R. I., Feinstein, M. B. 1985. Phorbol myristate acetate inhibits thrombin-stimulated Ca^{2+} mobilization and phosphatidylinositol 4,5-bisphosphate hydroysis in human platelets. *Proc. Natl. Acad. Sci. USA* 82:3859–62

91. Zschauer, A., Van Breemen, C., Buhler, F. R., Nelson, M. T. 1988. Calcium channels in thrombin-activated human platelet membrane. *Nature* 334:703–5

Annu. Rev. Physiol. 1990. 52:451–66

Ca²⁺ AS A SECOND MESSENGER WITHIN MITOCHONDRIA OF THE HEART AND OTHER TISSUES

R. M. Denton

Department of Biochemistry, School of Medical Sciences, University of Bristol, Bristol BS8 1TD, England

J. G. McCormack

Department of Biochemistry, The University of Leeds, Leeds LS2 9JT, England

KEY WORDS: dehydrogenases, citrate cycle, pyrophosphatase, ATP homeostasis, Ca²⁺-transport

INTRODUCTION

Many hormones and other external stimuli influence intramitochondrial metabolism (25). The mechanisms by which this occurs involve not only signal transmission across the plasma membrane but also across the inner membrane of mitochondria. This latter membrane is essentially impermeable to all charged molecules unless a specific carrier or transport system is present in the membrane. Of the known second-messenger molecules that act within the cytosolic compartment of mammalian cells, it appears that only Ca^{2+} is transferred into the mitochondrial matrix.

The Ca^{2+}-transport system in the inner membrane of mitochondria (Figure 1) has separate uptake and efflux components (for reviews see 9, 14, 70). Uptake of Ca^{2+} occurs via an electrophoretic uniporter driven by the large electrical potential across the inner membrane. This process is inhibited by the dye ruthenium red and also by Mg^{2+} at concentrations likely to be present in the cytoplasm of cells (i.e. about 1 mM). The transfer of Ca^{2+} out of the mitochondria in heart and many other tissues occurs mainly via an elec-

0066-4278/90/0315-0451$02.00

troneutral exchange of Ca^{2+} for $2Na^+$. There is also a sodium-independent pathway that probably involves the direct exchange of Ca^{2+} for $2H^+$ as well as a Ca^{2+}-dependent pore that may become open at high levels of matrix Ca^{2+} (14, 16, 40). The $Ca^{2+}/2Na^+$ antiporter is inhibited by introducing benzodiazipines such as diltiazem, which are perhaps better known as plasma membrane Ca^{2+}-channel blockers, and by increasing extramitochondrial concentrations of Ca^{2+} (14, 40). Distribution of Ca^{2+} across the inner membrane will depend on the relative activities of the separate uptake and efflux pathways.

Initially it was assumed that this system contributed to the regulation of the concentration of Ca^{2+} in the cytoplasm. Indeed, isolated mitochondria have been shown to effectively buffer the extramitochondrial concentration of Ca^{2+} at 1–3 μM, because above this concentration the efflux pathway becomes saturated. Net Ca^{2+}-uptake therefore occurs until the extramitochondrial concentration is decreased to that at which the rate of Ca^{2+} uptake matches that of the (saturated) efflux pathway (69). Mitochondria can only behave in this manner if the total content of Ca is greater than about 10 nmol per mg of protein (36, 69, 70). It was also suggested that hormones may cause the actual mobilization of Ca^{2+} from mitochondria (28, 77, 94).

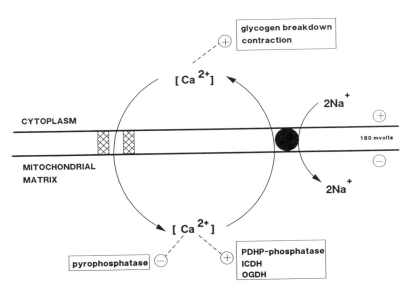

Figure 1   The calcium transport system in the inner mitochondrial membrane of vertebrates and its role in the relay of changes in the cytosolic concentration of Ca^{2+} into the mitochondrial matrix. Not shown are the Na^+ independent efflux pathway and the calcium dependent pore (1, 14, 15, 16).

However in 1980, we pointed out that this general emphasis on the possible role of mitochondria in the regulation of cytoplasmic Ca^{2+} was probably misplaced and instead that Ca^{2+} transport system in the inner membrane of mitochondria in vertebrates should be considered primarily as being involved with the regulation of the concentration of Ca^{2+} within mitochondria (23). This view followed recognition during the 1970s that three important dehydrogenases within mitochondria are sensitive to activation by Ca^{2+} in the approximate range of 0.1 to 10 μM. These are PDH (26), NAD-ICDH (27), and OGDH (56). Detailed studies on the kinetic properties of these enzymes using both purified preparations and intact mitochondria led us to propose that hormones and other external stimuli, which increase the cytosolic concentration of Ca^{2+}, may enhance rates of mitochondrial NADH formation and hence ATP synthesis through also increasing the mitochondrial concentration of Ca^{2+} (23, 25, 60). Such a mechanism may play a central role in ATP homeostasis, since supply may be increased to meet greater demand, for example for muscle contraction, without necessarily any decrease in the ATP/ADP ratio. It has been known for some time that stimulation of contraction in the heart can occur without any appreciable decrease in the ATP/ADP ratio (68), and this conclusion has been confirmed by more recent studies using NMR (6, 7, 29, 91).

Considerable support for these proposals has been obtained in a number of laboratories (8a, 18, 25, 39, 60). In this article, we concentrate on recent advances in the field with some emphasis on the heart.

KINETIC PROPERTIES OF INTRAMITOCHONDRIAL Ca^{2+}-SENSITIVE ENZYMES INFERRED FROM STUDIES ON THE ISOLATED ENZYMES AND ON MITOCHONDRIA

The Ca^{2+}-Sensitive Dehydrogenases

Ca^{2+} activates PDH by causing increases in the amount of the active, nonphosphorylated form of the enzyme (PDH_a), primarily through stimulation of PDHP-phosphatase activity (26). Studies with isolated enzymes suggest that Ca^{2+} may act as a bridging ligand between the phosphatase and the transacetylase (E_2) core of the PDH complex (88). Marked decreases in the apparent K_m for PDHP are also observed (74). However, more recent studies have focused on the kinetic properties of PDHP-phosphatase within mitochondria permeabilized to all small molecules by toluene treatment, or to divalent metal ions by the ionophore A23187. These studies suggest that when the components of the PDH system are located within their natural environment, the major effect of Ca^{2+} is a decrease in the K_m of the phosphatase for Mg^{2+} (64, 89, 90).

The activation of NAD-ICDH and OGDH by Ca^{2+} is exerted directly on the dehydrogenases, and the main effect is to greatly diminish the K_m values for their respective substrates, isocitrate and oxoglutarate (2, 26, 47, 48, 56).

Detailed comparisons, using both mitochondrial extracts and toluene-permeabilized mitochondria (Table 1), have been made of the Ca^{2+}-sensitivity of the three dehydrogenases from rat heart. The apparent sensitivity of each dehydrogenase in the two systems is broadly similar. The sensitivity of NAD-ICDH and OGDH to Ca^{2+} decreases as the ADP/ATP ratio diminishes, whereas that of the PDH-system remains unaltered (78, 79). In the presence of ADP and 1 mM Mg^{2+}, the sensitivity of OGDH appears to be slightly greater than that of the PDH-system, whereas that of NAD-ICDH is clearly less. The difference between the sensitivity of NAD-ICDH and that of OGDH and PDH is even more marked in the presence of ATP.

These results raise the question of the physiologic importance of the Ca^{2+}-activation of NAD-ICDH, since it would appear that the enzyme may only become appreciably activated when the Ca^{2+} concentration within mitochondria is sufficient to fully activate the other dehydrogenases (see below). It is possible that differential calcium sensitivity is a device for increasing the range of intramitochondrial Ca^{2+} concentrations, which can influence the rate of the citrate cycle. It should be noted that the in-

Table 1 Summary of the properties of the Ca^{2+}-sensitive enzymes from rat heart mitochondria

Enzyme	Effect of Ca^{2+}	Additions	$K_{0.5}$ value (μM) for Ca^{2+} of enzymes in	
			Mitochondrial extracts	Permeabilized mitochondria
PDHP-phosphatase	Activation	None	0.43[a]	—
		0.2mMADP	—	0.77[b]
		0.2mMATP	—	0.74[b]
NAD-ICDH	Activation	1.5mMADP	15[c]	5.4[c]
		1.5mMATP	43[c]	41[c]
OGDH	Activation	1.5mMADP	0.21[c]	0.28[c]
		1.5mMATP	2.12[c]	0.81[c]
Pyrophosphatase	Inhibition	None	3.2[d]	—

Values taken from the following sources:[a](71), [b](78), [c](79), [d](21). The Mg^{2+} concentrations were about 4, 0.07, 1, and 0.3 mM respectively.

Abbreviations: $K_{0.5}$ value, the concentration of effector required for half-maximal response; NAD-ICDH, NAD^+-linked isocitrate dehydrogenase; OGDH, the 2-oxoglutarate dehydrogenase complex; PDH, the pyruvate dehydrogenase complex; PDH$_a$, PDHP, the active non-phosphorylated and inactive phosphorylated forms of PDH respectively; Ca^{2+} refers exclusively to free calcium ions.

tramitochondrial Mg^{2+} concentration may have an important influence on the relative responses of the dehydrogenases to Ca^{2+}. Although the kinetic properties of OGDH are essentially unaffected by Mg^{2+}, as the concentration of Mg^{2+} increases both the Ca^{2+} response of PDHP-phosphatase (64) and the Ca^{2+} sensitivity of NAD-ICDH (80) decrease. Recent estimates of the concentration of Mg^{2+} in mitochondria suggest that the concentration is about 0.3 mM (13, 43), but little is known about the mechanisms that regulate its concentration.

Extensive studies have been made on the activation of the dehydrogenases within coupled mitochondria derived from rat heart (24, 35), rat liver (52), and several other tissues (3, 30, 39, 51, 54). These have clearly established that PDH and OGDH are activated in parallel when the extramitochondrial concentration of Ca^{2+} is increased within the expected physiologic range (i.e. between 0.5 and 2 μM. Figure 2 *(dashed line)* illustrates the activation of OGDH and PDH within rate heart mitochondria exposed to increases in

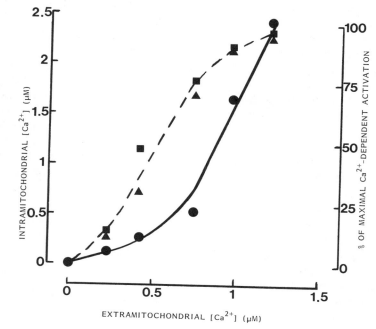

Figure 2 Relationships between the extramitochondrial and intramitochondrial concentrations (●) of Ca^{2+} in fura-2 loaded rat heart mitochondria incubated (at pH 7.0) with medium containing Na^+ (10 mM) and Mg^{2+} (2 mM). Also shown are the Ca^{2+}-dependent activations of PDH (▲) and OGDH (■) under the same conditions. Data adapted from McCormack et al (55) together with unpublished observations of J. G. McCormack.

extramitochondrial concentrations of Ca^{2+} in the presence of expected physiologic concentrations of Na^+ and Mg^{2+}. The $K_{0.5}$ values for the activation of both enzymes are close to 0.5 μM and similar results have been found in other studies.

There are considerable technical difficulties in the measurement of the activity of NAD-ICDH in intact mitochondria. These include the low activity of the tricarboxylate transporter in heart and some other mitochondria, the presence of high activities of NADP-ICDH, and the fact that the product of both NAD-ICDH and NADP-ICDH is oxoglutarate, which is metabolized by the Ca^{2+}-sensitive OGDH. This last aspect may be the explanation for why the apparent Ca^{2+} sensitivities of isocitrate oxidation by coupled mitochondria from adipose tissue, liver, or kidney are similar to those for oxoglutarate oxidation (51, 52, 54) and not rather less as might be expected from the relative Ca^{2+} sensitivities of the extracted dehydrogenases (see Table 1).

Studies on the activation of PDH and OGDH of the type illustrated in Figure 2 give an estimate of the relationship between extramitochondrial and intramitochondrial Ca^{2+} since the $K_{0.5}$ value of the two enzymes for Ca^{2+} is in the range of 0.2–0.8 μM (Table 1). Thus under such conditions, it is probable that little or no concentration gradient of Ca^{2+} can occur across the inner mitochondrial membrane when the extramitochondrial concentration is around 0.5 μM (Fig. 2) (24). Recently, excellent confirmation of this prediction employing isolated rat heart mitochondria (22, 49, 50, 55, 67) has been achieved with use of fluorescent Ca^{2+} indicators in much the same way as the indicators have previously been used with intact cells (see 11 for recent review). Figure 2 *(solid line)* shows the relationship between extramitochondrial and intramitochondrial concentrations of Ca^{2+}, with use of fura-2-loaded rat heart mitochondria; similar results are apparent using indo-1 (67). At low extramitochondrial concentrations of Ca^{2+} (below 0.25 μM and in the presence of Na^+ and Mg^{2+}), the concentration of Ca^{2+} within mitochondria is actually less than that outside the mitochondria, but as the extramitochondrial concentration is increased there is a much more marked increase in the intramitochondrial concentration such that the gradient becomes reversed above about 0.5 μM. The Ca^{2+}-transport system in the inner membrane thus appears to act as an amplifier so that changes in Ca^{2+} concentrations within mitochondria (occurring within the concentration range to which the dehydrogenases are sensitive) are greater than those occurring in the cytoplasm. This behavior was earlier predicted by Crompton (14) on the basis of the kinetic properties of the system.

Other Ca^{2+}-Sensitive Enzymes

A number of other intramitochondrial enzymes have been reported to be sensitive to Ca^{2+}, but in most cases the concentrations required appear to be in the mM range and hence too large to be of any physiologic relevance. Examples include the branched-chain oxoacid dehydrogenase complex (72), pyruvate carboxylase (95), and carbamyl phosphate synthetase (10, 63).

A more promising potential site for Ca^{2+} regulation is the H$^+$-ATP synthetase system. A small protein inhibitor of the system has been described that is apparently released with stimulation of ATPase activity in the presence of μM concentrations of Ca^{2+} (96, 97). It would certainly make sense to activate ATP synthesis at the same time as activating the Ca^{2+}-sensitive matrix dehydrogenases and hence the supply of NADH for the respiratory chain, but direct evidence for this attractive possibility remains elusive.

In contrast, there is now considerable evidence from the studies of Davidson & Halestrap (19–21) that increases in the intramitochondrial concentration of Ca^{2+} may inhibit matrix pyrophosphatase activity. The sensitivity of this enzyme to Ca^{2+} depends on the concentration of Mg^{2+}. At a Mg^{2+} concentration of 0.3 mM, which is presently the best estimate of the intramitochondrial concentration (13, 43), the $K_{0.5}$ for inhibition of the enzyme from both rat liver and heart mitochondria is about 3 μM. This inhibition probably underlies the increases in pyrophosphate concentration found on incubating mitochondria with increasing extramitochondrial concentrations of Ca^{2+} (19, 20). There is now mounting evidence from studies by Halestrap & colleagues that such increases, at least in liver mitochondria, may initiate a chain of events probably associated with enhanced uptake of K$^+$ and hence an enlargement of the mitochondrial matrix. This may result in further important changes in intramitochondrial metabolism, which include activation of the respiratory chain, fatty acid oxidation, and glutaminase activity (19, 34, 62, 75).

APPROACHES AVAILABLE TO EXPLORE THE ROLE OF CHANGES IN INTRAMITOCHONDRIAL CONCENTRATIONS OF Ca^{2+} WITHIN INTACT TISSUE AND CELL PREPARATIONS

The studies on isolated enzymes and intact mitochondria from rat heart, liver, and other mammalian sources are fully consistent with the notion that increases in the cytosolic Ca^{2+} concentration within the physiologic range would result in the activation of PDH, OGDH, and perhaps NAD-ICDH, together with the inhibition of intramitochondrial pyrophosphatase. Moreover, these studies suggest that the changes in enzyme activities could play a central role in the regulation of cell metabolism by allowing increases in mitochondrial ATP synthesis to occur without there necessarily being any increase in the concentration of ADP. Nevertheless it is of critical importance to obtain evidence on the role of intramitochondrial Ca^{2+} using intact tissue or cell preparations.

Only if all or most of the following approaches have been successively applied can a role for Ca^{2+} in the activation of mitochondrial oxidative metabolism and hence ATP formation be said to be established with some confidence. None of the approaches alone is sufficient. Convincing supportive data using the following approaches have been obtained in two well-studied and contrasting tissues, namely, the effects of positive inotropic stimulation on the rat heart and the effects of Ca^{2+}-mobilizing hormones (α-adrenergic agonists, vasopressin, and angiotensin) on rat liver cells.

Measurement of Total Calcium in the Mitochondria of Intact Cells

Studies on mitochondria isolated from rat heart (12, 38, 49), and liver (5, 12) indicate that about 0.1% of the total calcium content of mitochondria is present as free Ca^{2+} and that only increases in the total calcium content within the approximate range 0.2–4 nmol per mg of mitochondrial protein will lead to activation of PDH and OGDH. This value should be compared with the value of about 10 nmol per mg of mitochondrial protein, which is the minimum content compatible with the mitochondria acting as buffers of cytosolic Ca^{2+} (see introduction this chapter, 36, 70).

Total calcium content of mitochondria within intact cells can be measured either by atomic absorption of mitochondrial fractions following rapid cell fractionation under conditions where calcium uptake and egress from the mitochondria is inhibited (5, 17, 81), or by X-ray probe microanalysis of snap frozen tissue (8, 84, 85, 92, 93). When appropriate precautions are taken (25, 83), it is evident that both approaches yield similar values of ≈ 1–2 nmol per mg of mitochondrial protein in unstimulated cells of a wide variety of tissues. These values are near the level of detection of both methods; nevertheless they are consistent with Ca^{2+} regulation of the intramitochondrial enzymes and not with the mitochondria acting as buffers of cytoplasmic Ca^{2+}.

Following positive inotropic stimulation of the heart, increases in total mitochondrial calcium to about 2–4 nmol per mg protein have been reported using both methods (17, 92). Similar increases are also apparent in mitochondria isolated from livers perfused with a medium containing vasopressin or glucagon and are even more markedly apparent if both hormones are present (5). A recent study employing X-ray probe analysis failed to detect these increases in the liver mitochondria of rats previously injected with vasopressin plus glucagon (8). However in this study the stimulation of liver phosphorylase was very modest implying that the in vivo hormone treatment used may not have been optimal.

Measurement of PDH$_a$ and Citrate Cycle Flux and Concentrations of Key Intermediates Including the ATP/ADP and NADH/NAD$^+$ Ratios and Pyrophosphate

If Ca^{2+} is important in the stimulation of mitochondrial oxidative metabolism in any particular instance, then there should be increases in PDH$_a$ and citrate cycle flux (usually most simply inferred from an increase in O$_2$ uptake) without any decreases in the ATP/ADP and NADH/NAD$^+$ ratios. Indeed, if decreases are observed, it is possible that they may be responsible for the increases in PDH$_a$ and cycle flux since the activities of PDH, NAD-ICDH, and OGDH are all potentially regulated by these ratios (23, 25). This topic is discussed by Heineman & Balaban (this volume).

In rat heart and liver preparations it is well established that a range of conditions that lead to increases in cytoplasmic Ca^{2+} concentrations all result in increases in PDH$_a$ and citrate cycle flux (e.g. 4, 5, 41, 42, 57). These occur in most instances without any evidence of decreases in the ATP/ADP and NADH/NAD$^+$ ratios, consistent with activation of the respiratory chain by NADH supply rather than by increases in ADP concentration. In the liver, activation of OGDH is also suggested by marked decreases in cellular oxoglutarate and glutamate concentrations (82, 86).

Further evidence that the intramitochondrial concentration of Ca^{2+} increases in stimulated liver cells comes from recent findings of Halestrap & colleagues who find that the concentration of mitochondrial pyrophosphate is increased, and consistent with this, there is evidence from light-scattering and other studies that the volume of the mitochondria is greater (20, 34, 76). As mentioned above, studies with isolated mitochondria have demonstrated that such volume changes may initiate, at least in part, the activation of the respiratory chain, fatty acid oxidation, and glutaminase that occur under these conditions (19, 62, 75). In particular, activation of the respiratory chain may underlie the transient nature of the increases in NAD(P)H fluorescence observed in liver preparations exposed to phenylephrine or vasopressin, whereas the reduction state of cytochrome c and rate of respiration remains elevated (34, 75).

Use of Ruthenium Red

The use of ruthenium red represents a powerful extension of the above approach. This compound is a potent and apparently reasonably specific inhibitor of Ca^{2+} uptake into mitochondria (65). Despite being highly positively charged, it appears to enter a number of cell types and should therefore block any increases in PDH$_a$ activity that involve Ca^{2+} entry into mitochondria. This approach has been most extensively applied to the effects of a range of inotropic stimuli on the perfused rat heart. McCormack & England (61) showed that the increases in PDH$_a$ could be completely blocked by perfusion with a medium containing ruthenium red, whereas cytosolic Ca^{2+}-stimulated processes, such as contraction and phosphorylase a levels, were essentially unaffected. Subsequently, Hansford (37) showed that ruthenium red blocked the activation of PDH in quin-2 loaded myocytes subjected to various treatments designed to elicit increases in cytosolic Ca^{2+}, while the measured increases in cytosolic Ca^{2+} were largely unaffected. It seems probable that increased respiration and hence ATP formation may be largely achieved in the ruthenium red treated hearts through intrinsic control mechanisms, including an increase in ADP concentration (44, 45, 91) rather than activation of the dehydrogenases by an increase in the Ca^{2+} concentration.

Studies with ruthenium red have also demonstrated that increases in the intramitochondrial concentration of Ca^{2+} may be important in the activation of PDH (and by inference and the other Ca^{2+}-sensitive intramitochondrial enzymes) in skeletal muscle (32), synaptosomes (39, 73), and adipose tissue (51). Thus far it has not been a useful approach with liver preparations; this may be because the dye does not enter these cells, or that it is sequestered or metabolized within the cells.

Study of the Persistence of the Activation of PDH and OGDH in Mitochondria Prepared from Stimulated Tissue/Cells

Perhaps the most convincing evidence that hormones do act on intramitochondrial metabolism via changes in the intramitochondrial concentration of Ca^{2+} has come from studies of the type summarized in Table 2. This approach depends on the rapid disruption of tissues and the preparation of mitochondria under conditions where there is little loss or uptake of Ca^{2+} into these organelles. This can be achieved in both the rat heart and liver by the rapid extraction and preparation of mitochondria at 0°C in medium containing EGTA, but free of Na$^+$ (53, 59). Activation of PDH initiated by prior hormone treatment of the tissues is then found to persist not only during the preparation of the mitochondria, but also during their subsequent incubation at 30°C in Na$^+$-free medium containing EGTA and respiratory substrates. Parallel increases in the activity of OGDH measured at subsaturating concentrations of oxoglutarate are also apparent. However the increases in the activity of both dehydrogenases are lost if Na$^+$ is added to the mitochondrial incubation medium. Since these effects of Na$^+$ are absent in the presence of diltiazem, which inhibits the sodium dependent efflux pathway, one concludes that the increases in enzyme activity are the result of increases in Ca^{2+} concentration in the mitochondria from hormone-treated tissues. This conclusion is reinforced by the finding that incubation of the mitochondria with Ca^{2+} sufficient to elicit a maximum stimulation also results in the dis-

Table 2   Persistence of the activation of PDH and OGDH in mitochondria prepared from rat heart and liver previously exposed to adrenaline

Source of mitochondria	Additions to mitochondrial incubation medium	PDH$_a$ (as % total) after tissue treatment with		OGDH activity (as % V$_{max}$) after tissue treatment with	
		No hormone	Adrenaline	No hormone	Adrenaline
Rat heart[a] perfused	None	8	20	23	35
	NaCl	8	7	25	24
	NaCl plus diltiazem	8	20	23	32
	Ca^{2+}	45	47	65	—
Rat liver[b] in vivo	None	12	20	8	13
	NaCl	13	14	8	8
	NaCl plus diltiazem	13	23	9	18
	Ca^{2+}	49	51	33	35

Data taken from [a] (59) and [b] (53). After no hormone or adrenaline treatment, tissue was rapidly homogenized, mitochondria prepared, and then incubated at 30°C for 5 min in KCl-based medium containing respiratory substrates, EGTA, and where indicated additions of NaCl (10 mM), diltiazem (300 μM) and sufficient Ca^{2+} to maximally activate PDH. OGDH activity was measured at a suitable nonsaturating concentration of oxoglutarate.

appearance of the differences in the activities of both dehydrogenases in mitochondria from control and hormone-treated tissues (Table 2).

The application of this same approach has also shown that the activation of adipose tissue PDH by insulin is not brought about by any increase in the mitochondrial concentration of Ca^{2+} (51).

GENERAL DISCUSSION

Activation by μM concentrations of Ca^{2+} appears to be a common feature of PDHP-phosphatase, NAD-ICDH, and OGDH from all vertebrate sources so far studied; in contrast, the enzymes from nonvertebrate sources are not sensitive to Ca^{2+} (58). Indeed, mitochondria from nonvertebrate sources usually appear to lack the Ca^{2+}-uptake system characteristic of all vertebrate mitochondria (66), which lends general support to the view that in vertebrates the main role of the system is linked to the regulation of the dehydrogenases.

Overall there is good evidence that within the mitochondria of rat heart and liver Ca^{2+} acts as a second messenger to stimulate the formation of NADH formation and hence ATP synthesis. Detailed studies on other tissues, using the approaches described in the preceding section, are required before it can be conclusively stated that increases in intramitochondrial Ca^{2+} are invariably important in the stimulation of mitochondrial ATP formation under conditions where increases in cytoplasmic Ca^{2+} occur. A key question is the relative importance of changes in the mitochondrial concentration of Ca^{2+} to that of ADP in any particular circumstance. Much remains to be established concerning the role that inhibition of mitochondrial pyrophosphatase activity may play in tissues other than rat liver. In the heart and other tissues, it may provide a basis for increasing the supply of acetyl-CoA for the citrate cycle through the stimulation of fatty acid oxidation (33).

In the near future, it should be possible to measure the intramitochondrial concentration of Ca^{2+} through the use of high-resolution fluorescence imaging of intact cells loaded with a Ca^{2+}-sensitive indicator some of which is de-esterified within the mitochondria (87). This and other approaches should provide further insights into the relationship between changes in cytoplasmic and mitochondrial Ca^{2+}; in particular, the speed with which changes in cytoplasmic Ca^{2+} are relayed into mitochondria. For example, in the heart are there changes in intramitochondrial Ca^{2+} that follow the changes in the cytoplasm occurring within each heart beat, or is the mitochondrial concentration largely a reflection of the time-averaged concentration in the cytoplasm (14)? Small changes in PDH_a have recently been observed within the contractile cycle in dog heart (46), which suggests that the former may occur to an appreciable extent. There is also evidence that hormones may influence the activity of components of the mitochondrial calcium transport system (17, 31). The importance of this type of regulation within intact cells needs further investigation.

ACKNOWLEDGMENTS

Studies carried out in the authors' laboratories have been supported by grants from the Medical Research Council (U.K.), the British Diabetic Association, the British Heart Foundation, the Percival Waite Salmond Bequest, and the Lister Institute of Preventive Medicine. J. G. McC. is a Lister Institute Research Fellow.

Literature Cited

1. Al-Nasser, I., Crompton, M. 1986. The entrapment of the Ca^{2+}-indicator Arsenazo III in the matrix space of rat liver mitochondria by permeabilisation and resealing. *Biochem. J.* 239:31–40
2. Aogaichi, T., Evans, J., Gabriel, J. L., Plaut, G. W. E. 1980. The effects of calcium and lanthanide ions on the activity of bovine heart nicotinamide adenine dinucleotide-specific isocitrate dehydrogenase. *Arch. Biochem. Biophys.* 204: 350–60
3. Ashour, B., Hansford, R. G. 1983. Effect of fatty acids and ketones on the activity of pyruvate dehydrogenase in skeletal muscle mitochondria. *Biochem. J.* 214:725–36
4. Assimacopoulos-Jeannet, F., McCormack, J. G., Jeanrenaud, B. 1983. Effect of phenylephrine on pyruvate dehydrogenase activity in rat hepatocytes and its interaction with insulin and glucagon. *FEBS Lett.* 159:83–89
5. Assimacopoulos-Jeannet, F., McCormack, J. G., Jeanrenaud, B. 1986. Vasopressin and/or glucagon rapidly increases mitochondrial calcium and oxidative enzyme activities in the perfused rat liver. *J. Biol. Chem.* 261:8799–804
6. Deleted in proof

7. Balaban, R. S., Kantor, H. L, Katz, L. A., Briggs, R. W. 1986. Relation between work and phospho-metabolites in the *in vivo* placed mammalian heart. *Science* 232:1121–23

8. Bond, M., Vadasz, G., Somlyo, A. V., Somlyo, A. P. 1987. Subcellular calcium and magnesium mobilization in rat liver stimultated *in vivo* with vasopressin and glucagon. *J. Biol. Chem.* 262: 15630–36

8a. Brand, M. 1988. The signaling role of mitochondrial calcium transport. *ISI Atlas of Science: Biochem:* 1(4):350–54

9. Carafoli, E. 1987. Intracellular calcium homeostasis. *Annu. Rev. Biochem.* 56: 395–433

10. Cerdan, S., Lusty, C. J., Davis, K. N., Jacobsohn, J. A., Williamson, J. R. 1984. Role of calcium as an inhibitor of rat liver carbamyl phosphate synthetase. *J. Biol. Chem.* 259:323–31

11. Cobbold, P. H., Rink, T. J. 1987. Fluorescence and bioluminescence measurement of cystosolic free Ca^{2+}. *Biochem. J.* 248:313–28

12. Coll, K. E., Joseph, S. K., Corkey, B. E., Williamson, J. R. 1982. Determination of the matrix free Ca^{2+} concentration and kinetics of Ca^{2+} efflux in liver and heart mitochondria. *J. Biol. Chem.* 257:8696–704

13. Corkey, B. E., Duszynski, J., Rich, T. L., Matschinsky, B., Williamson, J. R. 1986. Regulation of free and bound magnesium in rat hepatocytes and isolated mitochondria. *J. Biol. Chem.* 261: 2567–74

14. Crompton, M. 1985. The regulation of mitochondrial calcium transport in heart. *Curr. Top. Membr. Transp.* 25:231–76

15. Crompton, M., Costi, A. 1988. Kinetic evidence for a heart mitochondrial pore activated by Ca^{2+}, inorganic phosphate and oxidative stress. *Eur. J. Biochem.* 178:489–501

16. Crompton, M., Costi, A., Hayat, L. 1987. Evidence for the presence of a reversible Ca^{2+}-dependent pore activated by oxidative stress in heart mitochondria. *Biochem. J.* 245:915–18

17. Crompton, M., Kessar, P., Al-Nassar, I. 1983. The α-adrenergic-mediated activation of the cardiac mitochondrial Ca^{2+} *in vivo*. *Biochem. J.* 216:333–42

18. Crompton, M., Roos, I. 1985. On the hormonal control of heart mitochondrial Ca^{2+}. *Biochem. Soc. Trans.* 13:667–69

19. Davidson, A. M., Halestrap, A. P. 1987. Liver mitochondrial pyrophosphate concentration is increased by Ca^{2+} and regulates the intramitochondrial

volume and adenine nucleotide content. *Biochem. J.* 246:715–23

20. Davidson, A. M., Halestrap, A. P. 1988. Inorganic pyrophosphate is located primarily in the mitochondria of the hepatocyte and increases in parallel with the decrease in light-scattering induced by gluconeogenic hormones, butyrate and ionophore A23187. *Biochem. J.* 254:379–84

21. Davidson, A. M., Halestrap, A. P. 1989. Inhibition of mitochondrial matrix inorganic pyrophosphatase by physiological [Ca^{2+}] and its role in the hormonal regulation of mitochondrial matrix volume. *Biochem. J.* 258:817–21

22. Davis, M. H., Altshuld, R. A., Jung, D. W., Brierley, G. P. 1987. Estimation of intramitochondrial pCa and pH by fura-2 and 2,7 biscarboxylethyl-5(6)-carboxyfluorescein (BCECF) fluorescence. *Biochem. Biophys. Res. Commun.* 149:40–45

23. Denton, R. M., McCormack, J. G. 1980. On the role of the calcium transport cycle in heart and other mammalian mitochondria. *FEBS Lett.* 119:1–8

24. Denton, R. M., McCormack, J. G., Edgell, N. J. 1980. Role of calcium ions in the regulation of intramitochondrial metabolism. Effects of Na$^+$, Mg^{2+} and ruthenium red on the Ca^{2+}-stimulated oxidation of oxoglutarate and on pyruvate dehydrogenase activity in intact rat heart mitochondria. *Biochem. J.* 190: 107–17

25. Denton, R. M., McCormack, J. G. 1985. Ca^{2+} transport by mammalian mitochondria and its role in hormone action. *Am. J. Physiol.* 249:E543–E554

26. Denton, R. M., Randle, P. J., Martin, B. R. 1972. Stimulation by calcium ions of pyruvate dehydrogenase phosphatase. *Biochem. J.* 128:161–63

27. Denton, R. M., Richards, D. A., Chin, J. G. 1978. Calcium ions and the regulation of NAD-linked isocitrate dehydrogenase from the mitochondria of rat heart and other tissues. *Biochem. J.* 176:894–906

28. Exton, J. H. 1981. Molecular mechanism involved in α-adrenergic responses. *Mol. Cell. Endocrinol.* 23: 233–64

29. From, A. H. L., Petein, M. A., Michurski, S. P., Zimmer, S. D., Ugurbil, K. 1986. ^{31}P-NMR studies of respiratory regulation in the intact myocardium. *FEBS. Lett.* 206:257–61

30. Fuller, S. J., Randle, P. J. 1984. Reversible phosphorylation of pyruvate dehydrogenase in rat skeletal muscle

mitochondria. Effects of starvation and diabetes. *Biochem J.* 219:635–46

31. Goldstone, T. P., Roos, I., Crompton, M. 1987. Effects of adrenergic agonists and mitochondrial energy state on the Ca^{2+} transport systems of mitochondria. *Biochemistry* 26:246–54

32. Hagg, S. A., Taylor, S. I., Ruderman, N. B. 1976. Glucose metabolism in perfused skeletal muscle. Pyruvate dehydrogenase activity in starvation, diabetes and exercise. *Biochem. J.* 158:203–10

33. Halestrap, A. P. 1987. The regulation of the oxidation of fatty acids and other substrates in rat heart mitochondria by changes in the matrix volume induced by osmotic strength, valinomycin and Ca^{2+}. *Biochem. J.* 244:159–64

34. Halestrap, A. P. 1989. The regulation of the matrix volume of mammalian mitochondria *in vivo* and *in vitro* and its role in the control of mitochondrial metabolism. *Biochim. Biophys. Acta* 973:355–82

35. Hansford, R. G. 1981. Effects of micromolar concentrations of free Ca^{2+} ions on pyruvate dehydrogenase interconversion in intact rat heart mitochondria. *Biochem. J.* 194:721–32

36. Hansford, R. G. 1985. Relation between mitochondrial calcium transport and control of energy metabolism. *Rev. Physiol. Biochem. Pharmacol.* 102:1–72

37. Hansford, R. G. 1987. Relation between cytosolic free Ca^{2+} concentration and the control of pyruvate dehydrogenase in isolated cardiac myocytes. *Biochem. J.* 241:145–51

38. Hansford, R. G., Castro, F. 1982. Intramitochondrial and extramitochondrial free calcium ion concentration of suspensions of heart mitochondria with very low, plausibly physiological contents of total calcium. *J. Bioenerg. Biomemb.* 14:361–76

39. Hansford, R. G., Castro, F. 1985. Roles of Ca^{2+} in pyruvate dehydrogenase interconversion in brain mitochondria and synaptosomes. *Biochem. J.* 227:129–53

40. Hayat, L. H., Crompton, M. 1987. The effects of Mg^{2+} and adenine nucelotides on the sensitivity of the heart mitochondrial Na^+/Ca^{2+} carrier to extramitochondrial Ca^{2+}. A study using Arsenazo III-loaded mitochondria. *Biochem. J.* 244:533–38

41. Hems, D. A., McCormack, J. G., Denton, R. M. 1978. Activation of pyruvate dehydrogenase in the perfused rat liver by vasopressin. *Biochem. J.* 176:627–29

42. Hiraoka, T., Debuysere, M., Olson, M.

S. 1980. Studies on the effects of β-adrenergic agonists on the regulation of pyruvate dehydrogenase in the perfused rat heart. *J. Biol. Chem.* 255:7604–9

43. Jung, D. W., Brierley, G. P. 1986. Matrix magnesium and the permeability of heart mitochondria to potassium ion. *J. Biol. Chem.* 261:6408–15

44. Katz, L. A., Koretsky, A. P., Balaban, R. S. 1987. Respiratory control in the glucose perfused heart. A ^{31}P NMR and NADH fluorescence study. *FEBS Lett.* 221:270–76

45. Katz, L. A., Koretsky, A. P., Balaban, R. S. 1988. Activation of dehydrogenase activity and cardiac respiration: a ^{31}P-NMR study. *Am. J. Physiol.* 255:H185–H88

46. Krause, E.-G., Beyerdorfer, I. 1988. Heart cycle-related activation of pyruvate dehydrogenase in canine myocardium *in vivo*. *J. Mol. Cell. Cardiol.* 20: (Suppl. V):S54

47. Lawlis, V. B., Roche, T. E. 1980. Effect of micromolar Ca^{2+} on NADH inhibition of bovine kidney α-ketoglutarate dehydrogenase complex and possible role of Ca^{2+} in signal amplification. *Mol. Cell. Biochem.* 32: 147–52

48. Lawlis, V. B., Roche, T. E. 1981. Inhibition of bovine kidney α-ketoglutarate dehydrogenase complex by reduced nicotinamide adenine dinucleotide in the presence or absence of calcium ion and effect of adenosine 5'-diphosphate on reduced nicotinamide adenine dinucleotide inhibition. *Biochemistry* 20:2519–24

49. Lukacs, G. L., Kapus, A. 1987. Measurement of the matrix free Ca^{2+} concentration in heart mitochondria by entrapped fura-2 and quin-2. *Biochem. J.* 248:609–13

50. Lukacs, G. L., Kapus, A., Fonyo, A. 1988. Parallel measurements of oxoglutarate dehydrogenase activity and matrix free Ca^{2+} in fura-2 loaded heart mitochondria. *FEBS Lett.* 229:219–23

51. Marshall, S. E., McCormack, J. G., Denton, R. M. 1984. Role of Ca^{2+} ions in the regulation of intramitochondrial metabolism in rat epididymal adipose tissue. Evidence against a role for Ca^{2+} in the activation of pyruvate dehydrogenase by insulin. *Biochem. J.* 218:249–60

52. McCormack, J. G. 1985. Characterization of the effects of Ca^{2+} on the intramitochondrial Ca^{2+}-sensitive enzymes from rat liver and within rat liver mitochondria. *Biochem. J.* 231:581–95

53. McCormack, J. G. 1985. Studies on the

activation of rat liver pyruvate dehydrogenase and 2-oxoglutarate dehydrogenase by adrenaline and glucagon. Role of increases in intramitochondrial Ca^{2+} concentration. *Biochem. J.* 231:597–608

54. McCormack, J. G., Bromidge, E. S., Dawes, N. J. 1988. Characterization of the effects of Ca^{2+} on the intramitochondrial Ca^{2+}-sensitive dehydrogenases within intact rat-kidney mitochondria. *Biochim. Biophys. Acta* 934:282–92

55. McCormack, J. G., Browne, H. M., Dawes, N. J. 1989. Studies on mitochondrial Ca^{2+}-transport and matrix Ca^{2+} using fura-2-loaded rat heart mitochondria. *Biochim. Biophys. Acta* 973:420–27

56. McCormack, J. G., Denton, R. M. 1979. The effects of calcium ions and adenine nucleotides on the activity of pig heart 2-oxoglutarate dehydrogenase complex. *Biochem. J.* 180:533–44

57. McCormack, J. G., Denton, R. M. 1981. The activation of pyruvate dehydrogenase in the perfused rat heart by adrenaline and other inotropic agents. *Biochem. J.* 194:639–43

58. McCormack, J. G., Denton, R. M. 1981. A comparative study of the regulation by Ca^{2+} of the activities of the 2-oxoglutarate dehydrogenase complex and NAD-isocitrate dehydrogenase from a variety of sources. *Biochem. J.* 196:619–24

59. McCormack, J. G., Denton, R. M. 1984. Role of Ca^{2+} ions in the regulation of intramitochondrial metabolism in rat heart. Evidence from studies with isolated mitochondria that adrenaline activates the pyruvate dehydrogenase and 2-oxoglutarate dehydrogenase complexes by increasing the intramitochondrial concentration of Ca^{2+}. *Biochem. J.* 218:235–47

60. McCormack, J. G., Denton, R. M. 1986. Ca^{2+} as a second messenger within mitochondria. *Trends Biochem. Sci.* 11:258–62

61. McCormack, J. G., England, P. J. 1983. Ruthenium red inhibits the activation of pyruvate dehydrogenase caused by positive inotropic agents in the perfused rat heart. *Biochem. J.* 214:581–85

62. McGiven, J., Vadher, M., Lacey, J., Bradford, N. 1985. Rat liver glutaminase. Regulation by reversible interaction with the mitochondrial membrane. *Eur. J. Biochem.* 148:323–27

63. Meijer, A. J., van Woerkom, G. M., Steinman, R., Williamson, J. R. 1981. Inhibition by Ca^{2+} of carbamoylphos-

phate synthetase (ammonia). *J. Biol. Chem.* 256:3443–46

64. Midgley, P. J. W., Rutter, G. A., Thomas, A. P., Denton, R. M. 1987. Effects of Ca^{2+} and Mg^{2+} on the activity of pyruvate dehydrogenase phosphate phosphatase within toluene-permeabilized mitochondria. *Biochem. J.* 241:371–77

65. Moore, C. L. 1971. Specific inhibition of mitochondrial calcium transport by ruthenium red. *Biochem. Biophys. Res. Commun.* 42:298–305

66. Moore, C. L., Akerman, K. E. O. 1984. Calcium and plant organelles. *Plant Cell Environ.* 7:423–40

67. Moreno-Sanchez, R., Hansford, R. G. 1988. Dependence of cardiac mitochondrial pyruvate dehydrogenase activity on intramitochondrial free Ca^{2+} concentration. *Biochem. J.* 256:403–412

68. Neely, J. R., Denton, R. M., England, P. J., Randle, P. J. 1972. The effects of increased heart work on the tricarboxylate cycle and its interactions with glycolysis in the perfused rat heart. *Biochem. J.* 128:147–59

69. Nicholls, D. G. 1978. The regulation of extra-mitochondrial free calcium ion concentration by rat liver mitochondria. *Biochem. J.* 176:463–74

70. Nicholls, D. G., Akerman, K. E. O. 1982. Mitochondrial calcium transport. *Biochim. Biophys. Acta* 683:57–88

71. Pask, H. T. 1976. The properties and regulation of pyruvate dehydrogenase phosphate phosphatase. *PhD thesis*, Univ. Bristol. 205 pp.

72. Patel, T. B., Olson, M. S. 1982. Evidence for the regulation of the branched chain α-keto acid dehydrogenase multienzyme complex by a phosphorylation/dephosphorylation mechanism. *Biochemistry* 21:4259–65

73. Patel, T. B., Sambasivarao, D., Rashed, H. M. 1988. Role of calcium in synaptosomal substrate oxidation. *Arch. Biochem. Biophys.* 264:368–75

74. Pettit, F. H., Roche, T. E., Reed, L. J. 1972. Function of calcium ions in pyruvate dehydrogenase phosphatase activity. *Biochem. Biophys. Res. Commun.* 49:563–71

75. Quinlan, P. T., Halestrap, A. P. 1986. The mechanism of the hormonal activation of respiration in isolated hepatocytes and its importance in the regulation of gluconeogenesis. *Biochem. J.* 236:789–800

76. Quinlan, P. T., Thomas, A. P., Armstrong, A. E., Halestrap, A. P. 1983. Measurement of the intramitochondrial volume in hepatocytes without cell dis-

ruption and its elevation by hormones and valinomycin. *Biochem. J.* 214:395–404

77. Reinhart, P. H., Taylor, W. M., Bygrave, F. L. 1984. The contribution of both extracellular and intracellular calcium to the action of α-adrenergic agonists in perfused rat liver. *Biochem. J.* 220:35–42

78. Rutter, G. A. 1988. Regulation of the Ca^{2+}-sensitive mitochondrial dehydrogenases within toluene-permeabilized rat heart mitochondria, and studies of the purified enzymes. *PhD thesis. Univ. Bristol.* 146 pp.

79. Rutter, G. A., Denton, R. M. 1988. Regulation of NAD^+-linked isocitrate dehydrogenase and 2-oxoglutarate dehydrogenase by Ca^{2+} ions within toluene-permeabilized rat heart mitochondria. Interactions with regulation by adenine nucleotides and $NADH/NAD^+$ ratios. *Biochem. J.* 252:181–89

80. Rutter, G. A., Denton, R. M. 1989. Rapid purification of pig heart NAD-isocitrate dehydrogenase. Regulation by Ca^{2+}. *Biochem. J.* 263:453–62

81. Severson, D. L., Denton, R. M., Bridges, B. J., Randle, P. J. 1976. Exchangeable and total calcium pools in mitochondria of rat epididymal fat cells: role in the regulation of pyruvate dehydrogenase activity. *Biochem. J.* 154:209–33

82. Siess, E. A., Brocks, D. G., Wieland, O. H. 1978. Comparative studies of the influence of hormones on the metabolic compartmentation of isolated liver cells during gluconeogenesis from lactate. *Biochem. Soc. Trans.* 6:1139–44

83. Somlyo, A. P. 1985. Cell calcium measurement with electron probe and electron energy loss analysis. *Cell Calcium* 6:197–222

84. Somlyo, A. P., Bond, M., Somlyo, A. V. 1985. Calcium content of mitochondria and endoplasmic reticulum in liver frozen rapidly *in vivo. Nature* 314:622–25

85. Somlyo, A. P., Somlyo, A. V. 1986. Electron probe analysis of calcium content, and movements in sarcoplasmic reticulum, endoplasmic reticulum, mitochondria and cytoplasm. *J. Cardiovasc. Pharmacol.* 8:542–47

86. Staddon, J. M., McGivan, J. D. 1985. Ca^{2+}-dependent activation of oxoglutarate dehydrogenase by vasopressin in isolated hepatocytes. *Biochem. J.* 225:327–33

87. Steinberg, S. F., Bilelzikian, J. P., Al-Awquati, Q. 1987. Fura-2 fluorescence is localized to mitochondria in endothelial cells. *Am. J. Physiol.* 253:C744–47

88. Teague, W. M., Pettit, F. H., Wu, T.-L., Silberman, S. R., Reed, L. J. 1982. Purification and properties of pyruvate dehydrogenase phosphatase from bovine heart and kidney. *Biochemistry* 21:5585–92

89. Thomas, A. P., Denton, R. M. 1986. Use of toluene-permeabilized mitochondria to study the regulation of adipose tissue pyruvate dehydrogenase *in situ. Biochem. J.* 238:93–101

90. Thomas, A. P., Diggle, T. A., Denton, R. M. 1986. Sensitivity of pyruvate dehydrogenase phosphate phosphatase to magnesium ions. Similar effects of spermine and insulin. *Biochem. J.* 238:83–91

91. Unitt, J. F., McCormack, J. G., Reid, D., Maclachlan, L. K., England, P. J. 1989. Direct evidence for a role of intramitochondrial Ca^{2+} in the regulation of oxidative phosphorylation in the stimulated rat heart. Studies using ^{31}P-n.m.r and ruthenium red. *Biochem. J.* 262:293–301

92. Wendt-Gallitelli, M. F. 1986. Ca-pools involved in the regulation of cardiac contraction under positive inotropy. X-ray microanalysis on rapidly-frozen ventricular muscle of guinea-pig. *Basic Res. Cardiol.* 81:25–32

93. Wendt-Gallitelli, M. F., Jacob, R. 1982. Rhythm-dependent role of different calcium stores in cardiac muscle: X-ray microanalysis. *J. Mol. Cell. Cardiol.* 14:487–92

94. Williamson, J. R., Cooper, R. H., Hoek, J. B. 1981. Role of calcium in the hormonal control of liver metabolism. *Biochim. Biophys. Acta* 639:243–95

95. Wimhurst, J. M., Manchester, K. L. 1970. Some aspects of the kinetics of rat liver pyruvate carboxylase. *Biochem. J.* 120:79–93

96. Yamada, E. W., Huzel, N. J. 1988. The calcium-binding ATPase inhibitor protein from bovine heart mitochondria. Purification and properties. *J. Biol. Chem.* 263:11498–503

97. Yamada, E. W., Shiffman, F. H., Huzel, N. J. 1980. Ca^{2+}-regulated release of an ATPase inhibitor protein from submitochondrial particles derived from skeletal muscles of the rat. *J. Biol. Chem.* 255:267–73

Annu. Rev. Physiol. 1990. 52:467–85

CYTOPLASMIC [Ca^{2+}] IN MAMMALIAN VENTRICLE: DYNAMIC CONTROL BY CELLULAR PROCESSES

W. G. Wier

Department of Physiology, University of Maryland School of Medicine, Baltimore, Maryland 21201

KEY WORDS: excitation-contraction coupling, sarcoplasmic reticulum, sarcolemma, fura-2, Ca^{2+} channels

INTRODUCTION

The role of intracellular calcium in signaling cellular functions is generally fulfilled by the chemical binding of the ion (Ca^{2+}) to a protein, such as troponin c or calmodulin. In the cytosolic environment the reaction between Ca^{2+} and its binding site can be described by the law of mass action, in which one of the terms is the cytosolic concentration of free calcium ions ([Ca^{2+}]$_i$). Because many cellular functions are steeply dependent on [Ca^{2+}]$_i$, the precise value of cytosolic [Ca^{2+}] is of critical importance in determining cell function. Thus the various cellular processes that determine [Ca^{2+}]$_i$ dynamically are of interest to the physiologist. This review will primarily discuss the available information on the quantitative contribution of these processes to control of cytosolic [Ca^{2+}] in mammalian heart muscle.

Previous quantitative studies of [Ca^{2+}]$_i$ transients in mammalian heart utilized aequorin and yielded estimates of peak [Ca^{2+}]$_i$ ranging from 0.7 to about 3 μM [for a previous review of these data, see (21)]. In aequorin-injected ferret papillary muscles, peak [Ca^{2+}]$_i$ transients varied from 0.5 to about 2 μM, over the range of an inotropic state spanning that of a closely

0066-4278/90/0315-0467$02.00

coupled extrasystole to that of a highly potentiated post-extrasystolic beat (71). In general, the use of voltage-clamp or control of intracellular ionic environment was not possible in those studies because of the requisite (for aequorin) use of multicellular preparations. Figures 1 and 2 illustrate the essential features of $[Ca^{2+}]_i$ transients as they have been revealed in recent studies. Individual guinea pig (8, 17, 18, 67) or rat ventricular cells (24–26) were perfused with the new fluorescent Ca^{2+} indicators (38). These types of studies, including those using digital imaging microscopy of Ca^{2+}-indicator signals in cardiac cells, have revealed substantial new information on $[Ca^{2+}]_i$ and this information is the focus of our review. Many other techniques, such as measurement of extracellular Ca^{2+} transients, and $^{45}Ca^{2+}$ flux measurements, have yielded valuable information, but space does not permit consideration of them here. Results obtained from cardiac cells loaded with Ca^{2+} indicator by exposure to the membrane permeant forms (fura-2/AM or indo-1/AM) or results obtained on suspensions of cardiac cells will generally not be considered in this review, since results from these studies are not yet quantifiable, and the measurement of cytosolic $[Ca^{2+}]_i$ is subject to artifacts associated with partial de-esterification (59) and the inevitable entry of the indicator into other cellular compartments (39).

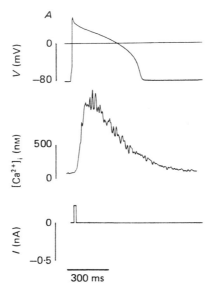

Figure 1   Representative action potential and $[Ca^{2+}]_i$ transient in a guinea pig ventricular myocyte at room temperature and physiologic ionic conditions. The cell was perfused internally with fura-2 and stimulated at 1 Hz. Voltage and $[Ca^{2+}]_i$ transient records are averaged (n=6). Resting potential is −81 mV, overshoot 55 mV. Resting $[Ca^{2+}]_i$ is 120 nM, peak $[Ca^{2+}]_i$ transient is 1100 nM (reproduced with permission from Reference 17).

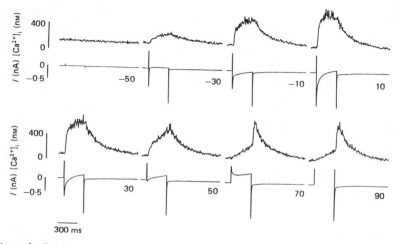

Figure 2   Representative [Ca^{2+}]$_i$ transients and membrane currents in a single guinea pig ventricular myocyte perfused internally with fura-2 at room temperature. Original current records and calculated [Ca^{2+}]$_i$ during depolarising pulses from a holding potential of −68 mV to various levels as indicated. TTX was present at a concentration of 30 μM (reproduced with permission from Reference 17).

As mentioned above, several experimental approaches to obtaining quantitative information on the processes controlling [Ca^{2+}]$_i$ dynamically are used. Here I will consider mainly, but not exclusively, results obtained with the new methods of direct measurement of [Ca^{2+}]$_i$ through the use of internal perfusion of single isolated cells with intracellular Ca^{2+} indicators. I begin by discussing the theory of this experimental approach. An explicit simple theory of the cytoplasmic [Ca^{2+}]$_i$ is explained in the next section.

THEORY OF CYTOPLASMIC [Ca^{2+}]$_i$-TRANSIENTS

The basic theoretical consideration is that, for an element of volume of the cytoplasm, the rate of change of [Ca^{2+}]$_i$ within the cytoplasm is determined by the sum of the fluxes of Ca^{2+} into and out of that element (30). Depending on the structures in that element, the fluxes are those occurring across surface or organellar membranes, the diffusional fluxes from neighboring elements of cytoplasm, and the fluxes onto or off of binding sites (ligands) within the element.

[Ca^{2+}]$_i$ can be observably non-uniform under some, abnormal conditions in mammalian heart cells (propagating [Ca^{2+}]$_i$ waves; Figure 3), (67, 69). During the [Ca^{2+}]$_i$ transients that accompany normal E-C coupling (Figures 1 and 2) [Ca^{2+}]$_i$ appears to be spatially uniform, insofar as it can be observed with digital imaging fluorescence microscopy (67, 68). The spatial resolution of these measurements is probably adequate to reject the possibility that gradients of $[Ca^{2+}]_i$ exist over several sarcomeres. Nevertheless, if $[Ca^{2+}]_i$ could be measured with high enough spatial and temporal resolution, it would almost certainly be found to be non-uniform during $[Ca^{2+}]_i$ transients; small gradients of $[Ca^{2+}]_i$ within each sarcomere are predicted (71) during $[Ca^{2+}]_i$ transients. Even in the steady-state, gradients of $[Ca^{2+}]_i$ at sub-micron distances from Ca^{2+} channels [65], Ca^{2+}-pumping ATPases, and ion-exchangers are expected from theory. Therefore reference to the cytoplasmic $[Ca^{2+}]_i$ transient should be a quantitative description of $[Ca^{2+}]_i$, at all points throughout the cytoplasm, over the period of time that is of interest. Measurement of $[Ca^{2+}]_i$ with the required degree of spatial and temporal resolution is not possible at present. For purposes of this review, I will make the assumption that the gradients of $[Ca^{2+}]_i$ that exist within each sarcomere of the cardiac cell during normal E-C coupling are negligible.

I will also assume that, to a first approximation, the published calculation of $[Ca^{2+}]_i$ from cardiac cells loaded with membrane impermeant forms of fluorescent Ca^{2+} indicators is acceptably accurate. The available data supports this assumption (8, 17, 26), and critical evaluation of this difficult issue is beyond the scope of this review. For this, the reader is referred to other sources (10, 22, 46).

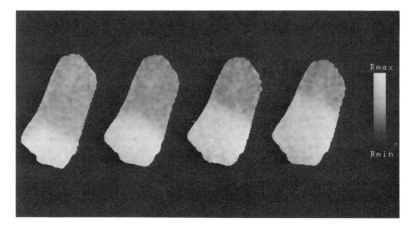

Figure 3 Images of a $[Ca^{2+}]_i$ wave in a single guinea pig ventricular myocyte exposed to sodium-free solution. The four images are separated in time from each other by 67 msec. The cell was perfused internally with indo-1 (pentapotassium salt 100 μM) and the membrane potential was clamped to -80 mV. Gray-level mapping as indicated; black corresponds to R_{min} ($[Ca^{2+}]_i =$ 0), and white corresponds to R_{max} (saturating $[Ca^{2+}]_i$) (reproduced with permission from Reference 67).

A mammalian ventricular cell is assumed in which Ca^{2+} can move across surface membrane (SL), sarcoplasmic reticulum membrane (SR), and mitochondrial membrane (M). SL contains Na/Ca exchanger, L-type Ca^{2+} channels, a Ca^{2+}-leak pathway, an ATP driven Ca^{2+} pump, and low-affinity Ca^{2+}-binding sites (SLb). SR contains Ca^{2+}-release channels, an ATP driven Ca^{2+}-pump, and Ca^{2+}-binding sites (SRb). The cytoplasm of each element contains calmodulin (Cm), troponin C (TnC), fura-2 (I), and phosphate (phos). Fluxes are denoted by J, with the appropriate subscript, and have the units, moles of Ca^{2+} per sec per cm^2 of membrane (SR or SL). Since it is assumed that $[Ca^{2+}]_i$ is uniform with the cell, there is no diffusional flux of Ca^{2+}. In the case of a cell subjected to internal perfusion, the rate of change of $[Ca^{2+}]_i$ at any instant in time will be given by Equation 1.

$$
\begin{aligned}
d[Ca^{2+}]_i/dt = \; & k_{SR} * (J_{SR_{rel}} + J_{SR_{pump}}) \\
& + k_{SL} * (J_{NaCa} + J_{I_{Ca}} + J_{Ca_{leak}} + J_{SL_{pump}}) \\
& + k_{Mito} * J_{Mito} \\
& - \text{Sum } \{d[CaL]_n/dt\} \\
& + J \text{ pipette}
\end{aligned} \qquad 1.
$$

where: $[CaL]_0 = [CaCm]$, $[CaL]_1 = [CaTnC]$, $[CaL]_2 = [CaI]$, $[CaL]_3 = [Caphos]$, $[CaL]_4 = [CaSLb]$, $[CaI]_5 = [CaSRb]$, $k_{SL} = $ (cell surface area)/(cell volume), $k_{SR} = $ (SR surface area)/(cell volume), $k_{Mito} = $ (mitochondrial surface area)/(cell volume), $d[CaL]n/dt = k_{on} * [Ca^{2+}]_i * [L]_n - k_{off} * [CaL]_n$.

Equation 1. or similar equations constitute the stated or unstated theoretical framework of much experimental work. It is certainly oversimplified as discussed above. I now assume that the flux of Ca^{2+} from the micropipette electrode is negligible on the time scale of the rapid $[Ca^{2+}]_i$ transient during E-C coupling and that Ca^{2+} fluxes into mitochondria are also negligible at this level of $[Ca^{2+}]_i$ (27). In this case Equation 1. reduces to 2.:

$$
\begin{aligned}
d[Ca^{2+}]_i/dt = \; & k_{SR} * (J_{SR_{rel}} + J_{SR_{pump}}) \\
& + k_{SL} * (J_{NaCa} + J_{I_{Ca}} + J_{Ca_{leak}} + J_{SL_{pump}}) \\
& - \text{Sum } \{d[CaL]_n/dt\}.
\end{aligned} \qquad 2.
$$

In general, experiments are done in which a simplified form of Equation 2. holds. (For example, the exclusion of Na^+ from the external solution and the filling solution of the micropipette electrode would be thought to create the experimental situation in which the term is zero that gives the flux through the Na/Ca exchanger.) This permits the observation, by dissection, of the various cellular processes. The ability to do this constitutes one of the chief advantages of the use of internally perfused, single ventricular cardiac cells.

DISSECTION OF $[Ca^{2+}]_i$ TRANSIENTS IN MAMMALIAN VENTRICLE

In this section I consider in detail the evidence on the quantitative contribution of the various cellular processes, as described in Equation 2., to the $[Ca^{2+}]_i$ transients that accompany normal excitation-contraction coupling in mammalian ventricular cells. In some instances, it is seen that through the use of single isolated cardiac cells experimental conditions have been arranged such that $[Ca^{2+}]_i$ transients have been reduced to highly simplified cases (i.e. many terms in Equation 2. have been eliminated). By appropriate manipulation of experimental conditions, information on the contribution of SL Ca^{2+} ATPase, Ca^{2+} current, Ca^{2+} leak, and Na-Ca exchange can be obtained.

Surface Membrane (SL)

SL Ca^{2+} ATPase   Numerous experimental observations, both physiologic (9) and biochemical (27, 28), indicate that SL Ca^{2+} ATPase plays a relatively minor role in removal of Ca^{2+} from ventricular cardiac cells.

A recent physiologic approach (64) that is helpful in determining more directly the role of SL Ca^{2+} ATPase is to impose a Ca^{2+} load by activating Ca^{2+} current and to observe the decline of that load in the absence of Ca^{2+} current, Na/Ca exchange, and SR function (Figure 4; see legend for details).

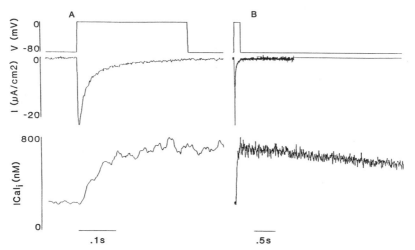

Figure 4 In the absence of sodium and SR function, $[Ca^{2+}]_i$ transients decline extremely slowly. (*A*) Verapamil-sensitive current and $[Ca^{2+}]_i$ transient in a guinea pig ventricular myocyte during a voltage step from -80 mV to 0 mV in the absence of sodium and in the presence of caffeine (10 mM). (*B*) Same record as in *A*, on smaller time scale to illustrate the extremely slow decay of the $[Ca^{2+}]_i$ transient under these conditions (reproduced with permission from Reference 64).

After repolarization, when Ca^{2+} current is no longer present, the experimental situation in Figure 4B can be described by Equation 3., a highly simplified form of Equation 2.

$$d[Ca^{2+}]_i/dt = k_{SL} * (J_{Ca_{leak}} + J_{SL_{pump}}) - Sum \{d[CaL]_n/dt\}$$ 3.

The result of this type of experiment is that the [Ca^{2+}]$_i$ declines extremely slowly. For example, the half-time of the fall in [Ca^{2+}]$_i$ from 0.7 μM back to the resting value of 0.3 μM is 8 sec. Thus is appears that in guinea pig ventricular cells, the SL Ca^{2+} ATPase contributes little to Ca^{2+} efflux on the time scale of the physiologic [Ca^{2+}]$_i$ transient.

The contribution of SL Ca^{2+}-pumping ATPase to the ventricular cell function has also been estimated by observing rapid cooling contractures (RCCs) in isolated ventricular cells (15) and in papillary muscles (14). It is well-known that the amount of Ca^{2+} in the SR of ventricular cells declines during a period of rest (13). The currently favored explanation is that during rest Ca^{2+} leaks from the SR into the cytoplasm and from there is extruded from the cell. It has been shown (D. Bers, J. Bridge, K. Spitzer, submitted for publication) that the rest decay of the rapid cooling contracture in guinea pig ventricular myocytes is almost completely prevented for periods up to five min by applying Na- and Ca-free solutions during the period of rest. By this procedure, both Na$_o$-dependent Ca efflux and Na$_i$-dependent Ca influx via Na/Ca exchange are eliminated. Thus these experiments show that the Ca^{2+} flux through the SL Ca^{2+}-pumping ATPase, at the low [Ca^{2+}]$_i$ existing during the period of rest, must be a very small fraction of that through the SR Ca^{2+}-pumping ATPase, since the loss of Ca^{2+} from the SR was too small to be detected.

Similar conclusions to those above have also been reached through biochemical observations. Carafoli (27) pointed out recently that although the Ca^{2+}-pumping ATPase has a relatively high affinity for Ca^{2+} (K_m = 0.5 μM), it is present in such small amounts that the V_{max} of Ca^{2+} transport (0.5 nM Ca^{2+}/mg membrane protein) is low relative to that of Na/Ca exchange (15–30 nM Ca^{2+}/mg membrane protein). This observation led Carafoli to suggest that the Ca^{2+}-pumping ATPase might be particularly important in pumping Ca^{2+} out of the cell during diastole, when Ca^{2+} is low (compared to the putative K_m of Na/Ca exchange).

The work cited above indicates that the SL Ca^{2+}-pumping ATPase plays a negligible role, both at high levels of [Ca^{2+}]$_i$ ([Ca^{2+}]$_i$ transients) and at low levels of [Ca^{2+}]$_i$ (diastole).

Ca^{2+} LEAK   Since [Ca^{2+}]$_i$ in an inactive ventricular cell at rest is not at the level that it would be if Na/Ca exchange were in equilibrium (20, 41, 61, 62) it is possible that there is a leak of Ca^{2+} into the cell. The physical pathway for Ca^{2+} leak is not known and almost no information on Ca^{2+} leak is available. Hilgemann (41) has calculated that such a leak would have to provide a current of 140 pA, in order to balance Ca^{2+} efflux by Na/Ca exchange, when the exchanger efflux was calculated from the studies of Kimura et al (45). Hilgemann noted that this large leak is inconsistent with certain other measurements and that the required Ca^{2+} leak would be smaller if the Na/Ca-exchanger becomes less activated as $[Ca^{2+}]_i$ fell below the K_m of its activating site (54) and that of calmodulin-stimulated SL Ca^{2+} ATPase (27).

In preliminary experiments of the type illustrated in Figure 4 (unpublished observations of K. Sipido, G. Wier), we have been unable to observe an effect of membrane potential on the decline of $[Ca^{2+}]_i$. On the assumption that the Ca^{2+} leak is ohmic, the fact that $[Ca^{2+}]_i$ does not change for many seconds when membrane potential changes by 100 mV suggests that a Ca^{2+} leak is not an important factor on the time scale of the physiologic $[Ca^{2+}]_i$ transient.

SL Ca^{2+} CHANNELS Ca^{2+} entering the cytoplasm via L-type Ca^{2+} channels makes a direct contribution to the $[Ca^{2+}]_i$ transient. Since Ca^{2+} channels are regulated biochemically (56) and are time- and voltage-dependent, Ca^{2+} flux through them will vary with cellular conditions. Under conditions in which Ca^{2+} entry via Na/Ca exchange was negligibly small, and SR Ca^{2+} release had been abolished with ryanodine, the running integral (for 100 ms) of the Ca^{2+} current in rat ventricular cells was almost superimposable with the running integral of the fura-2 fluorescence change (24). It was calculated that Ca^{2+} entering as current could have increased total $[Ca^{2+}]_i$ by 5–10 μM and that fura-2 alone bound $\sim$100μM of Ca^{2+} in the first 25 ms after depolarization.

The conclusion from these studies and others is that the amount of Ca^{2+} entering via SL Ca^{2+} current is probably less than 10% of the total in guinea pig and rat. This is an important number, since this amount of Ca^{2+} must be extruded each cycle by the Na/Ca exchange (since SL Ca^{2+} ATPase activity is negligible). Recent studies on internally perfused cells are providing new quantitative information on this issue by permitting the reliable measurement of $[Ca^{2+}]_i$ transients attributable primarily to Ca^{2+} entry. Optimal conditions for this are those illustrated in Figure 4A, in which Na/Ca exchange, SR release, and SR uptake have been eliminated.

Na/Ca EXCHANGE   The role of Na/Ca exchange in the $[Ca^{2+}]_i$ transient during each cardiac cycle has been reviewed extensively (6, 55). Mullins (52) was the first to point out that an electrogenic Na/Ca exchange could both bring Ca^{2+} into the cell during the action potential, making a direct contribution to the $[Ca^{2+}]_i$ transient, and also extrude Ca^{2+} from the cell when $[Ca^{2+}]_i$ is high and during the resting period (diastole). These two roles of the exchanger are considered below.

Components of physiologic $[Ca^{2+}]_i$ transients attributable to Na/Ca exchange (direct contribution)   In evaluating the experimental data on this issue, two factors need special consideration, the chemical activity of intracellular Na^+ (a^i_{Na}), and the species of mammalian heart cell.

Intracellular Na^+ is critically important in determining Na/Ca exchanger activity because 3 Na^+ must bind; the concentration of Na^+ required for half-maximal activation in heart is 20 mM (45), within the physiologic range of $[Na^+]_i$, and there is a steep dependence of the reversal potential (E_{NaCa}) on $[Na^+]_i$ (20). Thus Ca^{2+} influx through the exchanger is steeply dependent on physiologic $[Na^+]_i$. In experiments in which internally perfused cells are used (many of those considered here) a^i_{Na} is presumed to be influenced by the $[Na^+]$ in the micropipette electrode. At mammalian temperatures and normal $[Na^+]_i$, a^i_{Na} is about 7 mM (19). This corresponds to $[Na^+]_i$ of 10 mM, on the assumption of an activity coefficient for Na^+ in the pipette filling solution of 0.7. The a^i_{Na} of ferret papillary muscle has been determined to be ~11 mM at 22°C–24°C (19), or $[Na^+]_i$ of 16 mM. Thus the $[Na^+]$ in the micropipette electrode must be 16 and 10 mM to produce physiological a^i_{Na} at room temperature and normal mammalian temperatures, respectively.

In rat ventricular cells studied at 35°C, $[Ca^{2+}]_i$ did not increase during 100 msec depolarizing steps to +100 mV (26). The authors concluded that Ca^{2+} entry via Na/Ca exchange, which would be expected at +100 mV, was insufficient to activate Ca^{2+} release from SR. In a recent review of Na/Ca exchange (31), it was concluded from this result (26) that "under physiological conditions, any entry of Ca into the cell via Na/Ca exchange, which is produced solely by depolarization, is insufficient to materially affect $[Ca^{2+}]_i$". However, in the work cited (26) $[Na^+]$ in the micropipette electrode was far lower, 3.75 mM in the form of Na-phosphocreatine, than required for physiologic conditions (as discussed above). Similar results were obtained from rat heart cells at room temperature (20°C–25°C) (24) with $[Na^+]$ in the micropipette of 4.5 mM, in the form of 0.9mM Na_5 fura-2. Thus the $[Na^+]_i$ used in both these studies (24, 26) was substantially lower than that required to produce physiologic levels inside the cell. Mitchell et al (50) observed a bell-shaped dependence on membrane potential of shortening in rat ventricular cells. In this case, a single-electrode voltage clamp was used, and the micropipette electrode contained no Na^+. Since perfusion of the cell is slow with this method compared to tight-seal recording with a low resistance micropipette electrode, $[Na^+]_i$ is presumed to have been maintained close to physiologic levels.

Components of physiologic $[Ca^{2+}]_i$ transients attributable to Na/Ca exchange have been observed in guinea pig ventricular cells. Barcenas-Ruiz & Wier (8) were the first to observe slowly rising $[Ca^{2+}]_i$ transients at positive membrane potentials (see record of depolarization to $+90$ mV, Figure 2). In contrast to the rapidly rising component (depolarization to $+10$ mV, Figure 2), and the tail transient, (on repolarization from $+90$ mV, Figure 2), this component of the $[Ca^{2+}]_i$ transient was resistant to SL Ca^{2+}-channel block (verapamil) and SR Ca^{2+}-release block (ryanodine). Such transients were later shown to have a nearly exponential dependence on membrane potential (7, 18), increased by elevation of $[Na^+]_i$ (monensin) (7), and blocked by Ni^{2+}, a putative blocker of Na/Ca exchange (18).

Isenberg & colleagues (44) examined the influence of the $[Na^+]$ in the pipette on the voltage-dependence of the indo-1 fluorescence transient in voltage-clamped guinea pig ventricular myocytes. The cells had been loaded with indo-1 via exposure to indo-1/AM so quantification of $[Ca^{2+}]_i$ transients was not attempted. Nevertheless, the studies demonstrate clearly that the absence of Na^+ in the pipette filling solution is associated with a bell-shaped voltage-dependence of the fluorescence transient. In guinea pig cells clamped with micropipette electrodes containing Na^+ at 10 mM, slowly rising fluorescence transients that were not reduced at positive membrane potentials were observed.

It is reported that Ca^{2+} influx via Na/Ca exchange is insufficient to activate contraction directly in rabbit ventricular muscle unless a^i_{Na} is elevated (16).

Beuckelmann & Wier (18), from their study of Na/Ca exchange in guinea pig cells, point out that of the quantities known to affect Na/Ca exchange, the two that change significantly during each cardiac cycle are $[Ca^{2+}]_i$ and membrane potential. Therefore, the Ca^{2+}-fluxes through the exchanger can only be understood quantitatively by considering the relationship between $[Ca^{2+}]_i$ and exchange current [which is approximately linear in the physiologic range of $[Ca^{2+}]_i$ (7, 12, 18] and the effects of membrane potential on the exchanger [see Hilgemann, (41) for thorough discussion of this].

Clearly, the direct contribution of Ca^{2+} influx via Na/Ca exchanger to the $[Ca^{2+}]_i$ transient during E-C coupling is species-and condition-(membrane potential, $[Ca^{2+}]_i$, a^i_{Na}) dependent. A substantive contribution during the normal action potential seems likely, in the species studied so far, only in the guinea pig.

Contribution of Na/Ca exchange to Ca²⁺ efflux   The experiment illustrated in Figure 4 shows clearly that, in the absence of Na/Ca exchange, the Ca^{2+}

that enters the cell via L-type Ca^{2+} channels can be extruded only extremely slowly. Yet in the steady-state, the exact amount of Ca^{2+} that enters the cell via the current must be extruded from the cell.

Bridge et al (23) have shown that when Ca^{2+} sequestration by SR is inhibited by caffeine, increasing [Na$^+$]$_o$ from 0 to 144 mM, which permits Na/Ca exchange, increases the rate of relaxation of guinea pig myocytes six to eightfold. As discussed above, rest decay of rapid cooling contractures (RCCs) is prevented by Na-free, Ca-free solutions during rest (D. Bers, J. Bridge, K. Spitzer, submitted). Hilgemann (41) concluded that the Na/Ca exchanger cannot extrude more than about 6 μmol/l cell calcium per cycle. This is in rough agreement with the estimates of the amount of Ca^{2+} entering via L-type Ca^{2+} channels. I conclude, therefore, that in the steady-state Na/Ca exchange extrudes all the Ca^{2+} that enters via SL Ca^{2+} channels. Na/Ca exchange contributes to the decline of the [Ca^{2+}]$_i$ transient, but as will be seen below, it is not the major determinant.

Sarcoplasmic Reticulum (SR)

From the foregoing it can be inferred that SR Ca^{2+} release will have the major role in supplying Ca^{2+} for the [Ca^{2+}]$_i$ transient, since under normal conditions Ca^{2+} influx via Na/Ca exchange and SL Ca^{2+} channels is far too small to account for the total change in Ca^{2+} in the cytoplasm. Previous reviewers also have concluded that in mammalian ventricular muscle Ca^{2+} released from SR dominates the [Ca^{2+}]$_i$ transient (21, 29, 37). It is also recognized that a spectrum exists in this respect, with rat having the most contribution from SR and rabbit having the least (32).

Recent studies (8, 17, 24, 26, 44) utilizing fluorescent Ca^{2+} indicators in voltage-clamped single cardiac cells have produced new information as well as more reliable quantitative information on the contribution of SR to [Ca^{2+}]$_i$ transients. In general, the following points of agreement have emerged: (a) the initial rapid increase in [Ca^{2+}]$_i$ elicited by depolarization into the physiologic range of membrane potential arises primarily from Ca^{2+} released from SR (e.g. Figure 2); (b) release of Ca^{2+} from SR has a bell-shaped dependence on membrane potential, declining to low levels at positive membrane potentials; and (c) Ca^{2+} can also be released from SR upon repolarization from positive membrane potentials (Figure 2; depolarization to +90 mV).

SR RELEASE

Initial rise in [Ca^{2+}]$_i$ on depolarization is Ca^{2+} released from SR   A result common to all the recent studies is that depolarization into the plateau range of the action potential (+10 mV) elicits a large, rapidly rising [Ca^{2+}]$_i$ transient. This initial, rapid increase in [Ca^{2+}]$_i$ elicited by depolarization has been attributed primarily to Ca^{2+} released from the SR. The essential evidence in support of this is that, in both guinea pig (8, 17) and rat (24), ryanodine reduces this initial rise in $[Ca^{2+}]_i$ by up to 90%. Ryanodine is now known to lock the SR Ca^{2+}-release channel in a subconducting state (53). This seems to result in a more rapid loss of Ca^{2+} from the SR (40, 63) and to interfere with the normal release of Ca^{2+} from the SR (48). Thus, depending on experimental conditions, the reduction of the $[Ca^{2+}]_i$ transient upon depolarization in the presence of ryanodine may arise either from depletion of Ca^{2+} in the SR or from interference with the release mechanism. In either case, however, the conclusion is valid that the initial rapid rise in the $[Ca^{2+}]_i$ transient upon depolarization results from Ca^{2+} released from the SR.

Voltage dependence of Ca^{2+} release from SR on depolarization   The use of single isolated cardiac cells and fluorescent Ca^{2+} indicators permits the voltage-dependence of the $[Ca^{2+}]_i$ transient to be studied more reliably than in the past. Prior to 1986, only one such study existed (70). The voltage-dependence of Ca^{2+} release from SR is expected to be of importance in distinguishing mechanisms of E-C coupling in mammalian cardiac muscle. If, as in skeletal muscle (57), Ca^{2+} release from SR does not decline at positive membrane potentials, then it is unlikely that Ca^{2+}-induced release of Ca^{2+} (32–36) has a major role in E-C coupling. Ideally, it is the rate of Ca^{2+} release from SR as a function of the membrane voltage that is required, but this quantity has not yet been calculated in heart muscle. Instead, in heart the voltage-dependence of the peak of the ryanodine-sensitive $[Ca^{2+}]_i$ transient has been observed (17, 24) as an indication of SR Ca^{2+} release.

At least five studies (8, 17, 24, 26, 44) have now shown that the peak of the $[Ca^{2+}]_i$ transient in guinea pig or rat heart cells has a bell-shaped dependence on membrane potential. In all cases, these results have been interpreted to mean that release of Ca^{2+} from cardiac SR declines at positive potentials, a result that is distinctly different from that in skeletal muscle (57). All these studies have also shown that the voltage-dependence of the peak $[Ca^{2+}]_i$ transient is shifted slightly to the left of that of L-type Ca^{2+} current (cf Figure 3B of (26); Figure 15A of (17); Figure 2C of (24)]. The significance of this finding in distinguishing possible mechanisms of E-C coupling is not yet clear.

Ca^{2+} release from SR on repolarization   Increases in $[Ca^{2+}]_i$ upon repolarization (Figure 2) have been observed in guinea pig ventricular cells (8, 17, 44) and in rat ventricular cells [24, 26]. Such $[Ca^{2+}]_i$ transients have been termed repolarization transients (24) or tail transients (8, 17). The latter term is the one that will be used here since it reflects the putative connection

between the [Ca^{2+}]$_i$ transient and the tail of Ca^{2+} current that can occur upon repolarization from positive membrane potentials. Tail transients almost certainly arise from Ca^{2+} released from SR, since they are abolished by ryanodine [8, 17, 24]. Since tail transients have never been observed in skeletal muscle and since their occurrence is not predicted by charge-coupled release mechanisms, as formulated to explain E-C coupling in skeletal muscle (49), their existence in heart muscle is potentially revealing of the mechanism of E-C coupling in heart muscle. In particular, their existence offers a unique opportunity to examine the relationship between Ca^{2+} current and Ca^{2+} release from the SR, in the absence of depolarization, per se. This relationship has been examined in detail (17) in order to test the obvious hypothesis (8) that the release of Ca^{2+} from SR that underlies the tail transient is triggered, via Ca^{2+}-induced release of Ca^{2+}, by the tail of Ca^{2+} current that can occur upon repolarization from positive potentials. Briefly, the study showed that the amplitude of the tail transient does not correlate simply with the amplitude of the Ca^{2+}-current tail. Ca^{2+}-current tails increase with increasingly negative repolarization voltage, but tail transients do not. Upon repolarization to very negative membrane potentials, however, the Ca^{2+} current deactivates so quickly that the amount of Ca^{2+} entering during the tail is strongly reduced; it was suggested that this could account for the reduction of the tail transient. Upon further examination, it was concluded that the theory that Ca^{2+}-induced release of Ca^{2+} accounted for tail transients could not be rejected. It may be significant that the release of Ca^{2+} from SR on repolarization can be as large as that on depolarization. In rat heart cells particularly (24, 26), the magnitude of tail transients upon repolarization can be similar to that elicited by depolarization.

Mechanism of Ca^{2+} release from SR   The data discussed above have been interpreted (17, 24, 44) to support Ca^{2+}-induced release of Ca^{2+} (32–36) as an important mechanism of normal E-C coupling. Nevertheless, several authors (17, 26) have noted that some results, particularly the fact that early repolarization abbreviates the [Ca^{2+}]$_i$ transient (17, 26), are difficult to reconcile with the theory of Ca^{2+}-induced release of Ca^{2+}. The possibility that voltage-dependent mechanisms, different from those formulated for E-C coupling in skeletal muscle, modify SR Ca^{2+} release in cardiac muscle cannot be excluded (17).

Mechanism of inactivation of Ca^{2+} release from SR   It seems highly probable that SR Ca^{2+} release does inactivate, since [Ca^{2+}]$_i$ transients, attributable mainly to Ca^{2+} released from SR, decline from their peak during maintained depolarization. In skeletal muscle, a component of inactivation of

SR Ca^{2+} release is Ca^{2+}-dependent (10, 60). In skinned cardiac cells, SR Ca^{2+} release can be inactivated by Ca^{2+} (35). In intact cardiac cells, the $[Ca^{2+}]_i$ transient on repolarization (tail transient) begins to appear as a function of preceding depolarizing pulse voltage, only as the $[Ca^{2+}]_i$ transient on depolarization begins to decline [(cf Figure 11 of (17)]. This observation is consistent with the idea that Ca^{2+} release from SR is inactivated during a large $[Ca^{2+}]_i$ transient on depolarization but, again, other plausible explanations have not yet been excluded. This is an important issue because Ca^{2+}-dependent inactivation of SR Ca^{2+} release is an important component of Ca^{2+} release from SR in skinned cardiac cells (35).

Finally, I note that it should be possible to calculate the SR Ca^{2+}-release flux from observations of $[Ca^{2+}]_i$ transients and Equation 2 once adequate empirical mathematical descriptions of the other terms are obtained. The approach will be similar to that employed for calculating SR Ca^{2+} release in skeletal muscle (60).

SR Ca^{2+} PUMP   The biochemical evidence, summarized recently by Carafoli (27), supports the concept that the Ca^{2+} ATPase of the SR (43) will have the dominant role in determining the decline of the $[Ca^{2+}]_i$ transient once release of Ca^{2+} is over. The Ca^{2+} ATPase has a high affinity for Ca^{2+}, (K_m of O.5 μM) and a high V_{max}, relative to that of SL Ca^{2+} ATPase, which makes it suitable for this role.

The majority of the available physiologic evidence also supports the idea that the SR Ca^{2+}-pumping ATPase is, under physiologic conditions, the primary determinant of the rate of fall of the Ca^{2+} transient. Beta-adrenergic activation speeds the decline of the aequorin signal in rat ventricular muscle (47). Epinephrine increases the rate of decline of the fluorescence transients in rat heart cells (24). The most probable explanation of these effects is the AMP-dependent phosphorylation of phospholamban (66). Caffeine diminishes and prolongs the $[Ca^{2+}]_i$ transient (51). It is now known that caffeine activates SR Ca^{2+}-release channels by interacting with them directly; it increases both the open time of the SR Ca^{2+}-release channel and the sensitivity of the channel to activation by Ca^{2+} (58). The assumption is often made that caffeine inhibits sequestration of Ca^{2+} by the SR. It is becoming clear that the mechanism by which it does so is simply to render ineffective the transport of Ca^{2+} by SR Ca^{2+}-ATPase by allowing the Ca^{2+} to move immediately out of the SR again.

Intracellular Ligands

Fabiato (32) has provided the most complete set of estimates of concentration and affinities of Ca^{2+}-binding substances (ligands) in mammalian ventricular cells. The time course of the Ca^{2+}-bound form of these ligands may be computed readily, by well-known methods, from the experimentally recorded [Ca^{2+}]$_i$ transient. The major conclusion from this computation (not shown) is that the concentration and affinity of ligands can have a profound influence on the amplitude and time course of the [Ca^{2+}]$_i$ transient. Accurate determination of the SR Ca^{2+}-release flux will require accurate estimation of the amount of Ca^{2+} bound to ligands on each cycle. Most estimates of the total [Ca^{2+}]$_i$ change are in the range of several hundred micromolar (24).

The affinity of troponin c for Ca^{2+} may be influenced by cross-bridge attachment. Evidence for this is the occurrence of a rapid change in [Ca^{2+}]$_i$, attributed to release of Ca^{2+} from troponin c, when either skinned (2) or intact (2, 4, 42) cardiac muscle is allowed to shorten. [Ca^{2+}]$_i$ transients in muscle contracting isometrically from short length have a prolonged time course compared to those in muscle contracting isometrically from long lengths (2, 42). Affinity for Ca^{2+} of all these ligands may be influenced by intracellular pH, and several studies have demonstrated the dramatic changes in [Ca^{2+}]$_i$ transients that occur when intracellular pH is changed. Some of these issues have been discussed in more detail recently by Allen & colleagues (3, 5).

[Ca^{2+}]$_i$ WAVES

Some investigations have provided evidence that under certain conditions [Ca^{2+}]$_i$ in mammalian cardiac cells can oscillate spontaneously (11, 69). The use of high-temporal resolution Ca^{2+} imaging (67) has shown conclusively that these [Ca^{2+}]$_i$ oscillations are actually propagated waves of Ca^{2+}. [Ca^{2+}]$_i$ waves are of interest because it should be possible to use their characteristics (origin, velocity, and spatial profile) to infer characteristics of certain cellular phenomena, such as Ca^{2+}-induced release of Ca^{2+} from SR.

Figure 3 illustrates the fluorescence ratio in a guinea pig ventricular myocyte that had been exposed to a Na$^+$-free solution (67). Upon exposure to this solution cells rapidly developed Ca-overload, as judged by the appearance of spontaneous wavelike contractions, even when their membrane potential was clamped at −80 mV. The [Ca^{2+}]$_i$ transients accompanying these contractions were captured by manually recording images upon seeing a spontaneous change in fluorescence. The fluorescence ratio images shown in Figure 3 were produced from single frames captured every other frame. Thus the images are separated in time by 67 msec, beginning at the left of the figure. Under Na$^+$-free conditions, [Ca^{2+}]$_i$ waves tend to be very broad, presumably reflecting the inability of Na/Ca exchange to reduce cytoplasmic [Ca^{2+}]$_i$.

SUMMARY

A quantitative reconstruction of $[Ca^{2+}]_i$ transients is the desired goal, but that goal has yet to be reached. It will be reached by solving Equation 2., once an adequate mathematical description of all its terms is obtained. If computed $[Ca^{2+}]_i$ transients match closely those recorded under many experimental conditions, then we can be confident that our understanding of the cellular processes that control $[Ca^{2+}]_i$ is correct.

The SL Ca^{2+} ATPase and the SL Ca^{2+} leak do not make an important contribution on a given beat. All the available data, physiologic and biochemical, indicate clearly that the Ca^{2+} fluxes via the SL Ca^{2+}-ATPase and SL Ca^{2+}-leak pathways are small in comparison to others. Over many beats, however, the fluxes through these pathways will contribute to loading of the SR with Ca^{2+}. In the abnormal case of resting cardiac muscle, $[Ca^{2+}]_i$ will be determined by the balance between Ca^{2+} influx via leak and Ca^{2+} efflux via Na/Ca exchange and SL Ca^{2+} ATPase.

There is an emerging consensus that the amount of Ca^{2+} entering via Na/Ca exchange during normal activity is small. This consensus derives from direct observation of changes in $[Ca^{2+}]_i$ attributable to Na/Ca exchange, from computations that utilize new quantitative data on the current-voltage relation of the exchanger and on the quantitative relationship of exchanger current to $[Ca^{2+}]_i$. Clearly, the efflux of Ca^{2+} via Na/Ca exchange on each beat is significant. From theory and the fact that SL Ca^{2+} pumping is small, the efflux of Ca^{2+} via the exchanger must equal the Ca^{2+} influx through SL Ca^{2+} channels, but experimental studies have not yet verified this quantitatively.

All the studies, recent and older, indicate that the $[Ca^{2+}]_i$ transient in all mammalian species is dominated by Ca^{2+} released from SR. Even in the rat, widely believed to be the species most dependent on SR, the Ca^{2+} current contributes measurable Ca^{2+} (24). Provided that the SR is not depleted by rest, it is the major cellular entity that determines the $[Ca^{2+}]_i$ transient in mammalian ventricular tissue on a given beat. Quantitative knowledge of the flux of Ca^{2+} from it, required for evaluating theories of excitation-contraction coupling, still awaits determination.

Literature Cited

1. Allen, D. G., Kentish, J. C. 1988. Calcium concentration in the myoplasm of skinned ferret ventricular muscle following changes in muscle length. *J. Physiol.* 407:489–503
2. Allen, D. G., Kurihara, S. 1982. The effects of muscle length on intracellular calcium transients in mammalian cardiac muscle. *J. Physiol.* 327:79–94
3. Allen, D. G., Lee, J. A., Smith, G. L.

1989. The consequences of simulated ischaemia on intracellular Ca^{2+} and tension in isolated ventricular muscle. *J. Physiol.* 410:297–323
4. Allen, D. G., Nichols, C. G., Smith, G. L. 1988. The effects of changes in muscle length during diastole on the calcium transient in ferret ventricular muscle. *J. Physiol.* 406:359–70
5. Allen, D. G., Orchard, C. H. 1983. The

effects of changes of pH on intracellular calcium transients in mammaliam cardiac muscle. *J. Physiol.* 335:555–67

6. Allen, T. J. A., Noble, D., Reuter, H. 1989. *Sodium-Calcium Exchange.* Oxford: Oxford Press. In press

7. Barcenas-Ruiz, L., Beuckelmann, D. J., Wier, W. G. 1987. Sodium/calcium exchange in heart: membrane currents and changes in [Ca^{2+}]$_i$. *Science* 238:1720–22

8. Barcenas-Ruiz, L., Wier, W. G. 1987. Voltage dependence of intracellular [Ca^{2+}] transients in guinea pig ventricular myocytes. *Circ. Res.* 61:148–54

9. Barry, W. H., Rasmussen, C. A. F. Jr., Ishida, H., Bridge, J. H. B. 1986. External Na-independent Ca extrusion in cultured ventricular cells. *J. Gen. Physiol.* 88(3):393–411

10. Baylor, S. M., Hollingworth, S. 1988. Fura-2 calcium transients in frog skeletal muscle fibers. *J. Physiol.* 402:151–92

11. Berlin, J. R., Cannell, M. B., Lederer, W. J. 1989. Cellular origins of the transient inward current, I$_{TI}$, in cardiac myocytes: Role of fluctuations and waves of elevated intracellular calcium. *Circ. Res.* 65:115–26

12. Berlin, J. R., Hume, J. R., Lederer, W. J. 1988. [Ca^{2+}]$_i$-activated 'creep' currents in guinea-pig ventricular myocytes. *J. Physiol.* 407:128P (Abstr.)

13. Bers, D. M. 1989. SR Ca loading in cardiac muscle preparations based on rapid-cooling contractures. *Am. J. Physiol.* 256:C109–20

14. Bers, D. M., Bridge, J. H. B. 1989. Relaxation of rabbit ventricular muscle by Na-Ca exchange and sarcoplasmic reticulum Ca-pump: ryanodine and voltage sensitivity. *Circ. Res.* 65:334–42

15. Bers, D. M., Bridge, J. H. B., Spitzer, K. W. 1988. Intracellular [Ca] changes during rapid cooling contractures (RCCs) in isolated guinea-pig ventricular myocytes. *J. Physiol.* 407:133P (Abstr.)

16. Bers, D. M., Christensen, D. M., Nguyen, T. X. 1988. Can Ca entry via Na-Ca exchange directly activate cardiac muscle contraction? *J. Mol. Cell Cardiol.* 20:405–14

17. Beuckelmann, D. J., Wier, W. G. 1988. Mechanism of release of calcium from sarcoplasmic reticulum of guinea-pig cardiac cells. *J. Physiol.* 405:233–55

18. Beuckelmann, D. J., Wier, W. G. 1989. Sodium-calcium exchange in guinea-pig cardiac cells: exchange current and changes in intracellular Ca^{2+}. *J. Physiol.* 414:499–520

19. Blatter, L. A., McGuigan, J. A., Reverdin, E. C. 1986. Sodium/calcium exchange and calcium buffering in mammalian ventricular muscle. *Jpn. Heart J. Suppl.* 27:93–107

20. Blaustein, M. P. 1988. Sodium/calcium exchange and the control of contractility in cardiac muscle and vascular smooth muscle. *J. Cardiovasc. Pharmacol.* 12(5):S56–68 (Suppl.)

21. Blinks, J. R. 1986. See Ref. 37, pp. 671–701

22. Blinks, J. R., Wier, W. G., Hess, P., Prendergast, F. G. 1982. Measurement of Ca^{2+} concentration in living cells. *Prog. Biophys. Mol. Biol.* 40:1–114

23. Bridge, J. H. B., Spitzer, K. W., Ershler, P. R. 1988. Relaxation of isolated ventricular cardiomyocytes by a voltage-dependent process. *Science* 241:823–25

24. Callewaert, G., Cleemann, L., Morad, M. 1988. Epinephrine enhances Ca^{2+} current-regulated Ca^{2+} release and Ca^{2+} reuptake in rat ventricular myocytes. *Proc. Natl. Acad. Sci. USA* 85:2009–13

25. Cannell, M. B., Berlin, J. R., Lederer, W. J. 1987. *Cell Calcium and Control of Membrane Transport,* pp. 201–14. New York: Rockefeller Univ.

26. Cannell, M. B., Berlin, J. R., Lederer, W. J. 1987. Effect of membrane potential changes on the calcium transient in single rat cardiac muscle cells. *Science* 238:1419–23

27. Carafoli, E. 1988. Membrane transport of calcium: An Overview. *Methods Enzymol.* 157:3–11

28. Carafoli, W., Longoni, S. 1987. The plasma membrane in the control of the signaling function of calcium. In *Cell Calcium and Membrane Transport,* ed., pp. 21–29. New York: Rockefeller Univ.

29. Chapman, R. A. 1983. Control of cardiac contractility at the cellular level. *Am. J. Physiol.* 245:H535–52

30. Crank, J. 1975. *The Mathematics of Diffusion,* p. 3. Oxford: Clarendon

31. Eisner, D. A., Lederer, W. J. 1989. The electrogenic sodium-calcium exchange. In *Sodium-Calcium Exchange,* ed. T. H. A. Allen, D. Noble, H. Reuter, pp. 178–207. Oxford: Oxford Univ. Press

32. Fabiato, A. 1982. Calcium release in skinned cardiac cells: variations with species, tissues, and development. *Fed. Proc.* 41:2238–44

33. Fabiato, A. 1983. Calcium-induced release of calcium from the cardiac sarcoplasmic reticulum. *Am. J. Physiol.* 245:C1–14

34. Fabiato, A. 1985. Rapid ionic modification during the aequorin-detected cal-

cium transient in a skinned canine cardiac purkinje cell. *J. Gen. Physiol.* 85(2):189–246

35. Fabiato, A. 1985. Time and calcium dependence of activation and inactivation of calcium-induced release of calcium from the sarcoplasmic reticulum of a skinned canine cardiac purkinje cell. *J. Gen. Physiol.* 85(2):247–90

36. Fabiato, A. 1985. Simulated calcium current can both cause calcium loading in and trigger calcium release from the sarcoplasmic reticulum of a skinned canine cardiac purkinje cell. *J. Gen. Physiol.* 85(2):291–320

37. Fozzard, H. A. ed. 1986. *The Heart and Cardiovascular System.* New York: Raven

38. Grynkiewicz, G., Poenie, M., Tsien, R. W. 1985. A new generation of Ca^{2+} indicators with greatly improved fluorescence properties. *J. Biol. Chem.* 260(6):3440–50

39. Gunter, T. E., Restrepo, D., Gunter, K. K. 1988. Conversion of esterified fura-2 and indo-1 to Ca^{2+}-sensitive forms by mitochondria. *Am. J. Physiol.* 255: C340–10

40. Hansford, R. G., Lakatta, E. G. 1987. Ryanodine releases calcium from sarcoplasmic reticulum in calcium-tolerant rat cardiac myocytes. *J. Physiol.* 390:453–67

41. Hilgemann, D. W. 1989. "Best estimates" of physiological sodium-calcium exchange function: calcium conservation and the cardiac electrical cycle. In *Cardiac Electrophysiology: From Cell to Bedside,* ed. D. Zipes, J. Jalife, Philadelphia: Saunders

42. Housmans, P. K., Lee, N. K., Blinks, J. R. 1983. Active shortening retards the decline of the intracellular calcium transient in mammalian heart muscle. *Science* 221:159–61

43. Inesi, G. 1985. Mechanism of calcium transport. *Annu. Rev. Physiol.* 47:573–601

44. Isenberg, G., Spurgeon, H., Talo, A., Stern, M., Capogrossi, M., Lakatta, E. 1988. The voltage dependence of the myoplasmic calcium transient in guinea pig ventricular myocytes is modulated by sodium loading. In *Biology of Isolated Adult Cardiac Myocytes,* ed. W. A. Clark, R. S. Decker, T. K. Borg, pp. 354–57. Stowe: Elsevier Science

45. Kimura, J., Miyamae, S., Noma, A. 1987. Identification of sodium-calcium exchange current in single ventricular cells of guinea-pig. *J. Physiol.* 384:199–222

46. Konishi, M., Olson, A., Hollingworth, S., Baylor, S. M. 1988. Myoplasmic binding of Fura-2 investigated by steady-state fluorescence and absorbance measurements. *Biophys. J.* 54: 1089–1104

47. Kurihara, S., Konishi, M. 1987. Effects of β-adrenoceptor stimulation on intracellular Ca transients and tension in rat ventricular muscle. *Pflügers Arch.* 490:427–37

48. Marban, E., Wier, W. G. 1985. Ryanodine as a tool to determine the contributions of calcium entry and calcium release to the calcium transient and contraction of cardiac purkinje fibers. *Circ. Res.* 56:133–38

49. Miledi, R., Parker, I., Zhu, P. H. 1983. Calcium transients studied under voltage-clamp control in frog twitch muscle fibres. *J. Physiol.* 340:649–80

50. Mitchell, M. R., Powell, T., Terrar, D. A., Twist, V. W. 1987. Electrical activity and contraction in cells isolated from rat and guinea-pig ventricular muscle: a comparative study. *J. Physiol.* 391:527–44

51. Morgan, J. P., Blinks, J. R. 1982. Intracellular Ca^{2+} transients in the cat papillary muscle. *Can. J. Physiol. Pharmacol.* 60(4):524–28

52. Mullins, L. J. 1979. The generation of electric currents in cardiac fibers by Na/Ca exchange. *Am. J. Physiol.* 236: C103–10

53. Nagasaki, K., Fleischer, S. 1988. Ryanodine sensitivity of the calcium release channel of sarcoplasmic reticulum. *Cell Calcium* 9:1–7

54. Noda, M., Shepherd, N., Gadsby, D. C. 1988. Activation by $Ca[Ca^{2+}]_i$, and block by 3'-4'-dichlorobenzamil, of outward Na/Ca exchange current in guinea-pig ventricular myocytes. *Biophys. J.* 53:342a (Abstr.)

55. Reeves, J. P. 1989. Sodium-calcium exchange. In *Intracellular Calcium Regulation,* ed. F. Bronner. New York: Liss. In press

56. Reuter, H., Porzig, H., Kokubun, S., Prod'hom, B. 1988. Calcium channels in the heart. *Ann. NY Acad. Sci.* 522:16–24

57. Rios, E., Brum, G. 1987. Involvement of dihydropyridine receptors in excitation-contraction coupling in skeletal muscle. *Nature* 325:717–20

58. Rousseau, E., LaDine, J., Liu, Q.-Y., Meissner, G. 1988. Activation of the Ca^{2+} release channel of skeletal muscle sarcoplasmic reticulum by caffeine and related compounds. *Arch. Biochem. Biophys.* 267(1):75–86

59. Scanlon, M., Williams, D. A., Fay, F. S. 1987. A Ca^{2+}-insensitive form of Fura-2 associated with polymorphonuclear leukocytes. *J. Biol. Chem.* 262 (13):6308–12

60. Schneider, M. F., Simon, B. J. 1988. Inactivation of calcium release from the sarcoplasmic reticulum in frog skeletal muscle. *J. Physiol.* 405:727–45

61. Sheu, S.-S., Blaustein, M. P. 1986. See Ref. 37, pp. 509–35

62. Sheu, S.-S., Fozzard, H. A. 1982. Transmembrane Na^+ and Ca^{2+} electrochemical gradients in cardiac muscle and their relationship to force development. *J. Gen. Physiol.* 80:325–51

63. Silverman, H. S., Spurgeon, H. A., Capogrossi, M. C., Lakatta, E. G. 1988. Ryanodine depletes sarcoplasmic reticulum Ca^{2+} in single rat cardiac myocytes. *J. Mol. Cell Cardiol.* 20 (Suppl. III):S17 (Abstr.)

64. Sipido, K., Wier, W. G. 1989. $[Ca]_i$ transients in voltage clamped guinea pig ventricular myocytes in the presence of caffeine and the absence of sodium. *J. Physiol. (Abstr.)* In press

65. Smith, S. J., Augustine, G. J. 1988. Calcium ions, active zones and synaptic transmitter release. *Trends Neurosci.* 11(10):458–64

66. Tada, M., Katz, A. M. 1982. Phosphorylation of the sarcoplasmic reticulum and sarcolemma. *Annu. Rev. Physiol.* 44:401–23

67. Takamatsu, T., Wier, W. G. 1989. High temporal resolution video imaging of intracellular calcium. *Cell Calcium.* In press

68. Wier, W. G., Beuckelmann, D. J., Barcenas-Ruiz, L. 1989. $[Ca^{2+}]_i$ in single isolated cardiac cells: a review of recent results obtained with digital imaging microscopy and fura-2. *Can. J. Physiol. Pharmacol.* 66:1224–31

69. Wier, W. G., Cannell, M. B., Berlin, J. R., Marban, E., Lederer, W. J. 1987. Cellular and subcellular heterogeneity of $[Ca^{2+}]_i$ in single heart cells revealed by Fura-2. *Science* 235:325–28

70. Wier, W. G., Isenberg, G. 1982. Intracellular $[Ca^{2+}]$ transients in voltage clamped cardiac purkinje fibers. *Pflügers Arch.* 392:284–90

71. Wier, W. G., Yue, D. T. 1986. Intracellular calcium transients underlying the short-term force-interval relationship in ferret ventricular myocardium. *J. Physiol.* 376:507–30

Annu. Rev. Physiol. 1990. 52:487–504

FREE RADICALS AND THEIR INVOLVEMENT DURING LONG-TERM MYOCARDIAL ISCHEMIA AND REPERFUSION

J. M. Downey

Department of Physiology, University of South Alabama, Mobile, Alabama 36688

KEY WORDS: superoxide, dismutase, allopurinol, tetrazolium, collateral flow, reperfusion injury

INTRODUCTION

Much evidence has accumulated implicating cytotoxic free radicals as an underlying etiology of many clinical disorders. Prominent among these disorders has been ischemic heart disease (25, 57). The bulk of the incriminating evidence has been based on the ability of antioxidants to reduce injury in animal models of myocardial ischemia. Unfortunately, quantifying myocardial injury is still an imprecise science and, as a result, the performance of the various antioxidant interventions has varied widely in the different models. Because of the discrepant data, it has been impossible to determine the exact role that free radicals play in the ischemic heart or what long-term clinical benefit might be derived from an antioxidant intervention in the ischemic patient. Although it is well-established that some free radicals are produced on reperfusion of the ischemic heart, it is the magnitude of the injury that the radicals produce that remains in question. Although the in vitro work has established a theoretical framework for the free radical hypothesis, in the final analysis this question will only be answered by measuring the protection derived in a whole animal by an antioxidant intervention.

Unfortunately, the gaps in our understanding of any new theory have to be

0066-4278/90/0315-0487$02.00

filled with conjecture. In such a process it is often easy to lose sight of where fact ends and theory begins. In the following pages I will discuss the free radical hypothesis for ischemia/reperfusion injury in the heart and point out the critical pieces that are still missing from this puzzle. I will examine the limitations in the various animal models that are currently being used to address the above question and try to determine why the success of many of the antioxidants seems to be so model dependent. Finally, I will review the experience to date with the various trials to see if the recent wave of enthusiasm concerning the free radical hypothesis is warranted.

The Nature of Ischemic Injury

Three levels of ischemic cardiac injury are currently recognized, and all three are proposed to involve, at least in part, a free radical mechanism. The first detectable level of injury is the generation of reperfusion arrhythmias. Reperfusion, after an ischemic period of only several min, can result in ventricular tachycardia or fibrillation (4). Secondly, increasing the length of the ischemic period to between 5 and 15 min will result in a prolonged deficit in contractility following reperfusion. This state is often referred to as the stunned myocardium. All of the ischemic myocytes are still viable, and the heart will completely recover its function but such recovery may require several days (5, 20, 72). Finally, when the ischemic period is extended to 20 min or longer, some of the heart cells will be irreversibly injured and become infarcted (76). The greater the depth and duration of the ischemic insult, the more widespread the cell death. It is the latter form of injury, infarction, which has attracted the greatest attention from the clinical community. Because infarcted tissue is not contractile, pump function of the heart is greatly diminished in these patients, thus contributing to mortality and morbidity. Infarcted tissue is not regenerated and any deficit in contractile function caused by infarction will be permanent. In the early seventies it was proposed that one could intervene early after the onset of ischemia and promote survival of tissue that would otherwise have died (52). Such an intervention would have the effect of limiting the amount of infarction that, in turn, would preserve pump function. The early attempts at identifying such an intervention were primarily directed at improving energy balance in non-reperfused myocardium. Beta blockers (52), hyaluronidase (53), or glucose-insulin-potassium (GIK) (54) were typical examples of intervention agents. Unfortunately, none of those agents were ever convincingly shown to be capable of limiting infarct size in the animal models and interest in them has waned.

In the eighties it became clear that restoration of blood flow to the ischemic zone was a prerequisite to any tissue salvage, and several strategies were devised for effecting early reperfusion of the ischemic heart. Those strategies included emergency angioplasty and the use of thrombolytic agents. Clinical trials confirmed that both mortality and myocardial pump function were improved by early reperfusion (27, 86). Today few would doubt that the benefit was derived from infarct size reduction (10, 15), although technical limitations still prevent direct measurement of infarct size in man.

Reperfusion: Friend or Foe

Along with the obvious beneficial effects of reperfusion comes the possibility of reperfusion induced injury. In the seventies, Hearse & colleagues demonstrated that the reintroduction of oxygen to a hypoxic heart was accompanied by a rapid and profound disruption of the tissue as assessed by both release of cytosolic enzymes (33) and ultrastructure damage (34). Apparently some component of reoxygenation was responsible for the injury. Among the several possible explanations considered was the release of oxygen-derived free radicals (32). Several investigators subsequently found that a variety of free radical scavengers (antioxidants) could reduce the injury in the hypoxic heart model, which argued in favor of a free radical mechanism (30, 31, 58, 62). It should be noted, however, that not all investigators found the antioxidants to be protective in this model (35, 45).

The appearance of injury upon reoxygenation is not unique to the hypoxic heart preparation. Reperfusion of ischemic tissue also triggers a similar abrupt appearance of tissue disruption (8, 39, 41). It is currently a matter of intense debate as to whether the ischemic tissue is actually injured by reperfusion per se, or whether reperfusion is simply causing cells, killed by the ischemia, to suddenly disgorge their contents, perhaps through an osmotic effect (35, 40). Unfortunately, proof of reperfusion injury has been elusive because the only available test for viability of a myocyte in the ischemic phase is to observe whether it recovers on reperfusion, a test that itself would invoke the reperfusion injury. Proof of reperfusion injury will require either a complete understanding of all of the cellular events occurring in ischemia-reperfusion, an event not likely to occur in the near future, or the demonstration that some intervention administered only at the reperfusion period can promote cell survival. Reperfusion injury may prove to be real but may involve a mechanism unrelated to free radicals such as sodium-mediated calcium entry (29).

What are Free Radicals and Where Do They Come From?

Free radicals are compounds that have unpaired electrons in their outer shell. This unpaired state makes them very unstable and prone to react with other molecules to either gain or lose an electron. Although many compounds can exist as a radical species, most of the recent concern has been on the oxygen-derived free radicals, the superoxide anion and the hydroxy radical. Often included in this list is hydrogen peroxide, which although technically not a radical, is the primary precursor for the production of the hydroxyl radical.

Recent studies with spin-trap probes convincingly demonstrate that at least some free radicals are generated in the reperfused heart (3, 6, 26, 91, 92). Two questions must be asked, however: (a) Is there sufficient radical produced to actually injure the heart, and (b) Where are the radicals generated? The first question was recently addressed by Mitchell & colleagues (59). They examined glutathione in reperfused hearts and found that the reduced form, GSH, never approached depletion. They concluded that the oxidant stress at reperfusion was within the limits that endogenous scavengers could handle. As for the latter question, several sources for the oxyradicals in the reperfused myocyte have been proposed. One such source is xanthine oxidase (11, 57). Hypoxanthine released from the ischemic heart is oxidized by xanthine oxidase upon reperfusion, making both superoxide and hydrogen peroxide. The xanthine oxidase system is a highly mobilizable radical source where both purine and enzyme will be in place and active after occlusions as short as 5 min. Free radicals from this source seem to account almost fully for early reperfusion arrhythmias seen in the rat (51) as well as stunning in the dog (13).

Other sources or radicals could include oxidation of catecholamines, either through autoxidation (43), or enzymatic oxidation. Prostaglandin pathways also can generate radicals (50) and certainly are active during ischemia/reperfusion. Mitochondria have long been suspected of being a source of radical within the reperfused myocyte. Ischemia may induce a defect in the mitochondria to produce excess radical (82), or perhaps the loss of endogenous antioxidants during ischemia may leave the myocyte unable to cope with the normal mitochondrial leak of radical (21, 82).

Currently many investigators are proposing leukocytes as the source of free radical in the reperfused heart. Leukocytes, when activated, can generate, oxyradicals as part of their bacteriocidal mechanism via their NADPH oxidase pathway. It has been proposed that early after the onset of ischemia, leukocytes enter the ischemic tissue and attack viable myocytes (83) primarily through the release of radicals. There is no dispute that leukocytes concentrate in infarcted myocardium. The only question is, are leukocytes attacking viable cells in the reperfused tissue? Leukocytes are known to serve a role in scar healing by clearing the debris from tissue and their presence may be totally appropriate. Many doubt that leukocytes can be in place early enough to account for injury incurred at the time of reperfusion, although they could contribute to injury in the hours following reperfusion. Another problem with the leukocyte theory is that free radical-mediated injury has been shown to occur in many leukocyte free systems.

Measurement of Infarct Size in an Animal Model

The traditional approach to testing an agent's ability to limit necrosis has been to expose a heart to a standard ischemic insult and measure the resulting infarct size in both the presence and the absence of the agent. The problem lies both in achieving a standard insult and in measuring the infarct size. Consider the latter problem first. Infarction is a dynamic process with cells making the transition from living to dead in stages. Distinct changes in the myocyte's ultrastructure, with sarcolemmal defects and mitochondrial swelling with dense bodies, can be seen within an hr of coronary occlusion (38, 79). Under the light microscope, however, that tissue may appear perfectly normal. After 24 hr of occlusion, coagulation necrosis can be seen with the light microscope. In addition, there is often a heavy infiltration with leukocytes and petechial hemorrhages may be present. The exact borders where dead tissue meets living may still be indistinct, however.

Because histological evaluation of infarct size is tedious and requires that at least a day, and preferably three be included between the onset of ischemia and the evaluation, most investigators have sought an alternative that could be employed in a non-recovery type of animal model. The first of these was ST segment mapping (52). Unfortunately a large number of drugs were tested with this index before the validity of the index itself was carefully scrutinized and found to be an unreliable indicator of infarct size (36).

TETRAZOLIUM STAINING   Tetrazolium (TTC) staining soon emerged as the method to replace ST segment analysis. Dehydrogenase enzymes and the cofactor NADH react with TTC salts in living tissue to produce a formazan pigment that is intensely colored (64). Since enzyme and especially cofactor (49) are lost from the heart cells early after infarction, it was believed that the stain specifically differentiated living from dead tissue. In models of permanent occlusion, a coronary artery was typically occluded for 6 hr, the heart removed, sectioned and the slices incubated in TTC. While some reports found that this protocol accurately differentiated living from dead tissue (22, 68), others reported that some necrotic tissue still retained the ability to react with the stain at the six hr mark (19). More importantly, it was found that early evaluation of at least one drug in this model gave misleading results because infarct size limitation found six hr after occlusion was no longer apparent when the evaluation was performed a full 24 hr after occlusion (12).

When the focus of research shifted from permanent occlusion models to reperfusion, it was noted that reperfusion caused a much more rapid expression of cell death including the loss of TTC stainability (80). It has generally been found that TTC staining several hours after reperfusion yields essentially the same infarct size as seen by histology several days after reperfusion (37).

Based on those observations, TTC staining has become the method of choice for infarct size studies in this decade. Unfortunately, most investigators have relied entirely on the TTC measurements rather than instituting follow-up studies to see if the protection was reflected in either the mechanical function of the heart or the histology. This may have been a serious shortcoming, since a recent observation from this laboratory suggests that even in the setting of reperfusion, TTC may be prone to artifacts. Figure 1 shows that infarct size by histology was much larger than that by TTC following superoxide dismutase (SOD) treatment in rabbits (17). Thus while early evaluation with TTC reveals the ultimate infarct size in an untreated heart, drugs may interfere with that relationship. Since any intervention that actually limits infarct size should give a positive TTC result, it would seem that TTC still serves as an important screen for cardioprotective agents; yet follow-up tests such as histological evaluation must be performed to test for false positives. Those agents that fail to limit infarct size in an early TTC evaluation can probably be considered inactive at that point.

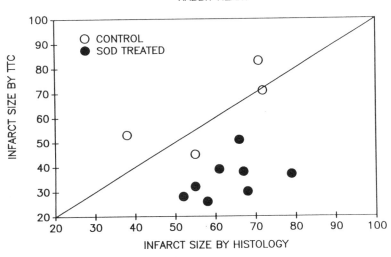

Figure 1 Rabbit hearts treated with SOD were analyzed by both histology and tetrazolium (TTC). Similar values were obtained by both methods in the untreated animals *(open circles)*. In the SOD-treated animals, however, infarcts were much smaller by TTC than by histology. It was concluded that SOD caused much dead tissue to retain the ability to react with tetrazolium. How many other agents possess the ability to cause a false positive result with TTC is not known at present (See reference 2).

Standardizing the Ischemic Insult

A second problem that has plagued investigators has been that of administering a standard ischemic insult. Dog hearts are quite variable in terms of their infarct size following a coronary occlusion (61). That variability both reduces the sensitivity of the model and increased the possibility of spurious conclusions. Reimer & Jennings, (75) studying the dog model, found that infarcts begin at the subendocardium and progress toward the subepicardium as the duration of ischemia increases. While the lateral border of the infarct was superimposed on the lateral boundary of the perfusion field, the transmural involvement was determined by two factors: the duration of ischemia, and the level of collateral flow. Figure 2 reveals that naturally occurring collateral flow significantly contributes to ischemic cell viability in both permanently occluded and reperfused dog hearts. Another feature of the dog heart is the wide variation of collateral flow from dog to dog. Figure 2 reveals that collateral flow may range from less than 5 to as high as 80% of the preocclusion value. The 20 to 1 range makes it virtually impossible to achieve a normal distribution of collateral flows with ten or less animals in a group. Thus the investigator can not assume that differences in collateral flow between groups will average themselves out, nor are the standard parametric tests for significance appropriate when a normal distribution has not been achieved. Most studies performed in the early eighties, including many from the author's laboratory, did not measure collateral flow and only expressed infarct size as a percentage of the field of the occluded artery. It is likely that many of those early studies were corrupted by unaccounted differences in collateral flow between the groups, especially where there was considerable overlap of data between the two groups. The best way to avoid a collateral flow artifact is to use an analysis of variance on the infarct sizes with collateral flow (measured by microspheres) as a covariate.

Unfortunately collateral flow does not account for all of the variability between animals either. In the rabbit, a species that has only a sparse native collateral circulation in its heart (56), collateral flow is too low to influence viability, but there is still unexplained variability in infarct size. We find that a 45 min occlusion will cause an average of 60% of the risk region to infarct, but with a standard deviation of $\pm 12\%$. This unaccountable variability still limits the resolution of the method.

ANTIOXIDANT INTERVENTIONS   The design of anti-free radical interventions has obviously been hampered by our lack of understanding as to which radical species mediates the injury or what is the radical source. One approach has been to employ a scavenger against one of the radical species. A scavenger removes free radicals directly and does not discriminate as to the source of the radical. Superoxide dismutase scavenges superoxide by dis-

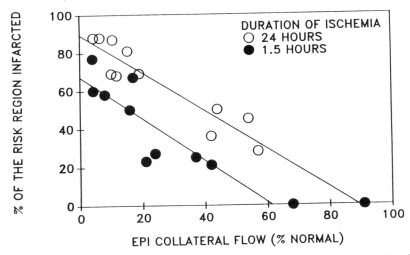

Figure 2 The extent of infarction of the ischemic zone (risk region) is plotted against collateral flow for both permanently occluded *(open circles)* and reperfused hearts *(solid circles)*. Note that infarct size is inversely related to collateral flow and that early reperfusion tends to shift that relationship down in a parallel fashion. Note the wide range of collateral flows seen in the dog population and the variability in infarct size it introduces. A cardioprotective drug could also cause a downward shift of the relationship. Source: unpublished data from the author's laboratory.

mutating it to oxygen and hydrogen peroxide. Catalase, reduced glutathione and glutathione peroxidase similarly scavenge hydrogen peroxide. The hydroxyl radical is the most difficult to scavenge. Because of its high reactivity, its probability of encountering a molecule other than the scavenger is high and the efficiency of a scavenger like DMSO or dimethylthiourea (DMTU) (23) to remove hydroxyl radical is thought to be limited at best. Therefore the strategy has been to try to eliminate the hydroxyl radical's precursors, hydrogen peroxide and superoxide. To be effective, the scavenger must get to the appropriate site of either production and/or attack, which may be inside the myocyte or in a cleft between a leukocyte and the sarcolemma. Obviously macromolecules like SOD and catalase may have a problem reaching such a site. The non-enzymatic scavengers are more adept at reaching intracellular sites because of their low molecular weights, but since scavenging consumes them they may be prematurely exhausted.

The second approach has been to try to intercept one of the above pathways at a key point. Examples of these interceptors include xanthine oxidase inhibitors or anti-leukocyte agents. The remainder of this review will summarize the available data on the performance of these antioxidants in models of experimental myocardial infarction. Choosing an antioxidant is further complicated by a total lack of agreement as to which free radical species is actually mediating the damage. While some reports implicate superoxide (11, 89), others implicate hydrogen peroxide (62), and still others implicate the hydroxyl radical (42).

SUPEROXIDE DISMUTASE (SOD) AND CATALASE   These two enzymes are the most widely studied of all of the antioxidant species. Jolly et al (44) were the first to employ them in an infarct size trial. They used open chest dogs, occluded a coronary branch for 90 min and then reperfused for 24 hr. Combined SOD and catalase were infused over a two hr period. Infarct size, which was expressed as a fraction of the region at risk, was smaller in groups that received the drug at the time of reperfusion over those that either did not receive drug or received it only 40 min after reperfusion. Shortly thereafter, Chambers et al (11) reported a positive effect in open chest, nephrectomized dogs receiving SOD only. The observation that SOD alone reduced infarct size in the dog model was confirmed by Werns et al (89). Finally SOD plus catalase was reported to limit infarct size in a rabbit (16) and a porcine model (66) of ischemia/reperfusion. TTC staining 24 hr or less following reperfusion was the end point for all of these studies and, unfortunately, no measurement of collateral flow was made in either of the dog studies.

Not all studies with these agents have been positive. Uraizee et al (87) found that the SOD plus catalase mixture did not affect infarct size in their model where the coronary artery was reperfused for four days; infarcts were sized by histology and analyzed according to their collateral flow. These authors ascribed their discrepant data to the refined methodology, particularly the attention to collateral flow. When critics argued that the 40 min of occlusion that Uraizee et al (87) employed may have been too short to evoke a free radical burst, the same laboratory repeated the study using a 90 min occlusion period (78). Again, no effect on infarct size was seen. In a similar study Nejima et al (67) also failed to demonstrate protection with SOD alone. Interestingly, they also used histology as the end point and included collateral flow in their analysis.

To add to the confusion, it must be mentioned that some studies using TTC as the end point have also failed to show protection. Patel at al (70) used SOD alone at two doses, 5mg/kg and 15mg/kg, and examined infarct size following 48 hr of reperfusion using TTC. Collateral flow was also incorporated in the analysis and again no effect on infarct size was seen. They repeated the study with only six hr of reperfusion and again could find no protection. Similarly, Klein et al (48) using the pig and Gallagher et al (24) using the dog have reported negative studies.

MANY EARLY SOD STUDIES HAVE BEEN CORRUPTED BY THEIR FAILURE TO MEASURE COLLATERAL FLOW   It is not fully understood why the early positive studies stand in such contrast to the latter negative studies but several explanations appear likely. One explanation suggests that the erroneous result might have resulted from the failure to take collateral flow into account in the first dog studies. To date there is only one positive study with the native SOD enzyme that incorporated collateral flow into the analysis and that is the study by Ambrosio et al (2). Human recombinant enzyme was administered just prior to reperfusion, and infarcts were examined 48 hr post reperfusion. Although there were only eight animals in each group, which reduces the statistical power of the study, the collateral flow analysis suggested that only animals with low collateral flow benefit from the SOD. Infarct size was, if anything, increased by the SOD over controls in animals having high collateral flow, and it was argued that SOD had changed the slope of the infarct-collateral flow relationship and only protected animals with low collateral flow. Preferential protection of the low collateral flow animals was not observed in two similar dog studies using native SOD (73) or PEG SOD (14). It is possible that there was not any real drug effect in the Ambrosio et al study and that chance variation in several critical animals lead them to their conclusion. Because of the expense of such trials, virtually all of the canine infarct size studies have had too few animals in each group, which greatly increases the chance of false interpretation.

SOD May Induce False Positives in the TTC Method

While the collateral flow argument might be sufficient to dismiss the early dog studies as unreliable, that argument can hardly can be applied to rabbit (16) or pig (65, 66) trials since neither of these species has significant coronary collateral circulations (56, 80). A possible source of the discrepancy could be the method used to estimate the infarct size. All of the positive studies involved TTC staining with 24 hr or less of reperfusion. Indeed, when the rabbit SOD plus catalase study (16) was repeated, but this time analyzing infarct size three days after reperfusion with histology, protection was no longer seen (89). We recently examined SOD alone in a rabbit model with three different reperfusion times. After 3 and 24 hr of reperfusion, TTC indicated very small infarcts, but at 72 hr no differences were found by TTC (81). Apparently SOD greatly retards the rate of loss of enzyme and cofactor from dead tissue to give the appearance of viability for a full day after reperfusion. SOD might be delaying the washout of enzymes by preserving capillary permeability as it does in other organs (28). The one report where cardiac permeability was measured following an ischemic insult, however, failed to find any protection from SOD plus catalase (84); thus the mechanism for the induced artifact with the tetrazolium method remains unclear.

The Short Plasma Half-Life of SOD May Have Prevented Protection

The original interpretation of reperfusion injury was that it resulted from a burst of free radical production confined to the reperfusion period. Indeed, Jolly et al (44) reported that the protection from SOD plus catalase was only seen when the drug was present at the time of reperfusion and that administration minutes after reperfusion did not confer protection. These enzymes have two distinct disadvantages, however. They are confined to the extracellular space, and they have a very short plasma half-life of only about 15 min. The former might not be a problem if the source of the free radical were extracellular as would be the case with leukocytes. The latter could be a major problem. Because of the short half-life and the expense of SOD, plasma levels can only be maintained for a relatively short period. It is possible that injurious free radicals are produced not just at reperfusion but long after and that the SOD was simply withdrawn too early in the above studies. Indeed spin-trap studies on reperfused dog hearts reveal that free radical production occurs as a burst in the first few min of reperfusion followed by a low level of production for several hr thereafter (6).

To achieve a longer half-life, SOD is conjugated to a polyethylene glycol polymer, which increases the molecular size to the point where it is not filtered by the kidney. At the time of this writing only two reports on PEG-SOD are available, both from the Ann Arbor group (14, 85). One important arm of those studies was done in dogs that were reperfused for 96 hr, and the analysis of infarct size incorporated collateral flow effects (six dogs in the intervention group); a 36% reduction in infarct size was seen (85).

Although the PEG-SOD results would appear encouraging, we have recently examined PEG-SOD in our rabbit model (69). A single dose of 1000 units of PEG-SOD were given 15 min prior to coronary occlusion, and infarct size was evaluated 72 hr after reperfusion by histology. The results, shown in Figure 3, indicate no change in infarct size. There are several possible explanations for the discrepant data, including species differences or methods used to delineate infarct size, but preliminary studies in our laboratories indicate that PED-SOD may simply be inappropriate for myocardial protection. Using the krebs perfused Langendorff model, protection as assessed by enzyme release could be induced by SOD but only if pretreatment was sufficiently long to allow SOD to become equilibrated in the cardiac lymph at reperfusion. PEG-SOD was not found in the lymph after 50 min of perfusion and could not confer protection in that model. Another interesting feature of those data are that SOD has a very narrow therapeutic range. Protection seen at 15 units/ml was lost at 150 units/ml. Because the very stringent dose and schedule considerations required for protection in the isolated heart were not

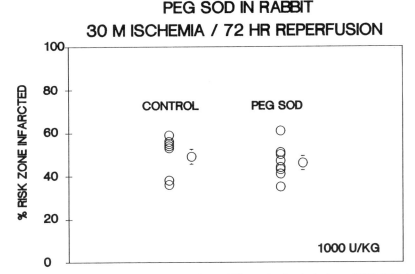

Figure 3   An infarct size trial in which open chest rabbits received a single dose of PEG-SOD 15 min prior to occlusion. Infarct size was determined by histology 72 hr post-reperfusion. Individual experiments are depicted by the open circles to the left while the mean and standard error appear to the right. Control animals received saline.

used in the previous animal trials, it is possible that SOD may still be effective but has been inappropriately administered.

The Xanthine Oxidase Inhibitors

Chambers et al (11) were the first to report a reduction in infarct size by allopurinol. Allopurinol was almost as effective as SOD in limiting infarct size in this canine model of one hr of ischemia followed by three hr of reperfusion. That observation was soon confirmed by Werns et al (88). Akizuki et al found that the allopurinol also could reduce infarct size in a canine model of permanent coronary occlusion for 24 hr (1). As was the case with SOD, the preliminary allopurinol trials using TTC could not be confirmed in a dog model where collateral flow was measured and infarct size was determined by histology (76). One might argue that inclusion of collateral flow measurements in the negative study confirms that allopurinol is ineffective, but there are other differences between the studies. Allopurinol was given as a 24 hr pretreatment in the positive studies but not the negative study, and pretreatment has been shown to be important (46). Allopurinol, a competitive xanthine oxidase inhibitor, is metabolized to oxypurinol, which is a non-competitive inhibitor, and it is thought that the accumulation of oxypurinol actually confers the protection. In a recent study from our laboratory allopurinol or oxypurinol was administered to dogs just prior to reperfusion and supplemented every eight hr thereafter (55). Infarct size was estimated by TTC 24 hr after reperfusion. As suspected, only oxypurinol shifted the collateral flow-infarct size relationship toward smaller infarcts in the absence of pretreatment.

Continued treatment also seems to be important. In a protocol virtually identical to the one just described, Peuet et al (74) failed to find protection with oxypurinol. Infarcts were measured with TTC 24 hr after reperfusion, and collateral flow was incorporated into the analysis. The only difference from the above study was that oxypurinol was administered as a single bolus and not supplemented thereafter. Because of the approximately three hr half-life of oxypurinol in the dog, the animal was unprotected through most of the reperfusion phase. Oxypurinol given as a single dose also failed to protect in an histological study (47). This would suggest that radical production is not just confined to the reperfusion period but may continue for hours or even days following reperfusion.

We still don't know if the 24 hr data with oxypurinol was a reflection of real protection or simply another artifact of TTC staining. The question may never be answered because recent work would indicate that unlike the dog or rat, human hearts contain undetectable amounts of xanthine oxidase (18). When allopurinol was given to the reperfused rabbit heart, which is also xanthine oxidase deficient, it had no effect on the TTC-indicated infarct size even though SOD plus catalase clearly reduced it (16). Until a clear demonstration of xanthine oxidase is made in the human heart or until an alternative mode of action of these drugs can be proven, it is unlikely that many future studies will be undertaken with these agents.

CONCLUDING COMMENTS

Historically models for assessing myocardial protection have been plagued with methodological problems and that situation has continued right up to the present time. Clearly we may have unwittingly relied too heavily on TTC staining to be the gold standard for infarct size. In the above discussion we saw how TTC staining in the first 24 hr of reperfusion may suffer from false positives and can only be considered as a first screen for cardioprotective drugs. Histology after prolonged reperfusion is probably the most reliable method of estimating infarct size, but because histology is tedious and expensive, few laboratories have chosen to use it. While most studies have concentrated on extracellular scavengers such as SOD and catalase, the data are sparse on intracellular species such as MPG (60, 63) and DMTU (7, 71), and none of these has been subjected to rigorous testing in a histological model. It is a sobering thought to realize that not one of the antioxidants, nor any other drug, for that matter, has been effective in a histological model. Another approach that could demonstrate long-term protection, but has been widely ignored to date, is the monitoring of long-term function in the ischemic region. Even though implantable sonnomicrometer crystals are inexpensive and easy to use, only a few studies have chosen to include them (9, 67).

After more than a decade of research on the free radical hypothesis, there is still little agreement on the role free radicals actually play in the reperfused myocardium. Since a sound theoretical basis for reperfusion injury does not appear to be forthcoming in the near future, we must continue to rely on drug screening with our animal models to identify active compounds with the hope that serendipidous discoveries will continue to provide insight into the cellular processes involved. The process has clearly been hampered by inadequate models, however. Until a simple, reliable, and inexpensive model of ischemic injury with good replication is developed, it is likely that progress in the cardioprotection field will continue to be slow.

Literature Cited

1. Akizuki, S., Yoshida, S., Chambers, D. E., Eddy, L. J., Parmley, L. F., et al. 1985. Infarct size reduction by the xanthine oxidase inhibitor, allopurinol, in closed chest dogs with small infarcts. *Cardiovasc. Res.* 19:686–92
2. Ambrosio, G., Becker, L. C., Hutchens, G. M., Weisman, H. F., Weisfeldt, M. L. 1986. Reduction in experimental infarct size by recombinant human superoxide dismutase: insights into the pathophysiology of reperfusion injury. *Circulation* 74:1424–33
3. Baker, J. E., Felix, C. C., Olinger, G. N., Kalyanaraman, B. 1988. Myocardial ischemia and reperfusion: Direct evidence for free radical generation by electron spin resonance spectroscopy. *Proc. Natl. Acad. Sci. USA* 85:2786–89
4. Bernier, M., Hearse, J. D., Manning, A. S. 1986. Reperfusion-induced arrhythmias and oxygen-derived free radicals. Studies with "anti-free radical" interventions and a free radical generating system in the isolated perfused rat heart. *Circ. Res.* 58:331–40
5. Bolli, R. 1988. Oxygen-derived free radicals and postischemic myocardial dysfunction ("stunned myocardium"). *J. Am. Coll. Cardiol.* 12(1):239–49
6. Bolli, R., Patel, B. S., Jeroudi, M. O., Lai, E. K., McCay, P. B. 1988. Demonstration of free radical generation in "stunned myocardium of intact dogs with the use of the spin trap alpha-phenyl N-tert-butyl nitrone. *J. Clin. Invest.* 82:476–85
7. Bolli, R., Zhu, W. X., Hartley, C. J., Michael, L. H., Repine, J. E., et al. 1987. Attenuation of dysfunction in the postischemic "stunned" heart by dimethylthiourea. *Circulation* 76:458–68
8. Braunwald, E. K., Kloner, R. A. 1985. Myocardial reperfusion: a double-edged sword? *J. Clin. Invest.* 76:1713–19
9. Bush, L. R., Buja, M., Tilton, G., Wathen, M., Apprill, P., et al. 1985. Effects of propranolol and diltiazem alone and in combination on the recovery of left ventricular segmental function after temporary coronary occlusion and long term reperfusion in dogs. *Circulation* 72:413–30
10. Campbell, C. A., Alker, K. J., Kloner, R. A. 1988. Does tissue plasminogen activating factor reduce infarct size in an experimental model of mechanical coronary artery occlusion and reperfusion in dogs. *J. Am. Coll. Cardiol.* 11:54A
11. Chambers, D. E., Parks, D. A., Patterson, G., Roy, R., McCord, J. M., et al. 1985. Xanthine oxidase as a source of free radical damage in myocardial ischemia. *J. Mol. Cell. Cardiol.* 17:145–52
12. Chambers, D. E., Yellon, D. M., Hearse, D. J. 1983. Effects of flurbiprofen in altering the size of myocardial infarcts in dogs: reduction or delay? *Am. J. Cardiol.* 51:884–90

13. Charlat, M. L., O'Neill, P. G., Egan, J. M., Abernathy, D. R., Michael, L. H., et al. 1987. Evidence for a pathogenetic role of xanthine oxidase in the "stunned" myocardium. *Am. J. Physiol.* 252: H566–77

14. Chi, L., Tamura, Y., Hoff, P. T., Macha, M., Gallagher, K. P., et al. 1989. Effect of superoxide dismutase on myocardial infarct size in the canine heart after 6 hours of regional ischemia and reperfusion: a demonstration of myocardial salvage. *Circ. Res.* 64:665–75

15. Darius, H., Yanagisawa, A., Brezinski, M. E., Lefer, A. M. 1986. Direct cardioprotective effect of tPA in feline ischemic myocardium. *Fed. Proc.* 45:808 (Abstr.)

16. Downey, J. M., Miura, T., Eddy, L. J., Chambers, D. E., Mellert, T., et al. 1987. Xanthine oxidase is not a source of free radicals in the ischemic rabbit heart. *J. Mol. Cell. Cardiol.* 19:1053–60

17. Downey, J. M., Shirato, C., Miura, T., Toyofuku, T. 1988. Tetrazolium is unreliable as an index of drug induced salvage. *J. Mol. Cell. Cardiol.* 20 (Suppl. 5):S70 (Abstr.)

18. Eddy, L. J., Stewart, J. R., Jones, H. P., Engerson, T. D., McCord, J. M., et al. 1987. Free radical producing enzyme, xanthine oxidase, is undetectable in human heart. *Am. J. Physiol.* 253: H709–711

19. Factor, S. M., Cho, S., Kirk, E. S. 1982. Non-specificity of triphenyl tetrazolium chloride (TTC) for the gross diagnosis of acute myocardial infarction. *Circulation* 66 (Suppl I):II333 (Abstr.)

20. Farber, N. E., Vercellotti, G. M., Jacob, H. S., Pieper, G. M., Gross, G. J. 1988. Evidence for a role of iron-catalyzed oxidants in functional and metabolic stunning in the canine heart. *Circ. Res.* 63:351–60

21. Ferrari, R., Ceconi, C., Curello, S., Cargnoni, A., Medici, D. 1985. Oxygen free radicals and reperfusion injury; the effect of ischemia and reperfusion on the cellular ability to neutralise oxygen toxicity. *J. Mol. Cell. Cardiol.* 18 (Suppl. 4):67–69

22. Fishbein, M. C., Meerbaum, S., Rit, J., Lando, U., Kanmatsuse, K., et al. 1981. Early phase acute myocardial infarct size quantification: validation of the triphenyl tetrazolium chloride staining technique. *Am. Heart J.* 101:593–99

23. Fox, R. B., Harada, R. N., Tate, R. M., Repine, J. E. 1983. Prevention of thiourea induced pulmonary edema by hydroxyl-radical scavengers. *J. Appl. Physiol.* 55:1456–59

24. Gallagher, K. P., Buda, A. J., Pace, D., Gerren, R. A., Shlafer, M. 1986. Failure of superoxide dismutase and catalase to alter size of infarction in conscious dogs after 3 hours of occlusion followed by reperfusion. *Circulation* 73(5):1065–76

25. Gardner, T. J., Stewart, J. R., Casale, A. S., Downey, J. M., Chambers, D. E. 1983. Reduction of myocardial ischemic injury with oxygen derived free radical scavengers. *Surgery* 94:423–27

26. Garlick, P. B., Davies, M. J., Hearse, D. J., Slater, T. F. 1987. Direct detection of free radicals in the reperfused rat heart using electron spin resonance spectroscopy. *Circ. Res.* 61:757–60

27. The GISSI study group. 1986. Effectiveness of intravenous thrombolytic treatment in acute myocardial infarction. *Lancet* 1:402–10

28. Granger, D. N., Hallworth, M., Parks, D. A. 1986. Ischemia-reperfusion injury: Role of oxygen derived free radicals. *Acta Physiol. Scand. Suppl.* 548:47–63

29. Grinwald, P. M. 1982. Calcium uptake during post-ischemic reperfusion in the isolated rat heart: influence of extracellular sodium. *J. Mol. Cell. Cardiol.* 14:359–65

30. Guaduel, Y., Duvelleroy, M. A. 1984. Role of oxygen radicals in cardiac injury due to reoxygenation. *J. Mol. Cell. Cardiol.* 16:459–70

31. Guarnieri, C., Ferrari, R., Visioli, O., Caldarera, C. M., Nayler, W. G. 1978. Effect of alpha-tocopheral on hypoxic-perfused and reoxygenated rabbit heart muscle. *J. Mol. Cell. Cardiol.* 10:893–906

32. Hearse, D. J., Humpherey, S. M. 1975. Enzyme release during myocardial anoxia: a study of metabolic protection. *J. Mol. Cell. Cardiol.* 7:463–82

33. Hearse, D. J., Humphrey, S. M., Chain, E. B. 1973. Abrupt reoxygenation of the anoxic potassium arrested perfused rat heart: a study of myocardial enzyme release. *J. Mol. Cell. Cardiol.* 5:395–407

34. Hearse, D. J., Humphrey, S. M., Nayler, W. G., Slade, A., Border, D. 1975. Ultrastructural damage associated with reoxygenation of the anoxic myocardium. *J. Mol. Cell. Cardiol.* 7:315–24

35. Heide, V., Sobotka, P. A., Ganote, C. E. 1987. Effect of free radical scavenger DMTU and manitol on the oxygen paradox in perfused rat hearts. *J. Mol. Cell. Cardiol.* 19:615–25

36. Holland, R., Brooks, H. 1977. T-Q ST

segment mapping: Critical review and analysis of current topics. *Am. J. Cardiol.* 40:110–28

37. Horneffer, P. J., Healy, B., Gott, V. L., Gardner, T. J. 1987. The rapid evolution of a myocardial infarction in an end-artery coronary preparation. *Circulation* 76(Suppl. 5):V39–42

38. Jennings, R. B., Ganote, C. E. 1974. Structural changes in myocardium during acute myocardial ischemia. *Circ. Res.* 34 (Suppl. III):III156–68

39. Jennings, R. B., Reimer, K. A. 1981. Lethal myocardial ischemic injury. *Am. J. Path.* 102:241–55

40. Jennings, R. B., Reimer, K. A. 1983. Factors involved in salvaging ischemic myocardium: effect of reperfusion of arterial blood. *Circulation* 68(Suppl. I):I25–36

41. Jennings, R. B., Sommers, H. M., Smyth, G. A., Flack, H. A. 1960. Myocardial necrosis induced by a temporary occlusion of a coronary artery. *Pathology* 70:68–78

42. Jeroudi, M. P., Patel, B., Bolli, R. 1988. Does superoxide dismutase or catalase alone attenuate myocardial stunning? *Circulation* (Suppl. I):78 (Abstr.)

43. Jewett, S. L., Eddy, L. J., Hochstein, P. 1989. Is the autoxidation of catecholamines involved in ischemia-reperfusion injury? *Free Radic. Biol. Med.* 6:323–26

44. Jolly, S. R., Kane, W. J., Bailie, M. B., Abrams, G. D., Lucchesi, B. R. 1984. Canine myocardial reperfusion injury: its reduction by the combined administration of superoxide dismutase and catalase. *Circ. Res.* 54:277–85

45. Kehrer, J. P., Piper, H. M., Sies, H. 1987. Xanthine oxidase is not responsible for reoxygenation injury in isolated-perfused rat heart. *Free Radic. Res. Commun.* 3:69–78

46. Kingma, J. G., Miura, T., Downey, J. M., Hearse, D. J., Yellon, D. M. 1988. Myocardial salvage with allopurinol during 24 h of permanent coronary occlusion: Importance of pretreatment. *Can. J. Cardiol.* 4:360–65

47. Kinsman, J. M., Murry, C. E., Richard, V. J., Jennings, R. B., Reimer, K. A. 1988. The xanthine oxidase inhibitor, oxypurinol, does not limit infarct size in a canine model of 40 minutes ischemia with reperfusion. *J. Am. Coll. Cardiol.* 12:209–17

48. Klein, H. H., Lindert, P. S., Buchwald, A., Nebendahl, K., Kreuzer, H. 1988. Intracoronary superoxide dismutase for the treatment of reperfusion injury. A blind randomized placebo-controlled trial in ischemic, reperfused porcine hearts. *Basic Res. Cardiol.* 83:141–48

49. Klein, H. H., Puschmann, S., Schaper, J., Schaper, W. 1981. The mechanism of the tetrazolium reaction in identifying myocardial infarction. *Virchows Arch. A* 393:287–97

50. Kontos, H. A., Wei, E. P., Ellis, E. F., Jenkins, L. W., Polvilshock, J. T., et al. 1985. Appearance of superoxide anion radical in cerebral extracellular space during increased prostaglandin synthesis in cats. *Circ. Res.* 57:142–51

51. Manning, A., Bernier, M., Crome, R., Little, S. H. D. 1988. Reperfusion arrhythmias: a study of the role of xanthine oxidase-derived free radicals in the rat heart. *J. Mol. Cell. Cardiol.* 20:35–40

52. Maroko, P. R., Kjekshus, J. K., Sobel, B. E., Watanabe, T., Covell, J. W., et al. 1971. Factors influencing infarct size following experimental coronary artery occlusions. *Circulation* 43:67–82

53. Maroko, P. R., Libby, P., Bloor, C. M., Sobel, B. E., Braunwald, E. 1972. Reduction by hyalurinidase of myocardial necrosis following coronary artery occlusion. *Circulation* 46:430–37

54. Maroko, P. R., Libby, P., Sobel, B. E., Bloor, C. M., Shell, W. E., et al. 1972. Effect of glucose-insulin-potassium infusion on myocardial infarction following experimental coronary artery occlusion. *Circulation* 45:1160–75

55. Matsuki, T., Shirato, C., Cohen, M. V., Downey, J. M. 1989. Oxypurinol limits myocardial infarct size without pretreatment. *Can. J. Cardiol.* In press

56. Maxwell, M. P., Hearse, D. J., Yellon, D. M. 1987. Species variation in the coronary collateral circulation during regional myocardial ischemia: a critical determinant of the rate of evolution and extent of myocardial infarction. *Cardiovasc. Res.* 21:737–46

57. McCord, J. M. 1985. Oxygen-derived free radicals in postischemic tissue injury. *New Engl. J. Med.* 312:159–63

58. McCord, J. M., Roy, R. S., Schaffer, S. W. 1985. Free radicals and myocardial ischemia: the role of xanthine oxidase. *Adv. Myocardiol.* 5:183–89

59. Mitchell, J. R., Smith, C. V., Hughes, H., Lenz, M. L., Jaeschke, H. et al. 1987. No evidence for reactive oxygen damage in ischemia-reflow injury. *Trans. Assoc. Am. Physicians* 100:54–61

60. Mitsos, S., Askew, T., Fantone, J., Kunkle S., Abrams, G., et al. 1986. Protective effects of N-2-mercapto-

propionyl glycine against myocardial reperfusion injury in the dog: evidence for the role of intracellular derived free radicals. *Circulation* 73:1077–86

61. Miura, T., Yellon, D. M., Hearse, D. J., Downey, J. M. 1987. Determinants of infarct size during permanent occlusion of a coronary artery in the closed chest dog. *J. Am. Col. Cardiol.* 9:647–654

62. Myers, C. L., Weiss, S. J., Kirsh, M. M., Shlafer, M. 1985. Involvement of hydrogen peroxide and hydroxyl radical in the oxygen paradox: reduction of creatine kinase release by catalase, allopurinol or desferoxamine, but not by superoxide dismutase. *J. Mol. Cell. Cardiol.* 17:675–84

63. Myers, M. L., Bolli, R., Lekich, R. F., Hartley, C. J., Roberts, R. 1986. N-2-mercaptopropionyl glycine improves recovery of myocardial function after reversible regional ischemia. *J. Am. Col. Cardiol.* 8:1161–68

64. Nachlas, M., Schnitka, T. 1963. Macroscopic identification of early myocardial infarcts by alterations in dehydrogenase activity. *Am. J. Path.* 42:379–406

65. Naslund, U., Haggmark, S., Johansson, G., Marklund, S., Reiz, S. 1988. The therapeutic window of SOD induced limitation of infarct size in a low-collateralized porcine reperfusion model. *J. Mol. Cell. Cardiol.* 20 (Suppl. 5):S25 (Abstr.)

66. Naslund, U., Haggmark, S., Johansson, G., Marklund, S. L., Reiz, S., et al. 1986. Superoxide dismutase and catalase reduce infarct size in a porcine myocardial ischemia/reperfusion model. *J. Mol. Cell. Cardiol.* 11:1077–84

67. Nejima, J., Knight, D. R., Fallon, J. T., Uemura, N., Manders, W. T., et al. 1989. Superoxide dismutase reduces reperfusion arrhythmias but fails to salvage regional function or myocardium at risk in conscious dogs. *Circulation* 79:143–53 Submitted

68. Nienaber, C., Gottwik, M., Winkler, B., Shaper, W. 1983. The relationship between the perfusion deficit, infarct size and time after experimental coronary occlusion. *Basic Res. Cardiol.* 78:210–26

69. Ooiwa, H., Jordan, M., Bylund-Fellanius, A. C., Downey, J. M. 1989. PEG SOD fails to limit infarct size in reperfused rabbit heart. *Circulation* 80:292. (Abstr.)

70. Patel, B., Jeroudi, M. O., O'Neill, P. G., Roberts, R., Bolli, R. 1988. Human superoxide dismutase fails to limit infarct size after 2-h ischemia and reperfusion. *Circulation* 78:II373 (Abstr.)

71. Portz, S. J., Van Benthuysen, K. M., Lesfnesky, E. J., McMurty, I. F., Horwitz, L. D., 1987. Dimethylthiourea but not dimethylsulfoxide reduces canine myocardial infarct size. *Circulation* 76:IV196 (Abstr.)

72. Przyklenk, K., Kloner, R. A. 1986. Superoxide dismutase plus catalase improve contractile function in the canine model of the "stunned myocardium". *Circ. Res.* 58:148–56

73. Przyklenk, K., Kloner, R. A. 1989. Reperfusion injury by oxygen free radicals? Effect of superoxide dismutase plus catalase, given at the time reperfusion, on myocardial infarct size, contractile function, coronary microvascular function. *Cir. Res.* 64:86–96

74. Puett, D. W., Forman, M. B., Cates, C. U., Wilson, B. H., Hande, K. R., et al. 1987. Oxypurinol limits myocardial stunning but does not reduce infarct size after reperfusion. *Circulation* 76:678–86

75. Reimer, K. A., Jennings, R. B. 1979. The wavefront phenomenon of myocardial ischemic cell death II. Transmural progression of necrosis within the framework of ischemic bed size (myocardium at risk) and collateral flow. *Lab. Invest.* 40:633–40

76. Reimer, K. A., Jennings, R. B. 1985. Failure of the xanthine oxidase inhibitor allopurinol to limit infarct size after acute ischemia and reperfusion in dogs. *Circulation* 71:1069–75

77. Reimer, K. A., Lowe, J. E., Rassmussen, M. M., Jennings, R. B. 1977. The wavefront phenomenon of ischemic cell death. 1. Myocardial infarct size vs. duration of coronary occlusion in dogs. *Circulation* 56:786–94

78. Richard, V. J., Murry, C. E., Jennings, R. B., Reimer, K. A. 1987. Superoxide dismutase and catalase do not limit infarct size after 90 minutes of ischemia and 4 days of reperfusion. *Circulation* 76: (Suppl. 4):IV199 (Abstr.)

79. Schaper, J., Mulch, J., Winkler, B., Schaper, W. 1979. Ultrastructural, functional and biochemical criteria for estimation of reversibility of ischemic injury: a study on the effects of global ischemia in the isolated dog heart. *J. Mol. Cell Cardiol.* 11:521–41

80. Schaper, W. 1984. Experimental infarcts and the microcirculation. In *Therapeutic Approaches to Myocardial Infarct Size Limitation,* ed. D. H. Hearse, D. M. Yellon, pp. 79–90. New York: Raven

81. Shirato, C., Miura, T., Downey, J. M. 1988. Superoxide dismutase (single dose) delays rather than prevents necrosis in reperfused rabbit hearts. *FASEB J.* 2:A918 (Abstr.)

82. Shlafer, M., Myers, C. L., Adkins, S. 1987. Mitochondrial hydrogen peroxide generation and activities of glutathione peroxidase and superoxide dismutase following global ischemia. *J. Mol. Cell. Cardiol.* 19:1195–1206

83. Simpson, P. J., Lucchesi, B. R. 1987. Free radicals and myocardial ischemia and reperfusion injury. *J. Lab. Clin. Invest.* 110:13–30

84. Sunnergren, K. P., Rovetto, M. J. 1987. Myocyte and endothelial injury with ischemia reperfusion in isolated rat hearts. *Am. J. Physiol.* 252:H1211–217

85. Tamura, Y., Chi, L., Driscoll, E. M., Hoff, P. T., Freeman, B. A., et al. 1988. Superoxide dismutase conjugated to polyethylene glycol provides sustained protection against myocardial ischemia/reperfusion injury in canine heart. *Circ. Res.* 63:944–59

86. The TIMI study group 1985. The thrombolysis in myocardial infarction (TIMI) trial: Phase one findings. *N. Engl. J. Med.* 312:832–936

87. Uraizee, A., Reimer, K. A., Murry, C. E., Jennings, R. B. 1987. Failure of superoxide dismutase to limit infarct size of myocardial infarction after 40 minutes of ischemia and 4 days of reperfusion in dogs. *Circulation* 75:1237–48

88. Wearns, S., Shea, M., Mitsos, S., Dysko, R., Fantone, F., et al. 1986. Reduction of the size of infarction by allopurinol in the ischemic-reperfused canine heart. *Circulation* 73:518–24

89. Werns, S. W., Shea, M. J., Driscoll, E. M., Cohen, C., Abrams, G. D., et al. 1985. The independent effects of oxygen radical scavengers on canine infarct size reduction by superoxide dismutase and not catalase. *Circ. Res.* 56:895–98

90. Yellon, D. M., Kingma, J. G., Hearse, D. J., Downey, J. M. 1989. Myocardial infarct size limitation with allopurinol during 24 hours of sustained coronary occlusion in the closed-chest dog: the importance of pre-treatment. *Can. J. Cardiol.* In press

91. Zweier, J. L. 1988. Measurement of superoxide-derived free radicals in the reperfused heart. *J. Biol. Chem.* 263 (3):1353–57

92. Zweier, J. L., Rayburn, B. K., Flaherty, J. T., Weisfeldt, M. L. 1987. Recombinant superoxide dismutase reduces oxygen free radical concentrations in reperfused myocardium. *J. Clin. Invest.* 80(6):1728–34

Annu. Rev. Physiol. 1990. 52:505–22

LOAD AND LENGTH REGULATION OF CARDIAC ENERGETICS[1]

George Cooper, IV

Cardiology Section of the Department of Medicine and the Department of Physiology, Gazes Cardiac Research Institute, Medical University of South Carolina, Veterans Administration Medical Center, Charleston, South Carolina 29425

KEY WORDS: oxygen consumption, heat production, length-dependent activation, Fenn effect, time-varying elastance

INTRODUCTION

Muscle is an engine whose production of force and shortening is continuously regulated by the ongoing results of its activity. The workings of this engine and the control of its output are based on events with obligatory energy requirements. Thus the study of energetics has been a valuable tool in elucidating the operating mechanisms both of this engine and of its regulatory controls.

Several decades have passed since the molecular workings of this engine began to be understood on the level of the sarcomere. More recently, a similar degree of understanding has been reached for the more numerous interrelated molecular events that regulate the mechanical output of the sarcomere. Energetic studies have been important at each step in reaching this present understanding, both of the output of the sarcomere and of its regulation on the molecular level.

The relation of cardiac mechanics to energetics has also been framed in terms of a succession of mathematical analogues of the heart, however, without necessary reference to the physical properties and control of the heart on the molecular level. As is usually the case for models of biological systems, each successive model, including the currently prevalent time-varying elastance model, has been useful in terms of simplifying descriptions

---

of complex biology, but each has been usurped by incompatible new data. Both because of this, and especially because striated muscle is the best present example of a mammalian tissue wherein structure and function can be causally interrelated at the molecular level, the future seems to belong to those approaches that do not interpose models, but instead directly attack the molecular basis of the workings and control of the heart.

ENERGETICS OF VENTRICULAR MYOCARDIUM

It has been more than 140 years since the initial demonstration that contraction is accompanied by chemical change (52) and heat production (53) in isolated striated muscle. These, and even earlier less direct observations, form the rationale for the use of energetic measurements both to define and to characterize the basis of the metabolic cost of muscle contraction. Since cardiac metabolism is almost entirely aerobic, with at least 85% of myocardial oxygen consumption (MVO_2) obligated by ATP generation which subserves contraction (14), and since understanding the control of MVO_2 is of immediate practical interest to both the physiologist and the clinician, the study of myocardial energetics has centered largely on elucidating the relationship of mechanical variables to MVO_2.

For the whole heart, where the chamber of interest has almost invariably been the left ventricle, even the earliest work (37, 95) showed a clear relation between tension generation and MVO_2. Subsequently a number of investigators confirmed that developed tension is the major determinant of left ventricular MVO_2 (80, 83, 94, 97, 117). By 1971 there was general agreement (11, 99) that this major determinant was primarily modified by inotropic state and heart rate, with lesser contributions to MVO_2 being made by shortening, by the ionic changes required for contractile activation, and by basal metabolism. Unfortunately, such a descriptive list provides little insight into either the interrelationship of these mechanical variables in determining the total MVO_2 of a ventricular contraction, or into the basic mechanisms by which contraction and energetics are coupled. Thus a simple description of ventricular mechanics that would encompass the various mechanical changes that occur during the heartbeat and allow such a net expression of mechanical output to be related directly to MVO_2 had obvious appeal.

As noted elsewhere (85), a time-varying compliance, or its inverse, which is elastance, was first used some time ago as a model for ventricular pump function (116). This concept was then formalized by Suga, who showed that characterizing left ventricular contraction in terms of a time-varying elastance results in a definition of total systolic mechanical energy that has little sensitivity either to diastolic (102) or to systolic load (103); i.e. cardiac contraction as defined by the time-varying elastance model consists of a pressure-volume relation that changes as a function of time during systole. This concept was then used to formulate the total mechanical energy of a ventricular contraction in terms of a systolic pressure-volume area, which is a specific area in the pressure-volume diagram circumscribed by the end-systolic pressure-volume line, the end-diastolic pressure-volume line, and the systolic segment of the pressure-volume trajectory (104). Given that both pressure-volume area and MVO_2 can be expressed in dimensions of energy, it is not surprising that the time-varying elastance model has proven successful in correlating contractile mechanics with energetics under a variety of ventricular loading conditions either in the excised or in the in situ heart (84, 106, 107). It is now clear, however, that the time-varying elastance model does not account for the molecular mechanisms that underlie the control and expression of either ventricular mechanics or energetics.

ENERGETICS OF ISOLATED LINEAR MYOCARDIUM

Largely because such preparations have far simpler geometry and allow much more direct control and interpretation of muscle mechanics than does the intact left ventricle, isolated linear myocardial segments, usually the right ventricular papillary muscles of small mammals, have been used extensively to relate cardiac mechanics to energetics. The excellent correlation of heat production with MVO_2, which has been established for the intact heart (24), has been confirmed in the isolated papillary muscle (15), and both types of energetic measurements have been used extensively. Such studies, which have been reviewed elsewhere in terms of both heat (44–46) and MVO_2 (17) measurements, have confirmed the major points established during the study of ventricular energetics; i.e. tension generation is the major determinant of energy demands during contraction, with shortening playing a lesser role. Further, for a given amount of tension generation, energy utilization varies directly with changes in contractile state, and the energy required for activation appears to be relatively low, especially when compared to that of fast skeletal muscle (20).

A series of studies from my laboratory, however, stands in contrast to this apparent congruence of the relation of cardiac mechanics to energetics when studied on the levels of ventricular and isolated linear myocardium. These studies (19–22, 61) had their genesis in the use of myocardial tetanus to define the MVO_2 cost of tension maintenance and then were extended to a definition of the extent and duration of MVO_2 during isometric and isotonic cat papillary muscle twitch contractions. Taken together, these studies demonstrated a load, length, and time dependence of energetics throughout the normal cardiac contraction, which was obviated by interventions that interfered with normal physiologic control of cardiac activation. The major findings were first, during myocardial tetanus, when activation is maximum and constant throughout contraction, the mechanical determinants that apply during twitch contractions are no longer important, and MVO_2 is linearly related to contraction duration during either isometric or isotonic tetanus (19); second, during the normally activated isometric twitch contraction, active tension is energy-dependent throughout contraction, and activation energy is both length- and tension-dependent (20); third, under conditions designed to maximize and prolong activation during the isometric twitch contraction, the time variation of energy utilization during contraction is far less apparent than it is during the normally activated isometric twitch contraction in that the normal length-dependent control of activation had been overridden (21); fourth, during the normally activated isotonic twitch contraction, MVO_2 is directly related to load and to the duration of contraction before shortening begins but is inversely related to the extent of shortening (22); fifth, while MVO_2 correlates very closely with force-length area, an analogue for linear myocardium of the ventricular pressure-volume area, time to end-systole is quite load-dependent during either isometric or isotonic twitch contractions, and substantial energy usage was, as before (20), shown to continue past the time of end-systole (61).

The energy dependence of active tension past the time of end-systole that I found (20, 61) in the isometric papillary muscle twitch contraction has subsequently been confirmed by myothermal techniques, with similar economy in terms of the ratio of tension-dependent heat to the time integral of active tension being found for normal muscle in both the tension generation and the relaxation phases of contraction (4). Further, the load dependence of the time to end-systole in isolated linear myocardium has also been seen by other investigators (32, 34).

Both the length- and tension-dependent modulation of MVO_2 throughout cardiac contraction and the load variation of the time to end-systole are consistent with the hypothesis that I generated during the course of my studies (19–22, 61). This hypothesis is that MVO_2, and the contractile processes that it subserves, are dynamically regulated by the level of length- and load-dependent activation in response to changing mechanical conditions throughout the cardiac contraction. This is similar to the formulation generated during studies of papillary muscle heat production, in which there is a mechanical feedback regulation during contraction of energy output (45), just as is the case in skeletal muscle. This concept of length-dependent modulation of energetics throughout contraction, with the time, rate, and extent of length change ultimately being responsible for the energy usage of any particular type of contraction, is incompatible with the time-varying elastance concept, wherein the energy requirements for contraction are fixed by the time that maximum elastance occurs at end-systole. These two conflicting views of the relation of cardiac mechanics to energetics are perhaps best resolved by considering other recent information about the length-dependent control of striated muscle contraction.

LOAD AND LENGTH EFFECTS ON MUSCLE ACTIVATION AND CROSSBRIDGE ACTIVITY

Hill, as early as 1922, showed that heat output varies directly with active force throughout skeletal muscle contraction when it is prolonged either pharmacologically or by tetanus (51), which implied that there might be regulation by changing mechanical conditions throughout contraction of the level of tension generation and thus of the rate of requisite energy usage. He then showed that for normal twitch contractions heat output is determined by muscle length at the beginning and throughout contraction and by external work (56). He showed later that during the isometric twitch, heat production continues until active tension has dissipated, while in the lightly loaded isotonic twitch, heat production ceases at the termination of shortening, which is at a time considerably earlier than the time of full relaxation in an isometric twitch (60). Edman then showed that the residual ability of cardiac muscle to produce motion or tension during contraction is a function of the amount of active shortening that had occurred previously during the same contraction (28).

The basis for such a length- and load-dependent modulation of mechanical output throughout striated muscle contraction became apparent with the finding that the contractile activation of skeletal myofibrils is diminished during shortening (111). Other data suggested that muscle stiffness varies directly with the number of attached crossbridges such that shortening reduces this number, and thus muscle stiffness, during contraction (72). The deactivating effect of shortening appears to depend not only on the load and thus the extent of shortening, but also on the time during contraction when the onset of shortening occurs; in the isometric twitch, shortening during the early rising phase of tension development was found by Edman to produce maximal deactivation (27). He also found that shortening deactivation occurs in both skeletal and cardiac muscle (29). Indeed, in heart muscle the shortening velocity for a given load appears to be related more to instantaneous length than to time during contraction, which suggests that length influences mechanical activity in all types of contraction and not just during isometric contractions (54). The length-dependent activation observed in isolated skeletal and cardiac muscle preparations has also been observed in the left ventricle (78, 109, 115). Here, changes in ventricular volume relate directly to changes in inotropic state that occur both immediately after the volume change and later when a new steady-state has been reached.

These load-, length-, and time-dependent deactivating effects of shortening might seem simply to be attributable to a change in sarcomere length from an initially more favorable to a subsequently less favorable length in terms of thick and thin filament overlap. The finding that very small changes in initial fiber length have marked effects on active tension in both cardiac (8) and skeletal (91) muscle however, provided compelling evidence that factors other than length-dependent effects on the number of crossbridge sites are important in determining length-dependent mechanical output during contraction. The fact that the length-tension curve of cardiac muscle shows a much steeper length dependence of tension generation than does that for skeletal muscle (1), together with the fact that cardiac muscle is not fully activated during contraction (38), suggests that there is substantial opportunity in cardiac muscle for factors other than myofilament overlap to modulate contractile behavior (100). Thus while muscle contractility and length were initially regarded as independent regulators of cardiac function, such a view is now untenable; it is clear that cardiac inotropic state is strongly length-dependent (69). Indeed, the length dependence of activation would appear to account almost entirely for the observed variation in tension generation over the ascending limb of the papillary muscle length-tension relationship (69).

Given the established role of calcium in regulating crossbridge activation, and the fact that the rate of force development for skeletal (5) and cardiac (121) muscle is closely paralleled in time by myoplasmic $[Ca^{2+}]_i$, bases for length-dependent effects on striated muscle mechanics and energetics and for the observed differences between cardiac and skeletal muscle in terms of their sensitivity to these length effects have been sought in studies of calcium metabolism (2). These studies have focused in two areas: the length dependence of myoplasmic $[Ca^{2+}]_i$ kinetics and the length dependence of myofibrillar calcium sensitivity and binding.

Changes in the amount and time variation of $[Ca^{2+}]_i$ in activated heart muscle appear to depend primarily on calcium entry across the sarcolemma (77, 118) and calcium release from the sarcoplasmic reticulum (118). Nevertheless, it appears that under basal conditions, with a physiologic level of extracellular calcium, substantial modulation of calcium influx across the sarcolemma is unlikely in mammalian myocardium, because the influence of calcium on inotropism is probably affected by loading or depletion of calcium stores in the sarcoplasmic reticulum (16, 114). Indeed, it was suggested that length-dependent cardiac inotropic effects may be partially explained by a direct relationship between muscle length and calcium-triggered calcium release from the sarcoplasmic reticulum (39).

Since the transsarcolemmal electrical potential affects the inward calcium current, a possible additional explanation for length dependence of myoplasmic $[Ca^{2+}]_i$ was suggested by observations that length changes affect skeletal muscle membrane potential (48) and the duration of the cardiac muscle action potential (74). However, it appears that changes in myoplasmic $[Ca^{2+}]_i$ may be a cause more than an effect of such electrophysiologic changes. Data showing that sarcomere shortening causes calcium to be displaced from the crossbridges (73) have been confirmed by aequorin measurements of $[Ca^{2+}]_i$, which show that the aequorin light signal declines later during isotonic than during isometric cardiac contractions (66); similar data have been obtained from skeletal muscle (92). Thus when cardiac muscle shortens extensively during contraction, mechanical activity is abbreviated, and the action potential duration is prolonged. It would appear that the explanation for this effect may be that shortening causes calcium release from troponin C, which then activates an inward current that is responsible for the action potential changes (76). In summary, there is good evidence that the relatively slow changes in contractile state following a length change are dependent on alterations in intracellular calcium stores (78, 109), but the evidence for immediate length-dependent effects, especially during the course of a single contraction, on calcium availability to the myofibrils is less compelling.

To reiterate, the paradoxical observation that elevated myoplasmic $[Ca^{2+}]_i$ persists longer during an isotonic cardiac contraction when shortening deactivation is occurring than during an isometric contraction (66) is apparently explained by the fact that this persistent myoplasmic calcium late in contraction is coming off of the myofilaments as the result of shortening induced deactivation rather than being used primarily for continuing activation. This, in turn, appears to relate to data that show that myofibrillar calcium sensitivity and the affinity of calcium binding increase in direct relation to sarcomere length within the ascending portion of the cardiac length-tension relationship (55). The finding that crossbridge interactions increase myofibrillar calcium sensitivity and that shortening or decreased active tension decrease calcium binding may well explain the general mechanism for shortening induced deactivation (49).

An early insight by Endo into the specific mechanisms for these effects in skeletal muscle showed that the level of myofibrillar activation by a given level of myoplasmic $[Ca^{2+}]_i$ increases with fiber length (35). This led him to suggest that Ca^{2+}-troponin C binding increases with muscle length and results in more active tension (36), as well as less myoplasmic free calcium. In addition, it was later found that myofibrillar calcium sensitivity varies directly with force development during contraction (93). The fact that troponin binding sites interact and that this interaction is increased by tropomyosin further suggested that this effect would cause the affinity of troponin for calcium to vary during contraction (65). Thus the length and time dependence of troponin C binding of calcium and the fact that troponin C calcium binding sites are at most half-saturated during cardiac systole (98) made it clear that length-and time-dependent changes in troponin C calcium sensitivity might well play a major role in length-dependent control of contractile mechanics and energetics, especially in heart muscle.

Further insight into the potential mechanisms for the length dependence of troponin C calcium binding showed that one of the troponin C calcium binding sites has a calcium sensitivity that varies directly with the extent of attachment via crossbridges between actin and myosin and thus with muscle length (43). These concepts are consistent with the finding in cardiac muscle that after an increase in length there is an immediate increase in developed tension coincident with an abbreviation of the myoplasmic calcium transient, while quick release during contraction causes a transient increase in $[Ca^{2+}]_i$ (3).

Evidence for mediation of these effects by the level of troponin C affinity for calcium was provided in reports on heart muscle where it was first shown that there is a length dependence over the rising portion of the length-tension relationship of calcium binding to the calcium-specific regulatory site of troponin C during rigor, which is dependent on the number of rigor crossbridges formed (62). It was then shown in ATP-induced contractions of skinned cardiac muscle bundles that at constant sarcomere length, the formation of crossbridges is associated with enhanced binding of calcium to the regulatory site of troponin C (63). Finally, it was shown that under similar conditions, a reduction in sarcomere length is correlated with a reduced binding of calcium to the regulatory site of troponin C (64). The same basic relationships were also described by an independent group of investigators (86).

The detailed physical chemistry of the Ca^{2+}-troponin C interaction is now being worked out (123, 124). It is well-known that active tension drops off at lengths less than the optimal length for force generation much more quickly for cardiac than for skeletal muscle (1), and it is also now known that for the troponin C calcium-specific binding sites, which regulate contraction, there are two for the troponin C isoform from fast skeletal muscle, while there is only one for the isoform from cardiac muscle (124). Interestingly, in skinned skeletal (82) and cardiac (6) muscle, the substitution of the native troponin C isoform in each case with that from the other tissue type causes contractile properties to change to those that are characteristic of the donor tissue type.

In summary, length, load, and time dependence of activation clearly exist in striated muscle and appear to be more marked in the cardiac form. The resultant dependence on these factors of mechanical output and energy utilization throughout contraction appears to be based to some extent on the interaction of these variables with myoplasmic calcium kinetics and to a major extent on the modulation by these variables of the affinity of troponin C for calcium.

Not only is the length-variable performance of the heart regulated by myofilament overlap, but these more newly formulated mechanisms relating mechanics and energetics to the level of activation throughout contraction play a critical and probably dominant role, especially within the physiologic length range for cardiac muscle. Finally, this load and length modulation of activation, especially if it obtains throughout contraction, is inconsistent with the time-varying elastance concept.

ENERGETICS OF ISOLATED LINEAR VERSUS VENTRICULAR MYOCARDIUM

As indicated above, studies of ventricular myocardium suggest that energy utilization is essentially complete at end-systole. Indeed, this is a requisite condition for the time-varying elastance model of ventricular mechanics and energetics. However, the studies from isolated linear myocardium reviewed in the first section demonstrate that myocardial energy utilization is length-, load-, and time-dependent throughout contraction. Further, the studies reviewed in the previous section provide a molecular basis for the effects of these variables on cardiac contraction and energetics. Since there is no reason a priori to think that most of these molecular events differ in kind rather than in degree during the onset as opposed to the offset of contraction, it is difficult to imagine what the molecular basis for an energy-independent relaxation phase of the cardiac contraction might be.

Hill, in 1949, envisioned relaxing muscle as having the same properties as active muscle, but at a continuously diminishing intensity (58). Jewell & Wilkie found evidence in 1960 for mechanical activity throughout the entirety of an isometric skeletal muscle twitch contraction, which was terminated more quickly by active shortening, and they suggested that the mechanical properties of relaxing muscle cannot be explained by means of a passive Maxwellian system of springs and dashpots (70). Similarly, while there are problems in precisely defining a muscle active state formulated as force development at constant contractile element length in terms of either mechanics (19, 71) or heat output (19, 59), it is of interest that Brady conceived of the active state for the isometric cardiac contraction as rising and falling in synchrony with the twitch tension curve when corrected for internal shortening (9, 10). It has also been suggested that relaxation requires energy for calcium reuptake into the relaxing system (25), which appears to be relatively small for cardiac muscle (20), and for residual crossbridge cycling (25), which appears to be relatively large for cardiac muscle (20). Lastly, data indicating that the rate of tension decay during relaxation is directly related to the rate limiting step of myofibrillar ATPase imply a dependence of relaxation kinetics on residual crossbridge cycling (30).

The finding that rapid shortening of isolated cardiac muscle diminishes subsequent force development during that contraction, with this effect becoming progressively more marked after the time of peak tension, also suggests length modulation of an active process during relaxation (113). Similar data regarding load variations gathered during the isotonic papillary muscle contraction (101) and the fact that left ventricular systolic load variations affect relaxation kinetics further support this view (122). Brutsaert, using similar data that demonstrated a dependency of cardiac relaxation kinetics on length and load, formulated a load-dependent relaxation process in terms of an interplay between load, length, and the number of active crossbridges during relaxation, which was thought to be reduced by shortening. Here, shortening-induced deactivation was seen in terms of a loss of load bearing capacity during relaxation, which reflected a reduced number of active crossbridges (13). Other data from his laboratory also suggested the modulation of an active process by length and load changes during cardiac relaxation (47, 110).

Data from skinned insect flight muscle suggests that the load and length dependence of mechanical output might be due not only to effects on calcium entry and myofibrillar calcium binding and sensitivity, but also to a direct mechanical effect on the crossbridges, since the probability of crossbridges being attached is thought to be greater when crossbridge strain is higher, such that unloading hastens crossbridge detachment and thus relaxation (50). As noted before, the load and length dependence of relaxation kinetics on calcium metabolism is also important in mammalian cardiac muscle, which has an active sarcoplasmic reticular calcium pump, since shortening causes release of myofibrillar calcium (66), which is taken up by the sarcoplasmic reticulum rather than reactivating crossbridges, and interventions, which prolong calcium uptake by the sarcoplasmic reticulum, tend to mask the load dependence of cardiac relaxation (89).

Nonetheless, whether by direct physical effects on the crossbridges or by effects on myofibrillar calcium release, shortening during relaxation appears to be modifying an active process; sarcomere stretch resistance, which probably reflects the number of attached crossbridges, is high at low velocity but becomes less as velocity increases, and relative to tension, stretch resistance does not decrease during relaxation (75). Pharmacological studies of cardiac muscle also suggest that relaxation is an active process. Agents that would be expected to affect crossbridge kinetics, but not passive muscle elastic properties, alter relaxation kinetics (87), even during the terminal 5% of force decay (88).

Real-time measurements of energetics by NMR during the heartbeat also provide some suggestion that high energy phosphate utilization continues throughout the entire cardiac contraction. The levels of myocardial ATP and creatine phosphate begin to decrease at the beginning of contraction and do not return to baseline until relaxation is complete (42, 119). The most compelling real-time evidence of crossbridge activity throughout contraction, however, is provided by X-ray diffraction studies that show that myosin heads transfer to the vicinity of the thin filament at the onset of the isometric cardiac twitch contraction and return to the vicinity of the thick filament with a time course that corresponds fully to that of the decay of isometric active tension (79). X-ray studies of skeletal muscle show similar crossbridge behavior throughout the isometric twitch contraction and further show that shortening results in a large number of these crossbridges detaching (68). Since both of these X-ray diffraction studies were done under conditions of metabolic support wherein the existence of rigor bridges would be extremely unlikely, it would seem virtually impossible that the crossbridges detected during relaxation could somehow be responsible for energy-independent mechanical output.

Nevertheless, the available evidence from ventricular myocardium would suggest that relaxation is indeed essentially energy-independent. It has been found that fully 90% of the MVO_2 of isovolumic ventricular contraction is accounted for by the time that peak systolic pressure is reached (81), and this finding has been confirmed in two more recent studies (26, 120). Indeed, these findings constitute the most decisive experimental support for the time-varying elastance model of ventricular contraction in terms of energetic measurements.

In terms of this model, energy usage past the time of end-systole would consist entirely of the dissipation of potential energy stored between the onset of activation and the time of end-systole (105), although the molecular mechanisms that might account for this being a dynamic process subject to regulation remain unknown and unaccountable thus far. It is important to reemphasize that in contrast to the ventricular data are those data that show in isolated cardiac muscle both that substantial energy utilization continues past the time of peak tension in the isometric twitch contraction, and that MVO_2 is length-, load-, and time-dependent throughout both isometric and isotonic cardiac contractions (20–22, 61). Further, another tenet of the time-varying elastance model, that the energy cost of a given mechanical output is constant through end-systole, has been contradicted both in isolated cardiac muscle (20) and in the left ventricle (112). Indeed, shortening-induced deactivation has been seen by Suga in the perfused in situ dog heart (108), and both Sagawa (96) and Suga (120) have identified difficulties of the time-varying elastance concept in dealing with the consequences of length changes during contraction. Finally, as stated before (32, 61), the time to end-systole is load-dependent in isolated heart muscle, which again is contrary to the tenets of the time-varying elastance model.

These data, and the preponderance of the other data reviewed herein, strongly suggest that the time-varying elastance model is fundamentally flawed. It cannot account for the load, length, and time dependence either of contractile and energetic processes or of regulatory processes during cardiac contraction, and this is true on both the tissue and the molecular levels. However, a dismissive approach to this model (31) serves little useful purpose. What is needed is an understanding both specifically of the contrasting data regarding isolated linear and ventricular myocardial energetics during relaxation and more generally of the reasons that the time-varying elastance model has been so successful pragmatically in describing most of the mechanical and energetic behavior of the intact heart.

With respect to the energetics of relaxation, comparisons of ventricular with isolated linear myocardial contraction are complicated by fact that in the ventricle there is considerable dispersion in time both of the onset of contraction and of the duration of mechanical activity within this large and architecturally complex chamber (12, 33). Such heterogeneity of geometric properties and of activation time, and thus of regional stiffness during contraction, may well account for the finding that for contractions in which there is no developed tension, the MVO_2 for the ventricle is fully 40% of that for an isovolumic contraction (26), while for a papillary muscle it is only 14% of that for an isometric contraction (20). Quick release deactivates the entire homogeneously activated papillary muscle, thereby terminating MVO_2 (20), but when quick release is used in studies of the time course of ventricular energetics (26, 81, 120) in an attempt to deactivate the ventricle, it apparently fails to do so, as is shown by the high residual MVO_2 (26). It would appear that the left ventricle, when externally unloaded during systole, continues to exhibit regional work and shortening imposed by regional differences in time-dependent stiffness and regional internal load. The fact that major shape changes and shortening-induced deactivation occur in the isovolumic left ventricle prior to the time of end-systole only compounds the problem of knowing when end-systole is for a given fiber within the left ventricular myocardium. Because of these considerations, while the time of end-systole is easily defined in terms of chamber mechanics, it is probably not possible to relate this to time-varying concepts of mechanics and energetics that assume myocardial homogeneity.

In order to understand the practical success of the time-varying elastance model in describing mechanics and energetics, it is useful to consider the contrast between the Fenn effect as observed in skeletal and cardiac muscle. Fenn originally described for skeletal muscle greater heat liberation during substantially afterloaded isotonic contractions than that for isometric contractions at optimum length (40); Fischer later confirmed this in terms of MVO_2 (41), thus vitiating concerns (19) about metabolic heat liberated during muscle movement being contaminated by degraded mechanical energy (57).

However, the Fenn effect, as observed in skeletal muscle has not been demonstrated in cardiac muscle (90), such that we are effectively returned to the finding of Beclard (7) in 1861 that isometric heat production is greater than isotonic. Instead, the increased energy liberation seen in isotonic as compared with isometric contractions is only observed in cardiac muscle when the two types of contraction are compared at equivalent loads and at initial lengths less than the optimal length for tension generation (18). For cardiac muscle, and indeed for skeletal muscle at physiologic temperatures, the importance of the Fenn effect lies not so much in its quantitative value but rather in its demonstration of the phenomenon of load regulation of muscle energetics during contraction.

In retrospect, given the greater slope of length-dependent tension generation in cardiac as opposed to skeletal muscle, and the apparent dependence of this difference largely on their respective troponin C isoforms, the reason for both the relatively minor expression of the Fenn effect in cardiac muscle and the pragmatic success of the time-varying elastance model when applied to cardiac muscle becomes apparent. In a manner analogous to the way in which opposing influences of ejection act via length-dependent activation effects to make ventricular end-systolic pressure relatively load-independent (67), shortening against a load causes increased energy utilization (18), but it also causes deactivation, and this effect is especially prominent in cardiac muscle. These two opposing energetic consequences of cardiac shortening may explain the relative constancy of ventricular energy utilization at end-systole for a given pressure-volume area despite differing systolic mechanical conditions. Further, this may explain both why the Fenn effect is not as prominent in cardiac muscle and, for the same reasons, why the time-varying elastance model works fairly well for describing, but not for explaining, the relation of cardiac mechanics to energetics.

SUMMARY

Crossbridge cycling and consequent energy utilization during contraction are subject to physiologic regulation by load and length; the length effect on the sensitivity of troponin C to a given $[Ca^{2+}]_i$ is an important, newly defined mechanism for this length regulation in cardiac muscle. Further, energy utilization persists throughout the cardiac contraction, demonstrably for isometric contractions initiated at optimal length, and is continuously modulated by length changes during variably loaded twitch contractions. The extent, rate, and time of load-induced length changes during myocardial contraction appear to be the primary variables affecting crossbridge activity and energetics.

Load and length regulation of the properties of the heart represents a remarkably simple and direct biological response to the physiologic input and role in this organ. This mechanism is utilized by the heart in response to its dynamic loading environment both for long-term adaptation of cardiac mass to chronic load alterations, as discussed here recently (23), and for short-term adaptation of cardiac mechanics and energetics to instantaneous load alterations, as discussed above. It is probably no coincidence, given their central physiologic importance, that both of these most basic adaptive responses of the heart are simultaneously coming to be understood at the molecular level.

ACKNOWLEDGMENTS

Support during the preparation of this review was provided by Grants HL29146, HL37196, and HL38124 from the National Institutes of Health, by a V.A. Clinical Investigator Award, and by V.A. research funds.

Literature Cited

1. Allen, D. G., Jewell, B. R., Murray, J. W. 1974. The contribution of activation processes to the length-tension relation of cardiac muscle. *Nature* 248:606–7
2. Allen, D. G., Kentish, J. C. 1985. The cellular basis of the length-tension relation in cardiac muscle. *J. Mol. Cell. Cardiol.* 17:821–40
3. Allen, D. G., Kurihara, S. 1982. The effects of muscle length on intracellular calcium transients in mammalian cardiac muscle. *J. Physiol.* 327:79–94
4. Alpert, N. R., Mulieri, L. A., Litten, R. Z. 1983. Isoenzyme contribution to economy of contraction and relaxation in normal and hypertrophied hearts. In *Cardiac Adaptation to Hemodynamic Overload, Training and Stress*, ed. R. Jacob, R. W. Gulch, G. Kissling, pp. 147–57. Darmstadt: Steinkopff Verlag. 373 pp.
5. Ashley, C. C., Ridgway, E. B. 1970. On the relationships between membrane potential, calcium transient and tension in single barnacle muscle fibers. *J. Physiol.* 209:105–30
6. Babu, A., Sonnenblick, E. H., Gulati, J. 1988. Molecular basis for the influence of muscle length on myocardial performance. *Science* 240:74–76
7. Beclard, J. 1861. De la contraction musculaire dans ses rapports avec la temperature animale. *Arch. Gen. Med.* 1:24–40, 157–80, 257–79
8. Bodem, R., Skelton, C. L., Sonnenblick, E. H. 1976. Inactivation of contraction as a determinant of the length-active tension relation in heart muscle of the cat. *Res. Exp. Med.* 168:1–13

9. Brady, A. J. 1968. Active state in cardiac muscle. *Physiol. Rev.* 48:570–600
10. Brady, A. J. 1971. A measurement of the active state in heart muscle. *Cardiovasc. Res.* 5(Suppl. 1):11–17
11. Braunwald, E. 1971. Control of myocardial oxygen consumption: Physiologic and clinical implications. *Am. J. Cardiol.* 27:416–32
12. Brutsaert, D. L. 1987. Nonuniformity: A physiologic modulator of contraction and relaxation of the normal heart. *J. Am. Coll. Cardiol.* 9:341–48
13. Brutsaert, D. L., De Clerck, N. M., Goethals, M. A., Housmans, P. R. 1978. Relaxation of ventricular cardiac muscle. *J. Physiol.* 283:469–80
14. Challoner, D. R. 1968. Respiration in myocardium. *Nature* 217:78–79
15. Chapman, J. B., Gibbs, C. L., Loiselle, D. S. 1982. Myothermic, polarographic, and fluorometric data from mammalian muscles. *Fed. Proc.* 41:176–84
16. Chuck, L. H. S., Parmley, W. W. 1980. Caffeine reversal of length-dependent changes in myocardial contractile state in the cat. *Circ. Res.* 47:592–98
17. Coleman, H. N. 1969. Mechanical determinants of oxygen consumption of isolated cat papillary muscle. *Ala. J. Med. Sci.* 6:121–34
18. Coleman, H. N., Sonnenblick, E H., Braunwald, E. 1969. Myocardial oxygen consumption associated with external work: The Fenn effect. *Am. J. Physiol.* 217:291–96
19. Cooper, G. 1976. The myocardial energetic active state: Oxygen consump-

tion during tetanus of cat papillary muscle. *Circ. Res.* 39:695–704

20. Cooper, G. 1979. Myocardial energetics during isometric twitch contractions of cat papillary muscle. *Am. J. Physiol.* 236:H244–53

21. Cooper, G. 1981. Influence of length changes on myocardial metabolism in the cat papillary muscle. *Circ. Res.* 49:423–33

22. Cooper, G. 1981. Length and load dependent metabolism during isotonic contraction of cat papillary muscle. *Fed. Proc.* 40:460 (Abstr.)

23. Cooper, G. 1987. Cardiocyte adaptation to chronically altered load. *Annu. Rev. Physiol.* 49:501–18

24. Coulson, R. L. 1976. Energetics of isovolumic contractions of the isolated rabbit heart. *J. Physiol.* 260:45–53

25. Curtin, N. A., Woledge, R. C. 1978. Energy changes and muscular contraction. *Physiol. Rev.* 58:690–761

26. Duwel, C. M. B., Westerhof, N. 1988. Feline left ventricular oxygen consumption is not affected by volume expansion, ejection or redevelopment of pressure during relaxation. *Pflügers Arch.* 412:409–16

27. Edman, K. A. P. 1975. Mechanical deactivation induced by active shortening in isolated muscle fibers of the frog. *J. Physiol.* 246:255–75

28. Edman, K. A. P., Nilsson, E. 1968. The mechanical parameters of myocardial contraction studied at a constant length of the contractile element. *Acta Physiol. Scand.* 72:205–19

29. Edman, K. A. P., Nilsson, E. 1971. Time course of the active state in relation to muscle length and movement: A comparative study on skeletal muscle and myocardium. *Cardiovasc. Res.* 5(Suppl.1):3–10

30. Edwards, R. H. T., Hill, D. K., Jones, D. A. 1975. Metabolic changes associated with the slowing of relaxation in fatigued mouse muscle. *J. Physiol.* 251:287–301

31. Elzinga, G., Mast, F., Westerhof, N. 1989. Left ventricular time varying elastance behavior does not reflect a basic property of cardiac muscle. *Circ. Res.* 64:629–30

32. Elzinga, G., Westerhof, N. 1981. "Pressure-volume" relations in isolated cat trabecula. *Circ. Res.* 49:388–94

33. Elzinga, G., Westerhof, N. 1982. Isolated cat trabeculae in a simulated feline heart and arterial system. *Circ. Res.* 51:430–38

34. Elzinga, G., Westerhof, N. 1984. Does the history of contraction affect the pressure-volume relationship? *Fed. Proc.* 43:2402–7

35. Endo, M. 1972. Length dependence of activation of skinned muscle fibers by calcium. *Cold Spring Harbor Symp. Quant. Biol.* 37:505–10

36. Endo, M. 1972. Stretch-induced increase in activation of skinned muscle fibers by calcium. *Nature New Biol.* 237:211–13

37. Evans, C. L., Matsuoka, Y. 1915. The effect of various mechanical conditions on the gaseous metabolism and efficiency of the mammalian heart. *J. Physiol.* 49:378–405

38. Fabiato, A. 1981. Myoplasmic free calcium concentration reached during the twitch of an intact isolated cardiac cell and during calcium-induced release of calcium from the sarcoplasmic reticulum of a skinned cardiac cell from the adult rat or rabbit ventricle. *J. Gen. Physiol.* 78:457–97

39. Fabiato, A., Fabiato, F. 1975. Dependence of the contractile activation of skinned cardiac cells on the sarcomere length. *Nature* 256:54–56

40. Fenn, W. O. 1923. A quantitative comparison between the energy liberated and the work performed by the isolated sartorius muscle of the frog. *J. Physiol.* 58:175–203

41. Fischer, E. 1931. The oxygen consumption of isolated muscles for isotonic and isometric twitches. *Am. J. Physiol.* 96:78–88

42. Fossel, E. T., Morgan, H. E., Ingwall, J. S. 1980. Measurement of changes in high energy phosphates in the cardiac cycle by using gated ^{31}P nuclear magnetic resonance. *Proc. Natl. Acad. Sci. USA* 77:3654–58

43. Fuchs, F. 1978. On the relation between filament overlap and the number of calcium binding sites on glycerinated muscle fibers. *Biophys. J.* 21:273–77

44. Gibbs, C. L. 1978. Cardiac energetics. *Physiol. Rev.* 58:174–254

45. Gibbs, C. L., Chapman, J. B. 1979. Cardiac heat production. *Annu. Rev. Physiol.* 41:507–19

46. Gibbs, C. L., Chapman, J. B. 1985. Cardiac mechanics and energetics: Chemomechanical transduction in cardiac muscle. *Am. J. Physiol.* 249:H199–206

47. Goethals, M. A., Housmans, P. R., Brutsaert, D. L. 1982. Loading determinants of relaxation in cat papillary muscle. *Am. J. Physiol.* 242:H303–9

48. Gordan, A. M., Ridgway, E. B. 1976. Length-dependent electromechanical coupling in single muscle fibers. *J. Gen. Physiol.* 68:653–69

49. Gordon, A. M., Ridgway, E. B., Martyn, D. A. 1984. Calcium sensitivity is modified by contraction. *Adv. Exp. Med. Biol.* 170:553–63

50. Guth, K., Kuhn, H. J., Tsuchiya, T., Ruegg, J. C. 1981. Length dependent state of activation—length change dependent kinetics of cross bridges in skinned insect flight muscle. *Biophys. Struct. Mech.* 7:139–69

51. Hartree, W., Hill, A. V. 1922. The heat-production and the mechanism of the veratrine contraction. *J. Physiol.* 56:294–300

52. Helmholtz, H. 1845. Ueber den stoffverbrauch bei der muskelaction. *Mueller's Arch. Anat. Physiol.* 72–83

53. Helmholtz, H. 1848. Ueber die warmeentwicklung der muskelaction. *Mueller's Arch. Anat. Physiol.* 144–64

54. Henderson, A. H., Cattell, M. R. 1976. Length-induced changes in activation during contraction. *Circ. Res.* 38:289–96

55. Hibberd, M. G., Jewell, B. R. 1982. Calcium- and length-dependent force production in rat ventricular muscle. *J. Physiol.* 329:527–40

56. Hill, A. V. 1930. The heat production in isometric and isotonic twitches. *Proc. R. Soc. London Ser. B* 107:115–31

57. Hill, A. V. 1938. The heat of shortening and the dynamic constants of muscle. *Proc. R. Soc. London Ser. B* 126:136–95

58. Hill, A. V. 1949. The abrupt transition from rest to activity in muscle. *Proc. R. Soc. London Ser. B* 136:399–420

59. Hill, A. V. 1961. The heat produced by a muscle after the last shock of a tetanus. *J. Physiol.* 159:518–45

60. Hill, A. V. 1964. The effect of tension in prolonging the active state in a twitch. *Proc. R. Soc. London Ser. B* 159:589–95

61. Hisano, R., Cooper, G. 1987. Correlation of force-length area with oxygen consumption in ferret papillary muscle. *Circ. Res.* 61:318–28

62. Hofmann, P. A., Fuchs, F. 1987. Effect of length and cross-bridge attachment on calcium binding to cardiac troponin C. *Am. J. Physiol.* 253:C90–96

63. Hofmann, P. A., Fuchs, F. 1987. Evidence for a force-dependent component of calcium binding to cardiac troponin C. *Am. J. Physiol.* 253:C541–46

64. Hofmann, P. A., Fuchs, F. 1988. Bound calcium and force development in skinned cardiac muscle bundles: Effect of sarcomere length. *J. Mol. Cell. Cardiol.* 20:667–77

65. Honig, C. R., Reddy, Y. S. 1975. Interaction of Ca^{++} binding sites of troponin: Significance for Ca^{++} movements. *Am. J. Physiol.* 228:172–78

66. Housmans, P. R., Lee, N. K. M., Blinks, J. R. 1983. Active shortening retards the decline of the intracellular calcium transient in mammalian heart muscle. *Science* 221:159–61

67. Hunter, W. C. 1989. End-systolic pressure as a balance between opposing effects of ejection. *Circ. Res.* 64:265–75

68. Huxley, H. E., Kress, M., Faruqi, A. F., Simmons, R. M. 1988. X-ray diffraction studies on muscle during rapid shortening and their implications concerning crossbridge behavior. *Adv. Exp. Med. Biol.* 226:347–52

69. Jewell, B. R. 1977. A reexamination of the influence of muscle length on myocardial performance. *Circ. Res.* 40:221–30

70. Jewell, B. R., Wilkie, D. R. 1960. The mechanical properties of relaxing muscle. *J. Physiol.* 152:30–47

71. Julian, F. J., Moss, R. L. 1976. The concept of active state in striated muscle. *Circ. Res.* 38:53–59

72. Julian, F. J., Sollins, M. R. 1975. Variation of muscle stiffness with force at increasing speeds of shortening. *J. Gen. Physiol.* 66:287–302

73. Kaufmann, R. L., Bayer, R. M., Harnasch, C. 1972. Autoregulation of contractility in the myocardial cell. *Pflügers Arch.* 332:96–116

74. Kaufmann, R. L., Lab, M. J., Hennekes, R., Krause, H. 1971. Feedback interaction of mechanical and electrical events in the isolated mammalian ventricular myocardium (cat papillary muscle). *Pflügers Arch.* 324:100–23

75. Krueger, J. W., Tsujioka, K., Okada, T., Peskin, C. S., Lacker, H. M. 1988. A "give" in tension and sarcomere dynamics in cardiac muscle relaxation. *Adv. Exp. Med. Biol.* 226:567–80

76. Lab, M. J., Allen, D. G., Orchard, C. H. 1984. The effects of shortening on myoplasmic calcium concentration and on the action potential in mammalian ventricular muscle. *Circ. Res.* 55:825–29

77. Lakatta, E. G., Jewell, B. R. 1977. Length-dependent activation: Its effect on the length-tension relation in cat ventricular muscle. *Circ. Res.* 40:251–57

78. Lew, W. Y. W. 1988. Time-dependent increase in left ventricular contractility following acute volume loading in the dog. *Circ. Res.* 63:635–47

79. Matsubara, I., Yagi, N., Endoh, M.

1979. Movement of myosin heads during a heart beat. *Nature* 278:474–76
80. McDonald, R. H., Taylor, R. R., Cingolani, H. E. 1966. Measurement of myocardial developed tension and its relation to oxygen consumption. *Am. J. Physiol.* 211:667–73
81. Monroe, R. G. 1964. Myocardial oxygen consumption during ventricular contraction and relaxation. *Circ. Res.* 14:294–300
82. Moss, R. L., Lauer, M. R., Giulian, G. G., Greaser, M. L. 1986. Altered Ca++ dependence of tension development in skinned skeletal muscle fibers following modification of troponin by partial substitution with cardiac troponin C. *J. Biol. Chem.* 261:6096–99
83. Neely, J. R., Liebermeister, H., Battersby, E. J., Morgan, H. E. 1967. Effect of pressure development on oxygen consumption by isolated rat heart. *Am. J. Physiol.* 212:804–14
84. Nozawa, T., Yasumura, Y., Futaki, S., Tanaka, N., Igarashi, Y., et al. 1987. Relation between oxygen consumption and pressure-volume area of in situ dog heart. *Am. J. Physiol.* 253:H31–40
85. Palladino, J. L., Porter, P. K., Melbin, J., Noordergraaf, A. 1987. An energy exchange-based theory of cardiac muscle contraction. In *Simulation and Control of the Cardiac System*, ed. S. Sideman, R. Beyar, 3:85–118. Boca Raton, Fla: CRC Press. 215 pp.
86. Pan, B., Solaro, R. J. 1987. Calcium-binding properties of troponin C in detergent-skinned heart muscle fibers. *J. Biol. Chem.* 262:7839–49
87. Parmley, W. W., Sonnenblick, E. H. 1969. Relation between mechanics of contraction and relaxation in mammalian cardiac muscle. *Am. J. Physiol.* 216:1084–91
88. Peterson, J. N. 1989. *A study of the mechanisms underlying relaxation in isolated mammalian cardiac muscle.* PhD thesis. Johns Hopkins Univ., Baltimore, Md. 275 pp.
89. Poggesi, C., Reggiani, C., Ricciardi, L., Minelli, R. 1982. Factors modulating the sensitivity of the relaxation to the loading conditions in rat cardiac muscle. *Pflügers Arch.* 394:338–46
90. Rall, J. A. 1982. Sense and nonsense about the Fenn effect. *Am. J. Physiol.* 242:H1–6
91. Ridgway, E. B., Gordon, A. M. 1975. Muscle activation: Effects of small length changes on calcium release in single fibers. *Science* 189:881–84
92. Ridgway, E. B., Gordon, A. M. 1984. Muscle calcium transient: Effect of post-

stimulus length changes in single fibers. *J. Gen. Physiol.* 83:75–103
93. Ridgway, E. B., Gordon, A. M., Martyn, D. A. 1983. Hysteresis in the force-calcium relation in muscle. *Science* 219:1075–77
94. Rodbard, S., Williams, C. B., Rodbard, D., Berglund, E. 1964. Myocardial tension and oxygen uptake. *Circ. Res.* 14:139–49
95. Rohde, E. 1912. Uber den einfluss der mechanischen bedingungen auf die tatigkeit und den sauerstoffverbrauch der warmbluterherzens. *Arch. Exp. Pathol. Pharmakol.* 68:401–34
96. Sagawa, K. 1978. The ventricular pressure-volume diagram revisited.. *Circ. Res.* 43:677–87
97. Sarnoff, S. J., Braunwald, E., Welch, G. H., Case, R. B., Stainsby, W. N., et al. 1958. Hemodynamic determinants of oxygen consumption of the heart with special reference to the tension-time index. *Am. J. Physiol.* 192:148–56
98. Solaro, R. J., Ruegg, J. C. 1982. Stimulation of Ca++ binding and ATPase activity of dog cardiac myofibrils by AR-L 115 BS, a novel cardiotonic agent. *Circ. Res.* 51:290–94
99. Sonnenblick, E. H., Skelton, C. L. 1971. Myocardial energetics: Basic principles and clinical implications. *New Engl. J. Med.* 285:668–75
100. Stephenson, D. G., Wendt, I. R. 1984. Length dependence of changes in sarcoplasmic calcium concentration and myofibrillar calcium sensitivity in striated muscle fibers. *J. Muscle Res. Cell Motil.* 5:243–72
101. Strauer, B. E. 1973. Force-velocity relations of isotonic relaxation in mammalian heart muscle. *Am. J. Physiol.* 224:431–34
102. Suga, H. 1969. Time course of left ventricular pressure-volume relationship under various end-diastolic volumes. *Jpn. Heart J.* 10:509–15
103. Suga, H. 1970. Time course of left ventricular pressure-volume relationship under various extents of aortic occlusion. *Jpn. Heart J.* 11:373–78
104. Suga, H. 1979. Total mechanical energy of a ventricle model and cardiac oxygen consumption. *Am. J. Physiol.* 236: H498–505
105. Suga, H. 1980. Relaxing ventricle performs more external mechanical work than quickly released elastic energy. *Eur. Heart J.* 1(Suppl. A):131–37
106. Suga, H., Hayashi, T., Suehiro, S., Hisano, R., Shirahata, M., et al. 1981. Equal oxygen consumption rates of isovolumic and ejecting contractions

with equal systolic pressure-volume areas in canine left ventricle. *Circ. Res.* 49:1082–91

107. Suga, H., Yamada, O., Goto, Y. 1984. Energetics of ventricular contraction as traced in the pressure-volume diagram. *Fed. Proc.* 43:2411–13

108. Suga, H., Yamakoshi, K. 1977. Reduction of the duration of isovolumic relaxation in the ejecting left ventricle of the dog: Residual volume clamping. *J. Physiol.* 267:63–74

109. Sugiura, S., Hunter, W. C., Sagawa, K. 1989. Long-term versus intrabeat history of ejection as determinants of canine ventricular end-systolic pressure. *Circ. Res.* 64:255–64

110. Sys, S. U., Paulus, W. J., Claes, V. A., Brutsaert, D. L. 1987. Post-reextension force decay of relaxing cardiac muscle. *Am. J. Physiol.* 253:H256–61

111. Taylor, S. R., Rudel, R. 1970. Striated muscle fibers: Inactivation of contraction induced by shortening. *Science* 167:882–84

112. Teplick, R., Haas, G. S., Trautman, E., Titus, J., Geffin, G., et al. 1986. Time dependence of the oxygen cost of force development during systole in the canine left ventricle. *Circ. Res.* 59:27–38

113. ter Keurs, H. E. D. J., Rijnsburger, W. H., Van Heuningen, R. 1980. Restoring forces and relaxation of rat cardiac muscle. *Eur. Heart J.* 1(Suppl. A):67–80

114. ter Keurs, H. E. D. J., Rijnsburger, W. H., Van Heuningen, R., Nagelsmit, M. J. 1980. Tension development and sarcomere length in rat cardiac trabeculae: Evidence of length-dependent activation. *Circ. Res.* 46:703–14

115. Tucci, P. J. F., Bregagnollo, E. A., Spadaro, J., Cicogna, A. C., Ribeiro, M. C. L. 1984. Length dependence of activation studied in the isovolumic blood-perfused dog heart. *Circ. Res.* 55:59–66

116. Warner, H. R. 1959. The use of an analog computer for analysis of control mechanisms in the circulation. *Proc. Inst. Radio Electron. Engs. Aust.* 47:1913–16

117. Weber, K. T., Janicki, J. S. 1977. Myocardial oxygen consumption: The role of wall force and shortening. *Am. J. Physiol.* 233:H421–30

118. Wier, W. G. 1980. Calcium transients during excitation-contraction coupling in mammalian heart: Aequorin signals of canine Purkinje fibers. *Science* 207: 1085–87

119. Wikman-Coffelt, J., Sievers, R., Coffelt, R. J., Parmley, W. W. 1983. The cardiac cycle: Regulation and energy oscillations. *Am. J. Physiol.* 245:H354–62

120. Yasumura, Y., Nozawa, T., Futaki, S., Tanaka, N., Suga, H. 1989. Time-invariant oxygen cost of mechanical energy in dog left ventricle: Consistency and inconsistency of time-varying elastance model with myocardial energetics. *Circ. Res.* 64:764–78

121. Yue, D. T. 1987. Intracellular [Ca^{++}] related to rate of force development in twitch contraction of heart. *Am. J. Physiol.* 252:H760–70

122. Zatko, F. J., Martin, P., Bahler, R. C. 1987. Time course of systolic loading is an important determinant of ventricular relaxation. *Am. J. Physiol.* 252:H461–66

123. Zot, A. S., Potter, J. D. 1987. Structural aspects of troponin-tropomyosin regulation of skeletal muscle contraction. *Annu. Rev. Biophys. Biophys. Chem.* 16:535–59

124. Zot, H. G., Guth, K., Potter, J. D. 1986. Fast skeletal muscle skinned fibers and myofibrils reconstituted with N-terminal fluorescent analogs of troponin C. *J. Biol. Chem.* 261:15883–90

Annu. Rev. Physiol. 1990. 52:523–42

CONTROL OF MITOCHONDRIAL RESPIRATION IN THE HEART IN VIVO[1]

F. W. Heineman and R. S. Balaban

Laboratory of Cardiac Energetics, National Institutes of Health/NHLBI, Bethesda, Maryland 20892

KEY WORDS: oxidative phosphorylation, myocardium, cardiac, control, metabolism

INTRODUCTION

Cardiac myocytes must respond rapidly to the wide variations of myosin ATPase activity associated with changes in workload. These demands are met by the continuous conversion of energy from highly reduced substrates to phosphate bonds. Adenosine triphosphate (ATP) constitutes the major cytosolic intermediate in this energy transducing process. ATP is produced by glycolysis and oxidative phosphorylation from the oxidation of fats, sugars, tricarboxylates, and peptides. Mitochondrial oxidative phosphorylation produces the majority of ATP necessary for cardiac function, whereas glycolysis plays a relatively minor role (60, 68). For this reason, the regulation of mitochondrial oxidative phosphorylation is vital for balancing cardiac ATP production and breakdown. Due to its high rate of ATP hydrolysis, the myocardium has a limited tolerance for a deficit in ATP production. Indeed, studies of work and respiration in the heart indicate that these two processes are closely linked (68). Thus an effective communication network must exist between mitochondrial ATP production and cytosolic ATP hydrolysis by myosin ATPase, which results in the coordination of energy supply and demand.

[1]The US Government has the right to retain a nonexclusive, royalty-free license in and to any copyright covering this paper.

Although it is accepted that the control of myocardial respiration plays a central role in cardiac energetics, the nature of this control has remained controversial (23, 28, 34, 56, 73, 80). The results of many studies applying recently developed techniques, particularly the adaptation of nuclear magnetic resonance (NMR) and optical spectroscopy to in vivo conditions, have questioned much of the dogma concerning this process. The objective of this review is to present the potential sites for feedback control of oxidative phosphorylation in the intact heart and the current experimental evidence concerning the possible role of these sites as mediators. As previous reviews of this topic have been based to a great extent on studies using isolated cells and mitochondria (out of a lack of other available data rather than by omission), we intend to focus on data from intact hearts and in vivo conditions wherever possible.

Overview of Oxidative Phosphorylation

The biochemical and thermodynamic details of ATP formation by oxidative phosphorylation have been discussed in several reviews (58, 61, 70) and the reader interested in the specifics of these reactions should refer to them. The major steps of the metabolic pathways as they apply to the possible regulatory mechanisms at our current level of understanding are schematically presented in Figure 1. We have arbitrarily divided ATP production into three general areas for the purpose of discussion: delivery of reducing equivalents to the electron transport chain; coupling of the oxidation/reduction free energy change (ΔG) at sites along the chain to proton ejection and subsequent phosphorylation of adenosine diphosphate (ADP); and the reduction of molecular oxygen to water.

The reducing equivalents used to drive coupled electron transport are provided by multiple biochemical pathways. In the general scheme of energy conservation, the electron transport chain serves as a point of convergence in catabolism. In the specific case of myocardial energy metabolism, however, cytosolic pyruvate and fatty acids are of primary importance (60). Figure 1 (I) summarizes the supply-side of the energy conversion process. Electrons from these compounds gain access to the electron transport chain via the pyridine-linked dehydrogenases (as, for example, with pyruvate) and flavin-linked dehydrogenases (such as fatty acyl-CoA and succinate). Since these enzymes are in a position to limit the flow of reducing equivalents to the phosphorylation sites, they are potentially capable of serving as modulators of the respiratory chain (27). Limiting the availability of substrates to these enzymes could function in a similar manner. These possibilities, along with the other potential regulatory sites, will be discussed later.

The next stage in ATP production by the mitochondria (Figure 1-II) is the actual coupling of the redox ΔG to the phosphorylation of ADP. According

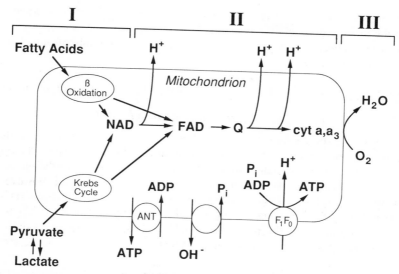

Figure 1 Major steps in oxidative phosphorylation. (I) Reducing equivalent supply from the Krebs Cycle and β-oxidation to the electron transport chain via pyridine- and flavin-linked dehydrogenases (NAD = nicotinamide adenine dinucleotide, FAD = flavin adenine di-nucleotide). (II) Steps involved in coupling the ΔG from extrusion of protons from the mitochondrion by the cytochrome chain to the formation of ATP (ATP = adenosine 5'-triphosphate, ADP = adenosine 5'-diphosphate, P_i = inorganic phosphorus, ANT = adenine nucleotide translocase, F_1F_O = F_1F_O proton-ATP synthase, Q = coenzyme Q (ubiquinone), cyt a,a_3 = cytochrome a,a_3). (III) Reduction of molecular oxygen to water.

to the chemiosmotic theory developed by Mitchell (58), reducing equivalents entering the respiratory chain are used to generate an electrochemical gradient (Δp) across the proton-impermeable inner mitochondrial membrane. The potential from this proton gradient is used, in turn, to drive ATP formation by the F_1F_O proton-ATPase. Clearly, there are numerous possibilities in this process that could influence the rate of ATP formation, which include modulation of Δp, the activity of the F_1F_O ATPase, and availability of ADP and inorganic phosphate (P_i).

Oxygen serves the electron transport chain as the terminal acceptor of electrons from the cytochrome aa_3 complex and, in doing so, is reduced to form water (Figure 1-III). Perhaps no other requirement of myocardial metabolism has been so clearly demonstrated in vivo as the need for an adequate supply of oxygen. Cardiac performance quickly deteriorates in the face of hypoxia, a fact that underlines the dependence of the heart on mitochondrial respiration as a means of ATP production (68). However, hypoxia and ischemia are pathologic conditions. The role of oxygen delivery as a regulator of respiration under normal conditions is more controversial

(11, 36, 87). Oxygen delivery to the cells, intracellular diffusion gradients, and the affinity of cytochrome aa$_3$ for O$_2$ could all alter the rate of electron transfer to molecular oxygen and, consequently, affect the rate of mitochondrial ATP formation.

REGULATION AT THE LEVEL OF PHOSPHORYLATION

ADP, ATP, and P$_i$ as Metabolic Feedback Signals

The results of studies on isolated mitochondria comprise the majority of the information available concerning the regulation of oxidative phosphorylation. This technique remains central to the study of oxidative phosphorylation as it allows many variables to be controlled. It should be remembered, however, that the composition of the medium surrounding isolated mitochondria is determined by the investigator, not the cell. Furthermore, the mitochondria have undergone rather drastic physical and environmental alterations during the isolation process, which potentially create a very nonphysiologic state (68).

Early experiments on isolated mitochondria demonstrated a direct relation of the concentrations of ATP hydrolysis products (ADP and P$_i$) to the rates of O$_2$ consumption and ATP production (10, 50). This observation resulted in an elegantly simple model of respiratory control that proposed that increases in cytosolic ADP and P$_i$, which result from the increase in ATP hydrolysis act as feedback between the energy demands of the cell and its rate of ATP production. A controversy arose after these initial in vitro observations about whether phosphate metabolites exert control over respiration through a kinetic or thermodynamic mechanism. The kinetic models propose that the ratio of ATP and ADP or the cytosolic concentrations of ADP and P$_i$ are the important controlling parameters (10, 28, 74), while thermodynamic models assign this role to the cytosolic phosphorylation potential (e.g. [ATP]/[ADP][P$_i$]) (28, 44, 62).

Kinetic control of oxidative phosphorylation by the ATP hydrolysis products was proposed by Lardy & Wellman (50) as well as by Chance & Williams (10). This mechanism attributes the balance between ATP formation and hydrolysis to the direct effects of ADP and P$_i$ concentrations on one or more of the reactions involved in ATP synthesis (Figure 1-II). This is an attractive hypothesis since the end-product feedback of ADP and P$_i$ on the mitochondria from the breakdown of ATP provides a plausible mechanism of respiratory control. Whether the effects of these metabolites act through a simple kinetic effect on the phosphorylation process, by altering the adenine nucleotide translocase activity (74, 78), or by participating in a creatine/PCr cytosolic shuttle (5, 34) or facilitated diffusion (57) is unclear. In support of the translocase being the site of kinetic control, there is evidence of an

[ATP]/[ADP] gradient across the inner mitochondrial membrane (26, 74). It has also been shown that gradual inhibition of this carrier quickly impinges on the respiratory capacity of the cells in vitro (1). While these findings are consistent with the translocase playing a role in mitochondrial regulation, their significance in terms of regulation in vivo is still under debate (72). Tissue extraction (88) and ^{31}P NMR (41, 42) data have placed the free cytosolic concentrations of cardiac ADP and P_i in vivo near their in vitro K_m values for oxidative phosphorylation (17, 18, 35). These findings also are consistent with, but not proof of, kinetic feedback by phosphate metabolites playing a role in regulating myocardial oxidative phosphorylation.

Thermodynamic control models of respiration hypothesize that the reactions of the cytochrome chain are near equilibrium (hence the name near equilibrium hypothesis) except for the reduction of oxygen by cytochrome aa$_3$, which is felt to be rate-limiting at steady-state (17). An increase in ATPase activity (i.e. work) is thought to cause a decrease in the cytosolic energy state ([ATP]/[ADP][P_i]), which displaces the equilibrium. The decrease in the energy state of the cytosolic phosphate compounds would, in this manner, draw reducing equivalents down the electron transport chain in order to reestablish an equilibrium. This decreases the cellular redox state and stimulates the oxidation of substrate. The net effect is to increase the rate of phosphorylation and delivery of reducing equivalents to the cytochrome chain. Criticisms of this model are based on evidence that the adenine nucleotide translocase (74) and the reactions at the first two sites of ATP formation are not near equilibrium (43, 49, 54), and that the cytosolic phosphate metabolites do not change concurrent with changes in respiration, as discussed below.

Both of these models predict that the relative or absolute cytosolic concentrations of the adenylates, PCr and P_i, should change with alterations in work. That is, an increase in ATP hydrolysis rate or work should increase the cytosolic concentrations of ADP and P_i and conversely, decrease PCr. Early studies using freeze-clamp/extraction techniques appeared to demonstrate appropriate changes in the phosphates with increases in work (24, 30, 62). Some freeze-clamp/extraction studies could not confirm these observations, but concluded that their results were atypical because of nonstandard conditions or variations in experimental technique (7, 59). Part of this discrepancy may be explained by the observation that the majority of cytosolic ADP is bound and presumably not directly influencing the respiratory reactions (2). Measurements of tissue extracts, however, generally include a large portion (or all) of the bound adenine nucleotide pool. Indeed, more recent investigations using ^{31}P NMR, which discriminates between free and unbound compounds, have found that the absolute or relative concentrations of the unbound phosphate metabolites do not change significantly over a wide range of work in isolated (13, 21, 39, 40, 55) and in vivo (4, 9, 42) hearts. Figure 2 illustrates the relationship in vivo of myocardial oxygen consumption (or work) to ^{31}P metabolites as detected by NMR. [ADP] and [PCR]/[ATP] do not change significantly despite the nearly fourfold change in ATP hydrolysis, as estimated from the myocardial oxygen consumption. No significant changes in ATP, ADP, P_i, or PCr were observed by Katz et al (42)

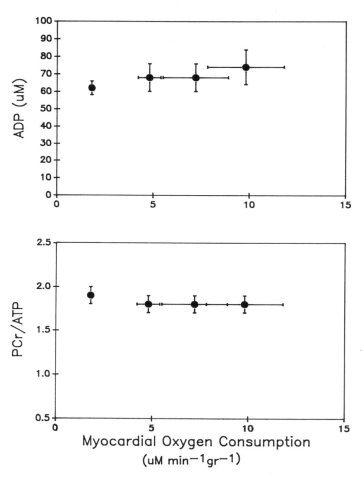

Figure 2   Relation between myocardial oxygen consumption and adenosine 5'-diphosphate *(top)* and phosphocreatine (PCr)/adenosine 5'-triphosphate (ATP) *(bottom)* in the canine heart in vivo. Illustration based on data from reference 42. Points, from left to right, represent the mean ± SEM where oxygen consumption was increased by phenylephrine infusion at rates of 0, 4, 6, and 10 μg/min/kg (n=5, 5, 5, and 4, respectively).

in the dog heart in vivo until the workload apparently out-stripped the ability of the heart to produce ATP, either because of limitations in coronary blood flow or oxidative phosphorylation capacity.

These data from intact organs demonstrate that neither the phosphorylation potential nor the absolute concentrations of ADP or P_i change significantly during physiologic increases in work in the intact heart. Are the changes in ADP and P_i that drive respiration too small to detect using these NMR techniques? Whole organ ^{31}P NMR is able to detect changes in these metabolites on the order of ten percent (42). Using a simple bireactant model and the in vitro K_m values for ADP and P_i, Katz et al (42) showed cytosolic [ADP] and $[P_i]$ would have to increase approximately fivefold in order to cause a threefold increase in myocardial respiration. Clearly, such changes would be well within the detection limits of the NMR experiment. Similar magnitudes of change would also be required for the near-equilibrium models (17).

It should be noted that both freeze-clamp and ^{31}P NMR data depend on the creatine kinase reaction to determine the concentration of unbound cytosolic ADP. This calculation assumes that the reaction is near equilibrium; its equilibrium constant is known and free tissue [creatine], [PCr], [ATP], and $[H^+]$ in vivo are known and not significantly compartmented (88). Creatine kinase has been shown to be near equilibrium in the intact working heart (6, 42), but currently it is not known if the in vivo K_m differs from that described in vitro. Furthermore, the degree to which myocardial creatine is bound (51, 69) or the phosphate compounds are compartmentalized (14, 64) has been questioned. If any of these occur, it could serve to amplify the feedback effects of changes in the phosphate metabolites on oxidative phosphorylation by lowering the free [ADP].

Considering developmental aspects of respiratory control, Portman et al (67) found that the ATP hydrolysis products change with increases in work in the neonatal sheep heart. This effect disappears by the time the animals reach two weeks of age, which suggests that the regulatory process is changing through development from one more dependent on cytosolic changes in [ADP] and $[P_i]$ in the neonate to one where these metabolites are buffered and do not change in the adult. A similar developmental change has been observed in chronically stimulated skeletal muscle (12), which, like the heart, has adapted to highly aerobic metabolism. In these studies, chronically stimulated skeletal muscle demonstrated little or no work-related change in cytosolic ADP and P_i, unlike normal skeletal muscle in which workload and ATP hydrolysis products are directly related (8, 12, 48, 76). These findings demonstrate that the metabolic events involved in the regulation of the high energy phosphates (and presumably the regulation of oxidative phosphorylation) can change with neonatal development or chronic perturbations.

From these observations it appears that the lack of change in ATP and its hydrolysis products during increases in work is specific for the adult heart in vivo and certain in vitro conditions. Appropriate substrate, perfusion, or pharmacologic manipulations in vitro appear to simplify the regulatory process, thus resulting in alterations of the phosphate metabolites with increases in work. These conditions include high pyruvate or acetate concentrations (40, 55) (which result in a highly reduced mitochondrial NADH redox state and an activation of pyruvate dehydrogenase), ischemia [either by hypotension (13) or constant flow in the face of increased work (31)], KCl arrest (30, 47), and the blockage of Ca^{2+} transport across the mitochondrial membranes by ruthenium red (40). These perturbations may decrease the importance of NADH, oxygen delivery, or other parameters in the regulation of oxidative phosphorylation and result in a system that may be primarily driven by the ATP hydrolysis products. Nevertheless, data acquired under more physiologic conditions in vivo argue against the normal occurrence of the fundamental requirement of both the thermodynamic and kinetic models—that changes in the phosphate metabolite concentrations are necessary for changes in the rate of oxidative phosphorylation. Thus, either the kinetics of the feedback process are much different in vivo than in vitro or other sites are contributing to the regulation of the mitochondrial respiratory rate.

Control of Phosphorylation at the Level F_1F_0 of Proton-ATPase

The binding of ADP and P_i at the F_1 protein on the inner mitochondrial membrane to form ATP is the goal of all the reactions of respiration. The energy requirement for these steps is met by coupling them to the electrochemical proton gradient across the inner mitochondrial membrane by the F_0 portion of the mitochondrial ATPase. Any factor that alters this process could affect the rate of oxidative phosphorylation (70). Direct regulation of the F_1F_0 proton-ATP synthase reaction rate has been proposed as a mechanism for affecting changes in oxidative phosphorylation. Possible mechanisms for this include modulation of the F_1F_0 ATPase by the ATPase inhibitor protein (49, 77) or site-site cooperativity at the F_1 ATPase (53). The evidence supporting this possibility, however, is primarily from submitochondrial particle experiments. It has not been determined if the F_1F_0 ATPase activity is varied as a means of respiratory regulation in intact organs.

Changes in the protonmotive force may influence the kinetics of mitochondrial F_1 and overall respiratory rate. Evidence from some studies in vitro show that changes of Δp are accompanied by alteration of the rate of mitochondrial respiration (20, 78), but this effect may be dependent on the experimental conditions (49, 53). Whether this mechanism, assuming Δp does correlate with O_2 consumption, contributes to the regulation of oxidative phosphorylation or simply serves to match F_1 ATPase activity to the rate at which reducing equivalents or phosphate metabolites are delivered remains to be clarified.

Summary—Phosphate Compounds in Respiratory Control

The most recent evidence concerning the adult myocardium in vivo indicates that ATP and its hydrolysis products are not solely responsible for matching the rates of ATP production and breakdown following an increase in work. However, these metabolites may be partially responsible for myocardial respiratory control, as evidenced by work-related changes in their concentrations under special conditions (as with excess substrate, KCl arrest, or limited O_2 supply). Whether this potential contribution to respiratory control by ATP, ADP, and P_i occurs through thermodynamic or kinetic mechanisms is still being debated, but the weight of current evidence favors a kinetic model.

ROLE OF REDUCING EQUIVALENT DELIVERY IN CONTROL

Cellular Redox State

The energy for the production of ATP ultimately comes from the energy in reduced metabolic substrates oxidized via intermediary metabolism. This energy, in the form of reducing equivalents, is delivered to the mitochondrial respiratory chain through NADH and FADH (see Figure 1-I). To increase ATP synthesis in the steady-state the delivery of reducing equivalents to the cytochrome chain must match its utilization in oxidative phosphorylation. Therefore, the flux of reducing equivalents into the cytochrome chain must be directly or indirectly regulated by the rate of ATP hydrolysis or work.

Can the delivery of reducing equivalents contribute to the control of the rate of oxidative phosphorylation? It has been shown that the maximum rate of respiration can be controlled by the delivery of reducing equivalents or the levels of mitochondrial NADH in liver mitochondria (46). In this study the mitochondria were also placed under more physiologic conditions by adding an external ATPase to drive oxidative phosphorylation at an intermediate rate [i.e. between state 3 and state 4 (10)]. Under these intermediate conditions the rate of respiration was also sensitive to the NADH levels, and the respiratory rate could be increased without an increase in the extra-mitochondrial [ADP] or [P_i] (46). Studies on perfused hearts also indicate that increases in mitochondrial NADH can stimulate the rate of oxidative phosphorylation (30, 63, 83). Thus, if the heart could modulate the reducing equivalent delivery to the mitochondria in concert with an increase in work, then an increase in ATP synthesis could occur without a significant change in the ATP hydrolysis products, consistent with observations in vivo (42).

The ultimate control of ATP synthesis in the steady-state must still be the rate of ATP hydrolysis. For respiration to be regulated by reducing equivalent delivery, or to simply match substrate supply with demand, a cytosolic communication system between the processes consuming ATP and the mechanism of reducing equivalent delivery must be present. There are numerous metabolic and transport processes that could be involved in the regulation of substrate delivery. Many of these enzymes and reactions have been demonstrated to be controlled by relevant factors in vitro, such as ADP, P_i, ATP, Ca^{2+}, Mg^{2+}, NAD, NADH, and numerous other metabolites.

The most extensively studied sites in this process are the dehydrogenases of intermediary metabolism, which have been shown to be activated by increases in cardiac work (32, 45). These enzymes are sensitive in vitro to Ca^{2+}, Mg^{2+}, NADH/NAD as well as other metabolites, which may make effective transducers between a work process and the dehydrogenases. This particular aspect of metabolic regulation is specifically addressed by Denton & McCormack (this volume) and will not be extensively described here. It has been suggested that mitochondrial Ca^{2+} concentrations can control the activity of several dehydrogenases regulating the delivery of NADH to the cytochrome chain (15, 27). This model is especially attractive since it uses the same effector, Ca^{2+}, to stimulate the ATPase activity as well as reducing equivalent delivery. Such simultaneous control would be extremely effective in keeping energy supply in pace with demand.

There are several other enzymatic or transport steps that could regulate reducing equivalent delivery. It is less clear, however, to what extent this regulation is important in the control of oxidative phosphorylation. One index of whether or not the delivery of reducing equivalents functions as a stimulant of oxidative phosphorylation is the redox state of mitochondrial NADH. If the reducing equivalent delivery simply follows the increased activity of the lower cytochrome chain through a mass action effect, then a net oxidation of mitochondrial NADH should accompany an increase in work. This has been demonstrated in isolated mitochondria and skeletal muscle (10). Conversely, if reducing equivalent delivery is directly stimulated, then the concentration of mitochondrial NADH should increase or remain the same when an increase in oxidative phosphorylation is induced by work. Enzymatic equilibrium studies on perfused hearts in vitro have demonstrated a net oxidation of mitochondrial NADH with increases in work (45, 59, 62). This has also been supported by NADH fluorescence studies on intact hearts (82). Other studies have demonstrated that the mitochondrial NADH increases in the glucose-perfused heart with moderate increases in work (39). Beta-adrenergic stimulation of the blood-perfused dog heart and isolated buffer-perfused rat heart (33, 83) have also been associated with net increases in mitochondrial NADH.

The lack of consistent results regarding the mitochondrial NADH redox state in response to work indicates that it is still unclear what role the activation of substrate delivery may play in the regulation of oxidative phosphorylation in vivo. There are many technical problems surrounding the interpretation of mitochondrial NADH measurements by both the classical enzymatic methods (81) and fluorescence techniques (16) that may account for the diversity of findings. Since multiple control sites may be involved in regulation, an interplay between the varying in vitro conditions used to study this process (such as differing substrates, hormones, temperature, and work-loads) could contribute to the confusion. The standard should be the heart in vivo, but very little information concerning its mitochondrial redox state is available.

Summary—Reducing Equivalent Delivery

An increase in the delivery of reducing equivalents to the cytochrome chain can increase the maximum rate of oxidative phosphorylation in isolated mitochondria as well as intact tissues. This supply of reducing equivalents to the cytochrome chain is increased or decreased in accordance with changes in work and oxidative phosphorylation, which indicates that the rate of substrate oxidation is coupled to ATP hydrolysis through some communication network. It is still unclear to what extent the modulation of reducing equivalent delivery is augmenting the oxidative phosphorylation capabilities of the tissue vs simply keeping up with demand.

THE REACTION BETWEEN CYTOCHROME AA_3 AND OXYGEN AS A REGULATOR

Kinetics of Cytochrome aa_3

Cytochrome c is oxidized by the copper-containing cytochrome aa_3 complex (cytochrome c oxidase) and the reducing equivalents are transferred to molecular oxygen, which forms the final reaction of the electron transport chain (Figure 1-III). The apparent K_m of cytochrome aa_3 for oxygen in isolated mitochondria is reported as 0.01 to 0.3 μM (36, 66), depending on conditions such as the rate of substrate oxidation, intramitochondrial pH, and the concentrations of P_i, ADP, and ATP (85). In contrast, the normal arterial and end-capillary pO_2s are roughly 100 torr ($\sim$160 μM) and 30 torr ($\sim$48 μM), respectively. In active tissue such as the heart the end-capillary pO_2 is probably maintained at >20 torr ($\sim$32 μM) under nonischemic conditions. Thus, for oxygen delivery to limit the rate of oxidative phosphorylation fairly large gradients in O_2 concentration must exist between the capillary and the mitochondria (36, 87) (see next section), or the in vitro estimates of the apparent cytochrome aa_3 K_m for oxygen do not apply to conditions in vivo. Since the reported in vitro K_m values vary over tenfold depending on experimental conditions (albeit still at very low absolute O_2 concentrations) (36), it appears that the K_{mO_2} is not necessarily the same under all conditions. Furthermore, some investigators find cytochrome aa_3 in intact hearts is far more reduced over a wide range of pO_2s (29, 30, 75) than would be predicted from in vitro results (see 87 for references), although there is not a consensus on this point (36, 84, 85). If the cytochrome aa_3 K_m for O_2 is considerably higher in vivo (71) than the in vitro data indicate (36, 87), oxidative phosphorylation could be influenced by intracellular O_2 concentrations much higher than what is commonly accepted. More work must be done before the discrepancies between reported values for the K_{mO_2} of cytochrome aa_3 and its effect on respiration in vivo are resolved.

O_2 Delivery

It is well established that oxygen can limit the rate of myocardial respiration under hypoxic or ischemic conditions (68) when O_2 delivery is compromised, either in vivo or in vitro. Whether or not the O_2 supply can limit electron transport during normoxic myocardial conditions remains controversial, as it implies that the O_2 gradient between the capillary and mitochondria is significant (87). Attempts to directly measure tissue pO_2 with oxygen electrodes in beating, intact hearts have resulted in values between 0 and 30 torr, with some studies consistently finding $pO_2 \sim 5$ torr (79). Even the high end of this range is considerably below arterial pO_2, yet the hearts maintained autoregulatory control over coronary flow. This suggests that a sizable blood to cell O_2 gradient is normal for the intact myocardium. Microelectrode studies have been criticized on the basis that even intracelluar electrodes cause some tissue disruption (particularly in a beating heart) and, consequently, may not accurately reflect the true cytosolic pO_2. Furthermore, there may be heterogenieties of pO_2 within the tissue that are not reflected by a point measurement. In support of a gradient, it has been observed that isolated cardiac myocytes require a media pO_2 several-fold higher than isolated mitochondria to attain the same level of respiratory function (36), although direct measurements of pO_2 in isolated myocytes and mitochondria have yielded data that generally indicate that there is only a small drop in the pO_2 between the external medium and the cytosol (38, 86, 87). The applicability of these observations to the intact heart is not necessarily clear. The process of isolating the cells may not only change their diffusion characteristics and the area available for diffusion, but such cells are frequently respiring at much lower rates than those in a working heart and therefore may not accurately reflect the metabolic conditions in vivo.

A variety of noninvasive techniques have been developed to estimate intracellular pO_2 and to determine if an oxygen gradient exists, including measurements of myoglobin and cytochrome redox states, mitochondrial monoamine oxidase activity, O_2-quenched fluorescence, and electron spin resonance (see 36 and 87 for references). Unfortunately they have not resolved whether or not significant O_2 gradients occur in cardiac myocytes under normal circumstances and the issue continues to be actively debated in the literature (11, 36, 87). Data based on optical measurements of cytosolic myoglobin redox states in intact hearts or isolated myocytes indicate that no physiologically significant gradients in cytosolic pO_2 exist (86, T. Gayeski, C. Honig, personal communication). In agreement with this, the O_2 saturation of myoglobin has been reported at greater than 50% in intact hearts (52), which implies a pO_2 well above the apparent K_m of cytochrome aa_3 in vitro. This conclusion assumes the in vivo affinity of cytochrome aa_3 for O_2 is much lower than that of myoglobin. The assumption may not be correct, as optical studies of crystalloid-perfused hearts have shown the level of cytochrome aa_3 reduction to be far greater than that predicted from the degree of simultaneous myoglobin saturation or arterial pO_2 (29, 75). The same study found cytochrome aa_3 redox state changed in parallel with myoglobin over a wide range of arterial pO_2 (75). Although optical spectra from intact hearts are difficult to interpret due to numerous sources of artifacts (87), these findings suggest that the oxygen gradient within the cardiac myocyte in buffer-perfused hearts is steep or that the affinity of cytochrome aa_3 for O_2 is much lower in vivo than in vitro. Optical measurements on rapidly frozen tissue from working, blood-perfused hearts (T. Gayeski, C. Honig, personal communication) demonstrate a relatively uniform level of myoglobin oxygenation ($\sim$50%) and pO_2 ($\sim$6 torr) throughout the myocyte. This suggests that the myoglobin P_{50} in vivo is considerably higher than the values reported for isolated myocytes (86) and that oxygen diffusion to the mitochondria in isolated cells may be very different from the conditions in intact hearts. Some reasons proposed to account for this apparent difference include lower rates of respiration in vitro (36) and the smaller cellular surface area in vivo directly exposed to the capillary (estimated at $\sim$20% of the cell surface) compared to the surface area in isolated cells exposed to the oxygenated medium (presumably 100%) (87).

Mathematical modeling of oxygen diffusion has not helped to settle the controversy over intracellular pO_2 gradients. Workers on both sides have defended their positions on theoretical grounds (11, 36), but such models are no more reliable than their assumptions. Disagreements over such factors as the influence of mitochondrial clustering on diffusion, the correct intracellular diffusion coefficient for oxygen, existence of an unstirred layer near the membranes, and mitochondrial and cellular geometry have not been resolved. Since models invariably rely on numbers generated through experimental work for verification, the discrepancy of reported values for the redox state of the cytochromes and myoglobin over the wide variety of experimental conditions used further confound the issue and guarantee that this will be an active area of research for some time.

Myocardial oxygen consumption and coronary blood flow are directly correlated over the range of physiologic workloads. Since coronary oxygen extraction is near maximal (19) even at low cardiac workloads, the primary mechanism for increasing oxygen delivery to the heart is blood flow. Thus there must be a metabolic link between flow and metabolism. While it is usually felt that changes in coronary flow follow the changes in cardiac metabolism (68), there has been no conclusive proof that flow (and O_2 delivery) cannot directly influence metabolism as well. The effect of increased myocardial O_2 consumption on coronary blood flow is well established and has been extensively investigated, although the mediator(s) of this feedback remain(s) controversial (19). This relationship involves the up-regulation of O_2 supply to the respiratory apparatus after (or during) an increase in work rather than the actual regulation of oxidative phosphorylation. Consequently, it falls outside the scope of this review and the reader is referred elsewhere for details (19). Conversely, if primary changes in coronary blood flow can induce changes in myocardial respiration, it is thought that the delivery of some constituent of blood may directly influence the respiratory rate in vivo.

Increased coronary flow has been shown to increase myocardial oxygen consumption (the Gregg phenomenon) in working and nonworking hearts. This effect can be induced whether flow is increased by increased perfusion pressure (25) or by vasodilators at constant pressure (65). It is not clear if this increase in oxygen consumption is due to a local mechanical effect on the heart or to an increase in the delivery of blood (and presumably O_2) to the myocytes. It is clear, however, that the increase in myocardial oxygen consumption is modest ($\sim$30%) compared to the increase in flow needed to induce it (100–200%) (65). In comparison, myocardial respiration would have to increase 100–200% (42) to cause a similar increase in coronary flow under normal circumstances. Although the finding that increased blood flow can cause small changes in myocardial respiration indicates that it could contribute to regulation, the magnitude of these changes relative to the normal wide range of myocardial O_2 consumption appears inconsistent with blood flow being a major determinant of the respiratory rate.

Summary—Cytochrome aa₃ and Oxygen

Although the oxygen-cytochrome aa_3 reaction in vivo can limit myocardial respiration under pathologic conditions, its contribution to regulation in normoxia is not clear. This is due in part to disagreement regarding the level of cytosolic pO_2. Technical aspects of both intact heart and in vitro myocyte and cell preparations used to study this problem make the results of these investigations difficult to extrapolate to conditions in vivo. Uncertainties regarding the K_m of cytochrome aa_3 for oxygen in the intact, working heart further confuse the issue since the intracellular pO_2 necessary to saturate this reaction will vary with the K_m. Physiologic evidence supports a possible direct influence by coronary flow on cardiac respiration, although the effect is small when compared to the normal range of myocardial oxygen consumption. Whether or not this implicates the delivery of oxygen, substrate, or some other blood-borne substance as a contributor to respiratory control in the heart has not been proven.

SUMMARY

After reviewing the controversies in the literature surrounding the regulation of oxidative phosphorylation, a unifying theory to integrate the disparate results would be welcome. Following the traditional biochemical approach to identifying sites of control, one searches for the rate-limiting step in a series of reactions (i.e. a biochemical pathway) that, presumably, will not be at equilibrium. This approach has not succeeded in locating a reaction in cardiac respiratory control that is singularly rate-limiting and may actually be contributing to, rather than clarifying, the problem. There are two major criticisms of this approach. First, even if the step is in disequilibrium, it does not prove that it is rate-limiting (26). Second, a reaction near equilibrium can contribute to regulation of a system (37).

In a complex, multiple-reaction integrated pathway such as mitochondrial respiration there are many steps that could potentially share the control of the overall system. Thus this pathway easily lends itself to the possibility of multiple sites of control, each of which could contribute by varying degrees to regulation. In Figure 3 we present one possible network (undoubtedly incomplete) for the distributed control of respiration, which incorporates contributions by the cellular redox state (supply), phosphate metabolite concentrations (either kinetic or thermodynamic), and oxygen. The coordination of the dehydrogenases, phosphate metabolites, and myosin ATPase activity (work) may be orchestrated by a second messenger. Calcium is an attractive candidate for this role (15) as it simultaneously can modulate reducing equivalent supply via the dehydrogenases and ATP use by the myofibrils.

The theory of shared control along the path of respiration is not new (37), and has been gaining support from a variety of laboratories (3, 9, 26). Applying this concept to the experimental setting, the relative control strengths for various steps in oxidative phosphorylation have been reported for isolated mitochondria (26). The control coefficients for respiration in isolated myocytes or hearts in vivo remain unknown at this time.

If control of respiration occurs at multiple sites, it could account for much

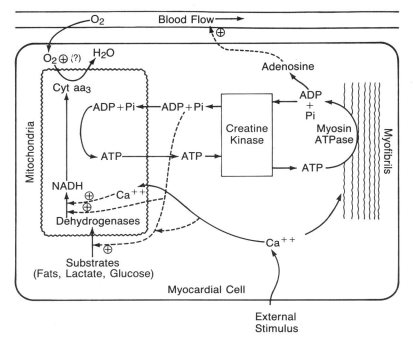

Figure 3   Schematic representation of the factors that influence the rate of myocardial oxidative phosphorylation (abbreviations as in Figure 1) (Adapted from Reference 4a).

of the disagreement in the literature. Experimental conditions, whether intentional or inadvertent, that saturate one or more control mechanisms will increase the relative effect of the other regulatory sites on the remaining range of mitochondrial function. If, for example, the medium surrounding isolated myocytes is such that the cytosolic redox state and pO_2 are very high, the phosphate metabolite concentrations could logically be expected to be a major factor influencing the observed rate of oxidative phosphorylation. This does not mean that measurements with other than in vivo conditions are ineffective for studying respiratory control. It is only under the highly controlled conditions attained in experiments in vitro that the individual sites for shared regulation and the conditions under which they contribute can be precisely identified. At the same time, our goal is not only to learn how oxidative phosphorylation is regulated in isolated hearts, myocytes or mitochondria, but ultimately to understand how this process occurs in the hearts of living, conscious mammals. The technical advances for studying energy metabolism in intact hearts have caused a recent surge of experiments conducted in vivo. This should permit a more complete integration of the many diverse findings in the field of myocardial respiratory control in the near future.

ACKNOWLEDGMENTS

The authors with to thank Dr. Teresa Fralix for review of the manuscript and Dr. John Eng for assistance with the illustrations.

Literature Cited

1. Akerboom, T. P. M., Bookelman, H., Tager, J. M. 1977. Control of ATP transport across the mitochondrial membrane in isolated rat liver cells. *FEBS Lett.* 74:50–54
2. Balaban, R. S. 1984. The application of nuclear magnetic resonance to the study of cellular physiology. *Am. J. Physiol.* 246:C10–C19
3. Balaban, R. S. 1989. Regulation of oxidative phosphorylation in the mammalian cell. *Am. J. Physiol.* In press
4. Balaban, R. S., Kantor, H. L., Katz, L. A., Briggs, R. W. 1986. Relation between work and phosphate metabolites in the in vivo paced mammalian heart. *Science* 232:1121–23
4a. Balaban, R. S., Heineman, F. W. 1989. Interaction of oxidative phosphorylation and work in the heart *in vivo. News Phys. Sci.* In press
5. Bessman, S. P., Geiger, P. J. 1981. Transport of energy in muscle: The phosphorylcreatine shuttle. *Science* 211:448–52
6. Bittl, J. A., Ingwall, J. S. 1985. Reaction rates of creatine kinase and ATP synthesis in the isolated heart. *J. Biol. Chem.* 260:3512–17
7. Boerth, R. C., Covell, J., Seagren, S. C., Pool, P. E. 1969. High-energy phosphate concentrations in dog myocardium during stress. *Am. J. Physiol.* 216:1103–6
8. Chance, B., Leigh, J. S., Clark, B. J., Maris, J., Kent, J., et al. 1985. Control of oxidative metabolism and oxygen delivery in human skeletal muscle: a steady-state analysis of the work/energy cost transfer function. *Proc. Natl. Acad. Sci. USA* 82:8384–88
9. Chance, B., Leigh, J. S., Kent, J., McCully, K., Nioka, S., et al. 1986. Multiple controls of oxidative metabolism in living tissues as studied by phosphorus magnetic resonance. *Proc. Natl. Acad. Sci. USA* 83:9458–62
10. Chance, B., Williams, C. M. 1956. The respiratory chain and oxidative phosphorylation. *Adv. Enzymol.* 17:65–134
11. Clark, A. Jr., Clark, P. A. A., Connett, R. J., Gayeski, T. E. J., Honig, C. R. 1987. How large is the drop in PO_2 be-

tween the cytosol and mitochondrion? *Am. J. Physiol.* 252:583–87
12. Clark, B. J. III, Acker, M. A., McCully, K., Subramanian, H. V., Hammond, R. L., et al. 1988. In vivo ^{31}P-NMR spectroscopy of chronically stimulated canine skeletal muscle. *Am. J. Physiol.* 254(Cell Physiol. 23):C258–66
13. Clarke, K., Willis, R. J. 1987. Energy metabolism and contractile function in rat heart during graded, isovolumic perfusion using ^{31}P nuclear magnetic resonance spectroscopy. *J. Mol. Cell. Cardiol.* 19:1153–60
14. Degani, H., Laughlin, M., Campbell, S., Shulman, R. G. 1985. Kinetics of creatine kinase in the heart: a ^{31}P NMR saturation- and inversion-transfer study. *Biochemistry* 24:5510–16
15. Denton, R. M., McCormack, J. G. 1980. On the role of the calcium transport cycle in heart and other mammalian mitochondria. *FEBS Lett.* 119:1–8
16. Eng, J., Lynch, R. M., Balaban, R. S. 1989. NADH fluorescence spectroscopy and imaging of isolated cardiac myocytes. *Biophys. J.* 55:621–30
17. Erecinska, M., Wilson, D. F. 1982. Regulation of cellular energy metabolism. *J. Memb. Biol.* 70:1–14
18. Ernster, L., Lee, C., Jnada, S. 1966. The reaction sequence in oxidative phosphorylation. In *Biochemistry of Mitochondria,* ed. E. Slater, Z. Kaniuga, L. Wojtczak, pp. 29–51. London: Academic
19. Feigl, E. O. 1983. Coronary Physiology. *Physiol. Rev.* 63:1–205
20. Feldman, R. I., Sigman, D. S. 1983. The synthesis of ATP by the membrane-bound ATP synthase complex from medium $^{32}P_i$ under completely uncoupled conditions. *J. Biol. Chem.* 258:12178–83
21. From, A. H. L., Petein, M. A., Michurski, S. P., Zimmer, S. D., Ugurbil, K. 1986. 31-P-NMR studies of respiratory regulations on the intact myocardium. *FEBS Lett.* 206:257–61
22. Deleted in proof
23. Gibbs, C. 1985. The cytoplasmic phosphorylation potential. Its possible role in the control of myocardial respira-

tion and cardiac contractility. *J. Mol. Cell. Cardiol.* 17:727–31

24. Giesen, J., Kammermeier, H. 1980. Relationship of phosphorylation potential and oxygen consumption in isolated perfused rat hearts. *J. Mol. Cell. Cardiol.* 12:891–907

25. Gregg, D. E. 1963. Effect of coronary perfusion pressure or coronary flow on oxygen usage of the myocardium. *Circ. Res.* 13:497–500

26. Groen, A. K., Wanders, R. J. A., Westerhoff, H. V., van der Meer, R., Tager, J. M. 1982. Quantification of the contribution of various steps to control mitochondrial respiration. *J. Biol. Chem.* 257:2754–57

27. Hansford, R. G. 1980. Control of mitochondrial substrate oxidation. *Curr. Top. Bioenerg.* 10:217–77

28. Hassinen, I. E. 1986. Mitochondrial respiratory control in the myocardium. *Biochim. Biophys. Acta.* 853:135–51

29. Hassinen, I. E., Hiltunen, J. K., Takala, T. E. S. 1981. Reflectance spectrophotometric monitoring of the isolated perfused heart as a method of measuring the oxidation-reduction state of cytochromes and oxygenation of myoglobin. *Cardiovasc. Res.* 15:86–91

30. Hassinen, I. E., Hiltunen, K. 1975. Respiratory control in isolated perfused rat heart. Role of the equilibrium relations between the mitochondrial electron carriers and the adenylate system. *Biochim. Biophys. Acta* 408:319–30

31. He, M.-X., Wangler, R. D., Dillion, P. F., Romig, G. D., Sparks, H. V. 1987. Phosphorylation potential and adenosine release during norepinephrine infusion in guinea pig heart. *Am. J. Physiol.* 253(Heart Circ. Physiol. 22):H1184–91

32. Illingworth, J., Mullins, R. 1976. Pyruvate dehydrogenase activation after an increase in cardiac output. *Biochem. Soc. Trans.* 4:291–92

33. Imai, S., Otorii, T., Takeda, K., Katano, Y., Nakagawa, Y. 1978. Effects of catecholamines on myocardial energy metabolism as studied by an organ redoximeter. In *Heart Function and Metabolism,* ed. T. Kobayashi, T. Sano, N. S. Dhalla, pp. 335–41. Baltimore: University Park Press

34. Jacobus, W. E. 1985. Respiratory control and the integration of heart high-energy phosphate metabolism by mitochondrial creatine kinase. *Annu. Rev. Physiol.* 47:707–25

35. Jacobus, W. E., Moreadith, R. W., Vandegaer, K. M. 1982. Mitochondrial respiratory control: Evidence against the regulation of respiration by extra-

mitochondrial phosphorylation potentials or by ATP/ADP ratios. *J. Biol. Chem.* 257:2397–2402

36. Jones, D. P. 1986. Intracellular diffusion gradients of O_2 and ATP. *Am. J. Physiol.* 250:C663–75

37. Kacser, H., Burns, J. A. 1973. The control of flux. *Symp. Soc. Exp. Biol.* 27: 65–104

38. Katz, I. R., Wittenberg, J. B., Wittenberg, B. A. 1984. Monoamine oxidase, an intracellular probe of oxygen pressure in isolated cardiac myocytes. *J. Biol. Chem.* 259:7504–9

39. Katz, L. A., Koretsky, A. P., Balaban, R. S. 1987. A mechanism of respiratory control in the heart: a ^{31}P NMR and NADH fluorescence study. *FEBS Lett.* 221:270–76

40. Katz, L. A., Koretsky, A. P., Balaban, R. S. 1988. The activation of dehydrogenase activity and cardiac respiration: A ^{31}P NMR study. *Am. J. Physiol.* 255:H185–88

41. Katz, L. A., Swain, J. A., Portman, M. A., Balaban, R. S. 1988. Intracellular pH and inorganic phosphate content of the heart *in vivo:* A ^{31}P NMR study. *Am. J. Physiol.* 255:H189–96

42. Katz, L. A., Swain, J. A., Portman, M. A., Balaban, R. S. 1989. Relation between phosphate metabolites and oxygen consumption of heart in vivo. *Am. J. Physiol.* 256:H265–74

43. Kingsley-Hickman, P. B., Sako, E. Y., Mohanakriahnan, P., Robitaille, P. M., From, A. H., et al. 1987. ^{31}P NMR studies of ATP synthesis and hydrolysis kinetics in the intact heart myocardium. *Biochemistry* 26:7501–10

44. Klingenberg, M. 1961. Zur reversibilitat der oxidativen phosphorylierung. *Biochem. Z.* 335:263–72

45. Kobayashi, K., Neely, J. R. 1979. Mechanism of pyruvate dehydrogenase activation by increased cardiac work. *J. Mol. Cell. Cardiol.* 15:369–82

46. Koretsky, A. P., Balaban, R. S. 1987. Changes in pyridine nucleotide levels alter oxygen consumption and extramitochondrial phosphates in isolated mitochondria: a ^{31}P NMR and fluorescence study. *Biochim. Biophys. Acta* 893:398–408

47. Kupriyanov, V. V., Steinschneider, A. Y., Ruuge, E. K., Kapel'ko, V. I., Zueva, M. Y., et al. 1984. Regulation of energy flux through the creatine kinase reaction in vitro and in perfused rat heart. *Biochim. Biophys. Acta* 805:319–31

48. Kushmerick, M. J., Meyer, R. A. 1985. Chemical changes in rat leg muscle by

phosphorus nuclear magnetic resonance. *Am. J. Physiol.* 248(Cell Physiol. 17): C542–49

49. LaNoue, K. F., Jefferies, F. M., Radda, G. K. 1986. Kinetic control of mitochondrial ATP synthesis. *Biochemistry* 25:7667–75

50. Lardy, H. A., Wellman, H. 1952. Oxidative phosphorylations: Role of inorganic phosphate as an acceptor systems in control of metabolic rate. *J. Biol. Chem.* 195:215–24

51. Lee, Y. C. P., Visscher, M. B. 1961. On the state of creatine in heart muscle. *Proc. Natl. Acad. Sci. USA* 47:1510–15

52. Makino, N., Kanaide, H., Yoshimura, R., Nakamura, M. 1983. Myoglobin oxygenation remains constant during the cardiac cycle. *Am. J. Physiol.* 245(Heart Circ. Physiol. 14):H237–43

53. Matsuno-Yagi, A., Hatefi, Y. 1986. Kinetic modalities of ATP synthesis. *J. Biol. Chem.* 261:14031–38

54. Matthews, P. M., Bland, J. L., Gadian, D. G., Radda, G. K. 1982. The steady state rate of ATP synthesis in the perfused rat heart measured by ^{31}P NMR saturation transfer. *Biochem. Biophys. Acta* 714:265–70

55. Matthews, P. M., Williams, S. R., Seymour, A. M., Schwartz, A., Dube, G., et al. 1982. A ^{31}P NMR study of some metabolic and functional effects of the inotropic agents epinephrine and ouabain, and the ionophore X537A in isolated perfused rat heart. *Biochem. Biophys. Acta* 720:163–71

56. Mela-Riker, L. M., Bukoski, R. D. 1985. Regulation of mitochondrial activity in cardiac cells. *Annu. Rev. Physiol.* 47:645–63

57. Meyer, R. A., Sweeney, H. L., Kushmerick, M. J. 1982. A simple analysis of the "Phosphocreatine Shuttle". *Am. J. Physiol.* 242:1–11

58. Mitchell, P. 1976. Vectorial chemistry and the molecular mechanics of chemiosmotic coupling: Power transmission by proticity. *Biochem. Soc. Trans.* 4:399–430

59. Neely, J. R., Denton, R. M., England, P. J., Randle, P. J. 1972. The effects of increased heart work on the tricarboxylate cycle and its interactions with glycolysis in the perfused rat heart. *Biochem. J.* 128:147–59

60. Neely, J. R., Rovetto, M. J., Oram, J. F. 1972. Myocardial utilization of carbohydrate and lipids. *Prog. Cardiovasc. Dis.* 15:289–329

61. Nicholls, D. G. 1982. *Bioenergetics.* New York: Academic

62. Nishiki, K., Erecinska, M., Wilson, D.

F. 1978. Energy relationships between cytosolic metabolism and mitochondrial respiration in rat heart. *Am. J. Physiol.* 234(Cell Physiol. 3):C73–81

63. Nuutinen, E. M. 1984. Subcellular origin of the surface fluorescence of nicotinamide in the isolated perfused rat heart. *Basic Res. Cardiol.* 79:49–58

64. Ogunro, E. A., Peters, T. J., Hearse, D. J. 1977. Subcellular compartmentation of creatine kinase isoenzymes in guinea pig heart. *Cardiovasc. Res.* 11:250–59

65. Oguro, K., Kubota, K., Kimura, T., Hashimoto, K. 1973. Effects of various coronary vasodilators on myocardial oxygen consumption. *Jpn. J. Pharmacol.* 23:459–66

66. Oshino, N., Jamieson, D., Sugano, T., Chance, B. 1974. Mitochondrial function under hypoxic conditions: the steady states of cytochrome a,a$_3$ and their relation to mitochondrial energy states. *Biochim. Biophys. Acta* 368:298–310

67. Portman, M. A., Heineman, F. W., Balaban, R. S. 1989. Developmental changes in the relation between phosphate metabolites and oxygen consumption in the sheep heart in vivo. *J. Clin. Invest.* 83:456–64

68. Reimer, K. A., Jennings, R. B. 1986. Myocardial ischemia, hypoxia, and infarction. In *The Heart and Cardiovascular System*, ed. H. A. Fozzard, E. Haber, R. B. Jennings, A. Katz, H. E. Morgan, 53:1133–1201. New York: Raven

69. Savabi, F. 1988. Free creatine available to the creatine phosphate energy shuttle in isolated rat atria. *Proc. Natl. Acad. Sci. USA* 85:7476–80

70. Senior, A. E. 1988. ATP synthesis by oxidative phosphorylation. *Physiol. Rev.* 68:177–231

71. Snow, T. R., Kleinman, L. H., Lamanna, J. C., Wichsler, A. S., Jobsis, F. F. 1981. Response of cytochrome a,a$_3$ in the in situ canine heart to transient ischemic episodes. *Basic Res. Cardiol.* 76:289–304

72. Stubbs, M. 1981. In *Inhibitors of Mitochondrial Function*, ed. M. Erecinska, D. F., Wilson, pp. 238–304. New York: Pergamon

73. Taegtmeyer, H. 1984. Six blind men explore an elephant: aspects of fuel metabolism and the control of tricarboxylic acid cycle activity in heart muscle. *Basic Res. Cardiol.* 79:322–36

74. Tager, J. M., Wanders, R. J. A., Groen, A. K., Kunz, W., Bohnensack, R., et al. 1983. Control of mitochondrial respiration. *FEBS Lett.* 151:1–9

75. Tamura, M., Oshino, N., Chance, B., Silver, I. A. 1978. Optical measurements of intracellular oxygen concentrations of rat heart *in vitro*. *Arch. Biochem. Biophys.* 191:8–22

76. Taylor, D. J., Styles, P., Matthews, P. M., Arnold, D. M., Gadian, D. G., et al. 1986. Energetics of human muscle: Exercise induced ATP depletion. *Magn. Res. Med.* 3:44–54

77. Tuena de Gomez-Puyou, M., Martins, O. B., Gomez-Puyou, A. 1988. Synthesis and hydrolysis of ATP by the mitochondrial ATP synthase. *Biochem. Cell Biol.* 66:677–82

78. Westerhoff, H. V., Plomp, P. J. A. M., Groen, A. K., Wanders, R. J. A., Bode, J. A., van Dam, K. 1987. On the origin of the limited control of mitochondrial respiration by the adenine nucleotide translocator. *Arch. Biochem. Biophys.* 257:154–69

79. Whalen, W. J ., Nair, P., Buerk, D. 1973. O$_2$ tension in the beating cat heart in situ. In *O$_2$ Supply*, ed. M. Kessler, D. F. Bruley, L. C. Clark Jr., D. W. Lubbers, I. A. Silver, J. Strauss. Baltimore: Univ. Park Press

80. Williamson, J. R. 1979. Mitochondrial function in the heart. *Annu. Rev. Physiol.* 41:485–506

81. Williamson, J. R. 1976. In *Gluconeogenesis,* ed. R. W. Hanson, M. A. Mehlman, pp. 194–204. New York: Wiley

82. Williamson, J. R., Ford, C., Illingworth, J., Safer, B. 1976. Coordination of citric acid cycle activity with electron transport flux. *Circ. Res.* 38:I39–I48

83. Williamson, J. R., Jamieson, D. 1966. Metabolic effects of epinephrine in the perfused rat heart. Comparison of intracellular redox states, tissue pO$_2$, and force of contraction. *Mol. Pharmacol.* 2:191–205

84. Wilson, D. F., Erecinska, M. 1980. The oxygen dependence of cellular energy metabolism. *Adv. Exp. Med. Biol.* 194:229–39

85. Wilson, D. F., Erecinska, M., Drown, C., Silver, I. A. 1979. The Oxygen dependence of cellular energy metabolism. *Arch. Biochem. Biophys.* 195:485–93

86. Wittenberg, B. A., Wittenberg, J. B. 1985. Oxygen pressure gradients in isolated cardiac myocytes. *J. Biol. Chem.* 260:6548–54

87. Wittenberg, B. A., Wittenberg, J. B. 1989. Transport of oxygen in muscle. *Annu. Rev. Physiol.* 51:857–78

88. Veech, R. L., Lawson, J. W. R., Cornell, N. W., Krebs, H. A. 1979. Cytosolic phosphorylation potential. *J. Biol. Chem.* 254:6538–47

Annu. Rev. Physiol. 1990. 52:543–59

MECHANISMS OF Ca²⁺ OVERLOAD IN REPERFUSED ISCHEMIC MYOCARDIUM

Masato Tani[1]

Weis Center for Research, Geisinger Clinic, Danville, Pennsylvania 17822

KEY WORDS: Na⁺/Ca²⁺ exchange, Na⁺/H⁺ exchange, Na⁺,K⁺ ATPase, Ca overload, reperfusion injury

INTRODUCTION

Both reperfusion (3, 26, 61, 73, 83, 89) and reoxygenation (14, 27, 28, 57, 58) after prolonged ischemia and hypoxia are associated with a large increase in Ca^{2+} content in severely damaged myocardium, however Ca^{2+} overload is not seen in the myocardium that is not irreversibly injured (36). Increased uptake of Ca^{2+} correlates with the depressed recovery of mechanical function of the myocardium (3, 83). Therefore excessive Ca^{2+} accumulation has been implicated as a primary event in irreversible myocardial injury and cell necrosis (20). Increased influx of Ca^{2+} during reperfusion in excess of the handling capacity of systems for Ca^{2+} extrusion from the cytosol results in elevation of cytosolic-free $[Ca^{2+}]$. Nevertheless, the exact mechanisms responsible for increased Ca^{2+} entry upon reperfusion have not been defined. Perturbations of ion transport systems in the sarcolemmal membrane appear to be responsible for increased Ca^{2+} accumulation in oxygen deficient myocytes because Ca^{2+} overload occurred without apparent ultrastructural changes in the membrane (14). The mechanisms involved in maintenance of Ca^{2+} homeostasis are complicated and interrelated with the regulatory systems of other cations. In addition, loss of membrane integrity and an increase in permeability can result from the action of endogenous enzymes (i.e. Ca^{2+}-dependent proteases or lipases) that are activated secondarily by an initial

---

[1]Present address: Cardiopulmonary Division, Department of Internal Medicine, Keio Gijuku University School of Medicine, 35 Shinanomachi, Shinjuku-ku, Tokyo 160, Japan

0066-4278/90/0315-0543$02.00

rise in cytosolic $[Ca^{2+}]$ (10, 61, 81; see Figure 1). Mechanical forces generated by contracture/rigor formation or cell swelling could also accelerate the disruption of the previously damaged sarcolemmal membrane. Although action of hydrolytic enzymes and mechanical forces are not trigger mechanisms for Ca^{2+} overload, they can aggravate its progression. Also, oxygen-derived free radicals may be involved in development of Ca^{2+} overload (30). In this article, the possible mechanisms that can initiate and accelerate the progression of Ca^{2+} overload in reperfused ischemic myocardium will be briefly reviewed.

PERTURBATIONS OF SARCOLEMMAL Ca^{2+} TRANSPORT SYSTEMS

Ca^{2+} Channels

In normal myocytes, the amount of Ca^{2+} influx through this channel is estimated to be less than 1 nmol/g of heart/beat or approximately 0.1 to 0.3 μmol/g/min (51). The maximal rate of Ca^{2+} uptake upon reperfusion rarely exceeded 0.5 μmol/g/min and averaged approximately 0.3 μmol/g/min for the first 30 min of reperfusion after 30 min of global ischemia in isolated rat hearts (84, 84a). Thus the Ca^{2+} channel may account, at least partially, for

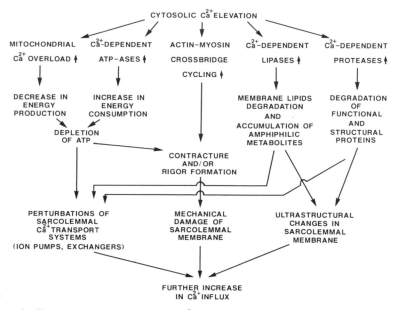

Figure 1   The role of elevated cytosolic $[Ca^{2+}]$ in irreversible myocardial injury.

the large increase in Ca^{2+} influx during reperfusion. Flux through the Ca^{2+} channel is modulated during ischemia by pH and ATP availability, however, and the channel was inactivated within 5 to 15 min after induction of ischemia because both pH and the intracellular ATP level decreased (80). These kinetic properties of the Ca^{2+} channel could lead to excessive accumulation of Ca^{2+} during reperfusion, but not during ischemia itself. If the hypothesis that the Ca^{2+} channel is the main pathway for Ca^{2+} entry during reperfusion is true, then inhibition by Ca^{2+} antagonists during reperfusion should prevent Ca^{2+} overload. Most investigators, however, have failed to demonstrate a reduction of Ca^{2+} overload when Ca^{2+} antagonists were employed either after the ischemic myocardium had ceased to contract or at the time of reperfusion (3, 49, 89). When Ca^{2+} antagonists were given prior to or at the onset of ischemia, accumulation of Ca^{2+} upon reperfusion was reduced (3, 49, 59, 73, 89). Recently, Murphy et al (57) found that binding sites for verapamil were still present and capable of interacting with it with high affinity, during reoxygenation and after hypoxia in heart cells. But they also suggested that the channels were inactive after reoxygenation. These circumstances may be due to high intracellular [Ca^{2+}] because an increase in cytosolic free [Ca^{2+}] can inhibit conductance of the slow Ca^{2+} channel (50). In fact, Steenbergen et al (82) found that cytosolic-free [Ca^{2+}] was elevated in ischemic myocytes. Therefore, the Ca^{2+} channel appears to be inactive during reoxygenation and presumably during reperfusion following ischemia, and it does not account for Ca^{2+} overload (3, 49, 50, 57, 89). Recently a novel type of the Ca^{2+} channel was reported that was less sensitive to Ca^{2+} antagonists. Its ion carrying capacity appeared to be far less than that of the slow Ca^{2+} channel (80), however, so it is unlikely that Ca^{2+} entry through this newly found channel is responsible for Ca^{2+} overload following ischemia.

The dependence of the protective effects of pretreatment with Ca^{2+} antagonists on myocardium prior to ischemia might be explained by several mechanisms other than direct blockade of the channels. First, Ca^{2+} antagonists can delay the depletion of high energy phosphates during ischemia by reduction of myocardial contractility (46). Second, better protection of the rate of mitochondrial oxidative phosphorylation during ischemia and reperfusion has been reported (59). These two mechanisms maintain high energy stores, preserve the function of energy-dependent subcellular processes during ischemia, and enhance functional recovery of these processes upon reperfusion. Indeed, some of these energy-dependent processes, such as the Na$^+$,K$^+$ or Ca$^+$ ATPases, are directly related to the maintenance of ion homeostasis. Third, Daly et al (16) reported that pretreatment with verapamil prevented reduction of sarcolemmal Na$^+$,K$^+$ ATPase activity in membrane vesicles from isolated perfused ischemic hearts. The maintenance of Na$^+$,K$^+$ ATPase activity favored the removal of intracellular Na$^+$ (Na$_i$) that accumulated during ischemia (2, 21, 71, 84, 84a). Fourth, Ca^{2+} antagonists can reduce the influx of Na^+ into myocytes (25). Direct interaction of Ca^{2+} antagonists with the Na^+ channel was demonstrated by the patch-clamp method in isolated myocytes (93) and by the binding of dihydropyridines to the cardiac Na^+ channel (94). Maintenance of Na^+,K^+ ATPase activity and inhibition of the Na^+ channel could lead to reduced Ca^{2+} influx via Na^+/Ca^{2+} exchange rather than a direct inhibition of the Ca^{2+} channel. Finally, Ca^{2+} antagonists have an anti-α_1-adrenergic effect (39) and inhibit the release of norepinephrine from ischemic myocardium (62).

Na^+/Ca^{2+} Exchanger

Several investigators have proposed that excessive Ca^{2+} entry occurred, in part, through Na^+/Ca^{2+} exchange during reperfusion following ischemia (26, 76, 84) or during reoxygenation after hypoxia (27, 57). This hypothesis was based primarily on the observation that tissue Na^+ content increased in ischemic myocardium (21, 36, 47, 83). Recently, elevation of cytosolic-free $[Na^+]$ was confirmed with nuclear magnetic resonance (NMR) (2, 71) and ion selective microelectrodes (91). If elevated intracellular Na^+ concentration ($[Na^+]_i$) is of importance for Ca^{2+} overload, increased $[Na^+]_i$ should be maintained for some time during reperfusion to allow the entry of a large amount of Ca^{2+} through Na^+/Ca^{2+} exchange. An elevated $[Na^+]_i$ is necessary to support the hypothesis, but the mechanisms responsible for changes in $[Na^+]_i$ have not been established.

The Na^+ ion is involved in several regulatory processes of ion homeostasis. The Na^+/Ca^{2+} exchanger links the Na^+ ion directly with cellular Ca^{2+} metabolism. The Na^+ ion is important in regulation of intracellular pH (pH_i) through Na^+/H^+ exchange (52). In addition, the Na^+ ion carries the rapid inward current which causes the upstroke of the action potential. This Na^+ flux is not coupled with the flux of other ions. Transport of Na^+ against its electrochemical gradient is dependent upon the Na^+,K^+ pump.

Influx of Na^+ through the fast Na^+ channel amounts to 20 to 40 nmol/g/beat or 3 to 6 μmol/g/min (12). Although the shift from beating to quiescence in ischemia abolished the Na^+ influx during the upstroke of the action potential after 10–20 min, velocity of the upstroke is hardly affected during early ischemia before cessation of beating, which suggests that the fast Na^+ channel is not influenced at this time (80). The fast Na^+ channel may preserve enough capacity for Na^+ influx to account for elevation of $[Na^+]_i$ during ischemia. Actually, elevation of $[Na^+]_i$ could be attenuated by pretreatment with lidocaine, a Na^+ channel blocker (71). These results suggest that the Na^+ channel, in contrast to the Ca^{2+} channel, is active during ischemia and that there is a continuous Na^+ leakage into myocytes through the Na^+ channel down its electrochemical gradient. In canine, guinea pig, or sheep hearts, an increase in the rate of beating raises $[Na^+]_i$ by over 30% and results in activation of Na^+,K^+ ATPase (12). Increased rate of stimulation did not appear to cause net gain in Na_i in adult rat ventricles (4), though inhibition of the Na^+,K^+ pump by reduction of extracellular K^+ ($[K^+]_o$) or addition of ouabain caused elevation of $[Na^+]_i$ and increased Ca^{2+} uptake (31). These studies suggest that there are species differences regarding the importance of the Na^+ channel relative to the Na^+,K^+ pump. Moreover, a large increase in $[Na^+]_i$ did not occur without inhibition of Na^+,K^+ pump activity. During reperfusion, following prolonged ischemia, beating does not start immediately after restoration of coronary flow, and when it does resume the rate is slow. Therefore, a further increase in Na^+ influx through the fast Na^+ channel would be small during early reperfusion.

Both a decrease in pH_i (11) and gain of Na^+ (2, 21, 71, 84, 84a) are observed in myocytes during ischemia. Based on these observations and the properties of the Na^+/H^+ exchanger, Lazdunski et al (47) proposed that stimulation of Na^+/H^+ exchange during ischemia accounted for the increase in $[Na^+]_i$. Neubauer et al (65) presented supportive evidence that $[Na^+]_i$ increased in proportion to the reduction of pH_i in ischemic and hypoxic myocardium. Based on this observation, they argued that much of the increase in $[Na^+]_i$ during ischemia was through Na^+/H^+ exchange that was driven by greater accumulation of H^+. Inhibition of Na^+,K^+ ATPase activity however, may be more important because severe acidosis and accumulation of metabolites, such as inorganic phosphate, are directly inhibitory for the enzyme (32). Moreover, the activity of the exchanger is very sensitive to extracellular pH and is greatly inhibited in a low pH range (47, 72). The extracellular pH may fall before pH_i during ischemia (64), and the value commonly seen in severe ischemic myocardium (11) is low enough to inhibit the exchanger. Upon reperfusion, extracellular fluid was replaced quickly by incoming perfusate with a normal pH, which resulted in rapid reactivation of the exchanger. Actually, we observed a further slight but significant increase in Na_i during the early reperfusion period after 30 min of global ischemia (Figure 2). This initial rise was not detected during reperfusion in myocardium subjected to a short period of ischemia (71, 84, 84a) in which accumulation of lactate, decrease in pH_i (11), and reduction of Na^+,K^+ ATPase activity (15) were less prominent. Anoxic preperfusion depleted endogenous glycogen stores (63) and reduced H^+ production during ischemia, thus resulting in smaller decrease in pH_i (44). When this procedure was performed prior to ischemia, the initial rise in Na_i during early reperfusion was prevented (84, 84a). Also, the reperfusion rise in Na_i was abolished by pretreatment with amiloride, a Na^+/H^+ exchange inhibitor (84, 84a). These two procedures had no effect on the accumulation of Na^+ during ischemia itself. The readjustment of pH_i following addition of extracellular Na^+ to acid-loaded heart cells had a $t_{1/2}$ of 2.9 min (72). This is comparable with the time course of the initial rise in Na$_i$ (Figure 2).

The Na$^+$,K$^+$ pump has a primary role in maintenance of a low and stable [Na$^+$]$_i$ in cardiac muscle cells. The pump mechanism involves a sarcolemmal Na$^+$,K$^+$ ATPase that requires the free energy of ATP hydrolysis (21) to transport three intracellular Na$^+$ ions out in exchange for two extracellular K$^+$ ions. The free-energy change of ATP hydrolysis (ΔG) is calculated as

$$\Delta = \Delta G^{\circ} + RT \ln ([ATP]/[ADP] [P_i]) \qquad\qquad 1.$$

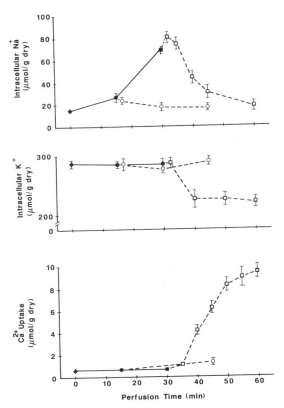

Figure 2   Changes in intracellular ion contents during ischemia and reperfusion.
Upper Panel: intracellular Na$^+$, Middle Panel: intracellular K$^+$, Lower Panel: Ca^{2+} uptake. The points and bars represent the mean ± S.E.M. of at least 6 hearts. ◆ = control; ● = 15 min of ischemia; ○ = 15 min of ischemia + reperfusion; ■ = 30 min of ischemia; □ = 30 min of ischemia + reperfusion. Data were taken from isolated perfused rat hearts subjected to normothermic global ischemia and/or reperfusion.

in which the concentration terms refer to the free cytosolic metabolite concentrations; ΔG° is the standard free-energy change; R is the gas constant; and T is the absolute temperature. During ischemia, inorganic phosphate increases and cytosolic [ATP] decreases. Therefore, the free energy available falls to a greater extent than the ATP level (21). Tani & Neely (85, 85a, 86, 86a, 86b) found that vascular washout by intermittent perfusion or maintained low coronary flow during global ischemia prevented the increase in Na$_i$ as long as myocardial ATP levels were preserved more than 30 to 40% of the preischemic value. The apparent K$_m$ of the enzyme for K$^+$ is in the lower mM range in isolated cell preparation with low [Na$^+$]$_i$ (22). In intact Purkinje fibers, however, much higher [K$^+$]$_o$ was needed for maximal pump rate if [Na$^+$]$_i$ was high (78). Since the Na$^+$,K$^+$ pump carries outward current, one of the intermediate reactions must be sensitive to the membrane potential. Gadsby et al (23) predicted that 40% of pump activity would be inhibited at the ordinary resting membrane potential when [K$^+$]$_o$ was in the physiologic range. Although an increase in [K$^+$]$_o$ (35, 42) and a decrease in membrane potential (42) counteract other inhibitory effects on the Na$^+$,K$^+$ pump, loss of the thermodynamic driving force caused by depletion of ATP (21) and accumulation of inorganic phosphate (32) impaired function of the Na$^+$,K$^+$ ATPase and led to elevation of [Na$^+$]$_i$. Restoration of mitochondrial oxidative phosphorylation, recovery from tissue acidosis, and washout of metabolites upon reperfusion together with increased [Na$^+$]$_i$ accelerated pump function. Sejersted et al (78) reported that the apparent K$_m$ of the enzyme for ionized Na$^+$ was about 10 to 11 mM and the maximum rate of fall of intracellular Na$^+$ activity was 6 to 7 mM/min at physiologic [K$^+$]$_o$. We observed that Na$_i$ declined about 30 μmol/g dry wt during a period of 8 min (Figure 2). Myocardial tissue contains 2 ml of intracellular water/g dry wt, which indicates that intracellular Na$^+$ activity fell about 2 mM/min. Even if total enzyme activity were reduced to 60 to 70% of the control value after 30 min of ischemia (15), the pump rate could still be 4 to 5 mM/min, based on the values given by Sejersted et al (78). Thus the Na$^+$,K$^+$ pump can account for the most of the decline in Na$_i$ during reperfusion. This hypothesis was further supported by the observation that ouabain (0.05, 0.1 or 0.2 mM) administered during reperfusion retarded abolished or even reversed the rapid decline of Na$_i$ in isolated rat hearts (M. Tani, unpublished data).

Na$^+$/Ca^{2+} exchange of myocytes can operate in either direction (68). The direction of ion flux is determined by the membrane potential because Na$^+$/Ca^{2+} exchange is electrogenic (18, 68). The reversal potential (V$_R$) for the exchanger is defined as follows:

$$V_R = (nV_{Na} - 2V_{Ca})/(n - 2)$$

2.

where n = the Na^+/Ca^{2+} coupling ratio, and V_{Na} and V_{Ca} are the equilibrium potentials for Na^+ and Ca^{2+}, respectively. They are defined as follows:

$$V_{Na} = RT/F \ln([Na^+]_o/[Na^+]_i); \hspace{3cm} 3.$$

$$V_{Ca} = RT/2F \ln([Ca^{2+}]_o/[Ca^{2+}]_i) \hspace{3cm} 4.$$

where R and T are the same as in equation 1, and F is the Faraday constant. When n = 3, V_R is between -10 and -30 mV (18). Thus, during the action potential, Ca^{2+} influx (Na^+ efflux) occurs, which contributes to elevation of cytosolic $[Ca^{2+}]$, whereas Ca^{2+} efflux (Na^+ influx) predominates during repolarization and contributes to relaxation of the myocardium. Although a moderate decrease in the total activity of Na^+/Ca^{2+} exchange was found in sarcolemmal preparations from ischemic and/or reperfused myocardium (15, 17), flux of both Na^+ and Ca^{2+} through this system still has a crucial effect on ion homeostasis because of the large transport capacity of the normal myocytes, as compared with other Ca^{2+} ion transport systems (6). The shorter duration of the action potential followed by cessation of beating in ischemia will decrease Na^+ efflux (Ca^{2+} influx) through Na^+/Ca^{2+} exchange. The resting membrane potential becomes less negative, but remains near the value of the K^+ equilibrium potential (V_K) (42). V_K is defined by an equation similar to that for V_{Na}. After an initial rise in $[K^+]_o$ at the onset of ischemia, both $[K^+]_i$ and $[K^+]_o$ (90) remain relatively constant between 15 and 30 min (Figure 2). As a result, it is unlikely that the resting membrane potential will exceed V_R for Na^+/Ca^{2+} exchange within 30 min after induction of ischemia unless V_{Na} and/or V_{Ca} are changed markedly during this period. Actually, elevation of $[Na^+]_i$ with longer duration of ischemia may decrease V_R and cause Na^+ efflux (Ca^{2+} influx). For any given $[Na^+]_i$ and membrane potential, there is an equilibrium value for cytosolic $[Ca^{2+}]$ at which the net exchange will cease. Steenbergen et al (82) reported that cytosolic-free $[Ca^{2+}]$ started to increase after 6 min of ischemia and reached 3 μM after 9 to 15 min. this value of cytosolic-free $[Ca^{2+}]$ is enough to restore V_R in ischemic myocytes. The amount of Ca^{2+} influx required to increase cytosolic-free $[Ca^{2+}]$ to 3 μM is at most 0.01 μmol/g dry, if intracellular water is assumed to be 2 ml/g dry. As a result a massive increase in cellular Ca^{2+} content will not occur unless cytosolic-free $[Ca^{2+}]$ is quickly sequestered by the mitochondria or sarcoplasmic reticulum and V_{Ca} is maintained near its original value.

The sarcoplasmic reticulum and mitochondria are not capable of accumulating Ca^{2+} under ischemic conditions (53, 92). Resumption of flow and delivery of oxygen, however, will restore energy production and pH_i and allow these intracellular buffers to take up Ca^{2+} (55, 58, 92). This mechanism is supported by the observation that reperfusion with an anoxic buffer or a buffer containing CN$^-$ decreased Ca^{2+} uptake after 30 min of global ischemia (9.7 $\pm$ 0.6 μmol/g dry down to 1.4 $\pm$ 0.1 μmol/g dry and 1.3 $\pm$ 0.3 μmol/g dry, respectively) which indicates that entry of Ca^{2+} during reperfusion is not the passive event predicted by the electrochemical gradient for Ca^{2+}, and massive Ca^{2+} uptake requires sequestration of intracellular Ca^{2+}.

The activity of the exchanger is inhibited during severe ischemia because pH$_i$ falls to approximately 6, a value at which exchange is blocked (68). The pH sensitivity of Na$^+$/Ca^{2+} exchange accounts for the reduced Ca^{2+} uptake during reperfusion with acidic buffer (61). In addition to the effects of pH, Na$^+$/Ca^{2+} exchange in a cardiac sarcolemmal preparation was also regulated by phosphorylation/dephosphorylation reactions and depended upon the ATP concentration in the incubation medium (7). When dephosphorylated, the affinity for Ca^{2+} and V$_{max}$ of the exchanger were reduced. The ATP concentration required for activation of the exchanger was in the micromolar range. Nevertheless, inhibition of Na$^+$/Ca^{2+} exchange by dephosphorylation of the exchanger was suggested in isolated heart cells with depleted cytosolic ATP (29). Reperfusion of ischemic myocardium could be expected to reactivate the exchanger by resumption of energy production and correction of tissue acidosis. Evidence for the involvement of Na$^+$/Ca^{2+} exchange was obtained when dichlorobenzamil (DCB), a Na$^+$/Ca^{2+} exchange inhibitor, was employed. Exposure of hearts to 40 μM DCB for 2 min before induction of ischemia had no effect on Na$^+$ accumulation during 30 min of ischemia, but reduced the reperfusion Ca^{2+} uptake by 50% (9.5 $\pm$ 0.4 μmol/g dry, down to 4.7 $\pm$ 0.4 μmol/g dry, n = 6). When DCB was added only during reperfusion, the effect was not as great as with pretreatment, but DCB still caused a significant reduction in reperfusion Ca^{2+} uptake. The data do not definitively show a direct effect of DCB on the exchanger because this agent also inhibited Ca^{2+} flux through the Ca^{2+} channel. DCB was effective during reperfusion, however, while other Ca^{2+} channel blockers were not (3, 49, 89), which suggests that DCB inhibited Na$^+$/Ca^{2+} exchange rather than a Ca^{2+} channel. Additional evidence for involvement of Na$^+$/Ca^{2+} exchange in reperfusion Ca^{2+} uptake was obtained in experiments employing a low [Ca^{2+}] (0.15 mM) perfusate. Reperfusion with the buffer containing the low Ca^{2+} concentration reduced reperfusion Ca^{2+} uptake and retarded the rapid decline in Na$_i$ (87a; M. Tani, unpublished data). Moreover, pretreatment with monensin, a Na$^+$ ionophore, resulted in a concentration-dependent elevation of Na$_i$ in hearts subjected to 15 min of global ischemia and a subsequent increase in reperfusion Ca^{2+} uptake and depression of ventricular function (84a) (Figure 3).

Sarcolemmal Ca^{2+} Pumps

A decrease in the capacity of the sarcolemmal Ca^{2+} ATPase leads to a reduction of Ca^{2+} efflux and net Ca^{2+} uptake. Sarcolemmal Ca^{2+} ATPase activity was reduced in membrane vesicles from ischemic myocardium (8,

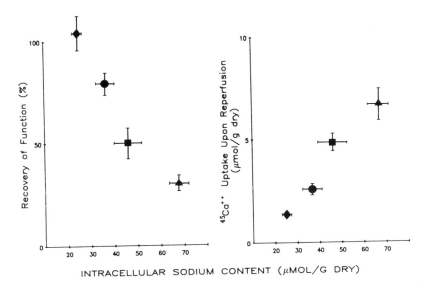

Figure 3 Effects of Na⁺ loading during 15 min of ischemia on recovery of function and reperfusion Ca²⁺ uptake. Left Panel: relationship between intracellular Na⁺ and recovery of function, Right Panel: relationship between intracellular Na⁺ and reperfusion Ca²⁺ uptake. The points and bars represent the mean ± S.E.M. of at least 6 hearts. ◆ = 0 monensin (a Na⁺ ionophore); ● = 1 M of monensin; ■ = 2 μM monensin; □ = 5 μM monensin. Monensin was added to the perfusate for 10 min before induction of 15 min of global ischemia in isolated perfused rat hearts.

17) and the reduction was enhanced upon reperfusion after prolonged ischemia (17). No changes in efflux of Ca^{2+} were detected during ischemia/hypoxia and reperfusion/reoxygenation in isolated perfused mycardium (5, 28). Under normal conditions, the rate of efflux is only about half-maximal because of the low $[Ca^{2+}]_i$ during diastole (6). Thus increased Ca^{2+} efflux in response to an elevation in cytosolic-free $[Ca^{2+}]$ under pathophysiologic conditions would mask the reduction of total enzyme activity. In addition, Na^+/Ca^{2+} exchange may be able to compensate for the loss of Ca^{2+} efflux by the Ca^{2+} pump because the amount of Ca^{2+} moved by the pump is relatively small as compared to the capacity of Na^+/Ca^{2+} exchange (6). In other words, even a complete loss of Ca^{2+} pump function would not result in a large increase in net Ca^{2+} uptake during reperfusion because of the limited role of the pump in moving Ca^{2+} out of the cell.

Possible Regulatory Factors for Excessive Ca^{2+} Influx

CATECHOLAMINES   Stimulation of either α or β adrenoreceptors has been reported to promote Ca^{2+} influx in the myocardium (19, 88). An increase in the density of both receptors was observed in ischemic myocardium (13, 56). Endogenous catecholamines were released during ischemia (77). These observations led to the hypothesis that some of the excessive gain in Ca^{2+} during reperfusion involved influx of Ca^{2+} through pathways controlled by the adrenoreceptors. Actually, pretreatment with adrenoreceptor blocking agents attenuated the reperfusion Ca^{2+} gain (60, 79). Activation of α_1-adrenoreceptor stimulates the phosphatidyl inositol cycle and the generation of diacylglycerol and inositol triphosphate in myocytes (66). Diacylglycerol activates protein kinase C, which may potentiate entry of Ca^{2+} through the slow channel (66). Moreover, activation of protein kinase C stimulates Na$^+$/H$^+$ exchange. Ikeda et al (34) suggested that stimulation of Na$^+$/H$^+$ exchange through activation of protein kinase C by phorbol esters caused an increase in Ca^{2+} influx via Na$^+$/Ca^{2+} exchange in cultured heart cells exposed to prolonged hypoxia. A similar process was suggested to be involved in Ca^{2+} uptake in reperfused ischemic myocardium (67).

Inhibition of β-adrenoreceptors may decrease Ca^{2+} accumulation in reperfused ischemic hearts (59, 79). The protective effects of the β-blocker may result from negative inotropism that reduces energy consumption during ischemia. Occupancy of the β-adrenoreceptor causes elevation of cAMP level by rapid activation of adenylate cyclase. Although cAMP increased Ca^{2+} influx through the slow Ca^{2+} channel, the effect of β-adrenergic blocking agents on Ca^{2+} overload does not appear to be mediated by inhibition of the slow Ca^{2+} channel as described earlier. β-adrenergic stimulation activates lipolysis in the myocardium, which may result from locally released catecholamines in oxygen deficient hearts (40). Since lipid degradation can cause a change to sarcolemmal membrane function even if membrane integrity is maintained, accelerated lipolytic activity may contribute to ischemic damage.

OXYGEN-DERIVED FREE RADICALS   Hess & Manson (30) proposed that oxygen-free radicals were involved in the development and progression of Ca^{2+} overload because reintroduction of molecular oxygen was temporally associated with the subsequent accumulation of Ca^{2+}. Two possible molecular processes can be proposed as major mechanisms of free radical-mediated increase in Ca^{2+} entry into myocytes. First, oxygen-free radicals cause peroxidation of lipids, essential components of biological membranes (54). The primary products of lipid peroxidation lead to perturbations of transmembrane ion transport and cause an increase in permeabilities for Ca^{2+} (48). Peroxidation of membrane lipids has been reported to modify sarcolemmal Na$^+$,K$^+$ and Ca^{2+} ATPase activities (28, 43). Second, oxidation of thiol (and probably methionine) residues of membrane-bound proteins related to ion homeostasis may be another mechanism (37). Reeves et al (75) showed that Na$^+$/Ca^{2+} exchange in the cardiac sarcolemmal membrane was activated by modification of thiol redox states induced by exogenous free radicals. Oxidation of protein thiols could result in conformational changes of proteins, that lead to alterations of the kinetic properties of membrane-bound proteins. The further reduction of Na^+,K^+ and Ca^{2+} ATPase activities upon reperfusion after prolonged ischemia (90 to 120 min) might be explained by this mechanism (17, 41), however, no further deterioration in enzyme activities was detected during reperfusion after shorter periods of ischemia (15, 17). Actually, continuous exposure to reactive oxygen metabolites generated by various exogenous systems was reported to modify sarcolemmal membrane function (33, 38, 43, 75); concentrations of the oxidant employed in these studies were between 0.05 and 5 mM (33, 38). A sudden burst of the oxygen-derived free radical production was detected by ESR with spin trap agents applied directly to the coronary effluent from ischemic myocardium during reperfusion of isolated hearts (24, 95). The burst lasted only a few minutes and quantitation of the peak signals for $\cdot OH$ and $R\cdot$ free radicals revealed that the concentrations were less than 1 μM (74, 95). Measurement of free radicals in frozen tissue gave values of 3 to 4 nmol/g wet (74), which would amount to less than 10 μM even when the free radicals were distributed only in the intracellular space. Therefore it is questionable whether free radicals produced endogenously in reperfused myocardium can account for the development of Ca^{2+} overload. We could detect only a slightly faster reduction of Na_i during the early reperfusion period after 30 min of global ischemia in hearts pretreated with superoxide dismutase and catalase (M. Tani; unpublished data). Furthermore, efforts to maintain the redox state of glutathione by administration of various sulfhydryl donors failed to accelerate restoration of Na^+ imbalance (M. Tani, unpublished data) or reduce reperfusion Ca^{2+} uptake in the same experimental model (87).

LIPID DEGRADATION   Direct application of phospholipases to cultured heart cells or sarcolemmal membrane vesicles can cause an increase in membrane permeability to Ca^{2+} and can stimulate Na^+/Ca^{2+} exchange (69). Amphiphilic metabolites produced by lipid degradation were also reported to increase Ca^{2+} permeability and to stimulate Na^+/Ca^{2+} exchange (45, 70) in sarcolemmal preparations. In the ischemia-reperfusion sequence, however, a decrease in membrane phospholipid content and accumulation of lipid degradation products were relatively late events and became evident only after prolonged ischemia (1–3 hr) (9), whereas Ca^{2+} overload was observed during reperfusion after 30 min of ischemia (83–85). In addition, a large amount of amphiphilic molecules was required to alter membrane function in sarcolemmal vesicles (1). The concentrations of these amphiphilic molecules at some specific loci in myocytes, especially the sarcolemmal membrane, might be high enough to cause dysfunction of membrane ion transport system because reacylation of fatty acids produced by lipolysis of membrane phospholipids was impaired (9).

CONCLUSION

Perturbations of Ca^{2+} ion transport systems in the sarcolemmal membrane are primarily responsible for the increased net influx of Ca^{2+} upon reperfusion. This is because modification of these membrane processes can lead to disruption of Ca^{2+} homeostasis in myocytes before ultrastructural damage to the sarcolemmal membrane becomes evident. Among these ion transport systems, Na$^+$/Ca^{2+} exchange most likely catalyzes the massive Ca^{2+} influx. Although many reports support this hypothesis, a final conclusion is not possible because the evidence is circumstantial. Future studies of the molecular mechanisms are needed. The possible role of catecholamines, oxygen-derived free radicals, and lipid degradation in excessive accumulation of Ca^{2+} is yet to be determined. These factors may accelerate the progression of Ca^{2+} overload by modification of function and/or structure of sarcolemmal membrane, however, their importance is still inconclusive.

ACKNOWLEDGMENTS

The author expresses sincere thanks to Dr. Howard E. Morgan for his valuable review and advice on the manuscript and to the late Dr. James R. Neely for his thoughtful suggestions and support. The author also thanks Madoka Tani for her secretarial assistance. This work was supported in part by Grant HL#37936 from the National Heart, Lung and Blood Institute.

Literature Cited

1. Ashavaid, T. F., Colvin, R. A., Messineo, F. C., MacAlister, T., Katz, A. M. 1985. Effects of fatty acids on Na/Ca exchange in cardiac sarcolemmal membranes. *J. Mol. Cell. Cardiol.* 17:851–61
2. Balschi, J. A., Frazer, J. C., Fetters, J. K., Clarke, K., Springer, C. S., et al. 1985. Shift reagent and Na-23 nuclear magnetic resonance discriminates between extra and intra cellular sodium pools in ischemic heart. *Circulation* 72 (Suppl. III):355 (Abstr.)
3. Bourdillon, P. D., Poole-Wilson, P. A. 1982. The effects of verapamil, quiescence, and cardioplegia on calcium exchange and mechanical function in ischemic rabbit myocardium. *Circ. Res.* 50:360–68
4. Blesa, E. S., Langer, G. A., Brady, A. J., Serena, S. D. 1970. Potassium exchange in rat ventricular myocardium:

its relation to rate of stimulation. *Am. J. Physiol.* 219:747–54
5. Bourdillon, P. D. V., Poole-Wilson, P. A. 1981. Effects of ischemia and reperfusion on calcium exchange and mechanical function in isolated rabbit myocardium. *Cardiovasc. Res.* 15:121–30
6. Carafoli, E. 1985. The homeostasis of calcium in heart cells. *J. Mol. Cell. Cardiol.* 17:203–12
7. Caroni, P., Carafoli, E. 1983. The regulation of the Na$^+$-Ca^{2+} exchanger of heart sarcolemma. *Eur. J. Biochem.* 132:451–60
8. Chemnitius, J. M., Sasaki, Y., Burger, W., Bing, R. J. 1985. The effects of ischemia and reperfusion on sarcolemmal function in perfused canine hearts. *J. Mol. Cell. Cardiol.* 17:1139–50
9. Chien, K. R., Han, A., Sen, A., Buja,

L. M., Willerson, J. T. 1984. Accumulation of unesterified arachidonic acid in ischemic canine myocardium. Relationship to a phosphatidylcholine deacylation-reacylation cycle and the depletion of membrane phospholipids. *Circ. Res.* 54:313–22

10. Chien, K. R., Sherman, C., Mittnacht, S., Farber, J. L. 1980. Microsomal membrane structure and functions subsequent to calcium activation of an endogenous phospholipase. *Arch. Biochem. Biophys.* 205:614–22

11. Cobbe, S. M., Poole-Wilson, P. A. 1980. The time of onset and severity of acidosis in myocardial ischemia. *J. Mol. Cell. Cardiol.* 12:745–60

12. Cohen, C. J., Fozzard, H. A., Sheu, S.-S. 1982. Increase in intracellular sodium ion activity during stimulation in mammalian cardiac muscle. *Circ. Res.* 50:651–62

13. Corr, P. B., Shayman, J. A., Kramer, J. B., Kipnis, R. J. 1981. Increased α adrenergic receptors in ischemic cat myocardium. *J. Clin. Invest.* 67:1232–36

14. Crake, T., Poole-Wilson, P. A. 1986. Evidence that calcium influx on reoxygenation is not due to cell membrane disruption in the isolated rabbit heart. *J. Mol. Cell. Cardiol.* 18 (Suppl. IV):31–36

15. Daly, M. J., Elz, J. S., Nayler, W. G. 1984. Sarcolemmal enzymes and Na^+-Ca^{2+} exchange in hypoxic, ischemic, and reperfused rat hearts. *Am. J. Physiol.* 247:H237–43

16. Daly, M. J., Elz, J. S., Nayler, W. G. 1985. The effects of verapamil on ischaemia-induced changes to the sarcolemma. *J. Mol. Cell. Cardiol.* 17:667–74

17. Dhalla, N. S., Panagia, V., Singal, P. K., Makino, N., Dixon, I. M. C., et al. 1988. Alterations in heart membrane calcium transport during the development of ischemia-reperfusion injury. *J. Mol. Cell. Cardiol.* 20:(Suppl. II):3–13

18. Eisner, D. A., Lederer, W. J. 1985. Na-Ca exchange: stoichiometry and electrogenicity. *Am. J. Physiol.* 248: C189–C202

19. Exton, J. H. 1981. Molecular mechanisms involved in α adrenergic responses. *Mol. Cell. Endocrinol.* 23: 233–64

20. Farber, J. L. 1982. Biology of disease: Membrane injury and calcium homeostasis in the pathogenesis of coagulative necrosis. *Lab. Invest.* 47:114–23

21. Fiolet, J. W. T., Baartscheer, A., Schumacher, C. A., Coronel, R., Ter Welle, H. F. 1984. The change of the free energy of ATP hydrolysis during global ischemia and anoxia in the rat heart. Its possible role in the regulation of transsarcolemmal sodium and potassium gradients. *J. Mol. Cell. Cardiol.* 16:1023–36

22. Gadsby, D. C. 1980. Activation of electrogenic Na^+/K^+ exchange by extracellular K^+ in canine cardiac Purkinje fibers. *Proc. Natl. Acad. Sci. USA* 77: 4035–39

23. Gadsby, D. C., Kimura, J., Noma, A. 1985. Voltage dependence of Na/K pump current in isolated heart cells. *Nature* 315:63–65

24. Garlick, P. B., Davies, M. J., Hearse, D. J., Slater, T. F. 1987. Direct detection of free radicals in the reperfused rat heart using electron spin resonance spectroscopy. *Circ. Res.* 61:757–60

25. Grima, M., Freyss-Beguin, M., Millanvoye-Van Brussel, E., Decker, N., Schwartz, J. 1987. Effects of various antianginal drugs on sodium influx in rat brain synaptosomes and in rat heart muscle cells in culture. *Eur. J. Pharmacol.* 138:1–8

26. Grinwald, P. M. 1982. Calcium uptake during post-ischemic reperfusion in the isolated rat heart: Influence of extracellular sodium. *J. Mol. Cell. Cardiol.* 14:359–65

27. Grinwald, P. M., Brosnahan, C. 1987. Sodium imbalance as a cause of calcium overload in post-hypoxic reoxygenation injury. *J. Mol. Cell. Cardiol.* 19:487–95

28. Harding, D. P., Poole-Wilson, P. A. 1980. Calcium exchange in rabbit myocardium during and after hypoxia: Effect of temperature and substrate. *Cardiovasc Res.* 14:435–45

29. Haworth, R. A., Goknur, A. B., Hunter, D. R., Hegge, J. O., Berkoff, H. A. 1987. Inhibition of calcium influx in isolated adult rat heart cells by ATP depletion. *Circ. Res.* 60:586–94

30. Hess, M. L., Manson, N. H. 1984. Molecular oxygen: Friend and foe. The role of the oxygen free radical system in the calcium paradox, the oxygen paradox and ischemia/reperfusion injury. *J. Mol. Cell. Cardiol.* 16:969–85

31. Hoerter, J. A., Miceli, M. V., Renlund, D. G., Jacobus, W. E., Gerstenblith, G., et al. 1986. A phosphorus-31 nuclear magnetic resonance study of the metabolic, contractile, and ionic consequences of induced calcium alterations in the isovolumic rat heart. *Circ. Res.* 58:539–51

32. Huang, W.-H., Askari, A. 1984. Regulation of $(Na^+ + K^+)$-ATPase by in-

organic phosphate: pH dependence and physiological implications. *Biochem. Biophys. Res. Commun.* 123:438–43

33. Hyslop, P. A., Hinshaw, D. B., Schraufstatter, I. U., Sklar, L. A., Spragg, R. G., et al. 1986. Intracellular calcium homeostasis during hydrogen peroxide injury to cultured P388D$_1$ cells. *J. Cell. Physiol.* 129:356–66

34. Ikeda, U., Arisaka, H., Takayasu, T., Takeda, K., Natsume, T., et al. 1988. Protein kinase C activation aggravates hypoxic myocardial injury by stimulating Na$^+$/H$^+$ exchange. *J. Mol. Cell. Cardiol.* 20:493–500

35. January, C. T., Fozzard, H. A. 1984. The effects of membrane potential, extracellular potassium, and tetrodotoxin on the intracellular sodium ion activity of sheep cardiac muscle. *Circ. Res.* 54:652–65

36. Jennings, R. B., Schaper, J., Hill, M. L., Steenbergen, C. Jr., Reimer, K. A. 1985. Effects of reperfusion late in the phase of reversible ischemic injury. *Circ. Res.* 56:262–78

37. Kako, K. J. 1987. Free radical effects on membrane protein in myocardial ischemia/reperfusion injury. *J. Mol. Cell. Cardiol.* 19:209–11

38. Kaneko, M., Beamish, R. E., Dhalla, N. S. 1989. Depression of heart sarcolemmal Ca^{2+}-pump activity by oxygen free radicals. *Am. J. Physiol.* 256:H368–74

39. Karliner, J. S., Motulsky, H. J., Dunlap, J., Brown, J. H., Insel, P. A. 1982. Verapamil competitively inhibits α_1-adrenergic and mauscarinic but not β-adrenergic receptors in rat myocardium. *J. Cardiovasc. Pharmacol.* 4:515–20

40. Karwatowska-Krynska, E., Beresewicz, A. 1983. Effect of locally released catecholamines on lipolysis and injury of the hypoxic isolated rabbit heart. *J. Mol. Cell. Cardiol.* 15:523–36

41. Kim, M.-S., Akera, T. 1987. O$_2$ free radicals: cause of ischemia-reperfusion injury to cardiac Na$^+$-K$^+$-ATPase. *Am. J. Physiol.* 252:H252–57

42. Kleber, A. G. 1983. Resting membrane potential, extracellular potassium activity, and intracellular sodium activity during acute global ischemia in isolated perfused guinea pig hearts. *Circ. Res.* 52:442–50

43. Kramer, J. H., Mak, I. T., Weglicki, W. B. 1984. Differential sensitivity of canine cardiac sarcolemmal and microsomal enzymes to inhibition by free-radical-induced lipid peroxidation. *Circ. Res.* 55:120–24

44. Kupriyanov, V. V., Lakomkin, V. L.,

Steinschneider, A. Ya., Severina, M. Yu., Kapelko, V. I., et al. 1988. Relationships between pre-ischemic ATP and glycogen content and post-ischemic recovery of rat heart. *J. Mol. Cell. Cardiol.* 20:1151–62

45. Lamers, J. M. J., Stinis, H. T., Montfoort, A., Hulsmann, W. C. 1984. The effect of lipid intermediates on Ca^{2+} and Na$^+$ permeability and (Na$^+$+K$^+$)-ATPase of cardiac sarcolemma. *Biochim. Biophys. Acta* 774:127–37

46. Lange, R., Ingwall, J., Hale, S. L., Alker, K. J., Braunwald, E., et al. 1984. Preservation of high-energy phosphates by verapamil in reperfused myocardium. *Circulation* 70:734–41

47. Lazdunski, M., Frelin, C., Vigne, P. 1985. The sodium/hydrogen exchange system in cardiac cells: Its biochemical and pharmacological properties and its role in regulating internal concentrations of sodium and internal pH. *J. Mol. Cell. Cardiol.* 17:1029–42

48. Lebedev, A. V., Levitsky, D. O., Loginov, V. A., Smirnov, V. N. 1982. The effect of primary products of lipid peroxidation on the transmembrane transport of calcium ions. *J. Mol. Cell. Cardiol.* 14 (Suppl. III):99–103

49. Lefer, A. M., Polansky, E. W., Bianchi, C. P., Narayan, S. 1979. Influence of verapamil on cellular integrity and electrolyte concentrations of ischemic myocardial tissue in the cat. *Basic Res. Cardiol.* 74:555–67

50. Linden, J., Brooker, G. 1980. Properties of cardiac contractions in zero sodium solutions: Intracellular free calcium controls slow channel conductance. *J. Mol. Cell. Cardiol.* 12:457–78

51. Lullmann, H., Peters, T., Preuner, J. 1983. Role of the plasmalemma for calcium homeostasis and for excitation-contraction coupling in cardiac muscle. In *Cardiac Metabolism*, ed. A. J. Drake-Holland, M. I. M. Noble, pp. 1–18. Chichester: Wiley

52. Mahnensmith, R. L., Aronson, P. S. 1985. The plasma membrane sodium hydrogen exchanger and its role in physiological and pathophysiological process. *Circ. Res.* 56:773–88

53. Mandel, F., Kranias, E. G., Grassi de Genede, A., Sumida, M., Schwartz, A. 1982. The Effect of pH on the transient-state kinetics of Ca^{2+}-Mg^{2+}-ATPase of cardiac sarcoplasmic reticulum. A comparison with skeletal sarcoplasmic reticulum. *Circ. Res.* 50:310–17

54. Marklund, S. L. 1988. Role of toxic effects of oxygen in reperfusion damage.

J. Mol. Cell. Cardiol. 20:(Suppl. II):23–30

55. Meno, H., Kanaide, H., Okada, M., Nakamura, M. 1984. Total adenine nucleotide stores and sarcoplasmic reticular Ca transport in ischemic rat heart. *Am. J. Physiol.* 247:H380–86

56. Mukherjee, A., Bush, L. R., McCoy, K. E., Duke, R. J., Hagler, H., et al. 1982. Relationship between β-adrenergic receptor numbers and physiological responses during experimental canine myocardial ischemia. *Circ. Res.* 50:735–41

57. Murphy, J. G., Smith, T. W., Marsh, J. D. 1988. Mechanisms of reoxygenation-induced calcium overload in cultured chick embryo heart cells. *Am. J. Physiol.* 254:H1133–41

58. Nakanishi, T., Nishioka, K., Jarmakani, J. M. 1982. Mechanism of tissue Ca^{2+} gain during reoxygenation after hypoxia in rabbit myocardium. *Am. J. Physiol.* 242:H437–49

59. Nayler, W. G., Ferrari, R., Williams, A. 1980. Protective effect of pretreatment with verapamil, nifedipine and propranolol on mitochondrial function in the ischemic and reperfused myocardium. *Am. J. Cardiol.* 46:242–48

60. Nayler, W. G., Gordon, M., Stephens, D. J., Sturrock, W. J. 1985. The protective effect of prazosin on the ischemic and reperfused myocardium. *J. Mol. Cell. Cardiol.* 17:685–99

61. Nayler, W. G., Papagiotopoulos, S., Elz, J. S., Daly, M. J. 1988. Calcium-mediated damage during post-ischemic reperfusion. *J. Mol. Cell. Cardiol.* 20 (Suppl. II):41–54

62. Nayler, W. G., Sturrock, W. J. 1985. Inhibitory effect of calcium antagonists on the depletion of cardiac norepinephrine during postischemic reperfusion. *J. Cardiovasc. Pharmacol.* 7:581–87

63. Neely, J. R., Grotyohann, L. W. 1984. Role of glycolytic products in damage to ischemic myocardium. Dissociation of adenosine triphosphate level and recovery of function of reperfused ischemic hearts. *Circ. Res.* 55:816–24

64. Neely, J. R., Whitmer, J. T., Rovetto, M. J. 1975. Effect of coronary blood flow on glycolytic flux and intracellular pH in isolated rat hearts. *Circ. Res.* 37:733–41

65. Neubauer, S., Balschi, J. A., Springer, C. S., Smith, T. W., Ingwall, J. S. 1987. Intracellular Na^+ accumulation in hypoxic vs. ischemic rat heart: Evidence for Na^+-H^+ exchange. *Circulation* 76 (Suppl. IV):IV–56 (Abstr.)

66. Otani, H., Otani, H., Das, D. K. 1988. α_1-adrenoreceptor-mediated phosphoinositide breakdown and inotropic response in rat left ventricular papillary muscles. *Circ. Res.* 62:8–17

67. Otani, H., Prasad, R., Engelman, R. M., Otani, H., Cordis, G. A., et al. 1988. Enhanced phosphodiesteratic breakdown and turnover of phosphoinositides during reperfusion of ischemic rat heart. *Circ. Res.* 63:930–36

68. Philipson, K. D. 1985. Sodium-calcium exchange in plasma membrane vesicles. *Annu. Rev. Physiol.* 47:561–71

69. Philipson, K. D., Frank, J. S., Nishimoto, A. Y. 1983. Effects of phospholipase C on the Na^+-Ca^{2+} exchange and Ca^{2+} permeability of cardiac sarcolemmal vesicles. *J. Biol. Chem.* 258:5905–10

70. Philipson, K. D., Ward, R. 1985. Effects of fatty acids on Na^+-Ca^{2+} exchange and Ca^{2+} permeability of cardiac sarcolemmal vesicles. *J. Biol. Chem.* 260:9666–71

71. Pike, M. M., Kitakaze, M., Marban, E. 1988. Increase in intracellular free sodium concentration during ischemia revealed by ^{23}Na NMR in perfused ferret hearts. *Circulation* 78 (Suppl. II):II–56 (Abstr.)

72. Piwnica-Worms, D., Jacob, R., Horres, C. R., Lieberman, M. 1985. Na/H exchange in cultured chick heart cells. pH_i regulation. *J. Gen. Physiol.* 85:43–64

73. Poole-Wilson, P. A., Harding, D. P., Bourdillon, P. D. V., Tones, M. A. 1984. Calcium out of control. *J. Mol. Cell. Cardiol.* 16:175–87

74. Rao, P. S., Cohen, M. V., Mueller, H. S. 1983. Production of free radicals and lipid peroxides in early experimental myocardial ischemia. *J. Mol. Cell. Cardiol.* 15:713–16

75. Reeves, J. P., Bailey, C. A., Hale, C. C. 1986. Redox modification of sodium-calcium exchange activity in cardiac sarcolemmal vesicles. *J. Biol. Chem.* 261:4948–55

76. Renlund, D. G., Gerstenblith, G., Lakatta, E. G., Jacobus, W. E., Kallman, C. H., et al. 1984. Perfusate sodium during ischemia modifies postischemic function and metabolic recovery in the rabbit heart. *J. Mol. Cell. Cardiol.* 16:795–801

77. Schomig, A., Dart, A. M., Dietz, R., Mayer, E., Kubler, W. 1984. Release of endogenous catecholamines in the ischemic myocardium of the rat. Part A: Locally mediated release. *Circ. Res.* 55:689–701

78. Sejersted, O. M., Wasserstrom, J. A., Fozzard, H. A. 1988. Na,K pump

stimulation by intracellular Na in isolated, intact sheep cardiac Purkinje fibers. *J. Gen. Physiol.* 91:445–66

79. Sharma, A. D., Saffitz, J. E., Lee, B. I., Sobel, B. E., Corr, P. B. 1983. Alpha-adrenergic-mediated accumulation of calcium in reperfused myocardium. *J. Clin. Invest.* 72:802–18

80. Sperelakis, N. 1988. Regulation of calcium slow channels of cardiac muscle by cyclic nucleotides and phosphorylation. *J. Mol. Cell. Cardiol.* 20 (Suppl. II):75–106

81. Steenbergen, C., Hill, M. L., Jennings, R. B. 1987. Cytoskeletal damage during myocardial ischemia: changes in vinculin immunofluorescence staining during total in vitro ischemia in canine heart. *Circ. Res.* 60:478–86

82. Steenbergen, C., Murphy, E., Levy, L., London, R.E. 1987. Elevation in cytosolic free calcium concentration early in myocardial ischemia in perfused rat heart. *Circ. Res.* 60:700–7

83. Tani, M., Neely, J. R. 1988. Hearts from diabetic rats are more resistant to in vitro ischemia: Possible role of altered Ca^{2+} metabolism. *Circ. Res.* 62:931–40

84. Tani, M., Neely, J. R. 1988. Intracellular Na (Na$_i$), calcium uptake and ventricular function of reperfused ischemic rat hearts. *Circulation* 78 (Suppl. II):II–642 (Abstr.)

84a. Tani, M., Neely, J. R. 1989. Role of intracellular Na$^+$ in Ca^{2+} overload and depressed recovery of ventricular function of reperfused ischemic rat hearts. Possible involvement of H$^+$-Na$^+$ and Na$^+$-Ca^{2+} exchange. *Circ. Res.* 15: In press

85. Tani, M., Neely, J. R. 1988. Intermittent perfusion of ischemic hearts lowers intracellular Na (Na$_i$) accumulation and improves recovery of function. *Circulation* 78 (Suppl. II):II–641 (Abstr.)

85a. Tani, M., Neely, J. R. 1990. Intermittant perfusion of ischemic myocardium: Possible mechanisms of the protective effects on mechanical function in isolated rat heart. *Circulation* 81: In press

86. Tani, M., Neely, J. R. 1988. Low flow anoxic perfusion of ischemic hearts reduces intracellular Na (Na$_i$) and attenu-

ates reperfusion Ca^{2+} overload and depressed ventricular function. *Circulation* 78 (Suppl. II):II–215 (Abstr.)

86a. Tani, M., Neely, J. R. 1990. Na$^+$ accumulation increases Ca^{2+} overload and impairs function in anoxic rat heart. *J. Mol. Cell. Cardiol.* 22: In press

86b. Tani, M., Neely, J. R. 1990. Vascular washout reduces Ca^{2+} overload and improves function of reperfused ischemic hearts. *Am. J. Physiol.* 258: In press

87. Tani, M., Neely, J. R. 1988. Failure of anti free-radical interventions to attenuates Ca^{2+} overload and depressed ventricular function of reperfused ischemic hearts. *Circulation* 78 (Suppl. II):II–343 (Abstr.)

87a. Tani, M., Neely, J. R. 1990. Mechanisms of reduced reperfusion injury by low Ca^{2+} and/or high K$^+$. *Am. J. Physiol.* 258: In press

88. Vanhoutte, P. M., Pinule, T. J. 1982. Calcium and α-adrenoreceptors in activation of vascular smooth muscle. *J. Cardiovasc. Pharmacol.* 4:S280–86

89. Watts, J. A., Koch, C. D., LaNoue, K. F. 1980. Effects of Ca^{2+} antagonism on energy metabolism: Ca^{2+} and heart function after ischemia. *Am. J. Physiol.* 238:H909–16

90. Weiss, J., Shine, K. I. 1982. [K$^+$]$_o$ accumulation and electrophysiological alterations during early myocardial ischemia. *Am. J. Physiol.* 243:H318–27

91. Wilde, A. A. M., Kleber, A. G. 1986. The combined effects of hypoxia, high K$^+$, and acidosis on the intracellular sodium activity and resting potential in guinea pig papillary muscle. *Circ. Res.* 58:249–56

92. Williams, A. 1983. Mitochondria. See Ref. 51, pp. 151–71

93. Yatani, A., Brown, A. M. 1985. The calcium channel blocker nitrendipine blocks sodium channels in neonatal rat cardiac myocytes. *Circ. Res.* 57:868–75

94. Yatani, A., Kunze, D. L., Brown, A. M. 1988. Effects of dihydropyridine calcium channel modulators on cardiac sodium channels. *Am. J. Physiol.* 254: H140–47

95. Zweier, J. L. 1988. Measurement of superoxide-derived free radicals in the reperfused heart. *J. Biol. Chem.* 263: 1353–57

Annu. Rev. Physiol. 1990. 52:561–76

MODULATION OF LEUKOCYTE-MEDIATED MYOCARDIAL REPERFUSION INJURY

Benedict R. Lucchesi

The University of Michigan Medical School, Department of Pharmacology, M6322 Medical Science Building I, Ann Arbor Michigan, 48109-0626

KEY WORDS: neutrophils, free radical, ischemic myocardium, inflammatory mediators, chemotactic stimuli

INTRODUCTION

New therapeutic interventions, such as coronary angioplasty or thrombolytic therapy, are directed towards the treatment of acute myocardial ischemia based upon the recognition that mortality among patients who are evolving a myocardial infarction is influenced by the extent of left ventricular dysfunction, which is directly related to the amount of myocardium that becomes infarcted and thus non-functional (1). Secondly, the size of the infarct that results is related directly to the severity and duration of the ischemic interval. Patients who are treated and reperfused early (<4 hr) after the onset of symptoms exhibit better functional recovery as measured by a larger ejection fraction and smaller infarct sizes as assessed on the basis of myocardial intracellular enzyme release (2). Third, reperfusion of the acutely ischemic myocardium results in a reduction in ultimate infarct size as determined in the experimental animal and presumably in patients. Proper aggressive treatment of acute myocardial infarction should involve attempts to recannalize the obstructed coronary vessels either by mechanical means or by thrombolytic therapy (3).

The size of the myocardial infarct resulting from a period of regional ischemia is related directly to the severity and duration of the ischemic insult (4). In the canine heart, coronary artery occlusion for more than 4 hr followed by reperfusion results in an infarct that is essentially identical to the extent of infarction that results after permanent coronary artery occlusion for 24 hr. Coronary occlusion less than 20 min is associated with prolonged ventricular dysfunction; a phenomenon referred to as the stunned myocardium (5) that eventually recovers without evidence of myocardial cell injury. Inasmuch as the degree of myocardial cellular necrosis increases with increasing duration of ischemia, it is apparent that early reperfusion of the ischemic myocardium will result in salvage of potentially viable tissue (6).

When the ischemic interval is extended to 40 min, the extent of irreversibly injured tissue (infarct size) is related directly to the duration of the ischemic event. Reimer & Jennings (4) described the "wavefront phenomenon" of advancing necrosis from the subendocardial to the subepicardial regions of the myocardium. The duration of protracted blood flow deprivation to the myocardium increased the extent of irreversibly injured myocardium and decreased the amount of tissue that could be salvaged by reperfusion. Most of the remaining viable tissue was confined to the subepicardial region, undoubtedly because of the maintenance of coronary blood flow provided by means of collateral vessels. It is clearly evident that early reperfusion of the ischemic cardiac muscle is essential if the goal is to prevent or reduce the extension of tissue damage associated with regional myocardial ischemia caused by a myocardial infarction.

THE CONCEPT OF MYOCARDIAL REOXYGENATION INJURY

Reperfusion of the ischemic myocardium results in an apparent acceleration of necrosis as manifested by cell swelling and the formation of contraction bands. This has been referred to as myocardial reperfusion injury. The sudden reintroduction of oxygenated whole blood reperfusion may be detrimental to the once ischemic myocyte, thereby giving rise to a paradoxical situation concerning the best approach to preserve the ischemic heart and the concept of myocardial reperfusion injury. Because the cellular morphologic changes observed with reperfusion are dependent upon the presence of molecular oxygen, it would be more appropriate to think in terms of reoxygenation injury (7).

As a simple definition, myocardial reperfusion (reoxygenation) injury refers to irreversible cellular damage (necrosis) resulting from the reintroduction of molecular oxygen at the time of organ reperfusion. This suggests that the reintroduction of oxygen itself causes injury that would not have occurred at all or at least not as rapidly as without perfusion. Injury to the myocardial cell upon whole blood reperfusion is characterized by a variety of events such as calcium overload into cells that have preexisting membrane defects, the influx of inflammatory cells (e.g. neutrophil), the generation of oxygen-derived free-radicals or other long-lived oxidants and the release of proteolytic enzymes associated with the acute inflammatory response. Reperfusion injury in vitro may be somewhat different under in vivo conditions, which involve the cumulative effects of one or more tissue or blood-borne factors. The alterations in myocardial cell viability observed under in vitro conditions may be a reflection of the intracellular generation of reactive species of oxygen and may differ significantly from what is observed in the intact heart perfused with oxygenated, whole blood. The tissue damage initiated with the reintroduction of whole blood will continue for an indeterminate period after reperfusion has been established. The subsequent regional myocardial inflammatory response to tissue injury and the accumulation of polymorphonuclear leukocytes at the site of injury secondary to the damage inflicted upon the myocardium due to the earlier ischemic insult is responsible for the extension of the tissue damage that occurs with reperfusion (8–10).

For the purpose of this presentation, we will employ a strict definition of reperfusion injury that considers the possibility that some or all of the ischemic myocytes that are not salvaged by reperfusion are viable at the time of reperfusion, but undergo a lethal explosive alteration because of an imposed oxidative stress that is associated with the reintroduction of oxygenated blood and the associated cellular components. Myocardial cells that were viable at the end of the ischemic interval are subjected to unfavorable conditions related to reperfusion, and it is the act of reperfusion itself that leads to cell death. This is the basis for the concept of reperfusion injury as used in this review. Myocardial cell death due to reperfusion injury may be different with respect to the mechanism of death than from that which occurs from prolonged myocardial ischemia.

POTENTIAL SOURCES FOR THE PRODUCTION OF REACTIVE SPECIES OF OXYGEN

There is a complex interrelationship among the various factors that contribute to reperfusion injury. Oxygen-derived free-radicals are produced by activated neutrophils that infiltrate the ischemic and reperfused myocardium. Free-radical scavengers as well as the oxygen-derived free-radical metabolizing enzyme, superoxide dismutase, and the hydrogen peroxide degrading enzyme, catalase, reduce the contribution to myocardial cell injury caused by superoxide anion and hydroxyl radical (11, 12). The polymorphonuclear neutrophil and other phagocytic cells possess the capacity to produce reactive species of oxygen when presented with appropriate stimuli (13) in a metabolic event that is referred to as the respiratory burst. The oxidants produced by the activated phagocytes consist of superoxide anion ($O_2^{\cdot-}$), hydrogen peroxide (H_2O_2), hypochlorous acid (HOCl), chloramines ($RNHCl^-$), and hydroxyl anion ($\cdot OH$). The primary function of these oxidants is to provide a defense mechanism against invading microorganisms. The killing of microorganisms occurs within the phagocytic vacuole in which oxidants are contained within an environment well-suited for such reactive products. The reactive species of oxygen become deleterious to surrounding cells when they are released into the extracellular environment. The primary reactant that serves as the ultimate source for each of the oxidants is $O_2^{\cdot-}$, which results from the one-electron reduction of oxygen catalyzed by the enzyme NADPH-oxidase. The oxidase, a membrane-bound flavoprotein, which is dormant in the resting phagocytic cell, becomes activated when stimulated by components of the complement system (C5a).

Neutrophils contain the enzyme myeloperoxidase, which catalyzes a H_2O_2-dependent oxidation of halide ions that involves both Cl^- and Br^- ions to give rise to OCl^- or OBr^-. Each of these hypohalite anions can act as a powerful oxidant capable of attacking a wide variety of biomolecules including α_1-antiproteinase.

An additional potential source of oxygen-derived free-radicals and oxidants is the enzyme, xanthine oxidase, which is localized within the vascular endothelium in many animal species studied to-date, but is not believed to be present in the myocyte of the human heart (14). Xanthine dehydrogenase undergoes a conversion from its dehydrogenase to its oxidase form because of the activation of a calcium-dependent protease (14, 15). Upon reperfusion, xanthine oxidase is believed to utilize hypoxanthine as a substrate and molecular oxygen as an electron acceptor, thereby leading to the production of superoxide anion ($O_2^{\cdot-}$). Support for this concept derives from the observation that allopurinol, an inhibitor of xanthine oxidase, has been reported to reduce tissue injury associated with myocardial reperfusion (15, 16).

Studies that demonstrate the protective effects of allopurinol in experimental models of myocardial ischemia provide evidence that xanthine oxidase may participate in the generation of oxygen-derived free-radicals during myocardial reperfusion (17). Under conditions of ischemia it appears that the enzyme xanthine dehydrogenase is converted by a calcium-activated protease to the oxidase form, xanthine oxidase, (D to O conversion) (18). Additionally, during ischemia there is an accumulation of purine metabolites from ATP and ADP (AMP, inosine, hypoxanthine). Upon reperfusion, the required substrates hypoxanthine and the necessary electron acceptor oxygen, are provided to the enzyme, which leads to the formation of uric acid and the generation of superoxide anion. The localization of xanthine oxidase, primarily in the endothelial cell (14), provides the xanthine with an important locus at which to induce tissue injury. Consistent with this premise is the reported observation that superoxide dismutase plus catalase administered one min before reperfusion reduced both the microvascular damage and the low reflow phenomenon in the endocardium of the canine heart subjected to regional ischemia for 2 hr followed by reperfusion for 4 hr (19).

Kehrer et al (20) were unable to detect any significant degree of conversion of xanthine dehydrogenase to xanthine oxidase in the rat heart, and pretreatment with allopurinol did not provide protection against the release of intracellular enzymes when the hearts were reoxygenated after a period of hypoxia. It was concluded that the tissue injury in the hypoxic reoxygenated rat heart was the result of a mechanism other than reactive oxygen generated by xanthine oxidase. A similar view was expressed by Bindoli et al (21), which indicated that the cardioprotective effect of allopurinol in the rat should be referred to as a mechanism that is unrelated to one based upon the inhibition of xanthine oxidase. Allopurinol does not prevent the formation of superoxide anion despite the fact that it can inhibit the production of uric acid by xanthine oxidase as opposed to its active metabolite oxypurinol, which can inhibit both functions of the enzyme (22). Some degree of caution is needed in interpreting data derived with allopurinol. The drug can not be regarded, when used in vivo, as a specific inhibitor of xanthine oxidase. According to more recent studies (16), it was suggested that metabolic conversion of allopurinol to oxypurinol may permit the active metabolite to exert an action to counteract the interaction of neutrophils with the coronary vasculature and/or with the cardiac myocytes.

THE ROLE OF REACTIVE OXYGEN METABOLITES IN REPERFUSION INJURY

The first suggestive evidence of the participation of oxygen-derived free-radicals in myocardial reperfusion injury in the intact animal developed from the work of Jolly et al (11). Given before reperfusion, the combined administration of the superoxide anion metabolizing enzyme, superoxide dismutase (SOD), and the H_2O_2 degrading enzyme, catalase, to anesthetized dogs subjected to 90 min of coronary artery occlusion followed by reperfusion was effective in reducing ultimate infarct size. In contrast, the antioxidant enzymes were without benefit if infused 40 min after reperfusion had begun. Werns et al (23) subsequently showed that the administration of SOD (5 mg/kg; 3800 U/mg) alone resulted in a 50% reduction in myocardial infarct size, whereas the administration of catalase alone was not accompanied with a significant degree of myocardial salvage. Ambrosio et al (24) demonstrated that recombinant human superoxide dismutase could reduce ultimate infarct size in the canine heart subjected to 90 min of regional ischemia followed by reperfusion, despite the fact that the enzyme was administered immediately upon reperfusion. The latter observation agrees with other similarly conducted studies (8, 11, 12, 25) and supports the contention that an extension of myocardial injury occurs coincident with the onset of reperfusion. It is of importance to note that not all studies are in agreement. The administration of superoxide dismutase plus catalase to the canine heart subjected to either 40 (26) or 90 (27) min ischemia followed by reperfusion for 4 days failed to provide evidence for a protective effect.

Several investigators who have employed the chronically instrumented canine heart also have failed to observe a reduction in ultimate infarct size with native superoxide dismutase (28, 29) given in combination with catalase. Gallagher & colleagues (28) employed a 3 hr period of ischemia followed by reperfusion for 24 hr, whereas Nejima et al (29) used a 90 min period of regional ischemia followed by 7 days of reperfusion.

One biological variable that could account for the differing results among the various studies with SOD is the duration of occlusion used to induce the infarcts. Studies reporting positive results employed durations of occlusion of 60 or 90 min. Those reporting negative results have used ischemic intervals of 40 min or 3 hr. Reperfusion injury may require an ischemic period of greater than 40 min and less than 3 hr. The failure to substantiate a protective effect in the above mentioned studies may be model dependent. The degree of myocardial cell death associated with a 3 hr ischemic interval may have resulted in far too little myocardium to be salvaged as a result of the applied intervention (30, 31). On the other hand, it is possible that an ischemic period of 40 min may be insufficient for the demonstration of myocardial injury due to a neutrophil-dependent, oxygen-radical-mediated mechanism.

Eng et al (32) provide an interesting insight into the relevance of the duration of coronary artery occlusion in studies designed to assess interventions for the protection of the ischemic heart. The latter investigators demonstrated that there is an explosive increase in the extent of necrosis between a narrow 50 to 60 min period of ischemia. Approximately 70% of the region at risk became necrotic when subjected to 90 min of severe blood flow deprivation, whereas only a limited extent of myocardial injury (approximately 10% of the risk region) was observed with a severe deprivation of coronary blood flow that lasted for 40 min. Short periods of ischemia (e.g. 40 min) may not be able to elicit a component of injury because of reperfusion, and most of the detected cellular damage is related to myocardial metabolism. Ischemia itself and the metabolic demands of the tissue at the time become the primary determinants of cell viability within the first 20 min. Necrosis was not detected as a result of 20 min of severe ischemia. Beginning at 30 min of blood flow deprivation, necrosis progressed from the endocardium toward the epicardium in a wave front pattern so that 90 min of ischemia resulted in 70% of the risk region undergoing irreversible injury.

There is support for the concept that myocardial ischemia and, in particular reperfusion injury, are accompanied by the formation of oxygen-derived free-radicals, which overwhelm diminished endogenous protective mechanisms to exacerbate cell injury. Cell death is probably a far more violent event than is often imagined, "an explosion rather than a dissolution", since the generation of free-radicals occurs rapidly, and the half-life of the reactive oxygen species, in most cases, is of relatively short duration. Recent studies utilizing electron spin resonance spectroscopy and spin trapping agents have provided direct evidence for the generation of oxygen-free radicals in myocardial tissue during the ischemic interval and particularly during reperfusion (33–35). Short durations of ischemia are not associated with irreversible cellular changes. The detection of free-radical production became apparent during the time of coronary occlusion and increased 100-fold during reperfusion (36). The burst of free-radical production peaked at 2–4 min after reperfusion and persisted for 3 hr after reflow. Relatively short periods of regional ischemia are accompanied by free-radical generation at the time of flow deprivation and by an explosive and prolonged period of free-radical production well into the period of reperfusion. The formation of both oxygen-centered and carbon-centered radical species appears to be a consequence of oxy-radical attack of cardiac membrane lipids and supports the idea of lipid peroxidation in the pathogenesis of ischemic heart damage, particularly during reperfusion (35). Free-radical production by endothelial cells, along with an inhibition of oxy-radical production by oxypurinol, provides additional support for the potential role of reactive oxygen products in ischemia and reperfusion injury (37).

The sustained generation of cytotoxic oxygen radicals (36) may explain why interventions such as superoxide dismutase with its relatively short pharmacologic half-life of 6–10 min may appear to be ineffective in experimental protocols designed to assess tissue damage 4 or more days after reperfusion (26, 39, 29). The scavenging action of the enzyme would have dissipated because of its short half-life, at a time when there is a continued production of lipid peroxidation because of oxygen-free radical attack on biological membranes. Przyklenk & Kloner (41) demonstrated significant protection by superoxide dismutase in the heart subjected to 6 hr of regional ischemia without reperfusion. If perfusion was instituted, the protective effect of the scavenger was no longer apparent at 30–48 hr post reperfusion. It was concluded that superoxide dismutase delayed rather than prevented the development of cell death. That this reasoning may be incorrect was suggested by a subsequent study in which polyethylene glycol conjugated superoxide dismutase, with a pharmacologic half-life of ca 30 hr, not only reduced infarct size in the heart subjected to 6 hr of regional ischemia, but continued to protect against cell death when infarct size was assessed 30 hr after reperfusion (42).

ROLE OF NEUTROPHILS AS A SOURCE OF REACTIVE OXYGEN METABOLITES AND PROTEOLYTIC ENZYMES AS POTENTIAL MEDIATORS OF MYOCARDIAL CELL INJURY

Neutrophils are capable of being activated upon attachment to the vascular endothelium with the subsequent generation of toxic oxygen products and the release of destructive proteases capable of altering vascular permeability. Acid and neutral proteases are also released that can alter the integrity of the vascular wall basement membrane (43). The neutrophil contains two latent metalloproteinases, collagenase and gelatinase, that are activated by hypochlorous acid and are capable of degrading collagen in addition to lysing endothelial cells (44). Mediators present during myocardial ischemia capable of activating neutrophils include complement activation products, leukotriene B_4, and platelet activating factor.

It was suggested that activation of neutrophils within the vascular space results in the formation of cellular aggregates that can physically impair blood flow to the myocardial capillary bed and thereby exacerbate the ischemic injury (45). Neutrophil accumulation in the vascular bed is thought to be the reason there is sometimes inadequate reflow or the no-reflow phenomenon after brief periods of ischemia (46) followed by reperfusion.

Associated with reperfusion of the ischemic myocardium is a cellular reaction characterized by the accumulation of inflammatory cells and the production of inflammatory mediators in the reperfused myocardium. The regional accumulation of inflammatory cells contributes, in part, to the extension of tissue injury associated with reperfusion of the previously ischemic myocardium (47–49). Leukocyte/endothelial cell interaction is essential for leukocyte migration across the endothelial surface, and superoxide anion, as well as C5a, have been demonstrated to increase adhesion of neutrophils to the endothelium (50).

Several studies have documented the correlation between infarct size resulting with reperfusion and the extent of neutrophil infiltration (48, 51, 52). Neutrophils have been observed to infiltrate the damaged myocardial region beginning with the onset of ischemic injury and to increase their numbers progressively for the first 24 hr post myocardial infarction (53). The infiltration of neutrophils within the early postischemic interval before the development of myocardial necrosis has been demonstrated (54–55). There is a direct relationship between the duration of myocardial ischemia and the extent of neutrophil infiltration and accumulation in the reperfused region (56). The formation of tissue edema, which accompanies cellular injury, involves interactions dependent upon the neutrophil for the full expression of the inflammatory response (57). The generation of oxygen-derived free-radicals represents one of the main mechanisms by which polymorphonuclear neutrophils can mediate tissue injury. The reactive products of oxygen are formed during the engulfment of particulate matter or when the neutrophils are activated by soluble stimuli, particularly C5a.

Romson et al (52) demonstrated that the myocardial protective effect of the non-steroidal anti-inflammatory agent, ibuprofen, was related to the inhibition of neutrophil accumulation in the reperfused myocardium or risk region. Evidently ibuprofen reduced myocardial infarct size in the dog subjected to 60 minutes of coronary occlusion followed by 24 hr of reperfusion. The anti-inflammatory effects of ibuprofen resulted in decreased neutrophil accumulation in the myocardial risk region with a concomitant salvage of tissue in the area subjected to reperfusion. The protective effects of ibuprofen are unrelated to its ability to inhibit cyclooxygenase since neither acetylsalicylic acid nor indomethacin reduced ultimate infarct size or inhibited the release of superoxide anion by activated neutrophils (58). Ibuprofen, in contrast to indomethacin and acetylsalicylic acid, provides a protective effect via a pharmacologic mechanism that does not involve its ability to inhibit the formation of prostanoids and most likely is acting by a direct action upon the inflammatory cells by impairing their chemoattraction to the region and impairing their ability to form and release cytotoxic derivatives.

Pharmacologic interventions capable of inhibiting the lipoxygenase pathway of arachidonic acid metabolism also reduce myocardial infarct size probably through a mechanism related to the inhibition of neutrophil accumulation within the myocardium. The dual cyclooxygenase-lipoxygenase inhibitor BW 755C (10 mg/kg) reduced myocardial infarct size by 50% as compared to non-treated controls when evaluated with a canine model of 90 min of coronary occlusion followed by 24 hr or reperfusion (55, 59) in association with a reduction in neutrophil accumulation in the reperfused myocardium (55).

CHEMOTACTIC STIMULI AND ACTIVATION OF NEUTROPHILS

In order for neutrophils to injure ischemic tissue, there must be a chemical signal or chemoattractant to direct the neutrophil to the affected myocardial region. Ischemic myocardial tissue gives rise to a tissue protease that activates the third component of complement (60). Extensive confirmation demonstrates that myocardial ischemia activates the complement system and that ischemia results in the migration of neutrophils into the jeopardized myocardium (61–63). Other chemotactic factors are generated in response to myocardial tissue injury, including leukotriene B_4. A chemotactic factor can be produced by a superoxide anion acting upon a plasma protein that has been characterized as a derivative of arachidonic acid (64). An increase in chemotactic activity is noted in the coronary sinus blood of dogs subjected to ligation of the left anterior descending coronary artery and correlates with the enzymatic and electrocardiographic indices of myocardial ischemia (65). Additional evidence for the participation of the complement system in the development of myocardial ischemic injury is obtained from studies in which complement depletion with cobra venom factor after coronary ligation resulted in a reduction in the amount of myocardium that eventually became infarcted (66). These observations were confirmed with the use of immunohistochemical methods demonstrating an extensive localization of complement components (C3, C4, and C5) within the ischemic myocardium which did not occur after decomplementation of the animal (61, 62). The membrane attack complex (MAC or attack sequence) of complement (C5b-9) is present within the ischemic myocardium of acutely infarcted humans as early as 6 hr after the onset of symptoms (67). The membrane attack complex consists of a stable macromolecular complex (C5b and C6, C7, and C8) that inserts into the membrane bilayer (with C9) and forms a pore or channel through the membrane that permits bidirectional flow of ions and macromolecules ultimately resulting in cell lysis. Thus, complement may have a direct as well as an indirect (neutrophil) effect on the sequential events associated with myocardial tissue injury and subsequent cell death.

THE ROLE OF THE ENDOTHELIAL CELL

A pathophysiologic finding in myocardial ischemic injury is the presence of endothelial damage to the coronary vascular bed, which leads to the extravasation of plasma and cellular components into the interstitial space. Polymorphonuclear leukocytes can adhere and migrate through the endothelial cell layer and are of pathophysiologic relevance with respect to their potential role in mediating myocardial injury. This latter event is a time-dependent process in the presence of total vessel occlusion. The inflammatory cells enter the damaged myocardium slowly and become apparent at 24 hr after the onset of injury. On the other hand, reperfusion of the once ischemic tissue allows for rapid access of the inflammatory cells to the jeopardized myocardial region (68). The movement of neutrophils and subsequent release of proteinases across the vascular wall may in itself be associated with permeability changes and injury to the vessel. The migration of the neutrophil across the connective tissue barrier of the blood vessel is dependent upon the action of proteolytic enzymes, which remain active even in the presence of plasma antiproteases (69). The adhesion of neutrophils to endothelial cells in culture is stimulated with endotoxin, interleukin-1 (IL-1), or tumor necrosis factor, which suggests that the endothelial cell plays an important role in regulating the entry of the inflammatory cells to sites of tissue injury. Bevilaqua & co-workers (70) have shown that there are subtle and profound interactions between leukocytes and the vascular endothelium that are under the influence of immune modulation. It was suggested that IL-1 can activate the vascular endothelium to increase the expression of its adherence molecules for leukocytes (71). These molecules are distinct from the CDw18, LFA (Mol, gp150,95) class of glycoproteins and appear to be independent of the leukocyte receptors for the formyl peptides such as f-Met-Leu-Phe or the complement receptors for C3b or C5a.

ADHERENCE PROMOTING CELL SURFACE GLYCOPROTEIN COMPLEXES

A group of neutrophil cell-surface glycoproteins mediates cell-cell interactions (72). The heterodimeric glycoprotein referred to as Mo1 and Mac-1 antigen consists of an alpha chain, CD 11b (165 kd); and a beta subunit, CD 18 (96 kd). The members of the leukocyte family each possess the same beta subunit that is covalently linked to the alpha subunit. The latter will vary, thereby giving rise to a family of membrane glycoproteins, LFA-1, Mo1 and gp150,95 (73). The alpha subunits dictate the molecular specificity. The expression of these molecules on the cell surface will be determined by the origin and stage of maturation of the leukocytes (74). Activation of leukocytes by con A, FMLP, zymosan-activated serum, C5a, or calcium ionophore results in an enhanced expression of cell-surface adhesion glycoprotein molecules in which upregulation is the result of a translocation of preformed receptors to the plasma membrane from an intracellular site. The process of expression on the cell surface is rapid and is not dependent upon new protein synthesis, which results in a 5–10-fold increase in the number of glycoprotein receptors from the resting state of 10,000 to 20,000 molecules per cell (75, 76).

Pathophysiologic conditions occur in which there is a chemoattraction and an enhanced binding of neutrophils to the surface of the affected cells. The localization of complement components may be a prerequisite for the attachment of neutrophils to the vascular endothelium after an ischemic insult to the tissue. Mo1 receptors on the neutrophil bind C3bi and thus promote the adherence to cells coated with C3bi. If neutrophil adhesion to the target tissue is prevented with an anti-Mo1 monoclonal antibody, there is an associated reduction in the extent of tissue injury (77). Neutrophil activation is accompanied by the expression of the adhesion promoting receptors, the net result of which is an amplification of the process of neutrophil accumulation at the endothelial surface. The resulting microenvironment at the neutrophil-endothelial cell-cell interface becomes the site at which the cytotoxic inflammatory mediators can exert their effects uninhibited by blood transported antioxidants and other cytoprotective factors.

THE INHIBITION OF NEUTROPHIL ADHESION

Administration of the anti-Mo1 antibody 45 min after the induction of regional myocardial ischemia results in a significant protection against reperfusion injury as measured by the size of the myocardial infarct that results after 6 hr of reperfusion (78). There was no effect of the antibody on arterial blood pressure, heart rate, or coronary artery blood flow that could account for the protective action. Anti-Mo1 administration in vivo significantly reduced neutrophil accumulation within the ischemic myocardial tissue as assessed by histological analysis of tissue sections. The specificity of the monoclonal antibody for the Mo1 receptor provides supportive evidence that the infiltrating neutrophil is a major contributor to the observed extension of myocardial injury at the time of reperfusion.

CONCLUSIONS

It is now accepted that early reperfusion of the once ischemic myocardium is an important consideration in an effort to reduce overall loss of functional tissue within the region of myocardium at risk. Thus reperfusion is essential for survival of the jeopardized heart muscle, and the reduction in ultimate infarct size is associated with a decrease in morbidity and mortality.

There will exist within the myocardial region at risk, a population of myocardial cells that are reversibly injured as a consequence of a period of (less than 3 hr) of ischemia. Within this population of cells, a fraction of the affected myocytes might undergo irreversible changes (cell death) associated with the onset of reperfusion. Reperfusion injury, therefore, refers to cell death caused by reperfusion. It is suggested that the lethal event may be reduced or prevented by appropriate measures directed against the cytotoxic effects of reactive species of oxygen and perhaps proteolytic products derived from inflammatory cells that are attracted to the injured area as a result of the influence of complement- and arachidonic-acid-derived chemoattractants, interleukin-1, and adhesion promoting neutrophil glycoproteins. Among the sites of production of the oxygen-derived free-radicals, one might include phagocytic cells, myocardial tissue, especially the mitochondria of the reperfused myocyte, and the vascular endothelial cells that possess the enzyme xanthine oxidase. Both oxygen metabolite-dependent and -independent processes may participate in the explosive tissue injury that is associated with the onset of reperfusion and additive to the myocardial damage that is secondary to the ischemic insult itself. The two events may be attributed to entirely different mechanisms of cell injury. This view may be at odds with the observations reported by others (79), and additional effort must be devoted towards a better understanding of the role of the inflammatory mediators that are attracted to the myocardial risk region within moments of the onset of reperfusion.

ACKNOWLEDGMENTS

The original work reported from the author's laboratory was supported by a grant from the National Institutes of Health, Heart, Lung and Blood Institute, HL-19782-10. The author acknowledges the valuable contributions of his colleagues Dr. Paul Simpson, Dr. Steven Werns, Dr. Robert Todd III, and Dr. Joseph Fantone.

Literature Cited

1. Rude, R. E., Muller, J. E., Braunwald, E. 1981. Efforts to limit the size of myocardial infarcts. *Ann. Intern. Med.* 95:736–61
2. Schwarz, F., Schuler, G., Katus, H., Hofman, M., Manthey, J., et al. 1982. Intracoronary thrombolysis in acute myocardial infarction: Duration of ischemia as a major determinant of late results after recanalization. *Am. J. Cardiol.* 50:933–37
3. Braunwald, E. 1985. The aggressive treatment of acute myocardial infarction. *Circulation* 71:1087–1092
4. Reimer, K., Jennings, R. 1979. The "wave-front phenomenon" of ischemic cell death. II. Transmural progression of necrosis within the framework of ischemic bed size (myocardium at risk) and collateral blood flow. *Lab. Invest.* 40:663–44
5. Heyndrickx, G. R., Millard, R. W., McRitchie, R. J., Maroko, P. R., Vatner, S. F. 1975. Regional myocardial functional and electrophysiological alterations after brief coronary artery occlusion in conscious dogs. *J. Clin. Invest.* 56:978–85
6. Koren, G., Weiss, A. T., Hasin, Y., Appelbaum, D., Wellber, S., et al. 1985. Prevention of myocardial damage in acute myocardial ischemia by early treatment with intravenous streptokinase. *New Engl. J. Med.* 313:1384–89
7. Hearse, D. J., Humphrey, S. M., Nayler, W. G., Slade, A., Bordu, D. 1975. Ultrastructural damage associated with reoxygenation of the anoxic myocardium. *J. Mol. Cell. Cardiol.* 7:315–24
8. Tamura, Y., Chi, L., Driscoll, E. M., Hoff, P. T., Freeman, B. A., et al. 1988. Superoxide dismutase conjugated to polyethylene glycol provides sustained protection against myocardial ischemia/reperfusion injury in the canine heart. *Circ. Res.* 63:944–59
9. Simpson, P. J., Fantone, J. C., Lucchesi, B. R. 1988. Myocardial ischemia and reperfusion injury: Oxygen radicals and the role of the neutrophil. In *Oxygen Radicals and Tissue Injury,* ed. B. Halliwell, pp. 63–77. Bethesda, Md: Fed. Am. Soc. Exp. Biol.
10. Jacob, H. S., Vercellotti, G. M. 1988. Granulocyte mediated endothelial injury: Oxidant damage amplified by lactorferrin and platelet activating factor. In *Oxygen Radicals and Tissue Injury,* ed. B. Halliwell, pp. 57–62. Bethesda, Md: Fed. Am. Soc. Exp. Biol.
11. Jolly, S. R., Kane, W. J., Bailie, M. B., Abrams, G. D., Lucchesi, B. R. 1984. Canine myocardial reperfusion injury: Its reduction by the combined administration of superoxide dismutase and catalase. *Circ. Res.* 54:277–85
12. Werns, S. W., Simpson, P. J., Mickelson, J. K., Shea, M. J., Pitt, B., Luc-

chesi, B. R. 1988. Sustained limitation by superoxide dismutase of canine myocardial injury due to regional ischemia followed by reperfusion. *J. Cardiovasc. Pharmacol.* 11:36–44

13. Babior, B. M. 1978. Oxygen-dependent microbial killing by phagocytes. *New Engl. J. Med.* 298:659–68

14. Jarasch, E.-D., Bruder, G., Heid, H. W. 1986. Significance of xanthine oxidase in capillary endothelial cells. *Acta Physiol. Scand.* 548(Suppl.):39–46

15. Parks, D. A., Granger, D. N. 1986. Xanthine oxidase: Biochemistry, distribution and physiology. *Acta Physiol. Scand.* 548(Suppl.):87–99

16. Werns, S. W., Shea, M. J., Mitsos, S. E., Dysko, R. C., Fantone, J. C., et al. 1986. Reduction of the size of infarction by allopurinol in the ischemic-reperfused canine heart. *Circulation* 73:518–24

17. DeWall, R. A., Vasko, K., Stanley, E., Kezdi, P. 1971. Responses of the ischemic myocardium to allopurinol. *Am. Heart. J.* 82:362–70

18. Battelli, M. G. 1980. Enzymic conversion of rat liver xanthine oxidase from dehydrogenase (D-form) to oxidase (O-form). *FEBS Lett.* 113:47–51

19. Przyklenk, K., Kloner, R. A. 1989. "Reperfusion injury" by oxygen-derived free radicals? Effect of superoxide dismutase plus catalase, given at the time of reperfusion, on myocardial infarct size, contractile function, coronary microvasculature and regional myocardial blood flow. *Circ. Res.* 64:86–96

20. Kehrer, J. P., Piper, H. M., Sies, H. 1987. Xanthine oxidase is not responsible for reoxygenation injury in isolated-perfused rat heart. *Free Radic. Res. Commun.* 3:69–71

21. Bindoli, A., Cavallini, L., Rigobello, M. P., Coassin, M., Di Lisa, F. 1988. Modification of the xanthine-converting enzyme of perfused rat heart during ischemia and oxidative stress. *J. Free Radic. Biol. Med.* 4:163–67

22. Spector, T. 1988. Oxypurinol as an inhibitor of xanthine oxidase-catalyzed production of superoxide radical. *Biochem. Pharmacol.* 37:349–52

23. Werns, S. W., Shea, M. J., Driscoll, E. M., Cohen, C., Abrams, G. D., et al. 1985. The independent effects of oxygen radical scavengers on canine infarct size. Reduction by superoxide dismutase and not catalase. *Circ. Res.* 56:895–98

24. Ambrosio, G., Becker, L. C., Hutchins, G. M., Weisman, H. F., Weisfeldt, M. L. 1986. Reduction in experimental infarct size by recombinant human superoxide dismutase: Insights into the pathophysiology of reperfusion injury. *Circulation* 74:1424–33

25. Tamura, Y., Saito, S., Hatano, M., Lucchesi, B. R. 1989. Limitation of myocardial infarct size by polyethylene glycol-conjugated superoxide dismutase in a canine model of 90 min coronary occlusion followed by 4 days of reperfusion. *Kokyu To Junkan* 37:201–8

26. Uraizee, A., Reimer, K. A., Murry, C. E., Jennings, R. B. 1987. Failure of superoxide dismutase to limit myocardial infarct size in a 40 minute ischemia/four days reperfusion model in dogs. *Circulation* 75:1237–48

27. Richard, V. J., Murry, C. E., Jennings, R. B., Reimer, K. A. 1988. Therapy to reduce free radicals during early reperfusion does not limit the size of myocardial infarcts caused by 90 minutes of ischemia in dogs. *Circulation* 78:473–80

28. Gallagher, K. P., Buda, A. J., Pace, D., Gerren, R. A., Shlafer, M. 1986. Failure of superoxide dismutase and catalase to alter size of infarction in dogs after 3 hours of occlusion followed by reperfusion. *Circulation* 73:1065–1076

29. Nejima, J., Canfield, D. R., Manders, W. T., Knight, D. R., Cohen, M. V., et al. 1989. Failure of superoxide dismutase and catalase to alter the size of infarcts and functional recovery in conscious dogs with reperfusion. *Circulation* 78:143–53

30. Jolly, S. R., Kane, W. J., Hook, B. G., Abrams, G. D., Kunkel, S. L., Lucchesi, B. R. 1986. Reduction of myocardial infarct size by neutrophil depletion: Effect of duration of occlusion. *Am. Heart J.* 112:682–90

31. Reimer, K. A., Jennings, R. B., Cobb, F. R., Murdock, R. H., Greenfield, J. C., et al. 1985. Animal models for protecting the ischemic myocardium: Results of the NHLBI cooperative study. *Circ. Res.* 56:651–65

32. Eng, C., Cho, S., Factor, S. M., Kirk, E. S. 1987. A nonflow basis for the vulnerability of the subendocardium. *J. Am. Coll. Cardiol.* 9:374–79

33. Blasig, I. E., Ebert, B., Lowe, H. 1986. Identification of free radicals trapped during myocardial ischemia *in vitro* by ESR. *Stud. Biophys.* 116:35–42

34. Zweier, J. L., Flaherty, J. T., Weisfeldt, M. L. 1987. Direct measurement of free radicals generated following reperfusion of ischemic myocardium. *Proc. Natl. Acad. Sci. USA* 84:1404–1407

35. Arroyo, C. M., Kramer, J. H., Leiboff, R. H., Mergner, G. W., Dickens, B. F.,

Weglicki, W. B. 1987. Spin trapping of oxygen and carbon-centered free radicals in ischemic canine myocardium. *J. Free Radic. Biol. Med.* 3:313–16

36. Bolli, R. 1988. Oxygen-derived free radicals and postischemic myocardial dysfunction ("Stunned Myocardium"). *J. Am. Coll. Cardiol.* 12:239–49

37. Zweier, J. L., Kuppusamy, P., Lutty, G. A. 1988. Measurement of endothelial cell free radical generation: Evidence for a central mechanism of free radical injury in post ischemic tissue. *Proc. Natl. Acad. Sci. USA* 85:4046–4050

38. Deleted in proof

39. Richard, V. J., Murry, C. E., Jennings, R. B., Reimer, K. A. 1988. Therapy to reduce free radicals during early reperfusion does not limit the size of myocardial infarcts caused by 90 minutes of ischemia in dogs. *Circulation* 78:473–80

40. Deleted in proof

41. Przyklenk, K., Kloner, R. A. 1987. Effect of oxygen-derived free radical scavengers on infarct size following six hours of permanent coronary artery occlusion: Salvage or delay of myocyte necrosis? *Basic Res. Cardiol.* 82:146–58

42. Chi, L., Tamura, Y., Hoff, P. T., Macha, M., Gallagher, K. P., et al. 1989. The effect of superoxide dismutase on myocardial infarct size in the canine heart after 6 hours of regional ischemia and reperfusion. A demonstration of myocardial salvage. *Circ. Res.* 64:665–75

43. Janoff, A., Zelig, J. D. 1968. Vascular injury and lysis of basement membrane in vitro by neutral protease of human leukocytes. *Science* 16:702–4

44. Smedly, L. A., Tonnesen, M. G., Haslett, C., Guthrie, L. A., Johnston, R. B. Jr. et al. 1986. Neutrophil-mediated injury to endothelial cells. Enhancement by endotoxin and essential role of neutrophil elastase. *J. Clin. Invest.* 77:1233–43

45. Jacob, H. 1981. The role of activated complement and granulocytes in shock states and myocardial infarction. *J. Lab. Clin. Med.* 98:645–53

46. Engler, R., Covell, J. W. 1987. Granulocytes cause reperfusion ventricular dysfunction after 15-minute ischemia in the dog. *Circ. Res.* 61:20–28

47. Lucchesi, B. R., Mullane, K. M. 1986. Leukocytes and ischemia-induced myocardial injury. *Annu. Rev. Pharmacol. Toxicol.* 26:201–24

48. Jolly, S. R., Kane, W. J., Hook, B. G., Abrams, G. D., Kunkel, S. L., Lucchesi, B. R. 1986. Reduction of myocardial infarct size by neutrophil depletion:

Effect of duration of occlusion. *Am. Heart. J.* 112:682–90

49. Hess, M. L., Rowe, G. T., Caplan, M., Romson, J. L., Lucchesi, B. 1985. Identification of hydrogen peroxide and hydroxyl radicals as mediators of leukocyte-induced myocardial dysfunction. Limitation of infarct size with neutrophil inhibition and depletion. *Adv. Myocardiol.* 5:159–75

50. Craddock, P. R., Hammerschmidt, D. E., Moldow, C. F., Yamada, O., Jacob, H. S. 1979. Granulocyte aggregation as a manifestation of membrane interactions with complement: Possible role in leukocyte margination, microvascular occlusion, and endothelial damage. *Semin. Hematol.* 16:14–147

51. Romson, J. L., Hook, B. G., Kunkel, S. L., Abrams, G. D., Schork, M. A., Lucchesi, B. R. 1983. Reduction of the extent of ischemic myocardial injury by neutrophil depletion in the dog. *Circulation* 67:1016–1023

52. Romson, J. L., Hook, B. G., Rigot, V. H., Schork, M. A., Swanson, D. P., Lucchesi, B. R. 1982. The effect of ibuprofen on accumulation of 111-indium labeled platelets and leukocytes in experimental myocardial infarction. *Circulation* 66:1002–1011

53. Fishbein, M. C., Maclean, D., Maroko, P. R. 1978. Histopathologic evolution of myocardial infarction. *Chest* 73:843–49

54. Engler, R. L., Dahlgren, M. D., Peterson, M. A., Dobbs, A., Schmid-Schonbein, G. W. 1986. Accumulation of polymorphonuclear leukocytes during 3-h experimental myocardial ischemia. *Am. J. Physiol.* 251:H93–H100

55. Mullane, K. M., Read, N., Salmon, J. A., Moncada, S. 1984. Role of leukocytes in acute myocardial infarction in anesthetized dogs: Relationship to myocardial salvage by antiinflammatory drugs. *J. Pharmacol. Exp. Ther.* 228:510–22

56. Go, L. O., Murry, C. E., Richard, V. J., Weischedel, G. R., Jennings, R. B., Reimer, K. A. 1988. Myocardial neutrophil accumulation during reperfusion and reversible or irreversible ischemic injury. *Am. J. Physiol.* 255:H1188–H1198

57. Wedmore, C. V., Williams, T. J. 1981. Control of vascular permeability by polymorphonuclear leukocytes in inflammation. *Nature* 289:646–50

58. Flynn, P. J., Becker, W. K., Vercellotti, G. M., Weisdorf, D. J., Craddock, P. R., et al. 1984. Ibuprofen inhibits granulocyte responses to inflammatory mediators: A proposed

mechanism for reduction of experimental myocardial infarct size. *Inflammation* 8:33–44

59. Jolly, S. R., Lucchesi, B. R. 1983. Effects of BW 755C in an occlusion reperfusion model of myocardial injury. *Am. Heart J.* 106:8–13

60. Giclas, P. C., Pinckard, R. N., Olson, M. S. 1979. In vitro activation of complement by isolated heart subcellular membranes. *J. Immunol.* 122:146–51

61. McManus, L. M., Kolb, W. P., Crawford, M. H., O'Rourke, R. A., Grover, F. L., Pinckard, R. N. 1983. Complement localization in ischemic baboon myocardium. *Lab. Invest.* 48:436–77

62. Pinckard, R. N., O'Rourke, R. A., Crawford, M. H. 1983. Complement localisation and mediation of ischemic injury in baboon myocardium. *J. Clin. Invest.* 66:1050–1056

63. Rossen, R. D., Michael, L. H., Kagiyama, A., Savage, H. H., Hanson, G., et al. 1988. Mechanism of complement activation after coronary artery occlusion: Evidence that myocardial ischemia in dogs causes release of constituents of myocardial subcellular origin that complex with human C1q in vivo. *Circ. Res.* 62:572–84

64. Perez, H. D., Goldstein, J. M. 1980. Generation of a chemotactic lipid from arachidonic acid by exposure to a superoxide generating system. *Fed. Proc.* 39:1170 (Abstr.)

65. Hartman, J. R., Robinson, J. A., Gunnar, R. M. 1977. Chemotactic activity in the coronary sinus after experimental myocardial infarction: Effects of pharmacologic interventions on ischemic injury. *Am. J. Cardiol.* 40:550–55

66. Maroko, P. R., Carpenter, C. B., Chiariello, M., Fishbein, M. C., Radvany, P., et al. 1978. Reduction by cobra venom factor of myocardial necrosis after coronary artery occlusion. *J. Clin. Invest.* 61:661–70

67. Mathey, D. G., Schafer, H., Schofer, J., Kruger, W., Langes, K., Bhakdi, S. 1986. Deposition of the terminal C5b-9 complement complex in infarcted areas of human myocardium. *Circulation* 74(Suppl. II):372 (Abstr.)

68. Mullane, K. M., Read, N., Salmon, J. A., Moncada, S. 1984. Role of leukocytes in acute myocardial infarction in anesthetized dogs: Relationship to myocardial salvage by anti-inflammatory drugs. *J. Pharmacol. Exp. Ther.* 228:510–22

69. Russo, R. G., Liotta, L. A., Thorgeirsson, U., Brundage, R., Schiffmann, E. 1981. Polymorphonuclear leukocyte migration through human amnion membrane. *J. Cell. Biol.* 91:459–67

70. Bevilaqua, M. P., Pober, J. S., Wheeler, M. E., Cotran, R. S., Gimbrone, M. A. 1985. Interleukin-1 acts on cultured human vascular endothelium to increase the adhesion of polymorphonuclear leukocytes, monocytes and related leukocyte cell lines. *J. Clin. Invest.* 769:2003–2011

71. Bevilaqua, M. P., Pober, J. S., Wheeler, M. E., Cotran, R. S., Gimbrone, M. A. 1985. Interleukin-1 activation of vascular endothelium. Effects on procoagulant activity and leukocyte adhesion. *Am. J. Pathol.* 121:394–403

72. Harlan, J. M. 1985. Leukocyte-endothelial interactions. *Blood* 65:513–25

73. Sanchez-Madrid, F., Nagy, J. A., Robbins, E., Simon, P., Springer, T. A. 1983. A human leukocyte differentiation antigen family with distinct alpha-subunits and a common beta-subunit: the lymphocyte function-associated antigen (LFA-1) and C3bi complement receptor (OKM1/Mac-1), and the p150,95 molecule. *J. Exp. Med.* 158:1785–1803

74. Miller, L. J., Schwarting, R., Springer, T. A. 1986. Regulated expression of the Mac-1, p150,95 glycoprotein family during leukocyte differentiation. *J. Immunol.* 137:2891–2900

75. Ross, G. D., Medof, M. E. 1985. Membrane complement receptors specific for bound fragments of C3. *Adv. Immunol.* 37:217–67

76. Berger, M., O'Shea, J., Cross, A. S., Folks, T. M., Chused, T. M., et al. 1984. Human neutrophils increase expression of C3bi as well as C3b receptors upon activation. *J. Clin. Invest.* 74:1566–71

77. Simon, R. H., DeHart, P. D., Todd, R. F. 1986. Neutrophil-induced injury of rat pulmonary alveolar epithelial cells. *J. Clin. Invest.* 78:1375–86

78. Simpson, P. J., Todd, R. F. III, Fantone, J. C., Mickelson, J. K., Griffin, J. D., Lucchesi, B. R. 1988. Reduction of experimental canine myocardial reperfusion injury by a monoclonal antibody (anti-Mo1, Anti-CD11b) that inhibits leukocyte adhesion. *J. Clin. Invest.* 81:624–29

79. Jennings, R. B., Reimer, K. A., Steenbergen, C. Jr. 1986. Myocardial ischemia revisited. The osmolar load, membrane damage, and reperfusion (Editorial). *J. Mol. Cell. Cardiol.* 18:769–80

Annu. Rev. Physiol. 1990. 52:577–90

CALCIUM-DEPENDENT REGULATION OF PROTEIN SYNTHESIS IN INTACT MAMMALIAN CELLS

Charles O. Brostrom and Margaret A. Brostrom

Department of Pharmacology, UMDNJ-Robert Wood Johnson Medical School, Piscataway, New Jersey 08854

KEY WORDS: mRNA translation, endoplasmic reticulum, BiP/GRP78, phorbol ester, GH$_3$ pituitary cells

INTRODUCTION

Protein synthesis is a complex process that involves a major expenditure of cellular energy and that affects all aspects of cellular performance. Rapidly acting mechanisms must therefore exist to coordinate protein synthesis with processes underpinning cellular responsiveness. It is clear that the synthesis of typical proteins is rapidly abolished in a variety of cell types exposed to certain types of stress including anoxia (60), heat shock or treatment with various chemicals (18, 25, 42, 60), and viral infection (39, 59) despite the existence of normal complements of mRNA within the cell and the continued ability of the cell to synthesize viral or stress proteins. These inhibitions are generally thought to involve changes in the activity of one or more of the initiation factors required for normal cellular mRNA translation (45, 49). While much data has been generated regarding the properties and interactions of the various initiation factors and other substances that configure the ribosome and mRNA such that peptide chain initiation and elongation can proceed, the mechanisms by which physiologic regulation of translation is achieved in intact cells remain subject to debate. Most regulatory schemes for

0066-4278/90/0315-0577$02.00

translation center on putative loci at initiation and include the binding of mRNA to the 43S ribosomal complex and modification of the association of specific initiation factors with the 40S or 60S ribosomal subunit. A number of proteins associated with the translational apparatus, including eIF-2_α (49), eIF-4B (29) and 4E (30, 57), EF-2 (48, 56), and ribosomal protein S6 (64) are subject to protein phosphorylation and, hence, potential regulation. Most of the current information regarding the details of translation in mammalian cells has been derived from cell-free systems, especially reticulocyte lysates. The value of using intact cells to study the regulation of translation has, in our judgment, been inadequately appreciated. Intact cells synthesize authentic proteins at sustained high rates and retain the organization and function of collateral processes underpinning putative regulatory interactions. In contrast, cell-free initiating systems derived from nucleated mammalian cells invariably operate with an extreme loss of activity and are subject to a variety of laboratory artifacts produced by disorganization, dilution, and disintegration of both regulatory and nonregulatory components. A broad body of literature attests to the central role of cytosolic free Ca^{2+} in the generation of cellular responses to a variety of extracellular stimuli. Continued improvements in methodology for measuring the cation have been accompanied by clearer understanding of the dynamics of Ca^{2+} homeostasis and the mechanisms by which cytosolic free Ca^{2+} participates in the generation of cellular responses to extracellular stimuli (9). Increased concentrations of free intracellular Ca^{2+} generated from influx of the cation across the plasmalemma and/or its release from internally sequestered stores are well-established to stimulate a series of Ca^{2+}-dependent enzymes that modify the phosphate content and activities of various regulatory enzymes (23, 36). For example, activation of a multifunctional Ca^{2+}/calmodulin-dependent protein kinase in response to Ca^{2+}-mobilizing hormones promotes the phosphorylation of a number of cytoplasmic proteins in isolated rat hepatocytes (36). Multi-enzymic foci of phosphorylation provide the potential for cytosolic free Ca^{2+} to coordinate diverse cell functions. Ca^{2+} is clearly required for stimulus secretion coupling and is interdigitated at a number of levels with the cAMP second messenger system.

While most of the Ca^{2+} in the cell is sequestered, Ca^{2+} in this state is not generally perceived to be regulatory. The prevailing view is that the bulk of intracellular sequestered Ca^{2+} resides in the endoplasmic reticulum (5, 44) and is subject to mobilization in response to such agents as various inositol phosphates (5, 44), Ca^{2+} ionophores (1, 2, 12), and fatty acids related to arachidonate (38, 68). Both the rough (4, 27) and the smooth (3) endoplasmic reticulum are reportedly capable of Ca^{2+} uptake, depending on which body of literature one surveys. The relationship of Ca^{2+} sequestration to broader functions of the endoplasmic reticulum, such as the synthesis and processing of nascent polypeptides, however, is currently undefined. Teleologically, it would seem reasonable that the endoplasmic reticulum should exert some governance on the rate of translation since it binds a large portion of the total ribosomal population of most cells and is intimately concerned with the disposal of a considerable fraction of newly synthesized protein. The subject of this review is the expanding data on intact cells that support the conclusion that mobilization of intracellular sequestered Ca^{2+} by pharmacologic procedures rapidly inhibits normal protein synthesis at translation.

THE GH$_3$ CELL AS A MODEL FOR THE MANIPULATION OF INTRACELLULAR Ca^{2+}

Relatively simple procedures are available by which the Ca^{2+} pools of most intact cells can be grossly adjusted. The first (control) condition is the Ca^{2+}-repleted state represented by cells equilibrated in Ca^{2+}-containing medium. Such preparations possess low (resting) cytosolic free Ca^{2+} concentrations and optimal stores of sequestered cation. A second condition is the Ca^{2+}-depleted state produced by exposure to low extracellular Ca^{2+} concentrations (1 mM EGTA with or without Ca^{2+} ionophore), which provide preparations possessing low cytosolic and low sequestered Ca^{2+} (1). A third condition is the Ca^{2+}-repleted state in combination with Ca^{2+} ionophore (A23187 or ionomycin), which produces cell preparations with high cytosolic but low sequestered Ca^{2+} (2). GH clonal strains of a functional rat pituitary tumor are particularly well-characterized with respect to such perturbations of Ca^{2+} homeostasis (1, 2, 13, 15, 58, 62, 70). The clonal strain GH$_3$ produces both prolactin and growth hormone (62a). Treatment of GH$_3$ cells with EGTA creates a reverse concentration gradient for free Ca^{2+} such that intracellular free Ca^{2+} is rapidly lost to the extracellular milieu as measured by Ca^{2+} fluorescent dye techniques (1). Sequestered stores are gradually depleted via release to the cytoplasm as determined by atomic absorption spectrophotometry (13, 15) or ^{45}Ca efflux (G. Kuznetsov, unpublished data). In effect, EGTA lowers free intracellular Ca^{2+} below the concentration required by active transport systems accumulating the cation at sequestering sites. Based on increasing degrees of inhibition of the rate of amino acid incorporation, Ca^{2+} depletion by EGTA is largely complete by 30 min and fully complete by 45 min (14, 16, 70). Cell viability as measured by dye exclusion, ATP content, and repleting efficiency is maintained during such treatment for many hours (13, 15).

Ca^{2+} ionophores are well-characterized agents (43, 51–53, 67) that are established to increase cytosolic free Ca^{2+} in numerous cell types by virtue of their ability to facilitate diffusion of the cation through biological membranes (51–53). The relative contributions of extracellular Ca^{2+} influx through the plasmalemma vs the release of Ca^{2+} from intracellular sites of sequestration in the ionophore-mediated increase in cytosolic free Ca^{2+} are not generally well defined. The prevailing view has been that Ca^{2+} influx is the more important of the two processes (52). Recent reports by Albert & Tashjian (1, 2) have questioned this view, at least with respect to GH pituitary cells. Based on extensive fluorescent dye measurements of free intracellular Ca^{2+} and Ca^{2+} mobilization for GH_3 and GH_4C_1 cells responding to a variety of agents, including EGTA, TRH, and ionomycin, these workers concluded that Ca^{2+} ionophores specifically released sequestered cellular Ca^{2+} with little effect on Ca^{2+} influx (1). Within 1 min of application ionomycin induced a release of 50–60% of cell-associated Ca^{2+} that paralleled an increase in intracellular free Ca^{2+} (2). In contrast to TRH, which appeared to mobilize Ca^{2+} through the agency of inositol trisphosphate (IP_3), Ca^{2+} ionophore acted directly. The effects of EGTA and Ca^{2+} ionophore are clearly complementary. Ionophore mobilizes Ca^{2+} to the cytosol and EGTA draws Ca^{2+} from the cytosol to the extracellular milieu. Combination of the two agents has been extremely effective in rapidly producing the Ca^{2+}-depleted state and in inhibiting amino acid incorporation in all nucleated mammalian cells studied to date (12).

Ca^{2+} REQUIREMENT FOR PROTEIN SYNTHESIS IN INTACT CELLS

Requirement of Sequestered Ca^{2+} for Amino Acid Incorporation

Expanding evidence supports the proposal that Ca^{2+}, in addition to its role as an intracellular mediator of cell surface humoral interactions, functions prominently in the regulation of translation in a variety of eukaryotic cell types (10, 11, 19, 31, 34, 55, 61). Effects of the cation on protein synthesis have been largely observed for intact cells or tissues exposed to low extracellular Ca^{2+} concentrations. Depletion of intracellular Ca^{2+} stores (in the better responding preparations) is accompanied by a concomitant 4–10fold reduction in the rate of amino acid incorporation. In our laboratories, amino acid incorporation into virtually all protein populations in normal rat hepatocytes (11), C6 glial tumor cells (10), and GH_3 pituitary cells (14, 69, 60) was found to be inhibited 80–90% following Ca^{2+} depletion with EGTA-buffered media over a period of approximately 30 min. Peptides synthesized for export, such as prolactin and growth hormone, were synthesized in a comparably Ca^{2+}-dependent manner to constitutive cell proteins (69). Addition of 1 mM Ca^{2+} in excess of chelator restored the rate of protein synthesis within 7–10 min to that of nondepleted control preparations. Ca^{2+} has proven to be uniquely potent and specific among physiologically occurring cations in conferring such stimulation over a broad range of Mg^{2+}, Na^+, and K^+ concentrations, pH, and osmolarity in both minimal and enriched media either with or without the addition of sera. The effects of Ca^{2+} depletion have not been traceable to changes in amino acid uptake, aminoacylation of transfer RNA including met-initiator tRNA, RNA synthesis, protein catabolism, the removal of cells from growth surfaces, or changes in purine nucleotide content or cell viability.

Various evidence supports the hypothesis that sequestered, rather than free cytosolic Ca^{2+}, maintains protein synthesis. As noted earlier, Ca^{2+} is rapidly drawn from the cytosolic pool when cells are exposed to EGTA, but amino acid incorporation is only slowly inhibited by the chelator. TRH, which has a modest ability to provoke release from sequestered sites in GH$_3$ cells via the agency of IP$_3$ (2), potentiated the action of EGTA at early times of exposure (14). Hormones, such as angiotensin II, vasopressin, and α-adrenergic agonists, which are widely believed to mobilize sequestered Ca^{2+} from the endoplasmic reticulum to the cytoplasm in hepatocytes, were found to inhibit amino acid incorporation in isolated hepatocytes and reduce the polysome contents of rat liver exposed to physiologic Ca^{2+} concentrations and pH (11, 22). These effects were largely reversible by the addition of supraphysiologic concentrations of Ca^{2+} to the extracellular medium. More recently, low concentrations of the Ca^{2+} ionophores, A23187 and ionomycin, were found to rapidly suppress the Ca^{2+}-dependent component of protein synthesis in GH$_3$ cells (12). More ionophore was required to inhibit amino acid incorporation into protein as extracellular Ca^{2+} was increased. Pre-existing inhibitions of protein synthesis produced by low concentrations of ionophore at low extracellular Ca^{2+} concentrations were reversed by adjustment to high extracellular Ca^{2+}. Ca^{2+} ionophores also revealed the strong underlying Ca^{2+} dependence of translation in cell types, such as HeLa and CHO, that display only a modest overt Ca^{2+}-dependent component following exposure to EGTA. Initial experiments with arachidonic acid, a reported mobilizing agent for sequestered Ca^{2+}, show strong inhibition of amino acid incorporation in GH$_3$, C6 glioma, and HeLa cells (E. Rotman, unpublished data).

Translational Initiation is a Ca^{2+}-Requiring Process in Nucleated Mammalian Cells

The translational phase of protein synthesis has been traditionally divided into three stages: peptide chain initiation, elongation, and termination. In studies of translation in intact GH$_3$ pituitary cells, Ca^{2+} depletion with EGTA resulted in the disappearance of polysomes and an accumulation of 80S monosomes and ribosomal subunits typical of slowed rates of initiation (21). Ca^{2+} repletion rapidly (min) restored cellular polysomal contents with an accompanying accumulation of 43S preinitiation complex (40S·eIF-2·Met-tRNA$_f$·GTP) as determined by [^{35}S]methionine pulse labeling experiments. As noted above, Ca^{2+} does not affect either the uptake of methionine or the aminoacylation of methionyl tRNA in either GH$_3$ (16) or C6 cells (10). When elongation was made rate limiting by the addition of the dissociable elongation inhibitor, cycloheximide, polysomal contents were comparable for both Ca^{2+}-depleted and restored cells. Average ribosomal transit times, as determined by the double isotope labeling procedure of Ledford & Davis (41), were the same for both Ca^{2+}-depleted and restored cells, which indicates that elongation per se is not directly affected by the cation under these conditions. Transit times were extended in parallel as a function of increasing cycloheximide concentration. Since the average ribosomal transit time was not altered by Ca^{2+}, it follows that noninitiator forms of transfer RNA are not affected in a limiting fashion by the cation. It is also apparent that peptide chain termination is not Ca^{2+}-dependent, since the procedure employed for determining transit time involves the measurement of radioactivity in ribosomal-bound nascent polypeptide vs released completed peptide. The mRNA content of the 80S monosomes is found to be identical for both Ca^{2+} depleted and restored cells as revealed by cDNA probing for the mRNA of prolactin, growth hormone, and tubulin, (C. Prostko, unpublished results), thus supporting the hypothesis that Ca^{2+} depletion slows the rate of late initiation. Lysates of GH_3 cells exhibited incorporation that was proportional to the polysomal contents derived from the original intact cell preparations. Such cell-free preparations did not possess the ability to initiate new peptide synthesis and were not affected by Ca^{2+} or EGTA. Ca^{2+}-depleted cells exposed to cycloheximide provided lysates with identical elongation activities to those of lysates prepared from either nontreated or cycloheximide-treated Ca^{2+}-restored cells.

Ca^{2+} ionophores induce a remarkably rapid and extensive inhibition of normal protein synthesis (12) comparable to that seen with traditional initiation blockers such as pactamycin and edeine (50). As noted above, within several min ionophores completely inhibited the Ca^{2+}-dependent component of post-transcriptional protein synthesis in Ca^{2+}-repleted GH_3 cells in a manner that mimicked Ca^{2+} depletion with EGTA. Treatment with A23187 reduced the cellular contents of polysomes and 43S preinitiation complex to values equivalent to those found for Ca^{2+}-depleted cells. Average ribosomal transit times were unaffected by ionophore, and treated cells retained the ability to accumulate polysomes when incubated with cycloheximide. Cell types, such as HeLa and CHO, that normally display only a modest Ca^{2+}-dependent component of protein synthesis in response to EGTA were rapidly and strongly inhibited at initiation by Ca^{2+} ionophores, apparently from the release of sequestered Ca^{2+} (12).

The exact mechanism whereby Ca^{2+} depletion or Ca^{2+} ionophores inhibit late initiation is not currently defined. Ca^{2+} depletion of GH_3 cells, as noted above, results in the accumulation of 80S monosomal units that appear to possess comparable association of specific mRNA to monosomes derived from Ca^{2+}-restored cells. The observed concomitant reduction in 43S pre-initiation complex may relate to a diminished recycling of eIF-2 that is required for the addition of initiator methionyl-tRNA to the 40S ribosomal subunit (6, 63). This initiation factor is normally released from 80S monosomes in very late initiation. It is conceivable that Ca^{2+} may trigger the release of eIF-2 from the 80S monosome while fostering entry of the ribosome into peptide chain elongation. A recently described 26-kd ribosome-associated protein that becomes dephosphorylated in response to Ca^{2+} ionophore or Ca^{2+} depletion is of potential interest to such a mechanism (32). Temporal correlation was observed between the phosphorylation/dephosphorylation state of the 26-kd protein and the stimulation/inhibition of protein synthesis by Ca^{2+} repletion/depletion, and between the dephosphorylation of the protein and inhibition of protein synthesis by ionophore. The subcellular distribution and antigenicity of this protein differed from those of the cap-binding protein, eIF-4E, which was not dephosphorylated in Ca^{2+}-depleted cells. The 26-kd protein was dephosphorylated following thermal stress. On this basis as well as size, it was distinguishable from hsp 30, a phosphoprotein rapidly induced in mammalian cells subjected to heat shock (66). In addition hsp 30 responds to Ca^{2+} ionophore with increased phosphorylation (66).

Special Considerations Regarding Reticulocyte Protein Synthesis

Translation in reticulocytes largely functions to saturate the cells with hemoglobin during their transformation to mature erythrocytes. Reticulocytes differ fundamentally from almost all other mammalian cells in possessing neither a nucleus nor an endoplasmic reticulum. Since the reticulocyte lysate retains most of the translational activity of the intact cells, it has been used extensively for characterizing the translational process for mammalian cells. In contrast to nucleated mammalian cells, intact reticulocytes do not display Ca^{2+}-dependent initiation (W. L. Wong, unpublished observations). Amino acid incorporation was identical for preparations exposed to either physiologic Ca^{2+} concentrations or 1 mM EGTA. Addition of Ca^{2+} ionophore was strongly inhibitory to intact reticulocytes in Ca^{2+} but not in EGTA-containing medium. Average ribosomal transit times were greatly extended with Ca^{2+} plus Ca^{2+} ionophore treatment. Elongation factor 2 is reported to be phosphorylated and inhibited in reticulocyte lysates by calmodulin-dependent protein kinase III (48, 56). This mechanism would produce inhibition of translation in response to elevation of cytosolic free Ca^{2+} and is presumably the basis for the inhibition seen above for intact reticulocytes exposed to a combination of Ca^{2+} and Ca^{2+} ionophore. The prevalence or physiologic significance of this mechanism in nucleated cells remains to be evaluated. As described earlier, analyses of average ribosomal transit times and polysomal size distributions following ionophore or hormonal mobilization of Ca^{2+} for several nucleated cell types have not revealed significant degrees of elongation block. It is conceivable that under some circumstances rapid mobilization of sequestered Ca^{2+} to the cytosol could produce inhibition of translation at both initiation and elongation.

ACCOMMODATION OF PROTEIN SYNTHESIS TO CHRONIC DEPLETION OF SEQUESTERED Ca^{2+}

Effects of Phorbol Esters and cAMP

The integrated process of protein synthesis including DNA transcription, mRNA translation, and post-translational protein processing by the endoplasmic reticulum and Golgi provides a wealth of sites potentially subject to phosphorylation and regulation by protein kinases activated by Ca^{2+}, phorbol esters, and cAMP. For example, cAMP has been frequently suggested to function in the induction of various enzyme activities; ribosomal protein S6 is well-established to be subject to phosphorylation mediated through both cAMP and phorbol ester (64). Accumulating evidence suggests that both cAMP and phorbol esters support a resumption of protein synthesis in GH3 cells exposed to protracted depletion of Ca^{2+}. This accommodation, as described below, proceeds in either Ca^{2+}-depleted cells or in cells treated with Ca^{2+} ionophore and is blocked by inhibitors of transcription.

Ca^{2+}-depleted GH3 cells maintain their viability with low, largely unchanged rates of amino acid incorporation throughout 8 hr incubation in serum-free medium. Upon exposure to phorbol myristate acetate (PMA), however, such preparations gain increased ability to incorporate amino acid as a function of treatment time, which culminates in a 4- to 6-fold stimulation after 2–3 hr (16). In contrast, Ca^{2+}-restored controls respond to phorbol ester with relatively slight increments in incorporation rates. Like Ca^{2+} restoration, PMA promotes incorporation into all detectable polypeptide species of Ca^{2+}-depleted preparations as determined by pulse labeling studies with [^{35}S]methionine. The ester fosters the accumulation of small polysomes without affecting average ribosomal transit times. Both the stimulation of incorporation and the accumulation of polysomes are suppressed by actinomycin D and are not attributable either to increased amino acid uptake or methionylation of tRNA. Substances that promote cAMP accumulation mimic the effects of PMA on protein synthesis. Exposure of Ca^{2+}-depleted cells to combinations of both types of agent stimulates amino acid incorporation maximally to rates approaching those achieved by Ca^{2+} restoration. Protein synthesis by dispersed normal anterior pituitary cells in low Ca^{2+} medium was also stimulated by PMA and cAMP-elevating substances.

The behavior of Ca^{2+}-deprived C6 glial tumor cells contrasts markedly with that of pituitary cells (16). C6 cells exposed to comparable low Ca^{2+} medium spontaneously increase their rate of amino acid incorporation with time of incubation in a manner that is suppressed by actinomycin D but not affected by either cAMP or PMA. In contrast to GH_3 cells that show increased phosphorylation of S6 ribosomal protein in response to PMA or elevation of cAMP, phosphorylation of the protein in C6 cells is not affected (C. Brostrom, unpublished results). Recovery of protein synthesis from the acute inhibitory effects of Ca^{2+} ionophore A23187 was also observed for C6 and GH_3 cells (M. Brostrom, unpublished results). In GH_3 but not C6 cells, recovery was dependent on the presence of phorbol ester or a cAMP-elevating agent.

Potential Role of BiP/GRP78 in Translational Accommodation

Inducible polypeptides were sought that were preferentially pulse-labeled with [^{35}S]methionine following Ca^{2+} depletion of GH_3 cells for periods of 90 min or less. Only one transcription-dependent inducible species was observed. On the bases of size, isoelectric point, subcellular distribution, and induction following exposure to reducing agents and glycosylation inhibitors, the poly-peptide was identical to a component of the endoplasmic reticulum most frequently termed BiP or GRP78 (33, 47, 65). Although present at constitutive levels in unstressed cells, BiP is known to be rapidly induced under conditions including exposure to inhibitors of glycosylation (40), EGTA or Ca^{2+} ionophores (28, 54), and reducing agents (37) that lead to accumulation of aberrant proteins within the endoplasmic reticulum. BiP is currently believed to function in control of protein processing and secretion through complex formation with incorrectly folded proteins within the lumen of the endoplasmic reticulum (26, 35, 40).

Three types of observations implicate BiP in the mechanism through which cells develop translational tolerance to Ca^{2+} deprivation. First, inductions of BiP and of translational tolerance to ionophore or EGTA in both GH_3 and C6 cells depend on active transcription. The mRNA for BiP in both cell types is rapidly induced (C. Prostko, unpublished results), but expressed spontaneously only in C6. Second, nascent BiP was detectable at incubation times preceding perceptible translational recovery, and the degree of labeling of BiP correlated with the subsequent extent of accommodation. In Ca^{2+}-depleted or ionophore treated GH_3 but not C6 cells, the synthesis of BiP was strongly promoted by phorbol ester and/or a cAMP-elevating substance. Third, acute exposure of either cell type to the BiP inducer, dithiothreitol (DTT), as observed earlier for EGTA or ionophore, inhibited protein synthesis at initiation. Upon continued exposure of cells to DTT, both induction of BiP and recovery of protein synthesis were observed. Cells pretreated with DTT, washed, and allowed to recover in fresh medium without the agent exhibited rates of amino acid incorporation identical to those of untreated controls and tolerance to the inhibitory effects of Ca^{2+} ionophore and EGTA. Correlative evidence of this nature is supportive without proving the hypothesis that nascent BiP functions in the recovery of protein synthesis during Ca^{2+} deprivation. The hypothesis, however, should be susceptible to testing with molecular biological techniques.

ABOLITION OF Ca^{2+}-DEPENDENT PROTEIN SYNTHESIS BY THERMAL AND CHEMICAL STRESS

Eukaryotic cells respond to brief thermal stress or exposure to various chemicals with an acute shutdown of normal protein synthesis and rapid induction of a number of specific proteins, termed heat shock proteins (hsp) (18, 25, 42, 60). The hsp are believed to function in the reassembly of cellular structures disrupted by stress (7, 20, 24). mRNAs for normal cellular proteins are not degraded in the cellular response to stress, but undergo translation at greatly reduced rates. In contrast, mRNAs for the hsp are readily translated. An analysis of GH_3 cells exposed to stress indicated that stress abolishes the Ca^{2+} input into translation of all cellular mRNAs.

Following thermal stress at 46°C or chemical stress from exposure to sodium arsenite or 8-hydroxyquinoline, rates of amino acid incorporation in Ca^{2+}-restored GH_3 cells were reduced acutely to those of unstressed, Ca^{2+}-depleted control preparations (17). Sodium arsenite treatment resulted in loss of ability to accumulate polysomes in response to Ca^{2+}. Stressed cells allowed to recover for 2–8 hr either with or without Ca^{2+} in the medium exhibited comparable, increasing rates of amino acid incorporation and the induction of a spectrum of hsp. Although rates of amino acid incorporation achieved during recovery were relatively high, such incorporation was only marginally dependent on Ca^{2+}. Abolition of the Ca^{2+}-dependent component of translation was proportional to the intensity of the stress. Mild thermal stress (41°C) resulted in good retention of Ca^{2+}-dependent protein synthesis. Under this condition at least one hsp, hsp 68, was induced and synthesized in a Ca^{2+}-dependent manner. After arsenite stress, restoration of the Ca^{2+} requirement for protein synthesis occurred by 24 hr, and was preceded by a transitional period during which polysomes accumulated in response to Ca^{2+} without concomitant increased rates of incorporation. Overall, responses to heat or chemical stress appear to include acute destruction of Ca^{2+}-stimulated initiation and a protracted period of recovery involving synthesis of the hsp accompanied by Ca^{2+}-independent amino acid incorporation and slowed peptide chain elongation.

Inactivation of the Ca^{2+} input into initiation could arise from a compromised ability to sequester intracellular Ca^{2+} and thereby to maintain Ca^{2+} homeostasis. Stressed GH_3 cells, however, do not exhibit mobilization of Ca^{2+} as determined by analytical fluorescence dye spectrophotometry or as measured by ^{45}Ca efflux (G. Kuznetsov, unpublished results). It is conceivable, therefore, that stress promotes uncoupling of Ca^{2+} stores from translational activity. The mechanisms responsible for slowed peptide chain elongation during recovery and the relationship of hsp induction to the ultimate restoration of the Ca^{2+} input into initiation remain to be defined.

SUMMARY AND CONCLUSIONS

Extensive bodies of literature describe protein synthesis and processing; the endocrinology and metabolic bases whereby a variety of hormonal, mechanical, and nutritional influences affect cell function and adaptive responses; and various regulatory mechanisms mediating concerted intracellular control. Nonetheless, our current understanding of the mechanisms responsible for the regulation and subordination of protein synthesis to the overall metabolic and stimulus-response status of the cell is inadequate. The endoplasmic reticulum is central to these concerns. Potential roles of the endoplasmic reticulum in the regulation of protein synthesis are largely unexplored. We have attempted in this rather speculative review, based largely on our own data, to project a view of the endoplasmic reticulum as moderating the rate of translation through a mechanism sensitive to sequestered Ca^{2+}. Compensatory routes whereby cells accommodate to Ca^{2+} deprivation so as to resume reasonable rates of protein synthesis are seen also to focus on the endoplasmic reticulum. With additional research, the underlying relationships that exist among reticular Ca^{2+} storage, protein processing, and mechanisms of translational control should become more broadly evident. The prevailing view of Ca^{2+} as a regulator of cytosolic processes may require some extension if sequestered Ca^{2+} participates in biological control mechanisms emanating from the endoplasmic reticulum. In effect, a reciprocal relationship would presumably exist among processes supported by cytosolic free Ca^{2+} vs those promoted by sequestered stores of the cation. Speculatively, such reciprocity would allow the rapid diversion of energy from one set of processes to the other. Conceivably, chronic Ca^{2+} loading at sequestered sites may be related to certain cellular adaptive Ca^{2+} loading involving tissue hypertrophy. Potential examples of stretch-induced responses that could be cited include thickening of arteriolar smooth muscle walls in hypertension (8) and cardiac hypertrophy in aortic stenosis (46).

ACKNOWLEDGMENTS

The preparation of this manuscript was supported by United States Public Health Service DK35393 and National Science Foundation BNS 86-06790.

Literature Cited

1. Albert, P. R., Tashjian, A. H. Jr. 1984. Relationship of thyrotropin-releasing hormone-induced spike and plateau phases in cytosolic free Ca^{2+} concentrations to hormone secretion. Selective blockade using ionomycin and nifedipine. *J. Biol. Chem.* 258:15350–63
2. Albert, P. R., Tashjian, A. H. Jr. 1986. Ionomycin acts as an ionophore to release TRH-regulated Ca^{2+} stores from GH_4C_1 cells. *Am. J. Physiol.* 251:C887–91
3. Andrews, S. B., Leapman, R. D., Landis, D. M. D., Reese, T. S. 1988. Activity-dependent accumulation of calcium in Purkinje cell dendritic spines. *Proc. Natl. Acad. Sci. USA* 85:1682–85
4. Bayerdorffer, E., Streb, H., Eckhardt, L., Haase, W., Schulz, I. 1984. Characterization of calcium uptake into rough endoplasmic reticulum of rat pancreas. *J. Membr. Biol.* 81:69–82
5. Berridge, M. J. 1987. Inositol trisphosphate and diacylglycerol: two interacting second messengers. *Annu. Rev. Biochem.* 56:159–93
6. Bienz, H. 1985. Properties and spatial arrangement of components in preinitiation complexes of eukaryotic protein synthesis. *Prog. Nucleic Acid Res. Mol. Biol.* 32:267–89
7. Bienz, M., Pelham, H. R. 1987. Mechanisms of heat-shock gene activation in higher eukaryotes. *Adv. Genet.* 24:31–72
8. Bohr, D. F., Webb, R. C. 1988. Vascular smooth muscle membrane in hypertension. *Annu. Rev. Pharmacol. Toxicol.* 28:389–409
9. Borle, A. B., Snowdowne, K. W. 1987. Methods for the measurement of intracellular ionized calcium in mammalian cells: comparison of four classes of Ca^{2+} indicators. *Calcium Cell Funct.* 6:159–200
10. Brostrom, C. O., Bocckino, S. B., Brostrom, M. A. 1983. Identification of a calcium requirement for protein synthesis in eukaryotic cells. *J. Biol. Chem.* 258:14390–99
11. Brostrom, C. O., Bocckino, S. B., Brostrom, M. A., Galuska, E. M. 1986. Regulation of protein synthesis in isolated hepatocytes by calcium-mobilizing hormones. *Mol. Pharmacol.* 29:104–11
12. Brostrom, C. O., Chin, K. V., Wong, W. L., Cade, C., Brostrom, M. A. 1989. Inhibition of translational initiation in eukaryotic cells by calcium ionophore. *J. Biol. Chem.* 254:1644–49
13. Brostrom, M. A., Brostrom, C. O. 1984. Calcium control of cyclic AMP metabolism in glial and pituitary tumor cells. *Calcium Cell Funct.* 5:165–208
14. Brostrom, M. A., Brostrom, C. O., Bocckino, S. B., Green, S. S. 1984. Ca^{2+} and hormones interact synergistically to stimulate rapidly both prolactin production and overall protein synthesis in pituitary tumor cells. *J. Cell. Physiol.* 121:391–401
15. Brostrom, M. A., Brostrom, C. O., Brotman, L. A., Green, S. S. 1983. Regulation of Ca^{2+}-dependent cAMP accumulation and Ca^{2+} metabolism in intact pituitary tumor cells by modulators of prolactin production. *Mol. Pharmacol.* 23:399–408
16. Brostrom, M. A., Chin, K. V., Cade, C., Gmitter, D., Brostrom, C. O. 1987. Stimulation of protein synthesis in pituitary cells by phorbol esters and cyclic AMP. Evidence for rapid induction of a component of translational initiation. *J. Biol. Chem.* 262:16515–23
17. Brostrom, M. A., Lin, X. J., Cade, C., Brostrom, C. O. 1989. Loss of a calcium requirement for protein synthesis in pituitary cells following thermal or chemical stress. *J. Biol. Chem.* 254:1638–43
18. Burdon, R. H. 1986. Heat shock and the heat shock proteins. *Biochem. J.* 240:313–24
19. Burton, D. N., Collins, J. M., Porter, J. W. 1969. Biosynthesis of the fatty acid synthetase by isolated rat liver cells. *J. Biol. Chem.* 244:1076–77
20. Carper, S. W., Duffy, J. J., Gerner, E. W. 1987. Heat shock proteins in thermotolerance and other cellular processes. *Cancer Res.* 47:5249–55
21. Chin, K. V., Cade, C., Brostrom, C. O., Galuska, E. M., Brostrom, M. A. 1987. Calcium dependent regulation of protein synthesis at translational initiation in eukaryotic cells. *J. Biol. Chem.* 262:16509–14
22. Chin, K. V., Cade, C., Brostrom, M. A., Brostrom, C. O. 1988. Regulation of protein synthesis in intact rat liver by calcium mobilizing agents. *Int. J. Biochem.* 20:1313–19
23. Cohen, P. 1985. The role of protein phosphorylation in the hormonal control of enzyme activity. *Eur. J. Biochem.* 151:439–48
24. Collier, N. C., Schlesinger, M. J. 1986. The dynamic state of heat shock proteins

in chicken embryo fibroblasts. *J. Cell Biol.* 103:1495–1507

25. Craig, E. 1985. The heat shock response. *CRC Crit. Rev. Biochem.* 18: 239–80

26. Dorner, A. J., Krane, M. G., Kaufman, R. J. 1988. Reduction of endogenous GRP78 levels improves secretion of a heterologous protein in CHO cells. *Mol. Cell. Biol.* 8:4063–70

27. Dorner, R. L., Brown, G. R., Doughney, C., McPherson, M. A. 1987. Intracellular Ca^{2+} in pancreatic acinar cells: regulation and role in stimulation of enzyme secretion. *Biosci. Rep.* 7: 333–44

28. Drummond, I. A. S., Lee, A. S., Resendez, E. Jr., Steinhardt, R. A. 1987. Depletion of intracellular calcium stores by calcium ionophore A23187 induces genes for glucose-regulated proteins in hamster fibroblasts. *J. Biol. Chem.* 262:12801–5

29. Duncan, R., Hershey, J. W. B. 1985. Regulation of initiation factors during translational repression caused by serum depletion. Covalent modification. *J. Biol. Chem.* 260:5493–97

30. Duncan, R., Milburn, S. C., Hershey, J. W. B. 1987. Regulated phosphorylation and low abundance of HeLa cell initiation factor eIF-4F suggest a role in translational control. Heat shock effects on eIF-4F. *J. Biol. Chem.* 262:380–88

31. Farese, R. V. 1971. Calcium as a mediator of adrenocorticotrophic hormone action on adrenal protein synthesis. *Science* 173:447–50

32. Fawell, E. H., Boyer, I. J., Brostrom, M. A., Brostrom, C. O. 1989. A novel calcium-dependent phosphorylation of a ribosomal-associated protein. *J. Biol. Chem.* 254:1650–55

33. Hendershot, L. M., Ting, J., Lee, A. S. 1988. Identity of the immunoglobulin heavy-chain-binding protein with the 78,000-dalton glucose-regulated protein and the role of posttranslational modifications in its binding function. *Mol. Cell. Biol.* 8:4250–56

34. Kaplan, E., Richman, H. G. 1973. Calcium stimulation of uridine-6-^{3}H incorporation into RNA of rat myocardium. *Can. J. Biochem.* 51:1331–34

35. Kassenbrock, C. K., Garcia, P. D., Walter, P., Kelly, R. B. 1988. Heavy-chain binding protein recognizes aberrant polypeptides translocated *in vitro*. *Nature* 333:90–93

36. Kennedy, M. B., Bennett, M. K., Erondu, N. E., Miller, S. G. 1987. Calcium/calmodulin dependent protein kinases. *Calcium Cell Funct.* 7:61–107

37. Kim, Y. K., Kim, K. S., Lee, A. S. 1987. Regulation of the glucose-regulated protein genes by β-mercaptoethanol requires *de novo* protein synthesis and correlates with inhibition of protein glycosylation. *J. Cell. Physiol.* 133:553–59

38. Kolesnick, R. N., Musacchio, I., Thaw, C., Gershengorn, M. C. 1984. Arachidonic acid mobilizes calcium and stimulates prolactin secretion from GH$_3$ cells. *Am. J. Physiol.* 246:E458–62

39. Kozak, M. 1986. Regulation of protein synthesis in virus-infected animal cells. *Adv. Virus Res.* 31:229–92

40. Kozutsumi, Y., Segal, M., Normington, K., Gething, M.-J., Sambrook, J. 1988. The presence of malfolded proteins in the endoplasmic reticulum signals the induction of glucose-regulated proteins. *Nature* 332:462–64

41. Ledford, B. E., Davis, D. F. 1978. Analysis of translational parameters in cultured cells. *Biochim. Biophys. Acta* 519:204–12

42. Lindquist, S. 1986. The heat shock response. *Annu. Rev. Biochem.* 55:1151–91

43. Liu, C., Herman, T. E. 1978. Characterization of ionomycin as a calcium ionophore. *J. Biol. Chem.* 253: 5892–94

44. Michell, R. H., Drummond, A. H., Downes, C. P., eds. 1989. *Inositol Lipids in Cell Signalling.* San Diego: Academic. 534 pp.

45. Moldave, K. 1985. Eukaryotic protein synthesis. *Annu. Rev. Biochem.* 54: 1109–49

46. Morgan, H. E., Gordon, E. E., Kira, Y., Chua, B. H. L., Russo, L. A., et al. 1987. Biochemical mechanisms of cardiac hypertrophy. *Annu. Rev. Physiol.* 49:533–44

47. Munro, S., Pelham, H. R. B. 1986. An hsp70-like protein in the ER: identity with the 78 kd glucose-regulated protein and immunoglobulin heavy chain binding protein. *Cell* 46:291–300

48. Nairn, A. C., Palfrey, H. C. 1987. Identification of the major Mr 100,000 substrate for calmodulin-dependent protein kinase III in mammalian cells as elongation factor-2. *J. Biol. Chem.* 262: 17299–303

49. Pain, V. M. 1986. Initiation of protein synthesis in mammalian cells. *Biochem. J.* 235:625–37

50. Pestka, S. 1977. Inhibitors of protein synthesis. In *Molecular Mechanisms of Protein Biosynthesis*, ed. H. Weissbach, S. Pestka, pp. 468–563. New York: Academic

51. Pfeiffer, D. T., Kaufman, R. F., Taylor, R. S. 1982. Cation complexation and transport by carboxylic acid ionophores. See Ref. 67, pp. 103–84

52. Reed, P. W. 1982. Biochemical and biological effects of carboxylic acid ionophores. See Ref. 67, pp. 183–302

53. Reed, P. W., Bokoch, G. M. 1982. Cardiovascular and renal effects of A23187 and monovalent polyether antibiotics. See Ref. 67, pp. 369–95

54. Resendez, E. Jr., Ting, J., Kim, K. S., Wooden, S. K., Lee, A. S. 1986. Calcium ionophore A23187 as a regulator of gene expression in mammalian cells. *J. Cell Biol.* 103:2145–52

55. Ruiz, N., Krauskopf, M. 1980. Calcium stimulation of polyphenylalanine synthesis in a bovine heart cell-free system. *Life Sci.* 27:2359–65

56. Ryazanov, A. G. 1987. Ca^{2+}/calmodulin-dependent phosphorylation of elongation factor 2. *FEBS Letts.* 214:331–34

57. Rychlik, W., Russ, M. A., Rhoads, R. E. 1987. Phosphorylation site of eukaryotic initiation factor 4E. *J. Biol. Chem.* 262:10434–37

58. Schlegel, W., Winiger, B. P., Mollard, P., Vacher, P., Wuarin, F., et al. 1987. Oscillations of cytosolic Ca^{2+} in pituitary cells due to action potentials. *Nature* 329:719–21

59. Schneider, R. J., Shenk, T. 1987. Impact of virus infection on host cell protein synthesis. *Annu. Rev. Biochem.* 56:317–32

60. Subjeck, J. R., Shyy, T.-T. 1986. Stress protein systems of mammalian cells. *Am. J. Physiol.* 250:C1–17

61. Takuma, T., Kuyatt, B. L., Baum, B. J. 1984. α_1-Adrenergic inhibition of protein synthesis in rat submandibular cells. *Am. J. Physiol.* 247:G284–89

62. Tan, K.-N., Tashjian, A. H. Jr. 1984. Voltage-dependent calcium channels in pituitary cells in culture. I. Characterization by $^{45}Ca^{2+}$ fluxes. *J. Biol. Chem.* 259:418–26

62a. Tashjian, A. H. Jr. 1979. Clonal strains of hormone-producing pituitary cells. *Methods Enzymol.* 58:527–35

63. Thomas, N. S. B., Matts, R. L., Levin, D. H., London, I. M. 1985. The 60S ribosomal subunit as a carrier of eukaryotic initiation factor 2 and site of reversing factor activity during protein synthesis. *J. Biol. Chem.* 260:9860–66

64. Traugh, J. A., Pendergast, A. M. 1986. Regulation of protein synthesis by phosphorylation of ribosomal protein S6 and aminoacyl-tRNA synthetases. *Prog. Nucleic Acid Res. Mol. Biol.* 33:195–230

65. Watowich, S. S., Morimoto, R. I. 1988. Complex regulation of heat shock- and glucose-regulated genes in human cells. *Mol. Cell. Biol.* 8:393–405

66. Welch, W. J. 1985. Phorbol ester, calcium ionophore, or serum added to quiescent rat embryo fibroblast cells all result in the elevated phosphorylation of two 28,000-dalton mammalian stress proteins. *J. Biol. Chem.* 260:3058–62

67. Westley, J. W., ed. 1982. *Polyether Antibiotics: Naturally Occurring Acid Ionophores, Biology,* Vol. 1. New York/Basel: Dekker. 465 pp.

68. Wolf, B. A., Turk, J., Sherman, W. R., McDaniel, M. L. 1986. Intracellular Ca^{2+} mobilization by arachidonic acid. Comparison with myo-inositol 1,4,5-trisphosphate on isolated pancreatic islets. *J. Biol. Chem.* 261:3501–11

69. Wolfe, S. E., Brostrom, C. O., Brostrom, M. A. 1986. Mechanisms of action of inhibitors of prolactin secretion in GH_3 pituitary cells. I. Ca^{2+}-dependent inhibition of amino acid incorporation. *Mol. Pharmacol.* 29:411–19

70. Wolfe, S. E., Brostrom, M. A. 1986. Mechanisms of action of inhibitors of prolactin secretion in GH_3 pituitary cells. II. Blockade of voltage-dependent Ca^{2+} channels. *Mol. Pharmacol.* 29:420–26

Annu. Rev. Physiol. 1990. 52:591–606

G$_E$: A GTP-BINDING PROTEIN MEDIATING EXOCYTOSIS

B. D. Gomperts

Department of Physiology, University College, London, University Street, London WC1E 6JJ, England

KEY WORDS: exocytosis, permeabilized cells, G proteins, mast cells, secretion

CELL PERMEABILIZATION

Recent advances in the field of exocytotic secretion have depended almost exclusively on the use of permeabilized cells that allow the composition of the cytosol to be precisely controlled. Many agents and strategies for plasma membrane permeabilization have been utilized (see Table 1), and it is important to appreciate that these generate, in the plasma membrane of individual cell types, lesions having widely differing dimensions and lifetimes. For example, the exocytotic release of catecholamines has been investigated using bovine adrenal chromaffin cells permeabilized by high voltage electric discharge (HVD) (37), by treatment with plant glycosides (19, 60), staphylococcal α-toxin (1, 4) and by streptolysin-O (SL-O) (64), and by capacitance measurement (to monitor the increase in plasma membrane surface area) using a patch-pipette in the whole cell mode (49). Two of these permeabilizing procedures (HVD and α-toxin) generate small membrane lesions allowing the dialysis but not full wash-out of the cytosol, while treatment with digitonin and SL-O (and presumably the patch-pipette) permit the release of cytosol proteins, though they do so at very different rates (60). It is not too surprising that there has been variability in the results obtained from experiments that are ostensibly the same.

In seeking to stimulate exocytosis from permeabilized cells, the main approach to date has been to control the concentrations of Ca^{2+} and nu-

Table 1 Methods of cell permeabilization

	Effective filtration diameter	Method of assessment	Reference
Sendai virus	Approximately 1 nm	Exclusion of fluorescent peptides	(34)
	Macromolecular dimensions	Protein leakage	(22)
		Electron microscopy	(20)
Staphylococcal α-toxin	2–3 nm	Rate of uptake and efflux of various markers in chromaffin cells	(37)
High voltage discharge	2–4 nm		
ATP^{4-}	Variable dimensions (α ATP^{4-})	Rate of ^{32}P-metabolite efflux and $^{57}Co.HEDTA$ uptake	(8, 14)
Lysolecithin	Variable dimensions	RNAase (M_r 14 kd) uptake and LDH efflux	(47)
		Slow leakage of LDH (M_r 140 kd)	(57)
Plant glycosides	Macromolecular dimensions	Efflux of urease (M_r 483 kd) from sheep red cell membrane vesicles	(10)
Streptolysin-0	Greater than 13 nm		
Patch-pipette	Micron dimensions	Measurement of tip resistance	(27, 44)

The filtration dimensions are given only as a rough guide. For any reagent or method there will be wide variation depending on membrane composition and other conditions. Furthermore, the different methods used to assess the filtration properties of membrane lesions must necessarily give different results.

cleotides. Discrepancies in the literature arise from variations in the composition of the different media used. For example, in our own work on mast cells permeabilized with SL-O, we find a total dependence for exocytosis on the presence of both Ca^{2+} and a guanine nucleotide (31); the bathing solution is comprised mainly of NaCl. By contrast, measurements of capacitance changes using patch-pipettes containing K glutamate indicate that guanine nucleotide (GTP-γ-S) is a sufficient stimulus (21) with Ca^{2+} serving mainly to accelerate the response (48).

Table 2 lists a number of tissues and cell types in which membrane permeabilization has been applied to investigate exocytosis. It is fair to say that we know most about the physiology of this process as it occurs in mast cells.

MAST CELLS

In comparison to other mammalian systems, the mast cells, easily isolated in a state of near homogeneity from rat peritoneal washings, offer a number of compelling advantages including the simple detection of degranulation (the morphological counterpart of exocytosis) under the light microscope. They represent a highly specialized secretory system, containing on average about 1000 granules (mean diameter 0.3 μm), and release upwards of 80% of their secretory products within minutes of stimulation.

Recent developments have depended largely on the exploitation of two permeabilization techniques. On the one hand, exocytosis has been monitored at the single cell level by measuring the increase in membrane area (manifested as an increase in electrical capacitance) by using patch-pipettes both as electrical probes and as a means for controlling the composition of the cytosol. Alternatively, mast cells in suspension have been permeabilized by treatment with SL-O. Each technique offers different advantages. We will mainly consider the experience of working with SL-O permeabilized cells; an extensive discussion of the exocytotic mechanism as perceived by capacitance measurement is the topic of a separate review in this volume (see W. Almers).

Mast cells leak approximately 75% of their lactate dehydrogenase (MW 150 kd) within five min of treatment with SL-O, yet they retain histamine (MW 100) and lysosomal enzymes unless also provided with Ca^{2+} together with a ligand (nucleotide) capable of interacting with and activating GTP-binding proteins (32). In our experiments we treat the cells prior to permeabilization with metabolic inhibitors to the point of total suppression of responsiveness to exogenous agonists such as compound 48/80 and IgE-directed crosslinkers. Under these conditions, exocytotic release of up to 90% of the contained histamine or lysosomal enzymes can be elicited by provision of Ca^{2+} (buffered at concentrations in the micromolar range) together with a guanine nucleotide (Figure 1).

Table 2 Secretory cells that have been investigated by the technique of membrane permeabilization

	Technique	Effectors	Reference
Mast cells	ATP^{4-}	Ca^{2+}	(8)
	Sendai virus	Ca^{2+}	(22)
	Digitonin	Ca^{2+}, guanine nucleotides, $[AlF_4]^-$	(65, 66)
	SL-0	Ca^{2+}-plus-guanine nucleotides	(31, 32)
	Patch-pipette	Ca^{2+}, guanine nucleotides	(21)
Adrenal chromaffin cells	Plant glycosides	Ca^{2+}, guanine nucleotides	(9)
	Staphylococcal α-toxin	Ca^{2+}	(1, 4)
	Digitonin	Ca^{2+}, guanine nucleotides, proteins	(19, 60)
	SL-0	Ca^{2+}	(64)
	HVD	Ca^{2+}, guanine nucleotides	(37, 38)
	Patch-pipette	Ca^{2+}	(49)
Nerve endings	Digitonin	Ca^{2+}	(12)
Platelets	HVD	Ca^{2+}	(28, 40)
Neutrophils	Plant glycosides	Ca^{2+}, guanine nucleotides	(62, 63)
	Sendai virus	Ca^{2+}, guanine nucleotides	(6, 7)
	Patch-pipette	Ca^{2+}, guanine nucleotides	(50)
Eosinophils	Patch-pipette	Ca^{2+}, guanine nucleotides	(51)
	SL-0	Ca^{2+}, guanine nucleotides	(51)
HL-60 cells	SL-0	Ca^{2+}, guanine nucleotides	(67)
Cytotoxic T cells	Staphylococcal α-toxin	Ca^{2+}, GTP	(61)
Islets of Langerhans	HVD	Ca^{2+}	(54, 77)
	Patch-pipette	Ca^{2+}, GTP-γ-S	(56)
RIN5mF cells	HVD	Ca^{2+}, guanine nucleotides	(72)
Pancreatic acinar cells	HVD	Ca^{2+}, cyclic nucleotides	(39)
Parotid cells	Saponin	cyclicAMP	(69)
Parathyroid cells	HVD	Ca^{2+}, guanine nucleotides	(53, 52)
Pituitary lactotrophs	Patch-pipette	Ca^{2+}	(45)
Pituitary melano-trophs	HVD	cyclicAMP, guanine nucleotides	(76)
Pituitary cells:			
ATt20	Digitonin	Ca^{2+}, guanine nucleotides	(42)
7315c	HVD	Ca^{2+}, cyclicAMP	(26)

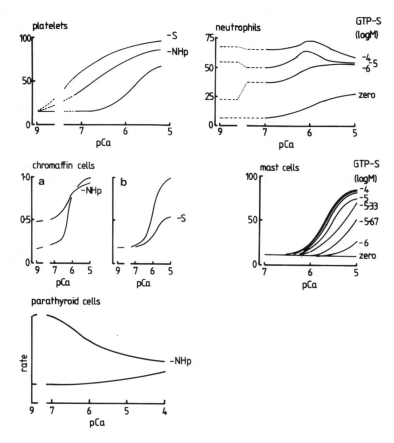

Figure 1 Diversity of interaction between guanine nucleotides and Ca²⁺ in the control of exocytosis from secretory cells. The graphs indicate the dependence of secretion on [Ca²⁺] from various secretory cells. [Ca²⁺] was regulated by the use of CaEGTA buffers; except for the mast cells, ATP was also provided. Platelets (HVD) (28, 40): effect of GppNHp (-NHp), 100 μM and GTP-γ-S (-S) 10 μM. Chromaffin cells (*a*) (digitonin permeabilization), effect of GppNHp (-NHp), 100 μM (9) (*b*) (HVD), effect of GTP-γ-S (-S), 80 μM (nb GppNHp (80μM) was without effect in this experiment) (38). Parathyroid cells (HVD): effect of GppNHp (10 μM) (53). Neutrophils (Sendai virus permeabilization) (7). Mast cells (SL-O permeabilization) (31).

Ca²⁺-plus-Guanine Nucleotide: Essential Effectors

We refer to the combination Ca²⁺-plus-guanine nucleotide as the essential effectors. Both are necessary, and together they are sufficient to elicit a maximal exocytotic response. Activation of protein kinase C is therefore superfluous; thus it follows that the essential action of GTP is exerted at a site other than G_P and is unconnected with the activation of (inositide specific) phospholipase C (15) (PPI-PDE, phosphodiesterase: see Figure 2). The reason for this is that ATP is not required; therefore protein phosphorylation does not comprise a step in the late stages of the exocytotic sequence. Further support for this conclusion comes from the observation that exocytosis stimulated by Ca^{2+}-plus-GTP-γ-S can be fully maintained under conditions in which G_P-linked phospholipase C is completely suppressed by neomycin (17). We refer to the late acting G protein mediating exocytosis as G_E.

This interpretation refers to the somewhat artificial situation of permeabilized cells. In intact cells, a role for a G protein in the stimulus-secretion pathway is indicated by the observation that mast cells microinjected with the constitutively activated product of the H-$ras^{val_{12}}$ oncogene undergo degranulation (5). The monomeric ras proteins have close structural homologies with the signal transducing α-subunits of the GTP-binding proteins (G_s, G_i, and so on) associated with receptor-controlled processes, although their effector function(s) are so far not known. The wild-type ras protein (i.e. the proto-oncogene product) is without comparable effect. Also, intact mast cells (and related rat basophilic leukemia cells), in which the level of endogenous GTP is selectively depressed by the antiviral drugs $ribavirin$ and mycophenolic acid, lose their ability to respond to ionophores (43, 74).

Role of ATP in Stimulus-Secretion Coupling

The finding of ATP-independent exocytosis flies in the face of overwhelming experience indicating that secretion only occurs from metabolically competent cells (35). There are at least three stages in the complete stimulus-secretion sequence (i.e. starting from the attachment of a receptor-directed ligand) at which ATP must play an indirect, but nonetheless, necessary role. (a) ATP is required to maintain the level of phosphatidylinositol-4,5-bisphosphate, the substrate of phospholipase C [e.g. in adrenal chromaffin cells (18)); (b) ATP is needed to maintain, by nucleotide trans-phosphorylation, the level of GTP required to control phospholipase C via G_P; (c) similarly, through maintenance of GTP, ATP allows for activation of G_E. In the permeabilized cells however, the reactions directly consequential to the activation of phospholipase C are obviated, and the levels of GTP and of Ca^{2+} are controlled. None of these actions of ATP is relevant to the exocytotic event itself.

ATP Modulates Exocytosis

Although not obligatory, ATP does play a number of important modulatory roles that reveal the sequence of steps in this pathway.

ATP REGULATES AFFINITY FOR Ca^{2+} AND GTP   When mast cells are permeabilized in the presence of ATP, the concentrations of Ca^{2+} and GTP-γ-S required to induce exocytosis are substantially reduced (16, 31). As

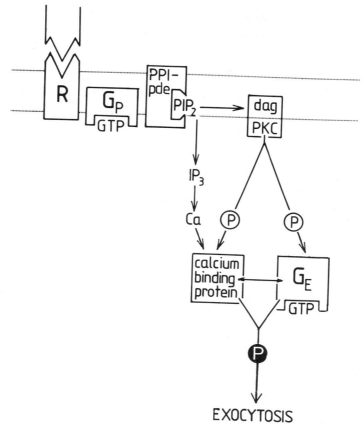

Figure 2 A schematic representation indicating the relationships between the early events in stimulus-secretion coupling and late events mediated by the GTP-binding protein G_E (70). Two GTP-binding proteins are understood to be involved in the complete stimulus-secretion pathway. The first, G_P, transduces receptor (R)-mediated signals and activates polyphosphoinositide-specific phosphodiesterase (PPI-pde, a phospholipase C) to generate inositol 1,4,5-trisphosphate (IP_3) and diglyceride (dag). To investigate the terminal stages of the pathway, permeabilized cells are used: IP_3 leaks out, and Ca^{2+} is controlled by the use of CaEGTA buffers. Diglyceride, which is retained in the plasma membrane, can activate protein kinase C only if ATP is provided, and this enhances the effective affinity for both Ca^{2+} and guanine nucleotide in the exocytotic reaction. ATP is not an absolute requirement for exocytosis to occur, however. Both Ca^{2+} and a guanine nucleotide are essential, but elevation of the one reduces the requirement for the other, which indicates that some form of communication between the Ca^{2+}-binding protein and the G protein G_E. ATP retards the onset of secretion following provision of Ca^{2+}-plus-GTP to the permeabilized cells, thus indicating that it inhibits reactions upstream of the terminal step. The duration of the ATP-induced delay can be reduced by increasing the concentration of either effector. These observations have led to the suggestion that the enabling reaction for exocytosis might involve protein dephosphorylation. In the absence of ATP the protein is rapidly de-phosphorylated; therefore onset of secretion is prompt (31, 17, 70, 25).

with other systems, the effective affinity for Ca^{2+} is controlled by phosphorylations catalyzed by protein kinase C (33). The enhancement by ATP of the effective affinity for the guanine nucleotide is even greater than for Ca^{2+} (10- to 30-fold) (23).

In the absence of ATP, responsiveness to the essential effectors during the period following permeabilization declines and is nonexistent at five min. Up to this time the dependence on $[Ca^{2+}]$ shifts systematically to higher concentrations (24, 32). It is likely that the decline in affinity observed following permeabilization is a reflection of a phosphorylation state of either a Ca^{2+}-binding protein, or of another protein that controls the affinity. If ATP is present, then the rate of decline is much reduced, and if ATP is provided alongside the essential effectors at five min post permeabilization (i.e. when the cells have become refractory), then full responsiveness can be restored (33). These observations indicate that a certain level of phosphorylation (i.e. a primed state) is required in order for exocytosis to occur.

ATP RETARDS ONSET OF EXOCYTOSIS   In a kinetic sense ATP is an inhibitor of exocytosis. In its absence, exocytosis is established at its maximal rate within three sec of applying the Ca^{2+} trigger to cells preloaded with GTP-γ-S and proceeds to completion in about two min. If ATP (or ATP-γ-S) is provided alongside GTP-γ-S at the time of permeabilization, then the onset of secretion is retarded (70). The duration of the ATP-induced delay (t) is related in a complex manner to the concentrations of both essentials (over a wide range) such that

$$1/t = k \cdot \{[Ca^{2+}] \cdot [GTP\text{-}\gamma\text{-S}]\}^{1/2} \ (25).$$

The delay in onset is characteristic of a reaction sequence that leads to the generation of a new steady-state that is permissive for exocytosis. Omission of ATP allows for a more rapid progression to the permissive state, which indicates that the reactions preceding onset might involve protein dephosphorylation and that the target enzyme of G_E might be a protein phosphatase.

In none of these modulatory effects can ATP be replaced by its nonphosphorylating analogue AppNHp; they are all fully expressed at concentrations of 100 μM with EC_{50} at or around 30 μM.

Figure 2 is a schematic representation of the main control steps of the exocytotic mechanism in mast cells. It is based mainly on our own observations using the SL-O method for membrane permeabilization, and it is undoubtedly a gross oversimplification. In particular there is the possibility that G_E may also be under direct control of the cell surface receptor for polycations such as compound 48/80 so that the G proteins G_P and G_E (and perhaps also G_S) may act both in series and also in parallel with each other (55).

OTHER SECRETORY SYSTEMS

Platelets

Exocytosis from human platelets can be fully supported by Ca^{2+} alone (Figure 1). Provision of GTP analogues alongside Ca^{2+} enhances the effective affinity for Ca^{2+} so that exocytosis of amines commences at concentrations of Ca^{2+} well below the normal physiologic resting level (28, 40). In contrast, guanine nucleotides have the effect of enhancing the extent of, but not the affinity for, Ca^{2+} in the exocytosis of lysosomal enzymes (3). At very high concentrations of GTP-γ-S there is evidence of Ca^{2+}-independent secretion from both systems, but GDP-β-S has no effect on Ca^{2+}-induced secretion. The action of guanine nucleotide appears to be expressed mainly by G_P, activation of phospholipase C, and consequent activation of protein kinase C, and there is no compelling evidence for involvement of G_E.

Neutrophils

Secretion of lysosomal enzymes from permeabilized neutrophils can be induced either by Ca^{2+} or by guanine nucleotides (Figure 1), and applied together, their effects are roughly additive (6). As with intact cells, this requires the provision of cytochalasin B. The extent of GTP-γ-S-induced secretion is actually enhanced as the level of Ca^{2+} is suppressed, which indicates Ca^{2+}-independent exocytosis. Since activation of phospholipase C does not occur under these conditions (13), protein kinase C is unlikely to be involved. GDP and its analogues, however, suppress the extent of Ca^{2+}-induced secretion, which suggests that a G protein is still involved in Ca^{2+}-induced secretion. Membrane capacitance measurements, using a patch-pipette in the whole cell configuration, are in full accord with these observations (50).

Since the concentration of Ca^{2+} required in a Ca^{2+} only stimulus far exceeds that which is achieved following agonist stimulation of intact cells (7, 16, 41), other signaling pathways are implicated, though whether these involve G_E, and whether G_E is under direct control of surface receptors (e.g. for formylmethionyl peptides) is not known.

HL-60 cells

As with the mast cells, exocytosis from HL-60 cells requires a pair of effectors, but here it has been shown that any two of Ca^{2+}, guanine nucleotide, or phorbol ester are supportive (67). The rank order of nucleotides in support of exocytosis is different from that which mediates activation of phospholipase C and supports the idea that G_E is distinct from G_P. As with mast cells, there is no requirement for ATP, though the extent of secretion is enhanced when it is provided.

Eosinophils

In many respects the exocytotic mechanism of guinea pig eosinophils resembles that of mast cells. Streptolysin-O permeabilized eosinophils release lysosomal enzymes (hexosaminidase) when provided with the combined effector system comprising Ca^{2+}-plus-GTP (or one of its analogues) (51). As with mast cells, these are both necessary and together they are sufficient. ATP is not necessary, which indicates that phosphorylation does not comprise a step in the release process. When ATP is provided to the permeabilized cells, the effective affinity for both effectors is enhanced.

Membrane capacitance measurements indicate the existence of two classes of secretory granules (51). In the initial stage of degranulation the capacitance increases smoothly without any interruption, which indicates fusion of granules too small to be resolved. Only after this phase has terminated do stepwise increments become manifest; these have a magnitude commensurate with the familiar peroxidase containing granules.

Neurosecretory Cells

ADRENAL CHROMAFFIN CELLS   These cells have been investigated by several groups using a variety of permeabilization methods and also using cells maintained under different conditions that may account for apparent discrepancies in published data. Thus, while GppNHp alone (i.e. at pCa9) induces Ca^{2+}-independent exocytosis in cultured cells (9), Ca^{2+}-induced exocytosis from both cultures and from freshly dispersed cells (permeabilized by HVD) is inhibited by guanine nucleotides (9, 38). Either way, there is some evidence for late acting G proteins. There is also disagreement concerning ATP, which is either obligatory [HVD permeabilization (37)) or modulatory, enhancing exocytosis [digitonin permeabilization (9, 29)]. These differences possibly arise from the necessity, when permeabilizing by the HVD method, to treat the cells in bulk thus incurring a delay before transfer to solutions of stimulating effectors. There appears to be no ATP requirement for secretion from the related (pheochromocytoma) PC12 cells following permeabilization with staphylococcal α-toxin (1).

The ability of digitonin and SL-O to generate membrane lesions of macromolecular dimensions has also been exploited to probe the exocytotic mechanism by introduction of lysate extracts, specific proteins (e.g. calmodulin, gelsolin) and antibodies (58), proteolytic enzymes (30), and phospholipase C (19). The aim is to discern proteins retained within the permeabilized cells that remain essential for exocytosis. As with mast cells, the propensity of chromaffin cells to undergo exocytosis declines with time, though the decline is much more rapid following permeabilization with digitonin (60) than with SL-O (64). Competence may be restored by provision of cytosolic extracts though neither calmodulin nor protein kinase C, both of which leak from the digitonin permeabilized cells, can by itself restore activity (60).

The role of retained enzymes or structures can be investigated by introduction of specific enzymes. The phosphatidylinositol-specific phospholipase C from *Bacillus thuringiensis* inhibits Ca^{2+}-induced exocytosis from digitonin-permeabilized chromaffin cells, which demonstrates a role for the inositol phospholipids that is quite independent of their role as substrates for the generation of IP_3 and diglyceride (19). The effects of inositide degradation and that of ATP depletion on these cells are quite similar, and this has provoked the suggestion that the enhancement of secretion by ATP reflects the need to maintain the phosphorylated inositol lipids.

NEUROPEPTIDE SECRETING NERVE ENDINGS   Digitonin-permeabilized nerve endings from rat neurohypophysis release vasopressin and oxytocin in response to Ca^{2+}. There is no absolute requirement for ATP, and thus a phosphorylation reaction does not comprise an essential step in the terminal stages of the exocytotic pathway. In this system however, GTP and its analogues are without apparent effect (12).

Parathyroid cells

Parathyroid cells respond to a decrease in the concentration of extracellular Ca^{2+}, which is reflected as a decline in the level of intracellular Ca^{2+}. Surprisingly (see Figure 1*f*), exocytosis from permeabilized cells is associated not with depletion, but with an elevation of cytosol Ca^{2+}, although the extent of Ca^{2+}-induced secretion is small (53). Non-metabolizable analogues of GTP (i.e. GTP-γ-S and GppNHp) induce exocytosis and do so, moreover, when the level of Ca^{2+} is reduced to pCa9. Indeed, when cells are loaded with GppNHp (10^{-5} M), exocytosis remains maximal as the level of Ca^{2+} is elevated to 200 nM, but above this it declines steeply to a nil response at pCa6 (52) exactly in line with the physiologic response of intact cells.

Insulin Secreting Cells

GTP-induced, Ca^{2+}-independent secretion of insulin has been demonstrated in RINm5F (insulinoma) cells and islet cells (HVD permeabilization) (73, 75). Under conditions of low Ca^{2+} (below pCa9), there was no release of IP_3 from the RIN5mF cells, so it is likely that GTP acts directly to cause exocytosis through reactions not involving activation of protein kinase C. The effects of Ca^{2+} and GTP (analogues) on insulin secretion are not additive, which suggests that they act at a common late stage in the exocytotic control pathway. Similar to the neutrophils, however, GDP and its analogues are inhibitory to Ca^{2+}-stimulated secretion.

GTP and presumably G protein, (G_{Ei}), also mediate the inhibition of insulin secretion at a late stage following activation of inhibitory α_2-adrenergic receptors. Although these remain coupled (through G_i) to adenylyl cyclase in permeabilized pancreatic islets (36) and RINm5F cells (72), there is no correlation between the amount of cAMP generated and the rate of secretion. When GTP is provided to permeabilized RINm5F cells, clonidine inhibits both Ca^{2+}- and diglyceride-induced secretion, an effect that is abolished by pretreatment with pertussis toxin (72).

Parotid

Secretion of amylase from parotid cells can be stimulated either by ligands, which initiate a normal inositide response leading to Ca^{2+} mobilization (such as carbachol), or alternatively by β-adrenergic agonists through elevation of cAMP. Stimulation by this latter pathway occurs without elevation of intracellular Ca^{2+} (46, 68). In saponin-permeabilized cells, amylase secretion can be induced by direct introduction of cAMP while maintaining a low concentration of Ca^{2+}. Although phosphorylation of protein kinase A substrates results, this appears to be unconnected to the secretory response, which is insensitive to provision of specific kinase inhibitors (69). The question of whether a late acting G protein controls exocytosis has not yet been addressed.

CONCLUSION

Figure 2 represents a physiologic view of exocytosis as it occurs in the rat mast cell, but it necessarily promotes biochemical arguments and terminology. Central to these are the definition of binding proteins for Ca^{2+} and guanine nucleotides. While Ca^{2+} has been known to be an agent in exocytosis for at least the past 30 years, there is still no agreement about the identity of the Ca^{2+}-binding protein that determines the exocytotic reaction. The definition of G_E is also conceptual, although in yeasts, a genetically defined GTP-binding protein having structural homology to the human *ras*-oncogene products (59) is implicated at a late stage in the constitutive secretory pathway leading to secretion of invertase. Whether G_E is a member of the low molecular weight class of monomeric G proteins as suggested by the ability of oncogenic *ras* to cause degranulation of mast cells (5), or whether it will turn out to be a high molecular weight heterotrimer as is hinted by experiments that indicate direct control by receptors [both stimulatory (55) or inhibitory (72)) is far from resolved. Both classes of G proteins are present on the membranes of chromaffin granules (11, 71). What does appear certain is that GTP-binding proteins are closely linked with the late stages of the exocytotic pathway; depending on the cell type and the conditions applied, they express their activities with bewildering variety. This reflects what has been known for a long time; exocytosis is a complex business, and there is an extensive repertoire of control mechanisms to match.

ACKNOWLEDGMENTS

Work in the author's laboratory has been supported by The Wellcome Trust, The Vandervell Foundation, and the Gower Street Secretory Mechanisms Group.

Literature Cited

1. Ahnert-Hilger, G., Bhakdi, S., Gratzl, M. 1985. Minimal requirements for exocytosis. A study using PC12 cells permeabilized with staphylococcal alpha toxin. *J. Biol. Chem.* 160:12730–34
2. Deleted in proof
3. Athayde, C. M., Scrutton, M. C. 1989. Guanine nucleotides and Ca^{2+}-dependent lysosomal secretion in electropermeabilised human platelets. *Eur. J. Biochem.* In press
4. Bader, M.-F., Thierse, D., Aunis, D., Ahnert-Hilger, G., Gratzl, M. 1986. Characterization of hormone and protein release from α-toxin-permeabilized chromaffin cells in primary culture. *J. Biol. Chem.* 261:5777–83
5. Bar-Sagi, D., Gomperts, B. D. 1988. Stimulation of exocytotic degranulation by microinjection of the *ras* oncogenic protein into rat mast cells. *Oncogene* 3:463–69
6. Barrowman, M. M., Cockcroft, S., Gomperts, B. D. 1986. Two roles for guanine nucleotides in the stimulus secretion sequence of neutrophils. *Nature* 319:504–7
7. Barrowman, M. M., Cockcroft, S., Gomperts, B. D. 1987. Differential control of azurophilic and specific granule exocytosis in Sendai virus permeabilized rabbit neutrophils. *J. Physiol. (London)* 383:115–24
8. Bennett, J. P., Cockcroft, S., Gomperts, B. D. 1981. Rat mast cells permeabilised with ATP secrete histamine in response to calcium ions buffered in the micromolar range. *J. Physiol. (London)* 317:335–45
9. Bittner, M. A., Holz, R. W., Neubig, R. R. 1986. Guanine nucleotide effects on catecholamine secretion from digitonin-permeabilized adrenal chromaffin cells. *J. Biol. Chem.* 261:10182–88
10. Buckingham, L., Duncan, J. L. 1983. Approximate dimensions of membrane lesions produced by streptolysin S and streptolysin O. *Biochim. Biophys. Acta.* 729:115–22
11. Burgoyne, R. D., Morgan, A. 1989. Low molecular weight GTP-binding proteins of adrenal chromaffin cells are present on the secretory granule. *FEBS Lett.* 245:122–26
12. Cazalis, M., Dayanithi, G., Nordmann, J. J. 1987. Requirements for hormone release from permeabilized nerve endings isolated from the rat neurohypophysis. *J. Physiol. (London)*. 390:71–91
13. Cockcroft, S. 1986. The dependence on Ca^{2+} of the guanine nucleotide-activated polyphosphoinositide phosphodiesterase in neutrophil plasma membranes. *Biochem. J.* 240:503–7
14. Cockcroft, S., Gomperts, B. D. 1979. ATP induces nucleotide permeability in rat mast cells. *Nature* 279:541–42
15. Cockcroft, S., Gomperts, B. D. 1985. Role of guanine nucleotide binding protein in the activation of polyphosphoinositide phosphodiesterase. *Nature* 314:534–36
16. Cockcroft, S., Gomperts, B. D. 1988. Some new questions concerning the role of calcium in exocytosis. In *Calcium and Drug Action*, ed. P. F. Baker, pp. 305–338. Heidelberg: Springer-Verlag
17. Cockcroft, S., Howell, T. W., Gomperts, B. D. 1987. Two G-proteins act in series to control stimulus-secretion coupling in mast cells: Use of neomycin to distinguish between G-proteins controlling polyphosphoinositide phosphodies-

terase and exocytosis. *J. Cell Biol.* 105:2745–50

18. Eberhard, D. A., Holz, R. W. 1989. Ca^{2+} and guanine nucleotide effects on inositol phospholipid metabolism: relationship between the production of inositol phosphates and inositol phospholipid levels. *J. Biol. Chem.* Submitted

19. Eberhard, D. A., Cooper, C. L., Low, M. G., Holz, R. W. 1989. Evidence that inositol phospholipids are necessary for exocytosis: Loss of inositol phospholipids and inhibition of secretion in permeabilized cells caused by a bacterial phospholipase C and removal of ATP. *Biochem. J.* In press

20. Füssle, R., Bhakdi, S., Sziegoleit, A., Tranum-Jensen, J., Kranz, T., Wellensiek, H. J. 1981. On the mechanism of membrane damage of Staphylococcus aureus alpha-toxin. *J. Biol. Chem.* 91:83–94

21. Fernandez, J. M., Neher, E., Gomperts, B. D. 1984. Capacitance measurements reveal stepwise fusion events in degranulating mast cells. *Nature* 312:453–55

22. Gomperts, B. D., Baldwin, J. M., Micklem, K. J. 1983. Rat mast cells permeabilized with Sendai virus secrete histamine in response to Ca^{2+} buffered in the micromolar range. *Biochem. J.* 210:737–45

23. Gomperts, B. D., Cockcroft, S., Howell, T. W., Nüsse, O., Tatham, P. E. R. 1987. The dual effector system for exocytosis in mast cells: Obligatory requirement for both Ca^{2+} and GTP. *Biosci. Rep.* 7:369–81

24. Gomperts, B. D., Cockcroft, S., Howell, T. W., Tatham, P. E. R. 1988. Intracellular Ca^{2+}, GTP and ATP as effectors and modulators of exocytotic secretion from rat mast cells. In *Molecular Mechanisms in Secretion*, ed. N. A. Thorn, M. Treiman, O. H. Petersen. pp. 248–261. Copenhagen: Munksgaard

25. Gomperts, B. D., Tatham, P. E. R. 1989. GTP-binding proteins in the control of exocytosis. *Molecular Biology of Signal Transduction. Cold Spring Harbor Symp. Quant. Biol.* (ed. M. Wigler, J. R. Feramisco, J. D. Watson. 53:983–92

26. Guild, S., Frey, E. A., Pocotte, S. L., Kebabian, J. W. 1988. Adenosine 3′,5′-monophosphate-mediated enhancement of calcium-evoked prolactin release from electrically permeabilised 7315c tumor cells. *Brit. J. Pharmacol.* 94:737–44

27. Hamill, O. P., Marty, A., Neher, E.,

Sakman, B., Sigworth, F. J. 1981. Improved patch-clamp techniques for high-resolution current recording from cells and cell-free membrane patches. *Eur. J. Physiol.* 391:85–100

28. Haslam, R. J., Davidson, M. M. L. 1984. Guanine nucleotides decrease the free $[Ca^{2+}]$ required for secretion of serotonin from permeabilized blood platelets: Evidence of a role for a GTP-binding-protein in platelet activation. *FEBS Lett.* 174:90–95

29. Holz, R. W., Bittner, M. A., Peppers, S. C., Senter, R. A., Eberhard, D. A. 1989. MgATP-independent and MgATP-dependent exocytosis: Evidence that MgATP primes adrenal chromaffin cells to undergo exocytosis. *J. Biol. Chem.* 264:5412–19

30. Holz, R. W., Senter, R. A. 1988. Effects of trypsin on secretion stimulated by micromolar Ca^{2+} and phorbol ester in digitonin-permeabilized adrenal chromaffin cells. *Cell. Mol. Neurobiol.* 8:115–28

31. Howell, T. W., Cockcroft, S., Gomperts, B. D. 1987. Essential synergy between Ca^{2+} and guanine nucleotides in exocytotic secretion from permeabilised mast cells. *J. Cell Biol.* 105:191–97

32. Howell, T. W., Gomperts, B. D. 1987. Rat mast cells permeabilised with streptolysin-O secrete histamine in response to Ca^{2+} at concentrations buffered in the micromolar range. *Biochim. Biophys. Acta.* 927:177–83

33. Howell, T. W., Kramer, I., Gomperts, B. D. 1988. Protein phosphorylation and the dependence on Ca^{2+} for GTP-γ-S stimulated exocytosis from permeabilized mast cells. *Cell. Signal.* 1:157–63

34. Impraim, C. C., Foster, K. A., Micklem, K. J., Pasternak, C. A. 1980. Nature of virally mediated changes in membrane permeability to small molecules. *Biochem. J.* 186:847–60

35. Johansen, T. 1987. Energy metabolism in rat mast cells in relation to histamine secretion. *Pharmacol. Toxicol.* 61:1–20(Suppl. II)

36. Jones, P. M., Fyles, J. M., Persaud, S. J., Howell, S. L. 1987. Catecholamine inhbition of Ca^{2+}-induced insulin secretion from electrically permeabilised islets of Langerhans. *FEBS Lett.* 219:139–44

37. Knight, D. E., Baker, P. F. 1982. Calcium-dependence of catecholamine release from bovine adrenal medullary cells after exposure to intense electric fields. *J. Membr. Biol.* 68:107–40

38. Knight, D. E., Baker, P. F. 1985.

Guanine nucleotides and Ca-dependent exocytosis. *FEBS Lett.* 189:345–49

39. Knight, D. E., Koh, E. 1984. Ca^{2+} and cyclic nucleotide dependence of amylase release from isolated rat pancreatic acinar cells rendered permeable by intense electric fields. *Cell Calcium* 5:401–18

40. Knight, D. E., Scrutton, M. C. 1986. Effects of guanine nucleotides on the properties of 5-hydroxytryptamine secretion from electro-permeabilised human platelets. *Eur. J. Biochem.* 160:183–90

41. Lew, P. D., Monod, A., Waldwogel, F. A., Dewald, B., Baggiolini, M., Pozzan, T. 1986. Quantitative analysis of the cytosolic free calcium dependency of exocytosis from three subcellular compartments in intact human neutrophils. *J. Cell Biol.* 102:2197–2204

42. Luini, A., De Matteis, M. A. 1988. Dual regulation of ACTH secretion by guanine nucleotides in permeabilized AtT-20 cells. *Cell. Mol. Neurobiol.* 8:129–38

43. Marquardt, D. L., Gruber, H. E., Walker, L. L. 1987. Ribavirin inhibits mast cell mediator release. *J. Pharmacol. Exp. Therap.* 240:145–49

44. Marty, A., Neher, E. 1983. Tight seal whole-cell recording. In *Single Channel Recording*, ed. B. Sakmann, E. Neher. pp. 107–121. New York: Plenum

45. Mason, W. T., Rawlings, S. R., Cobbett, P., Sikdar, S. K., Zorec, R., et al. 1988. Control of secretion in anterior pituitary cells: Linking ion channels, messengers and exocytosis. *J. Exp. Biol.* 139:287–316

46. McMillian, M. K., Soltoff, S. P., Talamo, B. R. 1988. Mediation of norepinephrine effects on free cytosolic calcium in rat parotid acinar cells by α_1 adrenergic receptors. *Biochem. Pharmacol.* 37:3790–93

47. Miller, M. T., Castellot, J. J., Pardee, A. B. 1978. A permeable animal cell preparation for studying macromolecular synthesis, DNA synthesis and the role of deoxy ribonucleotides in S phase initiation. *Biochemistry* 17:1073–80

48. Neher, E. 1987. The influence of intracellular calcium concentration on degranulation of dialysed mast cells from rat peritoneum. *J. Physiol. (London).* 395:193–214

49. Neher, E., Marty, A. 1982. Discrete changes of cell membrane capacitance observed under conditions of enhanced secretion in bovine adrenal chromaffin cells. *Proc. Nat. Acad. Sci. USA* 79:6712–16

50. Nüsse, O., Lindau, M. 1988. The dynamics of exocytosis in human neutrophils. *J. Cell Biol.* 107:2117–23

51. Nüsse, O., Lindau, M., Cromwell, O., Kay, A. B., Gomperts, B. D. 1990. Intracellular application of GTP-γ-S induces exocytotic granule fusion in guinea pig eosinophils. *J. Exp. Med.* In press

52. Oetting, M., LeBoff, M., Swiston, L., Preston, J., Brown, E. 1986. Guanine nucleotides are potent secretagogues in permeabilized parathyroid cells. *FEBS Lett.* 208:99–104

53. Oetting, M., Leboff, M. S., Levy, S., Swiston, L., Preston, J., et al. 1987. Permeabilization reveals classical stimulus-secretion coupling in bovine parathyroid cells. *Endocrinology* 121:1571–76

54. Pace, C. S., Tarvin, J. T., Neighbors, A. S., Pirkle, J. A., Greider, M. H. 1980. Use of a high voltage technique to determine the molecular requirements for exocytosis in islet cells. *Diabetes* 29:911–18

55. Penner, R. 1988. Multiple signaling pathways control stimulus-secretion coupling in rat peritoneal mast cells. *Proc. Nat. Acad. Sci. USA* 85:9856–60

56. Penner, R., Neher, E. 1988. The role of calcium in stimulus-secretion coupling in excitable and non-excitable cells. *J. Exp. Biol.* 139:329–45

57. Penner, R., Pusch, M., Neher, E. 1987. Washout phenomena in dialyzed mast cells allow discrimination of different steps in stimulus-secretion coupling. *Biosci. Rep.* 7:313–21

58. Perrin, D., Langley, O. K., Aunis, D. 1987. Anti-α-fodrin inhibits secretion from permeabilized chromaffin cells. *Nature* 326:498–501

59. Salminen, A., Novick, P. J. 1987. A *ras*-like protein is required for a post-Golgi event in yeast secretion. *Cell* 49:527–38

60. Sarafian, T., Aunis, D., Bader, M.-F. 1987. Loss of proteins from digitonin-permeabilized adrenal chromaffin cells essential for exocytosis. *J. Biol. Chem.* 262:16671–76

61. Schrezenmeier, H., Ahnert-Hilger, G., Fleischer, B. 1988. A T cell receptor-associated GTP-binding protein triggers T cell receptor-mediated granule exocytosis in cytotoxic T lymphocytes. *J. Immunol.* 141:3785–90

62. Smolen, J. E., Stoehr, S. J. 1985. Micromolar concentrations of free calcium provoke secretion of lysozyme from human neutrophils permeabilized with saponin. *J. Immunol.* 134:1859–65

63. Smolen, J. E., Stoehr, S. J. 1986. Guanine nucleotides reduce the free calcium requirement for secretion of granule constituents from permeabilized human neutrophils. *Biochim. Biophys. Acta.* 889–171–78

64. Sontag, J.-M., Aunis, D., Bader, M.-F. 1988. Peripheral actin filaments control calcium-mediated catecholamine release from streptolysin-O-permeabilized chromaffin cells. *Eur. J. Cell Biol.* 46:316–26

65. Sorimachi, M., Nishimura, S., Sadano, H. 1987. Role of guanine nucleotide regulatory protein in histamine secretion from digitonin-permeabilized rat mast cells. *Biomed. Res.* 8:205–9

66. Sorimachi, M., Nishimura, S., Yamagami, K., Yada, T. 1988. Fluoroaluminates stimulate histamine secretion in the digitonin-permeabilized rat mast cells. *Jpn. J. Physiol.* 38:227–32

67. Stutchfield, J., Cockcroft, S. 1988. Guanine nucleotides stimulate polyphosphoinositide phosphodiesterase and exocytotic secretion from HL-60 cells permeabilised with streptolysin O. *Biochem. J.* 250:375–82

68. Takemura, H. 1985. Changes in free cytosolic calcium concentration in isolated rat parotid cells by cholinergic and β-adrenergic agonists. *Biochem. Biophys. Res. Commun.* 131:1048–55

69. Takuma, T. 1988. Evidence against direct involvement of cyclic AMP-dependent protein phosphorylation in the exocytosis of amylase. *Biochem. J.* 256:867–71

70. Tatham, P. E. R., Gomperts, B. D. 1989. ATP inhibits onset of exocytosis in permeabilised mast cells. *Biosci. Rep.* 9:99–109

71. Toutant, M., Aunis, D., Bockaert, J., Homburger, V., Rouot, B. 1987. Presence of three pertussis substrates and $G_o\alpha$ immunoreactivity in both plasma and granule membranes of chromaffin cells. *FEBS Lett.* 215:339–44

72. Ullrich, S., Wollheim, C. B. 1988. GTP-dependent inhibition of insulin secretion by epinephrine in permeabilized RINm5F cells: Lack of correlation between insulin secretion and cyclic AMP levels. *J. Biol. Chem.* 263:8615–20

73. Vallar, L., Biden, T. J., Wollheim, C. B. 1987. Guanine nucleotides induce Ca^{2+} independent secretion from permeabilized RINm5F cells. *J. Biol. Chem.* 262:5049–56

74. Wilson, B., Deanin, G., Stump, R., Oliver, J. 1988. Depletion of guanine nucleotides suppresses IgE-mediated degranulation in rat basophilic leukemia cells. *FASEB J.* 2:A1236

75. Wollheim, C. B., Ullrich, S., Meda, P., Vallar, L. 1987. Regulation of exocytosis in electrically permeabilized insulin-secreting cells: Evidence for Ca^{2+} dependent and independent secretion. *Biosci. Rep.* 7:443–54

76. Yamamoto, T., Furuki, Y., Guild, S., Kebabian, J. W. 1987. Adenosine 3',5'-cyclic monophosphate stimulates secretion of alpha-melanocyte-stimulating hormone from permeabilized cells of the intermediate lobe of the rat pituitary gland. *Biochem. Biophys. Res. Commun.* 143:1076–84

77. Yaseen, M. A., Pedley, K. C., Howell, S. L. 1982. Regulation of insulin secretion from islets of Langerhans rendered permeable by electric discharge. *Biochem. J.* 206:81–87

Annu. Rev. Physiol. 1990. 52:607–24

EXOCYTOSIS

W. Almers

Department of Physiology and Biophysics, University of Washington, Seattle, Washington 98195

KEY WORDS: fusion pore, patch-clamp, fusion intermediates, membrane capacitance, fusion proteins

INTRODUCTION

All eukaryotic cells contain membrane-bounded vesicles that are destined for export. Molecular motors capture these vesicles in the cell interior and carry them to the plasma membrane; this requires metabolic energy. When the vesicle approaches the cell surface to within a few nanometers, it may undergo exocytosis, that is, the membrane surrounding the vesicle may fuse with the plasma membrane. The vesicle membrane then becomes a part of the cell membrane, and any material within the vesicle diffuses into the extracellular space. Eukaryotic cells undergo exocytosis either to insert new components into the plasma membrane or to export the membrane-impermeant substances stored within the vesicles. In constitutive exocytosis, vesicles exocytose approximately as soon as they reach the cell membrane, and no known mechanism controls the fusion event. In stimulated or regulated exocytosis, vesicles gather beneath the cell membrane in clusters and lie there waiting, until a signal reaching the cell membrane causes the appearance of a cytosolic messenger substance. The messenger then causes conformational changes in an unknown receptor protein on either the vesicle or the cell membrane, so that many or most of the vesicles undergo exocytosis in a burst. The regulatory processes vary among different cells; in some (neurons or eggs), an increase in cytosolic Ca^{2+} is enough to trigger exocytosis, while in others (e.g. mast cells; Gomperts, this volume), Ca^{2+} is merely a cofactor. The mechanisms of fusion also may vary. In this review, however, I make the

0066-4278/90/0315-0604$02.00

unproven assumption that fusion occurs in the same way in all cells, even when it is coupled to different control mechanisms.

One can imagine fusion to be regulated in two ways. (*a*) If secretory vesicles were innately eager to fuse with cell membranes, then regulating fusion would mean preventing it from happening in quiescent cells. (*b*) Alternatively, the fusion of biological membranes may be energetically difficult and require catalysis by specific fusion proteins. These would be continuously active in constitutive exocytosis and only occasionally active in regulated exocytosis. There are a number of reasons why the latter is probably correct. (*a*) Artificial bilayers made from biological lipids do not readily fuse with each other under the conditions found in most living cells (56). (*b*) The fusion of viral envelopes to host cell membranes is the only fusion process understood at the molecular level, and it requires catalysis by known fusion proteins (73). (*c*) In yeast, where secretion is constitutive, several gene products are required for vesicles to undergo exocytosis (46).

Previous articles have discussed why artificial lipid bilayers are so resistant to fusion (56), how this resistance may be overcome, and what the findings with pure lipid bilayers tell us about membrane fusion in living cells (7, 20, 55). The extensive work on pure lipid systems is important and exocytotic fusion clearly does involve the rearrangement of lipids. Nonetheless, it is difficult to disagree with Rand & Parsegian (55) that "in spite of heroic efforts, phospholipid bilayer models of fusion do not mimic the cellular processes closely enough to be confident that the cellular mechanism is being probed". The working hypothesis in this review will be that the earliest steps in membrane fusion are due to specific proteins that simultaneously interact with both the plasma and the vesicle membrane (8, 9, 32, 34, 53, 60, 79). Although the molecular basis of exocytotic membrane fusion is unknown, promising methods to study exocytosis in a controlled biochemical environment have been developed and reviewed [chromaffin cells (5), sea urchin eggs (28), *Paramecium* (51)].

Two Key Properties of Exocytotic Membrane Fusion

EXOCYTOSIS CAN BE FAST   After a stimulus reaches a cell, how long does it take before the first vesicles undergo exocytosis? In the examples listed in Table 1, this delay generally lasts seconds to tens of seconds. Most of this time is probably spent in generating the cytosolic messenger, in removing cytosolic barrier proteins (e.g. synapsin) or, in some cases, in conveying vesicles from the depth of the cell to the plasma membrane. To appreciate how rapidly exocytotic fusion can occur, it is instructive to consider neurons. In neurons, the vesicles containing the secreted product (i.e. the transmitter) are parked so close to the plasma membrane that they touch, and no chemical

Table 1   Speed of exocytosis

Cell type	Stimulus	Delay (s)	Duration (s)	Temperature °C	Method	Reference
Sea urchin egg	sperm	40	80	15	C	30
Neutrophils	GTP-γ-S	50	200	20[1]	C	47
Mast cells	GTP-γ-S	50	200	20[1]	C	19
	antigen	60	100	20[1]	C	36
	48/80	5	5	20[1]	C	38
Chromaffin cell	electrical	< 0.2	—	20[1]	C	44
Frog motor neuron	electrical	0.0005	—	19	psp	33
Cat afferent neurons	electrical	0.0002	—	38	psp	42
						13

Delay, time between application of stimulus and first signs of exocytosis; duration, time over which membrane area increased; C, capacitance measurement; psp, postsynaptic potential.
[1]Temperature given as room temperature.

reaction is required to generate the active cytosolic messenger, Ca^{2+}. Instead, Ca^{2+} enters the cytosol by crossing the plasma membrane through Ca channels. These Ca channels open during an action potential across the plasma membrane, and probably are 10–20 nm away from the vesicles. At the frog motor nerve terminal, the delay between the action potential and exocytosis (as assayed by the post-synaptic potential) is only 0.5 ms at 19°C (33). In mammalian neurons at 38°C, the delay is even less (0.2 ms; 13, 42). In this short time, several events must occur in sequence: first, Ca channels must open; then $[Ca^{2+}]$ near the synaptic vesicles must rise; Ca^{2+} must bind to its (unknown) receptor; the receptor must change conformation; the molecular rearrangements of membrane fusion must occur; and finally the transmitter must diffuse to its postsynaptic receptor, open ion channels, and produce the postsynaptic response. Even if all of the 0.5 ms synaptic delay in a frog neuromuscular junction were available for the triggering and execution of membrane fusion, it would suffice for at most one enzymatic reaction. Consider the rates of two enzymatic reactions that have been considered to start exocytosis: phosphorylation and dephosphorylation (23, 77). Some placental phosphatases (MW 40,000) have maximal rate constants of up to 45 μmol of substrate/min and per mg enzyme (67); this translates into one phosphate liberated by one enzyme molecule every 33 ms. One of the fastest known protein kinases, phosphorylase b kinase (MW 1,300,000) will phosphorylate 15 μmol substrate/min and per mg enzyme (65) at 30°C, or one substrate molecule every 12 ms per catalytic subunit. Both phosphorylation and dephosphorylation are rapid enough to play a role in signal transduction in many secretory cells and, indeed, in many aspects of neuronal secretion. Such reactions, however, are probably too slow to play a role in exocytosis at fast synapses. Judging by the enormous speed of transmitter release, exocytosis is probably triggered by a conformational change in a single macromolecule.

EXOCYTOSIS IS TIGHT   The fusion of lipid bilayers involves profound molecular rearrangements. Yet exocytotic membrane fusion causes damage to neither plasma nor vesicle membranes. As far as we know, exocytosis is alway tight; there is no morphologic evidence that exocytosis ever leads to the rupture of vesicles and to the discharge of their contents into the cytosol. The only connection that forms is between vesicle lumen and extracellular space, and no leaks form between the vesicle lumen and the cytosol, or between the extracellular space and the cytosol. Lindau & Fernandez (36) have reported an experiment where the electrical conductance between the cytosol and the extracellular space increased by less than 100 pS while about 1000 vesicles underwent exocytosis. Even if none of the vesicles contained open ion channels, each vesicle could have caused a leak of at most 0.1 pS, 100-fold less than the conductance of a typical ion channel. Clearly the exocytotic mechanism is highly successful in limiting leaks between cytosol and vesicle lumen or between cytosol and extracellular space. This success distinguishes exocytosis from known methods of fusing artificial lipid vesicles with other vesicles or with planar bilayers. It suggests that a highly specific macro-molecule must form the first connection between the lumen of an exocytosing vesicle and the cell exterior. The gap junction is a macromolecule that can achieve such a feat because it connects two aqueous compartments selectively without connecting them to a third compartment. Gap junctions do not, however, mediate fusion.

Morphology

EARLY STEPS IN EXOCYTOSIS   In thin sections, vesicles caught in the act of exocytosis are seen to form characteristic omega-figures, which show the vesicles united with the plasma membrane by a narrow neck of membrane. In freeze-fracture, the neck appears as a bump or a dip. The center of the larger bumps can be made into a pit by etching. It must therefore contain aqueous material and represent a pore (called fusion pore in this review) that connects the vesicle lumen with the extracellular space. Even in the same section, pore diameters vary over a wide range. Investigators infer that the pores are narrow at first and later dilate as fusion progresses.

The smallest pores seen under the electron microscope are generally about 20 nm in diameter; the preparations examined include posterior pituitary cells (18), mast cells (12), the neuromuscular junction (26), adrenal chromaffin cells (62), and *Paramecium* (41). In *Limulus* amoebocytes, an even smaller pore may have been seen. Thin sections of secreting amoebocytes show small areas where the two fusing membranes touch and form a sheet two membranes thick (50). Such "pedestals" are thought to form as a prelude to the fusion pore, and one of the pedestals was said to contain a small pore of 5 nm diameter. The pores seen in electron micrographs are comparable in diameter to the pores (17) formed by complement (10 nm) or perforin, the toxin of cytotoxic T-lymphocytes (16 nm). Both complement and perforin pores are assemblies of protein molecules. Whether or not fusion pores include proteins or protein complexes is not clear from electron micrographs.

Do the 20 nm pores arise suddenly and without a smaller precursor? Except possibly in amoebocytes, any such precursors are evidently too short-lived to be captured by present morphologic techniques. Unfortunately, it is precisely the early and short-lived forms of the fusion pore that will tell us the most about the mechanism of exocytosis. How does a fusion pore form? What are its molecular constituents? What are its properties at the instant of its formation? How does it expand, what is its fate, and ultimately how is it replaced by an apparently seamless neck of lipid bilayer connecting the vesicle to the plasma membrane? Some of these questions must be addressed with methods that can resolve fast events.

SPECIALIZATIONS NEAR EXOCYTOSIS SITES   At neuronal synapses and in some protozoa (such as *Paramecium*), exocytosis occurs at precisely determined sites, and one can search for membrane specializations that may be related to exocytosis. In both cell types, freeze-fracture reveals ordered arrays of plasma membrane macromolecules close to sites of exocytosis. In the frog neuromuscular junction, such sites (called active zones) are marked by double rows of intramembrane particles (11), and exocytosis occurs within a few tens of nm of these intramembrane particles. Large and sometimes ordered particles in the plasma membrane near active zones also occur at many other synapses, and it is likely that they play a role in exocytosis. In the neuromuscular junction, they cannot be fusion proteins, since exocytosis always occurs near but never exactly above the particles. The particles may represent voltage-sensitive Ca channels (25), but there is no experimental evidence concerning their role.

In *Tetrahymena* (60, 61) and *Paramecium* (52), each secretory vesicle docks beneath a set of some 10 plasma membrane particles. The particles form a radially symmetric cluster called a rosette that is probably related to exocytosis, since mutants without rosettes cannot exocytose their vesicles (6). In *Paramecium,* the tip of the secretory vesicle (trichocyst) just beneath the rosette shows an annular-shaped zone enriched with intramembrane particles; whether these particles interact with those of the rosette is unclear.

At first the rosette particles were thought to form the fusion pore (60). However, rare images probably representing early stages in membrane fusion (41) show a dispersing rosette, with a 10–20 nm diameter fusion pore forming in the middle. These images suggest that the rosette particles are not at the site of fusion when fusion occurs; hence the particles cannot be fusion proteins. It was later argued that the rosette particles were Ca channels providing the Ca influx thought to be necessary for triggering exocytosis (59). If so, they must be Ca channels of a new type previously unstudied. The voltage-sensitive Ca channels in *Paramecium* are associated with the cilia and not with the rosette (48), and both deciliated *Paramecia* and mutants lacking functional voltage-sensitive Ca channels are capable of exocytosis (51). In fact, it is unknown how much of the Ca needed for exocytosis comes from the outside in *Paramecium*. The role of rosettes in exocytosis remains a mystery.

In *Chlamydomonas* (72), an intracellular contractile vacuole gathers low-molecular-weight waste products and periodically discharges them into the extracellular environment. This discharge does not represent exocytosis in the strict sense, since the vacuole never fuses with the plasma membrane. Instead, the plasma and vacuole membranes approach each other to within a few nm and enclose between them a periodic array of electron-dense spots. The array of spots corresponds to an array of large intramembrane particles that appears in the cytosol-facing leaflets of both vacuole and plasma membranes. It has been suggested that the particles form aqueous channels connecting the vacuole lumen with the external medium and that the discharge mechanism of the contractile vacuole is an evolutionary precursor of exocytosis (72).

Where resting secretory vesicles bulge against the plasma membrane, the narrow cytoplasmic space between vesicle and plasma membrane is sometimes bridged by narrow filaments [e.g. in mast cells (12) or pancreatic beta cells (49)]. A recent review discusses the possible roles of cytoskeletal elements in exocytosis (34).

Electrophysiologic Assays of Exocytosis

Electrophysiologic assays allow one to monitor exocytosis at the level of single cells and even single secretory vesicles. At synapses, the postsynaptic potential reports the secretion of transmitter by a nerve terminal. In some synapses, miniature postsynaptic potentials can be recorded and provide, at submillisecond time resolution, an assay for exocytosis at the level of single synaptic vesicles (16). A more recent electrophysiologic assay relies on the fact that each exocytotic event increases the cell surface area. Since all biological membranes have an electrical capacitance of 1 $\mu F/cm^2$ one may monitor the cell surface area (and hence exocytosis) by measuring the plasma membrane capacitance (21, 30). The method was perfected by Neher & his collaborators (37, 44) and applied to most of the cells in Table 1. When secretion is sufficiently slow (no more than a few vesicles per second), the capacitance (C) can be seen to increase in small steps, each reporting the exocytosis of a single secretory vesicle. Such C steps have been seen in adrenal chromaffin cells (44), mast cells (19), pancreatic acinar cells (39), neutrophils (47), and pituitary lactotrophs (40). C steps as small as 2 fF can be resolved, which correspond to vesicles of 0.2 μm^2 surface area or 250 nm diameter (44, 47). Exocytosis of single synaptic vesicles containing a fast neurotransmitter (typically 50 nm in diameter) is still beyond the reach of this assay, but C changes due to the release of many synaptic vesicles can be detected (22). The method can also be used for monitoring episodes of endocytosis (2).

Mast cells have been useful for studying single exocytotic events because their secretory vesicles are large. Particularly convenient are mast cells from beige mice (strain C57BL/6J-bg^j/bg^j), which have a genetic defect resembling Chediak-Higashi syndrome in humans. Because of this defect, mast cells and other granulocytes of beige mice are unable to limit the size of their secretory vesicles. Instead of having some thousand vesicles of about 0.8 μm diameter, mast cells of beige mice have only 10–40 giant vesicles of 1–5 μm diameter. They secrete readily when stimulated by mast cell secretagogues (54) or intracellular GTP-γ-S (8, 78) and individual vesicles can be seen under the light microscope while they exocytose (15). Nowhere are the electric signals associated with the exocytosis of single vesicles as large as in mast cells of beige mice.

Time-Resolved Exocytosis of Single Vesicles

DO OSMOTIC FORCES DRIVE MEMBRANE FUSION?   Pure lipid bilayers can be fused to each other by placing them under mechanical stress. Secretory vesicles often swell as cells secrete, which suggests that swelling stretches the vesicle membrane and thereby causes membrane fusion [for a review of this hypothesis see (20)]. Mast cells of beige mice provide an opportunity to test this idea, because one can watch individual vesicles swell while one measures the capacitance (C) to monitor fusion. Two independent studies (1, 8, 78, 79) have shown that a step increase in C always precedes swelling. In these studies, the C step clearly represented fusion of the vesicle because when the vesicle's diameter was measured under the light microscope, the surface area calculated agreed well with the amplitude of the C step. Swelling followed the step with a mean delay of 0.4 s (8). Even in osmotically shrunk vesicles, fusion preceded swelling; hence even vesicles with a slack membrane can fuse. Work on chromaffin cells provides additional evidence that vesicle membranes can fuse without being stretched (27).

Swelling of the vesicle may have an important role in hastening extrusion of the contents from the vesicle cavity; the mechanism of swelling has been reviewed (Verdugo, this volume). It is likely, however, that vesicle swelling is a consequence rather than a cause of membrane fusion. In the search for early events in membrane fusion one must look elsewhere.

REVERSIBLE INTERMEDIATES IN MEMBRANE FUSION   It is widely believed that exocytosis is irreversible and that the subsequent retrieval of the exocytosed membrane occurs by a different mechanism. In agreement with this view, a plot of mast cell capacitance (i.e. mast cell surface) against time usually looks like a staircase, with each step building upon the previous one (9, 19). Occasionally, however, one obtains recordings as in Figure 1a, where C increases in a step, but then fluctuates for a second and once even returns to baseline. Since the step increase in C reports the formation of an electric connection between the exterior and the lumen of the exocytosing vesicle (the fusion pore), the experiment shows that this connection can form and break repeatedly. Only later does the step become stably established, which suggests that the vesicle has fused completely. Figure 1a is reminiscent of a single-channel recording. Just as the sudden appearance and disappearance of current through the single ion channel represents the sudden opening and closing of that channel, so do the flickering fluctuations in C represent the opening and closing of the fusion pore.

First seen by Fernandez et al (19), capacitance flicker as in Figure 1a has now been seen by several other groups in mast cells both from normal rats (1, 19) and from beige mice (4, 8, 9, 78). A flickering vesicle filled with a fluorescent dye will not readily release this dye, hence a flickering fusion pore must be narrow (8). The electrical conductance of a flickering pore (0.7–4 nS in giant vesicles) (4, 9) is consistent with a 4 to 10 nm diameter pore of 150 nm length (9). Unfortunately, we do not know why some vesicles flicker, and most do not.

Flicker suggests that a narrow pore is an early intermediate in exocytosis. Because flicker is rare, one imagines that the intermediate is usually short-lived and only occasionally survives for seconds. Indeed, even vesicles that do not flicker form transient pores of high electrical resistance. If one looks at C steps with high enough time resolution, one can often see that C grows gradually to a final value (Figure 1b). The time course reflects the increasing conductance of the dilating fusion pore (Figure 1c). Unfortunately, the initial phase of dilation is too rapid even for time-resolved capacitance recordings. Hence the method misses early steps in the formation of the pore.

THE EARLIEST FUSION PORE   The secretory vesicles of mast and chromaffin cells actively accumulate biogenic amines, and this active uptake is powered by a pH gradient across the vesicle membrane (31). The gradient is maintained by an electrogenic H^+ pump that generates a lumen-positive potential across the vesicle membrane (9, 58). As soon as the pore opens, the plasma and vesicle membrane become electrically connected. The difference between plasma and vesicle membrane potentials then drives an electric discharge through the fusion pore that adjusts the charge on the vesicle membrane

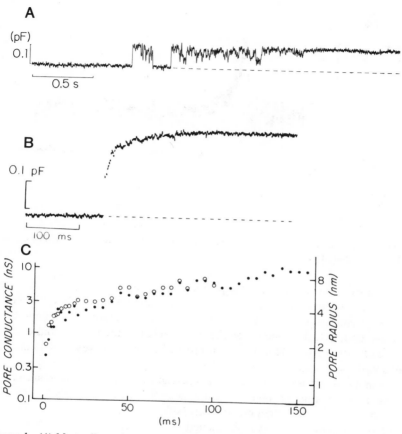

Figure 1 (*A*) Mast cell membrane capacitance during fusion of one secretory vesicle. (*B*) As above but from a different cell; note expanded time scale. (*C*) Conductance of the fusion pore calculated from trace B (*circles*) and from the real part (*dots*) of the electrical admittance to an 820 Hz sinusoid (not shown). Trace A from (8), B and C from (9).

capacitance until the two membranes have the same potential. In giant mast cell vesicles of beige mice, this discharge is large enough to be recorded as a current transient that precedes the C step (Figure 2a).

The current transient and subsequent C step allow one to calculate the membrane potential of an individual vesicle at the instant of exocytosis. To do this, one divides the charge carried by the transient (the amplitude of the transient's time integral, see Figure 2b) by the vesicle capacitance (C_v, the amplitude of the C step). The result is the difference between vesicle and plasma membrane potentials. Since the plasma membrane potential is known

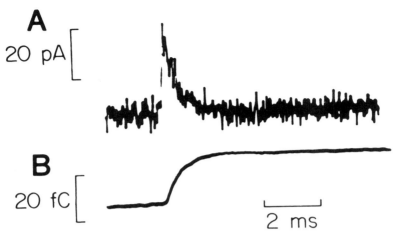

Figure 2   (A) Current transient due to discharge of vesicle capacitance through the fusion pore. (B) Time integral of A (from 9).

in these experiments, the vesicle potential is easily calculated. On average, the vesicle potential is between 70 and 80 mV and lumen positive (9), but it can be as small as 0 mV and as large as 160 mV. This large variation tells us that membrane fusion cannot require the vesicle membrane potential to have any particular value. Exocytosis can proceed even if the vesicle potential is collapsed by a proton ionophore (9).

From transients as in Figure 2 or 3a, one can calculate the conductance (and hence the size) of the fusion pore during the first millisecond of its existence if one knows $(E_c - E_v)$, the potential across the pore as a function of time. In trace b of Figure 3, this was calculated by subtracting the time integral of Figure 3a from its final value and dividing the result by C_v. The flat portion at the beginning of the trace shows the potential just before exocytosis, about 110 mV for this vesicle. Later, the potential declines in proportion to the charge passing through the pore. To get the conductance of the pore as a function of time (Figure 3c), one divides trace a point-for-point by trace b.

The conductance increases abruptly as the pore opens and reaches a value, g_o, that is about 270 pS in Figure 3c. Afterwards the conductance continues to increase more gradually, presumably because the pore dilates. When many experiments of this type are analyzed, the histogram of g_o values is found to have a broad peak between 200 and 300 pS (3). Figure 3 suggests that the first electrically observable event in exocytotic membrane fusion is the formation of an aqueous pore with a conductance of a few hundred pS. That the opening of the pore occurs so suddenly suggests that it represents a conformational change in a macromolecule; the sudden opening of an ion channel provides an obvious analogy.

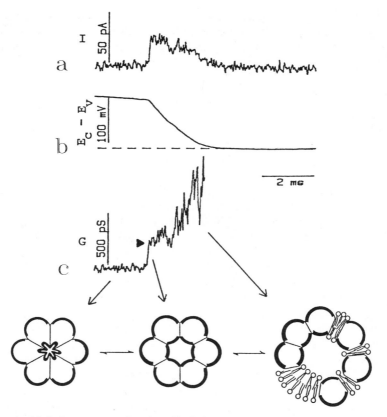

Figure 3 (*A*) I, the current transient through a fusion pore. (*B*) ($E_c - E_v$), the potential driving this current. It is calculated from the time integral of I and from the amplitude of the C step that followed. (*C*) G, the conductance of the fusion pore calculated by dividing I by ($E_c - E_v$). The arrow points to g_o, the initial conductance of the fusion pore. (*Bottom*) hypothetical drawings of the fusion pore corresponding to the three segments of the conductance trace. The drawing is a cross-section through the fusion pore made at a level midway between the two fusing membranes, e.g. Figure 4*b* or Figure 4*f*. Thick lines are hydrophilic and thin lines are hydrophobic surfaces (from 3).

What is the diameter of the pore when it first opens? The pore spans two membranes, namely the plasma membrane and the membrane of the vesicle. Hence one naturally compares it to the gap junction channel, the only other small pore known to span two membranes. The conductance of a single gap junction channel is variously given as 80 to 240 pS (45, 69, 70), and its inner diameter is less than 2 nm (68). The initial conductance of the fusion pore, g_o, is of similar size, hence its initial diameter is probably on the order of 2 nm or less. The fusion pore inferred from the analysis of transients is the smallest (and presumably the earliest) fusion intermediate thus far observed.

From traces as in Figure 1A, one can calculate that the conductance of flickering pores can be up to ten times larger than when the pore first opens (4, 9). Hence even after the pore has dilated, it can fluctuate in size or even close completely.

MECHANISM OF FUSION   Figure 4 illustrates how a pore-forming protein might lead to membrane fusion. The multimeric protein is imagined to reside in the vesicle membrane, but it could just as well reside in the plasma membrane. Fusion is considered to occur in five steps. (a) As the vesicle docks, the protein inserts itself into the plasma membrane (Figure 4a,b). This need not be a rapid event. (b) A cytosolic messenger activates the protein. In a neuron, activation would require only the binding of Ca to the protein, while in other slower secretory cells, the second messenger might cause a covalent change (phosphorylation or dephosphorylation). The activation of the protein causes a conformational change with two consequences, (c) and (d). (c) In the center of the macromolecule, a pore forms suddenly and connects the vesicle lumen with the external space, crossing two membranes much like a gap junction (Figure 4c,g). From the conductance of the pore (most often 200–300 pS) we infer that its diameter is on the order of 2 nm. The Ca-induced opening of the fusion pore in a synaptic vesicle might be analogous to the ligand-induced opening of a nicotinic acetylcholine receptor channel. As with ion channels, we imagine that the pore opens reversibly and may close again. (d) The affinity of the subunits for each other diminishes, so that lipid molecules can diffuse in and out between the subunits. The subunits drift apart and the pore dilates. This process is comparatively gradual, since it reflects the asynchronous participation of many relatively small lipid molecules (Figure 4d,h). (e) Usually the pore continues to dilate by recruitment of more lipid and soon becomes a seamless neck of lipid bilayer that connects the vesicle and plasma membrane and is large enough to appear in electron micrographs (Figure 4e). The observation of flicker suggests that occasionally even an expanded pore may narrow again and perhaps even close. What makes vesicles flicker is unknown.

The model in Figure 4 explains the following findings. (a) Since no hole is made across either the vesicle or plasma membrane, exocytosis can be tight enough to prevent movement of single molecules into or out of the cytoplasm. (b) If vesicles at a presynaptic terminal are docked as in Figure 4b or f, exocytosis can be triggered by a single conformational change, namely by the opening of the fusion pore complex. Hence exocytosis can be triggered and executed rapidly, as required at fast synapses. (c) The model explains the early dynamics of the fusion pore.

One wonders why fusion pores have not been seen in micrographs of vesicles docked at, for instance, the active zone of a synapse. Membrane-to-

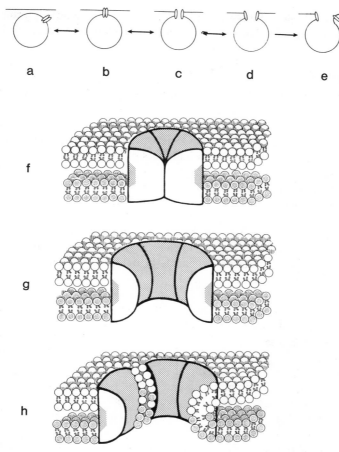

Figure 4 (*A–E*) Hypothetical steps in exocytosis as discussed in the text. *F, G, H* are more detailed representations of *B, C, D*. They show a section through the hypothetical fusion pore complex and the position of that complex in the two lipid bilayers of the plasma and vesicle membranes. Stippled surfaces of the protein are hydrophilic, clear surfaces are hydrophobic. Once the pore has opened, lipid molecules can diffuse along the amphipathic surfaces exposed between the fusion pore subunits. The entry of lipid molecules between the subunits causes the pore to dilate.

membrane junctions have been clearly identified only where they occur in a regular pattern: examples are gap junctions, the electron-dense "feet" connecting the sarcoplasmic reticulum of skeletal muscle with the transverse tubule membrane, and the channels connecting the vacuole with the extracellular space in *Chlamodymonas* (72). A docked secretory or synaptic vesicle may be connected with the plasma membrane by only a single fusion pore complex, and such solitary membrane-to-membrane junctions may be difficult to recognize. Furthermore, in the absence of structural information it is hard to predict whether or not a membrane protein will appear in freeze-fracture.

Candidates for Fusion Proteins

SYNEXIN   Synexin belongs to a large family of structurally related cytoplasmic proteins sometimes called annexins (21). The physiologic role of these proteins is poorly understood, and members of the family have been proposed to be mediators of exocytosis, substrates for tyrosine kinase, inhibitors of phospholipase A_2, and inhibitors of blood coagulation (24). Synexin causes a Ca-dependent aggregation of isolated chromaffin granules in cells of the adrenal medulla (14). It has been reported that synexin also causes Ca-dependent fusion of chromaffin granules. This fusion is leaky; about 15% of the vesicular contents escape from the vesicles during fusion (63). The mechanism of synexin-induced fusion is controversial (53, 76), and its relationship to exocytotic fusion is unclear. Synexin has been reported to form voltage-sensitive, Ca-selective channels in lipid bilayers (53). The primary structure of synexin is known (53).

SYNAPTOPHYSIN   Synaptophysin (38,000 dalton, also called p-38) is a membrane protein found in the vesicle membranes of many neurons and of some neuroendocrine cells (19, 43, 74, 75). The cytoplasmic portion of the molecule binds Ca (57). The primary structure of the molecule suggests that it has four membrane-spanning domains (20, 35, 64), as in the gap junction monomer. Synaptophysin monomers form homo-oligomers with the morphological appearance of channels (66). Furthermore, synaptophysin forms voltage-sensitive, 150 pS channels in lipid bilayers (66); their conductance is similar to that of gap junction channels. It has been suggested that synaptophysin oligomers in the vesicle membrane may couple to similar structures in the plasma membrane, thus creating channels connecting the vesicle lumen with the cell exterior (66, see also 8). It is unknown whether synaptophysin can cause fusion.

NSF   The posttranslational processing of secretory proteins requires their movement through successive layers (cisternae) of the Golgi stack. While moving through the Golgi stack, secretory proteins are conveyed by vesicles that pinch off one layer and then fuse with the next. Fusion requires several cytosolic proteins acting in sequence. One of these proteins (NEM-sensitive factor, NSF, 83000 dalton) has recently been cloned and sequenced (75a). It bears high homology to one of the gene products required for exocytosis in yeast (46) and has no hydrophobic domains. It is unknown whether the protein can cause fusion by itself; it could be a cofactor aiding the operation of another as yet unknown fusion protein.

CONCLUSION

New electrophysiologic techniques make it possible to study exocytosis with submillisecond time resolution at the level of single secretory vesicles. Such studies have shown that the 20 nm fusion pores seen in electron micrographs have short-lived precursors. The conductance of these early fusion pores suggests that they may have structural similarities to ion channels. In time-resolved electrical admittance measurements, one can track the dilation of the initial fusion pores until their diameters approach those observed in electron micrographs. These findings suggest molecular models that might explain two important features of exocytotic membrane fusion: tightness and speed. The molecular components of exocytotic membrane fusion remain to be identified. The methods to do this may be at hand.

ACKNOWLEDGMENTS

The author thanks Drs. A. Spruce, K. Houamed and P. Detwiler for their comments on the manuscript. His research was supported by National Institutes of Health grants AR17803 and GM39520.

Literature Cited

1. Almers, W., Breckenridge, L. J. 1988. Early steps in the exocytosis of secretory vesicles in mast cells. In *Molecular Mechanisms of Membrane Fusion Proc.*, eds. S. Ohki, D. Doyle, T. D. Flanagan, S. W. Hui, E. Mayhew, pp. 197–208. New York: Plenum
2. Almers, W., Breckenridge, L. J., Spruce, A. E. 1988. Time course of fusion pore conductance during exocytosis of secretory vesicles in beige mouse mast cells. *J. Physiol.* 407:96P
3. Almers, W., Neher, E. 1987. Gradual and stepwise changes in the membrane capacitance of rat peritoneal mast cells. *J. Physiol.* 386:205–17
4. Alvarez de Toledo, G., Fernandez, J. M. 1989. The events leading to secretory granule fusion. In *Cell Physiology of Blood,* ed. R. B. Gunn, J. C. Parker, New York: Rockefeller Univ. Press
5. Baker, P. F. 1986. Protein kinase C and exocytosis. *Progr. Zoology* 33:265–74
6. Beisson, J., Lefort-Tran, M., Pouphile, M., Rossignol, M., Satir, B. 1976. Genetic analysis of membrane differentiation in *Paramecium*. Freeze-fracture study of the trichocyst cycle in wild-type and mutant strains. *J. Cell Biol.* 69:126–43
7. Blumenthal, R. 1988. Membrane fusion. *Curr. Top. Membr. Transp.* 29:203–54
8. Breckenridge, L. J., Almers, W. 1987a. Final steps in exocytosis observed in a cell with giant secretory granules. *Proc. Natl. Acad. Sci. USA* 84:1945–49
9. Breckenridge, L. J., Almers, W. 1987b. Currents through the fusion pore that forms during exocytosis of a secretory vesicle. *Nature* 328:814–17
10. Buckley, K. M., Floor, E., Kelly, R. B. 1987. Cloning and sequence analysis of cDNA encoding p38, a major synaptic vesicle protein. *J. Cell Biol.* 105:2447–56
11. Cecarelli, B., Hurlbut, W. P. 1980. Vesicle hypothesis of the release of quanta of acetylcholine. *Physiol. Rev.* 60:396–441
12. Chandler, D. E., Heuser, J. E. 1980. Arrest of membrane fusion events in mast cells by quick-freezing. *J. Cell Biol.* 86:666–74
13. Cope, T. C., Mendell, L. M. 1982. Distributions of EPSP latency at different group Ia-fiber- alpha-motoneuron connections. *J. Neurosci.* 47:469–78
14. Creutz, C. E., Pazoles, C. H., Pollard, H. B. 1978. Identification and purification of an adrenal medullary protein (synexin) that causes Ca-dependent aggregation of isolated chromaffin granules. *Biol. Chem.* 253:2858–66
15. Curran, M. J., Brodwick, M. S., Edwards, C. 1984. Direct visualization of

exocytosis in mast cells. *Biophys. J.* 45:170a

16. Del Castillo, J., Katz, B. 1954. Quantal components of the end-plate potential. *J. Physiol.* 124:560–73

17. Dourmashkin, R. R., Deteix, P., Simone, C. B., Henkart, P. 1980. Electron microscopic demonstration of lesions in target cell membranes associated with antibody-dependent cellular cytotoxicity. *Clin. Exp. Immunol.* 42:554–60

18. Dreifuss, J. J., Akert, K., Sandri, C., Moor, H. Specific arrangements of membrane particles of sites of exoendocytosis in the freeze-etched neurohypophysis. *Cell Tissue Res.* 165:317–25

19. Fernandez, J. M., Neher, E., Gomperts, B. D. 1984. Capacitance measurements reveal stepwise fusion events in degranulating mast cells. *Nature* 312:453–55

20. Finkelstein, A., Zimmerberg, J., Cohen, F. S. 1986. Osmotic swelling of vesicles: its role in the fusion of vesicles with planar phospholipid bilayer membranes and its possible role in exocytosis. *Annu. Rev. Physiol.* 48:163–74

21. Geisow, M. J., Walker, J. H., Boustead, C., Taylor, W. 1987. Annexins—New family of Ca^{2+}-regulated phospholipid binding protein. *Biosci. Rep.* 7:289–98

22. Gillespie, J. I. 1979. The effect of repetitive stimulation on the passive electrical properties of the presynaptic terminal of the squid giant synapse. *Proc. R. Soc. London Ser B* 206:293–306

23. Gilligan, D. M., Satir, B. H. 1982. Protein phosphorylation/dephosphorylation and stimulus-secretion coupling in wild type and mutant. *Paramecium. J. Biol. Chem.* 257:13903–6

24. Haigler, H. T., Fitch, J. M., Jones, J. M., & Schlaepfer, D. D. 1989. Two lipocortin like proteins, endonexin II and anchorin CII, may be alternate splices of the same gene. *Trends Biochem. Sci.* 14:48–50

25. Heuser, J. 1976. Morphology of synaptic vesicle discharge and reformation at the frog neuromuscular junction. In *Motor Innervation of Muscle*, ed. by S. Thesleff, pp. 51–115. London: Academic

26. Heuser, J. E., Reese, T. S. 1981. Structural changes after transmitter release at the frog neuromuscular junction. *J. Cell Biol.* 88:564–580

27. Holtz, R. W., Senter, R. A. 1986. The effects of osmolarity and ionic strength on secretion from adrenal chromaffin

cells permeabilized with digitonin. *J. Neurochem.* 46:1835–42

28. Jackson, R. C., Crabb, J. H. 1988. Cortical exocytosis in the sea urchin egg. *Curr. Top. Membr. Transp.* 32:45–85

29. Jahn, R., Scheibler, W., Quimet, C., Greengard, P. 1985. A 38,000-dalton membrane protein (p38) present in synaptic vesicles. *Proc. Natl. Acad. Sci. USA* 82:4137–41

30. Jaffe, L. A., Hagiwara, S., Kado, R. T. 1978. The time course of cortical vesicle fusion in sea urchin eggs observed as membrane capacitance changes. *Dev. Biol.* 67:243–48

31. Johnson, R. G., Scarpa, A. 1984. Chemiosmotic coupling and its application to the accumulation of biological amines in secretory granules. In *Electrogenic Transport Fundamental Principles and Physiological Implications*, eds. M. P. Blaustein, M. Lieberman, pp. 71–91. New York: Raven

32. Katz, B. 1962. The transmission of impulses from nerve to muscle, and the subcellular unit of synaptic action. *Proc. R. Soc. London Ser. B* 155:455–77

33. Katz, B., Miledi, R. 1965. The effect of temperature on the synaptic delay at the neuromuscular junction. *J. Physiol.* 181:656–70

34. Kelly, R. B. 1988. The cell biology of the nerve terminal. *Neuron* 1:431–38

35. Leube, R. E., Kaiser, P., Seiter, A., Zimbelman, R., Franke, W. W., et al. 1987. Synaptophysin: molecular organization and mRNA expression as determined from cloned cDNA. *EMBO J.* 6:3261–65

36. Lindau, M., Fernandez, J. M. 1986. IgE-mediated degranulation of mast cells does not require opening of ion channels. *Nature* 319:150–53

37. Lindau, M., Neher, E. 1988. Patch-clamp techniques for time-resolved capacitance measurements in single cells. *Pflügers Arch.* 411:137–46

38. Lindau, M., Nüsse, O. 1987. Pertussin toxin does not affect the time course of exocytosis in mast cells stimulated by intracellular application of GTP-γ-S. *FEBS Lett.* 222:317–21

39. Maruyama, Y. 1986. Ca^{2+}-induced excess capacitance fluctuation studies by phase-sensitive detection method in exocrine pancreatic acinar cells. *Pflügers Arch.* 407:561–69

40. Mason, W. T., Sikdar, S. K., Zorac, R. 1988. Ca^{2+}-induced cell membrane capacitance increase in bovine lactotrophs in vitro. *J. Physiol.* 407:88p

41. Momayezi, M., Girwert, A., Wolf, C.,

Plattner, H. 1987. Inhibition of exocytosis in *Paramecium* cells by antibody-mediated cross-linking of cell membrane components. *Euro. J. Cell Biol.* 44:247–57

42. Munson, J. B., Sypert, G. W. 1979. Properties of single fibre excitatory postsynaptic potentials in triceps surae motoneurones. *J. Physiol.* 296:329–42

43. Navone, F., John, R., DiGioia, G., Stukenbrok, H., Greengard, P., De-Camilli, P. 1986. Protein p38: An integral membrane protein specific for small vesicles of neurons and neuroendocrine cells. *J. Cell Biol.* 103:2511–27

44. Neher, E., Marty, A. 1982. Discrete changes of cell membrane capacitance observed under conditions of enhanced secretion in bovine adrenal chromaffin cells. *Proc. Natl. Acad. Sci. USA* 79: 6712–16

45. Neyton, J., Trautman, A. 1985. Single channel currents of an intercellular junction. *Nature* 317:331–35

46. Novick, P., Ferro, S., Schekman, R. 1981. Order of events in the yeast secretory pathway. *Cell* 25:461–69

47. Nusse, O., Lindau, M. 1989. The dynamics of exocytosis in human neutrophils. *J. Cell Biol.* In press

48. Ogura, A., Takahashi, K. 1976. Artificial deciliation causes loss of calcium-dependent responses in *Paramecium*. *Nature* 264:170–72

49. Orci, L., Amherdt, M., Roth, J., Perrelet 1979. Inhomogeneity of surface labelling of B-cells at prospective sites of exocytosis. *Diabetologia* 16:135–38

50. Ornberg, R. L., Reese, T. S. 1981. Beginning of exocytosis captured by rapid-freezing of *Limulus* amebocytes. *J. Cell Biol.* 90:40–54

51. Plattner, H. 1987. Synchronous exocytosis in *Paramecium* cells. In *Cell Fusion*, ed. A. E. Sowers, pp. 69–98, New York: Plenum

52. Plattner, H., Miller, F., Bachmann, L. 1973. Membrane specializations in the form of regular membrane-to-membrane attachment sites in *Paramecium*. A correlated freeze-etching and ultrathin-sectioning analysis. *J. Cell. Sci.* 13: 687–719

53. Pollard, H. B., Burns, A. L., Rojas, E. 1988. A molecular basis for synexin-driven, calcium-dependent membrane fusion. *J. Exp. Biol.* 139:267–86

54. Poon, K. C., Liu, P. I., Spicer, S. S. 1981. Mast cell degranulation in beige mice with the Chediak-Higashi defect. *Am. J. Pathol.* 104:142–49

55. Rand, R. P., Parsegian, V. A. 1986. Mimicry and mechanism in phospholipid models of membrane fusion. *Annu. Rev. Physiol.* 48:201–12

56. Rand, R. P. 1981. Interacting phospholipid bilayers: Measured forces and induced structural changes. *Annu. Rev. Biophys. Bioeng.* 10:277–314

57. Rehm, H., Wiedenmann, B., Betz, H. 1986. Molecular characterization of synaptophysin, a major calcium-binding protein of the synaptic vesicle membrane. *EMBO J.* 5:535–41

58. Salama, G., Johnson, R. G., Scarpa, A. 1980. Spectrophotometric measurements of transmembrane potential and pH gradients in chromaffin granules. *J. Gen. Physiol.* 75:109–40

59. Satir, B. M., Oberg, S. G. 1978. *Paramecium* fusion rosettes: Possible function as Ca^{2+} gates. *Science* 199:536–38

60. Satir, B., Schooley, C., Satir, P. 1972. Membrane reorganization during secretion in *Tetrahymena*. *Nature* 235:53–54

61. Satir, B., Schooley, C., Satir, P. 1973. Membrane fusion in a model system. Mucocyst secretion in *Tetrahymena*. *J. Cell Biol.* 56:153–76

62. Schmidt, W., Patzak, A., Lingg, G., Winkler, H., Plattner, H. 1983. Membrane events in adrenal chromaffin cells during exocytosis: A freeze-etching analysis after rapid cryofixation. *Eur. J. Cell Biol.* 32:31–37

63. Stutzin, A. 1986. A fluorescence assay for monitoring and analyzing fusion of biological membrane vesicles in vitro. *FEBS Lett.* 197:274–80

64. Sudhof, T. C., Lottspeich, F., Greengard, P., Mehl, E., Jahn, R. 1987. A synaptic vesicle protein with a novel cytoplasmic domain and four transmembrane regions. *Science* 238:1142–44

65. Tessmer, G. W., Skuster, J. R., Tabatabai, L. B., Graves, D. J. 1977. Studies on the specificity of phosphorylase kinase using peptide substrates. *J. Biol. Chem.* 252:5666–71

66. Thomas, L., Hartung, K., Langosch, D., Rehm, H. R., Bamberg, E., et al. 1988. Identification of synaptophysin as a hexameric channel protein of the synaptic vesicle membrane. *Science* 242: 1050–53

67. Tonks, N. K., Dilta, C. D., Fischer, E. H. 1988. Characterization of the major protein-tyrosine-phosphatases of human placenta. *J. Biol. Chem.* 203:6731–36

68. Unwin, P. N. T., Zampighi, G. 1980. Structure of the junction between communicating cells. *Nature* 283:545–49

69. Veenstra, R. D., DeHaan, R. L. 1986. Measurement of single channel currents

from cardiac gap junctions. *Science* 233: 972–74

70. Veenstra, R. D., DeHaan, R. L. 1988. Cardiac gap junction channel activity in embryonic chick ventricle cells. *Am. J. Physiol.* 254:H170–H180

71. Deleted in proof

72. Weiss, R. L., Goodenough, D. A., Goodenough, U. W. 1977. Membrane particle arrays associated with the basal body and with contractile vacuole secretion in *Chlamydomonas. J. Cell Biol.* 72:133–43

73. White, J., Kielin, M., Helenius, A. 1983. Membrane fusion protein of enveloped animal viruses. *Quart. Rev. Biophys.* 16:151–95

74. Wiedenmann, B., Franke, W. W. 1985. Identification and localization of synaptophysin, an integral membrane glycoprotein of M_r 38,000 characteristic of presynaptic vesicles. *Cell* 41:1017–28

75. Wiedenmann, B., Franke, W. W., Kuhn, C., Moll, R., Gould, V. E. 1986. Synaptophysin: a marker protein for neuroendocrine cells and neoplasms. *Proc. Natl. Acad. Sci. USA* 83:3500–4

75a. Wilson, D. W., Wilcox, C. A., Flynn, G. C., Chen, E., Kuang, W. J., et al. 1989. A fusion protein required for vesicle mediated transport in both mammalian cells and yeast. *Nature* 339:355–59

76. Zak, W. J., Cruetz, C. E. 1988. Membrane fusion in model systems for exocytosis: characterization of chromaffin granule fusion mediated by synexin and calelectrin. In *Molecular Mechanisms of Membrane Fusion Proc.*, eds. S. Ohki, D. Doyle, T. D. Flanagan, S. W. Hui, E. Mayhew, pp. 325–40. New York: Plenum

77. Zieseniss, E., Plattner, H. 1985. Synchronous exocytosis in *Paramecium* cells involves very rapid ($< -$ 1s), reversible dephosphorylation of a 65-kD phosphoprotein in exocytosis-competent strains. *J. Cell Biol.* 101:2028–35

78. Zimmerberg, J. 1987. Fusion in biological and model membranes: similarities and differences. In *Molecular Mechanisms of Membrane Fusion Proc.*, eds. S. Ohki, D. Doyle, T-D. Flanagan, S. W. Hui, E. Mayhew, pp. 181–95, New York: Plenum

79. Zimmerberg, J., Curran, M., Cohen, S., Brodwick, M. 1987. Simultaneous electrical and optical measurements show that membrane fusion precedes secretory granule swelling during exocytosis of beige mouse mast cells. *Proc. Natl. Acad. Sci. USA* 84:1585–89

Annu. Rev. Physiol. 1990. 52:625–45

PATHWAYS TO REGULATED EXOCYTOSIS IN NEURONS

Pietro De Camilli

Department of Cell Biology and Section of Molecular Neurobiology, Yale University School of Medicine, New Haven, Connecticut 06510

Reinhard Jahn

Department of Neurochemistry, Max-Planck Institute for Psychiatry, Martinsried, West Germany

KEY WORDS: synaptic vesicles, secretory vesicles, synapses, neurotransmitters, endocrine cells

(This review is dedicated to the memory of Bruno Ceccarelli 1938–1988)

INTRODUCTION

Eukaryotic cells possess at least two different pathways for the delivery of secretory products by exocytosis to the extracellular space. They are referred to as constitutive and regulated pathways (15). The constitutive pathway is a basic feature of all cells. It operates by a constant flow of small vesicles from the *trans*-Golgi network. These vesicles move to the cell surface and undergo exocytosis without intermediate packaging or storage of the secretory material. The same pathway is responsible for the delivery of membrane components to the cell surface. In addition, many cells have a regulated pathway, primarily, although not exclusively, specialized for the secretion of proteins. It involves the concentration and packaging of the exported material in secretory granules, the storage of these granules in proximity to the release site, and finally exocytosis of the granules in response to an appropriate stimulus (see 15 for a review).

0066-4278/90/0315-0625$02.00

The concept of two different secretory pathways coexisting in the same cell has greatly advanced our understanding of molecular mechanisms involved in secretion. This concept, however, requires further elaboration to provide a comprehensive description of secretion from highly specialized cells such as neurons. Secretion of neurotransmitters and neuromodulators is mediated by regulated exocytosis, but this process involves at least two distinct regulated secretory pathways. In this short review, we will discuss pathways of regulated secretion from neurons in the context of established concepts of secretion from other cells.

Regulated Exocytosis from Neurons Involves at Least Two Types of Secretory Vesicles

Until 15 years ago it was generally believed that all nerve endings of a neuron release only a single neurotransmitter (40). Furthermore, it was believed that a single type of secretory organelle was involved in regulated secretion from a given neuron. In most neurons this organelle was thought to be the typical synaptic vesicle, i.e. the 50-nm diameter microvesicle [small synaptic vesicle (SSV)] (72). The property of SSVs to undergo repeated cycles of exo-endocytosis in nerve terminals (18, 36) was consistent with the nonpeptide nature of most neurotransmitters known at that time (40). These neurotransmitters, commonly referred to as classical neurotransmitters, can be loaded into vesicles in the nerve terminals without involvement of protein synthesis. A few highly specialized neurons were known to secrete peptides via secretory vesicles that are large enough to be seen in the light microscope (80). These neurons secrete into the blood rather than to adjacent neurons, and they were thought to represent an intermediate stage between neurons and endocrine cells: the so-called neuroscretory cells (80).

In recent years, many studies have conclusively established that each neuron can secrete a cocktail of peptide and nonpeptide neurotransmitter molecules via at least two types of secretory organelles (40). SSVs are involved in the release of classical neurotransmitters only, while peptides are secreted via larger vesicles with a dense core, the so-called large dense-core vesicles (LDCV) (21, 40). The known properties of these two organelles are summarized below.

Small Synaptic Vesicles (SSVs)

SSVs are the most characteristic features of nerve endings. They are highly homogeneous in size and are clustered near specialized regions of the plasmalemma in varicosities of peripheral axonal branches (72). The list of neurotransmitters that are concentrated and/or actively taken up by SSVs include acetylcholine (70), catecholamines (47), glutamate (14a, 60, 63), and GABA (28, 35). After each cycle of exo-endocytosis, SSVs are reloaded with neurotransmitters from a cytosolic pool by specific uptake systems that are driven by a proton gradient (28, 35, 47, 60, 63, 70). SSVs do not contain secretory proteins in concentrated form and have a clear core when observed by electron microscopy. SSVs that contain catecholamines, however, acquire an electron-opague core after certain fixation conditions and are often referred to as small dense-core vesicles (50).

The abundance of SSVs in the nervous tissue and their homogeneity in size and density have allowed their isolation with high yield and purity (35, 42, 97). Characterization of their protein composition has revealed a family of abundant proteins that are found on most, and perhaps all, SSVs irrespective of their neurotransmitter content (42). These proteins are prime candidates as mediators of some of the general functions of SSVs such as biogenesis of the vesicle, binding to the cytoskeleton, fusion with the plasmalemma, and so on. In addition, some proteins and enzymes found in other subcellular compartments were identified in purified SSVs. We will restrict our discussion to the major proteins of mammalian SSVs.

SYNAPSIN I AND II   Synapsin I and synapsin II (previously referred to as Protein III) represent a family of homologous proteins that were originally identified as substrates for endogenous phosphorylation present in mammalian brain. The family comprises four proteins, synapsin Ia, Ib, IIa and IIb (M_r 86,000, 80,000, 78,000, and 56,000 kd respectively) (12, 24, 87). The mRNAs encoding the four proteins are generated by differential splicing (a and b isoforms) of primary transcripts from two distinct genes (synapsin I and II). The amino-terminal and middle regions of the molecule are identical in the a and b isoforms and homologous in synapsin I and II. The carboxy-terminal region varies in the four proteins. No membrane-spanning segments are predicted from the primary structure, in agreement with other data suggesting that these proteins are localized at the cytoplasmic surface of SSVs (87). However, the central regions of the four proteins contain amphipathic motifs (87), and recent studies suggest that this region may interact with the hydrophobic core of the lipid bilayer (8). All synapsins can be phosphorylated by cAMP-dependent protein kinase and by Ca^{++}-calmodulin-dependent protein kinase type I at a homologous site located close to the amino-terminus. In addition, synapsin I can be phosphorylated by Ca^{++}-calmodulin-dependent protein kinase type II at two sites located on its highly basic carboxy-terminus. These sites are not present in the synapsin II molecule (24, 87).

Synapsin I has also been shown to interact with cytoskeletal proteins, particularly strongly with actin (5). These studies suggest that synapsin I may act as a link between SSVs and a specialized actin-based cytomatrix of the presynaptic compartment, thus allowing SSVs to cluster at release sites (24).

Recent electron microscopy studies using the quick-freezing/deep etching technique support this hypothesis (39).

Many studies have shown that all physiologic or pharmacologic manipulations that trigger or facilitate neurotransmitter release cause a rapid and reversible phosphorylation of the synapsins (reviewed in Reference 24). Thus it is thought that phosphorylation of the synapsins may play an important regulatory role in neurotransmitter release. The interactions of synapsin I with actin as well as with SSVs are weakened by phosphorylation (5, 42, 81). Phosphorylation of synapsin I may release SSVs from the actin-based cytomatrix and increase the SSV pool available for exocytosis. The homology of synapsin II with synapsin I suggests that synapsin II may have a similar role.

Recent studies involving antibodies specific for each of the four synapsins have shown that synapsin molecules are present on SSVs in all nerve terminals, but that their abundance ratio exhibits nerve terminal-specific variations (87). The synapsins are found in significant concentrations only in neurons, although low levels of some members of the family may be present in some endocrine cells and, in particular, in cultured endocrine cells (24, 34, P. De Camilli, R. Jahn, unpublished observations).

SYNAPTOPHYSIN   Synaptophysin (also referred to as protein p38) is an intrinsic membrane protein of 38 k (monomer) (44, 98). Its amino acid sequence suggests the presence of four transmembrane domains, with both ends of the molecule localized at the cytoplasmic side (53, 88). This orientation in the vesicle membrane has been confirmed with the aid of site-specific antibodies (46). The first extracellular loop is N-glycosylated. The cytoplasmic carboxy-tail contains the unique pentapeptide repeat YGP(Q)QG, binds Ca^{++}, and undergoes tyrosine phosphorylation by endogenous and exogenous tyrosine kinases (69, 74, 88). The protein is one of the major substrates for tyrosine kinases in the brain (37). Purified synaptophysin forms hexameric structures and a voltage-dependent ion channel when incorporated in planar lipid bilayers. The channel activity is partially inhibited by a tail-specific monoclonal antibody (89).

SYNAPTOBREVIN   Synaptobrevin is an integral membrane protein of 18 k (monomer) (7). Amino acid sequence analysis revealed that this protein is the mammalian homologue to VAMP-½, a protein recently identified in vesicles of *Torpedo* electric organ (94). A highly homologous protein was also identified in *Drosophila* (86). A comparison of the three amino acid sequences suggests that the protein has an unusual topology in the membrane. Four main domains exist in the molecule: (*a*) a cytoplasmic N-terminal domain of variable length and composition that is rich in proline in *Torpedo* and mammals, and rich in asparagine in *Drosophila;* (*b*) a hydrophilic central part that is highly conserved; (c) a well-conserved transmembrane region; and (d) an intravesicular domain that is very short (2–3 amino acids) in mammals and *Torpedo,* but is comprised of 20 amino acids in *Drosophila* (86, 94).

OTHER PROTEINS   Other proteins specific for SSVs that have been partially characterized, include p65, SV2, and p29 (7, 13, 59, M. Baumert et al, manuscript in preparation). They are all intrinsic membrane proteins and appear to be general components of SSVs irrespective of their specific neurotransmitter content. A proteoglycan has also been identified at the luminal side of the vesicle, which may be restricted to a subpopulation of SSVs (17).

In addition, some proteins and enzymes also present in other subcellular compartments of neurons have been identified in the membranes of purified SSVs. These include calmodulin (41), Ca^{++}/calmodulin-dependent protein kinase II (42), tubulin (35), a proton pump of the vacuolar type (35), and relatively high concentrations of the tyrosine kinase c-src (37). The presence of a tyrosine kinase and of at least one of its major substrates, synaptophysin (69), in the membranes of SSVs, suggests a central role of tyrosine phosphorylation in the life cycle of SSVs. Finally, proteins are present in the SSV membrane that are involved in neurotransmitter uptake and processing. These proteins are restricted to specific subpopulations of SSVs. One is cytochrome b561, which mediates electron transfer across the vesicle membrane, a process required for the enzyme dopamine β-hydroxylase (49). Thus far, none of the vesicle neurotransmitter carrier proteins has been thoroughly characterized.

Large Dense-Core Vesicles (LDCVs)

LDCVs are larger than SSVs and much more heterogeneous in size and appearance. The distinctive feature of LDCVs is the electron-dense core, which is formed primarily from condensed proteins, but may also include small nonpeptide molecules (50). LDCV content is similar in biochemical nature and in mechanism of packaging to that of secretory granules in the well-established secretory pathway of endocrine cells. Both LDCVs and endocrine granules contain a similar cocktail of proteins including regulatory peptides, processing enzymes, precursor fragments, and proteins of the chromogranin/secretogranin family [a group of acidic proteins with still unknown function (75)]. Finally, LDCVs and secretory granules of specific subpopulations of neurons and endocrine cells may also contain monoamines (see Reference 45 for reviews).

Because of their low abundance in most nerve terminals, purification of LDCV membranes in sufficient yield for biochemical analysis has been achieved only from specialized parts of the nervous system, such as the posterior pituitary and nerve trunks of the sympathetic nervous system (50, 78). It appears that some membrane proteins are shared by distinct sub-populations of LDCVs and endocrine granules (45). It is still unclear, however, whether a set of specific major membrane proteins is shared by all LDCVs, as in the case of SSVs. Functionally identified membrane proteins that appear to be common to a variety of endocrine granules and LDCVs include a proton pump of the vacuolar type (77), peptide α-amidase (27), cytochrome b561 [its electron transfer function is required for both dopamine β-hydroxylase and peptide α-amidase (49)] and, in the case of LDCVs and endocrine granules that store catecholamines in addition to peptides, the monoamine carrier (47), and a membrane form of dopamine β-hydroxylase (52). The primary structure of most of these enzymes has recently been elucidated (27, 52, 66, 71). In addition, families of proteins with unknown functions have been identified in the membrane of various types of endocrine granules (67).

Both SSVs and LDCVs May Be Present in All Nerve Terminals

SSVs are present in all presynaptic nerve endings. In addition, recent studies have shown that microvesicles morphologically and biochemically similar to SSVs are also present in other types of nerve endings. They have been found in sensory nerve endings (26, 79) and in nerve endings thought to be primarily specialized for the secretion of peptides into the blood, such as nerve endings of the neurohypophysis (63a) [the nerve endings of cells previously defined as neurosecretory cells (80) see above]. The function of SSVs at these non-conventional sites is unknown.

LDCVs, as well, are likely to be present in all nerve endings. The list of neuronal populations containing regulatory peptides in LDCVs has grown constantly over the last few years. The widespread distribution of LDCVs in the nervous tissue was demonstrated recently by the use of antibodies directed against secretory peptides common to a large number of neurons, such as the proteins of the secretogranin/chromogranin family (22, 75). In addition, the secretory granules of the neurosecretory cells can be considered as very large LDCVs (80). LDCVs are known to be present in sensory nerve endings (33, 79). Thus the coexistence of SSVs and LDCVs is likely to be an essential feature of all nerve endings.

Comparison of the Membrane Composition of SSVs and LDCVs

Both SSVs and LDCVs are components of a system of functionally intercon-nected vesicles involved in the cellular traffic between the Golgi complex and the plasmalemma. It is not surprising, therefore, that certain proteins are common to both types of vesicles. For example, membranes of both SSVs and LDCVs contain a proton pump of the vacuolar type (35, 77). Furthermore, in monoaminergic neurons, both membranes contain enzymes involved in the uptake and processing of monoamines (monoamine carrier, membrane form of dopamine β-hydroxylase, cytochrome b561) (45, 50).

LDCV membranes exhibit major differences, however, when compared to the membranes of SSVs. A survey by immunogold electron microscopy of central nervous system synapses reveals that the synapsins, synaptophysin, synaptobrevin, and p29 are not present at significant concentrations in the membranes of LDCVs (7, 64, 65, M. Baumert et al, in preparation). These findings were confirmed by subcellular fractionation of the neurohypophysis where an almost complete separation of SSV proteins (synapsin I, synapsin II, synaptophysin, p65, and p29) from LDCV markers was achieved (63a). The striking difference in the membrane composition between LDCVs and SSVs excludes the possibility that SSVs are formed from recycling LDCV membranes, without the involvement of extensive protein sorting, but rather suggests that they represent distinct organelles with an independent biogenesis.

SSVs are Biochemically Related to a Microvesicle Population of Endocrine Cells

SSVs represent a distinctive feature of nerve endings. All the major intrinsic membrane proteins of SSVs characterized so far, however, (with the exception of the synapsins, which are peripheral membrane proteins) are also present in at least some types of peptide-secreting endocrine cells, such as cells of the anterior pituitary, cells of the endocrine pancreas, chromaffin cells, C cells of the thyroid, and cells of the diffuse neuroendocrine system of the gut. The same proteins were not detected so far in any non-neuronal, non-endocrine cell (7, 13, 59, 65, P. De Camilli, R. Jahn, unpublished observations).

To identify the subcellular compartments enriched in SSV proteins, the intracellular localization of two of these proteins, synaptophysin and p29, has been analyzed in a variety of endocrine cells (65). Light microscopy immunofluorescence and immunogold electron microscopy have demonstrated that these proteins are highly concentrated in a population of microvesicles (henceforth defined as synaptic-like microvesicles, SLMVs) clearly distinct from secretory granules (Figure 1). SLMVs are pleomorphic (round, oval tubular) and somewhat larger than SSVs. They are distributed throughout the cytoplasm and are concentrated close to the microtubule organizing center, the area corresponding to the *trans*-side of the Golgi complex (65). In endocrine cells, which grow neurite-like processes in culture (chromaffin

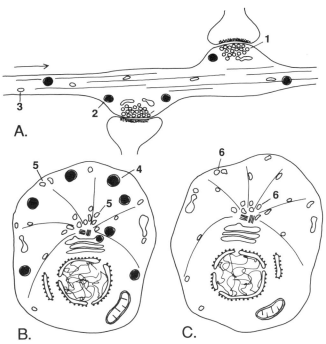

Figure 1   Schematic drawing illustrating the proposed relationship between secretory organelles of neurons and organelles of other cells. *A* is a terminal branch of an axon forming two synapses with dendritic spines. SSVs (*1*) are clustered at the synaptic junction. LDCVs (*2*) have a more scattered distribution in the axon. Pleomorphic vesicles visible in preterminal axons (*3*) may represent precursor organelles for SSVs. *B* is an endocrine cell. Secretory granules (*4*) are the equivalent organelles of LDCVs of neurons. SLMVs (*5*) are pleomorphic vesicles, somewhat larger than SSVs, whose membranes have major proteins in common with the membranes of neuronal SSVs. Whereas SSVs are clustered under specialized sites of the plasmalemma, SLMVs are concentrated at microtubule-organizing centers, i.e. the *trans*-region of the Golgi complex. They may be more closely related to the precursor membranes for SSVs (*3*) than to the SSVs themselves. *C* is a fibroblastic cell expressing (as a result of cDNA transfection) synaptophysin, an intrinsic membrane protein of SSVs and SLMVs. In these cells synaptophysin is localized in a population of pleomorphic vesicles that are similar in morphology and intracellular distribution to the SLMVs of endocrine cells (*6*). The ability of a fibroblastic cell line to target synaptophysin to a vesicle population with these characteristics raises the possibility that a pathway related to SSVs and SLMVs of endocrine cells may exist in all cells.

cells), SLMVs also accumulate in the distal portion of these processes (P. De Camilli, R. Jahn, unpublished observations). SLMVs are rapidly labeled by an extracellular tracer (peroxidase), which suggests that they are in functional continuity with the cell surface (46a). The preferential or selective association of synaptophysin with microvesicles and not with secretory granules has been confirmed by subcellular fractionation experiments (98, P. De Camilli, R. Jahn, unpublished observations). In addition, immunoisolation of SLMVs from endocrine cells suggests that at least some SSV proteins (synaptobrevin, p29) are colocalized on the same organelles (P. Burger, P. De Camilli, R. Jahn, unpublished observations).

It is still controversial whether a low concentration of SSV proteins is also present in the membranes of endocrine granules. Experiments carried out in other laboratories have suggested the presence of at least a small pool of synaptophysin, SV2, and p65 in secretory granules of chromaffin cells (55, 68). While these findings may be of functional importance, it is clear that the largest pool of SSV proteins in endocrine cells is not localized on secretory granules but on SLMVs.

In conclusion, SSVs appear to be biochemically related to a previously undefined microvesicle population of endocrine cells, the SLMVs. We have obtained evidence suggesting that SLMVs, like SSVs, may be recycling organelles (46a). Their precise function, however, remains to be determined. An interesting clue was obtained by the expression of synaptophysin (via cDNA transfection) in CHO cells, a fibroblastic cell line that normally does not express SSV proteins. In these cells synaptophysin was found in a population of recycling microvesicles that have the same morphology and intracellular distribution as SLMVs of endocrine cells (Figure 1) (46a). It is possible that SSVs and SLMVs may represent the neuronal and endocrine adaptation, respectively, of a membrane recycling pathway that operates in all cells. The fact that some of the neurotransmitters contained in SSVs are also metabolites in all cells raises the possibility that SSVs represent the adaptation of a pathway that has metabolic functions in other cells.

Biogenesis of SSVs

The biosynthesis of SSV membrane proteins occurs on the rough endoplasmic reticulum in the perikaryal-dendritic regions of neurons (6), but the precise cellular site at which newly synthesized SSV proteins are assembled into typical 50 nm SSVs is unclear. SSVs may be generated in nerve endings from large membranous intermediates. Following exocytosis, SSV membrane proteins are internalized from the plasmalemma and reused for other exo-endocytotic cycles (18, 36). After moderate stimulation, SSV reformation may take place directly from the plasmalemma without other intermediate vesicular stages (93, 96). Under these conditions, a stabilizing membrane-associated infrastructure may prevent the highly curved SSV membrane from flattening into the plasmalemma, and vesicles are thought to pinch off shortly after fusion (93, 96). After vigorous stimulation, however, SSV membranes clearly flatten into the plasmalemma, and SSV reformation is thought to involve coated vesicles and large membranous intermediates (endosomes ?) (36).

It is unclear whether newly synthesized SSV membrane proteins migrate down the axons as part of morphologically mature SSVs, or whether they travel as part of larger precursor membranes. In the latter case, they may be targeted by the same sorting process that operates in reforming SSVs after each round of exocytosis. Impressive images of SSVs aligned along microtubules in peripheral branches of lamprey axons have led to the suggestion that SSVs leave the perikaryon as mature organelles (83), but similar images were never observed in mammalian axons. In fact, when a focal block of organelle transport in axons is performed, no accumulation of SSVs is seen proximally to the block (91, 95) despite the accumulation of SSV protein immunoreactivity detectable by immunofluorescence (9). Organelles that accumulate at such sites include LDCVs and pleomorphic vesicles and tubules (91, 95), but the morphology of immunoreactive membranes has not yet been analyzed at the EM level. Thus the nature of the SSV transport form remains unclear. It is possible that the accumulations of SSVs observed on microtubules of peripheral lamprey axons (83) may represent SSVs in transit from one axonal varicosity to another rather than newly synthesized SSVs in transit from the perikaryon to axon endings.

In monoaminergic neurons, both SSV and LDCV membranes contain the proteins necessary for the uptake and processing of amines (45, 50). It was suggested that in such neurons LDCVs are the precursor of SSVs and that the latter originate by endocytosis from LDCV membranes (82). A similar mechanism was proposed for the generation of 50 nm microvesicles in nerve endings of the neurohypophysis (62). This idea was generalized to explain the origin of SSVs in all neurons (48, 55). The striking biochemical differences we observed between SSVs and LDCV membranes, however, make it highly unlikely that SSVs simply represent recycling LDCV membranes. We favor the hypothesis that at least some of the major membrane components of SSVs travel to nerve terminals independently of LDCVs. SSV precursor membranes may be a subpopulation of the pleomorphic vesicular structures that accumulate proximally to axonal blocks [another subpopulation of these pleomorphic vesicles is likely to be the elements of the axonal smooth endoplasmic reticulum (11)]. Interestingly, many of these vesicular structures have the same size range (around 80 nm) as reported for the carrier vesicles of the constitutive secretory pathway (15, 32). This does not exclude the possibility that a functional interconnection between membranes of LDCVs and membranes of SSVs may take place in nerve endings at the level of an endosomal compartment. Certain proteins common to the membranes of the two vesicles, such as the vacuolar proton pump, or the proteins involved in monoamine biosynthesis and uptake, may be selectively sorted into SSVs after retrieval from endocytosed LDCV membranes.

Studies on the biogenesis of SLMVs in endocrine cells may help to elucidate SSV biogenesis, since SLMVs and secretory granules of endocrine cells appear to be counterparts of SSVs and LDCVs of neurons, respectively. SLMVs, which are slightly larger and more pleomorphic than SSVs (see above), may correspond to the putative SSV precursor membranes that travel from the Golgi complex to the axon terminal (Figure 1) (see above). It is of interest that SLMVs are primarily concentrated in the Golgi-centrosomal area of the cell, while SSVs are primarily concentrated close to the release sites. Thus key aspects of the neuronal adaptation of the SLMV pathway are the ability of SSVs to interact with a specialized cytoskeletal matrix of nerve endings and their homogeneous size in the range of 50 nm (Figure 1). The remarkable size homogeneity of SSVs is important in ensuring a well-defined quantal content of neurotransmitter.

A different hypothesis concerning the origin of SLMVs was proposed by Lowe & coworkers (the same authors who proposed a precursor-product relationship between LDCV membranes and SSV membranes in nerve endings). These authors, who found evidence for a small pool of SSV membrane proteins in membranes of chromaffin granules (55), have hypothesized that in endocrine cells a precursor-product relationship exists between secretory granule membranes and SLMVs. According to this view, SLMVs originate from the plasmalemma as a result of a specific sorting of these proteins into a subclass of endocytic microvesicles (48, 55).

Biogenesis of LDCVs

LDCVs, like secretory granules of endocrine cells, are assembled at the *trans*-side of the Golgi complex (for recent reviews see References 15, 48). The biochemical mechanisms involved in their biogenesis are only partially understood. Granule formation begins with the condensation of the secretory material, which is promoted by a low pH and is associated with a reduction of its osmotic potential. The information for the sorting of certain proteins into the packaging pathway appears to be contained in the protein structure, though not just in the primary amino-acid sequence, since no common motifs have been identified. The mechanism of sorting is unclear. It may involve molecular sorting of individual secretory molecules (20), or, alternatively, bulk sorting of self-assembled secretory material (76). Clathrin-coated membranes are likely to be involved in this sorting, since clumps of condensed secretory products in the *trans*-Golgi network or in immature granules are often surrounded by clathrin-coated membrane patches (15).

After leaving the Golgi complex area, LDCVs are thought to be transported to the sites of release without further membrane sorting steps, although maturation of granule content by post-translational processing continues during this migration (78).

Traffic to the Release Sites and Neuronal Polarity

One of the key features of neurons is that the sites specialized for secretion are often very distant from the perikaryon. How are SSVs and LDCVs targeted to the release sites, and are the mechanisms of targeting different for the two organelles?

Neurons have two distinct types of processes, the axon and the dendrites. They differ in morphology, in biochemical characteristics, in organelle content, and in function. With few exceptions, axons are presynaptic structures, while dendrites are postsynaptic (6). Accordingly, SSVs are concentrated in axon endings where they are clustered at special sites that are an integral component of the synaptic junctional complex. Their exocytosis is thought to occur exclusively at the synaptic junction (active zones) (90, 93). (In nerve endings without a postsynaptic site, sites of contact between the axonal plasmalemma and components of the extracellular matrix may mimic a junctional contact and define sites for exocytosis). In contrast, LDCVs appear to have a more diffuse distribution in the neuronal cytoplasm. In many neurons, they are present at high concentration in the dendritic tree (25, 61), and exocytotic images of LDCVs have been observed at the dendritic surface (A. Thureson-Klein, personal communication). In peripheral branches of axons, LDCVs have a more sparse distribution than SSVs. They are often excluded from the clusters of SSVs, and their exocytosis takes place preferentially away from active zones (14, 21, 64, 90).

It is currently thought that microtubule-based motors play an important role in the intracellular translocation of organelles, particularly in neurons. It is also thought that a preferential affinity of organelles for anterograde (plus-end oriented) or retrograde (minus-end oriented) microtubule motors may be important in determining their localization. Thus the localization of many organelles in neurons, including the localization of LDCVs, may be partially explained by the homogeneous orientation of microtubules in axons (with the plus end pointing away from the perikaryon), and their mixed polarity in dendrites (with plus ends both towards and away from the perikaryon) (see Reference 1 for a review). Secretory granules, which are related to LDVCs, are thought to have a preference for anterograde movement (92). Binding of LDCVs to anterograde motors would concentrate them in the axonal periphery and would keep them more randomly distributed in dendrites where they can move in both directions. This corresponds to the distribution of LDCVs observed in many neurons.

Similarly, binding to anterograde motors is probably responsible for the transport of SSV precursor membranes from the perikaryon to axon endings. Yet, the selective concentration of SSVs in axon endings implies the participation of additional sorting/targeting mechanisms. Recent studies performed on cultured hippocampal neurons suggest that SSV-associated proteins (synapsin and synaptophysin) as well as other proteins (GAP-43) accumulate preferentially in axons from the very beginning of axonal and dendritic differentiation, i.e. before synaptic contacts are made (30, 54, T. Fletcher et al, unpublished observations). These findings support the existence of sorting mechanisms for the selective targeting of proteins and organelles to axons early on in neuronal development. During this phase, SSV marker proteins are sparsely distributed in the peripheral arbors of axons. However, when synaptic contacts are formed, they become rapidly clustered at these sites (54). This clustering is likely to be mediated by an actin-based cytoskeletal matrix that rapidly forms under microdomains of the plasmalemma involved in synaptic junctions. The synapsins probably play an important role in this aggregation, which may explain why LDCVs often appear to be excluded from SSV-clusters (64). Together these findings suggest that the accumulation of SSVs at presynaptic sites in nerve endings may result from both their specific targeting to the axonal periphery and their specific retention at release sites.

Exocytosis of SSVs and LDCVs: Differential Regulation and Distinct Exocytotic Sites

Both SSVs and LDCVs undergo regulated exocytosis. Physiologic and pharmacologic studies, however, indicate that exocytosis of the two organelles is differentially controlled. The relative proportion of peptide and classical neurotransmitters released from the same nerve ending varies with the frequency of stimulation; a high frequency of stimulation favors peptide secretion (3). Thus it is inferred that the ratio of LDCVs/SSVs that undergo exocytosis increases with the frequency of stimulation (3, 40).

An almost complete dissociation between exocytosis of SSVs and exocytosis of LDCVs was observed recently at the frog neuronmuscular junction after application of α-latrotoxin, the major toxin of black widow spider venom. Alpha-latrotoxin produces a massive, Ca^{++}-independent exocytosis of SSVs from motor nerve terminals. When applied at high doses, or at low doses in the absence of extracellular Ca^{++}, the toxin induces a rapid depletion of acetylcholine-containing SSVs. Under the same conditions the toxin did not produce any significant decrease in the number of LDCVs containing calcitonin gene-related peptide (CGRP) in the same nerve endings (58). Alpha-latrotoxin represents a non-physiologic stimulus. Yet its differential action on the two types of organelles suggests that exocytosis of LDCVs and SSVs is mediated by different biochemical mechanisms.

Additional evidence suggesting a difference in the stimulus-secretion coupling for SSVs and LDCVs was obtained by an analysis of the role of Ca^{++} and Ca^{++} channels in neurotransmitter release. For example, distinct types of Ca^{++} channels have been associated with the release of classical and peptide neurotransmitters from vertebrate neurons (38, 56, 73). L-channels are thought to be responsible for the Ca^{++} entry pathway controlling the release of endocrine secretory granules and of LDCVs from certain neurons, but not of SSVs (38, 73).

A differential exocytotic response of SSVs and LDCVs to Ca^{++} entry can be explained in several ways. Since the exocytotic sites of the two organelles appear to be distinct (see above), it is possible that SSVs and LDCVs have a distinct topological relationship to Ca^{++} channels or to different types of Ca^{++} channels. Furthermore, it is possible that the exocytotic machineries for the two organelles exhibit a different sensitivity to cytosolic Ca^{++} and/or to the rate of cytosolic Ca^{++} rise. This hypothesis has been thoroughly discussed in a recent review by Smith & Augustine (84). The model proposed is as follows: Exocytosis of SSVs is triggered by levels of cytosolic Ca^{++} much higher than those required for exocytosis of LDCVs. A subtype of voltage-dependent Ca^{++} channels [possibly the N type (38)] is concentrated at the active zone in close proximity to SSV clusters. Action potentials reaching the axon terminals induce synchronized opening of these channels which results in a strong (hundred(s) micromolar), but also very transient (hundreds of microseconds), increase of the cytosolic Ca^{++} concentration in close proximity to the channels. These Ca^{++} transients trigger SSV exocytosis. They are rapidly dissipated by dilution, by cytoplasmic Ca^{++} buffers, and by Ca^{++} extrusion mechanisms. High frequency stimulation would induce a slow build up of the overall Ca^{++} concentration (micromolar) in nerve terminals reaching the threshold for LDCV exocytosis (84). The mechanism of LDCV-exocytosis may be similar to that operating in the release of secretory granules from endocrine cells.

A differential regulation of excytosis of SSVs and LDCVs is fully consistent with the observed differences in the protein composition of the two membranes.

Mechanisms of Exocytosis

The molecular mechanisms underlying the fusion of cytoplasmic membranes, and in particular exocytosis, have been subject of intense studies over the last several years, but the key molecular components responsible for exocytosis have not yet been identified. The relevance to neuronal secretion of three fields that are currently the focus of intense investigation is discussed below.

G PROTEINS   It has been shown in a variety of systems that many fusion events of the secretory pathway require the participation of GTP-binding proteins (G proteins) (10, 29, 31). It has been proposed that specific G proteins (with molecular weight in the range of 20–25 kd) are involved in making the membrane of a given organelle competent for fusion with the membrane of the next compartment in the pathway. This mechanism would ensure the occurrence of fusion steps in a specific and sequential fashion (10, 31). A variety of 20–25-kd G proteins have been purified and/or sequenced, many of them from brain (19). Although their function is not known, they are prime candidates for proteins conferring the required specificity to membrane fusion events. Their involvement in SSV exocytosis is suggested by the recent finding that toxins that impair synaptic transmission by blocking SSV exocytosis are able to ADP-ribosylate G proteins (57). Involvement in LDCV exocytosis is suggested by the biochemical and functional similarity of LDCVs and secretory granules of endocrine cells, i.e. the cells in which the effect of G proteins on exocytosis had been first suggested (29).

THE TRANSIENT FUSION PORE MODEL   Recent studies in mast cells have shown that the first step in exocytosis is the formation of a fusion pore with conductance properties similar to those of gap junctions. The pore represents a transient and reversible stage of fusion that may open and close (flicker) without proceeding to full exocytosis. Low molecular weight components may be released from secretory organelles through such a pore even without complete fusion of the two apposed membranes (Almers, this volume). These results have stimulated a major interest in the field of neurobiology for two reasons. First, the major SSV protein synaptophysin has a structural similarity (same sequence of hydrophilic and hydrophobic segments) to connexon, the unit element of gap junctions, although no similarities are found in the amino acid sequence of the two proteins (53, 88). Like connexon, synaptophysin can assemble into hexamers to form high conductance channels in planar phospholipid bilayers, thus being a good candidate for pore formation (89). Second, a fusion pore allowing small neurotransmitter molecules to be released without full exocytosis could explain why, during moderate stimulation, components of SSV membranes and of the presynaptic plasma membrane do not intermix (96).

It is unlikely that secretion from SSV operates by a gap junction-like pore. At gap junctions, membrane contact is established by an homophilic interaction of the extracellular domains of the connexon proteins, whereas synaptophysin would bind with inverse polarity (cytoplasmic side-to cytoplasmic side) to an as yet unknown receptor at the inner surface of the plasma membrane. In addition, extracellular markers too large to pass through a gap junction channel are readily taken up by SSVs during exocytosis (18, 36), which rules out a release of classical neurotransmitters through a fusion pore without full exocytosis. Finally, the time-course of exocytosis mediated by the fusion pore in mast cells is much longer that of SSV exocytosis (Almers, this volume). In conclusion, the involvement of a transient fusion pore in exocytosis from SSVs remains highly hypothetical.

PERIPHERAL CYTOSKELETON   Several studies indicate that activation of regulated exocytosis in secretory cells correlates with a rapid reorganization of the actin-based peripheral cytoskeleton. These studies suggest the possibility that regulated exocytosis may be triggered by the removal of barriers to fusion rather than by, or in addition to, the activation of a fusogenic mechanism (4, 23, Burgoyne, this volume). The barrier to fusion may consist of a gel-like network of cytoskeletal proteins between the vesicles and the plasma membrane. The proteins of this matrix other than actin may vary from cell to cell, and in neurons these proteins may be different for LDCVs and SSVs. For chromaffin granules exocytosis, the involvement of spectrin and a class of Ca^{++}-binding peripheral granule proteins has been suggested (some of these peripheral granule proteins have also been implicated in the fusion event itself) (Burgoyne, this volume). Similar proteins may be involved in the release of neuronal LDCVs. In the case of SSV exocytosis, the synapsins may play a central role (see above).

CONCLUDING REMARKS: TWO PATHWAYS OF NEURONAL SIGNALING

Regulated secretion from neurons exhibits many features in common with regulated secretion from other cells, but it also exhibits some unique, neuron-specific properties. Secretion of neurotransmitters and neuromodulators involves at least two distinct regulated secretory pathways. In addition, constitutive secretion is likely to take place for other secretory products.

The regulated pathway involving SSVs is highly specialized for speed and topological precision (synaptic transmission). Like all recycling organelles, SSVs have both an exocytic and an endocytic phase. In many ways they are more closely related to vesicles generally regarded as endocytic organelles rather than to secretory granules. Exocytosis of SSVs occurs at active zones and a burst of SSV exocytosis is turned on and off in less than a millisecond. SSV exocytosis produces prominent, highly localized, and transient increases in the concentration of nonpeptide, fast neurotransmitters in the synaptic cleft. Most of these neurotransmitters act, at least in part, on fast-transducing receptors, i.e. neurotransmitter-gated ion channels (85). The close apposition of pre- and postsynaptic membranes define the pathways of signaling. This may explain why relatively few types of neurotransmitter molecules are used by SSVs in spite of the extremely high number of synapses present in the brain. However, neurotransmitters released from SSVs may also have nonsynaptic actions, for example in nerve terminals lacking a well-defined postsynaptic side (43).

The regulated pathway involving LDCVs is equivalent to the well-established regulated secretory pathway of non-neuronal cells, particularly of endocrine cells (15). The primary function of this pathway is the secretion of substances (mainly neuropeptides) that produce modulatory changes in target neurons. In most cases these changes appear to involve the generation of intracellular second messengers (40, 43). The relatively slow effects produced by this pathway in target cells (43, 51) are likely to be paralleled by an exocytotic mechanism that operates on a time scale much greater than that of SSV exocytosis. Also the extracellular half-life of peptide neurotransmitters is probably much longer than the half-life of neurotransmitters [consider, for example, the slow solubilization of LDCV content that is suggested by the presence of only partially dissolved cores of LDCVs in exocytotic pockets visible by EM (14, 90)]. The action of products secreted by LDCV is not confined to the immediate vicinity of sites of release. The multiplicity of neuropeptides secreted by neurons therefore may be required to define intercellular pathways of signaling.

In conclusion, neurons can be regarded as endocrine cells that have developed special adaptations for fast, point-to-point, chemically mediated intercellular communication. Key elements of this adaptation are the development of axons and the presence of a neuron-specific secretory mechanism in axon endings. This mechanism represents the modification of a recycling pathway present in endocrine cells and possibly in all cells. In addition, neurons secrete regulatory peptides as do endocrine cells. The ability of neurons to deliver chemical messages to target cells via two different modes of secretion is one of the elements allowing them to propagate signals at high speed and precision as well as to undergo plastic adaptive changes.

ACKNOWLEDGMENTS

We thank Drs. G. Palade and P. Maycox for discussion and critical reading of the manuscript. The work discussed in this review was partially supported by a grant from the Muscular Dystrophy Association to PDC.

Literature Cited

1. Allan, V. J., Vale, R. D., Navone, F. 1990. Microtubule-based organelle transport in neurons. In *The neuronal cytoskeleton*, ed. R. D. Burgoyne New York: Liss In press
2. Deleted in proof
3. Andersson, P. O., Bloom, S. R., Edwards, A. V., Järhult. 1982. Effects of stimulation of the chorda tympani in bursts on submaxillary responses in the cat. *J. Physiol.* 322:469–83
4. Aunis, D., Bader, M. F. 1988. The cytoskeleton as a barrier to exocytosis in secretory cells. *J. Exp. Biol.* 139:253–66
5. Bähler, M., Greengard, P. 1987. Synapsin I bundles F-actin in a phosphorylation-dependent manner. *Nature* 326:704–07
6. Banker, G. A., Waxman, A. B. 1988. Hippocampal neurons generate natural shapes in cell culture. In *Intrinsic determinants of neuronal form and function*, ed. R. Lasek, M. B. Black, pp. 61–82. New York: Liss
7. Baumert, M., Maycox, P. R., Navone, F., De Camilli, P., Jahn, R. 1989. Synaptobrevin: an integral membrane protein of 18,000 Daltons present in small synaptic vesicles of rat brain. *EMBO J.* 8:379–84
8. Benfenati, F., Bähler, M., Jahn, R., Greengard, P. 1989. Interactions of synapsin I with small synaptic vesicles: distinct sites in synapsin I bind to vesicle phospholipids and vesicle proteins. *J. Cell Biol.* 108:1863–72
9. Bööj, S., Dahlström, A. 1989. Biochemical composition of axonally transported organelles in motor neurons; immunofluorescence studies. *J. Neurochem.* 52:S22
10. Bourne, H. R. 1988. Do GTPases direct membrane traffic in secretion? *Cell* 53:669–71
11. Broadwell, R. D., Cataldo, A. M. 1984. The neuronal endoplasmic reticulum: Its cytochemistry and contribution to the endomembrane system. II. Axons and Terminals. *J. Comp. Neurol.* 230:231–48
12. Browning, M. D., Huang, C. K., Greengard, P. 1987. Similarities between protein IIIa and Protein IIIb, two prominent synaptic vesicle-associated phosphoproteins. *J. Neurosci.* 7:847–53
13. Buckley, K., Kelly, R. B. 1985. Identification of a transmembrane glycoprotein specific for secretory vesicles of neural and endocrine cells. *J. Cell Biol.* 100:1284–94

14. Buma, P., Roubos, E. W. 1986. Ultrastructural demonstration of nonsynaptic release sites in the central nervous system of the snail *Lymnea stagnalis*, the insect *Periplaneta americana*, and the rat. *Neuroscience* 17:867–79
14a. Burger, P. M., Mehl, E., Cameron, P. L., Maycox, P. R., Baumert, M., et al. 1989. Glutamate storage by synaptic vesicles is dependent on the preservation of an energy gradient. *Neuron* In press
15. Burgess, T. L., Kelly, R. B. 1987. Constitutive and regulated secretion of proteins. *Annu. Rev. Cell Biol.* 3:243–93
16. Deleted in proof
17. Carlson, S. S., Caroni, P., Kelly, R. B. 1986. A nerve terminal anchorage protein from electric organ. *J. Cell Biol.* 103:509–20
18. Ceccarelli, B., Hurlbut, W. P., Mauro, A. 1973. Turnover of transmitter and synaptic vesicles at the frog neuromuscular junction. *J. Cell Biol.* 57:499–524
19. Chardin, P. 1988. The RAS superfamily proteins. *Biochemie* 70:865–68
20. Chung, K. N., Walter, P., Aponte, G. W., Moore, H. P. H. 1989. Molecular sorting in the secretory pathway. *Science* 243:192–97
21. Coulter, H. D. 1988. Vesicular localization of immunoreactive (Met5) enkephalin in the globus pallidus. *Proc. Natl. Acad. Sci. USA* 85:7028–32
22. Cozzi, M. G., Rosa, P., Greco, A., Hille, A., Huttner, W. W., et al. 1989. Immunohistochemical localization of secretogranin II in the rat cerebellum. *Neuroscience* 28:423–41
23. Creutz, C., Drust, D. S., Martin, W. H., Kambouris, N. G., Snyder, S. L., Hamman, H. C. 1988. Calcium-dependent membrane-binding proteins as effectors of secretion in mammalian and fungal cells. *In Molecular mechanisms in secretion, Alfred Benzon Symp.* 25 ed., N. A. Thorn, M. Treiman, O. H. Petersen, 25:575–90. Copenhagen: Munksgaard
24. De Camilli, P., Greengard, P. 1986. Commentary: Synapsin I: A synaptic vesicle-associated neuronal phosphoprotein. *Biochem. Pharm.* 35:4349–57
25. De Camilli, P., Solimena, M., Moretti, M., Navone, F. 1988. Sites of action of second messengers in the neuronal cytomatrix. See Ref. 6, pp. 487–520
26. De Camilli, P., Vitadello, M., Canevini, M. P., Zanoni, R., Jahn, R., Gorio, A. 1988. The synaptic vesicle proteins synapsin I and synaptophysin (Protein

P38) are concentrated both in efferent and afferent nerve endings of the skeletal muscle. *J. Neurosci.* 8:1625–31

27. Eipper, B. A., Mains, R. E. 1988. Peptide alpha-amidation. *Annu. Rev. Physiol.* 50:333–44

28. Fyske, E., Fonnum, F. 1988. Uptake of gamma-aminobutyric acid by a synaptic vesicle fraction isolated from rat brain. *J. Neurochem.* 50:1237–42

29. Gomperts, B. 1986. Calcium shares the limelight in stimulus-secretion coupling. *Biol. Sci.* 11:290–92

30. Goslin, K., Schreyez, D. J., Skene, J. H. P., Banker, G. A. 1988. Development of neuronal polarity: GAP-43 distinguishes axonal from dendritic growth cones. *Nature* 339:672–74

31. Goud, B., Salminen, A., Walworth, N. C., Novick, P. J. 1988. A GTP-binding protein required for secretion rapidly associates with secretory vesicles and the plasma membrane in yeast. *Cell* 53:753–68

32. Griffiths, G., Pfeiffer, S., Simons, K., Matlin, K. 1985. Exit of newly synthesized membrane proteins from the *trans* cisterna of the Golgi complex to the plasma membrane. *J. Cell Biol.* 101:949–64

33. Gulbenkian, S., Merighi, A., Wharton, J., Varndell, I. M., Polak, J. M. 1986. Ultrastructural evidence for the coexistence of calcitonin gene-related peptide and substance P in secretory vesicles of peripheral nerves in the guinea pig. *J. Neurocytol.* 15:535–41

34. Haycock, J. W., Browning, M. D., Greengard, P. 1988. Cholinergic regulation of protein phosphorylation in bovine adrenal chromaffin cells. *Proc. Natl. Acad. Sci. USA* 85:1677–81

35. Hell, J. W., Maycox, P. R., Stadler, H., Jahn, R. 1988. Uptake of GABA by rat brain synaptic vesicles isolated by a new procedure. *EMBO J.* 7:3023–36

36. Heuser, J. E., Reese, T. S. 1973. Evidence for recycling synaptic vesicle membrane during transmitter release at the frog neuromuscular junction. *J. Cell Biol.* 57:315–44

37. Hirano, A. A., Greengard, P., Huganir, R. L. 1988. Protein tyrosine kinase activity and its endogenous substrates in rat brain: a subcellular and regional survey. *J. Neurochem.* 50:1447–55

38. Hirning, L. D., Fox, A. P., McCleskey, E. W., Olivera, B. M., Thayer, S. A., et al. 1988. Dominant role of N-type Ca^{++} channels in evoked release of norepinephrine from sympathetic neurons. *Science* 239:57–61

39. Hirokawa, N., Sobue, K., Kanda, K., Harada, A., Yorifuji, H. 1989. The cytoskeletal architecture of the presynaptic terminal and molecular structure of synapsin I. *J. Cell Biol.* 108:111–26

40. Hökfelt, T., Fuxe, K., Pernow, P., eds. 1986. Coexistence of neuronal messengers. *Progress Brain Res.* 68:1–411

41. Hooper, J. B., Kelly, R. B. 1984. Calmodulin is tightly associated with synaptic vesicles independent of calcium. *J. Biol. Chem.* 259:148–53

42. Huttner, W. B., Schlieber, W., Greengard, P., De Camilli, P. 1983. Synapsin I (Protein I), a nerve terminal-specific phosphoprotein: III. Its association with snyaptic vesicles studied in a highly-purified synaptic vesicles preparation. *J. Cell Biol.* 96:1374–88

43. Iversen, L. L., Goodman., E. C., eds. 1986. Fast and slow chemical signalling in the nervous system. *Oxford Univ. Press* 1–320

44. Jahn, R., Schiebler, W., Ouimet, C., Greengard, P. 1985. A 38,000-dalton membrane protein (p38) present in synaptic vesicles. *Proc. Natl. Acad. Sci. USA* 82:4137–41

45. Johnson, R. G. 1987. Cellular and molecular biology of hormone- and neurotransmitter-containing secretory vesicles. *Ann. N.Y. Acad. Sci.* 493:1–588

46. Johnston, P., Jahn, R., Südhof, T. C. 1989. Transmembrane topography and evolutionary conservation of synaptophysin. *J. Biol. Chem.* 264:1268–73

46a. Johnston, P. A., Cameron, P. A., Stukenbrok, H., Jahn, R., De Camilli, P., Sudhof, T. C. 1989. Synaptophysin is targeted to similar microvesicles in PC12 cells and CHO cells. *EMBO J.* 8:2836–72

47. Kanner, B. I., Schuldiner, S. 1987. Mechanism of transport and storage of neurotransmitters. *CRC Crit. Rev. Biochem.* 22:1–38

48. Kelly, R. B. 1988. The cell biology of nerve terminals. *Neuron* 1:431–38

49. Kent, U. M., Fleming, P. J. 1987. Purified cytochrome b561 catalyzes transmembrane electron transfer for dopamine beta-hydroxylase and peptidyl glycine alpha-amidating monooxygenase activities in reconstituted systems. *J. Biol. Chem.* 262:8174–78

50. Klein, R., Lagercrantz, H., Zimmermann, H. ed. 1982. *Neurotransmitter Vesicles,* New York: Academic. 375 pp.

51. Kuffler, S. W. 1980. Slow synaptic responses in autonomic ganglia and the pursuit of a peptidergic transmitter. *J. Expt. Biol.* 89:257–86

52. Lamoroux, A., Vigny, A., Fancon-Bignet, N., Darmon, M. C., Franck, R.,

et al. 1987. The primary structure of human dopamine-beta-hydroxylase. Insight into the relationship between the soluble and the membrane bound forms of the enzyme. *EMBO J.* 6:3931–37

53. Leube, R. E., Kaiser, P., Seiter, A., Zimbelmann, R., Franke, W. W., et al. 1987. Synaptophysin: molecular organization and mRNA expression as determined from cloned cDNA. *EMBO J.* 6:3261–68

54. Lindsley, T. P., De Camilli, P., Banker, G. A. 1987. The influence of cell-cell contact on the distribution of synapsin I in hippocampal neurons in culture. *Soc. Neurosci. Abstr.* 13:318

55. Lowe, A. W., Madeddu, L., Kelly, R. B. 1988. Endocrine secretory granules and neuronal synaptic vesicles have three integral membrane proteins in common. *J. Cell Biol.* 106:51–59

56. Martin, J. L., Magistretti, P. J. 1989. Pharmacological studies of the voltage-sensitive Ca^{2+} channels involved in the release of vasoactive intestinal peptide evoked by K^+ in mouse cerebral cortical slices. *Neuroscience* 30:423–31

57. Matsuoka, I., Sakuma, H., Syuto, B., Moriishi, K., Kubo, S., Kurihara, K. 1989. ADP-ribosylation of 24-26-kDa GTP-binding proteins localized in neuronal and non-neuronal cells by botulinus neurotoxin D. *J. Biol. Chem.* 264:706–12

58. Matteoli, M., Haimann, C., Torri-Tarelli, F., Polak, J. M., Ceccarelli, B., De Camilli, P. 1988. Differential effect of alpha-latrotoxin on exocytosis of acetylcholine-containing small synaptic vesicles and CGRP-containing large dense-core vesicles at the frog neuromuscular junction. *Proc. Natl. Acad. Sci. USA* 85:7366–70

59. Matthew, W. D., Tsavaler, L., Reichardt, L. F. 1981. Identification of a synaptic vesicle-specific membrane protein with a wide distribution in neuronal and neurosecretory tissue. *J. Cell Biol.* 91:257–69

60. Maycox, P. R., Deckwerth, T., Hell, J. W., Jahn, R. 1988. Glutamate uptake by brain synaptic vesicles. *J. Biol. Chem.* 263:15423–28

61. Morrison, J. H., Magistretti, P. J., Benoit, R., Bloom, F. E. 1984. The distribution and morphological characteristics of the intracortical VIP-positive cells: an immunohistochemical analysis. *Brain Res.* 292:269–82

62. Nagasawa, J., Douglas, W. W., Schulz, R. A. 1971. Micropinocytotic origin of coated and smooth microvesicles ("synaptic vesicles") in neurosecretory terminals of posterior pituitary glands

demonstrated by incorporation of horseradish peroxidase. *Nature* 232:341–42

63. Naito, S., Ueda, T. 1985. Characterization of glutamate uptake into synaptic vesicles. *J. Neurochem.* 44:99–109

63a. Navone, F., Di Gioia, G., Jahn, R., Browning, M., Greengard, P., De Camilli, P. 1989. Microvesicles of the neurohypophysis are biochemically related to small synaptic vesicles of presynaptic nerve terminals. *J. Cell Biol.* In press

64. Navone, F., Greengard, P., De Camilli, P. 1984. Synapsin I in nerve terminals: selective association with small synaptic vesicles. *Science* 226:1209–11

65. Navone, F., Jahn, R., DiGioia, G., Stukenbrok, H., Greengard, P., De Camilli, P. 1986. Protein p38: An integral membrane protein specific for small vesicles of neurons and neuroendocrine cells. *J. Cell Biol.* 103:2511–27

66. Nelson, N., Taiz, L. 1989. The evolution of H^+-ATPases. *Trends Biochem. Sci.* 14:113–16

67. Obendorf, D., Schwarzenbrunner, U., Fischer-Colbrie, R., Laslop, A., Winkler, H. 1988. Immunological characterization of a membrane glycoprotein of chromaffin granules: its presence in endocrine and exocrine tissues. *Neuroscience* 25:343

68. Obendorf, D., Schwarzebrunner, U., Fischer-Colbrie, R., Laslop, A., Winkler, H. 1988. In adrenal medulla synaptophysin (protein p38) is present in chromaffin granules and in a special vesicle population. *J. Neurochem.* 51:1573–80

69. Pang, D., Wang, J., Valtorta, F., Benfenati, F., Greengard, P. 1988. Protein tyrosine-phosphorylation in synaptic vesicles. *Proc. Natl. Acad. Sci. USA* 85:762–66

70. Parsons, S. M., Bahr, B. A., Gracz, L. M., Kaufman, R., Kornreich, W. D., et al. 1987. Acetylcholine transport: fundamental properties and effects of pharmacologic agents. *Ann. N.Y. Acad. Sci.* 493:220–33

71. Perin, M. S., Fried, V. A., Slaughter, C. A., Sudhof, T. C. 1988. The structure of cytochrome b561, A secretory vesicle-specific electron transport protein. *EMBO J.* 7:2697–2703

72. Peters, A., Palay, S. L., Webster, H. D. F. 1976. The neurons and supporting cells, in *The fine structure of the nervous system,* Philadelphia: Saunders. 406 pp.

73. Rane, S., Holz, G. G., Dunlap, K. 1987. Dihydropyridine inhibition of neuronal calcium current and substance P release. *Pflügers Arch.* 409:361–66

74. Rehm, H., Wiedenmann, B., Betz, H.

1986. Molecular characterization of synaptophysin, a major calcium-binding protein of the synaptic vesicle membrane. *EMBO J.* 5:535–41

75. Rosa, P., Hille, A., Lee, R. V. H., Zanini, A., De Camilli, P., Huttner, W. B. 1985. Secretogranins I and II: two tyrosine-sulfated secretory proteins common to a variety of cells secreting peptides by the regulated pathway. *J. Cell Biol.* 101:1999–2011

76. Rosa, P., Weiss, U., Pepperkok, R., Ansorge, W., Niehrs, C., et al. 1989. An antibody against secretogranin I (chromogranin B) is packaged into secretory granules. *J. Cell Biol.* 109:17–34

77. Rudnick, G. 1986. ATP-driven H^+ pumping into intracellular organelles. *Annu. Rev. Physiol.* 48:403–413

78. Russell, J. T. 1987. The secretory vesicle in processing and secretion of neuropeptides. *Curr. Top. Membr. Transp.* 31:277–312

79. Scarfone, E., Dememes D., Jahn, R., De Camilli, P., Sans, A. 1988. Secretory function of the vestibular nerve calix suggested by presence of vesicles, synapsin I and synaptophysin. *J. Neurosci.* 8:4640–45

80. Scharrer, E., Scharrer, B. 1954. Hormones produced by neurosecretory cells. *Recent Progr. Hormone Res.* 10:183–240

81. Schiebler, W. B., Jahn, R., Doucet, J. P., Rothlein, J., Greengard, P. 1986. Characterization of synapsin I binding to small synaptic vesicles. *J. Biol. Chem.* 261:8383–90

82. Smith, A. D. 1972. Mechanisms involved in the release of noradrenaline from sympathetic nerve. *Br. Med. Bull.* 29:123–29

83. Smith, D. S., Jarlfors, U., Beranek, R. 1970. The organization of synaptic axoplasm in the lamprey (petromyzon marinus) central nervous system. *J. Cell Biol.* 46:199–219

84. Smith, S., Augustine, G. J. 1988. Calcium ions, active zones and synaptic transmitter release. *Trends Neurosci.* 11:458–65

85. Stevens, C. 1987. Channels families in the brain. *Nature* 328:198–99

86. Südhof, T. C., Baumert, M., Perin, M. S., Jahn, R. 1989. A synaptic vesicle membrane protein is conserved from mammals to Drosophila. *Neuron* 2:1475–81

87. Südhof, T. C., Czernik, A. J., Kao, H., Takei, K., Johnston, P., et al. 1989. The synapsins: mosaics of shared and unique domains in a family of synaptic vesicle phosphoproteins. *Science* In press

88. Südhof, T. C., Lottspeich, F., Greengard, P., Mehl, E., Jahn, R. 1987. A synaptic vesicle protein with a novel cytoplasmic domain and four transmembrane regions. *Science* 238:1142–44

89. Thomas, L., Hartung, K., Langosch, D., Rehm, H., Bamberg, E., et al. 1988. Identification of synaptophysin as a hexameric channel protein of the synaptic vesicle membrane. *Science* 242:1050–53

90. Thureson-Klein, Å. K., Klein, R. L., Zhu, P. C., Kong, J. Y. 1988. Differential release of transmitters and neuropeptides co-stored in central and peripheral neurons. In *Cellular and molecular basis of synaptic transmission*, ed. H. Zimmermann, pp. 137–51. Berlin: Springer Verlag. 137–151

91. Tomlinson, D. R. 1975. Two populations of granular vesicles in constricted post-ganglionic sympathetic nerves. *J. Physiol.* 245:727–35

92. Tooze, J., Burke, B. 1987. Accumulation of adrenocorticotropin secretory granules in the midbody of telophase AtT20 cells: evidence that secretory granules move anterogradely along microtubules. *J. Cell Biol.* 104:1047–57

93. Torri-Tarelli, F., Grohovaz, F., Fesce, R., Ceccarelli, B. 1985. Temporal coincidence between synaptic vesicle fusion and quantal secretion of acetylcholine. *J. Cell Biol.* 101:1386–99

94. Trimble, W. S., Gray, T. S., Elferink, L. A., Wilson, N. C., Scheller, R. H. 1989. Distinct patterns of expression of two VAMP genes within the rat brain. *J. Neurosci.* In press

95. Tsukita, S., Ishikawa, H. 1980. The movement of membraneous organelles in axons. Electron microscopic identification of anterogradely and retrogradely transported organelles. *J. Cell Biol.* 84:513–30

96. Valtorta, F., Jahn, R., Fesce, R., Greengard, P., Ceccarelli, B. 1988. Synaptophysin (p38) at the frog neuromuscular junction: Its incorporation into the axolemma and recycling after intense quantal secretion. *J. Cell Biol.* 107:2717–27

97. Whittaker, V. P., Michaelson, I. A., Kirkland, R. J. A. 1964. The separation of synaptic vesicles from nerve-ending particles ('synaptosomes'). *Biochem. J.* 90:293–303

98. Wiedenmann, B., Franke, W. W. 1985. Identification and localization of synaptophysin, an integral membrane glycoprotein of M 38,000 characteristic of presynaptic vesicles. *Cell* 41:1017–28

Annu. Rev. Physiol. 1990. 52:647–59

SECRETORY VESICLE-ASSOCIATED PROTEINS AND THEIR ROLE IN EXOCYTOSIS

Robert D. Burgoyne

Department of Physiology, University of Liverpool, P.O. Box 147, Liverpool L69 3BX, England

KEY WORDS: cytoskeleton, annexins, calcium, secretion, G-proteins

INTRODUCTION

The process of exocytosis involves fusion of secretory vesicle membranes with the plasma membrane. Exocytosis can occur in a constitutive fashion as in normal plasma membrane turnover, or, for example, in the secretion of plasma proteins from hepatocytes. It can also occur in a regulated fashion in response to cell stimulation (45). In cells that secrete in a regulated fashion (professional secretory cells such as endocrine and exocrine cells, mast cells, platelets, neurons, and so on), secretory vesicles containing stored secretory products accumulate in the cytoplasm prior to release. Activation of surface receptors and a subsequent increase in the concentration of cytosolic calcium or cyclic AMP, or activation of protein kinase C leads to secretion from these cells. A great deal is known about the nature of the extracellular signals controlling secretion, and the calcium signal has been described in detail for some secretory cells (56). However the details of the molecular mechanisms involved in the late stages of the secretory process, namely the movement of secretory vesicles to the inner surface of the plasma membrane, docking of vesicles on the plasma membrane, and exocytotic membrane fusion and fission, are largely unknown.

The various aspects of the secretory process including exocytosis are likely to involve specific secretory vesicle proteins that mediate membrane/membrane and membrane/cytoskeletal interactions. In addition, the basic components of the exocytotic mechanisms are likely to be widespread and highly conserved given the essential nature of exocytosis even for normal cellular

0066-4278/90/0315-0647$02.00

growth. One approach used in an attempt to identify the molecular components of the exocytotic machinery has been to search for secretory vesicle proteins that are bona fide constituents of the secretory vesicle membrane, or that become associated with the secretory vesicle following cell stimulation. Information is becoming available on the nature of such proteins from studies on secretory vesicles of a variety of mammalian professional secretory cells and also from the study of nonmammalian systems including constitutive secretory mutants in yeast and cortical granule exocytosis in the sea urchin egg. The aim of this review is to summarize the available data on secretory vesicle-associated proteins and to discuss the possible roles of these proteins in exocytosis. A number of secretory vesicle proteins have been identified as biosynthetic enzymes or transport proteins. Since these proteins are unlikely to be directly involved in exocytosis, they have not been described in this review. Emphasis has been placed on information from studies on brain synaptic vesicles and on the best studied endocrine secretory vesicle, the chromaffin granule of the adrenal medullary chromaffin cell. In addition, the review concentrates on integral membrane proteins common to synaptic and secretory vesicles and proteins that are able to bind reversibly to the cytoplasmic surface of secretory vesicles.

INTEGRAL MEMBRANE PROTEINS OF SECRETORY VESICLES

Assuming that the basic mechanisms of exocytosis are likely to be common to all cell types, and with the expectation that exocytosis-specific proteins could be found (63) attempts have been made to dectect proteins common to a variety of secretory vesicle membranes. So far no membrane proteins have been found that are common to secretory vesicles from all types of secretory cells. With specific monoclonal antibodies, six proteins have been identified that were initially shown to be components of synaptic vesicles and subsequently of other, mainly endocrine, secretory vesicles (8, 10, 43, 51, 54, 72). The best characterized proteins of this group are SV2 (10), p65 (51), synaptophysin (43, 72), and synaptobrevin (8). All four are integral transmembrane proteins with some antigenic determinants on the cytoplasmic face of the vesicles. SV2 is a 100-kd glycoprotein present in synaptic vesicles, chromaffin granules of adrenal chromaffin cells, and secretory vesicles of pancreatic islet cells and various endocrine and neuronal cell lines, however it is absent from some secretory cells including exocrine cells (10, 49). A similar distribution was found for the 65-kd protein p65 (49, 51). p65 appears to be a major calmodulin-binding protein of chromaffin granules, synaptic vesicles, and posterior pituitary secretory vesicles (31).

Synaptophysin (also known as p38) was identified as a major synaptic vesicle membrane protein. Full sequence data are available for this protein, and a model with four transmembrane domains has been proposed (67). More recently it has been shown that native synaptophysin is a hexamer with a morphology very similar to channel-forming proteins and when incorporated into lipid bilayers shows voltage-dependent channel activity (69). The signficance of these findings is not yet clear, but it was suggested (69) on the basis of the similarity between the structure of synaptophysin and gap junction proteins that synaptophysin might be involved in the initial formation of a fusion pore that precedes exocytosis (9). It may be relevant that synaptophysin is a calcium-binding protein (61).

Immunocytochemical studies detected synaptophysin in adrenal chromaffin cells, pancreatic islet cells, endocrine cells of the stomach, anterior pituitary cells, and C cells of the thyroid. Low levels of immunoreactivity were also detected in one exocrine cell type, the acinar cells of the parotid gland (53). The 18-kd protein synaptobrevin has a similar distribution (8). From immunogold labeling, synaptophysin appeared to be present on small electron-lucent vesicles, but not on the dense-core secretory vesicles in rat anterior pituitary or the chromaffin granules of bovine adrenal chromaffin cells (53). The author's interpretation of these results was that these cells contain a novel secretory pathway whose vesicles contain synaptophysin, and that dense-core secretory vesicles differ fundamentally from the vesicles in this pathway and synaptic vesicles since they lack synaptophysin. However, another study using biochemical techniques has suggested that low levels of synaptophysin are present in chromaffin granules of bovine adrenal medulla (55). The presence of synaptophysin in chromaffin granules was also suggested by immunoprecipitation of the granules with anti-synaptophysin (49). These conflicting data may reflect the low sensitivity of the immuno-gold method.

The debate as to whether synaptophysin is or is not present on dense-core secretory vesicles continues (see De Camilli & Jahn, this volume). Nevertheless, even if synaptophysin turns out to be present on dense-core vesicles as well as synaptic-like vesicles in endocrine cells, an important point is its absence from certain (e.g. some exocrine) secretory cells. This restricted distribution is also the case with SV2, p 65, and synaptobrevin. The functions of these secretory-vesicle membrane proteins are unknown, but if they were involved in the fundamental mechanisms of exocytosis, their absence from exocrine cells would imply that these mechanisms differ in neurons/endocrine cells compared with exocrine cells. Alternatively, the data on distribution of these proteins may indicate that they do not have a fundamental role in the exocytotic mechanism itself, but perhaps have a regulatory role.

PROTEINS THAT BIND TO SECRETORY VESICLES

The failure to find proteins that are common integral membrane components of all types of secretory vesicles could have to one of four possible explanations: first, the essential exocytotic proteins have not yet been found; second, exocytosis in different tissues involves different secretory vesicle proteins; third, essential vesicle-associated proteins required for exocytosis are not integral membrane proteins of the secretory vesicle, but are loosely bound extrinsic proteins that can be lost during isolation of vesicles; fourth, the essential proteins are ones that only become associated with secretory vesicles following cell stimulation. A number of proteins including cytoskeletal proteins are known to be loosely associated with secretory vesicles and, in some cases, lost on isolation of vesicles. In addition, a number of proteins can reversibly associate with secretory vesicles in a manner regulated by protein phosphorylation or by calcium concentration.

Cytoskeletal Proteins of Secretory Vesicles

In nerve terminals that release fast neurotransmitters synaptic vesicles are held in close proximity to the presynaptic release sites, whereas in endocrine cells, such as the adrenal chromaffin cell, the secretory granules are prevented from reaching the plasma membrane prior to stimulation. Between these two extremes are certain synapses in the peripheral and the central nervous system (73) that contain both clear synaptic vesicles close to presynaptic release sites, and dense-core vesicles away from the active zone. It is likely that the positioning of secretory vesicles in nerve terminals or in endocrine cells is determined by the cytoskeleton. In nerve terminals synaptic vesicles are crosslinked to one another and to microtubules and actin filaments by the phosphoprotein synapsin I (see below), and they are linked to the presynaptic membrane by 100 nm filaments that may be fodrin molecules (41, 48). In the adrenal chromaffin the secretory granules are embedded in a three-dimensional cytoskeletal network (47). These morphological findings suggest that interactions between secretory vesicles and cytoskeletal elements may be important in the regulation of exocytosis either by holding vesicles at the plasma membrane ready for exocytosis (in nerve terminals), or, as in the adrenal chromaffin cell, by preventing access of the secretory granules to the plasma membrane until the cell is stimulated (14, 15, 22). Synapsin I may play an important role in vesicle/cytoskeletal interactions in nerve terminals and this is discussed below in relation to secretory vesicle phosphoproteins.

The interaction of cytoskeletal proteins with secretory vesicles has been studied in most detail with the adrenal chromaffin granule (11, 14). Isolated membranes of chromaffin granules contain actin as an extrinsic protein that can be removed by treatment with low ionic strength buffers (3, 44, 52), and the membranes can bind F-actin (21, 31). Binding of actin to these granule membranes occurs through the actin-binding proteins alpha-actinin (3, 44) and fodrin (2), which are also extrinsic components of the secretory granule membranes. Binding of F-actin to chromaffin granules results in the formation of a crosslinked gel, and, relevant to the control of exocytosis, the formation of this gel is inhibited by calcium concentrations in the micromolar range (30). These findings suggest that following cell stimulation and a rise in cytosolic calcium concentration the secretory granules would be released from the actin cytoskeleton and thus be able to reach exocytotic sites on the plasma membrane. The movement of chromaffin granules to the plasma membrane would also be facilitated by disassembly of the cortical actin network (22).

Other actin-binding proteins found associated with chromaffin granule membranes include tropomyosins (20) and caldesmon (16). Caldesmon is a calmodulin-regulated actin-binding protein. At low calcium concentration (0.1 μM) caldesmon binds to and can crosslink actin filaments. In the presence of micromolar calcium the binding of caldesmon to actin filaments is inhibited, and in these conditions caldesmon is able to bind reversibly to the chromaffin granule membrane (16). It is likely that increased cytosolic calcium following stimulation would result in solation of actin filaments crosslinked by caldesmon, and the subsequent binding of caldesmon to the chromaffin granule vesicle could regulate interactions of the granules with the plasma membrane or the plasma membrane cytoskeleton and lead to exocytosis. With regard to the last possibility, electron microscopy has shown that the granules in actively secreting chromaffin cells are often attached to the plasma membrane by filamentous structures (11); caldesmon or related proteins could be involved in such linkages. A direct role for caldesmon in exocytosis has yet to be demonstrated. The possibility that fodrin may play a similar role (15) has come from the observation that anti-fodrin inhibits calcium-dependent secretion when introduced into permeabilized chromaffin cells (59).

A possible involvement of cytoskeletal elements in the control of exocytosis has also been suggested from a study on secretory vesicles of the sea urchin egg. In these eggs the cortical secretory vesicles are docked on the plasma membrane in preparation for exocytosis. Isolated secretory vesicles from sea urchin eggs have been found to contain actin and also a 45-kd actin-severing protein (71). It may be that a rise in intracellular calcium initiates exocytosis by activating the actin-severing protein to remove actin from the cortical vesicle surface, thus allowing exocytotic fusion to occur.

Secretory Vesicle Phosphoproteins and Kinases

In many secretory cells and in synaptic terminals stimulation results in changes in the state of phosphorylation of many proteins concomitantly with exocytosis. Therefore attempts have been made to identify secretory vesicle-associated phosphoproteins that may be involved in exocytosis. Synapsin I (comprising synapsin Ia and Ib) is a major neuron-specific phosphoprotein. It is a substrate for cAMP- and calmodulin-dependent protein kinases, and its phosphorylation is increased by treatments that release neurotransmitters from nerve terminals (26). Synapsin I is synapse-specific and it is located exclusively on synaptic vesicles (27, 42). Synapsin I binds reversibly to synaptic vesicles in vitro, and significantly this binding is regulated by its phosphorylation. Synapsin I phosphorylated by calmodulin kinase II binds to synaptic vesicles with fivefold lower affinity than does the nonphosphorylated protein (66). It has also been shown that synapsin I will bind to cytoskeletal elements including spectrin (6) and actin filaments (5), and the ability of synapsin I to bundle actin filaments was reduced when it was phosphorylated (5).

The properties of synapsin I suggest a role for it in the control of neurotransmitter release (26). In the proposed scheme synaptic vesicles are normally crosslinked to the cytoskeleton through synapsin I, and phosphorylation of synapsin I results in its dissociation from the vesicles and cytoskeletal elements. Release of the vesicles from the cytoskeleton then would allow their movement to the active zone for exocytosis. Since neurotransmitter release from synapses is very fast, the proposed mechanism is unlikely to be part of the immediate control of neurotransmitter release. However, it may be important in allowing vesicles to move to the active zone in preparation for the next stimulus. In addition, it could provide a mechanism for modulation by neurotransmitters of the availability of vesicles ready for exocytosis following depolarization.

Synapsin I does not appear to play an essential role in exocytosis in all cell types, since it is absent from non-neuronal secretory cells such as chromaffin cells (13). Another related synaptic vesicle phosphoprotein known as protein III (consisting of related 74 and 55-kd polypeptides) is present in adrenal chromaffin cells, and its phosphorylation is increased on stimulation of these cells (40). However there is no confirmation that this phosphoprotein is present on the secretory granules in chromaffin cells, though phosphoproteins of the expected size are present (34).

A number of protein kinases are present as endogenous components of synaptic and secretory vesicle membranes. Recently, the tyrosine-kinase $p60^{c-src}$ was found to be a component of chromaffin granules (57), where it exists as a complex with a 38-kd protein of unknown identity (39). The significance of the presence of this kinase on chromaffin granules is that calpactin, which is a substrate for this kinase, binds to chromaffin granules in a calcium-dependent manner. Therefore stimulation of chromaffin cells and a rise in cytosolic calcium concentration could be followed by phosphorylation of calpactin after it has bound to the granule membrane. Since calpactin appears to be required for calcium-dependent secretion in chromaffin cells (see below), phosphorylation could be involved in switching exocytosis on or off, depending on the effect of phosphorylation on calpactin function.

Calcium-Dependent Vesicle-Binding Proteins

One approach used in attempts to identify proteins that may be involved in regulated exocytosis has been to search for soluble "cytosolic" proteins that bind to secretory vesicles, particularly chromaffin granules, when calcium is elevated to micromolar levels (32, 24). A number of proteins are able to bind reversibly to chromaffin granule membranes in vitro in a calcium-dependent fashion including calmodulin and members of the annexin family of calcium-binding proteins.

CALMODULIN Purified calmodulin has been shown to bind to isolated chromaffin granule membranes in a calcium-dependent fashion (4, 17, 31, 33, 35). In addition calmodulin is one of the proteins from a crude cytosol fraction that will bind to chromaffin granules in the presence of micromolar calcium (24). Calcium-dependent calmodulin binding involves, at least in part, specific proteins on the cytoplasmic surface of the chromaffin granule. The two major calcium-dependent calmodulin-binding proteins of the chromaffin granule membrane have molecular weights of 50–53 and 65–69 kd (4, 33), and the larger of these proteins has been identified as the integral membrane protein p65 (31). Calmodulin may be involved in exocytosis since anti-calmodulin antibodies introduced into chromaffin cells inhibit secretion (46). The significance of the granule membrane calmodulin-binding proteins to exocytosis is unknown. However the fact that p65 is present as a component of synaptic vesicles and secretory vesicles from several endocrine cell types suggests that calmodulin binding to this protein may be important in some aspect of the control of exocytosis in these cells.

THE ANNEXIN FAMILY Among those proteins from a crude adrenal medullary cytosol fraction that can bind to chromaffin granules in a calcium-dependent fashion are several members of the annexin family of calcium-and lipid-binding proteins (18). The annexins may be good candidates for proteins with a specific role in exocytosis since they have a wide tissue distribution and one or more members of the family have been detected in every mammalian tissue examined so far, including neurons, endocrine tissues, exocrine tissues, neutrophils, and platelets. At the last count seven distinct but related proteins of this family have been fully characterized (reviewed in 18). The major identified annexins for which full sequence data are available are lipocortin, calpactin, endonexin I, endonexin II (two forms), and p70 (also known as lipocortins I-VI respectively, Reference 58). The members of this family identified as present in adrenal medulla and able to bind to chromaffin granules are lipocortin, calpactin, endonexin I, and p70 (24, 25, 32, 34, 36). In addition, it has been reported that the protein synexin, which was isolated some years ago from adrenal medulla as a granule-aggregating protein, is also a member of the annexin family (60). The annexins contain four or, in the case of p70, eight conserved repeats that may form the calcium and lipid-binding domains of these proteins.

The ability of members of the annexin family to bind reversibly to chromaffin granules in the presence of micromolar calcium led to the suggestion that one or more of these proteins could be involved in calcium-dependent exocytosis (24, 32). In intact chromaffin cells, p70 and calpactin are located immediately beneath the plasma membrane (14), and biochemical measurements have shown that p70 and calpactin are bound to plasma membranes; in addition calpactin is present on chromaffin granules (29). Therefore p70 and calpactin are present at the correct sites within the cells for a role in exocytosis. Further evidence that calpactin may be involved in the control of exocytosis is provided by the observation that calpactin is phosphorylated during stimulation of chromaffin cells by nicotine (25).

All of the annexins are able to aggregate chromaffin granules in the presence of calcium (25, 28). It has been suggested that calpactin may be the most likely candidate for a calcium receptor in exocytosis since it caused aggregation of chromaffin granules at a calcium concentration closer to physiologic levels than any other annexin (28). In addition, aggregation due to calpactin was followed by membrane fusion if arachidonic acid was present. These results point towards calpactin as an effector protein in exocytosis.

Studies on the interaction of calpactin with chromaffin granules in vitro are not sufficient to establish a role for calpactin in exocytosis in the intact cell (12). Such data have come from the use of digitonin-permeabilized chromaffin cells. Following digitonin-permeabilization, exocytosis in chromaffin cells can be triggered by micromolar calcium, but the responsiveness of the cells declines as they lose cytosolic components (65). Calpactin leaks from the cells following permeabilization and the secretory responsiveness of these cells can be fully reconstituted by incubation with calpactin or its heavy chain p36(1). Further evidence for a role of calpactin or related protein in exocytosis comes from the finding that a synthetic peptide based on the conserved domain of the annexins inhibits secretion when introduced into permeabilized chromaffin cells (1). These results suggest that calpactin may be essential for calcium-dependent exocytosis in chromaffin cells, and it is possible that calpactin could act as the calcium receptor that activates exocytosis. However the details of the mode and site of action of calpactin are not yet known. Nor is it known whether calpactin is required for exocytosis in any other cell type.

OTHER CALCIUM-DEPENDENT VESICLE BINDING PROTEINS   Within the group of cytosolic proteins that bind in a calcium-dependent manner to chromaffin granules are the actin-binding protein caldesmon (see above), protein kinase C, which phosphorylates one of the annexins (68), a phosphatidylinositol-specific phospholipase C (23), and a novel ATP-regulated protein, chromobindin A (50). A number of other polypeptides that bind to chromaffin granule membranes have yet to be identified.

GTP-Binding Proteins

Studies of factors that regulate exocytosis in permeabilized cells have high-lighted the possible involvement of a novel GTP-binding protein in ex-ocytosis, since non-hydrolyzable GTP analogues stimulate exocytosis even in the absence of calcium (7). This GTP-binding protein (termed Ge) could be acting in signal transduction through generation of a second messenger, or, alternatively, more intimately in exocytosis as a secretory vesicle membrane protein (37). Members of the signal transducing G-protein family have been detected on the secretory granules of chromaffin cells and neutrophils (62, 70). In neutrophils the G-protein detected (Giα) was present on the specific granules, but not on the azurophilic granules. The absence of this G-protein from one class of secretory granule would rule out an essential role for it in exocytosis, however its presence on specific granules may provide an avail-able intracellular pool of the G-protein for insertion into the plasma membrane (62).

Information from the study of temperature-sensitive yeast mutants de-fective in constitutive secretion suggests that exocytosis requires distinct GTP-binding proteins that are related to the *ras* proto-oncogenes. A mutation in the SEC4 gene results in a block in exocytosis with a resultant accumula-tion of secretory vesicles in the cytoplasm (64). The SEC4 protein is a 23.5-kd GTP-binding protein with homology to the *ras* proteins. In the mutant, at the restrictive temperature, the SEC4 protein becomes bound to the secretory vesicles following posttranslational modification (38). It is not yet known whether SEC4-like proteins are present in mammalian cells, or whether they are involved in regulated as well as constitutive secretion. However similar low molecular weight GTP-binding proteins are present in adrenal chromaffin cells and are enriched in purified chromaffin granule fractions where they are tightly bound to the cytoplasmic surface (19). It will be of interest to determine whether any of these chromaffin granule GTP-binding proteins are related to the SEC4 protein and whether they are involved in exocytosis in these cells.

CONCLUSIONS

One major problem in attempting to identify the molecular machinery of exocytosis from the study of the regulated pathway of mammalian cells is the difficulty involved in distinguishing between those proteins actually involved in exocytosis and those involved in regulatory aspects of the secretory proc-ess. The regulatory proteins are likely to differ from cell to cell depending on the exact requirements for the physiology of that cell. Therefore many of the secretory vesicle components thus far identified, with some expressed in a limited subset of secretory cells, may turn out to be regulatory components.

Nevertheless significant progress has been made in determining the nature of the cytoskeletal control of exocytosis in neurons (involving synapsin I) and in the adrenal chromaffin cell that appears to be sub-served by different proteins in the two classes of cells. It is possible that some of the calcium-dependent vesicle-binding proteins (the annexins), which have a very widespread tissue distribution, may turn out to be essential for exocytosis. So far the only evidence from secretory competent cells rather than in vitro studies suggests a requirement for calpactin in secretion from chromaffin cells, though its site of action is unknown. Clues provided from systems such as the constitutive pathway in yeast and the exploitation of secretory mutants may point the way toward the identification of secretory vesicle components (such as the small GTP-binding proteins) that form a key part of the exocytotic machinery required for all forms of constitutive and regulated secretion. Regulated exocytosis is a complex process that is controlled at the level of secretory vesicle interaction with cytoskeletal elements and membrane fusion itself. This survey of the many known secretory vesicle-associated proteins illustrates the potential complexity of this process. Over the past few years a clearer picture of some aspects of the secretory process has begun to emerge but understanding the molecular basis of exocytotic membrane fusion remains as great a challenge as ever.

Literature Cited

1. Ali, S. M., Geisow, M. J., Burgoyne, R. D. 1989. A role for calpactin in calcium-dependent exocytosis in adrenal chromaffin cells. *Nature* 340:313–15
2. Aunis, D., Perrin, D. 1984. Chromaffin granule membrane-F-actin interactions and spectrin-like protein of subcellular organelles: a possible relationship. *J. Neurochem.* 42:1558–69
3. Bader, M.-F., Aunis, D. 1983. The 97-KD α-actinin-like protein in chromaffin granule membranes from adrenal medulla: evidence for localization on the cytoplasmic surface and for binding to actin filaments. *Neuroscience* 8:165–81
4. Bader, M.-F., Hikita, T., Trifaro, J. M. 1985. Calcium-dependent calmodulin binding to chromaffin granule membranes: presence of a 65-kilodalton calmodulin-binding protein. *J. Neurochem.* 44:526–39
5. Bahler, M., Greengard, P. 1987. Synapsin I bundles F-actin in a phosphorylation-dependent manner. *Nature* 326: 704–7
6. Baines, A. J., Bennett, V. 1985. Synapsin I is a spectrin-binding protein immunologically related to erythrocyte protein 4.1. *Nature* 315:410–13
7. Barrowman, M. M., Cockcroft, S., Gomperts, B. D. 1986. Two roles for guanine nucleotides in the stimulus-secretion sequence of neutrophils. *Nature* 319:504–7
8. Baumert, M., Maycox, P. R., Navone, F., De Camilli, P., Jahn, R. 1989. Synaptobrevin: an integral membrane protein of 18000 daltons present in small synaptic vesicles of rat brain. *EMBO J.* 8:379–84
9. Breckenridge, L. J., Almers, W. 1987. Currents through the fusion pore that forms during exocytosis of a secretory vesicle. *Nature* 328:814–17
10. Buckley, K., Kelly, R. B. 1985. Identification of a transmembrane glycoprotein specific for secretory vesicles of neural and endocrine cells. *J. Cell Biol.* 100:1284–94
11. Burgoyne, R. D. 1984. Mechanisms of secretion from adrenal chromaffin cells. *Biochim. Biophys. Acta* 779:201–16
12. Burgoyne, R. D. 1988. Calpactin in exocytosis? *Nature* 331:20
13. Burgoyne, R. D., Baines, A. J. 1987. Synapsin or protein 4.1 in chromaffin cells. *Nature* 330:115–16
14. Burgoyne, R. D., Cheek, T. R. 1987. Reorganisation of peripheral actin filaments as a prelude to exocytosis. *Biosci. Rep.* 7:281–88
15. Burgoyne, R. D., Cheek, T. R. 1987.

Role of fodrin in secretion. *Nature* 326:448

16. Burgoyne, R. D., Cheek, T. R., Norman, K. M. 1986. Identification of a secretory granule-binding protein as caldesmon. *Nature* 319:68–70

17. Burgoyne, R. D., Geisow, M. J. 1981. Specific binding of ^{125}I-calmodulin to and protein phosphorylation in adrenal chromaffin granule membranes. *FEBS Lett.* 131:127–31

18. Burgoyne, R. D., Geisow, M. J. 1989. The annexin family of calcium-binding proteins. *Cell Calcium* 10:1–10

19. Burgoyne, R. D., Morgan, A. 1989. Low molecular mass GTP-binding proteins of adrenal chromaffin cells are present on the secretory granule. *FEBS Lett.* 245:122–26

20. Burgoyne, R. D., Norman, K. M. 1985. Presence of tropomyosin in adrenal chromaffin cells and its association with chromaffin granule membranes. *FEBS Lett.* 179:25–28

21. Burridge, K., Phillips, J. H. 1975. Association of actin and myosin with secretory granule membranes. *Nature* 254:526–29

22. Cheek, T. R., Burgoyne, R. D. 1986. Nicotine-evoked disassembly of cortical actin filaments in adrenal chromaffin cells. *FEBS Lett.* 207:110–14

23. Creutz, C. E., Dowling, L. G. Kyger, E. M., Franson, R. C. 1985. Phosphatidylinositol-specific phospholipase C activity of chromaffin granule-binding proteins. *J. Biol. Chem.* 260:7171–73

24. Creutz, C. E., Dowling, L. G., Sando, J. J., Villar-Palasi, C., Whipple, J. H., Zaks, W. J. 1983. Characterization of the chromobindins. Soluble proteins that bind to the chromaffin granule membrane in the presence of Ca^{2+}. *J. Biol. Chem.* 258:14664–74

25. Creutz, C. E., Zaks, W. J., Hamman, H. C., Crane, S., Martin, W. H., et al. 1987. Identification of chromaffin granule-binding proteins. Relationship of the chromobindins to calelectrin, synhibin and the tyrosine kinase substrates p 35 and p36. *J. Biol. Chem.* 262:1860–68

26. De Camilli, P., Greengard, P. 1986. Synapsin I: a synaptic vesicle-associated neuronal phosphoprotein. *Biochem. Pharmacol.* 35:4349–57

27. De Camilli, P., Harris, S. M, Huttner, W. B., Greengard, P. 1983b. Synapsin I (protein I) a nerve terminal-specific phosphoprotein. II. Its specific association with synaptic vesicles demonstrated by immunocytochemistry in agarose-embedded synaptosomes. *J. Cell Biol.* 96:1355–73

28. Drust, D. S., Creutz, C. E. 1988. Aggregation of chromaffin granules by calpactin at micromolar levels of calcium. *Nature* 331:88–91

29. Drust, D. S., Creutz, C. E. 1988. Subcellular localization of calpactin and other annexins in chromaffin cells. *J. Cell Biol.* 107:339a

30. Fowler, V. M., Pollard, H. B. 1982. Chromaffin granule membrane-F-actin interactions are calcium sensitive. *Nature* 295:336–39

31. Fournier, S., Trifaro, J.-M. 1988. A similar calmodulin-binding protein expressed in chromaffin, synaptic, and neurohypophyseal secretory vesicles. *J. Neurochem.* 50:27–37

32. Geisow, M. J., Burgoyne, R. D. 1982. Calcium-dependent binding of cytosolic proteins by chromaffin granules from adrenal medulla. *J. Neurochem.* 38:1735–41

33. Geisow, M. J., Burgoyne, R. D. 1983. Recruitment of cytosolic proteins to a secretory granule membrane depends on Ca^{2+}-calmodulin. *Nature* 301:432–35

34. Geisow, M. J., Burgoyne, R. D. 1987. An integrated approach to secretion. Phosphorylation and Ca^{2+}-dependent binding of proteins associated with chromaffin granules. *Ann. NY Acad.Sci.* 493:563–76

35. Geisow, M. J., Burgoyne, R. D., Harris, A. 1982. Interaction of calmodulin with adrenal chromaffin granule membranes. *FEBS Lett.* 143:69–72

36. Geisow, M. J., Childs, J., Dash, B., Harris, A., Panayotou, G., et al. 1984. Cellular distribution of three mammalian Ca^{2+}-binding proteins related to Torpedo calelectrin. *EMBO J.* 3:2969–74

37. Gomperts, B. D. 1986. Calcium shares the limelight in stimulus-secretion coupling. *Trends Biochem.Sci.* 11:290–92

38. Goud, B., Salminen, A., Walworth, N. C., Novick, P. 1988. A GTP-binding protein required for secretion rapidly associates with secretory vesicles and the plasma membrane in yeast. *Cell* 53:753–68

39. Grandori, C., Hanafusa, H. 1988 p60^{c-src} is complexed with a cellular protein in subcellular compartments involved in exocytosis. *J. Cell Biol.* 107:2125–35

40. Haycock, J. W., Greengard, P., Browning, M. D. 1988. Cholinergic regulation of protein III phosphorylation in bovine adrenal chromaffin cells. *J. Neurosci.* 8:3233–39

41. Hirokawa, N., Sobue, K., Kanda, K., Harada, A., Yorifuji, H. 1989. The cytoskeletal architecture of the presynaptic terminal and the molecular

structure of synapsin I. *J. Cell Biol.* 108:111–26

42. Huttner, W. B., Schliebler, W., Greengard, P., De Camilli, P. 1983. Synapsin I (protein I) a nerve terminal-specific phosphoprotein. III. Its association with synaptic vesicles studied in a highly purified synaptic vesicle preparation. *J. Cell Biol.* 96:1374–88

43. Jahn, R., Schleiber, W., Ouimet, C., Greengard, P. 1985. A 38,000-dalton membrane protein (p38) present in synaptic vesicles. *Proc.Natl.Acad.Sci. USA* 82:4137–41

44. Jockusch, B. M., Burger, M. M., Da Prada, M., Richards, J. G., Chaponnier, C., Gabbiani, G. 1977. α-actinin attached to membranes of secretory vesicles. *Nature* 270:628–29

45. Kelly, R. B. 1985. Pathways of secretion in eukaryotes. *Science* 230:25–32

46. Kenigsberg, R. L., Trifaro, J. M. 1985. Microinjection of calmodulin antibodies into cultured chromaffin cells blocks catecholamine release in response to stimulation. *Neuroscience* 14:335–347

47. Kondo, H., Wolosewick, J. J., Pappas, G. D. 1982. The microtrabecular lattice of the adrenal medulla revealed by polyethylene glycol embedding and stereo electron microscopy. *J. Neurosci.* 2:57–65

48. Landis, D. M. D., Hall, A. K., Weinstein, L. A., Reese, T. S. 1988. The organization of cytoplasm at the presynaptic active zone of a central nervous system synapse. *Neuron* 1:201–9

49. Lowe, A. W., Madeddu, L., Kelly, R. B. 1988. Endocrine secretory granules and neuronal synaptic vesicles have three integral membrane proteins in common. *J. Cell Biol.* 106:51–59

50. Martin, W. H., Creutz, C. E. 1987. Chromobindin A. A Ca^{2+} and ATP regulated chromaffin granule binding protein. *J. Biol. Chem.* 262:2803–10

51. Matthew, W. D., Tsavaler, L., Reichardt, L. F. 1981. Identification of a synaptic vesicle-specific membrane protein with a wide distribution in neuronal and neurosecretory tissue. *J. Cell Biol.* 91:257–69

52. Meyer, D. I., Burger, M. M. 1979. The chromaffin granule surface: the presence of actin and the nature of its interaction with the membrane. *FEBS Lett.* 101:129–33

53. Navone, F., Jahn, R., Di Gioia, G., Stukenbrok, H., Greengard, P., De Camilli, P. 1986. Protein p38: an integral membrane protein specific for small vesicles of neurons and neuroendocrine cells. *J. Cell Biol.* 103:2511–27

54. Obata, K., Kojima, N., Nishiye, H., Inoue, H., Shirao, T., et al. 1987. Four synaptic vesicle-specific proteins: identification by monoclonal antibodies and distribution in the nervous tissue and the adrenal medulla. *Brain Res.* 404: 169–79

55. Obendorf, D., Schwarzenbrunner, U., Fischer-Colbrie, R., Laslop, A., Winkler, H. 1988. In adrenal medulla synaptophysin (protein p38) is present in chromaffin granules and in a special vesicle population. *J. Neurochem.* 51: 1573–80

56. O'Sullivan, A. J., Cheek, T. R., Moreton, R. B., Berridge, M. J., Burgoyne, R. D. 1989. Localization and heterogeneity of agonist-induced changes in cytosolic calcium concentration in single bovine adrenal chromaffin cells from video-imaging of fura-2. *EMBO J.* 8:401–11

57. Parsons, S. J., Creutz, C. E. 1986. p60^{c-src} activity detected in the chromaffin granule membrane. *Biochem. Biophys. Res. Commun.* 134:736–42

58. Pepinsky, R. B., Tizard, R., Mattaliano, R. J., Sinclair, L. K., Miller, G. T., et al. 1988. Five distinct calcium and phospholipid binding proteins share homology with lipocortin I. *J. Biol. Chem.* 263:10799–10811

59. Perrin, D., Langley, O. K., Aunis, D. 1987. Anti-α-fodrin inhibits secretion from permeabilized chromaffin cells. *Nature* 326:498–501

60. Pollard, H. B., Burns, A. L., Rojas, E. 1988. A molecular basis for synexin-driven calcium-dependent membrane fusion. *J. Exp. Biol.* 139:267–86

61. Rehm, H., Weidenmann, B., Betz, H. 1986. Molecular characterization of synaptophysin, a major calcium-binding protein of the synaptic vesicle membrane. *EMBO J.* 5:535–41

62. Rotrosen, D., Gallin, J. I., Spiegel, A. M., Malech, H. L. 1988. Subcellular localization of Giα in human neutrophils. *J. Biol. Chem.* 263:10958–64

63. Rubin, R. W., Lyubkin, A. K., Pressman, B. C. 1984. Comparison of the protein content of three different bovine secretory granule membrane types: a search for exocytosis-specific shared proteins. *J. Cell Biol.* 99:356–60

64. Salminen, A., Novick, P. J. 1987. A *ras*-like protein is required for a post-golgi event in yeast secretion. *Cell* 49:527–38

65. Sarafian, T., Aunis, D., Bader, M.-F. 1987. Loss of proteins from digitonin-permeabilised adrenal chromaffin cells

essential for exocytosis. *J. Biol. Chem.* 262:16671–76

66. Schlieber, W., Jahn, R., Doucet, J.-P., Rothlein, J. Greengard, P. 1986 Characterization of synapsin I binding to small synaptic vesicles. *J. Biol. Chem.* 261:8383–90

67. Sudhof, T. C., Lottspeich, F., Greengard, P., Mehl, E., Jahn, R. 1987. A synaptic vesicle protein with a novel cytoplasmic domain and four transmembrane regions. *Science* 238:1142–44

68. Summers, T. A., Creutz, C. E. 1985. Phosphorylation of a chromaffin granule-binding-protein by protein kinase C. *J. Biol. Chem.* 260:2437–43

69. Thomas, L., Hartung, K., Langosch, D., Rehm, H., Bamberg, E., et al. 1988. Identification of synaptophysin as a hexameric channel protein of the synaptic vesicle membrane. *Science* 242:1050–53

70. Toutant, M., Aunis, D., Bockaert, J., Homburger, V., Rouot, B. 1987. Presence of three pertussis toxin substrates and Goα immunoreactivity in both plasma and granule membranes of chromaffin cells. *FEBS Lett.* 215:339–44

71. Vater, C. A., Jackson, R. C. 1989. Purification and characterization of a cortical secretory vesicle membrane fraction. *Dev. Biol.* 135:111–35

72. Wiedenmann, B., Franke, W. W. 1985. Identification and localization of synaptophysin, and integral membrane glycoprotein of M_r 38,000 characteristic of presynaptic vesicles. *Cell* 42:1017–28

73. Zhu, P. C., Thureson-Klein, A., Klein, R. L. 1986 Exocytosis from large-dense cored vesicles outside the active synaptic zones of terminals within the trigeminal subnucleus caudalis: a possible mechanism for neuropeptide release. *Neuroscience* 19:43–54

Annu. Rev. Physiol. 1990. 52:661–74

STIMULUS-SECRETION COUPLING IN VASCULAR ENDOTHELIAL CELLS

Andrew C. Newby and Andrew H. Henderson

Department of Cardiology, University of Wales College of Medicine, Heath Park, Cardiff, CF4 4XN, Wales, UK

KEY WORDS: vasodilatation, calcium, prostaglandins, thrombosis, growth factors

INTRODUCTION: SECRETORY FUNCTIONS OF ENDOTHELIUM

Endothelium contributes to regulation of vasomotor tone through secretion of two well-characterized vasodilator substances, prostacyclin and endothelium-derived relaxing factor (EDRF). Endothelial cells may also secrete the endothelium-dependent vasodilators ATP, acetylcholine, and substance P, and at least one peptide vasoconstrictor substance, endothelin. Endothelium-derived vasoactive agents may be important in mediating the influence of flow on vasomotor tone, vascular geometry, and angiogenesis (35).

A second function of endothelium is regulation of intravascular thrombosis. This may be promoted by secretion of platelet adhesion proteins including thrombospondin, fibronectin, collagen, and von Willebrand factor (VWF), but prevented by the secretion of prostacyclin and EDRF, which inhibit platelet activation synergistically. Endothelium promotes coagulation through expression of tissue factor and secretion of factor V, and plasminogen activator inhibitor (PAI), but inhibits coagulation through secretion of thrombomodulin and tissue plasminogen activator (TPA).

Endothelial secretion of mitogens and growth inhibitors for vascular smooth muscle may be important in atherogenesis. Endothelial regulation of the extravasation of leucocytes by expression of adhesion proteins and secre-

0066-4278/90/0315-0661$02.00

tion of interleukin-1 (IL-1) and platelet activating factor (PAF) (21) is also relevant to atherogenesis and to the inflammatory response.

In this review, we concentrate on the regulation rather than the biochemical mechanisms of secretion. Our limited discussion cannot take into account the extensive and important functional diversity of endothelium through the vascular tree. The selection of agents for more detailed description is likewise not comprehensive, but is chosen to illustrate principles and experimental approaches.

SECOND-MESSENGER PATHWAYS

Phosphoinositidase

FORMATION OF INOSITOL PHOSPHATES AND DIACYLGLYCEROL   In many cell-types, activation of a phosphatidylinositol-specific phospholipase C ("phosphoinositidase") hydrolyses phosphatidylinositol 4,5-bisphosphate to yield the intracellular second-messengers inositol 1,4,5-trisphosphate [ins-(1,4,5)P$_3$] and diacylglycerol (4). A guanyl nucleotide transducing protein couples receptors to activation of phosphoinositidase, and in some cases this step is sensitive to inhibition by pertussis toxin (4). Once formed, ins-(1,4,5)P$_3$ causes mobilization of calcium from endoplasmic reticular intracellular stores, and diacylglycerol activates protein kinase C (4)—an action mimicked by tumor promoting phorbol esters.

In endothelial cells, prompt formation of ins(1,4,5)P$_3$ occurs in response to ADP and ATP (P$_{2y}$ receptor) (29, 79), bradykinin (B$_2$ receptor) (24, 51), endothelial cell growth factor (72), histamine (H$_1$ receptor) (58, 80, 83), thrombin (39, 71, 80), and mellitin, a direct activator of phosphoinositidase (59). A simultaneous decrease in phosphatidylinositol 4,5-bisphosphate (51) and an increase in diacylglycerol (71) have also been documented, albeit not as widely. Evidence that diacylglycerol may activate protein kinase C can be inferred from the actions of phorbol esters on endothelial cells (20, 22, 23, 56). Formation of ins(1,4,5)P$_3$ does not depend on elevation of intracellular calcium or on the presence of extracellular calcium (39), but probably involves a guanyl nucleotide transducing protein, since formation of ins-(1,4,5)P$_3$ in response to ATP (78) (although not bradykinin, 51) is inhibited by pertussis toxin.

Other phosphoinositide metabolites are also formed after agonist stimulation of endothelial cells. Inositol 4,5-bisphosphate is formed as rapidly as ins(1,4,5)P$_3$ while inositol monophosphate isomers and glycerophosphorylinositol are formed more slowly (24, 51, 71, 72, 80, 83). Inositol 1,3,4,5-tetrakisphosphate is also formed slowly (80), consistent with the presence of an active ins(1,4,5)P$_3$-3-kinase (71, 80), possibly activated by elevation of intracellular calcium (72). Rapid formation of its degradative product, inositol 1,3,4-trisphosphate, does not occur, however, in stimulated human or pig endothelial cells (71, 80), although it is the major isomer in unstimulated cells (80).

ELEVATION OF CYTOSOLIC CALCIUM   Endothelial cytoplasmic calcium concentration is elevated by acetylcholine (9), ADP or ATP (P_{2y} receptor) (38, 79), bradykinin (B_2 receptor) (12, 59, 70), histamine (H_1 receptor) (41, 46, 51, 80, 85), PAF (8), or thrombin (39, 41, 47, 80). This list contains all those agents known to promote endothelial ins(1,4,5)P_3 formation, which, in addition, is sufficiently rapid to explain the time-course of calcium elevation. Maximal concentrations of agonists typically raise intracellular calcium within seconds from about 0.1 μM to above 1 μM. Calcium concentration then declines rapidly to a lower value before returning more slowly to the resting level. The initial agonist-stimulated rise of calcium concentration is scarcely altered by removal of extracellular calcium, which suggests that it results from mobilization of intracellular stores (9a, 12, 38, 39, 41, 46, 70, 80, 85). The sustained phase of calcium elevation, by contrast, is abolished by removal of extracellular calcium or by addition of inorganic calcium antagonists such as Co^{2+} and Mn^{2+}, which strongly suggests that this phase results from calcium influx (9a, 38, 41, 70, 80, 85). The mechanism of agonist-stimulated calcium influx is uncertain. It might be mediated by ins(1,4,5)P_3 alone or together with its metabolite inositol 1,3,4,5-tetrakisphosphate (40). In other cells, however, calcium entry can be distinguished electrophysiologically, kinetically, and pharmacologically from calcium mobilization and hence from ins(1,4,5)P_3 formation (40, 69).

In single endothelial cells, histamine causes spikes of calcium elevation to almost 1 μM and of about 30 s duration (46), the frequency but not the magnitude of which increases with agonist concentration (46). In the absence of extracellular calcium, the spikes become progressively smaller and less frequent, apparently ceasing before the intracellular pool is depleted (46). This suggests that repletion of the intracellular pool to a critical level may be necessary before it can be discharged. It is unclear whether this repletion occurs via the cytoplasm or directly from the extracellular space (46).

Calcium elevation may be terminated by receptor desensitization (47) or feed-back inhibition of phosphoinositidase by activation of protein kinase C (4).

Ion Channels

CALCIUM CHANNELS   Functional and electrophysiologic studies of voltage-sensitive calcium channels with organic agonists or antagonists have provided evidence for (15, 86, 90) and against (5, 12, 68, 93, 100) their presence in endothelial cells. Depolarization with extracellular potassium does not elevate intracellular calcium concentration (12, 38, 46, 85), and electrophysiologic studies have uniformly failed to detect L-type calcium channels in freshly isolated (9, 75) or cultured (12, 52, 74, 93) endothelial cells. A stretch-activated single channel conductance with a modest $\sim$ sixfold preference for calcium over sodium has been detected in pig aortic endothelial cells (52), which suggests that it might be responsible for significant entry of calcium in response to increased shear force (5, 73).

POTASSIUM CHANNELS   Endothelial cells exposed to steady shear (5, 73, 74) or to acetylcholine (9, 74, 75), bradykinin (12), leucotrieneB$_4$ (LTB$_4$) (53), or PAF (53) undergo membrane hyperpolarization. Shear-activated and acetylcholine-operated potassium channels may mediate hyperpolarization directly (74, 75). Hyperpolarization may also occur secondarily to elevation of intracellular calcium concentration (5) via a calcium-activated potassium channel (9, 12).

CALCIUM/SODIUM AND SODIUM/PROTON EXCHANGE   ADP, ATP (P$_2$ purinoreceptor), or the calcium ionophore A23187 causes transient acidification and sustained alkalinization of the cytoplasm of bovine aortic endothelial cells (50). The pH changes depend on the extracellular calcium, sodium, and proton concentrations and are inhibited by amiloride (50), which suggests that they involve sequential calcium/sodium and sodium/proton exchange.

Adenylate and Guanylate Cyclases

Endothelial cells contain an adenylate cyclase that is activated by prostaglandins of the E and I series (2, 48, 99), β-adrenergic agonists (48), and the direct activator forskolin (48, 66, 99). Inhibition of the adenylate cyclase by α-adrenergic agonists has also been reported (48).

Endothelial cells contain soluble guanylate cyclase that is activated by NO, N$_3$, nitroprusside, *tert*-butylhydroperoxide, and glyceryltrinitrate and particulate guanylate cyclase that is activated by atriopeptins (1, 66).

In some cell types cyclic nucleotides modulate the activity of the phosphoinositidase pathway (4). In endothelial cells, however, cAMP elevation may not inhibit formation of ins(1,4,5)P$_3$ (78), and the effect of cGMP elevation on phosphoinositidase has not been studied directly.

EXAMPLES OF STIMULUS-SECRETION COUPLING MECHANISMS

Prostaglandins

Endothelial cells metabolize arachidonate mainly to prostacyclin and prostaglandin E$_2$ (26, 81, 83, 84, 99) with smaller amounts of thromboxane A$_2$

(TXA_2) (26, 83). Secretion of prostaglandins occurs spontaneously and in response to increased shear force (5). It is also rapidly stimulated by ATP (20), bradykinin (B_2 receptor) (1, 11, 15, 20, 24, 44, 62, 84, 98, 99), histamine (H_1 receptor) (1, 83, 84), and thrombin (1, 2, 39, 47, 81, 84, 99), all of which increase endothelial intracellular calcium, and also by the calcium ionophores A23187 and ionomycin (1, 2, 11, 22, 78, 81, 84, 98, 99). The agonist-stimulated formation of ins(1,4,5)P_3 and increase in intracellular calcium precede the initial stimulation of prostaglandin formation (24, 39, 62, 83). The rate of prostaglandin formation, however, then declines before intracellular calcium returns to resting levels (39, 62), which suggests that there may be a threshold intracellular calcium concentration (for example, 0.8 μM in human umbilical vein endothelial cells, 39) for stimulation of prostaglandin formation. Evidence for a calcium threshhold also comes from correlation of prostaglandin formation with the peak intracellular calcium response to different concentrations of agonist (ATP) or calcium ionophore (9a). Agonist-stimulated prostaglandin formation is only slightly inhibited by removal of extracellular calcium (1, 39, 62, 99), but it may be abolished by depletion of the intracellular calcium store (39). Such depletion of calcium does not affect formation of ins(1,4,5)P_3, therefore implying that calcium elevation is the essential consequence of receptor-stimulation that mediates prostaglandin formation. In further support of this, prostacyclin production may be inhibited by buffering of intracellular calcium concentration with quin-2 (5). It is also inhibited by TMB-8 (2, 62, 90, 97, but not 5), a supposed inhibitor of intracellular calcium mobilization, although this mechanism of action has been questioned (91).

The effects on prostaglandin formation of possible inhibitors of phosphoinositidase have also been investigated. These include direct inhibitors such as gentamycin and pertussis toxin and activators of protein kinase C (i.e. phorbol esters), which might cause feed-back inhibition (4). Gentamycin inhibits prostaglandin formation in bovine aortic endothelial cells (20) while pertussis toxin inhibits the response to LTC_4 and LTD_4 (11), but has no effect on the response to bradykinin (11). In the same cell-type, pertussis toxin potentiates prostaglandin release in response to ATP (and A23187), but partially inhibits ATP-stimulated ins(1,4,5)P_3 formation (78). These data suggest the participation of a second guanyl nucleotide transducing protein in regulation of prostaglandin formation (78). Phorbol 12-myristate 13-acetate (PMA) and R59022 (a diacylglyceride kinase inhibitor that may increase the concentration of endogenous diacylglyceride) also inhibit prostacyclin release from endothelial cells (9b, 20). However PMA alone can stimulate prostaglandin formation in endothelial cells (9b, 22) and acts synergistically with A23187, which suggests that it lowers the calcium threshold for prostaglandin production (9b). PMA might then, as in other cell-types (4), potentiate the effects of calcium elevation while reducing agonist-activated calcium mobilization by negative feed-back, thereby preserving the response while avoiding prolonged calcium elevation.

There is evidence in endothelial cells for both the phospholipase A_2 (and perhaps phospholipase A_1, 64) and phospholipase C/diacylglycerol lipase pathways (5, 44, 64, 81, 83) of prostaglandin formation. How these pathways are regulated by calcium is not clear, however.

Elevation of endothelial cell cAMP concentration with forskolin or addition of dibutyryl- or 8-bromo-cAMP had no effect on prostaglandin production in two studies (78, 98), but was inhibitory in one other (60). The cAMP phosphodiesterase inhibitor, isobutylmethylxanthine, and the inhibitor of soluble guanylate cyclase, methylene blue, inhibit prostaglandin formation (2, 65), but apparently by direct effects (65, 98). Elevation of endothelial cell cGMP concentration with atriopeptins, organic or inorganic nitrates, also did not inhibit prostaglandin production in four studies (1, 17, 18, 65) although a high concentration of NO was effective in one other (25).

A slow stimulation of prostacyclin production also occurs in endothelial cells in response to IL-1 (21) and tumor necrosis factor (TNF) (10). This takes place over a time-course of minutes or hours; it depends on both RNA and protein synthesis, and it may be mediated by induction of phospholipase A_2 (10). The mechanism of stimulus-secretion coupling has not been defined.

Endothelium-Derived Relaxing Factor (EDRF)

Chemical assays for EDRF have only recently become available since its identification as nitric oxide (45, 76). Most studies to date have therefore measured EDRF activity by bioassays (3, 35, 96). Secretion of EDRF occurs spontaneously and is accelerated by increased shear force (3, 35, 96). Its formation can also be stimulated by acetyl choline, ADP, ATP, bradykinin, histamine, 5-hydroxytryptamine, PAF, substance P, thrombin (a list which again includes all those agents that have been shown to increase endothelial intracellular calcium), and also by the calcium ionophore A23187 (3, 35, 96). Removal of extracellular calcium inhibits both spontaneous (61, 68, 97) and agonist-stimulated (34, 61, 68, 97) EDRF formation although, in some preparations, a transient stimulation of EDRF formation may still occur (59, 94, 97). Taken together, these data suggest that cytosolic calcium mediates stimulation of EDRF production. Stimulation of EDRF production by mellitin (59) and inhibition by phorbol esters (20, 56) further suggest that phosphoinositidase is involved.

Control of EDRF and prostaglandin production have been compared in the same cell preparations (62, 97). Stimulation of EDRF formation appears to be more sustained, which suggests that it continues during the lower plateau phase of calcium elevation and may thus have a lower calcium threshold. An alternative explanation is that EDRF production may be relatively more dependent on calcium derived from extracellular entry and that prostaglandin production may be more dependent on calcium from intracellular stores. Consistent with this, removal of extracellular calcium causes a greater inhibition of EDRF production whereas TMB-8, the supposed inhibitor of intracellular calcium mobilization, inhibits prostaglandin but not EDRF production. By contrast, elevation of cGMP concentration inhibits EDRF but not prostaglandin formation (28, 43). Since cGMP elevation may have a selective inhibitory effect on calcium entry, at least in platelets (69), inhibition by cGMP might further implicate calcium entry in EDRF production. Inhibition of EDRF production by an inhibitor of the sodium/hydrogen exchanger (100) suggests that (calcium-dependent) pH changes may also be involved.

The initial step in EDRF formation probably involves the metabolism of arginine to citrulline (77). The enzyme likely to be responsible has a divalent cation requirement (77), but whether this accounts for the calcium-activation of EDRF release is not yet clear. The dependence of stimulated (34) but not spontaneous (33) EDRF formation on mitochodrial ATP generation also remains to be explained.

Proteins and Growth Factors

VON WILLEBRAND FACTOR   Spontaneous secretion of von Willebrand factor (VWF) is dependent on protein synthesis (60), as is the case for the other adhesion proteins, fibronectin and thrombospondin (82), thus implying that newly synthesized material is secreted directly. Stimulated secretion, by contrast, is independent of protein synthesis (55, 88) and depletes the cellular content of VWF (in particular that localized in the Weibel-Palade bodies) (82, 88), which implies that it occurs by exocytosis of a stored pool. Secretion may be stimulated by agonists known to cause intracellular calcium elevation, namely thrombin (6, 19, 41, 55, 60, 82), histamine (H_1 receptor) (41), and epinephrine (6). The calcium ionophore A23187 (19, 41, 60, 82) and PMA (19, 60, 82) are also effective. Buffering of intracellular calcium with quin-2 inhibits secretion stimulated by histamine (41) and removal of extracellular calcium also attenuates responses to thrombin, histamine, and A23187 (but has no effect on spontaneous secretion) (41, 60). By comparison with secretion of prostaglandins, stimulation of VWF secretion is more prolonged (up to 24 hr), more dependent on extracellular calcium, more readily stimulated by PMA, and less readily inhibited by dibutyryl-cAMP (60). These data suggest that stimulation of VWF release requires a sustained rise in intracellular calcium and/or activation of protein kinase C.

Secretion of VWF is also stimulated by a number of agents not known to cause elevation of intracellular calcium, namely bacterial endotoxin (88), IL-1 (6, 88), and plasmin (6). The stimulus-secretion coupling mechanism involved has not been elucidated.

PLASMINOGEN ACTIVATORS AND INHIBITORS   Endothelial cells secrete urokinase-type and tissue-type plasminogen activator (TPA), and a number of plasminogen activator inhibitors, of which PAI-1 is the best characterized.

TPA is secreted spontaneously and in response to histamine (H_1 receptor) (54), thrombin (54), and PMA (36, 54). Unlike secretion of prostaglandins, EDRF and VWF, secretion of TPA is not stimulated by A23187 (67) and may therefore involve activation of protein kinase C independently of intracellular calcium elevation. Secretion of TPA requires a lag period of 4–8 hr and is inhibited by IL-1 and TNF (87).

Secretion of PAI, by contrast, is stimulated by IL-1 (21, 27, 87, 95), TNF (87, 95), and bacterial endotoxin (14, 27, 95), but not by PMA or A23187 (87, 95), and is accompanied by increased expression of PAI mRNA (87). Stimulation of PAI secretion requires a lag period of 2–12 hr (87, 95), and requires protein synthesis (27). The stimulus-secretion mechanism involved is as yet unknown but appears to be distinct from that for TPA, thereby allowing for their coordinated expression.

GROWTH FACTORS   Endothelial cells secrete several peptide mitogens for vascular smooth muscle, among which platelet-derived growth factor A (PDGFA) (13, 49, 57, 92) and PDGFB (17, 49, 57, 92) are the best characterized, though they may be only minor components of total mitogenic activity (32, 57). Secretion is stimulated by thrombin (16, 42, 92), which is known to elevate intracellular calcium, but also by bacterial endotoxin (30), IL-1 (37), transforming growth factor-beta (TGF-beta) (17), TNF (37, 92), and PMA (16, 30, 92), which do not elevate calcium. Stimulation leads to two phases of secretion with a first peak at 3–4 hr and a second at 15–17 hr (16, 31, 37). Secretion may not require either protein or RNA synthesis (31, 42), but neither does it appear to come from a stored precursor pool since endothelial cell lysates contain little growth factor activity (31, 42). This suggests that secretion may involve modification of an inactive, stored precursor. There may be two independent pathways for stimulus-secretion coupling. PMA, thrombin, and TNF all stimulate secretion of both PDGFA and PDGFB from human microvascular endothelial cells, but PMA is relatively more effective towards PDGFB and TNF towards PDGFA. Moreover, the stimulation by PMA or thrombin is inhibited by forskolin (i.e. cAMP elevation) whereas stimulation by TNF is not (49, 92). These data suggest that thrombin and PMA may act through one mechanism (most probably activation of protein kinase C) while TNF acts largely through a distinct but as yet unknown mechanism. Microvascular endothelial cells also secrete hemopoietic colony stimulating factors (63, 89), and this also may occur through two independent pathways of stimulus-secretion coupling (89).

CONCLUSIONS

Intracellular calcium appears to mediate the acute stimulation of endothelial secretion regardless of whether it occurs by synthesis from a precursor as in the case of prostaglandins and EDRF, or by release of a stored pool as in the case of VWF. The evidence for differential secretion of these agents in response to common agonists suggests either the involvement of different pools of intracellular calcium (e.g. derived from entry or intracellular release), or secondary regulation as for example by protein kinase C or cyclic nucleotide dependent protein kinases; the details of these mechanisms have yet to be elucidated. Protein kinase C may also be involved in the slow activation of TPA secretion and of a component of growth factor secretion, although this is not yet firmly established. Slow stimulation of prostaglandin, PAI, and the remaining component of growth factor secretion can not presently be explained by any second-messenger pathway known to occur in endothelial cells. Further studies of these pathways are particularly warranted. By analogy with activation of other cells, these pathways might possibly involve protein tyrosine kinase activity.

ACKNOWLEDGMENTS

A. H. Henderson holds the Sir Thomas Lewis Chair of Cardiology. The authors' work is supported by grants from the British Heart Foundation and the Medical Research Council.

Literature Cited

1. Adams Brotherton, A. F. 1986. Induction of prostacyclin biosynthesis is closely associated with increased guanosine 3',5'-cyclic monophosphate accumulation in cultured human endothelium. *J. Clin. Invest.* 78:1253–60
2. Adams Brotherton, A. F., Hoak, J. C. 1982. Role of Ca^{2+} and cyclic AMP in the regulation of the production of prostacyclin by the vascular endothelium. *Proc. Natl. Acad. Sci. USA* 79:495–99
3. Angus, J. A., Cocks, T. M. 1989. Endothelium-derived relaxing factor. *Pharmac. Ther.* 41:303–52
4. Berridge, M. J. 1987. Inositol trisphosphate and diacylglycerol: two interacting second messengers. *Annu. Rev. Biochem.* 56:159–93
5. Bhagyalakshmi, A., Frangos, J. A. 1989. Mechanism of shear-induced prostacyclin production in endothelial cells. *Biochem. Biophys. Res. Comm.* 158:31–37
6. Booth, F., Allington, M. J., Cederholm-Williams, S. A. 1987. An *in vitro* model for study of acute release of von Willebrand factor from human endothelial cells. *Br. J. Haem.* 67:71–78
7. Bordet, J.-C., Lagarde, M. 1988. Modulation of prostacyclin-thromboxane formation by molsidomine during platelet-endothelial cell interactions. *Biochem. Pharmacol.* 37:3911–14
8. Brock, T. A., Gimbrone, M. A. 1986. Platelet activating factor alters calcium homeostasis in cultured vascular endothelial cells. *Am. J. Physiol.* 250: H1086–92
9. Busse, R., Fichtner, H., Lückhoff, A., Kohlhardt, M. 1988. Hyperpolarization and increased free calcium in acetylcholine-stimulated endothelial cells. *Am. J. Physiol.* 255:H965–69
9a. Carter, T. D., Hallam, T. J., Cusack, N. J., Pearson, J. D. 1988. Regulation of P_{2y}-purinoreceptor-mediated pros-

tacyclin release from human endothelial cells by calcium concentration. *Br. J. Pharmacol.* 95:1181–90

9b. Carter, T. D., Hallam, T. J., Pearson, J. D. 1989. Protein kinase C activation alters the sensitivity of agonist-stimulated endothelial cell prostacyclin production to intracellular ionized calcium. *Biochem. J.* 262:431–37

10. Clark, M. A., Chen, M.-J., Crooke, S. T., Bamalaski, J. S. 1988. Tumour necrosis factor (cachetin) induces phospholipase A₂ activity and synthesis of a phospholipase A₂-activating protein in endothelial cells. *Biochem. J.* 250:125–32

11. Clark, M. A., Conway, T. M., Bennett, C. F., Crooke, S. T., Stadel, J. M. 1986. Islet-activating protein inhibits leukotriene D₄- and leukotriene C₄- but not bradykinin- or calcium ionophore-induced prostacyclin synthesis in bovine endothelial cells. *Proc. Natl. Acad. Sci. USA* 83:7320–24

12. Colden-Standfield, M., Schilling, W. P., Ritchie, A. K., Eskin, S. G., Navarro, L. T., et al. 1987. Bradykinin-induced increases in cytosolic calcium and ionic currents in cultured bovine aortic endothelial cells. *Cir. Res.* 61:632–40

13. Collins, T., Pober, J. S., Gimbrone, M. A., Hammacher, A., Betscholtz, C., et al. 1987. Cultured human endothelial cells express platelet-derived growth factor A chain. *Am. J. Pathol.* 127:7–12

14. Crutchley, D. J., Conanan, L. B., Ryan, U. S. 1987. Endotoxin-induced secretion of an active plasminogen activator inhibitor from bovine pulmonary arterial and aortic endothelial cells. *Biochem. Biophys. Res. Comm.* 148:1346–53

15. Crutchley, D. J., Ryan, J. W., Ryan, U. S., Fisher, G. H. 1983. Bradykinin-induced release of prostacyclin and thromboxanes from bovine pulmonary artery endothelial cells. *Biochim. Biophys. Acta* 751:99–107

16. Daniel, T. O., Gibbs, V. C., Milfay, D. F., Garovoy, M. R., Williams, L. T. 1986. Thrombin stimulates c-cis gene expression in microvascular endothelial cells. *J. Biol. Chem.* 261:9579–82

17. Daniel, T. O., Gibbs, V. C., Milfay, D. F., Williams, L. T. 1987. Agents that increase cAMP accumulation block endothelial c-cis induction by thrombin and transforming growth factor-β. *J. Biol. Chem.* 262:11893–96

18. De Caterina, R., Dorsol, C. R., Tack-Goldman, K., Weksler, B. B. 1985. Nitrates and endothelial prostacyclin production: studies *in vitro. Circulation.* 71:176–82

19. de Groot, P. G., Gonsalves, M. D., Loesberg, C., van Buul-Wortelboer, M. F., et al. 1984. Thrombin-induced release of von Willebrand factor from endothelial cells is mediated by phospholipid methylation. *J. Biol. Chem.* 259: 13329–33

20. De Nucci, G., Gryglewski, R. J., Warner, T. D., Vane, J. R. 1988. Receptor-mediated release of endothelium-derived relaxing factor and prostacyclin from bovine aortic endothelial cells is coupled. *Proc. Natl. Acad. Sci. USA* 85: 2334–38

21. Dejana, E., Breviario, F., Bussolino, F., Erroi, A., Mussoni, L., et al. 1987. Modulation of endothelial cell functions by different molecular species of interleukin 1. *Blood* 69:695–99

22. Demolle, D., Boeynaems, J.-M. 1988. Role of protein kinase C in the control of vascular prostacyclin: study of phorbol esters effect in bovine aortic endothelium and smooth muscle. *Prostaglandins* 35:243–55

23. Demolle, D., Lecomte, M., Boeynaems, J.-M. 1988. Pattern of protein phosphorylation in aortic endothelial cells. *J. Biol. Chem.* 263:18459–18465

24. Derian, C. K., Moskowitz, M. A. 1986. Polyphosphoinositide hydrolysis in endothelial cells and carotid artery segments. *J. Biol. Chem.* 261:3831–37

25. Doni, M. G., Whittle, B. J. R., Palmer, R. M. J., Moncada, S. 1988. Actions of nitric oxide on the release of prostacyclin from bovine endothelial cells in culture. *Eur. J. Pharmacol.* 151:19–25

26. Eldor, A., Vlodavsky, I., Hy-Am, E., Atzmon, R., Weksler, B. B., et al. 1983. Cultured endothelial cells increase their capacity to synthesize prostacyclin following the formation of a contact inhibited cell monlayer. *J. Cell. Physiol.* 114:179–83

27. Emeis, J. J., Kooistra, T. 1986. Interleukin 1 and lipopolysaccharide induce an inhibitor of tissue-type plasminogen activator *in vivo* and in cultured endothelial cells. *J. Exp. Med.* 163: 1260–66

28. Evans, H. G., Smith, J. A., Lewis, M. J. 1988. Release of endothelium-derived relaxing factor is inhibited by 8-bromocyclic guanosine monophospate. *J. Cardiovasc. Pharmacol.* 12:672–77

29. Forsberg, E. J., Feuerstein, G., Shohami, E., Pollard, H. B. 1987. Adenosine triphosphate stimulates inositol phos-

pholipid metabolism and prostacyclin formation in adrenal medullary endothelial cells by means of P2-purinergic receptors. *Proc. Natl. Acad. Sci. USA* 84:5630–34

30. Fox, P. L., DiCorleto, P. E. 1984. Regulation of production of a platelet-derived growth factor-like protein by cultured bovine aortic endothelial cells. *J. Cell. Physiol.* 121:298–308

31. Gajdusek, C., Carbon, S., Ross, R., Nawroth, P., Stern, D. 1986. Activation of coagulation releases endothelial cell mitogens. *J. Cell. Biol.* 103:419–28

32. Gajdusek, C., DiCorleto, P., Ross, R., Schwartz, S. M. 1980. An endothelial cell-derived growth factor. *J. Cell. Biol.* 85:467–72

33. Griffith, T. M., Edwards, D. H., Henderson, A. H. 1987. Unstimulated release of endothelium derived relaxing factor is independent of mitochondrial ATP generation. *Cardiovasc. Res.* 21:565–68

34. Griffith, T. M., Edwards, D. H., Newby, A. C., Lewis, M. J., Henderson, A. H. 1986. Production of endothelium derived relaxant factor is dependent on oxidative phosphorylation and extracellular calcium. *Cardiovasc. Res.* 20:7-12

35. Griffith, T. M., Lewis, M. J., Newby, A. C., Henderson, A H. 1988. Endothelium-derived relaxing factor. *J. Am. Coll. Cardiol.* 12:797–806

36. Gross, J. L., Moscatelli, D., Jaffe, E. A., Rifkin, D. B. 1982. Plasminogen activator and collagenase production by cultured capillary endothelial cells. *J. Cell Biol.* 95:974–81

37. Hajjar, K. A., Hajjar, D. P., Silverstein, R. L., Nachman, R. L. 1987. Tumor necrosis factor-mediated release of platelet-derived growth factor from cultured endothelial cells. *J. Exp. Med.* 166:235–45

38. Hallam, T. J., Pearson, J. D. 1986. Exogenous ATP raises cytoplasmic calcium in fura-2 loaded piglet aortic endothelial cells. *FEBS Lett.* 207:95–99

39. Hallam, T. J., Pearson, J. D., Needham, L. A. 1988. Thrombin-stimulated elevation of human endothelial-cell cytoplasmic free calcium concentration causes prostacyclin production. *Biochem. J.* 251:243–49

40. Hallam, T. J., Rink, T. J. 1989. Receptor-mediated Ca^{2+} entry: diversity of function and mechanism. *TIPS* 10:8–10

41. Hamilton, K. K., Sims, P. J. 1987. Changes in cytosolic Ca^{2+} associated with von Willebrand factor release in human endothelial cells exposed to histamine. *J. Clin. Invest.* 79:600–8

42. Harlan, J. M., Thompson, P. J., Ross, R. R., Bowen-Pope, D. F. 1986. Alpha-thrombin induces release of platelet-derived growth factor-like molecule(s) by cultured human endothelial cells. *J. Cell. Biol.* 103:1129–33

43. Hogan, J. C., Smith, J. A., Richards, A. C., Lewis, M. J. 1989. Atrial natriuretic peptide inhibits the release of endothelium-derived relaxing factor from blood vessels of the rabbit. *Eur. J. Pharmac.* 165:129–34

44. Hong, S. L., Deykin, D. 1982. Activation of phospholipases A_2 and C in pig aortic endothelial cells synthesizing prostacyclin. *J. Biol. Chem.* 257:7151–54

45. Ignarro, L. J., Buga, G. M., Wood, K. S., Byrns, R. E., Chaudhuri, G. 1987. Endothelium-derived relaxing factor produced and released from artery and vein is nitric oxide. *Proc. Natl. Acad. Sci. USA* 84:9265–69

46. Jacob, R., Merritt, J. E., Hallam, T. J., Rink, T. J. 1988. Repetitive spikes in cytoplasmic calcium evoked by histamine in human endothelial cells. *Nature* 335:40–45

47. Jaffe, E. A., Grulich, J., Weksler, B. B., Hampel, G., Watanabe, K. 1987. Correlation between thrombin-induced prostacyclin production and inositol trisphosphate and cytosolic free calcium levels in cultured human endothelial cells. *J. Biol. Chem.* 262:8557–65

48. Karnushina, I. L., Spatz, M., Bembry, J. 1983. Cerebral endothelial cell culture II. Adenylate cyclase response to prostaglandins and their interaction with the adrenergic system. *Life Sci.* 32:1427–35

49. Kavanaugh, W. M., Harsh, G. R., Starksen, N. F., Rocco, C. M., Williams, L. T. 1988. Transcriptional regulation of the A and B chain genes of platelet-derived growth factor in microvascular endothelial cells. *J. Biol. Chem.* 263:8470–72

50. Kitazono T., Takeshige, K., Cragoe, E. J., Minakami, S. 1988. Intracellular pH changes of cultured bovine aortic endothelial cells in response to ATP addition. *Biochem. Biophys. Res. Comm.* 152:1304–9

51. Lambert, T. L., Kent, R. S., Whorton, A. R. 1986. Bradykinin stimulation of inositol polyphosphate production in porcine aortic endothelial cells. *J. Biol. Chem.* 261:15288–93

52. Lansman, J. B., Hallam, T. J., Rink, T. J. 1987. Single stretch-activated ion channels in vascular endothelial cells as mechanotransducers? *Nature* 325:811–13

53. Lerner, R., Lindström, P., Palmblad, J. 1988. Platelet activating factor and leukotriene B induce hyperpolarisation of human endothelial cells but depolarization of neutrophils. *Biochem. Biophys. Res. Comm.* 153:805–10

54. Levin, E. G., Santell, L. 1988. Stimulation and desensitization of tissue plasminogen activator release from human endothelial cells. *J. Biol. Chem.* 263: 9360–65

55. Levine, J. D., Harlan, J. M., Harker, L. A., Joseph, M. L., Counts, R. B. 1982. Thrombin-mediated release of factor VIII antigen from human umbilical vein endothelial cells in culture *Blood* 60: 531–34

56. Lewis, M. J., Henderson, A. H. 1987. A phorbol ester inhibits the release of endothelium-derived relaxing factor. *Eur. J. Pharmacol.* 137:167–71

57. Limanni, A., Fleming, T., Molina, R., Hufnagel, H., Cunningham, R. E., et al. 1988. Expression of genes for platelet-derived growth factor in adult human venous endothelium. *J. Vasc. Surg.* 7: 10–20

58. Lo, W. W. Y., Fan, T.-P., D. 1987. Histamine stimulates inositol phosphate accumulation via the H_1-receptor in cultured human endothelial cells. *Biochem. Biphys. Res. Comm.* 148:47–53

59. Loeb, A. L., Izzo, N. J., Johnson, R. M., Garrison, J. C., Peach, M. J. 1988. Endothelium-derived relaxing factor release associated with increased endothelial cell inositol trisphosphate and intracellular calcium. *Am. J. Cardiol.* 62: 36G–40G

60. Loesberg, C., Gonsalves, M. D., Zandbergen, J., Willems, C., van Aken, W. G., et al. 1983. The effect of calcium on the secretion of factor VIII-related antigen by cultured human endothelial cells. *Biochim. Biophys. Acta* 763:160–68

61. Long, C. J., Stone, T. W. 1985. The release of endothelium-derived relaxant factor is calcium dependent. *Blood Vessels* 22:205–8

62. Lückhoff, A., Pohl, U., Mülsch, A., Busse, R. 1988. Differential role of extra- and intracellular calcium in the release of EDRF and prostacyclin from cultured endothelial cells. *Br. J. Pharmacol.* 95:189–96

63. Malone, D. G., Pierce, J. H., Falko, J. P., Metcalfe, D. D. 1988. Production of granulocyte-macrophage colony-stimulating factor by primary cultures of unstimulated rat mirovascular endothelial cells. *Blood* 71:684–89

64. Martin, T. W., Wysolmerski, R. B. 1987. Ca^{2+}-dependent and Ca^{2+}-independent pathways for release of arachidonic acid from phosphatidylinositol in endothelial cells. *J. Biol. Chem.* 262:13086–92

65. Martin, W., Drazan, K. M., Newby, A. C. 1989. Methylene blue but not changes in cyclic GMP inhibits resting and bradykinin-stimulated production of prostacyclin by pig aortic endothelial cells. *Br. J. Pharmacol.* 97:51–56

66. Martin, W., White, D. G., Henderson, A. H. 1988. Endothelium-derived relaxing factor and atriopeptin II elevate cyclic GMP levels in pig aortic endothelial cells. *Br. J. Pharmac.* 93:229–39

67. McArthur, M. M., MacGregor, I. R., Prowse, C. V., Hunter, N. R., Dawes, J., et al. 1986. The use of human endothelial cells cultured in flat wells and on microcarrier beads to assess tissue plasminogen activator and factor VIII related antigen release. *Thromb. Res.* 41:581–87

68. Miller, R. C., Schoeffter, P., Stoclet, J. C. 1985. Insensitivity of calcium-dependent endothelial stimulation in rat isolated aorta to the calcium entry blocker, flunarizine. *Br. J. Pharmac.* 85:481–87

69. Morgan, R. O., Newby, A. C. 1989. Nitroprusside differentially inhibits ADP-induced calcium influx and mobilization in human platelets. *Biochem. J.* 258:447–54

70. Morgan-Boyd, R., Stewart, J. M., Vavrek, R. J., Hassid, A. 1987. Effects of bradykinin and angiotensin II on intracellular Ca^{2+} dynamics in endothelial cells. *Am. J. Physiol.* 253:C588–98

71. Moscat, J., Moreno, F., Garcia-Barreno, P. 1987. Mitogenic activity and inositide metabolism in thrombin-stimulated pig aorta endothelial cells. *Biochem. Biophys. Res. Comm.* 145: 1302–9

72. Moscat, J., Moreno, F., Herrero, C., Lopez, C., Garcia-Barreno, P. 1988. Endothelial cell growth factor and ionophore A23187 stimulation of production of inositol phosphates in porcine aorta endothelial cells. *Proc. Natl. Acad. Sci. USA* 85:659–63

73. Nakache, M., Gaub, H. E. 1988. Hydrodynamic hyperpolarization of endothelial cells. *Proc. Natl. Acad. Sci. USA* 85:1841–43

74. Olesen, S.-P., Clapham, E. E., Davies, P. F. 1988. Haemodynamic shear stress activates a K^+ current in vascular endothelial cells. *Nature* 331:168–70

75. Olesen, S.-P., Davies, P. F., Clapham, D. E. 1988. Muscarinic-activated K^+ current in bovine aortic endothelial cells. *Circ. Res.* 62:1059–64

76. Palmer, R. M. J., Ashton, D. S., Moncada, S. 1988. Vascular endothelial cells synthesize nitric oxide from L-arginine. *Nature* 333:664–66

77. Palmer, R. M. J., Moncada, S. 1989. A novel citrulline-forming enzyme implicated in the formation of nitric oxide by vascular endothelial cells. *Biochem. Biophys. Res. Commun.* 158:348–52

78. Pirotton, S., Erneuz, C., Boeynaems, J. M. 1987. Dual role of GTP-binding proteins in the control of endothelial prostacyclin *Biochem. Biophys. Res. Comm.* 147:1113–20

79. Pirotton, S., Raspe, E., Demolle, D., Erneux, C., Boeynaems, J.-M. 1987. Involvement of inositol 1,4,5-trisphosphate and calcium in the action of adenine nucleotides on aortic endothelial cells. *J. Biol. Chem.* 262:17461–66

80. Pollock, W. K., Wreggett, K. A., Irvine, R. F. 1988. Inositol phosphate production and Ca^{2+} mobilization in human umbilical-vein endothelial cells stimulated by thrombin and histamine. *Biochem. J.* 256:371–76

81. Ragab-Thomas, J. M.-F., Hullin, F., Chap, H., Douste-Blazy, L. 1987. Pathways of arachidonic acid liberation in thrombin and calcium ionophore A23187-stimulated human endothelial cells: respective roles of phospholipids and triacylglycerol and evidence for diacylglycerol generation from phosphatidylcholine. *Biochim. Biophys. Acta* 917:388–97

82. Reinders, J. H., Groot, P. G., Dawes, J., Hunter, N. R., van Heugten, H. A. A., et al. 1985. Comparison of secretion and subcellular localization of von Willebrand protein with that of thrombospondin and fibronectin in cultured human vascular endothelial cells. *Biochim. Biophys. Acta* 844:306–13

83. Resink, T. J., Grigorian, G. Y., Moldabaeva, A. K., Danilov, S. M., Bühler, F. R. 1987. Histamine-induced phosphoinositide metabolism in cultured human umbilical vein endothelial cells. Association with thromboxane and prostacyclin release. *Biochem. Biophys. Res. Comm.* 144:438–46

84. Revtyak, G. E., Johnson, A. R., Campbell, W. B. 1988. Cultured bovine coronary arterial endothelial cells synthesize HETEs and prostacyclin. *Am. J. Physiol.* 254:C8–19

85. Rotrosen, D., Gallin, J. I. 1986. Histamine type I receptor occupancy increases endothelial cytosolic calcium, reduces F-actin, and promotes albumin diffusion across cultured endothelial monolayers. *J. Cell Biol.* 103:2379–87

86. Rubanyi, G. M., Schwartz, A., Vanhoutte, P. M. 1985. The calcium agonists BAY K 8644 and (+)202,891 stimulate the release of endothelial relaxing factor from canine femoral arteries. *Eur. J. Pharmacol.* 117:143–44

87. Schleef, R. R., Bevilacqua, M. P., Sawdey, M., Gimbrone, M. A., Loskutoff, D. J. 1988. Cytokine activation of vascular endothelium. *J. Biol. Chem.* 263:5797–5803

88. Schorer, A. E., Moldow, C. F., Rick, M. E. 1987. Interleukin 1 or endotoxin increases the release of von Willebrand factor from human endothelial cells. *Br. J. Haem.* 67:193–97

89. Seelentag, W. K., Mermod, J.-J., Montesano, R., Vassalli, P. 1987. Additive effects of interleukin 1 and tumor necrosis factor-on the accumulation of the three granulocyte and macrophage colony-stimulating factor mRNAs in human endothelial cells. *EMBO J.* 6:2261–65

90. Seid, J. M., Macneil, S., Tomlinson, S. 1983. Calcium, calmodulin, and the production of prostacyclin by cultured vascular endothelial cells. *Biosci. Reports* 3:1007–15

91. Simpson, A. W. M., Hallam, T. J., Rink, T. J. 1984. TMB-8 inhibits secretion evoked by phorbol ester at basal cytoplasmic free calcium in quin2-loaded platelets much more effectively than it inhibits thrombin-induced calcium mobilisation. *FEBS Lett.* 176:139–43

92. Starksen, N. F., Harsh, G. R., Gibbs, V. C., Williams, L. T. 1987. Regulated expression of the platelet-derived growth factor A chain gene in microvascular endothelial cells. *J. Biol. Chem.* 262:14381–84

93. Takeda, K., Schini, V., Stoeckel, H. 1987. Voltage-activated potassium, but not calcium currents in cultured bovine aortic endothelial cells. *Pflügers Arch.* 410:385–93

94. Tayo, F. M., Bevan, J. A. 1987. Extracellular calcium dependence of contraction and endothelium-dependent relaxation varies along the length of the aorta and its branches. *J. Pharmacol. Exp. Ther.* 240:594–601

95. van Hinsbergh, V. W. M., Kooistra, T., van den Berg, E. A., Princen, H. M. G., Fiers, W., et al. 1988. Tumor necrosis factor increases the production of plasminogen activator inhibitor in human endothelial cells *in vitro* and in rats *in vivo*. *Blood* 72:1467–73

96. Vanhoutte, P. M., Rubanyi, G. M.,

Miller, V. M., Houston, D. S. 1986. Modulation of vascular smooth muscle contraction by the endothelium. *Annu. Rev. Physiol.* 48:307–320

97. White, D. G., Martin, W. 1989. Differential control and calcium-dependence of endothelium-derived relaxing factor and prostacyclin production by pig aortic endothelial cells. *Br. J. Pharmacol.* 97:683–90

98. Whorton, A. R., Collawn, J. B., Montgomery, M. E., Young, S. L., Kent, R. S. 1985. Arachidonic acid metabolism in cultured aortic endothelial cells. *Biochem. Pharmacol.* 34:119–23

99. Whorton, A. R., Young, S. L., Data, J. L., Barchowsky, A., Kent, R. S. 1982. Mechanism of bradykinin-stimulated prostacyclin synthesis in porcine aortic endothelial cells. *Biochim. Biophys. Acta* 712:79–87

100. Winquist, R. J., Bunting, P. B., Schofield, T. L. 1985. Blockade of endothelium-dependent relaxation by the amiloride analog dichlorobenzamil: possible role of Na^+/Ca^{++} exchange in the release of endothelium-derived relaxant factor. *J. Pharmacol. Exp. Ther.* 235:644–50

Annu. Rev. Physiol. 1990. 52:675–97

VIRAL AND CELLULAR MEMBRANE FUSION PROTEINS

Judith M. White

Department of Pharmacology and the Cell Biology Program, University of California San Francisco, California 94143-0450

KEY WORDS: virus, cell, fusion, glycoprotein, membrane

INTRODUCTION

Membrane fusion reactions abound in the eukaryotic world. A staggering number and variety of intracellular fusion events occur each minute, mediating endocytosis, organelle formation, interorganelle traffic, and constitutive and regulated exocytosis. Important intercellular fusion events include sperm-egg fusion and myoblast fusion. The molecular mechanisms underlying cellular fusion reactions remain elusive. Since fusion is an energetically unfavorable process, however, and since enveloped viruses employ specific proteins to fuse with and thereby introduce their genetic material into host cells, it is likely that cellular fusion reactions are also protein-mediated. In recent years, the integrated application of biophysical, biochemical, immunological, and molecular biological techniques has advanced our understanding of the basic process of membrane fusion. The progress is documented in four recent books (29, 51, 91, 122) and in several recent review articles (8, 9, 128). The purpose of this review is to synthesize what is currently known about the structure and function of proteins that mediate viral and cellular membrane fusion reactions.

VIRAL FUSION REACTIONS

Our understanding of how viral membrane fusion proteins function has benefited from careful analysis of the reactions they mediate. Therefore, I begin with a review of the properties of viral fusion reactions.

675

0066-4278/90/0315-0675$02.00

pH Dependence

Viral fusion reactions fall into two classes, low pH-dependent and pH-independent (154). Viruses with low pH-dependent activity fuse with membranes of acidic endosomes; those with pH-independent activity fuse with the plasma membrane but may fuse with endosomes as well (4, 71). The pH dependence of fusion is a property of the virus family. All orthomyxo-, toga-, rhabdo- and bunyaviruses studied to date require low pH to fuse (71, 92). These viruses display sharp fusion pH profiles with midpoints ranging from pH 5.0 to 6.5, in good agreement with estimates for the pH of endosomes (77). Within this range the pH at which optimal fusion occurs varies for different family members (92). Viruses that display pH-independent activity include paramyxoviruses (83), herpesviruses (124) and coronaviruses (134). The retroviruses appear to be an exception to the stated generalization. Whereas mouse mammary tumor virus (MMTV) requires low pH (103), the human immunodeficiency virus (HIV) is capable of fusing at neutral pH (73, 121, 133). The pH requirements of other retroviruses are under investigation (42, 97).

The pH dependence of virus fusion is a property of the viral fusion protein. Cells expressing the fusion proteins of influenza, vesicular stomatitis virus (VSV) or Semliki forest virus (SFV) only fuse if exposed to low pH. Conversely, cells expressing the fusion proteins of simian virus 5, respiratory syncytial virus or HIV fuse at neutral pH (62, 66, 96, 128, 148, 154).

Syncytium Formation

The most dramatic visual manifestation of viral fusion activity is syncytium formation. Viruses that enter cells through a pH-independent path can form syncytia at neutral pH; those that require a low pH environment for infection require low pH to produce syncytia (154). It should be noted that lack of syncytium formation does not necessarily indicate lack of fusion activity. A combination of viral and host factors contribute to the syncytial (syn) phenotype (123). Variant influenza, herpes- and paramyxoviruses exist that do not yield syncytia even though they are fusion-competent. In some cases the syn phenotype maps to viral glycoproteins implicated in fusion (19, 41); in other cases, the syn phenotype maps to other viral genes (119, 145). Polykaryon production also depends on the density of the fusion protein at the cell surface. Considerably more influenza virus hemagglutinin (HA) is needed to generate syncytia than to cause fusion with red blood cells (RBCs) or liposomes (33, 41). The lipid composition and other properties of the target cell membrane can influence the ability of a virus to produce polykaryons (2, 22, 107).

Role of Target Membrane Lipids and Proteins

LIPIDS   The lipid composition of the target membrane can affect the rate, extent, and pH dependence of fusion (44, 132). Although no absolute requirement for any specific phospholipid has been observed, phosphatidylethanolamine (67, 116) and *cis*-unsaturated phospholipids (159) have modest enhancing effects for several viruses. With respect to phospholipids, an important principle recently gleaned is that high concentrations of negatively charged lipids (e.g. cardiolipin or phosphatidylserine) can artifactually enhance the rate and extent of fusion by allowing non-physiologic fusion reactions to occur (128, 129, 132). In contrast to any specific phospholipid, cholesterol is found to be absolutely required for the fusion reactions of Semliki forest and Sindbis viruses. Although not absolutely required, the presence of cholesterol has been shown to affect the rate, extent, and/or pH dependence of other viral fusion reactions (28, 44, 53, 58, 67, 116, 128, 132, 154, 159).

VIRUS RECEPTORS   Orthomyxo-, paramyxo-, rhabdo- and togaviruses can fuse with liposomes that lack functional receptors (21, 44, 53, 67, 116, 132, 159). Although the presence of a receptor enhances the rate of aggregation between virus and target membranes, it does not affect the fusion rate for influenza and Sendai viruses per se (88, 132). It will be interesting to see whether viruses, such as HIV, that bind with high affinity to specific proteinaceous receptors (69) actually require these receptors for membrane fusion.

OTHER HOST CELL FACTORS   HIV binds to both mouse and human CD4$^+$ cells but only infects certain CD4$^+$ human cells. Based on this observation and the fact that the HIV genome can replicate in mouse cells, it has been proposed that the block to infection of CD4$^+$ mouse cells may be at the level of fusion (69, 135). Similar host cell restrictions have been observed for other viruses (61, 89). In the case of Sendai virus, both the rate and extent of fusion with erythrocyte ghosts are considerably higher than with liposomes containing virus receptors (113). Collectively these data suggest that some viruses, notably those with pH-independent fusion activity, may require host cell factors distinct from the virus receptor for optimal fusion.

Kinetics, Temperature Dependence, and Other Properties

KINETICS   Low pH-dependent viruses fuse rapidly. At the pH optimum and at 37°C, the half-times are generally $\leq$ 30 sec, and fusion is usually complete within 2 to 5 min (44, 82, 116, 129, 132, 152). Sendai virus, a virus with pH-independent activity, fuses ~30–200-fold more slowly (48, 49, 50, 87, 113, 128). Detailed analyses have shown that the fusion reactions of Sendai and influenza viruses consist of two sequential reactions: a second order aggregation step followed by a first order fusion step. In the overall process, the aggregation step is rate-limiting (8, 88, 132, 137).

TEMPERATURE DEPENDENCE   The fusion reactions of enveloped viruses are temperature dependent. With Sendai virus, the initial rate of fusion is virtually zero at $T \leq 22°C$ and then increases about 25-fold between 25 and 37°C (49, 50). Although not as strict in terms of the 22°C threshold, the fusion reactions of all other viruses tested have also been found to be temperature-dependent (10, 42, 44, 49, 56, 116, 128, 154). Viral as well as cellular factors probably contribute to the overall temperature dependence (50, 56, 65, 155).

OTHER PROPERTIES   Fusion of viruses with low pH-dependent activity is highly efficient. Under optimal conditions 60–90% of virions in this class fuse with liposomes (44, 58, 154, 159), and ~30–50% fuse with cells (10, 131). Fusion of Sendai virus, a virus with pH-independent activity, appears to be less efficient (128). In all cases studied, viral fusion is independent of divalent cations (44, 128, 154). Gradients of ions or osmotic pressure are not required (58, 82). Viral fusion reactions are not leaky to macromolecules or, at least in their initial stages, to small molecules and ions (125, 128).

VIRAL MEMBRANE FUSION PROTEINS

Over the past ten years many viral membrane fusion proteins have been identified. These include the fusion proteins from eight of the thirteen known families of enveloped animal viruses and encompass viruses with both RNA and DNA genomes. The strongest evidence that a particular protein is the viral fusion protein has involved demonstrating fusion activity following expression of the cloned gene (96, 148, 154) or following reconstitution of the purified fusion protein into artificial vesicles (79, 117, 130). Suggestive evidence has come from genetic analyses (23) and the use of antibodies that inhibit fusion without inhibiting virus binding (37, 38, 80, 104). The genes encoding the fusion proteins from many members of over 25 genera of enveloped viruses have now been cloned and sequenced. What is clear is that many distinct viral polypeptides are able to carry out the same basic function of membrane fusion.

General Motifs

All viral membrane fusion proteins studied to date are class I integral membrane proteins (i.e. their N-termini are external and their C-termini internal to the viral membrane). In all cases, > 85% of the protein mass is external to the viral membrane. All of the well-characterized fusion proteins are products of a single mRNA. They are synthesized and oligomerize in the rough endoplasmic reticulum. Most, but not all (147), contain N-linked oligosaccharides and many are fatty acylated. Although the carbohydrate and fatty acyl groups may influence protein folding and/or stability, these post-translational modifications are not strictly required for fusion (40, 63, 108, 141). Despite general similarities, the fusion proteins differ in many important respects.

Oligomeric Structures

All known viral fusion proteins are oligomers; many are trimers. Crystallographic studies (156) have proven that the influenza hemagglutinin is a trimer of identical disulfide-linked subunits (HA1-S-S-HA2). All three subunits are involved in fusion (12). The trimeric nature of togavirus and rhabdovirus fusion proteins has been strongly indicated by high resolution image reconstruction analysis and by a combination of sedimentation and crosslinking analysis (27, 39, 142, 147). However, not all fusion proteins are trimers. The prototypic paramyxovirus fusion protein, the F protein of Sendai virus, appears to be a tetramer (118). Although some retroviral fusion proteins are reported to be trimers (31, 101), the *env* glycoprotein of HIV is reported to be a tetramer (98, 115). In all cases enumerated so far, the fusion protein is a single oligomeric spike that projects from the viral envelope. For other viruses, additional viral proteins may play a role in fusion. The paramyxovirus HN glycoprotein, although not formally required (96, 148), appears to modulate the viral fusion activity (54). Fusion of viruses with more complex genomes, such as herpesviruses, may actually require the coordinate participation of several distinct oligomeric spike glycoproteins (1, 20, 37, 126, 161).

Processing/Activation

Many viral fusion proteins are made as larger precursors. Cleavage occurs late in the biosynthetic pathway and generates two polypeptide chains; the C-terminal product anchors the protein in the viral membrane; the N-terminal product remains associated through disulfide bonds or through non-covalent interactions (see Figure 1 for examples). Proteins that fall into this category include orthomyxovirus HA, paramyxovirus F, retroviral *env*, and coronavirus E2 proteins. Processing is necessary to activate the fusion function and hence infectivity of virus particles containing these proteins (83, 92, 123, 128, 134, 154). Fusion proteins requiring processing can be divided into two groups depending on the new amino terminal sequence generated by the cleavage. Those of influenza HAs, paramyxovirus F, and *env* glycoproteins of HIV, MMTV, and murine and feline leukemia viruses (36, 74, 83, 92,

123, 128, 154), are apolar sequences termed fusion peptides (Figure 1, see next section). In contrast, the sequences adjacent to the cleavage sites of the RSV *env* glycoprotein (55) and the coronavirus E2 protein (68) do not have the characteristic features of amino terminal fusion peptides (Table 1). Although one of the subunits of the togavirus fusion spike is made as a larger precursor, processing of this precursor does not appear to be required for fusion (99, 111). Fusion proteins that are not made as precursors include the G protein of VSV and the fusogenic spike glycoprotein of Uukuniemi virus (106, 128, 154).

Fusion Peptides

A striking feature of most, but not all, viral fusion proteins is the presence of a fusion peptide, a stretch of apolar amino acids (distinct from the signal sequence and transmembrane domain) that is conserved within, but not between, virus families. Based on these criteria, two types of fusion peptides have been identified, amino terminal and internal. All orthomyxovirus HAs, all paramyxovirus F proteins, and the *env* glycoproteins of HIV and several other retroviruses contain amino terminal fusion peptides (74, 83, 92, 123, 128, 154). As noted above, these proteins are made as larger precursors, and cleavage places the fusion peptide at the amino terminal of the membrane-anchoring chain (Figure 1). Putative internal fusion peptides are found in the fusion proteins of two togaviruses, SFV and Sindbis, and in one retrovirus, RSV (55, 154). There is no correlation between the pH dependence of fusion

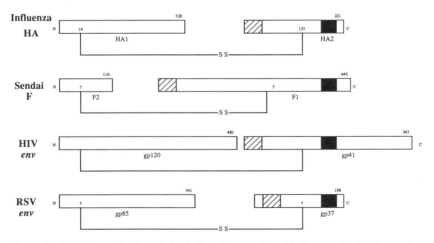

Figure 1 Subunit organization of the fusion glycoproteins of influenza, Sendai, human immunodeficiency, and Rous Sarcoma viruses. Hatched boxes represent fusion peptides. Filled black boxes represent transmembrane domains.

Table 1 General motifs of viral fusion proteins

pH Dependence	Fusion peptide	Example	Oligomer	Binding	Processing
Low pH	N-terminal	Influenza HA	3[HA1-S-S-HA2]	Yes	Yes
	N-terminal	MMTV env	3[gp52-gp36]	Yes	n.d.
	Internal	SFV spike	3[E1-E2-E3]	Yes	No
	Not obvious	VSV G	3[G]	Yes	No
Neutral pH	N-terminal	Sendai F	4[F1-S-S-F2]	No	Yes
	N-terminal	HIV env	4[gp120-gp41]	Yes	Yes
	Internal	RSV env	3[gp85-S-S-gp37]	Yes	Yes
	Not obvious	Corona E2	n.d.	Yes	Yes

For sources of information, see references contained within the text. The oligomeric structures are established for the influenza HA, the SFV spike glycoprotein, and the VSV G and suggested for the others. Fusion proteins that also house the receptor binding activity of the virus are indicated with a Yes in column 5. Those that require proteolytic processing for fusion activity are indicated with a Yes in column 6. n.d., not determined.

and the location of the fusion peptide (Table 1). Table 2 contains a list of representative amino terminal and internal fusion peptides. Most of these assignments are tentative. Mutagenesis studies (11, 36, 41) and hydrophobic photoaffinity labeling experiments (47) have demonstrated involvement of the amino terminal fusion peptides of the influenza HA and the HIV env glycoprotein in mediating fusion. Conversely, none of the putative internal fusion peptides have yet been shown, based on functional criteria, to participate in the fusion process.

Some of the general properties of fusion peptides are listed in Table 3. Amino terminal fusion peptides range in length from 24 to 36 amino acids, the termination point being identified, tentatively, as the first positively charged residue. The amino terminal fusion peptides of paramyxoviruses (and most retroviruses) are exclusively apolar. The corresponding peptides of influenza HAs contain 2 to 3 negatively charged amino acids. The putative internal fusion peptides are tentatively defined as stretches of 16 or 17 apolar amino acids. They are bounded on the amino terminal end by a positively charged amino acid and on the C-terminal end by either a positively or a negatively charged amino acid. Both amino terminal and internal fusion peptides are relatively hydrophobic. Their hydrophobicity values range from 0.5 to 0.8, the approximate range between the averages of those of their signal sequences and their transmembrane domains. Fusion peptides are rich in alanine and glycine residues (Table 3).

Based on a predictive analysis (35), the fusion peptides of influenza virus HAs show a propensity to form amphipathic helices (J. Finer-Moore, J. White, unpublished). Although the other fusion peptides analyzed (Table 2) are not predicted to form amphipathic helices, most show a tendency

Table 2 Representative fusion peptides

		10		20		30	
Influenza HA2 (X:31)	G L F G A I A G F I	E N G W E G M I D G W Y G F R					
Influenza HA2 (C/Calif.)	I F G I D D L I I G L L F V A I V E A G I G G Y L L G S R						
Influenza HA2 (Japan)	G L F G A I A G F I E G G W Q G M V D G W Y G F R						
MMTV gp36	F V A A I I L G I S A L I A I I T S F A V A T T A L V K						
Simian virus 5F1	F A G V V I G L A A L G V A T A A Q V T A A V A L V K						
NDV F1	F I G A I I G S V A L G V A T A A Q I T A A S A L I Q A N Q N A A N I L R						
HIV env gp41	A V G I G A L F L G F L G A A G S T M G A A S M T L T V Q A R						
MuLV env p15E	E P V S L T L A L L L G G L T M G G I A A G V G T G T T A L V A T K						
SFV E1	K V Y T G V Y P F M W G G A Y C F C D						
Sindbis E1	K V F G G V Y P F M W G G A Q C F C D						
RSV env gp 37	R I F A S I L A P G V A A A Q A L R						

For sources of sequences, see references within the text and the EMBL nucleotide sequence data library. Charged residues are underlined. Numbers above line one indicate residue numbers for the amino terminal fusion peptides (first eight sequences).

Table 3 Properties of viral fusion peptides

Virus	Protein	Peptide	Length	Hydrophobicity	Ala/Gly (%)
Influenza (X:31)	HA	N-HA2	24	.53	38
Influenza (Japan)	HA	N-HA2	24	.57	42
Influenza (C/Calif.)	HA	N-HA2	28	.71	29
MMTV	*env*	N-gp36	27	.79	30
SV5	F	N-F1	26	.70	42
NDV	F	N-F1	36	.49	39
HIV	*env*	N-gp41	30	.58	43
MuLV	*env*	N-p15E	33	.55	36
SFV	E1·E2·E3	Int-E1	17	.56	24
Sindbis	E1·E2	Int-E1	17	.58	29
RSV	*env*	Int-gp37	16	.65	44
	Average Fusion Peptide		17/28[1]	.61 ± .09	36 ± 7
	Average Signal Sequence		22	.44 ± .27	16 ± 5
	Average Transm. Domain		29	.70 ± .09	16 ± 8

The fusion peptide sequences analyzed are those listed in Table 2. The signal and transmembrane domain sequences from the same proteins were analyzed. Hydrophobicities were calculated using the normalized consensus scale of Eisenberg (32). The signal sequences of the *env* glycoproteins of MMTV, SFV, Sindbis, and RSV were not included in this analysis as they are unusually long (≥60 amino acids). The average hydrophobicity of an independent set of signal sequences (those listed in Figure 3 of reference 143) was calculated to be .46 ± .17. [1]The average length of the putative internal (Int) fusion peptides is 17 residues. That of amino (N-) terminal fusion peptides is 28 residues.

to form sided helices, with most of the bulkier, more hydrophobic amino acids falling on one face of the helix (encircled residues in Figure 2) and most of the smaller, apolar amino acids, including the majority (75–100%) of the alanine and glycine residues, falling on the opposite face of the helix (Figure 2). Although it is presently unclear whether these peptides adopt helical configurations during the act of fusion, two lines of evidence support such a possibility for the influenza HA. Firstly, a synthetic HA fusion peptide adopts a helical configuration in the presence of liposomes (64), consistent with the correlation, albeit not strict, between the helicity of synthetic fusion peptides from HA variants and their membrane interactive properties (150). Secondly, when the bromelain-released fragment of the influenza HA (BHA) interacts with liposomes at low pH, residues on the bulky hydrophobic face of the proposed helix are labeled with hydrophobic labeling reagents (47).

As noted above, fusion peptides are always found in a polypeptide chain with a transmembrane anchoring segment (Figure 1). It is thought that the presence of two apolar sequences within a single polypeptide allows the fusion protein to interact simultaneously and hydrophobically with both the viral and the target membrane (25, 128, 153), thereby promoting rapid and efficient fusion. Support for this hypothesis is the observation that fusion mediated by the influenza virus HA is most efficient when HA is membrane-anchored. BHA, which lacks the transmembrane segment, is not fusogenic (128, 152, 154). Although non-membrane anchored aggregates of the HA (rosettes) can fuse small liposomes, they do so less rapidly than membrane-anchored HA. Fusion presumably occurs because the rosettes are polyvalent and therefore able to bridge two fusing membranes (152). The reported ability of synthetic HA fusion peptides to promote fusion of small and/or negatively charged liposomes (30, 64, 85, 150) probably reflects the inherent tendency of amphipathic helices to interact with these types of liposomes (95, 128).

Conformational Changes

For viruses with low pH-dependent activity, exposure to mildly acidic pH converts the protein to its fusion-active state. Fusion-associated conformational changes are best characterized in the case of the X:31 HA. Two interrelated reasons account for success with this HA. The first is the availability of a water soluble ectodomain fragment that mimics the initial

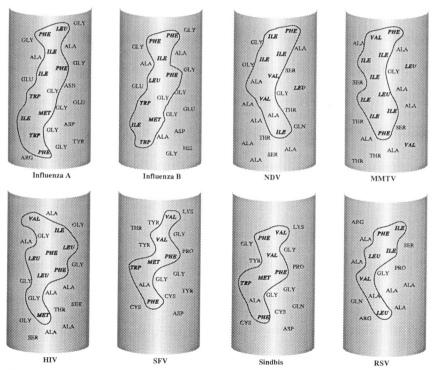

Figure 2 Helix net analysis of representative fusion peptides. Several sequences listed in Table 2 were analyzed according to the method of Finer-Moore & Stroud (35). Bulky apolar amino acids (Ile, Leu, Met, Phe, Trp, Val) are in bold and italic.

stages of HA-mediated fusion. The second is the fact that the structure of this fragment (at neutral pH) is known to high resolution. Although the structure of the HA in its low pH conformation is not known, insight into fusion-activating conformational changes has been obtained from biochemical, biophysical, immunological, morphological and genetic studies (25, 26, 47, 110, 127, 128, 149, 151, 154–156). The collective findings can be summarized as follows: (a) Changes occur throughout the molecule. (b) The protein does not denature; no changes in secondary structure are observed. (c) The stem region remains trimeric but elements of it change their relative positions. (d) The globular heads dissociate from one another apparently by bending about a hinge region. (e) The conserved and apolar amino terminal fusion peptide is released from the molecular interior. (f) The molecule acquires new amphipathic properties. (g) The moiety primarily responsible for the increased hydrophobicity is the fusion peptide.

A study employing anti-peptide antibodies suggests that the conformational change (in isolated HA) occurs in two major steps: changes in the stem region, which include release of the fusion peptide, preceding the dissociation of the globular heads. Based on the observation that the fusion pH dependence more closely parallels that for separation of the globular heads than for release of the fusion peptide, it was proposed that liberation of the fusion peptide, although necessary, is not sufficient for fusion, and that dissociation of the globular heads may be a key step in the reaction (155). Three lines of evidence support this hypothesis. Firstly, after exposure to low pH at 4°C, influenza virions become hydrophobic but do not fuse with RBC ghosts. Under these conditions, the HA spike morphology remains unchanged, which suggests that the heads have not separated (127). Secondly, a genetically engineered mutant HA in which an aspartic acid has been introduced into the interface between the globular heads induces fusion at a higher pH than the wild type HA. Thirdly, another mutant in which the globular heads are locked together with disulfide bonds appears to be unable to induce fusion at least under the conditions tested. (L. Godley, J. Pfeifer, S. Wharton et al, in preparation).

The HA is the only membrane fusion protein for which a crystal structure is known. Nevertheless, studies using specific proteases, antibodies, and chemical modifying reagents have suggested that conformational changes occur in other fusion glycoproteins coincident with their acquisition of fusion potential (10, 16, 25, 27, 45, 52, 59, 94, 128, 154). Interestingly, the conformational change in the SFV spike glycoprotein requires cholesterol (58), a lipid that is absolutely required for the fusion activity of this virus. The fusion-associated conformational changes in the influenza virus HA, and in the spike glycoproteins of SFV, Sindbis, and La Crosse viruses appear to be irreversible. In contrast, the G protein of VSV appears to undergo a reversible conformational change at low pH (10, 16, 27). Potentially relevant to the fusion mechanism of VSV is the recent observation that, at low pH, the G protein spikes reversibly aggregate at the ends of virus particles (16).

Since we do not yet know if there is a specific trigger for fusion proteins that act at neutral pH and, if so, what constitutes the trigger, it has been more difficult to analyze fusion-inducing conformational changes in these proteins. What is known is that the fusion protein of Sendai virus displays increased hydrophobicity following cleavage of its precursor, F_o, and that its conformation at neutral pH appears to differ from those at elevated or reduced pH (52).

Hydrophobic Interactions

A key feature of the fusion-inducing conformational change in the influenza virus HA is release of the fusion peptide from the molecular interior (110, 155). Concomitantly, HA acquires amphipathic properties (25, 26, 128, 149, 153). Several lines of evidence indicate that the fusion peptide is the major determinant of the observed increased hydrophobicity: (a) An HA with a site-specific mutation in this peptide (glycine 1 to glutamic acid) is impaired in its ability to interact with membranes and has no detectable fusion activity at pH $\geq$ 4.8 (41). (b) The HA precursor does not acquire amphipathic properties when exposed to low pH (26). (c) BHA aggregates if treated at low pH; thermolysin resolubilizes these aggregates by digesting the fusion peptide (110). (d) The fusion peptide is the only sequence labeled with hydrophobic photoaffinity labels when BHA is added to preformed liposomes at low pH (47).

Information on the interaction of other viral fusion proteins with target membranes is not as detailed. Nevertheless, the acquisition of hydrophobic properties may be a general prerequisite to fusion. Studies employing hydrophobic interaction chromatography suggest that, in response to low pH, the SFV spike glycoprotein becomes more hydrophobic (93). Upon interaction of Sendai virus with negatively charged liposomes, the F1 protein, which houses the fusion peptide, can be labeled with a hydrophobic photoaffinity reagent (90). It will be interesting to see whether a similar result is obtained with zwitterionic liposomes. Asano & Asano (3) have suggested a specific interaction between cholesterol and the Sendai fusion peptide.

THE FUSION SITE

Ultimately, the two fusing bilayers must come into molecular contact and their lipid components must mix. Since the major barrier to fusion is a strong short-range repulsive hydration force, it has been proposed that fusion starts at a dehydrated interbilayer contact site. Local defects in lipid packing with resultant exposure of hydrophobic surfaces are probably also required (8, 91, 102, 120, 128, 157).

It is still not known how any fusion protein induces the perturbation of lipid bilayer structure necessary to cause membrane fusion. In the case of the influenza HA, it has been proposed that more than one trimer may be necessary (25, 82, 128). Preliminary data from our laboratory support this notion; the relative fusion efficiency of two cell lines that stably express HA at different surface densities is not linearly proportional to their relative HA surface density (33). A highly schematic model incorporating this idea is shown in Figure 3. In this model, the fusion peptide does not actually embed in either the target (47, 128, 153) or in the viral (110) membrane. Rather, after it is liberated from the molecular interior, it provides a hydrophobic surface along the HA for flow of lipids between the viral and target membranes. The model further proposes that the outer leaflets of the fusing bilayers mix first, followed by the inner leaflets, and that fusion starts as a small pore. Electrophysiologic (125) and enhanced video microscopical (113a) studies also suggest that, like an exocytic fusion reaction (15), HA-mediated fusion begins with the formation of a small pore. The proposed highly schematic model is consistent with a focal point fusion mechanism suggested previously on the basis of freeze-fracture images (60). The extent to which this model reflects reality must now be tested. Furthermore, it is important to keep in mind that other viral fusion proteins may use different mechanisms (16, 17).

CELLULAR FUSION REACTIONS

A present challenge is to identify endogenous proteins that mediate cellular fusion reactions. In retrospect, it has been relatively easy to identify the fusion proteins of simple enveloped viruses, such as influenza and SFV, that contain

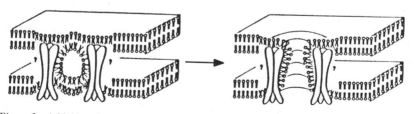

Figure 3 A highly schematic model of the postulated fusion site created during influenza virus HA-mediated fusion. *Left;* the association of several unfolded HA trimers is proposed to dehydrate the intermediate space, thereby forming an intermembrane intermediate (120). *Right;* rupture of the intermembrane intermediately perpendicular to the plane of the membranes would create a small pore, or interlamellar attachment site (8, 120), and thereby cause bilayer fusion.

only one or two glycoprotein spikes. It has proven more difficult, however, to identify the fusion proteins of viruses with more complex envelopes. For the latter viruses (e.g. herpes- and vacciniaviruses), several distinct glycoprotein spikes may be required. Therefore, given the complexity of cellular membranes, it is anticipated that the identification of cellular fusion proteins will be a difficult task. Several candidate cellular fusion proteins have now been identified. Proof that any of these constitutes a bona fide membrane fusion protein is eagerly awaited. As established with the viruses, confirmation of the fusion function will require satisfaction of at least one of the following criteria: (*a*) reconstitution of the fusion activity in vitro from the purified candidate protein(s); and (*b*) expression of fusion activity following transfection of the cloned gene(s) encoding the candidate fusion proteins.

In discussing cellular fusion events, endoplasmic and exoplasmic reactions constitute useful general categories. Endoplasmic fusion events are those in which cytoplasmically-oriented leaflets make initial contact. Exoplasmic fusion events are those in which the leaflets exposed to the extracellular surface (or the lumen of intracellular organelles) make initial contact (128). Given the differences between the extracellular/luminal and the cytoplasmic environments, the proteins and mechanisms involved in endo- and exoplasmic fusion events may be very different. The ionic compositions of the cytoplasm and extracellular/luminal environments vary considerably. The two membrane surfaces have different lipid and protein compositions. Proteins facing the endoplasmic space generally do not contain disulfide bonds, whereas those facing the extracellular/luminal space do. Exoplasmically-oriented proteins commonly contain N-linked carbohydrate groups; cytoplasmically oriented proteins do not. Since endoplasmic fusion events occur repeatedly (e.g. fusion of transport vesicles between the ER and Golgi), at least some of the proteins involved in endoplasmic fusion events may be reutilized. Since many different endoplasmic fusion events occur concomitantly in the cytoplasm, special mechanisms must exist to ensure rapid and specific targeting of the fusion partners. Exoplasmic fusion events (e.g. sperm-egg fusion) are single-time events. Nevertheless, they too exhibit exquisite target specificity. Extrapolating from the virus systems, it is important to keep in mind that the proteins that dictate target specificity may be distinct from those that mediate fusion.

Endoplasmic Fusion Events

Many endoplasmic fusion events are under study. These include fusion of early endocytic vesicles (14, 24, 46) and fusion of vesicles transporting materials from ER to Golgi apparatus (6), between Golgi stacks (146), and from endosomes to Golgi (43). Several regulated exocytic events are also being studied (15, 81, 114, 138, 140). It appears that many distinct proteins are involved in each endoplasmic fusion event. For example, 11 yeast gene products have been identified that are involved in ER to Golgi transport (86). Which of these are regulatory molecules and which are involved in the final fusion reaction remain to be clarified.

Several classes of proteins involved in the regulation of endoplasmic fusion events have been recognized. Signal transducing G proteins (18), specific phosphorylated proteins (7, 81, 114), and metalloendoproteases (84) have all been implicated as controlling molecules in regulated exocytosis. GTP binding proteins have been implicated in the control of a variety of interorganelle fusion reactions (5, 43, 76, 112). An attractive hypothesis is that hydrolysis of GTP by these GTP binding proteins insures the vectoriality of interorganelle fusion events (13).

No protein that solely mediates an endoplasmic fusion event has yet been identified. A large class of calcium binding proteins, collectively called annexins, are involved in exocytosis of secretory vesicles. However, synexin, a well-studied member of this group, appears to be involved in a prefusion vesicle binding step rather than in the actual membrane mixing reaction (75). An NEM-sensitive factor (NSF) that is conserved between yeast and higher eukaryotes (158) has recently been shown to be involved in several distinct interorganelle fusion events, including endosome-endosome fusion (24), ER to Golgi transport (6), and inter-Golgi transport (70). As NSF requires at least two other components in order to bind to target membranes, it is thought to be a component of an intracellular fusion machine (70, 146). Whether NSF, either alone or as part of the fusion machine, actually engages in the final membrane perturbation leading to fusion remains to be determined.

Exoplasmic Fusion Events

The fusion reactions of enveloped viruses are, by definition, exoplasmic fusion events. Therefore, the proteins that mediate exoplasmic fusion events may more closely resemble viral fusion proteins (especially ones that function at neutral pH) than those involved in endoplasmic fusion events. Cellular exoplasmic fusion events include fertilization, myoblast fusion, fusion of monocytes to form osteoclasts, and fusion of cytotrophoblasts to form the placental syncytiotrophoblast. The two cellular exoplasmic fusion reactions most actively investigated, myoblast fusion and fertilization, share several features including developmental regulation, a requirement for calcium influx, and inhibition by metalloendoprotease inhibitors (105, 144, 160).

Numerous cell surface proteins have been implicated in myoblast fusion based on their developmental appearance or modification (57, 109, 144). Physiologic studies suggest roles for the acetylcholine receptor (34) and calcium channels (Franco, J. B. Lansman, submitted) in regulating myoblast fusion. Proteins that control myoblast differentiation, such as the fibronectin receptor, indirectly influence myoblast fusion (78). If a specific myoblast membrane fusion protein exists, however, its molecular identity has not yet been revealed.

Several proteins have been implicated in mating reactions in a number of systems (139, 160). Two yeast genes have been identified, FUS1 and FUS2, whose products are involved in a post gamete attachment step leading to fusion. Fus1 is a highly glycosylated integral membrane protein that localizes to the gamete attachment site (72, 136). Characterization of fus2 is in progress. Whether either or both of these molecules are involved in the actual membrane fusion event has not yet been determined. An attractive candidate fusion protein is PH30, an integral membrane protein present in the sperm plasma membrane. Of two monoclonal antibodies that bind to PH30, one inhibits fusion (without preventing sperm building), whereas the other does not (100). Preliminary data from our lab suggest that proteolytic processing of PH-30 correlates with acquisition of sperm fusion competence.

CONCLUSIONS AND PERSPECTIVES

Presently many viral fusion proteins have been identified, cloned and sequenced. The mechanisms of certain viral fusion proteins have begun to be elucidated. Several proteins involved in cellular fusion reactions have been recognized, and a requirement for multisubunit complexes in intracellular fusion reactions has been established. The overall picture emerging is that a large group of highly divergent proteins and protein assemblies can carry out the fundamental process of bilayer fusion.

Many questions remain unanswered. In the arena of viral membrane fusion proteins present challenges include: (a) determining whether the mechanism of the influenza virus HA can be generalized to other low pH-activated viral fusion proteins; (b) elucidating the triggers and mechanisms of viral fusion proteins that function at neutral pH; (c) identifying the membrane-interactive domains of fusion proteins that lack characteristic amino terminal fusion peptides; (d) elucidating the mechanisms of more complex viruses, such as herpesviruses, where several glycoprotein spikes may be involved; and (e) clarifying the molecular architecture of the fusion site. In the area of cellular fusion proteins, candidate fusion proteins must now be scrutinized to determine their precise roles in the overall fusion process. Further studies are necessary to identify the constituents and to elucidate the mechanism(s) of multisubunit intracellular fusion machines. The mechanisms imparting target specificity to cellular fusion reactions must now be investigated. In order to elucidate the basic principles governing proteins that mediate biological fusion reactions, careful attention must be given to the similarities and differences among various viral and cellular fusion proteins and between proteins that mediate exoplasmic and those that mediate endoplasmic fusion reactions. Our minds should be kept open to the possibility of multiple and unexpected mechanisms.

ACKNOWLEDGMENTS

I would like to thank Samuel Green, Janet Finer-Moore, Vishu Lingappa, and the members of my laboratory for helpful discussions and for critical assessment of the manuscript. The work in my laboratory was supported by grants from the National Institutes of Health (AI22470) and the Muscular Dystrophy Association and an award from the Pew Scholars Program in the Biomedical Sciences.

Literature Cited

1. Ali, M., Butcher, M., Ghosh, H. P. 1987. Expression and nuclear envelope localization of biologically active fusion glycoprotein gB of herpes simplex virus in mammalian cells using cloned DNA. *Proc. Natl. Acad. Sci. USA* 84:5675–79

2. Aroeti, B., Henis, Y. 1988. Effects of fusion temperature on the lateral mobility of Sendai virus glycoproteins in erythrocyte membranes and on cell fusion indicate that glycoprotein mobilization is required for cell fusion. *Biochemistry* 27:5654–61

3. Asano, K., Asano, A. 1988. Binding of cholesterol and inhibitory peptide derivatives with the fusogenic hydrophobic sequence of F-glycoprotein of HVJ (Sendai virus): Possible implications in the fusion reaction. *Biochemistry* 27:1321–29

4. Bächi, T. 1988. Direct observation of the budding and fusion of an enveloped virus by video microscopy of viable cells. *J. Cell Biol.* 107:1689–95

5. Beckers, C. J., Balch, W. E. 1989. Calcium and GTP: Essential components of vesicular trafficking between the endoplasmic reticulum and Golgi apparatus. *J. Cell Biol.* 108:1245–56

6. Beckers, C. J., Block, M. R., Glick, B. S., Rothman, J. E., Balch, W. E. 1989. Vesicular transport between the endoplasmic reticulum and the Golgi stack requires the NEM-sensitive fusion protein. *Nature* 339:397–98

7. Benfenati, F., Greengard, P., Brunner, J., Bahler, M. 1989. Electrostatic and hydrophobic interactions of synapsin I and synapsin I fragments with phospholipid bilayers. *J. Cell Biol.* 108:1851–62

8. Bentz, J., Ellens, H. 1988. Membrane fusion: Kinetics and mechanisms. *Colloids Surf.* 30:65–112

9. Blumenthal, R. 1987. Membrane fusion. *Curr. Top. Membr. Transp.* 29:203–54

10. Blumenthal, R., Bali-Puri, A., Walter, A., Covell, D., Eidelman, O. 1987. pH-dependent fusion of vesicular stomatitis virus with vero cells. *J. Biol. Chem.* 262:13614–19

11. Bosch, M. L., Earl, P. L., Fargnoli, K., Picciafuoco, S., Giombini, F., et al. 1989. Identification of the fusion peptide of primate immunodeficiency viruses. *Science* 244:694–97

12. Boulay, F., Doms, R. W., Webster, R. G., Helenius, A. 1988. Posttranslational oligomerization and cooperative acid activation of mixed influenza hemagglutinin trimers. *J. Cell Biol.* 106:629–39

13. Bourne, H. 1988. Do GTPases direct membrane traffic in secretion? *Cell* 53:669–71

14. Braell, W. A. 1987. Fusion between endocytic vesicles in a cell-free system. *Proc. Natl. Acad. Sci. USA* 84:1137–41

15. Breckenridge, L. J., Almers, W. 1987. Final steps in exocytosis observed in a cell with giant secretory granules. *Proc. Natl. Acad. Sci. USA* 84:1945–49

16. Brown, J. C., Newcomb, W. W., Lawrenz-Smith, S. 1988. pH-dependent accumulation of the vesicular stomatitis virus glycoprotein at the ends of intact virions. *Virology* 167:625–29

17. Bundo-Morita, K., Gibson, S., Lenard, J. 1988. Radiation inactivation analysis of fusion and hemolysis by vesicular stomatitis virus. *Virology* 163:622–24

18. Burgoyne, R. D. 1987. Control of exocytosis. *Nature* 328:112–13

19. Cai, W., Gu, B., Person, S. 1988. Role of glycoprotein gB of Herpes simplex virus type I in viral entry and cell fusion. *J. Virol.* 62:2596–2604

20. Campadelli-Fiume, G., Avitabile, E., Fini, S., Stirpe, D., Arsenakis, M., et al. 1988. Herpes simplex virus glycoprotein D is sufficient to induce spontaneous pH-independent fusion in a cell line that constitutively expresses the glycoprotein. *Virology* 166:598–602

21. Citovsky, V., Laster, Y., Schuldiner, S., Loyter, A. 1987. Osmotic swelling allows fusion of Sendai virions with membranes of desialized erythrocytes and chromaffin granules. *Biochemistry* 26:3856–64

22. Daya, M., Cervin, M., Anderson, R. 1988. Cholesterol enhances mouse hepatitis virus-mediated cell fusion. *Virology* 163:276–83

23. Desai, P. J., Schaffer, P. A., Minson, A. C. 1988. Excretion of non-infectious virus particles lacking glycoprotein H by a temperature-sensitive mutant of herpes simplex virus type 1; evidence that gH is essential for virion infectivity. *J. Gen. Virol.* 69:1147–56

24. Diaz, R., Mayorga, L., Weidman, P. J., Rothman, J. E., Stahl, P. D. 1989. Vesicle fusion following receptor-mediated endocytosis requires a protein active in Golgi transport. *Nature* 339:398–400

25. Doms, R., White, J., Boulay, F., Helenius, A. 1990. Influenza virus hemagglutinin and membrane fusion. In *Cellular Membrane Fusion: Fundamental Mechanisms and Applications of Membrane Fusion Techniques,* ed. D. Hoekstra, J. Wilschut, New York: Dekker

26. Doms, R. W., Helenius, A. 1988. Properties of a viral fusion protein. In *Molecular Mechanisms of Membrane Fusion,* ed. S. Ohki, D. Doyle, T. D. Flanagan, S. W. Hui, E. Mayhew pp. 385–398. New York: Plenum

27. Doms, R. W., Keller, D. S., Helenius, A., Balch, W. E. 1987. Role for adenosine triphosphate in regulating the assembly and transport of vesicular stomatitis virus G protein trimers. *J. Cell. Biol.* 105:1957–69

28. Duzgunes, N. 1988. Cholesterol and membrane fusion. In *Biology of Cholesterol,* ed. P. L. Yeagle pp. 197–212. Press, Boca Raton: CRC

29. Duzgunes, N., Bronner, F. 1988. Membrane fusion in fertilization, cellular transport, and viral infection. *Curr. Top. Membr. Transp.* 32: 1–384.

30. Duzgunes, N., Gambale, F. 1988. Membrane action of synthetic N-terminal peptides of influenza virus hemagglutinin and its mutants. *FEBS Lett.* 227:110–14

31. Einfeld, D., Hunter, E. 1988. Oligomeric structure of a prototypic retrovirus glycoprotein. *Proc. Natl. Acad. Sci. USA* 85:8688–92

32. Eisenberg, D. 1984. Three-dimensional structure of membrane and surface proteins. *Annu. Rev. Biochem.* 53:595–623

33. Ellens, H., Bentz, J., Mason, D., White, J. 1989. The fusion site of influenza hemagglutinin -expressing fibroblasts requires more than one hemagglutinin trimer. *Am. Soc. Cell Biol.* 159a. (Abstr.)

34. Entwistle, A., Zalin, R. J., Warner, A. E., Bevan, S. 1988. A role for acetylcholine receptors in the fusion of chick myoblasts. *J. Cell Biol.* 106:1703–12

35. Finer-Moore, J., Bazan, F., Rubin, J., Stroud, R. M. 1989. Identification of membrane proteins and soluble secondary structural elements, domain structure, and packing arrangements by Fourier-transform amphipathic analysis. In *Prediction of Protein Structure and the Principles of Protein Conformation,* ed. G. Fasman pp. New York: Plenum

36. Freed, E. O., Risser, R. 1989. Mutational analysis of the precursor, fusion and cytotoxic domains of the HIV-1 envelope glycoprotein. *Cold Spring Harbor RNA Tumor Virus Meet.* p. 202. (Abstr.)

37. Fuller, A. O., Santos, R. E., Spear, P. G. 1989. Neutralizing antibodies specific for glycoprotein H of herpes simplex virus permit viral attachment to cells but prevent penetration. *J. Virol.* 63:3435–43

38. Fuller, A. O., Spear, P. G. 1987. Antiglycoprotein D antibodies that permit adsorption but block infection by herpes simplex virus 1 prevent virion-cell fusion at the cell surface. *Proc. Natl. Acad. Sci. USA* 84:5454–58

39. Fuller, S. D. 1987. The T = 4 envelope of Sindbis virus is organized by interactions with a complementary T = 3 capsid. *Cell* 48:923–34

40. Gallagher, P., Henneberry, J., Wilson, I., Sambrook, J., Gething, M.-J. 1988. Addition of carbohydrate side chains at novel sites on influenza virus hemagglutinin can modulate the folding, transport, and activity of the molecule. *J. Cell Biol.* 107:2059–73

41. Gething, M.-J., Doms, R. W., York, D., White, J. 1986. Studies on the mechanism of membrane fusion: site-specific mutagenesis of the hemagglutinin of influenza virus. *J. Cell Biol.* 102:11–23

42. Gilbert, J., White, J. 1989. Fusion of Rous sarcoma virus with host cells is

pH-independent. *Cold Spring Harbor RNA Tumor Virus Meet.* p. 33. (Abstrst.)

43. Goda, Y., Pfeffer, S. R. 1988. Selective recycling of the mannose 6-phosphate/ IGF-II receptor to the *trans* Golgi network in vitro. *Cell* 55:309–20

44. Gollins, S. W., Porterfield, J. S. 1986. pH-dependent fusion between the flavivirus West Nile and liposomal model membranes. *J. Gen. Virol.* 67:157–66

45. Gonzalez-Scarano, F. 1985. La Crosse virus G1 glycoprotein undergoes a conformational change at the pH of fusion. *Virology* 140:209–16

46. Gruenberg, J., Howell, K. 1987. An internalized transmembrane protein resides in a fusion-competent endosome for less than 5 minutes. *Proc. Natl. Acad. Sci. USA* 84:5758–62

47. Harter, C., James, P., Bächi, T., Semenza, G., Brunner, J. 1989. Hydrophobic binding of the ectodomain of influenza hemagglutinin to membranes occurs through the "fusion peptide". *J. Biol. Chem.* 264:6459–64

48. Hoekstra, D., Klappe, K. 1986. Sendai virus-erythrocyte membrane interaction: quantitative and kinetic analysis of viral binding, dissociation, and fusion. *J. Virol.* 58:87–95

49. Hoekstra, D., Klappe, K., de Boer, T., Wilschut, J. 1985. Characterization of the fusogenic properties of Sendai virus: Kinetics of fusion with erythrocyte membranes. *Biochemistry* 24:4739–46

50. Hoekstra, D., Klappe, K., Hoff, H., Nir, S. 1989. Mechanism of fusion of Sendai virus: Role of hydrophobic interactions and mobility constraints of viral membrane proteins. Effects of polyethylene glycol. *J. Biol. Chem.* 264:6786–92

51. Hoekstra, D., Wilschut, J. 1990. See Ref. 25.

52. Hsu, M.-C., Scheid, A., Choppin, P. W. 1982. Enhancement of membrane-fusing activity of Sendai virus by exposure of the virus to basic pH is correlated with a conformational change in the fusion protein. *Proc. Natl. Acad. Sci. USA* 79:5862–66

53. Hsu, M.-C., Scheid, A., Choppin, P. W. 1983. Fusion of Sendai virus with liposomes: Dependence on the viral fusion protein (F) and the lipid composition of liposomes. *Virology* 126:361–69

54. Huang, R. T. C., Dietsch, E., Rott, R. 1985. Further studies on the role of neuraminidase and the mechanism of low pH dependence in influenza virus-induced membrane fusion. *J. Gen. Virol.* 66:295–301

55. Hunter, E., Hill, E., Hardwick, M., Bhown, A., Schwartz, D. E., et al. 1983. Complete sequence of the *Rous* sarcoma virus *env* gene: identification of structural and functional regions of its product. *J. Virol.* 46:920–36

56. Junankar, P. R., Cherry, R. J. 1986. Temperature and pH dependence of the haemolytic activity of influenza virus and of the rotational mobility of the spike glycoproteins. *Biochim. Biophys. Acta* 854:198–206

57. Kaufman, S. J., Foster, R. F., Haye, K. R., Faiman, L. E. 1985. Expression of a developmentally regulated antigen on the surface of skeletal and cardiac muscle cells. *J. Cell Biol.* 100:1977–87

58. Kielian, M., Helenius, A. 1984. Role of cholesterol in fusion of Semliki forest virus with membranes. *J. Virol.* 52:281–83

59. Kimura, T., Ohyama, A. 1988. Association between the pH-dependent conformational change of West Nile flavivirus E protein and virus-mediated membrane fusion. *J. Gen. Virol.* 69:1247–54

60. Knoll, G., Burger, K. N. J., Bron, R., van Meer, G., Verkleij, A. J. 1988. Fusion of liposomes with the plasma membrane of epithelial cells: Fate of incorporated lipids as followed by freeze fracture and autoradiography of plastic sections. *J. Cell Biol.* 107:2511–21

61. Kooi, C., Mizzen, L., Alderson, C., Daya, M., Anderson, R. 1988. Early events of importance in determining host cell permissiveness to mouse hepatitis virus infection. *J. Gen. Virol.* 69:1125–35

62. Kowalski, M., Potz, J., Basiripour, L., Dorfman, T., Goh, W. C., et al. 1987. Functional regions of the envelope glycoprotein of human immunodeficiency virus type 1. *Science* 237:1351–55

63. Lambrecht, B., Schmidt, F. G. 1986. Membrane fusion induced by influenza virus hemagglutinin requires protein bound fatty acids. *FEBS Lett.* 202:127–32

64. Lear, J. D., DeGrado, W. F. 1987. Membrane binding and conformational properties of peptides representing the NH2 terminus of influenza HA-2. *J. Biol. Chem.* 262:6500–5

65. Lee, P. M., Cherry, R. J., Bächi, T. 1983. Correlation of rotational mobility and flexibility of Sendai virus spike glycoproteins with fusion activity. *Virology* 128:65–76

66. Lifson, J., Feinberg, M., Reyes, G., Rabin, L., Banapour, B., et al. 1986. Induction of CD4-dependent cell fusion

by the HTLV-III/LAV envelope glycoprotein. *Nature* 323:725–28

67. Lorge, P., Cabiaux, V., Long, L., Ruysschaert, J. 1986. Fusion of Newcastle disease virus with liposomes: role of the lipid composition of liposomes. *Biochim. Biophys. Acta* 858:312–16

68. Luytjes, W., Sturman, L. S., Bredenbeek, P. J., Charite, J., van der Zeijst, B. A., et al. 1987. Primary structure of the glycoprotein E2 of Coronavirus MHV-A59 and identification of the trypsin cleavage site. *Virology* 161:479–87

69. Maddon, P. J., Dalgleish, A. G., McDougal, J. S., Clapham, P. R., Weiss, R. A., Axel, R. 1986. The T4 gene encodes the AIDS virus receptor and is expressed in the immune system and the brain. *Cell* 47:333–48

70. Malhotra, V., Orci, L., Glick, B. S., Block, M. R., Rothman, J. E. 1988. Role of an N-ethylmaleimide-sensitive transport component in promoting fusion of transport vesicles with cisternae of the Golgi stack. *Cell* 54:221–27

71. Marsh, M., Helenius, A. 1989. Virus entry into animal cells. *Adv. Vir. Res.* 36:107–51

72. McCaffrey, G., Clay, F. J., Kelsay, K., Sprague, G. F. 1987. Identification and regulation of a gene required for cell fusion during mating of the yeast *Saccharomyces cerevisiae. Mol. Cell. Biol.* 7:2680–90

73. McClure, M. O., Marsh, M., Weiss, R. A. 1988. Human immunodeficiency virus infection of CD4-bearing cells occurs by a pH-independent mechanism. *EMBO J.* 7:513–18

74. McCune, J. M., Rabin, L. B., Feinberg, M. B., Lieberman, M., Kosek, J. C., et al. 1988. Endoproteolytic cleavage of gp160 is required for the activation of Human immunodeficiency virus. *Cell* 53:55–67

75. Meers, P., Bentz, J., Alford, D., Nir, S., Papahadjopoulos, D., et al. 1988. Synexin enhances the aggregation rate but not the fusion rate of liposomes. *Biochem.* 27:4430–38

76. Melancon, P., Glick, B. S., Malhotra, V., Weidman, P. J., Serafini, T., et al. 1987. Involvement of GTP-binding "G" proteins in transport through the Golgi stack. *Cell* 51:1053–62

77. Mellman, I., Fuchs, R., Helenius, A. 1986. Acidification of the endocytic and exocytic pathways. *Annu. Rev. Biochem.* 55:663–700

78. Menko, A. S., Boettiger, D. 1987. Occupation of the extracellular matrix receptor, integrin, is a control point for myogenic differentiation. *Cell* 51:51–57

79. Metsikko, K., van Meer, G., Simons, K. 1986. Reconstitution of the fusogenic activity of vesicular stomatitis virus. *EMBO J.* 5:3429–35

80. Miller, N., Hutt-Fletcher, L. M. 1988. A monoclonal antibody to glycoprotein gp85 inhibits fusion but not attachment of Epstein-Barr virus. *J. Virol.* 62:2366–72

81. Momayezi, M., Lumpert, C. J., Kersken, H., Gras, U., Plattner, H., et al. 1987. Exocytosis induction in *Paramecium tetraurelia* cells by exogenous phosphoprotein phosphatase in vivo and in vitro: possible involvement of calcineurin in exocytic membrane fusion. *J. Cell Biol.* 105:181–89

82. Morris, S., Sarkar, D., White, J., Blumenthal, R. 1989. Kinetics of pH-dependent fusion between 3T3 fibroblasts expressing influenza hemagglutinin and red blood cells. Measurement by dequenching of fluorescence. *J. Biol. Chem.* 264:3972–78

83. Morrison, T. 1988. Structure, function, and intracellular processing of paramyxovirus membrane proteins. *Vir. Res.* 10:113–36

84. Mundy, D. I., Strittmatter, W. J. 1985. Requirement for metalloendoprotease in exocytosis: evidence in mast cells and adrenal chromaffin cells. *Cell* 40:645–56

85. Murata, M., Sugahara, Y., Takahashi, S., Ohnishi, S. I. 1987. pH-dependent membrane fusion activity of a synthetic twenty amino acid peptide with the same sequence as that of the hydrophobic segment of influenza virus hemagglutinin. *J. Biochem.* 102:957–62

86. Newman, A. P., Ferro-Novick, S. 1987. Characterization of new mutants in the early part of the yeast secretory pathway isolated by a 3[H] mannose suicide selection. *J. Cell Biol.* 105:1587–94

87. Nir, S. 1986. Kinetics and extent of fusion between Sendai virus and erythrocyte ghosts: Application of a mass action kinetic model. *Biochemistry* 25:2155–61

88. Nir, S., Klappe, K., Hoekstra, D. 1986. Mass action analysis of kinetics and extent of fusion between Sendai virus and phospholipid vesicles. *Biochemistry* 25:8261–66

89. Notter, M., Leary, J., Balduzzi, P. 1982. Adsorption of Rous sarcoma virus to genetically susceptible and resistant chicken cells studied by laser flow cytometry. *J. Virol.* 41:958–64

90. Novick, S. L., Hoekstra, D. 1988.

Membrane penetration of Sendai virus glycoproteins during the early stages of fusion with liposomes as determined by hydrophobic photoaffinity labeling. *Proc. Natl. Acad. Sci. USA* 85:7433–37

91. Ohki, S., Doyle, D., Flanagan, T., Hui, S. W., Mayhew, E., eds. 1988. *Molecular Mechanisms of Membrane Fusion.* New York: Plenum

92. Ohnishi, S.-I. 1988. Fusion of viral envelopes with cellular membranes. See Ref. 29, pp. 257–96

93. Omar, A., Koblet, H. 1988. Semliki forest virus particles containing only the E1 envelope glycoprotein are infectious and can induce cell-cell fusion. *Virology* 166:17–23

94. Omar, A., Koblet, H. 1989. The use of sulfite to study the mechanism of membrane fusion induced by E1 of Semliki forest virus. *Virology* 168:177–79

95. Parente, R. A., Nir, S., Szoka, F. C. 1988. pH-dependent fusion of phosphatidylcholine small vesicles. Induction by a synthetic amphipathic peptide. *J. Biol. Chem.* 263:4724–30

96. Paterson, R. G., Hiebert, S. W., Lamb, R. A. 1985. Expression at the cell surface of biologically active fusion and hemagglutinin/neuraminidase proteins of the paramyxovirus simian virus 5 from cloned cDNA. *Proc. Natl. Acad. Sci. USA* 82:7520–24

97. Pinter, A., Chen, T.-E., Lowry, A., Cortez, N., Silagi, S. 1986. Ecotropic murine leukemia virus-induced fusion of murine cells. *J. Virol.* 57:1048–54

98. Pinter, A., Honnen, W., Tilley, S., Bona, C., Zaghouani, H., et al. 1989. Oligomeric structure of gp41, the transmembrane protein of human immunodeficiency virus type 1. *J. Virol.* 63:2674–79

99. Presley, J. F., Brown, D. T. 1989. The proteolytic cleavage of pE2 to envelope glycoprotein E2 is not strictly required for maturation of Sindbis virus. *J. Virol.* 63:1975–80

100. Primakoff, P., Hyatt, H., Tredick-Kline, J. 1987. Identification and purification of a sperm surface protein with a potential role in sperm-egg membrane fusion. *J. Cell Biol.* 104:141–49

101. Racevskis, J., Sarkar, N. 1980. Murine mammary tumor virus structural protein interactions: formation of oligomeric complexes with cleavable cross-linking agents. *J. Virol.* 35:937–948

102. Rand, R. P. 1981. Interacting phospholipid bilayers: measured forces and induced structural changes. *Annu. Rev. Biophys. Bioeng.* 10:277–314

103. Redmond, S., Peters, G., Dickson, C. 1984. Mouse mammary tumor virus can mediate cell fusion at reduced pH. *Virology* 133:393–402

104. Rodiguez, J. F., Paez, E., Esteban, M. 1987. A 14,000-Mr envelope protein of vaccinia virus is involved in cell fusion and forms covalently linked trimers. *J. Virol.* 61:395–404

105. Roe, J. L., Farach, H., Strittmatter, W. J., Lennarz, W. J. 1988. Evidence for involvement of metalloendoproteases in a step in sea urchin gamete fusion. *J. Cell Biol.* 107:539–44

106. Ronnholm, R., Pettersson, R. F. 1987. Complete nucleotide sequence of the M RNA segment of Uukuniemi virus encoding the membrane glycoproteins G1 and G2. *Virology* 160:191–202

107. Roos, D. S., Davidson, R., Choppin, P. 1987. Control of membrane fusion in polyethylene glycol-resistant cell mutants: application to fusion technology. In *Cell Fusion*, ed. A. E. Sowers pp. 123–44. New York: Plenum

108. Rose, J. K., Doms, R. W. 1988. Regulation of protein export from the endoplasmic reticulum. *Annu. Rev. Cell Biol.* 4:257–88

109. Rosenberg, J., Szabo, A., Rheuark, D., Kayalar, C. 1985. Correlation between fusion and the developmental regulation of membrane glycoproteins in L6 myoblasts. *Proc. Natl. Acad. Sci. USA* 82: 8409–13

110. Ruigrok, R. W. H., Aitken, A., Calder, L. J., Martin, S. R., Skehel, J. J., et al. 1988. Studies on the structure of the influenza virus haemagglutinin at the pH of membrane fusion. *J. Gen. Virol.* 69:2785–95

111. Russell, D. L., Dalrymple, J. M., Johnston, R. E. 1989. Sindbis virus mutations which coordinately affect glycoprotein processing, penetration, and virulence in mice. *J. Virol.* 63:1619–29

112. Salminen, A., Novick, P. 1987. A *ras*-like protein is required for a post-Golgi event in yeast secretion. *Cell* 49:527–38

113. Sarkar, D. P., Blumenthal, R. 1989. The role of the target membrane structure in fusion with Sendai virus. *Membr. Biochem.* in press

113a. Sarkar, D. P., Morris, S. J., Eidelman, O., Zimmerberg, J., Blumenthal, R. 1989. Initial stages of influenza hemagglutinin-induced cell fusion monitored simultaneously by two fluorescent events: cytoplasmic continuity and lipid mixing. *J. Cell Biol.* 109:113–22

114. Satir, B. H., Hamasaki, T., Reichman, M., Murtaugh, T. J. 1989. Species dis-

tribution of a phosphoprotein (parafusin) involved in exocytosis. *Proc. Natl. Acad. Sci. USA* 86:930–32

115. Schawaller, M., Smith, G. E., Skehel, J. J., Wiley, D. C. 1989. Studies with crosslinking reagents on the oligometric structure of the env glycoprotein of HIV. *Virology* 172:367–69

116. Scheule, R. K. 1987. Fusion of Sindbis virus with model membranes containing phosphatidylethanolamine: implications for protein-induced membrane fusion. *Biochim. Biophys. Acta* 899:185–95

117. Sechoy, O., Philippot, J. R., Bienvenue, A. 1986. Preparation and characterization of F-protein vesicles isolated from Sendai virus by means of octyl glucoside. *Biochim. Biophys. Acta* 857:1–12

118. Sechoy, O., Philippot, J. R., Bienvenue, A. 1987. F protein-F protein interaction within the Sendai virus identified by native bonding or chemical cross-linking. *J. Biol. Chem.* 262:11519–23

119. Shioda, T., Wakao, S., Suzu, S., Shibuta, H. 1988. Differences in bovine parainfluenza 3 virus variants studied by sequencing of the genes of viral envelope proteins. *Virology* 162:388–96

120. Siegel, D. P. 1986. Inverted micellar intermediates and the transition between lamellar, cubic and inverted hexagonal amphiphile phases. III. Isotropic and inverted cube state formation via intermediates in transitions between L and H-II phases. *Chem. Phys. Lipids* 42:279–301

121. Sinangil, F., Loyter, A., Volsky, D. J. 1988. Quantitative measurement of fusion between human immunodeficiency virus and cultured cells using membrane fluorescence dequenching. *FEBS* 239:88–92

122. Sowers, A., ed 1987. (ed.), Cell Fusion. New York: Plenum

123. Spear, P. 1987. Virus-induced cell fusion. See Ref. 122, pp. 3–32

124. Spear, P., Wittels, M., Fuller, A., WuDunn, D., Johnson, R. 1989. Herpes simplex virus: pathway of entry into cells. In *Cell Biology of Virus Entry, Replication, and Pathogenesis*, ed. R. Compans, A. Helenius, M. Oldstone 90:163–75. New York: Liss

125. Spruce, A. E., Iwata, A., White, J. M., Almers, W. 1989. Patch clamp studies of single cell fusion events mediated by a viral fusion protein. *Nature* In press

126. Stannard, L., Oveta-Fuller, A., Spear, P. G. 1987. Herpes simplex virus glycoproteins associated with different morphological entities projecting from the virion envelope. *J. Gen. Virol.* 68:715–25

127. Stegmann, T., Booy, F. P., Wilschut, J. 1987. Effects of low pH on influenza virus. Activation and inactivation of the membrane fusion capacity of the hemagglutinin. *J. Biol. Chem.* 262:17744–49

128. Stegmann, T., Doms, R. W., Helenius, A. 1989. Protein-mediated membrane fusion. *Annu. Rev. Biophys. Biophys. Chem.* 18:187–211

129. Stegmann, T., Hoekstra, D., Scherphof, G., Wilschut, J. 1986. Fusion activity of influenza virus: a comparison between biological and artificial target membrane vesicles. *J. Biol. Chem.* 261:10966–69

130. Stegmann, T., Morselt, H. W. M., Booy, F. P., van Breemen, J. F. L., Scherphof, G., et al. 1987. Functional reconstitution of influenza virus envelopes. *EMBO J.* 6:2651–59

131. Stegmann, T., Morselt, W., Scholma, J., Wilschut, J. 1987. Fusion of influenza virus in an intracellular acidic compartment measured by fluorescence dequenching. *Biochim. Biophys. Acta* 904:165–70

132. Stegmann, T., Nir, S., Wilschut, J. 1989. Membrane fusion activity of influenza virus. Effects of gangliosides and negatively charged phospholipids in target liposomes. *Biochemistry* 28:1698–1704

133. Stein, B. S., Gowda, S. D., Lifson, J. D., Penhallow, R. C., Bensch, K. G., et al. 1987. pH-independent HIV entry into CD4-positive T cells via virus envelope fusion to the plasma membrane. *Cell* 49:659–68

134. Sturman, L. S., Ricard, C. S., Holmes, K. V. 1985. Proteolytic cleavage of the E2 glycoprotein of murine coronavirus: Activation of cell-fusing activity of virions by trypsin and separation of two different 90K cleavage fragments. *J. Virol.* 56:904–11

135. Tersmette, M., van Dongen, J. J., Clapham, P. R., de Goede, R. E., Wolvers-Tettero, I. L., et al. 1989. Human immunodeficiency virus infection studied in CD4-expressing human-murine T-cell hybrids. *Virology* 168:267–73

136. Trueheart, J., Boeke, J. D., Fink, G. R. 1987. Two genes required for cell fusion during yeast conjugation: evidence for a pheromone-induced surface protein. *Mol. Cell. Biol.* 7:2316–28

137. Tsao. Y. S., Huang, L. 1986. Kinetic studies of Sendai virus-target membrane interactions: Independent analysis of

binding and fusion. *Biochemistry* 25: 3971–76

138. Turner, P. R., Jaffe, L., Fein, A. 1986. Regulation of cortical vesicle exocytosis in sea urchin eggs by inositol 1, 4, 5-trisphosphate and GTP-binding protein. *J. Cell Biol.* 102:70–76

139. Urushihara, H., Habata, Y., Yanagisawa, K. 1988. A membrane protein with possible relevance to sexual cell fusion in Dictyostelium discoideum. *Cell Diff. Dev.* 25:81–88

140. Vater, C. A., Jackson, R. C. 1989. Purification and characterization of a cortical secretory vesicle membrane fraction. *Dev. Biol.* In press

141. Veit, M., Schmidt, M. F., Rott, R. 1989. Different palmitoylation of paramyxovirus glycoproteins. *Virology* 168:173–76

142. Vogel, H. H., Provencher, S. W., von Bonsdorff, C. H., Adrian, M., Dubochet, J. 1986. Envelope structure of Semliki Forest virus reconstructed from cryoelectron micrographs. *Nature* 320:533–35

143. von Heijne, G. 1985. Signal sequences The limits of variation. *J. Mol. Biol.* 184:99–105

144. Wakelam, M. J. 1988. Myoblast fusion. A mechanistic approach. *Curr. Top. Membr. Transp.* 32:87–112

145. Waxham, M. N., Wolinsky, J. S. 1986. A fusing Mumps virus variant selected from a nonfusing parent with the neuraminidase inhibitor 2-deoxy-2,3-dehyrdro-N-acetylneuraminic acid. *Virology* 151:286–95

146. Weidman, P. J., Melancon, P., Block, M. R., Rothman, J. E. 1989. Binding of an N-ethylmaleimide-sensitive fusion protein to Golgi membranes requires both a soluble protein(s) and an integral membrane receptor. *J. Cell Biol.* 108:1589–96

147. Wengler, G., Wengler, G., Nowak, T., Wahn, K. 1987. Analysis of the influence of proteolytic cleavage on the structural organization of the surface of the West Nile flavivirus leads to the isolation of a protease-resistant E protein oligomer from the viral surface. *Virology* 160:210–19

148. Wertz, G. W., Stott, E. J., Young, K. K. Y., Anderson, K., Ball, L. A. 1987. Expression of the fusion protein of human respiratory syncytial virus from recombinant vaccinia virus vectors and protection of vaccinated mice. *J. Virol.* 61:293–301

149. Wharton, S. A. 1987. The role of influenza virus haemagglutinin in membrane fusion. *Microbiol. Sci.* 4:119–24

150. Wharton, S. A., Martin, S. R., Ruigrok, R. W., Skehel, J. J., Wiley, D. C. 1988. Membrane fusion by peptide analogues of influenza virus haemagglutinin. *J. Gen. Virol.* 69:1847–57

151. Wharton, S. A., Ruigrok, R. W. H., Martin, S. R., Skehel, J. J., Bayley, P. M., et al. 1988. Conformational aspects of the acid-induced fusion mechanism of influenza virus hemagglutinin. *J. Biol. Chem.* 263:4474–80

152. Wharton, S. A., Skehel, J. J., Wiley, D. C. 1986. Studies of influenza haemagglutinin-mediated membrane fusion. *Virology* 149:27–35

153. White, J., Doms, R., Gething, M.-J., Kielian, M., Helenius, A. 1986. Viral membrane fusion proteins. In *Virus Attachment and Entry into Cells,* ed. R. L. Crowell, K. Lonberg-Holm, pp. 54–59. Am. Soc. Microbiol., Washington, DC

154. White, J., Kielian, M., Helenius, A. 1983. Membrane fusion proteins of enveloped animal viruses. *Q. Rev. Biophys.* 16:151–95

155. White, J. M., Wilson, I. A. 1987. Antipeptide antibodies detect steps in a protein conformational change: Low-pH activation of the influenza virus hemagglutinin. *J. Cell Biol.* 105:2887–96

156. Wiley, D. C., Skehel, J. J. 1987. The structure and function of the hemagglutinin membrane glycoprotein of influenza virus. *Annu. Rev. Biochem.* 56:365–94

157. Wilschut, J. 1988. Membrane interactions and fusion. In *Energetics of the Secretion Response,* ed. J. W. Akkerman, II: 63–80. Boca Raton, Fla: CRC

158. Wilson, D. W., Wilcox, C. A., Flynn, G. C., Chen, E., Kuang, W.-J., et al. 1989. A fusion protein required for vesicle-mediated transport in both mammalian cells and yeast. *Nature* 339:355–59

159. Yamada, S., Ohnishi, S. 1986. Vesicular stomatitis virus binds and fuses with phospholipid domain in target cell membranes. *Biochemistry* 25:3703–8

160. Yanagimachi, Y. 1988. Sperm-egg fusion. *Curr. Top. Membr. Transp.* 32:3–43

161. Zhu, Q., Courtney, R. J. 1988. Chemical crosslinking of glycoproteins on the envelope of herpes simplex virus. *Virology* 167:377–84

Annu. Rev. Phsyiol. 1990. 52:699–708

RENAL EFFECTS OF ATRIAL NATRIURETIC FACTOR

Martin G. Cogan

Division of Nephrology, Veterans Administration Medical Center and University of California, San Francisco, California

KEY WORDS: glomerular filtration rate, renal hemodynamics, tubular transport, cyclic GMP, diuretic

INTRODUCTION

A prominent effect of atrial natriuretic factor (ANF), indeed that for which it is named, is the ability to effect a solute and water diuresis. The renal mechanisms responsible for this natriuresis and diuresis have been subjects of intensive inquiry since the hormone's discovery in 1981.

The following sections summarize direct and indirect means by which ANF alters renal electrolyte handling. For the direct effects, three primary criteria have been used to define nephron sites that respond to ANF: a nephron segment should (*a*) have biological ANF receptors; (*b*) generate ANF's second messenger 3',5'-cyclic guanosine monophosphate (cGMP) in response to ANF; and (*c*) respond functionally when exposed to ANF. For physiologic responses, only studies that have examined tubular transport directly and specifically through use of micropuncture or microperfusion will be reviewed. Indirect techniques (e.g., free water clearance or lithium clearance) will not be considered, since they are insufficiently rigorous with respect to site-specificity definition.

DIRECT EFFECTS OF ANF ON RENAL CIRCULATION

Glomerular Filtration Rate

The renal glomerulus is a rich repository of ANF receptors (4, 7, 10, 23, 30, 38, 42) and generates cGMP in response to ANF (9, 26, 44, 56, 58), as summarized in Table 1. Consonant with the presence of a cell signaling

0066-4278/90/0315-0699$02.00

Table 1 Nephron sites of action of ANF

Nephron site	Receptor density	cGMP generation	Physiologic response
Glomerulus	+ + + +	+ + + +	+ + + +
Proximal	0	0	0[a]
Loop	0	+	0
CCT	0	+	+
MCT	+ + +	+ + +	+ + +

[a] Conflicting information regarding antagonism of angiotensin II.

system, ANF markedly affects glomerular hemodynamics, by augmenting glomerular filtration rate (GFR) (5, 12, 16, 17, 25–27, 33, 36, 37).

The principal mechanism by which ANF increases GFR is by raising the glomerular hydraulic pressure (16, 17, 25, 52). The intraglomerular capillary pressure in both superficial and juxtamedullary nephrons is increased primarily by afferent arteriolar dilatation (16, 17, 39, 47, 60). In addition, there is a tendency for ANF to induce efferent arteriolar constriction (16, 39), thereby maintaining total renal vascular resistance relatively constant. ANF also increases the glomerular permeability coefficient (K_f) (16, 17), probably because of relaxation of mesangial cells (2). Glomerular hyperfiltration is sustained because tubulo-glomerular feedback is inhibited by ANF (25).

The glomerulus was one of the first sites documented in vivo in which a functional change induced by ANF was correlated with a rise in intracellular cGMP. A marked increase in cGMP production by glomerular mesangial cells accompanies the ANF-induced increment in GFR. Some of the cGMP egresses from the cells into the glomerular ultrafiltrate within Bowman's space (26) and ultimately is excreted into the urine (26, 62). This glomerulogenous cGMP is an excellent biochemical marker of the natriuretic response attributable to ANF (62). Administration of a permeable cGMP analogue without ANF faithfully recapitulates the renal hemodynamic effects of ANF (26). These findings identify cGMP as the second messenger for ANF's actions on glomerular function in vivo.

Renal Blood Flow

Several methods have shown that ANF does not change absolute or regional distribution of renal blood flow. Although a brief and mild increase in total renal blood flow can occur during the initial two min following continuous ANF administration (6, 37), the natriuresis is sustained despite return of renal blood flow to a control level (6, 28, 37, 57). ANF differs from glucagon and other vasodilators that augment GFR by increasing renal blood flow and depressing filtration fraction. Indeed, ANF is a unique hormone in being able to increase GFR above a normal value without altering total renal blood flow and causing filtration fraction to increase. When ANF is infused, the relative cortical/medullary distribution of blood flow has been reported to be decreased (19, 24), unaltered (28, 57), or increased (27a). The functional significance of relative renal blood flow distributional alteration is controversial even when documented.

DIRECT EFFECTS OF ANF ON SEGMENTAL TUBULAR TRANSPORT

Proximal Tubule

The proximal tubule lacks ANF biologic receptors, has no particulate guanylate cyclase, and does not generate cGMP in response to ANF (4, 7, 9, 10, 23, 26, 38, 42, 44, 56, 58). Consistent with this lack of biochemical signaling capacity, most functional studies have demonstrated that ANF is devoid of transport effects in the proximal nephron. Four in vivo and in vitro microperfusion studies of the S_1, S_2, and S_3 subsegments of proximal convoluted and straight tubules in the rat or rabbit have failed to find any effect by ANF on sodium, bicarbonate, and chloride transport (1, 3, 35, 40). ANF also does not alter phosphate absorption or organic acid secretion by the proximal tubule (1, 20, 40).

In the free-flow state in vivo, five micropuncture studies have failed to show any effect by ANF on sodium, bicarbonate, and chloride transport in the rat proximal convoluted tubule (5, 12, 27, 33, 54), which confirms the microperfusion studies. In these free-flow studies, absolute rates of solute and water transport increased appropriately for the increment in delivery attributable to the rise in single nephron GFR (i.e. glomerulo-tubular balance was unaffected by ANF).

A provocative report suggested that ANF had no effect on proximal sodium transport unless there was pre-stimulation with angiotensin II (22). The results of this study, which used the sometimes problematic technique of the shrinking split-droplet, could not be confirmed when the more reliable technique of in vivo microperfusion was utilized (35). Other indirect neurohumoral interactions of ANF and angiotensin II might account for changes in proximal transport (see below).

Loop Of Henle

Cells of the loop of Henle lack ANF receptors (7) and respond with little cGMP generation when ANF is administered (9, 44, 58). In vivo and in vitro microperfusion studies have found no effect of ANF on cortical or medullary thick ascending limb sodium chloride transport in the rat and rabbit (29, 48). Changes in medullary solute concentration consequent to the high luminal flow rate and vasa recta hydraulic pressure (41) can alter transport of solutes and water in the thin limbs of Henle, but these effects in the free-flow state are small (49).

Collecting Ducts

Relatively low levels of biologic receptors and cGMP generation exist in the cortical collecting duct (7, 44). In vitro microperfusion studies have shown that ANF inhibits sodium chloride and vasopressin-stimulated water absorption in the cortical collecting duct and that these effects are mediated by cGMP (15, 46).

The highest density of receptors and of cGMP generation in the collecting system occurs in the inner medullary collecting duct (4, 10, 23, 30, 38, 42, 44), as summarized in Table 1. Studies using inner medullary collecting duct cells in culture have shown that sodium uptake is depressed by ANF (63). This process is effected via cGMP-mediated inhibition of a sodium channel resident in the cell membrane (31). ANF does not change NaCl permeability of the tubule (50). ANF also inhibits vasopressin-stimulated osmotic water permeability in this segment (45). ANF-induced reduction in sodium and water transport by the inner medullary and papillary collecting duct has been confirmed in vivo using micropuncture and microcatheterization techniques (18, 54, 55, 59).

INDIRECT TRANSPORT EFFECTS BY ANF CAUSED BY ALTERED NEUROENDOCRINE FUNCTION

ANF inhibits biosynthesis of both renin and aldosterone (6, 37) and antagonizes the action of angiotensin II on cells bearing receptors for both hormones (2). ANF also decreases the activity of the sympathetic nervous system and inhibits vasopressin release and action (15, 45). These neuroendocrine-mediated effects of ANF can affect transport along the entire length of the nephron: glomerulus (angiotensin II, nerve activity, and vasopressin); proximal tubule (angiotensin II and nerve activity); loop of Henle (vasopressin and nerve activity); and collecting tubule (aldosterone, vasopressin, and nerve activity). These secondary transport inhibitory responses due to change in hormone levels may be additive to those caused by direct alteration in GFR and epithelial function effected by ANF.

INTEGRATED EFFECTS BY ANF ON RENAL SOLUTE EXCRETION

Relative Importance of Glomerular vs Collecting Duct Actions of ANF

There is substantial evidence that the primary sites of action of ANF are the beginning and end of the nephron; the glomerulus and the inner medullary collecting duct (see above). Substantial controversy persists regarding the relative importance of these two effects.

The possibility that a rise in GFR can effect a natriuresis is not a new concept, but one that has fallen into disfavor in recent years. Previous protocols used to examine this issue, in which GFR rises slowly because of protein feeding (32), are not directly comparable to the marked, acute rise in GFR uniquely provoked by ANF. The argument that an increase in GFR can in itself be responsible for substantial natriuresis rests on the observation from in vivo microperfusion and micropuncture studies that load-dependence of sodium chloride transport in the proximal nephron (as distinguished from load-dependence of sodium bicarbonate transport) is very poor; i. e. there is little or no proximal glomerulo-tubular balance for sodium chloride (21, 33). When GFR acutely rises above a normal euvolemic value, virtually the entire increment in filtered sodium chloride load is transmitted out of the proximal tubule (33). Although load-dependence of sodium chloride transport in the loop of Henle and the rest of the distal nephron is good, it is not perfect (43, 51). Indeed, only ~10% of the increment in sodium chloride delivery to the distal nephron need be unreabsorbed to account for the magnitude of natriuresis and chloruresis observed following ANF.

Several strategies have been employed to evaluate the relative potencies of the glomerular vs tubular effects of ANF. One approach has been to prevent the normal ANF-induced increase in GFR to occur by partial clamping of the aorta above the origin of the renal artery. When GFR is restrained from rising during ANF infusion, there is either no change in urinary sodium excretion or the subsequent natriuresis is greatly attenuated to ≤ 10% of the control value (8, 12, 14, 53). The selective direct tubular (non-GFR) transport effects were therefore concluded to play only a minor role in the natriuresis usually observed with ANF.

Another approach to settle the GFR/tubule controversy surrounding ANF has been to compare the magnitude of natriuresis when glomerular hyperfiltration is induced by an agent (glucagon) that stimulates rather than inhibits sodium transport in the distal nephron. Despite hormonally-mediated changes in distal sodium transport in opposite directions, comparable glomerular hyperfiltration induced by either ANF or by glucagon elicited a similar magnitude of natriuresis (61). The primacy of GFR vs the tubular response was again supported.

A final approach has been to compare the degree of natriuresis induced by ANF with a drug that does not change GFR but mimics ANF's ability to inhibit the medullary collecting duct sodium channel. Such a drug, amiloride, is known to be an impotent diuretic and natriuretic agent and is thus qualitatively dissimilar in mechanism to ANF, which is a powerful diuretic.

Thus these three approaches have led to the conclusion that ANF acts primarily hemodynamically, by increasing GFR, to render a natriuresis. The impact of inhibiting sodium transport in the inner medullary collecting duct is minor compared to changes in sodium handling that occur when ANF augments filtered sodium load. The literature, however, is replete with reports stating that ANF can increase urinary sodium excretion even when there has been no change in GFR. Such studies have been difficult to rigorously interpret, since they frequently suffer from technical problems in measuring GFR accurately under dynamic conditions (36). GFR measurement requires multiple determinations under steady-state conditions, often very difficult to achieve given the rapidly changing hemodynamics and urine flow rate encountered with ANF. Even under the best of conditions, GFR measurements frequently suffer from >5–10% inaccuracy. In general, these studies still show a directionally upward trend in GFR when ANF is administered, associated with a relatively small natriuretic response (36).

Influence of Acid-Base Status on Renal Response to ANF

As noted above, the increment in GFR and filtered solute load induced by ANF usually results in increased sodium chloride but not in sodium bicarbonate delivered out of the proximal tubule to the distal nephron. This differential anion handling occurs because the proximal nephron is adept in adjusting transport to changed delivery of sodium bicarbonate but not sodium chloride (33).

In metabolic alkalosis, however, reabsorption of sodium bicarbonate is rendered static and unresponsive to load (33, 34). With metabolic alkalosis, the basal level of GFR is usually low so that the high bicarbonate concentration is accompanied by a normal filtered bicarbonate load. When GFR is normalized by ANF administration, the increment in sodium bicarbonate load cannot be reabsorbed because of suppressed proximal acidification by alkalemia, so it is transmitted out of the proximal tubule into the distal tubule (11). Since the loop and distal nephron are relatively poor at reabsorbing bicarbonate, bicarbonate escapes into the urine. The low filtered concentration and load of chloride explain the relatively low urinary chloride excretion rate. Thus metabolic alkalosis acts to change the anionic composition of the urine following ANF, which results in a sodium bicarbonate rather than sodium chloride diuresis (11, 13).

Impact of Renal Perfusion Pressure and Other Determinants of Sodium Reabsorption on Renal Response to ANF

The complexity of sites and control systems responsible for regulating renal sodium excretion makes it inevitable that a single factor never acts in an independent, unregulated fashion. Since an important mechanism by which ANF effects a natriuresis is by increasing GFR through augmentation of glomerular capillary pressure, it is not surprising that anything that reduces renal perfusion pressure counteracts effects of ANF (8, 12, 14, 53). In this regard, the systemic hemodynamic effects of ANF act in a negative feedback fashion to blunt its own natriuretic response. By causing significant systemic vasodilation and hypotension, ANF attenuates its ability to cause glomerular hypertension and hyperfiltration.

Similarly, administration of ANF in the setting of any antinatriuretic stimulus predictably results in diminished natriuresis. Such depressed functional responses to ANF have been recorded in many conditions of high renin-angiotensin-aldosterone and/or sympathetic nervous system activities, as in congestive heart failure, cirrhosis, nephrosis, and some forms of hypertension. Blunting of ANF's effects due to a concurrent antinatriuretic stimulant gives no insight, however, into the sites and/or mechanisms of interaction.

Literature Cited

1. Ando, R., Sasaki, S., Shiigai, T., Takeuchi, J. 1987. Lack of effect of alpha-human atrial natriuretic polypeptide on volume reabsorption and p-aminohippuric acid secretion in the rabbit proximal straight tubule. *Jpn. J. Physiol.* 37:81–91

2. Appel, R. G., Wang, J., Simonson, M. S., Dunn, M. J. 1986. A mechanism by which atrial natriuretic factor mediates its glomerular actions. *Am. J. Physiol.* (Renal Fluid Electrolyte Physiol. 20) 251:F1036–42

3. Baum, M., Toto, R. D. 1986. Lack of a direct effect of atrial natriuretic factor in the rabbit proximal tubule. *Am. J. Physiol.* (Renal Fluid Electrolyte Physiol. 19) 250:F66–69

4. Bianchi, G., Gutkowska, J., Thibault, G., Garcia, R., Genest, J., Cantin, M. 1985. Radioautographic localization of ^{125}I-atrial natriuretic factor (ANF) in rat tissues. *Histochemistry* 82:441–52

5. Briggs, J. P., Steipe, B., Schubert, G., Schnermann, J. 1982. Micropuncture studies of the renal effects of atrial natriuretic substance. *Pflügers Arch.* 395:271–76

6. Burnett, J. C. Jr., Granger, J. P., Opgenorth, T. J. 1984. Effects of synthetic atrial natriuretic factor on renal function and renin release. *Am. J. Physiol.* (Renal Fluid Electrolyte Physiol. 16) 247:F863–66

7. Butlen, D., Mistaoui, M., Morel, F. 1987. Atrial natriuretic peptide receptors along the rat and rabbit nephrons: [^{125}I]alpha-rat atrial natriuretic peptide binding in microdissected glomeruli and tubules. *Pflügers Arch.* 408:356–65

8. Camargo, M. J. F., Atlas, S. A., Maack, T. 1986. Role of increased glomerular filtration rate in atrial natriuretic factor-induced natriuresis in the rat. *Life Sci.* 38:2397–2404

9. Chabardes, D., Montegut, M., Mistaoui, M., Butlen, D., Morel, F. 1987. Atrial natriuretic peptide effects on cGMP and cAMP contents in microdissected glomeruli and segments of the rat and rabbit nephrons. *Pflügers Arch.* 408:366–72

10. Chai, S. Y., Sexton, P. M., Allen, A. M., Figdor, R., Mendelsohn, F. A. O. 1986. In vitro autoradiographic localization of ANP receptors in rat kidney and adrenal gland. *Am. J. Physiol.* (Renal Fluid Electrolyte Physiol. 19) 250: F753–57

11. Cogan, M. G. 1985. Atrial natriuretic factor ameliorates chronic metabolic alkalosis by increasing glomerular filtration. *Science* 229:1405–7

12. Cogan, M. G. 1986. Atrial natriuretic factor can increase renal solute excretion primarily by raising glomerular filtration. *Am. J. Physiol.* (Renal Fluid Electrolyte Physiol. 19) 250:F22–26

13. Cogan, M. G., Huang, C.-L., Liu, F.-Y., Madden, D., Wong, K. 1986. Effect of atrial natriuretic factor on acid-base homeostasis. *J. Hypertension* 4(Suppl. 2)S31–34

14. Davis, C. L., Briggs, J. P. 1987. Effect of reduction in renal artery pressure on atrial natriuretic peptide-induced natriuresis. *Am. J. Physiol.* (Renal Fluid Electrolyte Physiol. 21) 252:F146–53

15. Dillingham, M. A., Anderson, R. J. 1986. Inhibition of vasopressin action by

atrial natriuretic factor. *Science* 231: 1572–73

16. Dunn, B. R., Ichikawa, I., Pfeffer, J. M., Troy, J. L., Brenner, B. M. 1986. Renal and systemic hemodynamic effects of synthetic atrial natriuretic peptide in the anesthetized rat. *Circ. Res.* 59:237–46

17. Fried, T. A., McCoy, R. N., Osgood, R. W., Stein, J. H. 1986. Effect of atriopeptin II on determinants of glomerular filtration rate in the in vitro perfused dog glomerulus. *Am. J. Physiol.* (Renal Fluid Electrolyte Physiol. 19) 250: F1119–22

18. Fried, T. A., Osgood, R. W., Stein, J. H. 1988. Tubular site(s) of action of atrial natriuretic peptide in the rat. *Am. J. Physiol.* (Renal Fluid Electrolyte Physiol. 24) 255:F313–16

19. Fujioka, S., Tamaki, T., Fukui, K., Okahara, T., Abe, Y. 1985. Effects of a synthetic human atrial natriuretic polypeptide on regional blood flow in rats. *Eur. J. Pharmacol.* 109:301–4

20. Goldinger, J. M., Hong, R. B., Lee, S. H., DeBold, A. J., Hong, S. K. 1986. Lack of interaction between atrial natriuretic factor and renal organic anion transport system. *Fed. Proc. Soc. Exp. Biol. Med.* 182:358–63

21. Green, R., Moriarity, R. J., Giebisch, G. 1981. Ionic requirements of proximal tubular fluid reabsorption: Flow dependence of fluid transport. *Kidney Int.* 20:580–87

22. Harris, P. J., Thomas, D., Morgan, T. O. 1987. Atrial natriuretic peptide inhibits angiotensin-stimulated proximal tubular sodium and water reabsorption. *Nature* 326:697–98

23. Healy, E. P., Fanestil, D. D. 1986. Localization of atrial natriuretic peptide binding sites within the rat kidney. *Am. J. Physiol.* (Renal Fluid Electrolyte Physiol. 19) 250:F573–78

24. Hirata, Y., Ganguli, M., Tobian, L., Iwai, J. 1984. Dahl S rats have increased natriuretic factor in atria but are markedly hyporesponsive to it. *Hypertension* 6 (Suppl. I):I-148-I-155

25. Huang, C.-L., Cogan, M. G. 1987. Atrial natriuretic factor inhibits maximal tubuloglomerular feedback response. *Am. J. Physiol.* (Renal Fluid Electrolyte Physiol. 21) 252:F825–28

26. Huang, C.-L., Ives, H. E., Cogan, M. G. 1986. *In vivo* evidence that cGMP is the second messenger for atrial natriuretic factor. *Proc. Natl. Acad. Sci. USA.* 83:8015–18

27. Huang, C.-L., Lewicki, J., Johnson, L. K., Cogan, M. G. 1985. Renal mech-

anism of action of rat atrial natriuretic factor. *J. Clin. Invest.* 75:769–73

27a. Jaschke, W., Sievers, R. E., Lipton, M. J., Cogan, M. G. 1989. Cine-computed tomographic assessment of regional renal blood flow. *Acta Radiol.* In press

28. Kiberd, B., Larson, T., Jamison, R. L. 1987. Effect of atrial natriuretic factor on medullary blood flow. *Am. J. Physiol.* (Renal Fluid Electrolyte Physiol. 21): 252:F1112–17

29. Kondo, Y., Imai, M., Kangawa, K., Matsuo, H. 1986. Lack of direct action of alpha-human atrial natriuretic polypeptide on the in vitro perfused segments of Henle's loop isolated from rabbit kidney. *Pflügers Arch.* 406:273–78

30. Koseki, C., Hayashi, Y., Torikai, S., Furuya, M., Ohnuma, N., Imai, M. 1986. Localization of binding sites for alpha-rat atrial natriuretic polypeptide in rat kidney. *Am. J. Physiol.* (Renal Fluid Electrolyte Physiol. 19) 250:F210–16

31. Light, D. B., Schwiebert, E. M., Karlson, K. H., Stanton, B. A. 1989. Atrial natriuretic peptide inhibits a cation channel in renal inner medullary collecting duct cells. *Science* 243:383–85

32. Lindheimer, M. D., Lalone, R. C., Levinsky, N. G. 1967. Evidence that an acute increase in glomerular filtration has little effect on sodium excretion in the dog unless extracellular volume is expanded. *J. Clin. Invest.* 46:256–65

33. Liu, F.-Y., Cogan, M. G. 1986. Axial heterogeneity of bicarbonate, chloride and water transport in the rat proximal convoluted tubule. Effects of change in luminal flow rate and of alkalemia. *J. Clin. Invest.* 78:1547–57

34. Liu, F.-Y., Cogan, M. G. 1988. Acidification is inhibited in the late proximal convoluted tubule during chronic metabolic alkalosis. *Am. J. Physiol.* (Renal Fluid Electrolyte Physiol. 22) 253:F89–94

35. Liu, F.-Y., Cogan, M.G. 1988. Atrial natriuretic factor does not inhibit basal or angiotensin II-stimulated proximal transport. *Am. J. Physiol.* (Renal Fluid Electrolyte Physiol. 24) 255:F434–37

36. Maack, T., Atlas, S. A., Camargo, M. J. F., Cogan, M. G. 1986. Renal hemodynamic and natriuretic effects of atrial natriuretic factor. *Fed. Proc. Soc. Exp. Biol. Med.* 45:2128–2132

37. Maack, T., Marion, D. N., Camargo, M. J. F., Kleinert, H. D., Laragh, J. H., et al. 1984. Effects of auriculin (atrial natriuretic factor) on blood pressure, renal function, and the renin-aldosterone

system in dogs. *Am. J. Med.* 77:1069–75

38. Mantyh, C. R., Kruger, L., Brecha, N. C., Mantyh, P. W. 1986. Localization of specific binding sites for atrial natriuretic factor in peripheral tissues of the guinea pig, rat, and human. *Hypertension* 8:712–21

39. Marin-Grez, M., Fleming, J. T., Steinhausen, M. 1986. Atrial natriuretic peptide causes pre-glomerular vasodilatation and post-glomerular vasoconstriction in rat kidney. *Nature* 324:472–76

40. McGowan, J. A., Pitts, T. O., Rose, M. E., Puschett, J. B. 1987. The effects of atrial natriuretic peptide on whole-kidney and proximal straight tubular function in the rabbit. *Fed. Proc. Soc. Exp. Biol. Med.* 185:62–68

41. Mendez, R. E., Dunn, B. R., Troy, J. L., Brenner, B. M. 1988. Atrial natriuretic peptide and furosemide effects on hydraulic pressure in the renal papilla. *Kidney Int.* 34:36–42

42. Murphy, K. M. M., McLaughlin, L. L., Michener, M. L., Needleman, P. 1985. Autoradiographic localization of atriopeptin III receptors in rat kidney. *Eur. J. Pharmacol.* 111:291–92

43. Morgan, T., Berliner, R. W. 1969. A study of continuous microperfusion of water and electrolyte movements in the loop of Henle and distal tubule of the rat. *Nephron* 6:388–405

44. Nonoguchi, H., Knepper, M. A., Manganiello. 1987. Effects of atrial natriuretic factor on cyclic guanosine monophosphate and cyclic adenosine monophosphate accumulation in microdissected nephron segments from rats. *J. Clin. Invest.* 79:500–7

45. Nonoguchi, H., Sands, J. M., Knepper, M. A. 1988. Atrial natriuretic factor inhibits vasopressin-stimulated osmotic water permeability in rat inner medullary collecting duct. *J. Clin. Invest.* 82:1383–90

46. Nonoguchi, H., Sands, J. M., Knepper, M. A. 1989. ANF inhibits NaCl and fluid absorption in cortical collecting duct of rat kidney. *Am. J. Physiol.* (Renal Fluid Electrolyte Physiol. 25) 256:F179–86

47. Ohishi, K., Hishida, A., Honda, N. 1988. Direct vasodilatory action of atrial natriuretic factor on canine glomerular afferent arterioles. *Am. J. Physiol.* (Renal Fluid Electrolyte Physiol. 24) 255:F415–20

48. Peterson, L. N., De Rouffignac, C., Sonnenberg, H., Levine, D. Z. 1987. Thick ascending limb response to dDAVP and atrial natriuretic factor in vivo. *Am. J. Physiol.* (Renal Fluid Electrolyte Physiol. 21) 252:F374–81

49. Roy, D. R. 1986. Effect of synthetic ANP on renal and loop of Henle function in the young rat. *Am. J. Physiol.* (Renal Fluid Electrolyte Physiol. 20) 251:F220–25

50. Sands, J. M., Nonoguchi, H., Knepper, M. A. 1988. Hormone effects on NaCl permeability of rat inner medullary collecting duct. *Am. J. Physiol.* (Renal Fluid Electrolyte Physiol. 24) 255:F421–28

51. Schnermann, J. 1968. Microperfusion study of single short loops of Henle in the rat kidney. *Pflügers Arch.* 300:255–62

52. Schnermann, J., Marin-Grez, M., Briggs, J. P. 1986. Filtration pressure response to infusion of atrial natriuretic peptides. *Pflügers Arch.* 406:237–39

53. Seymour, A. A., Smith, S. G. III, Mazack, E. K. 1987. Effects of renal perfusion pressure on the natriuresis induced by atrial natriuretic factor. *Am. J. Physiol.* (Renal Fluid Electrolyte Physiol. 22) 253:F234–38

54. Sonnenberg, H., Cupples, W. A., De-Bold, A. J., Veress, A. T. 1982. Intrarenal localization of the natriuretic effect of cardiac atrial extract. *Can. J. Physiol. Pharmacol.* 60:1149–52

55. Sonnenberg, H., Honrath, U., Chong, C. K., Wilson, D. R. 1986. Atrial natriuretic factor inhibits sodium transport in medullary collecting duct. *Am. J. Physiol.* (Renal Fluid Electrolyte Physiol. 19) 250:F963–66

56. Stokes, T. J. Jr., McConkey, C. L. Jr., Martin, K. J. 1986. Atriopeptin III increases cGMP in glomeruli but not in proximal tubules of dog kidney. *Am. J. Physiol.* (Renal Fluid Electrolyte Physiol. 19) 250:F27–F31

57. Takezawa, K., Cowley, A. W. Jr., Skelton, M., Roman, R. J. 1987. Atriopeptin III alters renal medullary hemodynamics and the pressure-diuresis response in rats. *Am. J. Physiol.* (Renal Fluid Electrolyte Physiol. 21) 252:F992–F1002

58. Tremblay, J., Gerzer, R., Vinay, P., Pang, S. C., Beliveau, R., Hamet, P. 1985. The increase in cGMP by atrial natriuretic factor correlates with the distribution of particulate guanylate cyclase. *FEBS* 181:17–22

59. Van de Stolpe, A., Jamison, R. L. 1988. Micropuncture study of the effect of ANP on the papillary collecting duct in the rat. *Am. J. Physiol.* (Renal Fluid Electrolyte Physiol. 23) 254:F477–83

60. Veldkamp, P. J., Carmines, P. K., Inscho, E. W., Navar, L. G. 1988. Direct evaluation of the microvascular actions of ANP in juxtamedullary nephrons. *Am. J. Physiol.* (Renal Fluid Electrolyte Physiol. 23) 254:F440–44

61. Wong, K. R., Cogan, M. G. 1987. Comparison of the natriuresis and chloruresis associated with glomerular hyperfiltration induced by atrial natriuretic factor or glucagon. *Life Sci.* 40:1595–1600

62. Wong, K. R., Xie, M.-H., Shi, L.-B., Liu, F.-Y., Huang, C.-L., et al. 1988. Urinary cGMP as biological marker of the renal activity of atrial natriuretic factor. *Am. J. Physiol.* (Renal Fluid Electrolyte Physiol. 24) 255:F1220–24

63. Zeidel, M. L., Kikeri, D., Silva, P., Burrowes, M., Brenner, B. M. 1988. Atrial natriuretic peptides inhibit conductive sodium uptake by rabbit inner medullary collecting duct cells. *J. Clin. Invest.* 82:1067–74

Annu. Rev. Physiol. 1990. 52:709–26

TRANSEPITHELIAL OSMOLALITY DIFFERENCES, HYDRAULIC CONDUCTIVITIES, AND VOLUME ABSORPTION IN THE PROXIMAL TUBULE

James A. Schafer

Nephrology Research and Training Center, Departments of Physiology and Biophysics, and Medicine, University of Alabama at Birmingham, Birmingham, Alabama 35294

KEY WORDS: water permeability, water channels, renal interstitium, water transport, solute transport

INTRODUCTION

Volume absorption in leaky epithelia such as the proximal tubule has posed the difficult problem of identifying the location and magnitude of a small osmotic driving force that is responsible for a large volume flow. The traditional explanation for volume flow in the absence of any apparent transepithelial driving force has been the existence of a hyperosmotic compartment in the lateral intercellular spaces produced by active solute transport (17). In the case of the mammalian proximal tubule, however, it is now generally accepted that the diffusion resistance of the lateral intercellular spaces is too small to allow the development of a significant solute concentration gradient. As described by the Wellings & their collaborators (51a–54a), the lateral intercellular space is wrapped around the proximal tubule like a very full skirt with a ruffle at the hemline. But the distance from the tight junction (waist of the skirt) to the basal membrane (ruffled hemline) is no more than the height of the cell, 7–8 μm (53, 54), and one can calculate that diffusion would prevent the development of any osmolality gradient in excess of 1 mOsM (42, 43, 54).

If the spaces cannot be sufficiently hyperosmotic in the proximal tubule, then the osmolality difference required to drive the water absorption must exist between the bulk solution compartments on either side of the epithelium. The challenge has been to demonstrate this previously unmeasured small osmolality difference and to explain how it can result in the rapid rates of volume flow. The first requirement for rapid water flow in the presence of a small driving force is a high transepithelial hydraulic conductivity, which has been demonstrated and has some interesting characteristics.

OSMOTIC WATER PERMEABILITY OF THE PROXIMAL TUBULE

The hydraulic conductivity (e.g. units of ml min^{-1} mm Hg^{-1}) of the proximal tubule is most often expressed in terms of the osmotic water permeability (P_f, μm/sec) for easier comparison to diffusional water permeabilities (19). P_f has been measured in the proximal tubule both in vivo and in vitro, but the values obtained have been quite variable even in the same preparation. As discussed in the excellent review of Berry (7), P_f measurements in both the rat proximal convoluted tubule and in the isolated perfused rabbit proximal convoluted and straight tubules have varied from 400 to 20,000 μm/sec, although most values are in the range of 1,000 to 3,000 μm/sec. It should be noted that these permeability values are based on the apparent area of the luminal membrane, i.e. the surface area of a right circular cylinder having the same radius as the tubule lumen. When one takes into account the amplification of luminal membrane surface area produced by the microvilli, P_f normalized for the true luminal membrane area is in the range of 50–180 μm/sec, which is comparable to that observed for the plasma membrane of many cells including red blood cells (21).

Berry & Verkman (9) recently examined the source of this variability in more detail in isolated rabbit proximal convoluted tubules by measuring P_f with varying osmolality differences produced by adding raffinose to the perfusate or bathing solution. When the bathing solution was 20 mOsM hyperosmotic to the lumen, P_f was 5000 μm/sec, but it fell with increasing bath osmolality to 800 μm/sec at a 100 mOsM difference (9). In earlier studies in the gallbladder, Diamond (18) observed a similar nonlinearity of osmotic water flow with driving force, which he ascribed to the presence of water channels that altered their resistance to flow with changes in extracellular osmolality. Berry & Verkman (9) considered additional explanations for the nonlinear osmosis. Since changes in perfusate osmolality had no effect on the measured P_f, there was no evidence for solute polarization due to external unstirred layers. (One of the primary advantages of working with isolated perfused nephron segments is the absence of significant unstirred layers due to the small luminal diameter and the ability to flow the bathing solution past the basement membrane with no intervening tissue layers.) Berry & Verkman (9) also determined that a simple intracellular unstirred layer between the apical and basolateral membranes would not explain the anomalous behavior if that unstirred layer remained unchanged with differing transepithelial osmolality differences (9). They were forced to conclude that there was a complex intracellular unstirred layer that increased resistance to solute diffusion and/or decreased the area for volume flow with an increasing osmolality difference, although this unstirred layer could reside in another compartment within the epithelium.

Based on these observations, Berry & Verkman (9) examined previously reported P_f values from isolated perfused tubules and plotted them together with their data as shown in Figure 1. They interpreted the resulting plot to indicate that P_f increased exponentially as the imposed osmotic gradient decreased. Since most investigators believe that any transepithelial osmolality difference would be much less than 20 mOsM, this plot would suggest that P_f could be extremely high under normal in vivo conditions. Upon further examination however, it appears as if the data fall in two groups: those in which the imposed osmolality difference is $\leq$20 mOsM have a P_f in the range 3500–7500 μm/sec, whereas those at $>$20 mOsM all have P_f values less than 1000 μm/sec. Thus the effect may be a discontinuous one with an abrupt decrease in water permeability when the osmolality difference exceeds a certain threshold. In our studies to determine P_f (3, 44), we specifically chose an osmolality difference of 20 mOsM, because we had observed that with differences of 30 mOsM or greater the proximal end of the perfused tubule segment took on a dark granular appearance. We have examined this phenomenon more thoroughly in recent studies using Nomarski and transmission electron microscopy with the isolated rabbit proximal straight tubule perfused with an imposed osmotic gradient of 20 mOsM (58). We found that when the 6 g/dl albumin normally present in the bathing solution was removed large, clear, fluid-filled vacuoles rapidly began to appear in the cells, especially near the perfusion end of the tubule. No such vacuolation was observed in the absence of an osmolality difference. These vacuoles produced the granular appearance often observed in proximal tubule segments, and the lumen was obscured in a short period of time. The granularity was distributed along the tubule in rough approximation to the expected osmolality difference, being more intense at the perfusion end and moderate to absent at the collection end where most of the osmolality difference had been dissipated by water flow. The vacuolation disappeared when albumin or high molecular weight dextran was re-added to the bathing solution (58). We do not know why colloid has a protective effect, but it is possible that similar structural changes may be involved in the fall in P_f at higher osmolality differences. The bathing solution contained protein in each of the studies shown in Figure 1, but it seems likely that vacuoles could form at the higher osmolality differences as indicated by the granularity we observed even in the presence of albumin at osmolality differences in excess of 30 mOsM.

Such structural changes could well involve the very complex microanatomy near the base of proximal tubule cells where 75% of the total basolateral membrane area is concentrated (54a). Welling et al (51a, 54a) have proposed that the majority of the volume flow occurs across this basal membrane complex because of its large area. These investigators have also hypothesized that peritubular interstitial proteins could exert a transmembrane oncotic pressure in this region, which would contribute to the driving force for volume absorption (51a, 54a). Changes in the peritubular protein concentration could cause a change in volume absorption as well as changes in the area of the basal microvilli themselves (54a).

The results of Berry & Verkman (9) indicate that high rates of volume flow would be produced with a very small transepithelial osmolality difference. Even if the actual P_f were only 4000 μm/sec (and from the appearance of the

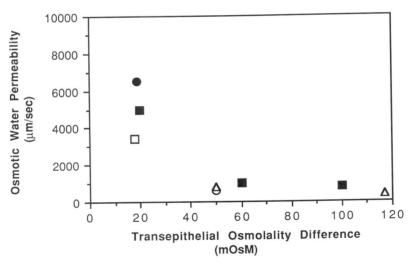

Figure 1   Effect of imposed osmolality difference on measured osmotic water permeability (P_f) in proximal tubule. □, data of Andreoli et al (3); ■, data of Berry & Verkman (9); ○, data of Corman & DiStefano (16); △, data of Kokko et al (30); ●, data of Schafer et al (44). Adapted from Figure 3 in Berry & Verkman (9).

plot in Figure 1, it could be much higher), volume absorption rates of 0.5 to 4 nl min^{-1} mm^{-1} (the range observed in the rat proximal convoluted tubule in vivo) could be produced with transepithelial osmolality differences in the range of 1 to 10 mOsM.

TRANSEPITHELIAL OSMOLALITY DIFFERENCES

A high hydraulic conductivity (P_f) is an essential component of the hypothesis that volume absorption in the proximal tubule depends on a small transepithelial osmolality difference (1, 2), but the demonstration of that small difference presents a formidable technical obstacle. The model of Andreoli & Schafer (1, 2) showed that solute absorption by the proximal tubule would result in slight dilution of the lumen because of its limited volume, as implied much earlier by Homer Smith (46). Smith had drawn on the free flow micropuncture observations of Walker et al (49), in which there was a trend for lower osmolalities of the tubular fluid samples compared to plasma. But these observations were compromised by the relatively large standard error (± 20 mOsM) in the microanalytical methods used. Bishop et al (10) also observed that when rat proximal tubules were microperfused, the osmolality of the absorbate significantly exceeded that of the original perfusate, thus implying that a transepithelial osmolality gradient would develop. Using careful measurements of luminal fluid osmolality, Liu et al (31) have more recently shown that the osmolality of the tubular fluid obtained from the Munich-Wistar rat proximal tubule by free flow micropuncture was significantly less than the plasma. In the early proximal tubule, the fluid was dilute by 2.8 mOsM and the hypotonicity increased progressively with distance from the glomerulus to a maximum of 7.5 mOsM lower than plasma. The rising osmolality difference was interpreted to indicate that P_f was lower in the more distal regions (31).

Although highly suggestive of a transepithelial osmolality difference, all of the above observations were complicated by the fact that the tubular fluid osmolality was compared to that of the systemic plasma, which was presumed to be the same as that of the interstitium. As shown by Atherton (5) however, the composition of plasma in the peritubular capillaries differs from systemic plasma. Furthermore, as discussed in more detail below, there are indications that the interstitial fluid is not in diffusion equilibrium with the peritubular capillary plasma (35, 60). Thus one would need to determine the interstitial osmolality in order to ensure that the observed luminal hypotonicity reflected a transepithelial osmolality difference. Green & Giebisch (27, 28) approached this problem by perfusing both the peritubular capillaries and the lumen with isosmotic NaCl solution. They observed that the tubular fluid collected from the distal end of the perfused segment was dilute compared to the original perfusate. Furthermore, the collected osmolality was lower when volume absorption was more rapid: the tubular fluid became dilute by 1.7 mOsM at a volume absorption rate of 0.4 nl min^{-1} mm^{-1} and increased to 3.9 mOsM at 0.9 nl min^{-1} mm^{-1}. Adding cyanide to the perfusate dropped the absorption rate to zero, and no luminal hypotonicity developed (27).

The volume absorption rates in the studies of Green & Giebisch (27) were relatively low because of the simple perfusate solution used. The use of a more natural perfusate introduces other complications, however. When the tubular fluid contains glucose, bicarbonate, amino acids, and other substrates, the composition of the tubular fluid changes dramatically and may be quite different from the interstitial fluid as these solutes are preferentially reabsorbed by active transport. If these solutes have different reflection coefficients, the actual or effective osmotic pressure across the epithelium may be different than predicted from the cryoscopically determined osmolality difference (2, 41). In other words, if the preferentially absorbed solutes have higher reflection coefficients than the NaCl remaining in the lumen, then the effective osmolality difference may be greater than that measured. Thus the presence of these solutes in the original perfusate would enhance the rate of volume absorption as observed in several studies (see 2, 41, 45). The present debate considers whether the reflection coefficient of NaCl is less than that of the preferentially absorbed solutes (see below).

Evaluation of the Adequacy of the Transepithelial Driving Force

The above studies have demonstrated that the presence of cyroscopic hypotonicity of the luminal fluid would serve as a driving force for volume absorption; however, Weinstein (50) has questioned whether the resulting osmolality difference is sufficient to produce the observed rates of volume absorption. Using a modeling approach based on irreversible thermodynamics, Weinstein & Stephenson (51) examined the coupling of solute and solvent transport in leaky epithelia such as the proximal tubule. In this work they developed a parameter referred to as the strength of transport ($\hat{C}$) to describe apparent active water transport due to solute-solvent coupling within an intraepithelial compartment. In the proximal tubule, $\hat{C}$ can be defined as the increment in luminal osmolality that would be required to bring the rate of volume absorption to zero. Weinstein (50) used currently available parameters of proximal tubule transport and calculated that the $\hat{C}$ required for observed rates of volume absorption was 8 to 23 mOsM. In other words, either the osmolality difference was inadequate by this degree, or P_f had to exceed the values of 1200 and 2400 μm/sec used in the model.

Weinstein (50) interpreted these observations to indicate the presence of solute-solvent coupling because of hyperosmolality in the lateral intercellular spaces. This explanation may be correct in the case of amphibian proximal tubules. Using an electrophysiologic approach, Sackin (38, 39) has shown that the intracellular spaces in the *Abystoma* proximal tubule may be 2 to 5 mOsM hyperosmotic compared to the lumen, which approaches the $\hat{C}$ calculated for the *Necturus* by Weinstein (50). The epithelial cell layer of these amphibia is much thicker than the mammalian proximal tubule, and thus the diffusion constraints preventing dissipation of the intercellular osmolality are significantly greater.

A high $\hat{C}$ in the mammalian proximal tubule is also supported by the data of Bomsztyk & Wright (11), who observed that volume absorption in the rat proximal tubule could be brought to zero only with the addition of 30 mM mannitol to the luminal perfusate. It must be remembered that P_f is markedly lower at osmolality differences of this magnitude. Therefore, it may be impossible to assess $\hat{C}$ by raising luminal osmolality. The apparent inadequacy of the observed degree of luminal hypotonicity to drive volume absorption according to Weinstein's analysis (50) may be explained in two ways. First, the experimentally measured P_f values used in the analysis may be lower than the actual values because of the complications introduced by the use of large osmolality differences in their determination (see above; 9). Second, if the intercellular space cannot be sufficiently hyperosmotic to explain $\hat{C}$, it is possible that the interstitial compartment itself becomes hyperosmotic during absorption.

This latter explanation becomes particularly intriguing when one compares the results from the in vivo and in vitro proximal tubule preparations. In contrast to the predicted shortfall of the transepithelial osmotic difference in the rat in vivo, Weinstein (50) found that the observed rates of volume absorption in isolated perfused rabbit proximal tubules could be explained by the measured P_f and luminal hypotonicity; in in vivo but not in vitro there appeared to be a missing osmotic driving force. The primary difference between the two preparations is the presence of an interstitial compartment of limited volume between the basement membrane and the peritubular capillaries in vivo compared to a large well-stirred bathing solution in vitro. In vivo, one measures the transepithelial osmolality difference between the lumen and plasma, and it has been tacitly assumed that the interstitial fluid is in diffusion equilibrium with the plasma because of the presumed high permeability of the capillaries. We have recently questioned these assumptions (60).

Using a previously developed mathematical model of transepithelial solute and water transport (59), we examined the effect of adding a third compartment corresponding to the interstitium and found that that compartment could become significantly hyperosmotic as a consequence of solute absorption (60). The essence of this argument is best appreciated if one considers the case of an actively absorbed solute such as glucose, shown in Figure 2. This

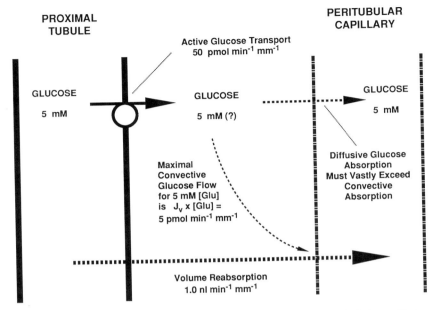

Figure 2   Diffusional and convective components of glucose uptake into peritubular capillaries. For the purposes of illustration, an average rate of glucose absorption of 50 pmol min^{-1} mm^{-1} has been assumed. Because this solute is preferentially absorbed, its rate of convectional uptake into the capillaries must be much less than the rate of transepithelial transport, which necessitates diffusional movement in the steady-state as described in the text.

figure illustrates the transport of glucose across the proximal tubule and the peritubular capillary. In the early proximal tubule a reasonable average rate of glucose absorption would be 50 pmol min^{-1} mm^{-1} with a volume absorption rate of 1.0 nl min^{-1} mm^{-1}. In the steady-state the uptake of glucose and volume by the peritubular capillary must occur at exactly this same rate. Volume absorption is driven by the Starling forces, but the maximal rate of glucose absorption by this convective process is equal to the product of the volume absorption rate (1.0 nl min^{-1} mm^{-1}) and the glucose concentration in the interstitium. If the glucose concentration in the interstitium is the same as in plasma, 5 mM, then the maximal rate of convective glucose uptake by the capillaries (assuming a reflection coefficient of zero) is 5 pmol min^{-1} mm^{-1}, i.e. for a preferentially absorbed solute such as glucose, the primary mechanism of peritubular capillary uptake must occur by diffusion. Therefore there must be a gradient of solute concentration between the interstitial fluid and the plasma that drives the diffusion process. The question is how much higher the interstitial solute concentration must be in order for the combined rates of diffusional and convective uptake to equal the rate of transepithelial transport, and this depends on the capillary permeability (60).

Unfortunately, there are no direct measurements of peritubular capillary permeabilities, and it is unlikely that they can be measured by existing methods. Therefore, in our model we were forced to use permeability values obtained in similar fenestrated diaphragmated capillaries found in other tissues. Using permeabilities in this range (1–10 μm/sec), the model predicted that, given the rapid rates of solute and water absorption by the proximal tubule, the capillary endothelium would constitute a significant diffusion barrier resulting in an interstitial osmolality that is higher than the plasma as a consequence of the influx of hyperosmotic absorbate from the early segments of the proximal tubule (60).

There is some limited support for this hypothesis from investigations of the composition of renal lymph, which is thought to reflect the composition of the interstitial fluid in the regions it drains. O'Morchoe et al (35) compared the composition of hilar lymph, which drains the renal medulla, with the composition of capsular lymph, which derives primarily from the cortex. They showed that the glucose concentration of the capsular lymph was higher than that of the renal venous or arterial plasma, and higher than the hilar lymph. In contrast, the Na$^+$ and Cl$^-$ concentrations were higher in hilar than in capsular lymph. O'Morchoe et al (35) interpreted their results to show that the composition of the capsular lymph is intermediate between that of systemic plasma and the absorbate from renal tubules. As shown by Barfuss & Schafer (6), absorbate collected from the surface of isolated rabbit proximal convoluted tubules perfused under oil has a far higher glucose concentration than the luminal perfusate, whereas the NaCl concentration of the absorbate is lower, which would explain the findings of O'Morchoe et al (35).

In summary, the observation of luminal fluid hypotonicity was an important step in the demonstration of a transepithelial osmolality difference. Whether luminal hypotonicity alone is responsible for this osmotic driving force depends on the true value of the osmotic water permeability in the proximal tubule. Even if P_f is at the lower end of the observed range, the effective transepithelial osmolality difference may be augmented by interstitial fluid hyperosmolality due primarily to the preferentially absorbed solutes such as glucose.

PATHWAYS OF WATER FLOW ACROSS THE PROXIMAL TUBULE

There has been a long standing debate about whether the primary route of water flow across the epithelium of the proximal tubule is transcellular or paracellular. At present, most investigators in this area fall into two camps: those maintaining that the flow is exclusively transcellular, and those maintaining that it is approximately equally divided between the two routes. One approach to this problem is to compare the osmotic water permeabilities of the individual plasma membranes to the transepithelial P_f.

In order to measure P_f in the individual membranes, it is necessary to resolve the initial rate of cell volume change when the osmolality of either the luminal or basolateral bathing solution is changed rapidly. In order for the method to be successful in measuring a high P_f, the solution change must be virtually instantaneous and volume changes of less than 1% of the total cell volume must be resolved by measuring the diameter of the tubule at sampling intervals of less than 10 msec. Appreciably, technical limitations would most likely lead to underestimates of the rate of volume change and thus of P_f. The earliest studies used optical and video methods, but the relatively subjective criteria used for edge detection in the determination of the tubule diameter, resulted in P_f values at the lower end of the ranges reported in Table 1. Subsequently, more sophisticated analysis of video images has been employed to obtain very rapid and unbiased resolution of tubule diameter changes, and better methods for rapid solution changes and their verification have been developed (14, 56). The resulting P_f values are higher than the previous estimates and probably reliable. Although Table 1 shows differences in the P_f determined for luminal and basolateral membranes, when expressed in terms of the true membrane area, the values for both membranes are quite comparable even with the different methodologies used to measure them.

In a technical tour de force, Carpi-Medina & Whittembury (15) have applied this methodology to the measurement of P_f for both the luminal and basolateral membranes of the rabbit proximal straight tubule. The high P_f values obtained are shown in Figure 3. In these same experiments, the investigators also measured the initial rate of transepithelial water flow after a step change in bathing solution osmolality to obtain a transepithelial P_f estimate of ~ 4300 μm/sec. From the two membrane P_f values in series, they calculated a total transcellular P_f of 1800 μm/sec and a paracellular P_f of 2500 μm/sec (15). Their estimates indicate that, in the presence of a transepithelial osmolality difference, approximately equal rates of volume flow would occur through the cell and between cells.

Other investigators question such high values for the paracellular P_f based on the limited area for water flow across the junctional complexes between cells (7, 8, 51a, 54). As summarized in the review of Berry (7), it would appear that a high paracellular water permeability would require that the junctions have quite large pores to give a sufficiently high P_f. Yet large pores would not discriminate between water and small solutes, and they would result in much higher solute permeabilities than have been observed. This conclusion is based on analyzing the junctional complexes as a collection of conventional right circular cylindrical or slit pores (7). Fraser & Baines (23)

Table 1 Water permeabilities of individual proximal tubule membranes

PREPARATION	P_f (μm/sec)	P_f' (μm/sec)	P_D (μm/sec)	P_D' (μm/sec)	Method
S_1 Segment basolateral membrane—rabbit	2300–5500	140–300	—	—	Isolated nonperfused; Optical methods (12, 55, 56)
S_2 Segment luminal membrane—rabbit	1260–4500	70–250	—	—	Isolated perfused; Optical methods (15, 25)
S_2 Segment basolateral membrane—rabbit	1400–5000	100–375	—	—	Isolated nonperfused; Optical methods (14, 15, 26, 55, 56, 57)
S_3 Segment basolateral membrane—rabbit	3000	380	—	—	Isolated nonperfused; Optical methods (55)
Brush border membrane vesicles—rat	—	240–600	—	—	Stop-flow Light Scattering (37, 47)
Brush border membrane vesicles—rabbit	—	730	—	—	Stop-flow Light Scattering (33)
Basolateral membrane vesicles—rabbit	—	190	—	—	Stop-flow Light Scattering (33)
Isolated proximal tubule cells—rabbit	—	—	200–600	22–32	^{1}H-NMR (13, 33)
Proximal tubule suspension—rabbit	—	—	300–400	20	^{1}H-NMR (48)

Osmotic water permeabilities and diffusional water permeabilities are presented either normalized for the apparent membrane area (P_f and P_D, respectively), or in terms of the actual membrane area (P_f' and P_D', respectively). The apparent luminal membrane area is calculated as the surface area of a right circular cylinder with the same diameter as the lumen; the apparent basolateral membrane area is equivalent to the basement membrane area. The actual membrane area takes into account the amplification of the surface area that is produced by the luminal microvilli and the basolateral invaginations as described by Welling & Welling (52, 54). In some cases, one or the other parameter was calculated from the data presented in the referenced work using the surface amplification factors of Welling & Welling (54). S_1, S_2, and S_3 refer to the standard proximal tubule segments. Most experiments reported were conducted at 37°C with the exception of some studies in membrane vesicles and proximal tubule cells.

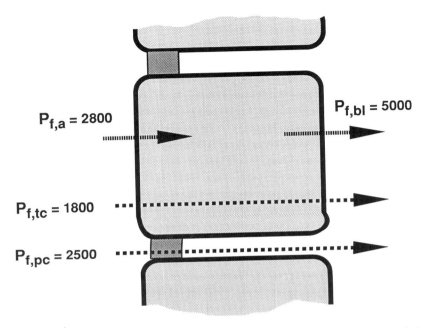

Figure 3 Water permeabilities of individual barriers in the rabbit proximal straight tubule. Osmotic water permeabilities of the luminal ($P_{f,a}$) and basolateral ($P_{f,bl}$) cell membranes are those reported in the study of Carpi-Medina & Whittembury (15), and from which they calculated the transcellular osmotic water permeability ($P_{f,tc}$). (The luminal P_f was re-normalized per cm² of basement membrane area rather than apparent luminal membrane area in order to calculate $P_{f,tc}$.) These investigators also measured the transepithelial P_f in the same tubules in order to derive an estimate for the paracellular pathway ($P_{f,pc}$).

recently proposed that the junctional complexes might more logically resemble a fiber-matrix barrier with a large aqueous void volume. They have demonstrated that for void volumes in excess of 90% such a model is consistent with a high P_f yet low solute permeabilities, and thus would allow for non-unity reflection coefficients and significant water flow through the junctional complexes. Obviously, firm conclusions regarding the quantitative role of the paracellular pathway in water and solute absorption must await further experimental and modeling work.

The high P_f values of both luminal and basolateral membranes in proximal tubules are comparable to those of the red blood cell and toad bladder apical membrane, and higher than expected for diffusional water movement through an unmodified lipid bilayer (see 20 for references) As in the red blood cell and toad bladder (see 22, 32 for references), several investigators maintain that water transport across the proximal tubule membranes is mediated by water channels that allow single file movement of the water molecules. This conclusion is supported by three lines of evidence: inhibition of water permeability by sulfhydryl reagents, the activation energy of water permeability, and the difference in diffusional and osmotic water permeabilities.

Berry (8) has estimated the transepithelial diffusional water permeability (P_D, μm/sec) in the rabbit proximal convoluted tubule by THO diffusion to be at least 125 μm/sec, which is still considerably less than P_f. More accurate measurements of P_D in individual cell membranes have been made using ^{1}H-NMR (see Table 1). This method allows the water permeability to be measured under conditions of diffusion equilibrium so that the resistances of unstirred layers, which complicate measurements using THO, are avoided. Values obtained both in intact tubules and tubule cells (Table 1) are actually some average of the P_D for apical and basolateral membranes, but are much less than corresponding P_f values; thus the P_f/P_D ratio calculated from the values in Table 1 ranges from 10 to 20.

As described in detail by Finkelstein (19), a P_f/P_D ratio in excess of 1.0 can be due either to the presence of pores that allow quasilaminar convective water flow, or channels that allow only single file water movement. Since much lower solute permeabilities are observed for proximal tubule membranes, the latter explanation seems the more likely (15). The existence of proteinaceous water channels is also indicated by the fact that P_f and P_D are reversibly inhibited by sulfhydryl reagents. Para-chloromercuribenzene sulfonate (pCMBS), $HgCl_2$, and mersalyl have been found to inhibit both P_f and P_D by 50–100% in intact tubules (8, 57), proximal tubule suspensions (48), isolated proximal tubule cells (13, 33), and isolated brush border and basolateral membrane vesicles (33, 37, 47), and the inhibitory effect of these sulfhydryl agents is prevented or reversed by the reducing agent dithiothreitol. As in the red blood cell, these effects have been attributed to blockage of water channels by the reagents (see references in 22, 32), but it should also be recognized that these reagents can produce nonspecific and irreversible damage to the cells that could cause high solute permeabilities (15).

Activation energy data is also consistent with water movement through such channels. Under normal conditions, the activation energy for both P_f and P_D is very low, on the order of 1–5 kcal/mol (8, 13, 47, 48, 57). Such a low activation energy is generally attributed to movement through a specialized channel in which the diffusing water molecules scarcely interact with the membrane (13). In the presence of pCMBS however, the activation energy rises to 9–10 kcal/mol (13, 57), which is taken to indicate that the remaining water movement occurs through the lipid membrane itself.

Non-unity Reflection Coefficients

The possibility that NaCl and other small solutes have non-unity reflection coefficients across the proximal tubule provides a further indication that the paracellular pathway is a common route for a portion of transepithelial salt and water transport and thus a site of solute-solvent interaction. The reflection coefficient for NaCl has been estimated by comparing osmotic water flows induced by equal gradients of NaCl and poorly permeant solutes such as mannitol and raffinose. Both in the rat proximal convoluted tubule in vivo (24, 28, 34, 40) and in isolated rabbit proximal tubule segments (40, 42, 43, 45), the reflection coefficient has been estimated from this approach to be 0.5 to 0.8. A significant difference between the reflection coefficients for Cl^- and HCO_3^- has also been demonstrated by the presence of flow-dependent net volume absorption in the absence of active transport in isolated perfused rabbit proximal convoluted and straight tubule segments with opposing transepithelial concentration gradients of the two anions (42, 43, 45). The inequality in reflection coefficients has been suggested to form a driving force for passive volume absorption in the late proximal tubule and would give rise to an underestimate of the true effective transepithelial osmolality difference as discussed above (41–43).

The presence of a non-unity reflection coefficient for Cl^- has been disputed from experimental attempts to measure the solvent drag component of Cl^- transport. Although some investigators have observed apparent Cl^- solvent drag (4), others have not (16, 29). The latter results appear to indicate that most solutes have unity reflection coefficients across the epithelium and that there is little water flow through junctional complexes between cells. It must be recognized, however, that the measurements of changes in net Cl^- movement when osmotic water flow is imposed, as employed to assess Cl^- solvent drag, are inherently insensitive and would be unlikely to resolve the small changes expected in the net flux [see (41)]. On the basis of most evidence, it would appear that the reflection coefficient for NaCl is significantly less than that for $NaHCO_3$ and other preferentially absorbed solutes such as sugars and amino acids.

It is also debated whether a non-unity reflection coefficient for NaCl unequivocally indicates a paracellular pathway for solute-solvent coupling. The apparent solvent drag of small electrolytes (11) and sucrose (57a) has been taken to indicate such paracellular coupling in the rat proximal convoluted tubule. Welling et al (56) have used video methods to compare the apparent P_f of the basolateral membrane of isolated, nonperfused proximal tubule segments when osmotic water flow is produced by NaCl and by raffinose. From their analysis, they calculate that the NaCl reflection coefficient of the basolateral membrane is ~0.5, which indicates that solvent drag must be occurring within the water channels in this membrane. If this were true, the water channels would be quite different from the pCMBS-inhibitable ones described in the red blood cell, which have unity reflection coefficients for solutes as small as urea [see (32)]. The low reflection coefficient for NaCl has been questioned by more recent measurements in isolated brush border and basolateral membrane vesicles by Pearce & Verkman (36). Using both osmotic water flow and solvent drag approaches, these investigators have determined that the NaCl reflection coefficient is not significantly different from unity. The contradiction between these results and those of Welling & Welling (56) may relate to the different preparations used. Certainly the issue needs further exploration.

SUMMARY

The weight of current evidence indicates that the proximal tubule has a high transepithelial osmotic water permeability in the range of 3500–6000 μm/sec, which is attributable in large part to the high water permeabilities of the cell membranes. Water movement through these membranes may occur through specialized, proteinaceous channels that can be blocked by sulfhydryl reagents. The water channels probably exclude even the smallest solutes and allow only single file movement of the water molecules as do the water channels previously described in the red blood cell and vasopressin-responsive epithelia.

If a significant fraction of the water flow also occurs through the junctional complexes, it seems likely that these junctions could be a site for solute solvent coupling which would contribute to solute absorption by solvent drag and which would be responsible for non-unity reflection coefficients for some solutes such as Na^+ and Cl^-. This possibility is still a matter of vigorous debate.

Since the transepithelial water permeability is high, only a very small osmolality difference (1–10 mOsM) is required to drive normally observed rates of volume absorption both in vivo and in vitro. The osmolality difference is produced at least in part by dilution of the luminal fluid and is possibly augmented by the development of intersitial hyperosmolality because of the rapid transport of preferentially absorbed solutes.

In the future it is likely that the most important work in this field will relate to the factors that alter transepithelial water permeability and the solute and water permeabilities of the junctional complexes. Investigation in this area is essential in understanding how changes in capillary and interstitial hydrostatic and colloid osmotic pressure may affect volume absorption.

ACKNOWLEDGMENTS

I would like to give special thanks to collaborators who have been so essential for many of the ideas and experiments from our laboratory reported herein. They include T.E. Andreoli, D.W. Barfuss, C.S. Patlak, S. L. Troutman, M. L. Watkins, and J. C. Williams Jr. Research support for recent work in our laboratory, which has been described in this article, came from National Institutes of Health Grants 5-RO1-DK25519-10 and 1-P50-DK39258-02.

Literature Cited

1. Andreoli, T. E., Schafer, J. A. 1978. Volume absorption in the pars recta. III. Luminal hypotonicity as a driving force for isotonic volume absorption. *Am. J. Physiol.* 234:F349–55
2. Andreoli, T. E., Schafer, J. A. 1979. Effective luminal hypotonicity: the driving force for isotonic proximal tubular fluid absorption. *Am. J. Physiol.* 236: F89–96
3. Andreoli, T. E., Schafer, J. A., Troutman, S. L. 1978. Perfusion rate dependence of transepithelial osmosis in isolated proximal convoluted tubules: Estimation of the hydraulic conductance. *Kidney Int.* 14:263–69
4. Andreoli, T. E., Schafer, J. A., Troutman, S. L., Watkins M. L. 1979. Solvent drag component of Cl⁻ flux in superficial proximal straight tubules: evidence for a paracellular component of isotonic fluid absorption. *Am. J. Physiol.* 237:F455-62
5. Atherton, J. C. 1977. Comparison of chloride concentration and osmolality in proximal tubular fluid, peritubular capillary plasma and systemic plasma in the rat. *J. Physiol.* 273:765–73
6. Barfuss, D. W., Schafer, J. A. 1984. Rate of formation and composition of absorbate from proximal nephron segments. *Am. J. Physiol.* 247:F117–29
7. Berry, C. A. 1983. Water permeability and pathways in the proximal tubule. *Am. J. Physiol.* 245:F279–94
8. Berry, C. A. 1985. Characteristics of water diffusion of the rabbit proximal convoluted tubule. *Am. J. Physiol.* 249: F729–38
9. Berry, C. A., Verkamn, A. S. 1988. Osmotic gradient dependence of water permeability in rabbit proximal convoluted tubule. *J. Membr. Biol.* 105:33–43
10. Bishop, J. H. V., Green, R., Thomas, S. 1979. Free-flow reabsorption of glucose, sodium, osmoles and water in rat proximal convoluted tubule. *J. Physiol.* 288:331–51
11. Bomsztyk, K., Wright, F. S. 1986. Dependence of ion fluxes on fluid transport by rat proximal tubule. *Am. J. Physiol.* 250:F680–89
12. Carpi-Medina, P., González, E., Whittembury, G. 1983. Cell osmotic water permeability of isolated rabbit proximal convoluted tubules. *Am. J. Physiol.* 244:F554–63
13. Carpi-Medina, P., Leon, V., Espidel, J., Whittembury, G. 1988. Diffusive water permeability in isolated kidney proximal tubular cells: nature of the cellular water pathways. *J. Membr. Biol.* 105:35–43
14. Carpi-Medina, P., Lindemann, B., González, E., Whittembury, G. 1984. The continuous measurement of tubular volume changes in response to step changes in contraluminal osmolality. *Pflügers Arch.* 400:343–48
15. Carpi-Medina, P. E., Whittembury, G. 1988. Comparison of transcellular and transepithelial water osmotic permeabilities (Pos) in the isolated proximal straight tubule (PST) of the rabbit kidney *Pflügers Arch.* 412:66–74
16. Corman, B., DiStefano, A. 1983. Does water drag solutes through kidney proximal tubule? *Pflügers Arch.* 397:35–41
17. Diamond, J. M. 1979. Osmotic water flow in leaky epithelia. *J. Membr. Biol.* 51:195–216
18. Diamond, J. M. 1966. Non-Linear osmosis. *J. Physiol.* 183:58–82
19. Finkelstein, A. 1987. *Water movement through lipid bilayers, pores, and plasma membranes. Theory and Reality.* New York: Wiley. 228 pp.
20. Finkelstein, A. 1987. See Ref. 19, pp. 102–6
21. Finkelstein, A. 1987. See Ref. 19, pp. 153–65
22. Finkelstein, A. 1987. See Ref. 19, pp. 166–84
23. Fraser, W. D., Baines, A. D. 1989. Application of a fiber matrix model to transport in renal tubules. *J. Gen. Physiol.* 94:
24. Frömter, E., Rumrich, G., Ullrich, K. J. 1973. Phenomenologic description of Na⁺, Cl⁻ and HCO₃⁻ absorption from proximal tubules of the rat kidney. *Pflügers Arch.* 343:189–220
25. González, E., Carpi-Medina, P., Linares, H., Whittembury, G. 1984. Water osmotic permeability of the apical membrane of proximal straight tubular (PST) cells. *Pflügers Arch.* 402:337–39
26. González, E., Carpi-Medina, P., Whittembury, G. 1982. Cell osmotic water permeability of isolated rabbit proximal straight tubules. *Am. J. Physiol.* 242: F321–30
27. Green, R., Giebisch, G. 1984. Luminal hypotonicity: a driving force for fluid absorption from the proximal tubule. *Am. J. Physiol.* 246:F167–74
28. Green, R., Giebisch, G. 1989. Reflection coefficients and water permeability in the proximal tubule. *Am. J. Physiol.* 257:F658–68

29. Jacobson, H. R., Kokko, J. P., Seldin, D. W., Holmberg, C. 1982. Lack of solvent drag of NaCl and NaHCO$_3$ in rabbit proximal tubules. *Am. J. Physiol.* 243:F342–48

30. Kokko, J, P., Burg, M. B., Orloff, J. 1971. Characteristics of NaCl and water transport in the renal proximal tubule. *J. Clin. Invest.* 50:69–76

31. Liu, F.-Y., Cogan, M. G., Rector, F. C. Jr. 1984. Axial heterogeneity in the rat proximal convoluted tubule II. Osmolality and osmotic water permeability. *Am. J. Physiol.* 247:F822–26

32. Macey, R. I. 1984. Transport of water and urea in red blood cells. *Am. J. Physiol.* 246:C195–C203

33. Meyer, M. M., Verkman, A. S. 1987. Evidence for water channels in renal proximal tubule cell membranes. *J. Membr. Biol.* 96:107–19

34. Neumann, K. H., Rector, F. C. Jr. 1976. Mechanism of NaCl and water reabsorption in the proximal convoluted tubule of rat kidney. *J. Clin. Invest.* 58:1110–18

35. O'Morchoe, C. C. C., O'Morchoe, P. J., Donati, E. J. 1975. Comparison of hilar and capsular lymph. *Am. J. Physiol.* 229:416–21

36. Pearce, D., Verkman, A. S. 1989. NaCl reflection coefficients in proximal tubule apical and basolateral membrane vesicles: Measurement by induced osmosis and solvent drag. *Biophys. J.* 55:1251–59

37. Pratz, J, Ripoche, P., Corman, B. 1986. Evidence for proteic water pathways in the luminal membrane of kidney proximal tubule. *Biochim. Biophys. Acta.* 856:259–66

38. Sackin, H. 1986. Electrophysiology of salamander proximal tubule I. Effects of rapid cooling. *Am. J. Physiol.* 251: F319–33

39. Sackin, H. 1986. Electrophysiology of salamander proximal tubule II. Interspace NaCl concentrations and solute-coupled water transport. *Am. J. Physiol.* 251:F334–47

40. Sansom, S. C., Senekjian, H. O., Knight, T. F., Frommer, P., Weinman, E. J. 1983. Water absorption in the proximal tubule: effect of bicarbonate, chloride gradient, and organic solutes. *Proc. Soc. Exp. Biol. Med.* 172:111–17

41. Schafer, J. A. 1984. Mechanisms coupling the absorption of solute and water in the proximal nephron. *Kidney Int.* 25:708–16

42. Schafer, J. A., Patlak, C. S., Andreoli, T. E. 1975. A component of fluid absorption linked to passive ion flows in the superficial pars recta. *J. Gen. Physiol.* 66:445–71

43. Schafer, J. A., Patlak, C. S., Andreoli, T. E. 1977. Fluid absorption and active and passive ion flows in the rabbit superficial pars recta. *Am. J. Physiol.* 233: F154–67

44. Schafer, J. A., Patlak, C. S., Troutman, S. L., Andreoli, T. E. 1978. Volume absorption in the pars recta. II. Hydraulic conductivity coefficient. *Am. J. Physiol.* 234:F340–48

45. Schafer, J. A., Troutman, S. L., Watkins, M. L., Andreoli, T. E. 1981. Flow dependence of fluid transport in the isolated superficial pars recta: Evidence that osmotic disequilibrium between external solutions drives isotonic fluid absorption. *Kidney Int.* 20:588–97

46. Smith, H. W. 1951. *The kidney. Structure and function in health and disease,* pp. 309. New York: Oxford Univ. Press.

47. van Heeswijk, M. P. E., van Os, C. H. 1987. Osmotic water permeability of brush border and basolateral membrane vesicles from rat renal cortex and small intestine. *J. Membr. Biol.* 92:183–93

48. Verkman, A. S., Wong, K. R. 1987. Proton nuclear magnetic resonance measurement of diffusional water permeability in suspended renal proximal tubules. *Biophys. J.* 51:717–23

49. Walker, A. M., Bott, P. A., Oliver, J., MacDowell, M. C. 1941. The collection and analysis of fluid from single nephrons of the mammalian kidney. *Am. J. Physiol.* 134:580–95

50. Weinstein, A. M. 1988. Modeling the proximal tubule: complications of the paracellular pathway. *Am. J. Physiol.* 254:F297–F305

51. Weinstein, A. M., Stephenson, J. L. 1981. Coupled water transport in standing gradient models of the lateral intercellular space. *Biophys. J.* 35:167–91

51a. Welling, D. J., Welling, L. W., Hill, J. J. 1978. Phenomenological model relating cell shape to water reabsorption in the proximal nephron. *Am. J. Physiol.* 234:308–17

52. Welling, L. W., Welling, D. J. 1975. Surface areas of brush border and lateral cell walls in the rabbit proximal nephron. *Kidney Int.* 8:343–48

53. Welling, L. W., Wellng, D. J. 1976. Shape of epithelial cells and intercellular channels in the rabbit proximal nephron. *Kidney Int.* 9:385–94

54. Welling, L. W., Welling, D. J. 1988. Relationship between structure and func-

tion in renal proximal tubule. *J. Electron Microsc.* 9:171–85

54a. Welling, L. W., Welling, D. J., Holsapple, J. W., Evan, A. P. 1987. Morphometric analysis of distinct microanatomy near the base of proximal tubule cells. *Am. J. Physiol.* 253:F126–40

55. Welling, L. W., Welling, D. J. Ochs, T J. 1983. Video measurement of basolateral membrane hydraulic conductivity in the proximal tubule. *Am. J. Physiol.* 245:F123–29

56. Welling, L. W., Welling, D. J., Ochs, T. J. 1987. Video measurement of basolateral NaCl reflection coefficient in proximal tubule. *Am. J. Physiol.* 253:F290–98

57. Whittembury, G., Carpi-Medina, P., González, E., Linares, H. 1984. Effect of para-chloromercuribenzenesulfonic acid and temperature on cell water osmotic permeability of proximal straight tubules. *Biochim. Biophys. Acta* 775:365–73

57a. Whittembury, G., Malnic, G., Mello-Aires, M., Amorena, C. 1988. Solvent drag of sucrose during absorption indicates paracellular water flow in the rat kidney proximal tubule. *Pflügers Arch.* 412:541–47

58. Williams, J. C. Jr., Abrahamson, D. R., Schafer, J. A. 1989. Bath colloid prevents vacuolization induced by osmotic water flow in proximal tubule. *Kidney Int.* 35:504 (Abstr)

59. Williams, J. C. Jr., Schafer, J. A. 1987. A model of osmotic and hydrostatic pressure effects on volume absorption in the proximal tubule. *Am. J. Physiol.* 253:F563–75

60. Williams, J. C. Jr., Schafer, J. A. 1988. The cortical interstitium as a site for solute polarization during tubular absorption. *Am. J. Physiol.* 254:F813–23

Annu. Rev. Physiol. 1990. 52:727–46

REGULATION OF THE PREDOMINANT RENAL MEDULLARY ORGANIC SOLUTES IN VIVO[1]

S. D. Wolff and R. S. Balaban

Laboratory of Cardiac Energetics, National Heart Lung and Blood Institute, Bethesda, Maryland 20892

KEY WORDS: sorbitol, inositol, glycerolphosphorylcholine, betaine, osmoregulation

INTRODUCTION

Cells in the renal inner medulla are unique in that they are the only mammalian cells that are normally exposed to high concentrations of NaCl and urea. In addition, these concentrations change dramatically with the diuretic state of the animal. Most mammalian cells could not survive, let alone function, in such a hostile and dynamically changing environment. Recently it has been proposed that renal medullary cells adapt to their environment by accumulating high concentrations of organic solutes (8). We will review the predominant organic solutes of the renal medulla with special emphasis on their physiologic significance in vivo. The role metabolism and transport might play in the regulation of organic solute content is also discussed.

It has long been known that high concentrations of NaCl or urea are harmful to the function of proteins and enzymes. Urea, specifically, has been shown to inhibit embryological development (52), collagen fiber assembly (30), muscle contraction (1, 64), and the in vitro activity of numerous enzymes (79). It has also been shown to be highly permeable to medullary cells, such as those from the thin ascending limb and inner medullary collecting duct (58). In light of its high permeability, urea is generally assumed to equilibrate across renal inner medullary cell membranes (10). Thus in the renal medulla, where the urea concentration can exceed 1 M, intracellular and

---

extracellular urea concentrations are believed to be approximately equal. This concentration of urea is well above the level considered to be inhibitory for the function of many enzymes; nevertheless, renal medullary cells function regularly under these conditions, although it should be noted that normally functioning renal medullary cells are relatively inactive metabolically with a minimal aerobic respiratory capacity (20) and a slow rate of cell division (65).

Sodium chloride is also in high concentration in the renal medulla. However electron microprobe studies have demonstrated that the intracellular concentration of NaCl is much less than that found extracellularly (9). Indeed, the intracellular concentrations of all of the major electrolytes are similar to values found in most mammalian cells. It has been suggested that renal medullary cells limit their intracellular concentration of electrolytes to avoid the adverse effects of high ionic strength on enzyme function (3, 8). In light of the fact that cells cannot maintain significant osmotic pressure differences across their semifluid membranes and that the intracellular concentration of electrolytes is limited, renal medullary cells accumulate organic solutes that osmotically retain water and therefore can control cell volume. Because in vitro studies have shown that certain organic solutes affect enzyme function less than comparable concentrations of electrolytes, these organic solutes have been termed compatible or nonperturbing.

A variety of marine creatures (such as elasmobranchs, crabs, and hagfish) adopt a similar strategy to cope with exposure to the high salinity of the ocean (79). Although plasma electrolyte concentrations are high in these animals, intracellular values are much lower. As in the case of the renal medulla, cells from these organisms accumulate nonperturbing organic solutes that osmotically balance high extracellular concentrations of NaCl. Interestingly, despite the wide variety of organisms studied, the same types of organic solutes accumulated. The organic solutes were found to comprise three general groups: amino acids and their derivatives, polyhydric alcohols, and methylamines. In vitro studies have shown, in general, that in contrast to inorganic ions, high concentrations of the nonperturbing solutes do not adversely affect protein structure or function as assessed by a variety of parameters including V_{max}, K_m, thiol group reactivity, and rate of renaturation (79). In addition to their osmotic role, intracellular organic solutes have also been proposed to protect macromolecular structure and function from the adverse effects of urea (79). These claims are based in part on reports that some marine vertebrates maintain an intracellular concentration ratio of urea to methylamine of approximately 2. Subsequent studies in vitro showed that the adverse effects of urea on enzyme function can be completely counteracted by methylamines, when the ratio of urea to methylamine is ~2. Thus in the strictest sense methylamines are not nonperturbing since they do modify the kinetic aspects of various enzymes. On the basis of the above observations it was proposed that methylamines not only serve an osmotic role but also reduce the disruptive effects of high urea concentrations in marine animals. However it should be mentioned that the counterbalancing effect of methylamines is not observed for all enzymes and that some marine organisms have enzymes that function properly only when urea is present (80).

Can organic solutes play an osmotic and urea-protective role in renal medullary cells in vivo? In the past there have been reports of various organic solutes concentrated in the renal medulla, which include glycerolphosphorylcholine (GPC) (68), inositol (21), sorbitol (33), and lactate (26). However the first suggestion that high concentrations of organic solutes play a role in the regulation of renal medullary cell intracellular milieu was made by Balaban & Knepper (8) who proposed that, as in the marine animals, high concentrations of GPC and other methylamines could protect macromolecules from the adverse effects of urea. Bagnasco et al (3) later measured the content of four predominant organic solutes in rat and rabbit whose total concentration in renal medullary cells could fill the osmotic gap described by the electron microprobe studies (9) (See Figure 1a). The four predominant organic solutes identified were the polyhydric alcohols, inositol and sorbitol, and the methylamines, GPC and betaine. Of interest is that polyhydric alcohols and methylamines are two of the three general groups of organic solutes observed in the marine organisms.

The third group, amino acids and their derivatives, are also present in relatively high concentration in the renal medulla (measured as ninhydrin-positive substances); however their osmotic role is only significant when they are considered as a group because no single solute is in high concentration. Amino acids have been implicated in the volume regulation of numerous marine invertebrate cells (79) and Ehrlich ascites tumor cells (42). Law et al (48) reported that in papillary slices ninhydrin-positive substances increase in concentration when incubated in hypertonic NaCl solutions. However, as pointed out by these investigators, this increase can only explain a small fraction of the total osmotic gap. In contrast, Gullans et al (35) did not detect any change in ninhyrin-positive substances in the rat inner medulla in vivo with increased antidiuretic state. Thus the role of the ninhydrin-positive substances in the osmoregulation of the renal medulla is unclear.

Since the connection between the predominant organic solutes and renal medullary intracelluluar milieu was first made, numerous studies have been directed at evaluating the role of the four predominant organic solutes to cell function. Before these studies are reviewed the renal distribution, metabolism, and transport of the four predominant organic solutes will be discussed.

RENAL DISTRIBUTION OF ORGANIC SOLUTES

Each of the four organic solutes is present in higher concentration in the renal medulla than in the cortex. However studies have demonstrated that their

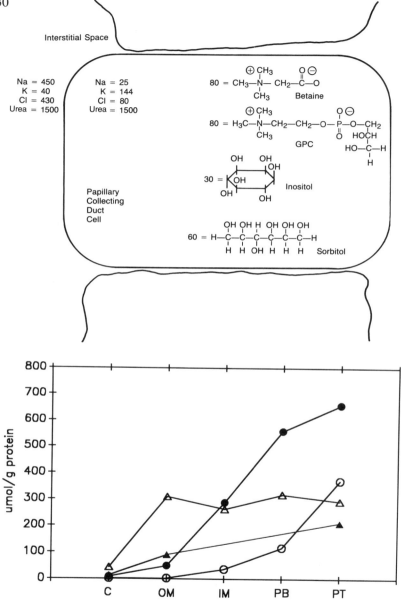

Figure 1 Inorganic and organic solute contents of the mammalian kidney. (*A*) Schematic diagram of the solutes in the papillary collecting duct. All values are reported as mMoles/Kg wet wt. Ion data is from reference 9 in rats, organic solute data from reference 3 in rabbits. (*B*) Distribution of organic solutes in the rat kidney. C-cortex, OM-outer medulla, IM-inner medulla, PB Papilla base, PT Papillary tip. Sorbitol, inositol, and GPC data is from reference (73) in Spraque Dawly rats. Betaine data is from the deer mouse (78).

intrarenal distributions differ and do not necessarily parallel the concentration gradients for NaCl or urea. For example, Cohen et al (21) first showed that in the dog the inositol concentration increased from cortex to outer medulla, but then slightly decreased in the inner medulla. This profile was also reproduced in the rat kidney (73) and in mice (78). In contrast, the concentration gradients for GPC, sorbitol, and betaine increase along the corticomedullary axis to the papillary tip as one might expect if these solutes were playing a role in maintaining the intracellular milieu. These studies of rats and mice also suggest that sorbitol exhibits a significantly steeper concentration gradient along the corticomedullary axis than the other three organic solutes. Reports to date have not provided enough information to determine if the organic solutes linearly increase in concentration along the medullopapillary axis as do sodium and urea (2). Figure 1b shows the distribution of the predominant organic solutes in the rat kidney.

Although the same four predominant organic solutes have been found in the renal medullas of rats, rabbits, mice, and vole, some interspecies differences are noted with regard to their relative concentrations. For example, in rabbits betaine content (3) is much higher than in rats (35) where this lower betaine content is made up by a higher concentration of GPC. The differences in the polyols is within experimental error. The reasons for these differences may be species or diet related. It is also unclear whether all of the cells at the same level in the renal medulla have the same organic contents. Studies on cell cultures have shown a wide variety in the distribution of the osmolytes in different cell lines (54), which suggests that different medullary cell types may be utilizing different organic solutes. In addition, the intracellular distribution (i.e. mitochondria, vesicles, and so on) of these solutes is also unknown. Although no information on the organic solute content of human kidneys has been reported, betaine and proline-betaine have been measured in human urine (15) and therefore are likely to be present in the human renal medulla. Human intrarenal distribution of these solutes may be obtained using noninvasive NMR techniques (13, 75–77).

RENAL ORGANIC SOLUTE METABOLISM AND TRANSPORT

Although all four organic solutes are hypothesized to play a role in maintaining a favorable intracellular milieu, each solute has its own biochemistry and cellular transport characteristics. The content of each organic solute will depend on many factors including rate of influx and efflux and rate of biosynthesis and catabolism. The general biochemical pathways involving the organic solutes have been elucidated largely in nonrenal tissues. For the purposes of discussion, each solute will be briefly discussed with regard to its metabolism and transport.

Myo-Inositol

MYO-INOSITOL METABOLISM   Myo-inositol is a polyhydric cyclitol. Numerous mammalian organs, including kidney, brain, liver, and testis, can synthesize inositol de novo (27). In fasting humans, for example, each kidney synthesizes ~2g/day of myo-inositol from glucose (19). This amount is more than the normal dietary intake of ~1g/day (18). As shown in Figure 2a, inositol is produced by the oxidation of glucose 6-phosphate to L-inositol 1-phosphate, which is then converted to free myo-inositol.

The rate limiting step in de novo synthesis is thought to be the formation of L-inositol 1-phosphate, since in the whole kidney the activity of the synthase is half that of the phosphatase (27). In addition, there is some evidence that in rat liver and testis the activity of this enzyme is under hormonal control (27, 38, 70). However no hormonally induced changes in synthase activity have been obseved in the kidney. Figure 2a also shows that inositol can be produced from phosphatidylinositol, which results in D-inositol 1-phosphate that can then be converted to myo-inositol. Because de novo synthesis produces L-inositol 1-phosphate and phosphoinositide breakdown produces D-inositol 1-phosphate, the rate of de novo synthesis can be compared to the rate of phosphoinositide breakdown. In whole kidney, the rate of de novo inositol synthesis is ~4 times greater than its formation from phosphatidylinositol (61).

In contrast to myo-inositol synthesis, which occurs in many organs, myo-inositol catabolism occurs only in the kidney (43, 49). Slices of rat renal cortex and outer medulla catabolize exogenously applied myo-inositol at a 200-fold greater rate than do papillary slices (43). The first step in myo-inositol catabolism is its conversion to D-glucuronate by myo-inositol oxygenase, an enzyme found only present in kidney (Figure 2a). In subsequent steps the D-glucuronate is converted to D-xylulose-5-phosphate, which then enters the pentose phosphate cycle (37, 69).

MYO-INOSITOL TRANSPORT   At physiologic plasma concentrations myo-inositol is almost completely reabsorbed by the rat and human kidney, with only about 2% of the filtered load being found in the urine (23, 24). Studies using rabbit renal brush border membranes demonstrate electrogenic, sodium-dependent inositol transport (36). Glucose inhibits myo-inositol uptake, but myo-inositol does not inhibit glucose uptake, which suggests that myo-inositol has a separate transporter from that used for the majority of glucose transport (36).

It is unknown to what extent renal medullary cells can transport myo-inositol and whether the high extracellular concentration of sodium found in this region during antidiuresis could provide an increased driving force for myo-inositol cotransport. The fact that the highest concentration of myo-inositol is present in the outer medulla suggests that the accumulation of myo-inositol may be related to factors other than simply extracellular Na.

Sorbitol

SORBITOL METABOLISM   Sorbitol is a polyhydric alcohol that has been widely studied because of its pathologic accumulation in mammalian tissues in diabetes mellitus. The normal concentration of sorbitol in systemic plasma is low, ~30 μM in rat and ~2 μM in man (44). Although in many tissues the normal concentration of sorbitol is also low, some tissues such as the renal medulla, placenta, and seminal fluid normally have high concentrations of sorbitol. In placenta and seminal fluid the high concentrations of sorbitol are thought to result as a metabolic intermediate from active fructose production (71).

As shown in Figure 2b, aldose reductase (AR) catalyzes the synthesis of sorbitol from glucose. Gabbay & O'Sullivan (33) were the first to report that in the kidney AR activity is highest in the papilla. Since then, immunohistochemical staining of the rat (50) and dog (47) kidney for AR shows that the enzyme is located primarily in cells comprising the thin limbs of the loop of Henle, the inner medullary collecting ducts, and the pelvic epithelial lining. The amount of AR in other regions of the kidney is much lower. Sands et al (59) studied the activity of AR in isolated segments of the rat kidney and found a similar distribution. These findings suggest that sorbitol synthesis may play an important role in the regulation of renal sorbitol content.

Studies of renal cells in culture also suggest that AR may play an important role in sorbitol accumulation. The amount of AR protein (and as a result, AR activity) increased with a time course on the order of days when cells were exposed to a medium of high osmolarity (11). The sorbitol accumulation observed in this cell line was attributed to increased expression of AR and may be a long-term regulatory mechanism in the regulation of sorbitol levels (7).

Sorbitol biosynthesis is also affected by the concentration of glucose and by the concentration of $NADP^+$. In many tissues AR's, K_M for glucose is much higher than the intracellular glucose concentration. Bovine kidney AR has a K_M of 56 mM (32) and rat renal medullary AR has a K_M of 72 mM (16). Thus, in the kidney, as in most other tissues, the rate of sorbitol synthesis should be regulated by the intracellular glucose concentration. This conclusion is supported by studies that show a twofold increase in papillary sorbitol in rats seven days after induction of diabetes, despite no change in AR or sorbitol dehydrogenase (SDH) activity (16).

All the enzymes necessary for sorbitol catabolism are present in significant activity in the human kidney (40) (see Figure 2b). Sorbitol is first oxidized to fructose by SDH. Fructose is then phosphorylated to fructose 1-phosphate,

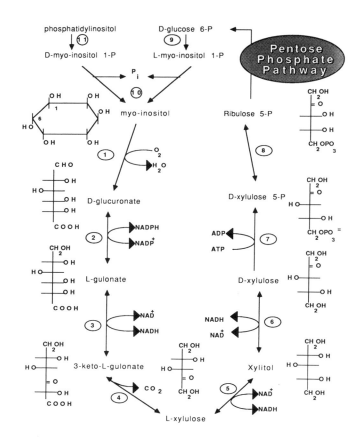

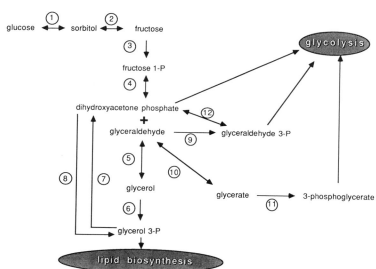

which is split into dihydroxyacetone phosphate and glyceraldehyde. These products can be used eventually in glycolysis, gluconeogenesis, and lipid biosynthesis.

SDH is present in a variety of mammalian tissues but, in general, it is found in highest activity in liver and kidney (17). Renal SDH activity per wet weight is roughly tenfold higher in the cortex than in the medulla (16, 17, 40). The activities of the other enzymes involved in the metabolism of fructose are all generally much higher in the renal cortex than in the renal medulla (40). Tracer studies using 3-^{19}F-deoxyglucose in vivo have demonstrated that sorbitol catabolism is mostly limited to the renal cortex (12). The reciprocal relation in the kidney with regard to the locations and activities of AR and enzymes that catabolize sorbitol explains the observed high concentration of sorbitol in renal medulla and its low concentration in renal cortex (16, 55).

SORBITOL TRANSPORT   Little is known about sorbitol transport in renal tissue; indeed, it has occasionally been used as an extracellular space marker. However cultured renal cells, as well as isolated medullary tubules (73), rapidly and selectively release sorbitol when exposed to isotonic media after adaptation to hypertonic conditions. Recent data suggest that a specific transport pathway for sorbitol exists in the cultured papillary cells (A. W. Siebens & K. Spring, personal communication). However the precise selectivity and mechanism of activation of this transport process is presently unknown. Thus both metabolism (for accumulation) and transport (for acute exit) may be involved in the regulation of sorbitol levels in vivo.

Betaine

BETAINE METABOLISM   Betaine (also called glycine-betaine or N,N,N-trimethylglycine) is present in many plants and, therefore, is present in the

---

Figure 2   Metabolism of inositol and sorbitol. (A) myo-inositol. The numbers in circles refer to the enzymes that catalyze each reaction: 1) myo-inositol oxygenase (EC 1.13.99.1); 2) glucuronate reductase (EC 1.1.1.19); 3) L-3-aldonate dehydrogenase (EC 1.1.1.45); 4) Keto-L-gulonate decarboxylase (EC 4.1.1.34); 5) L-xylulose reductase (EC 1.1.1.10); 6) L-iditol dehdrogenase (EC 1.1.1.14) and D-xylulose reductase (EC 1.1.1.9); 7) xylulokinase (EC 2.7.1.17); 8) ribulose-phosphate 3-epimerase (EC 5.1.3.1); 9) myo-inositol 1-phosphate synthase (EC 5.5.1.4); 10) 1-L-myo-inositol-1-phosphatase (EC 3.1.3.25), and 11) phospholipase C (EC 3.1.4.3). Carbons 1 and 6 of myo-inositol are labeled to highlight the fact that it is the 1–6 bond that is cleaved in the first step of its catabolism. (B) Sorbitol. The numbers in circles refer to the enzymes that catalyze each reaction: 1) aldose reductase (EC 1.1.1.21); 2) L-iditol dehydrogenase (EC 1.1.1.14); 3) ketohexokinase (EC 2.7.1.3); 4) aldolase B (EC 4.1.2.13); 5) aldose reductase (EC 1.1.1.21); 6) glycerol kinase (EC 2.7.1.30); 7) glycero-3-phosphate dehydrogenase (NAD$^+$) (EC 1.1.1.8); 8) glycero-3-phosphate dehydrogenase (EC 1.1.99.5); 9) triose kinase (EC 2.7.1.28); 10) aldehyde dehydrogenase (EC 1.2.1.3); 11) glycerate kinase (EC 2.7.1.31); 12) triose phosphate isomerase (EC 5.3.1.1).

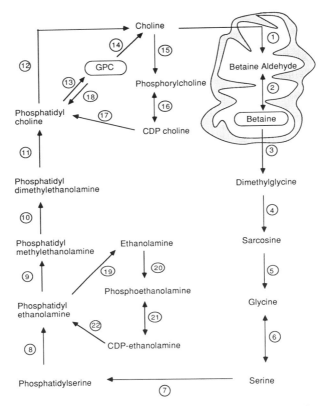

Figure 3 Metabolism of betaine and GPC. The numbers in circles refer to the enzymes that catalyze each reaction: 1) choline dehydrogenase (EC 1.1.99.1); 2) betaine aldehyde dehydrogenase (EC 1.2.1.8); 3) betaine-homocyseine transmethylase (EC 2.1.1.5); 4) dimethylglycine dehydrogenase (EC 1.5.99.2); 5) sarcosine oxidase (EC 1.5.3.1); 6) serine hydroxymethyl transferase (EC 2.1.2.1); 7) base exchange reaction with another phospholipid; 8) phosphatidyl serine decarboxylase (EC 4.1.1.65); 9) phosphotidylethanolamine methyltransferase (EC 2.1.1.17); 10) phosphotidyl-N-methylethanolamine methyltransferase (EC 2.1.1.71); 11) phosphotidyl-N-methylethanolamine methyltransferase (EC 2.1.1.71); 12) phospholipase D (EC 3.1.4.4); 13) phospholipase A$_2$ (EC 3.1.1.4); 14) phospholipase B (EC 3.1.1.5); 15) choline kinase (EC 2.7.1.32); 16) choline-phosphate cytidylytransferase (EC 2.7.7.15); 17) cholinephosphotransferase (EC 2.7.8.2); 18) reacylation of GPC to phosphatidylcholine; 19) base exchange reaction with serine; 20) choline kinase (EC 2.7.1.32); 21) ethanolamine phosphate cytidylyl transferase (EC 2.7.7.14); 22) ethanolamine phosphotransferase (EC 2.7.8.1). The mitochondrion drawn around betaine aldehyde and betaine serves as a reminder that choline and betaine aldehyde are oxidized in the mitochondrial matrix.

diet of most animals. However, the major dietary source for betaine is probably choline, which is oxidized to betaine in the liver and kidney (39). The metabolic pathways involving betaine biosynthesis are shown in Figure 3. Choline is a substrate for betaine synthesis. It is oxidized in the mitochondria to betaine aldehyde, which in turn is then oxidized to betaine (22). The ability to oxidize choline to betaine has been identified in the proximal convoluted and pars recta tubule (74) and the inner medulla of the rat kidney (34). Interestingly, no choline dehydrogenase is present in the outer medulla (74). Studies using radioactive (39) and ^{2}H tracers (28) have demonstrated that the major short-term (1 to 2 hr) metabolite or infused choline is betaine, and it is present in the kidney in high concentration.

As shown in Figure 3, only after choline is oxidized to betaine can the methyl groups be removed. Betaine is catabolized to dimethylglycine then to sarcosine, and finally to glycine. Only one methyl group is recovered to generate methionine; the other two are converted to formate.

BETAINE TRANSPORT   Although there have been no reports of betaine transport by renal medullary cells, active transport of betaine has been demonstrated in both small intestine and renal cortex (29). Imino acids such as proline and hydroxyproline are transported by the same system and can competitively inhibit betaine transport (29, 31). It appears that renal cortical cells have a separate transporter for choline (63).

Betaine transport has also been demonstrated in rat liver mitochondria where it is believed to be a rate limiting step in its synthesis (26a). The rate of betaine efflux from mitochondria has also been observed to decrease with an increase in the concentration of inorganic ions in the medium (26a). Although this in vitro observation suggests that the production of betaine would be inhibited by an increase in the inorganic ion content of the cytosol, it is consistent with the mitochondrial matrix retaining betaine as a nonperturbing solute upon its exposure to hypertonic environments.

Studies of betaine transport with regard to osmoregulation have been conducted in E. coli and show induction of uptake mechanisms when the bacterium is exposed to a hypertonic environment (41). These studies also showed that the enzymes responsible for synthesizing betaine from choline were also induced in hyperosmotic environments. In bacteria a long-term exposure to a hypertonic external medium causes an increase in intracellular ionic strength which, through an as yet undefined mechanism, appropriately regulates gene expression. DNA supercoiling in high ionic strength has been suggested as a mechanism (41).

Glycerophosphorylcholine (GPC)

GPC METABOLISM   GPC is a lipid metabolite present in a variety of tissues (e.g. liver, muscle, brain, and testis) in concentrations of 0.1–1 mM (14, 72). It has not been previously described as an osmoregulatory solute in any marine organisms. However, because it has structural similarities to both polyhydric alcohols and methylamines, it has been proposed to have similar properties with regard to protecting the intracellular milieu (8, 62). Despite the fact that GPC was originally discovered to be in high concentration in the renal medulla [the 1950s (68)], little is known about its metabolism and transport.

As shown in Figure 3, GPC can accumulate intracellularly via its synthesis that depends on the rate of phosphatidylcholine (lecithin) catabolism. Phosphatidylcholine can be de-acylated via sequential action of phospholipase A (A_1 or A_2) and phospholipase B (lysophospholipase) to leave free GPC. However, the precise pathway utilized by renal medullary cells to produce GPC remains to be elucidated.

Catabolism of GPC can potentially occur via its hydrolysis, although the activity of GPC hydrolizing enzymes in the rat renal papilla is low ($\sim$100-fold lower than in the cortex) (72). Alternatively, GPC can potentially be incorporated into phosphatidylcholine, since acyltransferases have been demonstrated in this region of the kidney (66).

GPC TRANSPORT   It is possible that GPC accumulates in the renal medulla via active transport. The potential for GPC transport has been shown by the recent finding of a GPC transporter in preparations of rat liver microsomes (46). However to date there have been no reports of transport of GPC by renal medullary cells.

PHYSIOLOGIC SIGNIFICANCE OF ORGANIC SOLUTES

To play a significant role in volume regulation and in protection of the normal intracellular milieu, the organic solutes must be intracellular, osmotically active in the cytosol (i.e. not bound), and appropriately regulated by changes in the extracellular space (i.e. responsive to the diuretic state). Evidence supporting their osmoregulatory role is presented below.

Are They Intracellular?

The organic solutes must be located within the cell if they are to osmotically balance extracellular NaCl and protect macromolecular function from the adverse effects of urea. However in vivo studies of medullary organic solutes that rely on measurements obtained from nuclear magnetic resonance (NMR) or analysis of renal extracts are unable to determine to what extent these organic solutes are located intracellularly. The strongest evidence for intracellular localization comes from the finding that medullary tubule suspensions contain high concentrations of GPC, sorbitol, and inositol, and that these concentrations are not significantly different from those found in intact medullary tissue in vivo (6, 73). Although betaine was not measured in these studies, it is likely that it too is located intracellularly. Support for this notion comes from cell culture studies that show that hypertonic media can cause betaine to accumulate to high intracellular concentrations (54) and in vivo studies that show that the concentration of betaine and the other organic solutes in antidiuretic urine is low (3).

Are They Osmotically Active?

There have been no reports of studies specifically designed to determine osmotic activity of the organic solutes in renal cells. However studies of skeletal muscle suggest that myo-inositol is bound intracellularly in this tissue and that this process serves as the mechanism by which myo-inositol is concentrated in the cell (53). But, it should be noted that the concentration of myo-inositol in skeletal muscle is roughly 100-fold less than that found in the renal medulla (25, 53).

The problem of measuring the activity of these solutes in renal medullary cells is complicated by the fact that there are no selective microelectrodes to determine the intracellular activity of these solutes, although a K^+ sensitive electrode could possibly be used to determine total trimethylamine content (3). Nevertheless, ^1H and ^{31}P NMR spectroscopic studies indicate that the organic solutes are osmotically active in the kidney in vivo. Myo-inositol, GPC, and total trimethylamines have relatively narrow ^1H and ^{31}P NMR resonances, which dictate a maximum rotational correlation time for these solutes on the order of 10^{-10} s for these simple dipole nuclides (13, 76, 77). These narrow NMR lines and calculated short correlation times suggest that little or no macromolecular binding of these solutes occurs in vivo. In addition, studies of cell cultures adapted to hypertonic media domonstrate that cellular sorbitol balances most of the electrolytic osmotic gap, thus suggesting that sorbitol is not significantly bound in this system as well (5).

Do They Change Appropriately with Diuretic State?

Physiologists have known for years that the concentrations of NaCl and urea in the inner medulla change as a function of diuretic state. Thus if the medullary organic solutes are present in response to high concentrations of NaCl and urea, then one might also expect them to change with diuretic state. Several laboratories have tested this theory in vivo to investigate the physiologic importance of the medullary organic solutes. Studies have examined both the long-term (> 1 hr) and short-term (≤ 1 hr) effects of the diuretic state on medullary organic solute content.

LONG-TERM STUDIES   Philippson (56) was the first to demonstrate changes in an organic solute concentration as a function of diuretic state when he reported that compared to antidiuretic rats, medullary GPC content decreased by ~80% after 2 hr of diuresis. These findings were confirmed by Wolff et al (77) in rabbit, where renal GPC content decreased 30% after 20 hr of continual water diuresis. Cohen et al (21) demonstrated changes in inositol content as a function of diuretic state when they found that diuresis resulted in a 30% decrease in myo-inositol in canine inner medulla. Subsequent studies of rabbit (3), rat (35), and mouse (78) have monitored all four organic solutes and found that, in general, each organic solute changes in content as a function of diuretic state. In these studies, organic solute content was monitored 18–72 hr after a change in diuretic state. Therefore, these data are consistent with the notion that the organic solutes play a physiologically significant role in the renal medulla, at least over the long term.

SHORT-TERM STUDIES   Additional studies of the medullary organic solutes have been conducted to determine their acute physiologic significance. Using ^{31}P NMR in vivo Wolff et al (77) showed that renal GPC content did not change within 1 hr after antidiuretic rabbits underwent saline and or furosemide-induced diuresis. The effectiveness of the diuresis in diluting the medullary interstitium was demonstrated by a decrease in medullary sodium as assessed by ^{23}Na NMR imaging, an increase in urine output, and decreases in urinary sodium and urea. These findings are in apparent conflict with similar studies on rat that showed GPC content to decline substantially after 1 hr of water diuresis and 4 hr of furosemide diuresis (72).

Later studies that measured all the organic solutes in rabbit medullary extracts (75) showed that 40 min after furosemide diuresis, the three organic solutes other than GPC decreased by 50–80%. In contrast, infusion of isotonic mannitol caused all four organic solutes to decrease significantly, which indicates that each of the organic solutes can decrease acutely with diuresis. Administration of isotonic glucose caused a significant decrease in the three organic solutes other than sorbitol. Notably, glucose infusion also caused a decrease in phosphorylethanolamine, an organic solute primarily located in the renal cortex (77).

The above data show that the organic solutes respond differently with different modes of diuresis and medullary dilution. This finding suggests that the organic solutes may be regulated separately, respond to different signals, and/or be predominantly located in different cell types. The exact function of each organic solute and the precise signals involved in their regulation are still unknown.

Shorter time course studies (75) showed that organic solutes significantly decreased in content 20 min after the start of saline and furosemide infusion. Although shorter time points were not collected, the data suggest that the decrease in organic solute content can take place with a time course similar to that observed for inorganic ion fluxes. Later time points demonstrated that after diuresis the sodium and urea gradients returned to prediuresis levels, but the organic solutes did not similarly increase in content (over ~2 hr). Therefore the renal medullary cells had to increase their intracellular concentration of inorganic ions or lose cell water because of the lower organic solute content present after recovery of the sodium gradient. The data suggest that the organic solutes are physiologically significant in the short term in vivo with regard to their acute efflux from the cell to prevent damage from osmotic swelling, and they may share similar signals, such as intracellular Ca^{2+} that can trigger KCl efflux during volume regulatory decreases. However organic solutes may not be physiologically significant in the short term with regard to their osmotically balancing extracellular NaCl or protecting macromolecular function from the adverse effects of urea. This conclusion is based on the fact that despite the rapid decrease in organic solute content that accompanies diuresis, organic solute reaccumulation does not parallel the recovery of the NaCl and urea gradient. Similar results have also been obtained in Brattleboro rats after treatment with ADH, where the sodium and urea gradients are established much faster than the organic solutes accumulate (60).

There are no reports of short-term studies in vivo demonstrating the fate of the organic solutes that are no longer present in the kidney after the onset of diuresis. Studies involving suspensions of medullary tubules demonstrate that inositol, sorbitol, and GPC (betaine was not measured) are released from the cells when they are incubated in isotonic media (73). Similar findings were obtained from cell culture studies involving renal epithelial cell lines that demonstrate a rapid efflux of sorbitol when hypertonically adapted cells are placed in isotonic media (4). These findings suggest that during diuresis in vivo the organic solutes are released into the circulation and possibly the urine and are not catabolized acutely by the renal medullary cells.

Reason for Maintaining Intracellular Milieu

A relationship between organic solute content and long-term medullary sodium chloride and urea has been established in intact animals as well as in cell culture systems. Thus these solutes may play a long-term role in the maintenance of the intracellular milieu. In the short term, the organic solutes can decrease rapidly just as has been observed for the inorganic constituents of the cell. However the medullary gradient of NaCl and urea can reform much faster than the organic solutes accumulate after diuresis or with ADH, which indicates that the organic solutes may not be critical to the short-term physiologic function of the renal medulla. The organic solutes may be more important to the long-term function or survival of the renal medulla (i.e. cell division or growth). For example, cell culture studies have shown that the inhibition of organic solute accumulation during hypertonic challenges inhibits cloning efficiency (P. Yancy, S. Bagnaseco, M. Burg, personal communication). In the kidney in vivo the epithelial cellular proliferation rate of the renal medulla is one of the slowest in the body (65), which might be influenced by the high concentrations of extracellular urea and NaCl, as discussed earlier, that may be only partially corrected by the organic solutes. Thus in the short term the renal medulla could still function with a significantly reduced content of the prominent organic solutes. Over the long term these solutes do adjust appropriately to the extracellular environment and, based mostly on cell culture data, these solutes are necessary for the long-term survival of these cells. Clearly more studies are needed to evaluate the short- and long-term physiologic significance of the organic solutes to normal renal function and to observe how they relate to human renal disease and pathology.

Other Physiologic Functions

Although the predominent organic solutes are hypothesized to be present because of the elevated NaCl and urea concentrations in the renal medulla, the possibility still exists that they could serve other physiologic functions. They could serve alternate functions in renal medullary cells or potentially in cells of other organs, if the organic solutes were released into the circulation with diuresis.

MYO-INOSITOL   Others have proposed that high concentrations of myo-inositol are present in the kidney to favor the formation of phosphatidylinositol (67) which, among other things, has been implicated as an endogenous activator of the $(Na^+ + K^+)$-ATPase in microsomes of the rabbit kidney (51). This suggestion is based on the observation that phosphatidylinositol synthase (which uses myo-inositol and CDP-diacylglycerol to synthesize phosphatidylinositol) has a relatively high K_M (1.5 mM) for myo-inositol.

It is possible that in the kidney myo-inositol has two functions: serving an osmotic role in the inner medulla and serving as a precursor to phosphatidylinositol in the outer medulla. Consistent with an alternate role for myo-inositol is the fact that its concentration does not increase linearly to the papillary tip as one might expect if it were playing solely an osmotic role (21). The highest concentration appears to be in the outer medulla, which suggests perhaps that high concentrations of myo-inositol are in cells active in transport like those from the thick ascending limb and straight proximal tubule. In the dog the concentration of myo-inositol in this outer medullary region did not decrease with a decrease in the corticomedullary sodium and urea gradients that accompanies diuresis (21). However, inner medullary myo-inositol content did decrease in response to a decrease in inner medullary osmolarity, a finding consistent with myo-inositol's role as an osmotic determinent in cells in this region of the kidney.

SORBITOL   The physiologic role of the polyol pathway in mammalian tissues is largely undefined except for the case of the seminal vesicle that uses it to generate fructose, the preferred substrate for glycolysis in spermatazoa (71). While there is no evidence for the accumulation of fructose in renal medullary cells, flux though the polyol pathway has been described as an alternative pathway to glycolysis (45). The alternative pathway, which is favored when glycolysis is active, can produce glycerol, a metabolite involved in lipid synthesis. Thus, besides being a nonperturbing solute, sorbitol and its metabolism could be serving a metabolic role in the renal medulla.

SUMMARY AND CONCLUSION

The predominant organic solutes of the renal medulla have been hypothesized to osmotically balance extracellular NaCl and protect macromolecular function from the adverse effects of urea. The evidence for their long- and short-term physiologic significance in vivo has been reviewed. The organic solutes decrease acutely in response to diuresis with a time course similar to that observed for inorganic ion fluxes and therefore probably play an important role in short-term volume regulation. However, because organic solutes are slow to accumulate (even in the presence of high urea and sodium concentrations), their significance to the short-term physiologic function of renal medullary epithelia is in doubt and needs further investigation. The organic solutes may be more important to the long-term function and survival of renal medullary cells.

ACKNOWLEDGMENTS

The authors would like to thank M.B. Burg, P. Yancey, K. Spring, and W. G. Guder for stimulating discussions and continuing exchange of unpublished data. Dr. Wolff was a Howard Hughes Medical Institute—National Institutes of Health Research Scholar during the preparation of this review.

Literature Cited

1. Altringham, J. D., Yancey, P. H., Johnston, I. A. 1982. The effects of osmoregulatory solutes on tension generation by dogfish skinned muscle fibers. *J. Exp. Biol.* 96:443–45
2. Atherton, J. C., Green, R., Thomas, S. 1970. Effects of 0.9% saline infusion on urinary and renal tissue composition in the hydropaenic, normal, and hydrated conscious rat. *J. Physiol.* 210:45–71
3. Bagnasco, S., Balaban, R., Fales, H. M., Yang, Y., Burg, M. 1986. Predominant osmotically active organic solutes in rat and rabbit renal medullas. *J. Biol. Chem.* 261:5872–5877
4. Bagnasco, S., Bedford, J., Burg, M. 1988. Slow changes in aldose reductase

and rapid changes in sorbitol flux mediate osmoregulation by renal medullary cells. *Fed. Proc.* 46:1229
5. Bagnasco, S. M., Uchida, S., Balaban, R. S., Kador, P. F., Burg, M. B. 1987. Induction of aldose reductase and sorbitol in renal inner medullary cells by elevated extracellular NaCl. *Proc. Natl. Acad. Sci. USA* 84:1718–20
6. Balaban, R. S. 1983. The Application of Nuclear Magnetic Resonance to the Study of Epithelial Tissues. In *Membrane Biophysics II: Physical Methods in the Study of Epithelia*, pp. 73–86. New York: Liss
7. Balaban, R. S., Burg, M. B. 1987. Osmotically active organic solutes in the

renal inner medulla. *Kidney Int.* 31:562–64

8. Balaban, R. S., Knepper, M. A. 1983. Nitrogen-14 nuclear magnetic resonance spectroscopy of mammalian tissues. *Am. J. Physiol.* 245 (*Cell Physiol.* 14):C439–44

9. Beck, F., Dorge, A., Rick, R., Thurau, K. 1984. Intra- and extracellular element concentrations of rat renal papilla in antidiuresis. *Kidney Int.* 25:397–403

10. Beck, F., Dorge, A., Rick, R., Thurau, K. 1985. Osmoregulation of renal papillary cells. *Pflügers. Arch.* 405:528–32

11. Bedord, J. J., Bagnasco, S. M., Kador, P. F., Harris, H. W. Jr., Burg, M. B. 1987. Characterization and purification of a mammalian osmoregulatory protein, aldose reductase, induced in renal medullary cells by high extracellular NaCl. *J. Biol. Chem.* 262(29):14255–59

12. Berkowitz, B. A., Moriyama, T., Balaban, R. S. 1989. Distribution and metabolic fate of 3F3Deoxy glucose in vivo. *Eighth Ann. Mtg. Soc. Magn. Reson. Med.* 1:383

13. Berkowitz, B. A., Wolff, S. D., Balaban, R. S. 1988. Detection of metabolites in vivo using 2D proton homonuclear correlated spectroscopy. *J. Magn. Reson.* 79:547–53

14. Chalovich, J. M., Burt, C. T., Danon, M. J., Glonek, T., Barany, M. 1979. Phosphodiesters in muscular dystrophies. *Ann. NY. Acad. Sci.* 317:614–57

15. Chambers, S. T., Kunin, C. M. 1987. Isolation of glycine betaine and proline betaine from human urine: assessment of their role as osmoprotective agents for bacteria and the kidney. *J. Clin. Invest.* 79:731–37

16. Chauncey, B., Leite, M. V., Goldstein, L. 1988. Renal sorbitol accumulation and associated enzyme activities in diabetes. *Enzyme* 39:231–34

17. Clampitt, R. B., Hart, R. J. 1978. The tissue activities of some diagnostic enzymes in ten mammalian species. *J. Comp. Path.* 88:607–21

18. Clements, R. S. Jr., Reynertson, R. 1977. Myoinsoitol metabolism in diabetes mellitus. *Diabetes* 26:215–21

19. Clements, R. S. Jr., Diethelm, A. G. 1979. The metabolism of myo-inositol by the human kidney. *J. Lab. Clin. Med.* 93:210–19

20. Cohen, J. J. 1979. Is the function of the renal papilla coupled exclusively to an anaerobic pattern of metabolism? *Am. J. Physiol.* 236:F423–33

21. Cohen, M. A. H., Hruska, K. A.,

Daughaday, W. H. 1982. Free myo-inositol in canine kidneys: selective concentration in the renal medulla. *Proc. Soc. Exp. Biol. Med.* 169:380–85

22. Dagley, S., Nicholson, D. E. 1970. In *An introduction to metabolic pathways.* Oxford: Blackwell

23. Daughaday, W. H., Larner, J. 1954a. The renal excretion of inositol in normal and diabetic human beings. *J. Clin. Invest.* 23:326–32

24. Daughaday, W. H., Larner, J. 1954b. The renal excretion of inositol by normal and diabetic rats. *J. Clin. Invest.* 23: 1075–80

25. Dawson, R. M. C., Freinkel, N. 1961. The distribution of free mesoinositol in mammalian tissues, including some observations on the lactating rat. *Biochem. J.* 78:606–10

26. Dell, R. B., Winters, R. W. 1967. Lactate gardients in the kidney of the dog. *Am. J. Physiol.* 213:301–7

26a. deRidder, J. J. M., van Dam, K. 1973. The efflux of betaine from rat-liver mitochondria a possible regulating step in choline oxidation. *Biochim. Biophys. Acta.* 291:557–63

27. Eisenberg, F. Jr. 1967. D-Myoinositol 1-phosphate as product of cyclization of glucose 6-phosphate and substrate for a specific phosphatase in rat testis. *J. Biol. Chem.* 242(7):1375–82

28. Eng, J., Berkowitz, B. A., Balaban, R. S. 1990. Renal distribution and metabolism of 2Hg-choline: a 2H NMR and MRI study. *NMR Biomed.* In press

29. Evered, D. F., Nunn, P. B. 1970. Transport pathway for glycine betaine in rat kidney cortex *in vitro. Biochem. J.* 118:40P–41P

30. Fessler, J. H., Tandberg, W. D. 1975. Interactions between collagen chains and fiber formation. *J. Supramol. Struct.* 3:17–23

31. Franklin, C. S., Evered, D. F., Nunn, P. B. 1970. Transport pathway for glycine betaine in rabbit kidney *in vivo. Biochem. J.* 118:41P

32. Gabbay, K. H., Cathcart, E. S. 1974. Purification and immunologic identification of aldose reductase. *Diabetes* 23:460–68

33. Gabbay, K. H., O'Sullivan, J. B. 1968. The sorbitol pathway in diabetes and galactosemia: enzyme and substrate localization and changes in the kidney. *Diabetes* 17:300

34. Grossman, E. B., Hebert, S. C. 1989. Renal inner medullary choline dehydrogenase activity: characterization and modulation. *Amer. J. Physiol.* 256:F107–11

35. Gullans, S. R., Blumenfeld, J. D., Balaschi, J. A., Kaleta, M., Brenner, R. M., et al. 1988. Accumulation of major organic osmolytes in rat renal inner medulla in dehydration. *Am. J. Physiol.* 255 (*Ren. Fluid Electrolyte Physiol.* 24):F626–34

36. Hammerman, M. R., Sacktor, B., Daughaday, W. H. 1980. Myo-inositol transport in renal brush border vesicles and its inhibition by D-glucose. *Am. J. Physiol.* 239 (*Ren. Fluid Electrolyte Physiol.* 8):F113–20

37. Hankes, L. V., Politzer, W. M., Touster, O., Anderson, L. 1969. Myo-Inositol catabolism in human pentosurics: the predominant role of the glucuronate-xylulose-pentose phosphate pathway. *Ann. N.Y. Acad. Sci.* 165:564–76

38. Hasegawa, R., Eisenberg, F. Jr. 1981. Selective hormonal control of myo-inositol biosynthesis in reproductive organs and liver of the male rat. *Proc. Natl. Acad. Sci. USA* 78(8):4863–66

39. Haubrich, D. R., Wang, P. F. L., Wedeking, P. W. 1975. Distribution and metabolism of intravenously administered choline[methyl-^{3}H] and sythesis in vivo of acetylcholine in various tissues of guinea pigs. *J. Pharm. Exp. Ther.* 193:246–55

40. Heinz, F., Schlegel, F., Krause, P. H. 1975. Enzymes of fructose metabolism in human kidney. *Enzyme* 19:85–92

41. Higgins, C. F., Cairney, J., Stirling, D. A., Sutherland, L., and Booth, R. 1987. Osmotic regulation of gene expression: ionic strength as an intracellular signal? *Trends Biol. Sci.* 12:339–44

42. Hoffmann, E. K., Lambert, I. H. 1983. Amino acid transport and cell volume regulation in Ehrlich ascites tumor cells. *J. Physiol.* 338:613–25

43. Howard, C. F., Anderson, L. 1967. Metabolism of myo-inositol in animals. II. complete catabolism of myo-inositol-^{14}C by rat kidney slices. *Arch. Biochem. Biophys.* 118:332–39

44. Jeffrey, J., Jornvall, H. 1988. Sorbitol dehydrogenase. In *Adv. Enzym. and Rel. Mol. Biol,* ed. A. Meister, pp. 47–106. New York: Wiley Vol. 61

45. Jeffrey, J., Jornvall, H. 1983. Enzyme relationships in a sorbitol pathway that bypasses glycolysis and pentose phosphates in glucose metabolism. *Proc. Natl. Acad. Sci. USA* 80:901–5

46. Kawashima, Y., Bell, R. M. 1987. Assembly of the endoplasmic reticulum phospholipid bilayer. Transporters for phosphatidylcholine metabolites. *J. Biol. Chem.* 262(34):16495–502

47. Kern, T. S., Engerman, R. L. 1982.

Immunohistochemical distribution of aldose reductase. *Histochem. J.* 14: 507–15

48. Law, R. O., Turner, D. P. J. 1987. Are ninhydrin-positive substances volume regulatory osmolytes in rat renal papillary cells? *J. Physiol.* 386:45–61

49. Lewin, L. M., Yannai, Y., Sulimovici, S., Kraicer, P. F. 1976. Studies on the metabolic role of myo-inositol. Distribution of radioactive myo-inositol in the male rat. *Biochem. J.* 156:375–80

50. Ludvigson, M. A., Sorenson, R. L. 1980. Immunohistochemical localization of aldose reductase. II. rat eye and kidney. *Diabetes* 29:450–59

51. Mandersloot, J. G., Roelofsen, B., de Gier, J. 1978. Phosphatidylinositol as the endogenous activator of the $(Na^+ + K^+)$-ATPase in microsomes of the rabbit kidney. *Biochim. Biophys. Acta.* 508:478–85

52. McMillan, D. B., Battle, H. I. 1954. Effects of ethyl carbonate and related compounds on early developmental processes in the Leopard frog *Rana pipiens. Cancer. Res.* 14:319–23

53. Molitoris, B. A., Karl, I. E., Daughaday, W. H. 1980. Concentration of myo-inositol in skeletal muscle of the rat occurs without active transport. *J. Clin. Invest.* 65:783–88

54. Nakanishi, T., Balaban, R. S., Burg, M. B. 1988. Survey of osmolytes in renal cell lines. *Am. J. Physiol.* 255 (*Cell Physiol.* 24):C181–91

55. Oates, J., Goddu, K. J. 1987. A sorbitol gradient in rat renal medulla. *Kidney Int.* 31:448

56. Philippson, C. 1964. Der Gehalt an Glycerylphosphorylcholin und Glyceryl phosphorylaethanolamin von Nierenmark und Nierenrinde hochreiner Wistarratten während forcierter Wasserdiurese und extrem langer Durstantidiurese. *Pflügers Archiv.* 280:30–37

57. Deleted in proof

58. Sands, J. M., Nonoguchi, H., Knepper, M. A. 1987. Vasopressin effects on urea and H_2O transport in inner medullary collecting duct subsegments. *Am. J. Physiol.* 253 (*Ren. Fluid Electrolyte Physiol.* 22):F823–32

59. Sands, J. M., Terada, Y., Bernard, L. M., Knepper, M. A. 1989. Aldose reductase activities in microdissected rat nephron segments. *Amer. J. Physiol.* (*Renal Fluid Electrolyte Physiol.*) 256:F179–86

60. Schmolke, M., Beck, F., Guder, W. G. 1989. Effect of antidiuretic hormone on renal organic osmolytes in Brattleboro rats. *Am. J. Physiol.* 257F: In press

61. Sherman, W. R., Munsell, L. Y., Gish, B. G., Honchar, M. P. 1985. Effects of systematically administered lithium on phosphoinositide metabolism in rat brain, kidney, and testis. *J. Neurochem.* 44:798–807
62. Somero, G. N. 1986. Protons, osmolytes, and fitness of internal milieu for protein function. *Am. J. Physiol.* 251 (*Reg. Integrative Comp. Physiol.* 20): R197–13
63. Sung, C. P., Johnstone, R. M. 1969. Evidence for the existence of separate transport mechanisms for choline and betaine in rat kidney. *Biochim. Biophys. Acta.* 173:548–53
64. Thesleffs, S., Schmidt-Nielsen, K. 1962. Osmotic tolerance of the muscles of the crab-eating frog, *Rana cancriooria. J. Cell. Comp. Physiol.* 59:31–34
65. Threlfall, G. 1968. Cell proliferation in the rat kidney induced by folic acid. *Cell Tissue Kinet.* 1:383–92
66. Tou, J. S., Huggins, C. G. 1977. Lipid metabolism in mammals. In *Kidney,* ed. F. Snyder, p. 39. New York: Plenum Vol. 2
67. Troyer, D. A., Schwertz, D. W., Kreisberg, J. I., Venkatachalam, M. A. 1986. Inositol phospholipid metabolism in the kidney. *Annu. Rev. Physiol.* 48:51–71
68. Ullrich, K. J. 1956. Uber das Vorkommen von Phosphorverbindungen in verschiedenern Nierenabschnitten und Änderumgen ihrer Konzentration in Abhangigkeit vom Diuresezustad. *Pflügers Arch.* 262:551–61
69. Wang, Y., van Eys, J. 1981. Nutritional significance of fructose and sugar alcohols. *Annu. Rev. Nutr.* 1:437–75
70. Whiting, P. H., Palmano, K. P., Hawthorne, J. N. 1979. Enzymes of myoinositol and inositol lipid metabolism in rats with streptozotocin-induced diabetes. *Biochem. J.* 179:549–53
71. Winegrad, A. I., Clements, R. S. Jr., Morrison, A. D. 1972. Insulin-independent pathways of carbohydrate metabolism. In *Handbook of Physiology, Endocrinology 1,* ed. D. F. Steiner, N. Frenkel, pp. 457–71. Washington, DC: Amer. Physiol. Soc.
72. Wirthensohn, G., Beck, F. X., Guder, W. G. 1987. Role and regulation of glycerophosphorylcholine in rat renal papilla. *Pflügers Arch.* 409:411–15
73. Wirthensohn, G., Lefrank, S., Schmolke, M., Guder, W. G. 1989. Regulation of organic osmolyte concentrations in tubules from rat renal inner medulla. *Am. J. Physiol.* 256 (*Ren. Fluid Electrolyte Physiol.* 25):F128–35
74. Wirthensohn, G. Vandewalle, A., Guder, W. G. 1982. Choline kinase activity along the rabbit nephron. *Kidney Int.* 21:877–79
75. Wolff, S. D., Stanton, T. S., James, S. L., Balaban, R. S. 1990. Acute regulation of the predominant organic solutes of the rabbit renal inner medulla. *Am. J. Physiol.* 257:F676–81
76. Wolff, S. D., Balaban, R. S. 1987. Proton NMR spectroscopy and imaging of the rabbit kidney, in vivo, at 4.7 tesla. *J. Magn. Reson.* 75:190–92
77. Wolff, S. D., Eng, C., Balaban, R. S. 1988. NMR Studies of phosphate metabolites in vivo: Effects of hydration and dehydration. *Am. J. Physiol.* 255 (*Ren. Fluid Electrolyte Physiol.*):F581–89
78. Yancey, P. H. 1988. Osmotic effectors in kidneys of xeric and mesic rodents: corticomedullary distributions and changes with water availability. *J. Comp. Physiol.* [B] 158(3):369–80
79. Yancey, P. H., Clark, M. E., Hand, S. C., Bowlus, R. D., Somero, G. N. 1982. Living with water stress: evolution of osmolyte systems. *Science* 217: 1214–22
80. Yancey, P. H., Somero, G. N. 1978. Urea-requiring lactate dehydrogenases of marine elasmobranch fishes. *J. Comp. Physiol.* [B] 125:135–41

Annu. Rev. Physiol. 1990. 52:747–59

RENAL ACTIONS OF ATRIAL NATRIURETIC PEPTIDE: REGULATION OF COLLECTING DUCT SODIUM AND WATER TRANSPORT[1]

Mark L. Zeidel

Department of Medicine, Brockton-West Roxbury Veterans Administration Medical Center and Brigham and Women's Hospital, Harvard Medical School, Boston, Massachusetts, 02115

KEY WORDS: kidney collecting duct, sodium transport, hormonal regulation, cyclic GMP, epithelial transport

INTRODUCTION

Atrial natriuretic peptide (ANP) is a hormone secreted primarily by the cardiac atria in response to increased intravascular volume (1, 28). Actions of this peptide on the vasculature, adrenals, and kidneys cause reduction in intravascular volume and a decrease in blood pressure. In the vasculature, ANP reduces blood pressure by a combination of reduced sympathetic outflow, extravasation of intravascular fluid into the extravascular space, and ANP-receptor-mediated relaxation of vascular smooth muscle cells (1). ANP inhibits renin and aldosterone secretion, reduces renin secretion, lowers levels of angiotensin II, leading to reduced vascular tone and reduced aldosterone secretion. ANP also directly inhibits aldosterone secretion; reduced aldosterone levels diminish renal sodium retention (1, 28, 55). In the kidney, ANP, by concerted action both on renal vasculature and renal epithelial cells, stimulates a profound natriuresis and diuresis (51).

747

RENAL ACTIONS OF ANP

As outlined in Figure 1, ANP augments glomerular filtration rate (GFR) by increasing hydraulic pressures within glomerular capillaries and, perhaps by a direct action, relaxing glomerular mesangial cells, which leads to increased surface area for filtration (1, 51). The increased delivery of filtrate to the proximal tubule is not totally reabsorbed, perhaps owing to some effect of ANP on the proximal tubule epithelium (14, 18), although such an action is controversial (11, 19, 26). An increased load of sodium and volume is passed on through the descending and ascending limbs of Henle's loop and the distal convoluted tubule. In the cortical collecting duct, ANP appears to reduce vasopressin-dependent free water reabsorption and sodium absorption. The increased load of sodium and water is then presented to the inner medullary collecting duct where ANP inhibits the normal compensatory increase in solute reabsorption and antagonizes the action of vasopressin, leading to profound natriuresis and diuresis. In this review, we will examine the actions of ANP along the collecting duct and describe what is known about the signal transduction mechanisms involved.

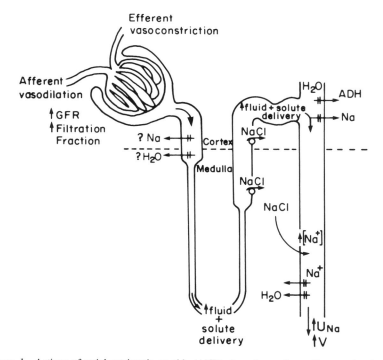

Figure 1   Actions of atrial natriuretic peptide (ANP) along the nephron. See text for details.

Role of Increased GFR in Natriuretic and Diuretic Actions of ANP

The relative contributions of hemodynamic (increased GFR) and epithelial (collecting duct) actions of ANP in the natriuretic and diuretic response remain a major controversy in the study of the renal mechanism of action of this hormone. Several investigators have proposed that the increase in GFR alone can account for the natriuresis (7, 11, 19, 28) while others have argued that ANP also directly alters tubule sodium and water reabsorption (4, 18, 25, 32, 34, 41, 42, 49, 53). In many studies, ANP has stimulated natriuresis and diuresis without producing a detectable alteration of GFR (4, 41, 42). In several of these studies, infusion of ANP at doses low enough to simulate the variations encountered in endogenous ANP levels results in natriuresis and diuresis without a detectable change in GFR; at higher doses, the increase in GFR is noted (5, 30, 35, 40, 55). These studies suggest that the natriuresis at these lower doses occurs independently of changes in GFR. However, since the filtered load of sodium and water is very large compared with the amount excreted in the urine, even during natriuresis, it has been argued that undetectable changes in GFR could in themselves lead to the natriuresis observed with ANP (27).

Several observations, however, indicate that changes in GFR cannot alone account for the bulk of the natriuresis and diuresis in response to ANP. First, in toadfish, a species that lacks glomeruli, ANP induces a striking natriuresis. This result indicates the antiquity of responsiveness to ANP in phylogeny, and it demonstrates that in the absence of glomeruli ANP can mediate a natriuresis (23). In addition, increases in sodium delivery to the distal nephron following ANP administration are insufficient to explain the observed natriuresis and diuresis (4, 41, 42). Finally, there is now considerable evidence for direct effects of ANP on collecting duct sodium and water handling (13, 25, 33, 34, 41, 42, 49, 52–54), thus indicating that increases in GFR contribute to but do not totally account for ANP-induced natriuresis and diuresis. Since the nephron consists of several highly specialized structures acting in series, it is far more fruitful to consider how actions of a hormone at several nephron sites may amplify the effect on the kidney in toto than to dwell on the issue of which nephron site is most important.

ACTIONS OF ANP ALONG THE COLLECTING DUCT: STUDIES IN VIVO

There is currently strong evidence that ANP effects natriuresis and diuresis in part by inhibiting net sodium and water reabsorption in the collecting duct. In early microcatheterization studies (41) in which collecting duct fluid was sampled by passing thin catheters retrograde for varying distances up individual collecting ducts, infusion of atrial extracts did not alter delivery of Na^+ and water to the loop of Henle, but led to increases in sodium and water delivery out of the outer medullary collecting duct. Between the outer medullary collecting duct and the final urine there was a large increment in fractional sodium excretion (41). The increased delivery out of the outer medullary collecting duct was consistent with inhibition of net salt and water reabsorption in the cortical collecting duct. Furthermore, since both micropuncture and microcatheterization studies had shown that the inner medullary collecting duct (IMCD) is capable of reabsorbing large increments in outer medullary collecting duct solute load (20), it appeared that atrial extract had interfered with the normal load-dependent increase in reabsorption in this segment. Use of pure ANP in similar microcatheterization studies has given similar results (42). To determine the contribution of increased solute load to the natriuretic response to ANP, KCl was infused. This maneuver increased sodium delivery to the IMCD to a rate similar to that achieved with ANP; however, in the animals subjected to KCl infusion, the collecting duct increased sodium reabsorption normally, thus minimizing the natriuresis observed (41, 42).

Micropuncture studies of the late distal convoluted tubule and papillary tip have demonstrated that ANP infusion augments sodium or chloride delivery to the base of the accessible papilla without altering delivery out of the late distal convoluted tubule (3, 49). In addition, reabsorption of sodium or chloride between the puncture site and the tip of the papilla was significantly decreased in ANP-treated compared to the control animals (3, 49). Because the length of the collecting duct accessible to micropuncture is a small fraction of the entire inner medullary collecting duct (20), the increment in delivery to the "papillary base" may reflect decreased reabsorption along the length of the inaccessible portions of the cortical and medullary collecting ducts (20). It is also possible, of course, that this increased delivery represents the contribution of deep nephrons to the collecting duct fluid.

Effect of ANP on Transepithelial Driving Forces

These in vivo studies demonstrate that administration of ANP inhibits net sodium and water reabsorption in the collecting duct, but do not determine whether the hormone acts directly on the epithelial cells or alters the transepithelial driving forces regulating transport. There is some evidence that in the renal medulla ANP alters transepithelial driving forces; there is no information available pertaining to the cortical collecting duct. Papillary micropuncture demonstrated that ANP increased hydraulic pressures in loops of Henle, collecting ducts, and vasa recta (29). Because pressures in the vasa recta increased more markedly than pressures within the lumina of the collecting ducts, ANP created unfavorable hydraulic gradients for net sodium reabsorption in the IMCD. The sensitivity of ANP-induced natriuresis to transepithelial gradients is further emphasized by observing the effects of altering peritubular hydraulic and oncotic pressures. Administration of hyperoncotic albumin increases peritubular oncotic pressure, thus favoring net reabsorption of sodium. In the presence of hyperoncotic albumin, ANP-induced natriuresis was markedly attenuated (29). Administration of angiotensin II increases peritubular capillary hydraulic pressure, which favors net sodium excretion. Although angiotensin II alone did not induce a natriuresis, this peptide markedly potentiated the natriuretic effect of ANP (29). Taken together, these results indicate that ANP can increase the hydrostatic gradient from vasa recta to collecting duct, which favors reduced net volume reabsorption in the inner medullary collecting duct.

Another proposed action of ANP to alter transepithelial driving forces in the IMCD is medullary washout (19, 28, 50). It has been suggested that ANP increases vasa recta blood flow, leading to dissipation of medullary solute gradients. With the loss of medullary solute, water abstraction from the descending loop of Henle would be reduced, leading to decreased luminal concentration of salt delivered to the thick ascending limb and reduced NaCl transport in this segment. Reduced thick ascending limb NaCl transport would explain, in part, the natriuretic actions of ANP. A problem with this hypothesis is the fact that medullary washout would also lead to diminished backleak of solute from interstitium to lumen along the inner medullary collecting duct, thus reducing natriuresis (12). Measurement of medullary solute contents during administration of ANP indicates that solute is, indeed, lost in the medulla (12). At issue is whether this solute is lost by increased medullary blood flow or by excretion in the urine. Measurement of medullary and vasa recta blood flow indicates that ANP increases these parameters, but only after a significant diuresis and natriuresis has ensued (21). Thus medullary washout appears to be a consequence of, and not a cause of, the natriuresis and diuresis stimulated by ANP; increased medullary blood flow may further reduce medullary solute content, thus acting to sustain the natriuretic response.

There is now strong evidence that the natriuretic and diuretic effects of ANP on the collecting duct are mediated in large part by direct effects of the peptide on cellular transport processes.

DIRECT EFFECTS OF ANP ON CORTICAL COLLECTING DUCT SODIUM AND WATER REABSORPTION

Mechanisms of Sodium and Water Reabsorption in the Cortical Collecting Duct

In the cortical collecting duct (CCD), Na^+ reabsorption is thought to occur primarily across principal cells. Na^+ enters the cell from the lumen by crossing apical Na^+ channels; the Na^+ is then pumped against an electrochemical gradient from the cytoplasm to the basolateral side by the Na/K-ATPase (44). Since aldosterone stimulates Na^+ reabsorption in the CCD, inhibition of aldosterone secretion by ANP will, over hours to days, reduce Na^+ reabsorption in this segment (44). Water reabsorption also occurs via the principal cells; in response to vasopressin, cAMP is elevated, increasing the permeability of the apical membrane to water.

Effects of ANP on Water Transport in the CCD

In the rabbit CCD perfused in vitro, ANP applied to the basolateral membrane inhibited the hydraulic conductivity response to vasopressin, but not to forskolin, which stimulates the catalytic subunit of adenylate cyclase or exogenous cAMP (13). These results suggest that ANP inhibits the increase in cAMP in response to vasopressin, which results in inhibition of the hydroosmotic response. This inhibition of water transport may account for some of the diuresis observed during administration of ANP. The mechanisms involved in ANP inhibition of water flow remain unclear, however. It has not been possible to demonstrate that ANP in any way alters basal or vasopressin-stimulated cAMP accumulation in microdissected cortical collecting ducts of rats or rabbits (48), or in primary cultures of rabbit CCD cells (31). These results are difficult to reconcile with the in vitro perfused cortical collecting tubule data (13). Possibly ANP inhibits the hydroosmotic response to vasopressin, by stimulating cGMP. Whether this inhibition involves reduction of adenylate cyclase activity or a step beyond, formation of cAMP remains unclear.

Effects of ANP on Sodium Transport in the CCD

ANP can also reduce net sodium reabsorption in perfused cortical collecting ducts isolated from rats pretreated with mineralocorticoid (33). Inhibition of CCD sodium reabsorption would result in natriuresis, and this may account for the increased delivery of sodium to the medullary collecting duct observed by Sonnenberg (41, 42). It is important to note that tubules isolated from animals pretreated with mineralocorticoids may differ significantly from those from untreated animals. The transport pathways involved in ANP inhibition of sodium transport in the cortical collecting tubule have not been rigorously defined.

It is notable that no ANP receptors were observed in rat cortical collecting tubule in autoradiograms or in vitro (6, 22). ANP has been shown to increase cGMP levels to some extent in freshly obtained cortical collecting tubules (9, 32, 46), however. In addition, in primary cultures of cortical collecting tubule cells, ANP markedly stimulated cGMP accumulation, at concentrations at which the peptide inhibits sodium and water transport (31). Addition of cGMP analogues to the basolateral solution, like ANP, reduced Na^+

reabsorption (33). Taken together, these results suggest that the inhibitory effect of ANP on CCD Na^+ transport is mediated by cGMP.

DIRECT EFFECTS OF ANP ON INNER MEDULLARY COLLECTING DUCT SODIUM AND WATER TRANSPORT

Mechanisms of Sodium and Water Reabsorption in the Inner Medullary Collecting Duct

Because the mechanisms of Na^+ transport in the IMCD are so poorly understood, it is important to review the evidence that Na^+ reabsorption is effected in this segment, as in the CCT, by apical Na^+ channels and basolateral Na/K-ATPase (see Figure 2). (a) In vivo micropuncture studies demonstrated that luminal amiloride markedly reduced volume reabsorption in the IMCD (47). Microcatheterization studies demonstrated that intravenous amiloride inhibits net sodium reabsorption in the IMCD (43). Sensitivity of sodium or volume reabsorption to amiloride is consistent with a role for an apical Na^+ channel in sodium reabsorption in this segment. (b) In freshly prepared suspensions of rabbit IMCD cells, oxygen consumption, a measure of the activity of Na/K-ATPase, was inhibited by amiloride at concentrations in the submicromolar range, which suggests that this diuretic inhibited conductive Na^+ entry in these cells, thus leading to secondary reduction in pump activity (53). Recent studies of isotopic Na^+ uptake into these cells have confirmed this hypothesis, demonstrating that Na^+ entry carries positive charge into the cell, that hyperpolarization of membrane potential markedly stimulates Na^+ entry, and that Na^+ uptake is sensitive to 10^{-7} M amiloride (52). Thus these cells appear to possess an amiloride-sensitive conductive Na^+ entry pathway or channel (52). (c) Electrical measurements in isolated perfused rat IMCD demonstrate that luminal amiloride reduces transepithelial potential and increases transepithelial resistance, consistent with inhibition of an apical conductive sodium pathway (43). (d) In primary cultures of rat IMCD cells grown on glass coverslips, patch-clamp studies demonstrate the activity of a nonselective cation channel, which is inhibited by submicromolar concentrations of amiloride (24). (e) An amiloride-sensitive Na^+ channel has been reconstituted and purified to apparent homogeneity from bovine inner medulla and the toad kidney cell line, A6 (2, 38). Thus the available experimental evidence strongly supports the model of transepithelial Na^+ reabsorption shown in Figure 2.

Effects of ANP on Sodium Transport in the IMCD

Because the IMCD is highly branched and difficult to perfuse in vitro, the earliest mechanistic studies of the regulation of Na^+ transport by ANP in this segment were performed on freshly prepared suspensions of rabbit IMCD

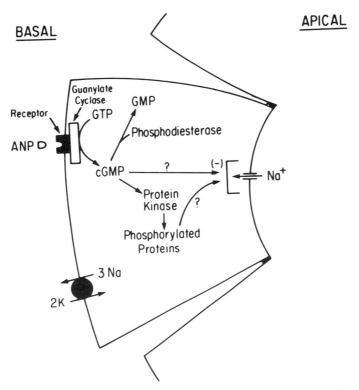

Figure 2   Direct inhibition of collecting duct sodium transport by ANP. See text for details.

cells (53). In this preparation, ANP inhibited transport-dependent oxygen consumption (QO_2) without altering this parameter in cells derived from the outer medullary collecting duct or thick ascending limb (53). Measurable responses to ANP occurred at $10^{-11}-10^{-10}$ M, levels achieved in the plasma of animals under basal and volume expanded conditions. Examination of the interaction of ANP with amiloride, ouabain, and amphotericin in QO_2 measurements suggested that the peptide was inhibiting Na^+ entry into these cells (53). Recent studies of isotopic Na^+ uptake in these suspensions demonstrate that ANP reduces the rate of Na^+ entry via the conductive pathway by two-thirds, at concentrations identical to those which were effective in oxygen consumption studies (52). In primary cultures of rat IMCD, application of ANP to the cell-attached patch preparation reduced the open time of the amiloride-sensitive cation channel, which provided direct confirmation that ANP acts in this tissue by reducing Na^+ flux across conductive cation channels (25). Inhibition of Na^+ channels by ANP has also been shown in LLCPK$_1$ cells, a renal epithelial cell line that exhibits characteristics of proximal and distal renal epithelia (8, 15). Thus, as shown in Figure 2, ANP inhibits a sodium or cation[2] channel, probably located on the luminal surface of the collecting duct cell. This inhibition probably contributes significantly to the natriuretic effect of this peptide in the inner medullary collecting duct.

Because of the magnitude of the natriuretic response of the IMCD to ANP, it has been suggested that this peptide not only reduces reabsorptive flux of Na^+ in this segment, but also stimulates a secretory flux (42), possibly mediated by a basolateral Na/K/2Cl cotransporter. In fresh suspensions of rat IMCD, a furosemide-sensitive Na^+ entry pathway has been identified (45). In addition, preliminary measurements of isotopic sodium transport in isolated perfused rat IMCD suggest that a basolateral furosemide-sensitive pathway may mediate net secretion of Na^+; this pathway appears to be stimulated by vasopressin (36). In rabbit IMCD cells, however, furosemide has no effect on oxygen consumption, isotopic sodium uptake, or potassium fluxes, which suggests that Na/K/2Cl cotransport is not an important pathway for Na^+ transport in this segment in the rabbit (52, 53). In support of an action of ANP to stimulate Na^+ secretion, preliminary measurements of isotopic sodium fluxes in isolated perfused rat IMCD indicate that ANP has dual effects on sodium transport, inhibiting lumen to bath sodium flux and stimulating a furosemide-sensitive and vasopressin-stimulated bath to lumen sodium flux (36). These results suggest that in the rat inner medullary collecting duct, ANP inhibits net sodium reabsorption by reducing entry of sodium into the cell from the lumen and stimulating a basolateral Na/K/2Cl cotransporter. In apparent contradiction to the hypothesis that ANP stimulates sodium secretion in this segment, Sands et al (37) demonstrated in isolated perfused rat IMCD that ANP did not alter passive sodium permeability. Thus an effect of ANP to stimulate a secretory Na^+ flux in the IMCD remains unproven.

Thus there is strong evidence from many laboratories that ANP interacts directly with cells of the inner medullary collecting duct to interfere with Na^+ reabsorption via luminal Na^+ or cation channels. These direct effects on epithelial transport, combined with alterations in transepithelial driving forces governing net transport, result in striking natriuresis and diuresis in the IMCD in response to ANP. Since aldosterone stimulates Na^+ reabsorption in the IMCD (20), reductions in aldosterone secretion by ANP serve to augment the other natriuretic effects of this peptide in this segment.

---

[2]Unlike the Na^+ channels of cortical collecting duct and amphibian bladder, which exhibit 10-fold or greater selectivity for Na^+ over other cations such as K^+, these cation channels are not selective or only partly selective for Na^+. The relationship between the amiloride-sensitive nonselective cation channel and the amiloride-sensitive Na^+-selective channel of amphibian bladder and cortical collecting duct remains unclear. It is possible that the channel changes its properties in culture, or that this nonselective cation channel is a different protein from the Na^+-selective channel. Evidence for the latter possibility comes from the fact that ANP and cGMP do not alter Na^+ transport (as measured by short circuit current) in several epithelia known to possess Na^+-selective channels, such as the toad bladder, frog skin, and A6 cells.

Signal Transduction Mechanisms of ANP Inhibition of IMCD Sodium Transport

The signal transduction mechanisms mediating ANP inhibition of conductive Na^+ entry into IMCD cells have been most thoroughly characterized in the IMCD; a model of ANP action is outlined in Figure 2. Freshly prepared suspensions of intact rabbit IMCD cells express a single class of cell surface ANP receptors [using affinity crosslinking techniques (16)] with an apparent kd of 10^{-10} M and a molecular weight of 120–130 kd. This class of receptors is known, in other tissues such as vascular smooth muscle, to be tightly linked with a membrane-associated or particulate guanylate cyclase. Indeed, a single peptide sharing guanylate cyclase and ANP-binding activity has recently been cloned and sequenced (10); it is likely that the IMCD ANP receptor is either identical or homologous to this peptide.

There is strong evidence that cGMP is the mediator of the effects of ANP on Na^+ transport in this segment. Several laboratories have demonstrated that ANP increases intracellular cGMP with a concentration-response relationship and time-course congruent with the actions of this peptide on transport (32, 46, 54). Indeed, ANP stimulates particulate guanylate cyclase prepared from IMCD cells by tripling the Vmax of the enzyme at levels of ANP that effect inhibition of Na^+ transport (17). Several studies have also shown that cGMP can reproduce the transport effects of ANP. In freshly prepared IMCD cells, increasing cGMP by exposure to nitroprusside (which stimulates a soluble guanylate cyclase), by inhibition of phosphodiesterase with isobutylmethylxanthine, or by addition of the cGMP analogue, 8-Br-cGMP, mimics the inhibitory effect of ANP on transport-dependent oxygen consumption and on the uptake of Na^+ via the conductive channel (52, 54). In primary cultures of rat IMCD cells, patch-clamp studies have demonstrated that cGMP applied to the cell-detached membrane reduces the open time of the amiloride-sensitive cation channel (25). Taken together, these results fulfill Sutherland's criteria for demonstrating that a response to a peptide hormone is mediated by synthesis of a cyclic nucleotide. This has established cGMP as the mediator of ANP regulation of Na^+ transport in the IMCD.

Whether the cGMP acts by binding to the channel, as occurs in the rod outer segment of the retina, or by stimulating a membrane-associated protein kinase remains unclear. The patch-clamp data (25) suggest that cGMP binds directly to the cation channel, but do not rule out the activity on the plasma membrane of a cGMP-dependent protein kinase.

Effects of ANP on Water Transport in the IMCD

As is the case in the CCD, ANP antagonizes the hydroosmotic action of vasopressin, which accounts, in part, for the diuretic action of ANP. In isolated perfused rat inner medullary collecting duct, application of ANP to the basolateral, but not apical, surface has been shown to inhibit vasopressin-stimulated water flow (33); ANP did not alter cAMP accumulation in response to vasopressin at concentrations of 10^{-11}–10^{-10}M in this segment (32, 33). ANP also inhibited the osmotic water permeability response to an analogue of cAMP (33). Thus ANP inhibits ADH-stimulated water reabsorption, apparently at a site distal to the increase in cAMP. Since cGMP duplicated the action of ANP on vasopressin-stimulated water flow, it is likely that cGMP also mediates the diuretic effects of ANP in IMCD.

SUMMARY

ANP stimulates a profound natriuresis and diuresis by a series of concerted actions along the nephron, including stimulation of glomerular filtration and inhibition of net salt and water reabsorption in the cortical and inner medullary collecting ducts. Several actions of ANP contribute to its natriuretic and diuretic effects in the collecting duct. These include reductions in aldosterone secretion, increases in hydrostatic pressures opposing Na^+ reabsorption, possible stimulation of medullary washout, and direct inhibition of salt and water transport. In both CCD and IMCD, ANP antagonizes the hydroosmotic actions of vasopressin, which leads to diuresis. The mechanisms by which ANP inhibits response to vasopressin remain unclear, although in IMCD, cGMP can duplicate the response to ANP. In CCD, ANP can inhibit Na^+ reabsorption via cGMP; the transport pathway regulated by ANP is unknown. In IMCD, ANP acting via cGMP inhibits a conductive Na^+ or cation channel, which appears to be on the luminal membrane.

ACKNOWLEDGMENTS

Dr. Zeidel is supported by a Veterans Administration Career Development Award, as well as grants from the National Institutes of Health (DK-38690, and DK-70651).

Literature Cited

1. Ballermann, B. J., Brenner, B. M. 1986. Role of atrial peptides in body fluid homeostasis. Circ. Res. 58:619–30
2. Benos, D. J., Saccomani, G., Brenner, B. M., Sariban-Sohraby, S. 1986. Purification and characterization of the amiloride-sensitive sodium channel from A6 cultured cells and bovine renal papilla. Proc. Natl. Acad. Sci. USA 83:8525–29
3. Briggs, J. P., Soejima, H., Schnermann, J. 1988. Effect of atrial natriuretic peptide on chloride absorption along papillary collecting duct. Proc. Tenth Int. Congr. Nephrol. 10:218
4. Briggs, J. P., Steipe, B., Schubert, G., Schnermann, J. 1982. Micropuncture studies of the renal effects of atrial natriuretic substance. Pflügers Arch. 395:271–76
5. Burnett, J. C., Granger, J. P., Opgenorth, T. J. 1984. Effects of synthetic atrial natriuretic factor on renal function and renin release. Am. J. Physiol. 247: F863–66
6. Butlen, D., Mistaoui, M., Morel, F. 1987. Atrial natriuretic peptide receptors along rat and rabbit nephrons: rat atrial natriuretic peptide binding in microdissected glomeruli and tubules. Pflügers Arch. 408:356–65

7. Camargo, M. J. F., Kleinert, H. D., Atlas, S. A., Sealey, J. E., Laragh, J. H., Maack, T. 1984. Calcium-dependent hemodynamic and natriuretic effects of atrial extract in isolated rat kidney. *Am. J. Physiol.* 246:F447–56

8. Cantiello, H. F., Ausiello, D. A. 1986. Atrial natriuretic factor and cGMP inhibit amiloride-sensitive Na transport in the cultured renal epithelial cell line, LLC-PK1. *Biochem. Biophys. Res. Comm.* 134:852–60

9. Chabardes, D., Montegut, M., Mistaoui, M., Butlen, D., Morel, F. 1987. Atrial natriuretic peptide effects on cGMP and cAMP contents in microdissected glomeruli and segments of the rat and rabbit nephrons. *Pflügers Arch.* 408:366–72

10. Chinkers, M., Garbers, D. L., Chang, M., Lowe, D. G., Chin, H., et al. 1989. A membrane form of guanylate cyclase is an atrial natriuretic peptide receptor. *Nature* 338:78–83

11. Cogan, M. G. 1986. Atrial natriuretic factor can increase renal solute excretion primarily by raising glomerular filtration. *Am. J. Physiol.* 250:F710–14

12. Davis, C. L., Briggs, J. P. 1987. Effect of atrial natriuretic peptides on renal medullary solute gradients. *Am. J. Physiol.* 253:F679–84

13. Dillingham, M. A., Anderson, R. J. 1986. Inhibition of vasopressin action by atrial natriuretic factor. *Science* 231:1572–73

14. Garvin, J. L. 1989. ANF inhibits transport in the isolated, perfused rat proximal straight tubule (PST). *FASEB J.* 3:A247

15. Gologorski, M. S., Duncan, R. L., Westbrook, S., Reinach, P., Hruska, K. A. 1987. Demonstration of a direct effect of atrial natriuretic factor on epithelium: study in cultured pig kidney cells. *Miner. Electrol. Metab.* 13:51–56

16. Gunning, M. E., Ballermann, B. J., Silva, P., Brenner, B. M., Zeidel, M. L. 1988. Characterization of ANP receptors in rabbit inner medullary collecting duct cells. *Am. J. Physiol.* 255:F324–30

17. Gunning, M. E., Silva, P., Brenner, B. M., Zeidel, M. L. 1989. Characteristics of ANP-sensitive guanylate cyclase in inner medullary collecting duct cells. *Am. J. Physiol.* In press: 256:F766–75

18. Harris, P. J., Thomas, D., Morgan, T. O. 1987. Atrial natriuretic peptide inhibits angiotensin-stimulated proximal tubular sodium and water reabsorption. *Nature* 326:697–98

19. Huang, C. K., Lewicki, J., Johnson, L. K., Cogan, M. G. 1985. Renal mechanism of action of rat atrial natriuretic factor. *J. Clin. Invest.* 75:769–73

20. Jamison, R. L., Sonnenberg, H. H., Stein, J. H. 1979. Questions and replies: role of the collecting duct in fluid, sodium, and potassium balance. *Am. J. Physiol.* 237:F247–61

21. Kiberd, B. A., Larson, T. S., Robertson, C. R., Jamison, R. L. 1987. Effect of atrial natriuretic peptide on vasa recta blood flow in the rat. *Am. J. Physiol.* 252:F1112–17

22. Kosecki, C., Hayashi, Y., Torikai, S., Furuya, N., Ohnuma, N., Imai, M. 1986. Localization of binding sites for rat atrial natriuretic polypeptide in rat kidney. *Am. J. Physiol.* 250:F210–16

23. Lee, J., Malvin, R. L. 1987. Natriuretic response to homologous heart extract in aglomerular toadfish. *Am. J. Physiol.* 252:R1055–58

24. Light, D. B., McCann, F. V., Keller, T. M., Stanton, B. A. 1988. Amiloride-sensitive cation channel in rat inner medullary collecting duct. *Am. J. Physiol.* 255:F278–86

25. Light, D. B., Schwiebert, E. M., Karlson, K. H., Stanton, B. A. 1989. Atrial natriuretic peptide inhibits a cation channel in renal inner medullary collecting duct cells. *Science* 243:383–85

26. Liu, F. Y., Cogan, M. G. 1988. Atrial natriuretic factor does not inhibit basal or angiotensin II-stimulated transport. *Am. J. Physiol.* 255:F434–37

27. Maack, T. 1986. Renal clearance and isolated kidney perfusion techniques. *Kidney Int.* 30:142–51

28. Maack, T., Camargo, M. J. F., Kleinert, H. D., Laragh, J. H., Atlas, S. A. 1985. Atrial natriuretic factor: structure and functional properties. *Kidney Int.* 27:607–15

29. Mendez, R. E., Dunn, B. R., Troy, J. L., Brenner, B. M. 1986. Modulation of the natriuretic response to atrial natriuretic peptide by alterations in peritubular Starling forces in the rat. *Circ. Res.* 59:605–11

30. Murray, R. D., Itoh, S., Inagami, T., Misono, K., Seto, S., et al. 1985. Effects of synthetic atrial natriuretic factor in the isolated perfused rat kidney. *Am. J. Physiol.* 249:F603–9

31. Naray-Fejes-Toth, A., Carretero, O. A., Fejes-Toth, G. 1988. Effects of atrial natriuretic factor and vasopressin on cyclic nucleotides in cultured kidney cells. *Hypertension* 11:392–96

32. Nonoguchi, H., Knepper, M. A., Manganiello, V. C. 1987. Effects of atrial natriuretic factor on cyclic guanosine monophosphate and cyclic adenosine

monophosphate accumulation in micro-dissected nephron segments from rats. *J. Clin. Invest.* 79:500–7

33. Nonoguchi, H., Sands, J. M., Knepper, M. A. 1988. Atrial natriuretic factor inhibits vasopressin-stimulated osmotic water permeability in rat inner medullary collecting duct. *J. Clin. Invest.* 82:1383–90

34. Nonoguchi, H., Sands, J. M., Knepper, M. A. 1989. ANF inhibits NaCl and fluid absorption in cortical collecting duct of rat kidney. *Am. J. Physiol.* 256:F179–86

35. Pamnani, M. B., Clough, D. L., Chen, J. S., Link, W. T., Haddy, F. J. 1984. Effects of rat atrial extract on sodium transport and blood pressure in the rat. *Proc. Soc. Exp. Biol. Med.* 176:123–31

36. Rocha, A. S., Kudo, L. H. 1988. Direct effect of atrial natriuretic factor on Na, Cl, and water transport in the papillary collecting duct. *Proc. Tenth Int. Congr. Nephrol.* 10:218

37. Sands, J. M., Nonoguchi, H., Knepper, M. A. 1988. Hormone effects on NaCl permeability of rat inner medullary collecting duct. *Am. J. Physiol.* 255:F421–28

38. Sariban-Sohraby, S., Benos, D. J. 1986. Detergent solubilization, functional reconstitution, and partial purification of epithelial amiloride-binding protein. *Biochemistry* 25:4639–46

39. Sariban-Sohraby, S., Brenner, B. M., Benos, D. J. 1988. Phosphorylation of a single subunit of the epithelial sodium channel protein following vasopressin treatment of A6 cells. *J. Biol. Chem.* 263:13875–79

40. Seymour, A. A., Blaine, E. H., Macack, E. K., Smith, S. G., Stabilito, I. I., et al. 1985. Renal and systemic effects of synthetic atrial natriuretic factor. *Life Sci.* 36:33–44

41. Sonnenberg, H., Cupples, W. A., De Bold, A. J., Veress, A. T. 1982. Intrarenal localization of the natriuretic effects of cardiac atrial extract. *Can. J. Physiol. Pharmacol.* 60:1149–52

42. Sonnenberg, H., Honrath, U., Chong, C. K., Wilson, D. R. 1986. Atrial natriuretic factor inhibits sodium transport in medullary collecting duct. *Am. J. Physiol.* 250:F963–66

43. Sonnenberg, H., Honrath, U., Wilson, D. R. 1987. Effects of amiloride in the medullary collecting duct of rat kidney. *Kidney Int.* 31:1121–25

44. Stokes, J. B. 1982. Ion transport by the cortical and outer medullary collecting tubule. *Kidney Int.* 22:473–84

45. Stokes, J. B., Grupp, C., Kinne, R. H. 1987. Purification of rat papillary collecting duct cells: functional and metabolic assessment. *Am. J. Physiol.* 253:F251–62

46. Tremblay, J., Gertzer, R., Vinay, P., Pang, S. C., Beliveau, R., Hamet, P. 1985. The increase of cGMP by atrial natriuretic factor correlates with the distribution of particulate guanylate cyclase. *FEBS Lett.* 181:17–22

47. Ullrich, K. J., Papavassiliou, F. 1979. Effect of adrenalectomy, low sodium diet, acetazolamide, bicarbonate-free solutions, and of amiloride on medullary collecting duct transport. *Pflügers Arch.* 3799:49–52

48. Umemura, S., Smyth, D. D., Pettinger, W. A. 1985. Lack of inhibition by atrial natriuretic factor on cyclic AMP levels in single nephron segments and the glomerulus. *Biochem. Biophys. Res. Comm.* 127:943–49

49. Van De Stolpe, A., Jamison, R. L. 1988. Micropuncture study of the effect of ANP on papillary collecting duct in the rat. *Am. J. Physiol.* 254:F477–83

50. Wakitani, K., Cole, B. R., Geller, D. M., Currie, M. G., Adams, S. P., et al. 1985. Atriopeptins: correlation between renal vasodilation and natriuresis. *Am. J. Physiol.* 249:F49–53

51. Zeidel, M. L., Brenner, B. M. 1987. Actions of atrial natriuretic peptides on the kidney. *Semin. Nephrol.* 7:91–97

52. Zeidel, M. L., Kikeri, D., Silva, P., Burrowes, M., Brenner, B. M. 1988. Atrial natriuretic peptides inhibit conductive sodium uptake by rabbit inner medullary collecting duct cells. *J. Clin. Invest.* 82:1067–74

53. Zeidel, M. L., Seifter, J. L., Lear, S., Brenner, B. M., Silva, P. 1986. Atrial peptides inhibit oxygen consumption in kidney medullary collecting duct cells. *Am. J. Physiol.* 251:F379–83

54. Zeidel, M. L., Silva, P., Brenner, B. M., Seifter, J. L. 1987. Cyclic GMP mediates effects of atrial peptides on medullary collecting duct cells. *Am. J. Physiol.* 252:F551–59

55. Zimmerman, R. S., Schirger, J. A., Edwards, B. S., Schwab, T. R., Heublein, D. M., Burnett, J. C. 1987. Cardiorenal-endocrine dynamics during stepwise infusion of physiologic and pharmacologic concentrations of atrial natriuretic factor in the dog. *Circ. Res.* 60:63–69

Annu. Rev. Physiol. 1990. 52:761–72

CELL VOLUME REGULATION IN THE NEPHRON

Chahrzad Montrose-Rafizadeh and William B. Guggino

Department of Physiology, Johns Hopkins University, Baltimore, Maryland 21205

KEY WORDS: regulatory volume increase, regulatory volume decrease, RVI and RVD, organic osmolyte, kidney

INTRODUCTION

Most cells control their volume when exposed to changes in extracellular fluid osmolarity. Epithelial cells, such as renal tubular cells, have the additional stress of having to survive in the presence of transcellular flow during transepithelial transport. Medullary and papillary portions of the mammalian nephron experience large variations in osmolarity during changes from a diuretic to an antidiuretic state. For this reason cells of medullary segments have to be adapted to survive in osmolarity both higher and lower than plasma. In contrast, cortical osmolarity is not modified by the diuretic status of the organism. Thus it is not necessary for cells from cortical regions of the kidney to be adapted for survival in extreme media osmolarities. Hence, volume regulatory mechanisms in these cells probably function to minimize cell volume changes in isosmotic conditions during acute changes in membrane transport.

Cell volume regulation is a complicated process that involves at least several fundamental processes. First, the cell must be able to detect changes in cell volume. This can be accomplished by sensing the degree of membrane stretch (5, 28, 31, 37, 38) or by detecting changes in the total concentration of solutes or changes in a particular substance such as intracellular Ca^{2+} concentration (46). Second, the cell must initiate regulatory processes that alter intracellular solute content. Finally, the cell must remember its initial volume

761

0066-4278/90/0315-0761$02.00

and shut down the volume regulatory process when the cell reaches its original volume. An epithelial cell such as a renal cell, which is normally transporting solutes and balancing input and output of solutes across individual cell membranes, must upset this balance in anisotonic conditions and induce a change in intracellular solute content (10, 29). Recent studies have begun to shed some light on each of these processes.

REGULATORY VOLUME INCREASE

General Characteristics

When exposed to an abrupt increase in extracellular fluid osmolarity, cells shrink initially. This initial response is followed by an increase in intracellular solute and water content, which restores the cells to their original volume. This secondary response is termed regulatory volume increase (RVI). Volume regulation in hyperosmotic solutions has been demonstrated in both proximal and distal nephron segments (1–4, 8, 9, 14–16, 18, 20, 23, 24, 26, 27, 29, 30, 32–34, 36, 40). For example, *Necturus* proximal tubule cells shrink initially when exposed to a hyperosmotic fluid (26). The initial shrinking is followed by a gradual return toward the original volume (RVI). Re-exposure to normal osmolarity causes the cells to swell to a larger volume than before the exposure to the hyperosmotic solutions. This overshoot, upon return of the cells to their original osmolarity, indicates that the intracellular solute content increased during RVI (Figure 1).

A complete RVI response following exposure to hyperosmolarity does not occur in all nephron segments. For example, rabbit proximal tubule cells (9, 20), rabbit cortical collecting duct cells (36), mouse cortical ascending limb cells (14), Madin-Darby canine kidney and opossum kidney (MDCK) (OK) cultured cell lines (33, 30, 27) shrink but fail to return back to their original volume when exposed to a large increase in osmolarity. Most of the renal cells that lack a complete RVI response have the ability to gain solutes in hyperosmotic solutions. Often when these cells are exposed to hyperosmotic media and then re-exposed to their original osmolarity (9, 20), they swell to a volume greater than the starting volume. The presence of this overshoot suggests that a net increase in intracellular solute content has occurred during the exposure to hyperosmotic solutions, but that the increase in cell solute content was too small to produce a full RVI response.

One possible explanation is that some cells cannot regulate their volume if exposed to a hyperosmotic solution too quickly. For example, nonperfused proximal tubule cells do not display the typical RVI response if the osmolarity is changed abruptly (23), but if it is increased slowly (for example at 1.5 milliosmole/min), the cells maintain a constant volume presumably by in-

Effect of Hyper-osmotic Lumen and Bath Solutions

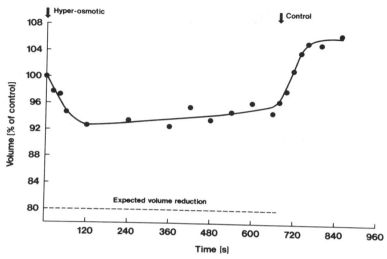

Figure 1 Volume regulation in the early proximal tubule of *Necturus* kidney. Cell volume relative to control following an increase in osmolarity of the perfusion solutions. The perfusion solution osmolarity was switched from control at time zero *(left arrow)* and changed back to control *(the right arrow)* (from 26).

creasing intracellular solute content. This phenomenon is called isovolumetric regulation because it does not involve an initial shrinking followed by RVI. Thus RVI mechanisms in some cells may operate slowly and can only respond to gradual changes in extracellular fluid osmolarity.

Another explanation is that transport mechanisms may have to be activated prior to an abrupt increase in osmolarity. Two different sets of observations show that RVI mechanisms, in some cases, fail to operate unless they are activated prior to an abrupt increase in osmolarity.

First, rabbit proximal tubule cells (20) or cultured MDCK cells (30) exposed to hyposmotic solutions undergo a regulatory volume decrease (RVD) that returns them to their original volume. As discussed below RVD involves a decrease in intracellular solute content. When re-exposed to an isosmotic medium, they shrink below their original volume followed by a post-RVD RVI. It is unknown why some cells must first be exposed to hyposmotic solutions to induce RVI abilities. It appears that the loss of ions or solutes during the RVD phase is important in some renal cells to stimulate RVI mechanisms.

Second, when the mouse medullary thick ascending limb (TAL) cells (14,

15) are exposed to a hyperosmotic extracellular bath, in the absence of antidiuretic hormone (ADH), they shrink as a perfect osmometer without regulating their volume. In sharp contrast, if the cells are exposed to hypertonic solutions in the presence of ADH, the initial shrinking is followed by a rapid RVI. The effect of ADH can be mimicked by 8-bromo cAMP. Thus in the TAL, RVI mechanisms must be activated by ADH to control cell volume via cellular regulatory pathways.

Clearly, most renal cells regulate their volume in hyperosmotic solutions, but it appears that RVI mechanisms in some cells must be activated prior to exposure to hyperosmotic solutions. Recent evidence suggests that RVI following a hyperosmotic challenge occurs either by increasing NaCl influx or by increasing the organic osmolyte content.

NaCl Influx via Parallel Na^+-H^+ and $Cl^--HCO_3^-$ Exchangers

In the thick ascending limb, furosemide, which is a potent inhibitor of luminal $Na^+-K^+-2Cl^-$ cotransport and net NaCl reabsorption, has no effect on ADH-activated RVI (14, 15). Hence, volume control and net NaCl reabsorption are separate processes in the TAL. Studies to identify the exact nature of transporters involved have shown that RVI does not occur in the absence of HCO_3^-, bath Na^+, or bath Cl^-. In addition, RVI is inhibited by amiloride and SITS applied to the basolateral cell membrane and by the carbonic anhydrase inhibitor, ethoxzolamide. Taken together, the evidence suggests that basolateral Na^+-H^+ and $Cl^--HCO_3^-$ exchangers are involved in RVI in the TAL. Because parallel operation of these exchangers results in net influx of NaCl across the basolateral membrane, RVI probably lowers the efficiency of net NaCl reabsorption in the TAL. NaCl influx via Na^+-H^+ and $Cl^--HCO_3^-$ exchangers also occurs in rabbit isolated nonperfused proximal tubule (24) during isovolumetric regulation in hyperosmotic solutions.

RVI-Induced Solute Influx via the $Na^+-K^+-2Cl^-$ Cotransporter

Rabbit medullary thick ascending limb cells lack carbonic anhydrase activity (7) and possess a completely different mechanism for RVI than the same segment in the mouse kidney (15, 8). For example (8), the uptake of ^{22}Na and ^{86}Rb increased, became interdependent, and was furosemide-sensitive in hyperosmotic media. The data suggest that transport via $Na^+-K^+-2Cl^-$ cotransporters is enhanced in hyperosmotic conditions.

Cultured opossum kidney (OK) cells (27) exposed to hyperosmotic media shrink without any RVI. However, if they are first exposed to a hyposmotic media and then returned to their original osmolarity the cells shrink below their original volume. This secondary shrinking is followed by a post-RVD RVI which is Na-dependent, furosemide-sensitive, but amiloride-insensitive.

Thus in these cells as well as rabbit medullary thick ascending limb cells, Na^+-K^+-$2Cl^-$ cotransporters are involved in RVI.

Role of Organic Solutes in RVI

Cells in the renal medulla and papilla that are exposed to a hyperosmotic environment contain high levels of organic osmolytes such as polyols (sorbitol, inositol) and trimethylamines (betaine, glycerophosphorylcholine (1, 3, 32). Increased levels of sorbitol, inositol, glycerophosphorylcholine, and betaine are present in renal cultured cell lines (such as MDCK, LLC-PK1, LLC-PK3, A6, and GRB-MAL1) after exposure to hyperosmotic media (29).

It has been suggested that increased organic osmolyte content in the renal medulla in antidiuretic states or following exposure of papillary cells to hyperosmotic media enables cells to survive in high osmolarity. The increased organic osmolyte content occurs both by uptake from the bath (29) and by de novo synthesis stimulated by the high osmolarity (2). For example, the activity of aldose reductase, an enzyme that catalyses the conversion of glucose to sorbitol, increases in the papillary cell line, GRB-PAP1, exposed to hyperosmotic media (2). The induction of aldose reductase and sorbitol production is slow and takes at least 24 hr after exposure to hyperosmotic media for a detectable amount of sorbitol to be observed (40, 1, 2). The slowness of the induction suggests that stimulation of inorganic and organic osmolyte uptake may occur first when medullary cells are exposed to hyperosmotic media, followed by induction of enzymes that increase organic osmolyte content by de novo synthesis (34, 4).

VOLUME REGULATION IN HYPOTONIC SOLUTIONS

General Characteristics

Most cells in the nephron regulate their volume in hyposmotic solutions (6, 9, 10, 12, 17, 19, 20, 25, 33, 35, 43–45). Most renal cells swell initially following an abrupt decrease in extracellular fluid osmolarity (see Figure 2). The swelling is followed by a RVD back to their original volume. Although the typical RVD response in hyposmotic solutions is very common in the nephron, it is not universal. For example, early distal tubule cells of the *Amphiuma* kidney, which share many of the properties of the mammalian thick ascending limb, swell in hyposmotic solutions and do not exhibit any tendency to return to control volume (13). These cells possess transport systems that can affect net solute loss in response to an increase in volume, but only after the apical Na^+-K^+-Cl^- cotransporter is blocked with furosemide (13). It is likely that in the absence of furosemide, transport systems that are moving solute out of the cell are stimulated by a decrease in bath osmolarity; however, net loss of solute does not occur because of a matched stimulation of solute influx through the apical Na^+-K^+-Cl^- cotransporter. Thus these cells are not able to stimulate solute exit pathways selectively to reduce intracellular solute content.

When it occurs in kidney cells, RVD is commonly associated with a reduction in both intracellular K^+ and Cl^- content (10). However, reductions in the content of other cations such as Na^+ (9, 10), anions such as HCO_3^- (26, 42, 43), or organic osmolytes (2) may occur during RVD.

RVD-Induced Increase in K^+ Conductance and Stimulation of K^+ Channel Activity

RVD-induced loss of K^+ occurs most commonly via conductive pathways (6, 9, 10, 12, 19, 20–22, 25, 26, 33, 41–43, 45). For example, in *Necturus* proximal tubules, reducing osmolarity from 200 to 150 mosM induces cells to swell (26). Associated with cell swelling is an increase in the relative K^+ conductance of the basolateral cell membrane and an increase in the ratio of apical to basolateral resistances (R_a/R_b) from 5.0 to 7.2 consistent with an increase in the magnitude of the basolateral K^+ conductance. Since intracellular K^+ is much higher than extracellular K^+ in the *Necturus* proximal tubule (26), an increased K^+ conductance would cause increased K^+ loss from the cell and play an important role in RVD.

Evidence for an involvement of basolateral K^+ conductance in RVD in the mouse and rabbit proximal tubules comes from two sources. First, the rate of RVD is decreased both by application of basolateral ouabain and by raising basolateral K^+ concentrations, maneuvers that reduce the electrochemical potential difference for K^+ across the basolateral cell membrane (19). Second, Ba^{2+} and quinine, well-known inhibitors of K^+ channels, applied to the basolateral cell membrane slow RVD (19, 26, 43, 45).

In the rabbit thin descending limb (TDL), RVD is slowed in the presence of Ba^{2+} in the basolateral solution. Ba^{2+} blocks basolateral K^+ channels, thus reducing both K^+ loss and RVD. Prior exposure of the TDL to ouabain, which inhibits the basolateral Na-K pump (25), abolishes RVD (see Figure 2). Ouabain is effective because RVD in the TDL is a dissipative process involving K^+ loss from the cell. The pump functions to establish the concentration differences across TDL cell membranes necessary for RVD to occur.

Recent experiments using the patch-clamp technique have characterized the properties of K^+ channels that are activated in hyposmotic solutions. In general, there are two classes of K^+ channels that are activated in hyposmotic solutions: stretch-activated K^+ channels (SAK), and Ca^{2+}-activated K^+ channels (5, 28, 33, 37, 38).

Channels directly activated by membrane stretch are present in the basolateral cell membrane of the *Necturus* proximal tubule (31). These channels, which have a single-channel conductance of about 42 pS, display a low open

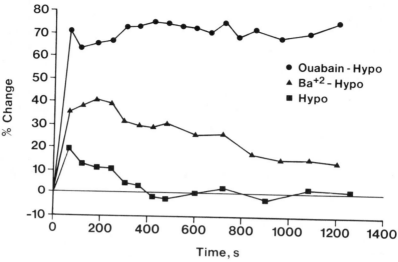

Figure 2   Volume regulation in the rabbit thin descending limb of Henle's loop. Cell volume relative to control following a reduction of lumen and bath osmolarity by 85 mosM. Solutions were made hyposmotic at time zero. Either Ba^{2+} (9 mM) or ouabain (10^{-4} M) was applied in the bath before the solution were made hyposmotic (from 25).

time probability in isosmotic solutions. Channel open probability can be increased at negative membrane potentials, but it is insensitive to changes in either intracellular or extracellular Ca^{2+}. Exposing *Necturus* proximal tubule cells to hyposmotic solutions stimulates the open probability of these channels dramatically. Since the magnitude of the K^+ current through SAK channels in the basolateral cell membrane is a direct function of $N \times P_o \times i$ (n = the number of channels in the basolateral cell membrane, P_o = the probability of opening and i = the single-channel conductance), an increased P_o results in enhanced K^+ loss across the basolateral cell membrane. Activation of P_o in hyposmotic solutions is via the direct influence of membrane stretch on the gating mechanism of the SAK channel. Another type of K^+ channel, sensitive to mechanical stress, is present in opossum kidney cells (38). This channel has a conductance of 22 pS and is permeable to Na^+, K^+, and Cl^-. Thus one mechanism for an enhanced K^+ loss during RVD occurs directly by the physical process of stretching the cell membrane.

Ca^{2+}-activated K^+ channels are activated indirectly during RVD (5, 28, 33, 37, 39). At least two types of Ca^{+2}-activated K^+ channels are sensitive to reductions in extracellular fluid osmolarity. One type, identified in opossum kidney cells (39) has a single-channel conductance of 15 pS at depolarized voltages. Another, maxi-K^+ channels, have a relatively large single-channel conductance of about 100 pS (11). The open probability of maxi-K^+ channels becomes greater at increasing intracellular Ca^{2+} concentrations and at depolarizing cell membrane potentials (11, 37). Interestingly, in unstimulated conditions Ca^{+2}-activated maxi-K^+ channels spend only a very small fraction of the time open and most likely do not contribute significantly to resting K^+ conductance of the apical cell membrane (28). In cultured medullary thick ascending limb cells, P_o of maxi-Ca^{+2}-activated K^+ channels can be increased dramatically when the cells are exposed to hyposmotic solutions (see Figure 3).

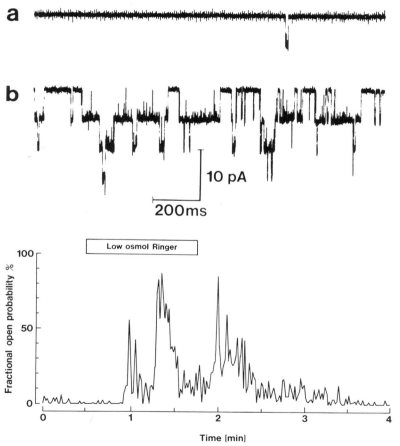

Figure 3 Low osmotic activation of a Ca^{2+}-activated-K^+ channel in rabbit medullary thick ascending limb cells. Top panel: Recording from a cell attached patch in control Ringer (*a*) and in low osmotic Ringer in which the NaCl concentration was reduced by 50 mM (*b*). Bottom panel: The effect of low osmotic Ringer solution on the open probability of K^+ channel (from 37).

In contrast to the SAK channels, Ca^{2+}-activated K^+ channels are not intrinsically sensitive to membrane stretch. Activation in hyposmotic solutions occurs instead via an increase in intracellular Ca^{2+}. It appears that hyposmotic cell swelling stretches the apical cell membrane, which increases Ca^{2+} entry. The increase in intracellular Ca^{2+} activates Ca^{2+}-activated K^+ channels. In the choroid plexus, the Ca^{2+} entry pathway [that is stretch-sensitive has been shown to be a large Ca^{2+} channel of about 200 pS (5). In kidney, the nature of the Ca^{2+} entry pathway] has not been determined.

Clearly, two methods can increase K^+ conductances either in the apical or basolateral cell membrane, one involving a stretch receptor K^+ channel that responds directly to stretch and another involving a stretch-sensitive Ca^{2+} channel that indirectly activates Ca^{2+}-activated K^+ channels via a rise in intracellular Ca^{2+}.

RVD-Induced Loss of Anions

The exact nature of the anion pathways activated during RVD is different among the different nephron segments and among species. In *Necturus* proximal tubule, removal of HCO_3^- from both apical and basolateral solutions inhibits volume regulation (26). In the mouse proximal tubule, RVD is not affected by prior removal of bath Cl^-, but like the *Necturus* proximal tubule is inhibited by removal of extracellular HCO_3^- (42, 43). RVD in the mouse proximal tubule is associated with an increase in the relative conductance of the basolateral cell membrane to HCO_3^- (42). Thus it is likely that in these two nephron segments HCO_3^- is the major anion involved in RVD.

In contrast, in the rabbit proximal tubule, Cl^- depletion partially inhibits RVD. It appears that Cl^- is the principle anion involved in RVD in the rabbit proximal tubule with anion loss occurring via the parallel operation of KCl cotransporters and a basolateral Cl^- conductance. RVD is unaffected by either HCO_3^- removal or application of the anion exchange inhibitor SITS (44). In cultured opossum kidney cells (OK continuous cell line), RVD is also reduced in Cl^--free solutions. In these cells, anion loss in RVD occurs via a Cl^- conductance pathway (21). Finally, in the TAL it has been demonstrated that both Cl^- and HCO_3^--dependent anion exit pathways are involved in RVD (25). Clearly, either Cl^--dependent or HCO_3^--dependent or a combination of both pathways participate in RVD in the kidney. The precise nature of the carrier-mediated transporters or ion channels that participate in anion loss in RVD in the kidney is not well-characterized.

Role of Organic Solutes in RVD

In principal and intercalated cells of the cortical collecting tubule of rabbit (35), RVD is not sensitive to maneuvers that alter K^+, Cl^-, or HCO_3^- concentration differences across either the apical or basolateral cell membranes. In addition, RVD is not affected by inhibitors that block K^+ conductances such as Ba^{2+}, or anion pathways such as SITS. Even blockade of the basolateral Na-K pump with ouabain does not alter RVD in these cells. These results argue against a significant role of passive KCl efflux in RVD in the cortical collecting duct, but suggest a role for other solutes such as organic solutes.

A mechanism of efflux of organic solutes has been described in the papillary cell line, PAP-HT25 (1). These cells derive from the papillary cell line, GRB-PAP1, that have been exposed to high osmolarity medium for three years. When these cells (PAP-HT25) are exposed to a hyposmotic medium, the intracellular sorbitol content decreases because of an enormous increase of organic solute efflux. In about 15 min after reduction of media osmolarity, the intracellular sorbitol content is reduced by 50%. This suggests that the efflux of this organic solute could be the mechanism by which the papillary cells regulate the volume in hyposmotic conditions.

SUMMARY

Nearly every cell in the kidney can volume regulate in response to a hypertonic challenge. Some are able to respond immediately to hyperosmotic media by a RVI. Other cells require stimulation prior to exposure to hyperosmolarity to demonstrate RVI. An increase of intracellular osmolytes during RVI usually occurs by an increase of NaCl influx either via the activation of parallel Na^+-H^+ and Cl^--HCO_3^- exchangers, or Na^+-K^+-$2Cl^-$ cotransporters. Medullary and papillary cells use organic solutes as well to increase the intracellular concentration of osmolytes.

In response to a hypotonic challenge, a RVD response has been demonstrated in the majority of the kidney cells. The efflux of solute during RVD is usually via K^+ loss by activation of conductance pathways. Stretch-activated K^+ channels and Ca^{2+}-activated-K^+ channels have been shown to be stimulated in cells exposed in hyposmotic solutions and could thus be involved in RVD. The accompanying anion loss is less well-defined but could be either Cl^- or HCO_3^- in different segments of the nephron. In some cells, the reduction of intracellular solute content is via an efflux of organic osmolytes.

Thus it appears that cells in all segments of the nephron volume regulate in response to osmotic stresses. This regulation may be an essential part of transepithelial transport since the cells have to survive transcellular fluxes of osmolytes. It may be particularly important in the kidney to control cell volume both in response to changes in osmolarity and transcellular fluxes of solute in order to maintain proper flow of fluid through the nephron.

ACKNOWLEDGMENTS

We thank Dr. Joseph Handler for reading the manuscript and Lisa Maddox for secretarial assistance. This work was supported by a National Institutes of Health Grant #DK32753.

Literature Cited

1. Bagnasco, S., Balaban, R., Fales, H. M., Yang, Y.-M., Burg, M. 1986. Predominant osmotically active organic solutes in rat and rabbit renal medullas. *J. Biol. Chem.* 261:5872–77

2. Bagnasco, S. M., Murphy, H. R., Bedford, J. J., Burg, M. B. 1988. Osmoregulation by slow changes in aldose reductase and rapid changes in sorbitol flux. *Am. J. Physiol.* 254:C788–92

3. Balaban, R. S., Burg, M. B. 1987. Osmotically active organic solutes in the renal inner medulla. *Kidney Int.* 31:562–64

4. Burg, M. B. 1988. Role of aldose reductase and sorbitol in maintaining the medullary intracellular milieu. *Kidney Int.* 33:635–41

5. Christensen, O. 1987. Mediation of cell volume regulation by Ca^{2+} influx through stretch-activated channels. *Nature* 330:66–68

6. Dellasega, M., Grantham, J. J. 1973. Regulation of renal tubule cell volume in hypotonic media. *Am. J. Physiol.* 224(6):1288–94

7. Dobyan, D. C., Magill, L. S., Friedman, P. A., Hebert, S. C., Bulger, R. E. 1982. Carbonic anhydrase histochemistry in rabbit and mouse kidneys. *Anat. Rec.* 204:185–97

8. Eveloff, J. L., Calamia, J. 1986. Effect of osmolarity on cation fluxes in medullary thick ascending limb cells. *Am. J. Physiol.* 250:F176–80

9. Gagnon, J., Ouimet, D., Nguyen, H., Laprade, R., Le Grimellec, C., et al. 1982. Cell volume regulation in the proximal convoluted tubule. *Am. J. Physiol.* 243:F408–15

10. Grantham, J. J., Lowe, C. M., Dellasega, M., Cole, B. R. 1977. Effect of hypotonic medium on K and Na content of proximal renal tubules. *Am. J. Physiol.* 232(1):F42–49

11. Guggino, S. E., Guggino, W. B., Green, N., Sacktor, B. 1987. Ca^{2+} activated K^+ channels in cultured medullary thick ascending limb cells. *Am. J. Physiol.* 252:C121–27

12. Guggino, W. B. 1989. Potassium and cell volume. In *The Regulation of Potassium Balance*, ed. D. W. Seldin, G. Giebisch. pp. 121–37. New York: Raven

13. Guggino, W. B., Oberleithner, H., Giebisch, G. 1985. Relationship between cell volume and ion transport in the early distal tubule of the amphiuma kidney. *J. Gen. Physiol.* 86:31–58

14. Hebert, S. C. 1986. Hypertonic cell volume regulation in mouse thick limbs I. ADH dependency and nephron heterogeneity. *Am. J. Physiol.* 250:C907–19

15. Hebert, S. C. 1986. Hypertonic cell volume regulation in mouse thick limbs II. Na^+-H^+ and Cl^--HCO_3^- exchange in basolateral membranes. *Am. J. Physiol.* 250:C920–31

16. Hebert, S. C. 1987. Volume regulation in renal epithelial cells. *Semin. Nephrol.* 7:48–60

17. Hebert, S. C., Sun, A. 1988. Hypotonic cell volume regulation in mouse medullary thick ascending limb: effects of ADH. *Am. J. Physiol.* 255:F962–69

18. Hoffmann, E. K., Simonsen, L. O. 1989. Membrane mechanisms in volume and pH regulation in vertebrate cells. *Physiol. Rev.* 69:315–82

19. Kirk, K. L., DiBona, D. R., Schafer, J. A. 1987. Regulatory volume decrease in perfused proximal nephron: evidence for a dumping of cell K^+. *Am. J. Physiol.* 252:F933–42

20. Kirk, K. L., Schafer, J. A., DiBona, D. R. 1987. Cell volume regulation in rabbit proximal straight tubule perfused in vitro. *Am. J. Physiol.* 252:F922–32

21. Knoblauch, C., Montrose, M. H., Murer, H. 1989. Regulatory volume decrease by cultured renal cells. *Am. J. Physiol.* 256:C252–59

22. Law, R. 1985. Volume regulation by mammalian renal cells exposed to anisosmotic media. *Mol. Physiol.* 8:143–60

23. Lohr, J. W., Grantham, J. J. 1986. Isovolumetric regulation of isolated S2 proximal tubules in anisotonic media. *J. Clin. Invest.* 78:1165–72

24. Lohr, J. W., Sullivan, L. P., Cragoe, E. J. Jr., Grantham, J. J. 1989. Volume regulation determinants in isolated proximal tubules in hypertonic medium. *Am. J. Physiol.* 256:F622–31

25. Lopes, A. G., Amzel, L. M., Markakis, D., Guggino, W. B. 1988. Cell volume regulation by the thin descending limb of Henle's loop. *Proc. Natl. Acad. Sci. USA* 85:2873–77

26. Lopes, A. G., Guggino, W. B. 1987. Volume regulation in the early proximal tubule of the *Necturus* kidney. *J. Membr. Biol.* 97:117–25

27. Montrose, M. H., Knoblauch, C., Murer, H. 1988. Separate control of regulatory volume increase and Na^+-H^+ exchange by cultured renal cells. *Am. J. Physiol.* 255:C76–85

28. Morris, C. E., Sigurdson, W. J. 1989. Stretch-inactivated ion channels coexist with stretch-activated ion channels. *Science* 243:807–9

29. Nakanishi, T., Balaban, R. S., Burg, M. B. 1988. Survey of osmolytes in renal cell lines. *Am. J. Physiol.* 255: C181–91

30. Roy, G., Sauve, R. 1987. Effect of anisotonic media on volume, ion and amino-acid content and membrane potential of kidney cells (MDCK) in culture. *J. Membr. Biol.* 100:83–96

31. Sackin, H. 1989. A stretch-activated K^+ channel sensitive to cell volume. *Proc. Natl. Acad. Sci. USA* 86:1731–35

32. Sands, J. M., Terada, Y., Bernard, L. M., Knepper, M. A. 1989. Aldose reductase activities in microdissected rat renal tubule segments. *Am. J. Physiol.* 256:F563–69

33. Simmons, N. L. 1984. Epithelial cell volume regulation in hypotonic fluids: studies using a model tissue culture renal epithelial cell system. *Q. J. Exp. Physiol.* 69:83–95

34. Spring, K. R., Siebens, A. W. 1988. Solute transport and epithelial cell volume regulation. *Comp. Biochem. Physiol.* 90A:557–60

35. Strange, K. 1988. RVD in principal and intercalated cells of rabbit cortical collecting tubule. *Am. J. Physiol.* 255: C612–21

36. Strange, K., Spring, K. R. 1987. Cell membrane water permeability of rabbit cortical collecting duct. *J. Membr. Biol.* 96:27–43

37. Taniguchi, J., Guggino, W. B. 1989. Membrane stretch: a physiological stimulator of Ca^{2+}-activated K^+ channels in medullary thick ascending limb cells. *Am J. Physiol.* 257:F347–52

38. Ubl, J., Murer, H., Kolb, H.-A. 1988a. Ion channels activated by osmotic and mechanical stress in membranes of opossum kidney cells. *J. Membr. Biol.* 104:223–32

39. Ubl, J., Murer, H., Kolb, H.-A. 1988b. Hypotonic shock evokes opening of Ca^{2+}-activated K channels in opossum kidney cells. *Pflügers Arch.* 412:551–53

40. Uchida, S., Garcia-Perez, A., Burg, M. 1987. Mechanism by which high NaCl induces aldose reductase activity in cells cultured from kidney medulla. *Fed. Proc.* 46:1229 (Abstr.)

41. Volkl, H., Lang, F. 1988. Effect of amiloride on cell volume regulation in renal straight proximal tubules. *Biochim. Biophys. Acta* 946:5–10

42. Volkl, H., Lang, F. 1988. Electrophysiology of cell volume regulation in proximal tubules of the mouse kidney. *Pflügers Arch.* 411:514–19

43. Volkl, H., Lang, F. 1988. Ionic requirement for regulatory cell volume decrease in renal straight proximal tubules. *Pflügers Arch.* 412:1–6

44. Welling, P. A., Linshaw, M. A. 1988. Importance of anion in hypotonic volume regulation of rabbit proximal straight tubule. *Am. J. Physiol.* 255: F853–60

45. Welling, P. A., Linshaw, M. A., Sullivan, L. P. 1985. Effect of barium on cell volume regulation in rabbit proximal straight tubules. *Am. J. Physiol.* 249: F20–27

46. Wong, S. M. E., Chase, H. S. 1986. Role of intracellular calcium in cellular volume regulation. *Am. J. Physiol.* 250: C841–52

Annu. Rev. Physiol. 1990. 52:773–91

A FAMILY OF POU-DOMAIN AND PIT-1 TISSUE-SPECIFIC TRANSCRIPTION FACTORS IN PITUITARY AND NEUROENDOCRINE DEVELOPMENT

Holly A. Ingraham, Vivian R. Albert, Ruoping Chen, E. Bryan Crenshaw III, Harry P. Elsholtz, Xi He, Michael S. Kapiloff, Harry J. Mangalam, Larry W. Swanson, Maurice N. Treacy and Michael G. Rosenfeld

Howard Hughes Medical Institute and Eukaryotic Regulatory Biology Program, School of Medicine, University of California, San Diego, La Jolla, California 92093

KEY WORDS: development, somatotroph, lactotroph, gene expression, DNA-binding proteins

INTRODUCTION

The sequential activation of a hierarchy of regulatory genes is a prominent mechanism for dictating the precise temporal and spatial patterns of development (23, 50) and the specific patterns of gene expression that will ultimately dictate organ identity. Considerable evidence has supported the existence of tissue-specific factors critical for the transcriptional activation of the genes that define cellular phenotype in mammals (e.g. 58, 55, 47, 6, 27, 28, 15, 14, 46, 53). We have utilized the development of the anterior pituitary gland as an excellent model system in which to study cell-specific gene activation. Pituitary development results in the temporally precise appearance of five distinct cell types derived from a common lineage that are distinguished on the basis of the trophic hormone elaborated. Somatotrophs and lactotrophs are the last

0066-4278/90/0315-0773$02.00

two phenotypically distinct cell types to appear during development, which produce the recently diverged hormones, growth hormone and prolactin, respectively (10, 59, 13, 32). Transient co-expression of prolactin and growth hormone occurs in a subset of somatotrophs during pituitary development prior to the appearance of lactotrophs (10, 59, 32), which suggests a common lineage for somatotrophs and lactotrophs; a variable number of such cells (somatomammotrophs) persist in the developed gland. Understanding the molecular basis of the binary decisions that ultimately lead to generation of distinct cell types is critical to understanding pituitary development.

Cell-specific expression of the rat prolactin gene is dictated by two separate regions, a distal enhancer (-1831 to -1530) (46) and a proximal region (-422 to $+33$) (see Figure 1) (47, 26, 7, 41, 46). Transfectional analyses of various pituitary cell lines in our laboratory have indicated that the distal enhancer is predominately responsible for the high levels of cell-specific expression, which suggests that both the distal and promoter regions are critical (46, 47), while others have suggested that cell-specific expression in cell culture reflects the actions of only the promoter proximal region (26, 41). Based on studies of DNA-mediated gene transfer into pituitary cells (GC or GH_3 cells), mutagenesis revealed that both the distal and proximal regulatory regions contained multiple related sequences that appeared to bind tissue-specific, nuclear protein(s) and exhibit synergistic interactions (46).

Determinants of Development Patterns of Prolactin and Growth Hormone Gene Expression

Because of the potential action of two discrete genomic regions in vitro, a critical issue was the basis for determination of physiologic patterning expression during normal development. This question has been tested in physiologic development by the introduction of prolactin fusion genes into fertilized

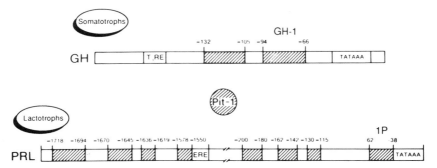

Figure 1   Schematic diagram of cell-specific *cis*-active elements present in rat prolactin and growth hormone 5'-flanking genomic sequences.

mouse oocytes and analysis of the resultant transgenic animals. Fusion genes containing three kb of 5' flanking region or the proximal region (-422 to $+33$ bp) alone directed strict cell-type specific expression (16). Prolactin proximal elements alone conferred low levels of reporter gene expression in a small percentage of the transgenic pedigrees that were established. Inclusion of both the distal enhancer and the proximal promoter region dramatically increased the expression of the transgene. The distal enhancer was also capable of directing tissue-specific expression when fused to the herpes virus thymidine kinase (tk) promoter, but the reporter gene expression in the pituitary was low, and thyrotroph as well as lactotroph expression was observed (16). The distal enhancer, therefore, specifically directed expression to the correct tissue, but it apparently required specific flanking sequences to restrict its expression to the correct cell type within the pituitary of transgenic mice. These results indicated that while the distal and proximal regions were each capable of directing tissue-specific expression, they acted synergistically to generate high penetrance and high expression levels of rat prolactin fusion genes in transgenic mice (16) (Figure 2). Transgenes containing prolactin promoter constructs showed strict tissue specificity of expression with no detectable expression (< 3 orders of magnitude) outside of the pituitary gland. Mutation of even single *cis*-active elements of the distal enhancer reduced prolactin gene expression by 80–90% (46). Expression of growth hormone in somatotrophs of transgenic mice (4, 40) was specified by as little as 180 bp of rat growth hormone 5'-flanking genomic information (40). This region contained two *cis*-active elements required for cell-specific expression in vitro (47, 61, 63, 46). The possibility that a single or two related cell-specific positive transcription factors could bind to sites in both the rat

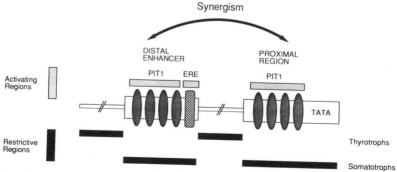

Figure 2   Model of the determinants of pituitary-specific and lactotroph-specific expression of the prolactin gene based on transgenic animal analyses. Prolactin distal enhancer and proximal region are synergistic, and additional sequences appear to restrict expression out of thyrotrophs.

prolactin and growth hormone genes was suggested by competition analyses of DNase 1 footprints and in vitro transcription (46). In examining the role of the distal and proximal regions in prolactin expression, it was established that the context of the distal enhancer was important for the strict cell-type specific expression of the prolactin gene (16).

Pit-1, a Pituitary Specific Transcription Factor

To characterize factors responsible for prolactin and growth hormone gene activation, purification employing conventional separation techniques combined with DNA affinity chromatography was performed using nuclear extracts from a rat pituitary cell line (GC). A highly purified (> 4000-fold) preparation of biologically active protein (Pit-1) (33,000, 31,000 M_r protein doublet) that activated both prolactin and growth hormone fusion genes (35, 42) was obtained. The ability of the purified Pit-1 to bind to cell-specific *cis*-active elements of the prolactin and growth hormone genes permitted successful utilization of this property for screening of rat pituitary and GC cell cDNA expression libraries (35). Pit-1 had similar properties to proteins isolated in other laboratories, referred to as PUF-1 or GHF-1 (7, 6).

The coding sequence for Pit-1 (Figure 3) predicted an 873 nucleotide open reading frame corresponding to an encoded protein of 291 amino acids and a

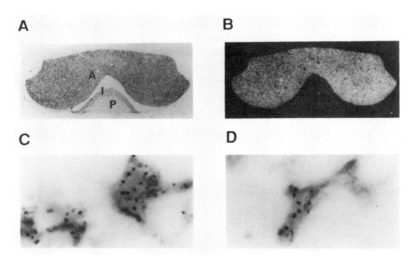

Figure 3 Expression of Pit-1 transcripts in the pituitary gland. In situ hybridization histochemistry reveals selective expression in the anterior pituitary *(panel B)*, but not in intermediate *(I)* or posterior *(P)* lobes. Pit-1 is expressed in somatotrophs and lactotrophs, colocalizing with growth hormone *(panel C)* and prolactin *(panel D)*.

predicted $M_r=32,900$ (35). Pit-1 mRNA is expressed only in the anterior pituitary gland and is present in lactotrophs and somatotrophs (35, 42) (Figure 3). Cotransfectional analyses using Pit-1 transcription units in HeLa cells resulted in expression of both prolactin and growth hormone fusion genes (Figure 4). A critical issue was whether, at physiologic levels of expression, Pit-1 was capable of activating prolactin or growth hormone fusion gene expression in heterologous cells; in permanent HeLa cell transfectants expressing levels of Pit-1 at tenfold less than those present in pituitary cells, preferential transcriptional activation of the prolactin gene promoter was observed (42). In contrast to reported results with a fusion GHF (Pit-1) protein (6) or in a partially purified protein preparation (9), Pit-1 expressed in bacteria effectively bound to and activated in vitro transcription of both the prolactin and growth hormone promoters (42).

Unexpectedly, Pit-1 shared significant homology with a 60 amino acid region, referred to as the homeodomain, initially described in three gene products regulating early development in *Drosophila antennapedia, Ultrabithorax,* and *fushi tarazu* (51, 43) and present in over 20 related gene

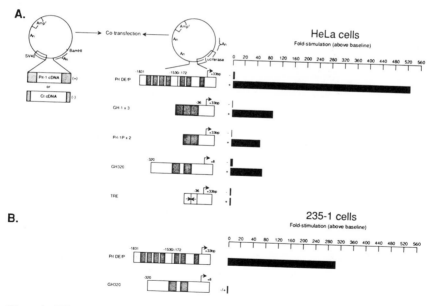

Figure 4 Effects of Pit-1 on prolactin and growth hormone fusion genes in HeLa cells and the 235-1 putative lactotroph cell line show similar results.

products that dictate position-specific determination in *Drosophila* (1, 23, 51) (Figure 4). Multigene families containing highly conserved homeobox domains appear to direct early developmental events and have been described in *C. elegans,* amphibians, mice, and humans (8, 39, 12, 1). Their shared homology with the yeast a_1 and a_2 regulatory gene products, known to individually and in combination with other transcription factors regulate gene expression that determines yeast cell mating type (52; see review 45), suggested similar functional roles for the homeotic genes. It was observed that Pit-1 directly activated prolactin and growth hormone fusion gene transcription as a consequence of binding to *cis*-active elements, and in heterologous cells in mammals formally linked homeodomain-containing proteins to tissue-specific transcriptional activation; subsequently, data confirming a transcriptional role for *Drosophila* homeodomain proteins have been reported (e.g. 17, 36, 29).

Pit-1 exhibited an identity of 7 of the 9 invariant and 15 of the 20 most highly conserved amino acids present in the *Drosophila* homeodomains (see Figure 5). The sequence variations modify only several of the conserved amino acids predicted to be on one side of the putative α helical regions (44, 49). An apparently critical divergence is observed in the putative recognition region where cysteine, glutamine, and glutamic acid are uniquely present in residues 50, 54, 56. Recently a number of genes with highly diverged homeobox domains, and often exhibiting tissue-specific and cell-specific patterns of expression, have been identified (e.g. 60, 2, 5); however, the WFC motif is unique to the POU-domain gene family.

A lymphoid B cell-specific factor that activates the transcription of immunoglobulin genes (Oct-2) as a consequence of binding to an octamer recognition element and a more generally distributed octamer binding protein (Oct-1) have recently been sequenced based on cDNA analysis (11, 56). A comparison of Pit-1, Oct-2, and Oct-1 with a *C. elegans* regulatory gene

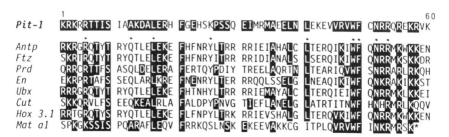

Figure 5   Pit-1: Identification of a 60 amino acid region similar to homeodomains of several *Drosophila* regulatory proteins.

product, unc-86 (21) genetically defined as a determinant of cell-specific development fate, revealed that the four proteins share an extended region of homology (see Figure 6a). Amino-terminal to the 60 amino acid divergent homeodomain, referred to as the POU-homeodomain, is a 76–78 amino acid region that is unique to these four proteins, referred to as the POU-specific domain (31). These two regions, together with a nonconserved region between them, constitute the POU-domain (Figure 6); the evolutionary conservation suggests critical functions are subserved by each region.

POU-Domain Protein Recognition Sites

The Pit-1 DNA recognition element is an A,T-rich sequence (T/A T/A T/A ATANCAT); a core sequence differing by only a single nucleotide from the

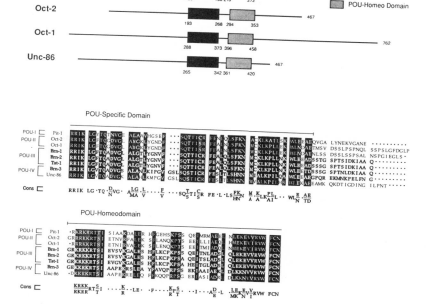

Figure 6 Identification of four new mammalian POU-domain regulatory genes expressed in the neuroendocrine system. The POU-specific and POU homeodomains encoded by four transcripts expressed in brain and endocrine tissues (Brn-1, Brn-2, Tst-1, and Brn-3). Tst-1 is expressed in both brain and testes. Brn-1 is expressed in both the central nervous system and medulla of kidney. The eight POU-domain proteins appears to fall into four classes (I–IV).

octamer sequence (ATTTGCAT) that binds different factors in lymphoid and non-lymphoid cells. This binding site is sufficient to impart lymphoid-specific promoter activity (58, 62, 53). While Pit-1 can bind at tenfold lower affinity to the octamer sequence, Pit-1 fails to activate transcription units containing the octamer, rather than Pit-1 elements. The binding sites for *Drosophila* homeodomain gene products are A/T-rich (33), and the consensus yeast MATa$_2$ product binding site (37) is remarkably similar to the Pit-1 recognition element. Therefore, it is possible that the members of the homeodomain and POU-domain families responsible for developmental activation of gene transcription bind to highly related A/T-rich elements. This would be analogous to the steroid hormone T$_3$ receptor gene family that exhibits remarkable similarity of their binding sites (reviewed in 3; 20, 24, 25).

The presence of multiple required elements, many of which bind Pit-1 in the prolactin gene, appears to be an important aspect of its developmental activation because a single element is insufficient to produce marked increases in gene expression. Therefore, combinatorial effects of multiple Pit-1 elements and sites for other transcription factors must constitute the code responsible for the temporal and quantitative patterns of prolactin gene expression. In lactotrophs, additional factors may also bind to Pit-1 sites and functionally effect prolactin gene transcription.

Ontogeny of Pit-1 Expression in Somatotrophs, Lactotrophs, and Thyrotrophs

Because the distal enhancer contains Pit-1 binding sites, at least two of which are necessary for expression in prolactin-producing cells (46), possibly Pit-1 was responsible for the activation of the distal enhancer-containing fusion genes in thyrotrophs (16). Hybridization histochemistry of sections immunostained for the TSH peptide revealed that Pit-1 mRNA colocalized with TSH immunostaining in some thyrotrophs (Figure 7). The ontogeny of Pit-1 expression correlates with the appearance of pituitary cell types during development. Expression of Pit-1 appears to be restricted to the developing anterior pituitary on embryonic day (16) (e16) with hybridization for Pit-1 more difficult to detect in e15 embryos. Pit-1 gene expression is, therefore, found early in the ontogeny of the pituitary prior to the reported appearance of TSH, growth hormone, and prolactin. Many reports suggest that prolactin is expressed postnatally many days after the initial expression of Pit-1, but reports vary widely in the initial appearance of prolactin from e21 to just after birth in the rat (59, 10) and 8 days postpartum in the mouse (54). This apparent discrepancy between the appearance of Pit-1 and the initial expression of prolactin might indicate that low levels of prolactin expression could be activated by Pit-1 very early in development, but that other factors either cooperate with or replace Pit-1 to generate detectable levels of expression at

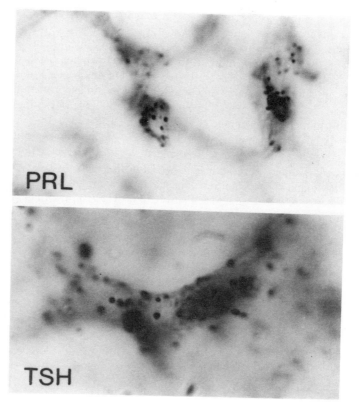

Figure 7 Expression of Pit-1 in lactotrophs and thyrotrophs based on colocalization of Pit-1, by hybridization histochemistry with immunostaining for PRL and TSH.

later times coincident with birth of the lactotroph. Consistent with this explanation, we found the expression of prolactin transgenes on mouse day e16 (rat day e17) (16). These analyses indicated that prolactin gene expression was activated at low levels in the rodent fetus, coordinate with or closely following the expression of Pit-1 during ontogeny. The progressive increase in expression of two orders of magnitude, however, suggests that additional factors must be involved in establishing the patterns of cell-specific restriction and physiologic levels of gene expression.

Because Pit-1 at levels tenfold lower than those in pituitary cells (42) is capable of activating the expression of both the growth hormone and prolactin fusion genes and because the Pit-1 gene is expressed in somatotrophs, lacto-trophs (35, 6), and thyrotrophs (16), there are likely to be restrictive mech-anisms that prevent the expression of growth hormone and prolactin genes in

lactotrophs and thyrotrophs, respectively. Sequences flanking the distal enhancer are likely to be required for restricting prolactin gene expression from
thyrotrophs. Restrictive mechanisms could represent either negative regulation or the lack of complementing factors that interact with or displace Pit-1 to
give physiologic levels of prolactin expression. On this basis, it is expected
that there are additional factors that bind to the prolactin and growth hormone
5' flanking regions and play pivotal roles in regulating the physiologic levels
of prolactin and growth hormone gene expression. The role of Pit-1 during the
organogenesis of the pituitary may be to activate initial transcription of
specific genes in a pituitary-specific manner, while additional activation and
restrictive mechanisms are responsible for delineating specific cell type within
the pituitary gland. These additional mechanisms that regulate the differentiation into lactotrophs and somatotrophs should provide an important paradigm
for differentiation during mammalian development.

A Large Family of POU-Domain Regulatory Genes in Mammalian Brain Development

Brain development involves an intricate program of gene expression that leads
to the establishment of many neuronal phenotypes and a precise complex
pattern of connections between them. The nuclear events underlying neuronal
development and the accompanying diverse patterns of specific gene expression remain largely unknown. It is likely, however, that the precise temporal
and spatial patterns characteristic of mammalian brain development reflect
sequential activation of a complex network of regulatory factors similar to
those presumed to account for establishing structural patterns in *Drosophila*
(51, 23). The specification of a variety of neuronal phenotypes derived from
an apparently homogeneous population of neuroepithelial cells are pre-
requisites for brain development.

The possibility that novel POU-domain proteins were expressed during
establishment of the nervous system with distinct spatial and temporal patterns, potentially exerting some roles in specifying neuronal phenotypes, was
investigated using a strategy based on the structure of the initial four members
of the POU-domain gene family. Degenerate oligonucleotides based on two
highly conserved amino sequences in the A region of the POU-specific
domain and in the C-terminal portion of the POU homeodomain were used as
primers for the polymerase chain reaction employing DNA complementary to
brain and testes mRNAs as templates. Four new members of the POU-domain
gene family were identified; three from brain cDNA (Brn-1, Brn-2, and
Brn-3) and one from rat testes cDNA (Tst-1), although this gene is predominantly expressed in the brain. Predicted amino acid residues for each
new member are shown in Figure 6*b*.

Structural comparisons of the four new POU-domain proteins revealed that they are all highly related to Pit-1, Oct-1, Oct-2, and unc-86. Recently another POU-protein has also been identified in *C. elegans* (ceh-6) (6a). These nine proteins constitute a distinct POU-domain protein family. Three of the new proteins (Brn-1, Brn-2, and Tst-1) are highly homologous, with > 94% of the amino acid residues being identical among them throughout the entire POU-domain. Even the variable region between the POU-specific domain and the POU-homeodomain is well conserved among these proteins. Brn-3 is highly related to unc-86, including three characteristic additional amino acid residues in the region between the A and B portions of the POU-specific domain. Pit-1 is distinct from the other eight proteins in the POU-family domain at several amino acid positions that otherwise would be totally conserved, and it is thus far the most divergent member of the family. The known POU-domain proteins appear to segregate into four classes arbitrarily referred to as POU-1 (Pit-1), POU-2 (Oct-1, Oct-2), POU-3 (Brn-1, Brn-2, Tst-1), and POU-4 (Brn-3, unc-86). The N' terminal basic part of the POU-homeodomain is identical for the first 11 or 12 amino acids, and 15–18 amino acids in the C-terminal WFC region (see Figure 5) are particularly well-conserved between all members of each class. A consensus sequence for the POU-domain emphasizes the degree of primary amino acid sequence conservation among all nine family members. It is predicted that the POU III gene family will contain the most members.

Each gene is expressed in at least one tissue other than brain and generates transcripts of different size. Thus Brn-1 and Brn-2 exhibit virtually identical patterns of expression in the central nervous system, but Brn-1 is clearly expressed in the medullary zone of the kidney, while Brn-2 is not (30). Hybridization for Brn-1 and Brn-2 is found in at least some classes of neurons at all levels of the neuraxis. Almost all regions of the cerebral (layers II–V) and cerebellar (Purkinje cells) cortices are labeled, as are the basal forebrain cholinergic system, ventral midbrain dopamine system, paraventricular and supraoptic neuroendocrine system, somatic motoneurons in the cranial nerve nuclei and ventral horn, and tectum (Figure 8). In contrast, the Brn-3 gene transcript exhibits a considerably more restricted pattern with relatively dense hybridization limited to the habenula, posterior hypothalamic area, inferior olive, inferior colliculus, and nucleus ambiguus. Brn-3 transcripts are uniquely present in sensory ganglion cells (in the trigeminal and dorsal root ganglia), which are derived from the neural crest. The Tst-1 gene, while expressed in testes, is particularly well-expressed in brain and displays a characteristic pattern of expression in the cerebral (layers V–VI) and cerebellar (granule cells) cortices, as well as in the striatum, medial habenula, superior colliculus and parabigeminal nucleus, and dorsal motor nucleus of the vagus nerve. Thus each POU-domain gene exhibits a unique, restricted pattern of expression, though not obviously correlated with known de-

Table 1 Distribution of POU-domain mRNA expression in the adult rat nervous system determined by *in situ* hybridization

	Pit-1	Brn-1	Brn-2	Brn-3	Tst-1	Oct-1	Oct-2
SENSORY GANGLIA	−	−	−	+ + + +	−	−	−
CORTEX							
isocortex, layers 2-5	−	+	+	−	−	−	−
layers 5-6	−	−	−	−	+	−	−
olfactory bulb, mitral	−	+	+	−	+	−	−
periglomerular	−	+	+	−	−	−	−
islands of Calleja	−	+ + +	+ +	−	−	−	−
piriform	−	+	+	−	+	−	−
presubiculum, layer 2	−	+ +	+ +	−	−	−	−
CA1/subiculum	−	+ +	+ +	−	+ + +	−	−
dentate gyrus	−	+	+	−	−	−	−
subependymal zone	−	+ +	+ +	−	−	−	−
AMYGDALA							
n. lateral olfactory tract	−	+	+	−	+ +	−	−
SEPTUM							
medial n./n. diagonal band	−	+	+	−	−	−	−
bed n. stria terminalis	−	+	+	−	−	−	−
BASAL GANGLIA							
striatum	−	−	−	−	+	−	−
substantia innominata	−	+	+	−	−	−	−
s. nigra/ventral tegmental a.	−	+	+ +	−	+	−	−
THALAMUS							
medial habenula	−	+ + +	+ +	+ + +	+ +	+ +	−
lateral habenula	−	−	−	+ +	−	−	−
parafascicular n.	−	+	+	−	−	−	−
reticular n.	−	+	+	−	−	−	−
zona incerta	−	+	+	−	−	−	−
HYPOTHALAMUS							
suprachiasmatic n.	−	−	−	−	−	−	+ +
supraoptic/paraventricular n.	−	+ +	+ + +	−	−	−	✝
medial preoptic n.	−	+	+	−	−	−	−
tuberomammillary n.	−	+	+	−	−	−	−
lateral mammillary n.	−	+	+	−	−	−	−
medial mammillary n.	−	−	−	−	−	+	+ +
posterior hypothalamic a.	−	+	+	+ +	−	−	−
BRAINSTEM - SENSORY							
superior colliculus, inter. gray	−	+	+	+	+	−	−
parabigeminal n.	−	+ +	+ + +	−	+ + +	−	−
superior olive	−	−	−	+	−	−	−
inferior colliculus, dorsal n.	−	+	+	+ +	−	−	−
area postrema	−	+	+ +	−	−	+	−
BRAINSTEM - MOTOR							
motor n. trigeminal	−	+	+	−	−	−	−
facial n.	−	+	+	−	−	−	−
hypoglossal n.	−	+	+	−	−	−	−
n. ambiguus	−	−	−	+ +	−	−	−
dorsal motor n. vagus	−	−	−	−	+ +	−	−
BRAINSTEM - CORE							
periaqueductal gray	−	+	+	+	−	−	−
n. incertus	−	+ +	+ +	−	−	−	−
interpeduncular n.	−	−	−	+	−	−	−
CEREBELLUM & RELATED							
deep nuclei	−	+	+	−	−	−	−
Purkinje	−	+ +	+ +	−	−	−	−
granule	−	−	−	−	+ +	+ + +	+ +
red n.	−	−	−	−	−	−	+
inferior olive	−	+	+	+ + + +	−	−	−
SPINAL CORD							
ventral horn	−	+	+	−	−	−	−

Relative density of **in situ** hybridization indicated as follows:−; not detected; +: low; + +: moderate; + + +: high; + + + +: very high. Sense-strand control hybridization was (−) for all regions indicated.

Figure 8 Distributors of POU-domain mRNA expression in the adult rat nervous system determined by *in situ* hybridization. The hypothalmic pattern of expression is noted.

velopmental, functional, or neurotransmitter-related systems in the nervous system. All four new POU-domain proteins are widely expressed in all levels of the neural tube during at least some part of this period. The anatomical restriction for each gene product in the developing neural tube is distinct however, and reflects the adult loci of expression. Expression is observed in the ventricular (proliferative) zone of the neuroepithelium, the mantle layer, the early cortical plate (Brn-1, Brn-2), and external granular layer of the cerebellum (Tst-1) (Figure 9). These data suggest that the genes are expressed

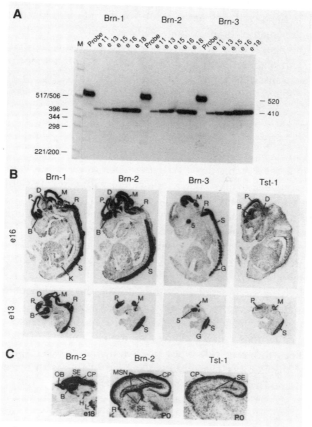

Figure 9 Developmental patterns of expression of Brn-1, Brn-2, Brn-3, and Tst-1. Panel A uses a RNase protection assay to document the ontogeny of transcript expression during embryogenesis. Panel B shows examples of localization on embryonic days 13 and 16 (e13, e16). Panel C reveals expression of Brn-2 and Tst-1 during cortical plate development (CP), showing expression of Brn-2 in migrating superficial neurons (MSN) that will ultimately become the superficial layers of the adult cortex.

during the migratory phase of at least some types of young neurons. RNase protection analyses confirm the temporal expression pattern of these cloned genes.

Neuronal Expression of Pit-1, Oct-1, and Oct-2 Transcripts Overlapping Patterns of POU-Domain Gene Expression

Pit-1 transcripts identical to those expressed in the anterior pituitary are detected in the neural plate and tube on embryonic days 10 through 13 and disappear thereafter until embryonic day 16, when Pit-1 transcripts reappear exclusively in the developing anterior lobe of the pituitary gland. Pit-1 is not detected in any mature brain region. Although Pit-1 is initially widely expressed in the neural tube, it is subsequently restricted completely from the nervous system and reappears in a novel location, the anterior pituitary.

Oct-2 gene transcripts are also found widely in the developing neural tube, in the diencephalon, brainstem, spinal cord, and sensory ganglia. In contrast to Pit-1, however, Oct-2 transcripts continue to be expressed in the brain of the adult animal with expression limited to the suprachiasmatic and medial mammillary nuclei of the hypothalamus as well as to cerebellar granule cells and the red nucleus. The Oct-1 gene is also found to be widely expressed in the neural tube (embryonic day 13), but at much lower levels than any of the other POU-domain proteins. Later, coincident with cerebellar development, Oct-1 expression is highly restricted to cerebellar granule cells, and to the medial habenula, medial mammillary nucleus, and area postrema.

When the pattern of expression for the six mammalian POU-domain genes that are present in the mature nervous system (all but Pit-1) is compared (Figure 8), several intriguing features emerge. First, none of the patterns for individual members of the family corresponds entirely to any known topographical division or functional system, to the distribution of any known neurotransmitter or receptor, or to any one cell type. Second, some regions of the nervous system appear to express only one of the members examined here, whereas other regions clearly express multiple members of the family. In some instances different cell types in a particular region express different members of the family. The clearest example of this is in the cerebellum, where Brn-1 and Brn-2 are expressed in Purkinje cells while Tst-1, Oct-1, and Oct-2 are expressed in granule cells. Only one of the known POU-domain proteins, Oct-2, is expressed in the suprachiasmatic nucleus, while Brn-1, Brn-2, Brn-3, Tst-1, and Oct-1 are all expressed in the medial habenula. It would appear that neurons in a region such as the medial habenula may express as many as five of the seven mammalian POU-domain genes identified thus far, whereas there are many brain regions where no expression of any known POU-domain protein is detected. One of the new POU-domain proteins, Brn-3, is highly similar to unc-86, and interestingly it is the only known member of the mammalian POU-domain gene family expressed in sensory ganglion cells. The similarity between the protein sequence and the patterns of expression in such divergent organisms as nematodes and mammals suggests highly conserved roles for these two proteins. By analogy with Pit-1 and Oct-1, it seems likely that all members of the POU-domain gene family exert their effects by modulating specific patterns of gene transcription.

The observation that POU-domain proteins are co-expressed in certain parts of the developing and mature brain suggests that a combinatorial code may be important for the mature phenotypes observed and that these gene products may cross-regulate, analogous to the proposed interactions of homeodomain proteins in *Drosophila* (50). In fact, the pattern of expression of POU-domain genes also overlaps with that for several mouse homeodomain genes that display discrete positional and temporal patterns of expression during spinal cord or brain development (19, 30, 22, 34, 38, 48); however, in contrast to known homeodomain gene products, the POU-domain transcripts are expressed in the forebrain. Recently it has been shown that the variant homeodomain proteins are involved in sensory organ development in *Drosophila (cut)* (18) and *C. elegans* (mec-3) (5), as well as ommatidia assembly in *Drosophila (rough)* (57). It is likely that while classic homeodomain genes play broad roles in development, from pattern formation to tissue-specific delineation, POU-domain genes may exert their critical functions in tissue-specific cell-type diversification and organogenesis. Because of the unusually high degree of conservation from *Drosophila* and nematodes to human, their distinct functions must be essential for the organism. The potential interactions between the POU-domain proteins and the other homeodomain proteins are yet to be investigated.

SUMMARY

The anterior pituitary gland provides a model for investigating the molecular basis for the appearance of phenotypically distinct cell types, within an organ, a central question in development. The rat prolactin and growth hormone genes are selectively expressed in distinct cell types (lactotrophs and somatotrophs) of the anterior pituitary gland, which reflect differential mechanisms of gene activation or restriction because of interactions of multiple factors binding to these genes. We find that the pituitary-specific 33,000 dalton transcription factor, Pit-1, normally expressed in somatotrophs, lactotrophs, and thyrotrophs, can bind to and activate both growth hormone and prolactin promoters in vitro at levels even tenfold lower than those normally present in pituitary cells. In the case of the prolactin gene, high levels of expression in transgenic animals required two *cis*-active regions; a distal enhancer (−1.8 to

−1.5 kb) and a proximal region (−422 to +33 bp). Each of these regions alone can direct low levels of fusion gene expression to prolactin-producing cell types in transgenic mice, but a synergistic interaction between these regions is necessary for high levels of expression. The initial appearance of the prolactin transgene expression closely follows the appearance of high levels of Pit-1, but later increases in expression coincident with appearance of mature lactotrophs suggest the operation of additional, critical positive factor(s). Unexpectedly, transgenes containing the distal enhancer removed from its normal context are expressed in both the prolactin-producing lactotrophs and the TSH-producing thyrotrophs, thereby suggesting that sequences flanking this enhancer are necessary to restrict expression to the correct cell type within the pituitary. These data indicate that distinct processes of gene activation and restriction are necessary for the fidelity of cell-type specific expression within an organ. Consistent with this model, we find that lactotroph cell lines that cannot express the growth hormone gene contain high levels of functional Pit-1. We suggest a large, highly related POU-domain gene family, potentially exceeding 100 members, has been conserved and expanded in evolution to meet the increasing requirements for more intricate patterns of cell phenotypes. The POU-domain subgroup of the homeodomain gene family, in concert with other homeodomain proteins and with other classes of transcription factors, is likely to contribute to the establishment of the mammalian neuroendocrine system.

Literature Cited

1. Awgulewitsch, A., Utset, M. F., Hart, C. P., McGinnis, W., Ruddle, F. H. 1986. Spatial restriction in expression of a mouse homeobox locus within the central nervous system. *Nature* 320:328–35
2. Barad, M., Jack, T., Chadwick, R., McGinnis, W. 1988. A novel, tissue-specific, *Drosophila* homeobox gene. *EMBO J.* 7:2151–61
3. Beato, M. 1989. Gene regulation by steroid hormones. *Cell* 56:335–44
4. Behringer, R. R., Mathews, L. S., Palmiter, R. D., Brinster, R. L. 1988. Dwarf mice produced by genetic ablation of growth hormone-expressing cells. *Genes Dev.* 2:453–60
5. Blochinger, K., Bodner, R., Jack, J., Jan, L. Y., Jan, Y. N. 1988. Primary structure and expression of a product from *cut*, a locus involved in specifying sensory organ identity in *Drosophila*. *Nature* 333:629–35
6. Bodner, M., Castrillo, J. L., Theill, L. E., Deerinck, T., Ellisman, M., Karin, M. 1988. The pituitary-specific transcription factor GHF-1 is a homeobox-containing protein. *Cell* 50:267–75
6a. Burglin, T. R., Finney, M., Coulson, A., Ruvkun, S. 1989. *Caenorhabditis elegans* has scores of homeobox-containing genes. *Nature* 341:239–43
7. Cao, Z., Barron, E. A., Carrillo, A. J., Sharp, Z. D. 1987. Reconstitution of cell-type-specific transcription of the rat prolactin gene in vitro. *Mol. Cell Biol.* 7:3402–8
8. Carrasco, A. E., McGinnis, W., Gehring, W. J., De Robertis, E. M. 1984. Cloning of a *X. laevis* gene expressed during early embryogenesis that codes for a peptide region homologous to *Drosophila* homeotic genes. *Cell* 37:409–14
9. Castrillo, J.-L., Bodner, M., Karin, M. 1987. Purification of growth hormone-specific transcription factor GHF-1 containing homeobox. *Science* 243:814–17
10. Chatelain, A., Dupuoy, J. P., Dubois, M. P. 1979. Ontogenesis of cells producing polypeptide hormones in the fetal hypophysis of the rats: Influence of the

hypothalamus. *Cell Tissue Res.* 196: 409–27

11. Clerc, R. G., Corcoran, L. M., Le-Bowitz, J. H., Baltimore, D., Sharp, P. A. 1988. The B-cell specific Oct-2 protein contains POU box and homeo box-type domains. *Genes Dev.* 2:1570–81

12. Colberg-Poley, A. M., Voss, S. D., Chowdhury, K., Gruss, P. 1985. Structural analysis of murine genes containing homeobox sequences and their expression in embryonal carcinoma cells. *Nature* 314:713–18

13. Cooke, N. E., Coit, D., Weiner, R. I., Baxter, J. D., Martial, J. A. 1981. Human prolactin: structural analysis and evolutionary comparisons. *J. Biol. Chem.* 256:4007–16

14. Costa, R. H., Grayson, D. R., Xanthopoulos, K. G., Darnell, J. E. 1988. A liver-specific DNA binding protein recognizes multiple nucleotide sites in regulatory regions of transthyretin, α1-antitrypsin, albumin, and simian virus 40 genes. *Proc. Natl. Acad Sci. USA* 85:3840–44

15. Courtois, G., Morgan, J. G., Campbell, L. A., Fourel, G., Crabtree, G. R. 1987. Interaction of a liver-specific nuclear factor with the fibrinogen and α1-antitrypsin promoters. *Science* 238:688–92

16. Crenshaw, E. B. III, Kalla, K., Simmons, D. W., Swanson, L. W., Rosenfeld, M. G. 1989. Cell-specific expression of the prolactin gene in transgenic mice is controlled by synergistic interactions between enhancer and promoter elements. *Genes Dev.* 3:959–72

17. Desplan, C., Theis, J., O'Farrell, P. H. 1988. The sequence specificity of homeodomain-DNA interaction. *Cell* 54:1081–90

18. Doe, C. Q., Hiromi, Y., Gehring, W. J., Goodman, C. S. 1988. Expression and function of the segmentation gene *fushi tarazu* during *Drosophila* neurogenesis. *Science* 239:170–75

19. Dony, C., Gross, P. 1987. Specific expression of the Hox 1.3 homeo box gene in murine embryonic structures originating from or induced by the mesoderm. *EMBO J.* 6:2965–75

20. Evans, R. M. 1988. Steroid and thyroid hormone receptors as transcriptional regulators of development and physiology. *Science* 240:889–95

21. Finney, M., Ruvkun, G., Horvitz, H. R. 1988. The *C. elegans* cell lineage and differentiation gene *unc* 86 encodes a protein containing a homeodomain and extended sequence similarity to mammalian transcription factors. *Cell:* 55:757–69

22. Gaunt, S. J. 1987. Homeobox gene *Hox-1.5* expression in mouse embryos: earliest detection by *in situ* hybridization is during gastrulation. *Development* 101:51–60

23. Gehring, W. J. 1987. Homeoboxes in the study of development. *Science* 236: 1245–52

24. Glass, C. K., Franco, R., Weinberger, C., Albert, V. R., Evans, R. M., Rosenfeld, M. G. 1987. A *c-erb-A* binding site in rat growth hormone gene mediates *trans*-activation by thyroid hormone. *Nature* 329:738–41

25. Glass, C. K., Holloway, J. M., Devary, O. V., Rosenfeld, M. G. 1988. The thyroid hormone receptor binds with opposite transcriptional effects to a common sequence motif in thyroid hormone and estrogen response elements. *Cell* 54:313–23

26. Guitierrez-Hartmann, A., Siddiqui, S., Loukin, S. 1987. Selective transcription and DNAase I protection of the rat prolactin gene by GH3 pituitary cell-free extracts. *Proc. Natl. Acad. Sci. USA* 84:5211–15

27. Hammer, R. E., Krumlauf, R., Camper, S. A., Brinster, R. L., Tilghman, S. M. 1987. Diversity of α-fetoprotein gene expression in mice is generated by a combination of separate enhancer elements. *Science* 235:53–58

28. Hammer, R. E., Swift, G. H., Ornitz, D. M., Quaife, C. J., Palmiter, R. D., et al. 1987. The rat elastase 1 regulatory element is an enhancer that directs correct cell specificity and developmental onset of expression in transgenic mice. *Mol. Cell Biol.* 7:2956–67

29. Han, K., Levine, M. S., Manley, J. 1989. Synergistic activation and repression of transcription by *Drosophila* homeobox proteins. *Cell* 56:573–83

30. He, X., Treacy, M. N., Simmons, D. M., Ingraham, H. A., Swanson, L. W., Rosenfeld, M. G. 1989. Expression of a large family of POU-domain regulatory genes in mammalian brain development. *Nature* 340:35–42

31. Herr, W., Sturm, R. A., Clerc, R. G., Corcoran, L. M., Baltimore, D., et al. 1988. The POU domain: A large conserved region in the mammalian *Pit-1, Oct-2,* and *Caenorhabditis elegans unc-86* gene products. *Genes Dev.* 2:1513–16

32. Hoeffler, J. P., Boockfor, F. R., Frawley, L. S. 1985. Ontogeny of prolactin cells in neonatal rats: Initial prolactin secretors also release growth hormone. *Endocrinology* 117:187–95

33. Hoey, T., Levine, M. 1988. Divergent homeo box proteins recognize similar DNA sequences in *Drosophila*. *Nature* 332:858–61

34. Holland, P. W. H., Hogan, B. L. M. 1986. Phylogenetic distribution of *Antennapedia*-like homeo boxes. *Nature* 321:251–53

35. Ingraham, H. A., Chen, R., Mangalam, H. J., Elsholtz, H. P., Flynn, S. E., et al. 1988. A tissue-specific transcription factor containing a homeodomain specifies a pituitary phenotype. *Cell* 55:519–29

36. Jaynes, J. B., O'Farrell, P. H. 1988. Activation and repression of transcription by homeodomain-containing proteins that bind a common site. *Nature* 336:744–49

37. Johnson, A. D., Herskovitz, I. 1985. A repressor (*MAT* α2 product) and its operator control expression of a set of cell type specific genes in yeast. *Cell* 42:237–47

38. Krumlauf, R., Holland, P. W. H., McVey, J. H., Hogan, B. L. M. 1987. Developmental and spatial patterns of expression of the mouse homeobox gene, *Hox 2.1*. *Development* 99:603–17

39. Levine, M., Rubin, G. M., Tjian, R. 1984. Human DNA sequences homologous to a protein coding region conserved between homeotic genes of *Drosophila*. *Cell* 38:667–73

40. Lira, S. A., Crenshaw, E. B. III, Glass, C. K., Swanson, L. W., Rosenfeld, M. G. 1988. Identification of rat growth hormone genomic sequences targeting pituitary expression in transgenic mice. *Proc. Natl. Acad. Sci. USA* 85:4755–59

41. Lufkin, T., Bancroft, C. 1987. Identification by cell fusion of gene sequences that interact with positive *trans*-acting factors. *Science* 237:283–86

42. Mangalam, H. J., Albert, V. R., Ingraham, H. A., Kapiloff, M., Wilson, L., et al. 1989. A pituitary POU domain protein, Pit-1, activates both growth hormone and prolactin promoters transcriptionally. *Genes Dev.* 3:946–58

43. McGinnis, W., Levine, M. S., Hafen, E., Kuroiwa, A., Gehring, W. J. 1984. A conserved DNA sequence in homeotic genes of the *Drosophila Antennapedia* and *bithorax* complexes. *Nature* 308:428–33

44. McKay, D. B., Steitz, T. A. 1981. Structure of catabolite gene activator protein at 2.9 A° resolution suggests binding to the left-handed B-DNA. *Nature* 290:744–49

45. Naysmyth, K., Shore, D. 1987. Transcriptional regulation in the yeast life cycle. *Science* 237:1162–70

46. Nelson, C., Albert, V. R., Elsholtz, H. P., Lu, L. E.-W., Rosenfeld, M. G. 1988. Activation of cell-specific expression of rat growth hormone and prolactin genes by a common transcription factor. *Science* 239:1400

47. Nelson, C., Crenshaw, E. B. III, Franco, R., Lira, S. A., Albert, V. R., et al. 1986. Discrete *cis*-active genomic sequences dictate the pituitary cell type-specific expression in rat prolactin and growth hormone genes. *Nature* 322:557–62

48. Odenwald, W. F., Taylor, C. F., Palmer-Hill, F. J., Freidrich, V. Jr., Tani, M., Lazzarini, R. A. 1987. Expression of a homeo domain protein in noncontact-inhibited cultured cells and postmitotic neurons. *Genes Dev.* 1:482–96

49. Ohlendorf, D. H., Anderson, W. F., Matthews, B. W. 1983. Many gene-regulatory proteins appear to have a similar α-helical fold that binds DNA and evolved from a common precursor. *J. Mol. Evol.* 19:109–14

50. Scott, M. P., Carroll, S. B. 1987. The segmentation and homeotic gene network in early *Drosophila* development. *Cell* 51:689–98

51. Scott, M. P., Weiner, A. J. 1984. Structural relationships among genes that control development: sequence homology between the *Antennapedia*, *Ultrabithorax*, and *fushi tarazu* loci of *Drosophila*. *Proc. Natl. Acad. Sci. USA* 81:4115–19

52. Shephard, J. C. W., McGinnis, W., Carrasco, A. E., DeRobertis, E. M., Gehring, W. J. 1984. Fly and frog homeodomains show homologies with yeast mating type regulatory proteins. *Nature* 310:70–71

53. Singh, H., LeBowitz, J. H., Baldwin, A. S. Jr., Sharp, P. A. 1988. Molecular cloning of an enhancer binding protein: isolation by screening of an expression library with a recognition site DNA. *Cell* 52:415–29

54. Slabaugh, M. B., Lieberman, M. E., Rutledge, J. J., Gorski, J. 1982. Ontogeny of growth hormone and prolactin gene expression in mice. *Endocrinology* 110:1489–97

55. Staudt, L. M., Singh, H., Sen, R., Wirth, T., Sharp, P. A., Baltimore, D. 1986. A lymphoid-specific protein binding to the octomer motif of immunoglobulin genes. *Nature* 323:640–43

56. Sturm, R. A., Das, G., Herr, W. 1988.

The ubiquitous octamer binding protein Oct-1 contains a POU domain with a homeobox subdomain. *Genes Dev.* 2: 1582–99

57. Tomlinson, A., Kimmel, B. E., Rubin, G. M. 1988. *rough*, a Drosophila homeobox gene required in photoreceptors R2 and R5 for inductive interactions in the developing eye. *Cell* 55:771–84

58. Walker, M., Edlund, T., Boulet, A. M., Rutter, W. J. 1983. Cell-specific expression controlled by the 5'-flanking region of insulin and chymotrypsin genes. *Nature* 306:557–61

59. Watanabe, Y. G., Daikoku, S. 1979. An immunohistochemical study on the cytogenesis of adenohypophysial cells in fetal rats. *Dev. Biol.* 68:557–67

60. Way, J. C., Chalfie, M. 1988. *mec-3*, a homeobox-containing gene that specifies differentiation of the touch receptor neurons in *C. elegans*. *Cell* 54:5–16

61. West, B. L., Catanzaro, D. F., Mellon, S. H., Cattini, P. A., Baxter, J. D., Reudelhuber, T. L. 1987. Interaction of a tissue-specific factor with an essential rat growth hormone gene promoter element. *Mol. Cell. Biol.* 7:1193–97

62. Wirth, T., Staudt, L., Baltimore, D. 1987. An octamer oligonucleotide upstream of the TATA motif is sufficient for lymphoid-specific promoter activity. *Nature* 329:174–78

63. Ye, Z. S., Samuels, H. H. 1987. Cell- and sequence-specific binding of nuclear proteins to 5'-flanking DNA of the rat growth hormone gene. *J. Biol. Chem.* 262:6313–17

Annu. Rev. Physiol. 1990. 52:793–806

SOMATOSTATIN GENE REGULATION

O. M. Andrisani and J. E. Dixon

Biochemistry Department, Purdue University, West Lafayette, Indiana 47907

KEY WORDS: cAMP, cAMP-responsive element (CRE), CRE-binding (CREB), transactivator, cloning of CREB

INTRODUCTION

Somatostatin gene regulation is important not only because of the wide-spread biological activities of the gene product, but also because it was one of the first genes shown to be regulated by cAMP (33). Recently, the somatostatin gene has taken on added interest because a protein important in recognizing the DNA sequences responsible for cAMP regulation has been cloned by the research groups of Habener et al (22) and Montminy et al (13). This review will briefly cover the background associated with somatostatin gene structure and will focus primarily on recent developments associated with somatostatin gene regulation.

The structure and functions of the polypeptide hormone somatostatin have been studied for many years in several species (37, 51). The 14-residue form of somatostatin has been conserved in all organisms examined. In addition, several other members of the somatostatin family have been identified, which include a 28-residue somatostatin from the anglerfish (21) and a 22-residue somatostatin from the catfish (35, 1). cDNAs have been isolated and se-quenced that encode each of these peptides (12, 14, 15, 21, 29, 30, 44, 50). The gene encoding somatostatin-14 has been isolated from a human gene library by Shen & Rutter (45) and from a rat gene library both by Montminy et al (32) and our laboratory (49).

The transcriptional unit of the rat somatostatin gene includes exons of 238 and 367 base pairs (bp) separated by one intron of 621 bp. The intron is located between the codons for Gln (−57) and Glu (−56) of pre-prosomatostatin. Analysis of the nucleotide sequence 5' to the start of transcription reveals a number of sequences that may be involved in the expression of the somatostatin gene. A variant of the TATA box, TTTAAA, lies 26 bp upstream from the start of transcription, and a sequence homologous to the CAAT box, GGCTAAT, occurs 92 bp upstream from the transcription initiation site. A long alternating purine-pyrimidine stretch, $(GT)_{25}$, which is similar to Z-DNA-forming sequences in other genes, lies 628 bp 5' to the start of transcription (20). Southern blot analysis of rat DNA suggests that a single gene is present that codes for the preprohormone that is ultimately processed into somatostatin-14. The human gene also consists of two exons separated by an intron of 877 bp. The exon-intron junctions are conserved in the rat and human genes.

AN OVERVIEW OF TRANSCRIPTION

The past several years have witnessed a tremendous increase in our knowledge of how genetic elements of eukaryotic genes regulate transcription through their interaction with cellular transcription factors. Genetic elements (promoters and enhancers) of eukaryotic genes have been defined by a combination of in vitro mutagenesis and gene transfer studies. These genetic elements, which are modular in nature, function through sequence-specific interactions with cellular protein factors. The sequence-specific nature of the interaction of the cellular factors with the genetic cis-acting elements is a powerful property of this class of proteins. Based on the sequence-specific binding of the transcription factors, a number of assays have been developed that have led to the identification and purification of a number of these proteins, also termed transactivators. The general principle that appears to be consistently reinforced is that protein-DNA interactions as well as protein-protein interactions will play dominant roles in defining the course of events that result in the expression and regulation of eukaryotic genes.

DEFINITION OF THE *CIS*-ACTING ELEMENT REQUIRED FOR SOMATOSTATIN GENE TRANSCRIPTION

In order to define the cis-acting elements required for expression of the rat somatostatin gene, deletions of the 5' non-transcribed region of the gene were cloned in front of a reporter gene, and the activity of these deletions was determined by gene transfer experiments in the appropriate cell lines. Ideally, the host cell line should express the endogenous gene of interest; thus agents modulating expression of the transfected gene should also modulate expression of the endogenous promoter.

Andrisani et al (2) utilized the CA-77 cell line system to introduce 5' deletions of the rat somatostatin promoter aligned to transcribe the chloramphenicol acetyltransferase (CAT) reporter gene. The CA-77 cell line established by Roos & colleagues (5) is a neuronally derived cell line that originated from a rat medullary thyroid carcinoma. This cell line expresses elevated levels of somatostatin mRNA and has been utilized as the mRNA source for the isolation of somatostatin cDNA clones (12, 15). The *cis*-acting element required for maximal expression of the somatostatin gene was localized between position -60 to -43 of the promoter. Deletion of the sequences between nucleotide positions -47 and -42 reduced the activity of the promoter to 9% of the wild-type level in CA-77 cells, which suggests that the deleted sequences constitute an important element required for expression of the somatostatin promoter.

Montminy et al (34) introduced similar 5'-end deletions into PC12 cells, a neuronally derived pheochromocytoma cell line. Although PC12 cells do not express the endogenous somatostatin gene, they are cAMP-responsive, thereby providing a system for the study of cAMP effects on neuropeptide gene transcription. Also, a mutant PC12 cell line exists that is deficient in cAMP-dependent protein kinase. These investigators (34) demonstrated that transcription from the somatostatin promoter of the transfected SST-CAT plasmid is inducible by cAMP. This cAMP-induced transcription from the somatostatin promoter requires the presence of a genetic element located between position -71 to -48 of the somatostatin promoter. These are the same sequences required for expression of the somatostatin gene in CA-77 cells (2), although the observed transcription from the somatostatin promoter in the CA-77 cell line does not require nor respond to cAMP induction. Montminy et al (33) showed that the sequences of the somatostatin promoter between nucleotide positions -60 to -29, when placed in front of the *SV40* promoter (which is cAMP non-responsive), confer cAMP-responsiveness in the SST-SV40-CAT construct. The cAMP response occurs only in wild-type PC12 cells and not in the kinase A-deficient PC12 cell line. These results demonstrate the involvement of the cAMP pathway in the transcriptional effect of cAMP on the somatostatin promoter.

Comparison of the cAMP-responsive element present within the somatostatin gene to sequences near the promoters of other genes known to be regulated by cAMP (8, 10, 47, 53) suggest the TGACGTCA sequence as the cAMP consensus (Table 1). The TGACGTCA sequence is referred to as CRE for cAMP-responsive element.

The TGACGTCA module is also present and required for function in viral

TABLE 1   Genes containing the TGACGTCA (CRE) consensus

Gene	Sequence	Distance to the 5' cap site in bp
Somatostatin	TTGGCTGACGTCAGAGAGAGAG	−48
PEPCK	GCCCCTTACGTCAGAGGCGAGC	−90
VIP	TACTGTGACGTCTTTCAGAGCA	−75
Proenkephalin	GGGCCTG CGTCAGC	−92
α-Chorionic gonadotrophin	AAAATTGACGTCATGG	−122
c-Fos	CCCAGTGACGTAGGA	−66
Fibronectin	ACAGTCCCCCGTGACGTCACCCGGGAGCCC	−173
Cytomegalovirus enhancer	CCCATTGACGTCAATGGGAGTT	−140
HTLV-II LTR	GGCCCTGACGTCCCTCCCCCCC	−178
Bovine leukemia virus LTR	GACAGAGACGTCAGCTGCCAGA	−159
Adenovirus 5 (Ad5) E$_4$	GGAAGTGACGTAACGTGGGAAAACGG	−163
Ad2 E$_4$	AAATGGGAAGTGACGTATCGTGGGAAAAC	−163
Ad2 E$_3$	GCGGGCGGCTTTCGTCACAGGGTGCGGTC	−61
Ad2 E$_2$	CTGGAGATGACGTAGTTTTCGCGCTTAAATTT	−76
Ad2 E1A	ATAGTCAGCTGACGTGTAGTGTATTTATACCC	−43
Ad2,5 E1A	ACTTTGACCGTTTACGTGGAGACTCGC	−117

promoters such as the E1A inducible early (E1A, E$_2$a, E$_3$, E$_4$) *adenovirus* promoters (6, Table 1). Sassoni-Corsi (41) utilized deletion mutants of the E$_2$a and E$_3$ *adenovirus* promoters to show by transient expression assays in PC12 cells that a related CRE-like sequence, TACGTCA, is required for both cAMP-responsiveness and E1A transactivation. An interesting observation reported in this study is that the action of the E1A protein in transactivating the E$_2$a and E$_3$ promoters is maintained in the mutant PC12 cell line, which is deficient in cAMP-dependent protein kinase.

Engel et al (11) utilized the cAMP-responsive S49 cell line to study cAMP induction of the viral E1A-inducible early promoters during the course of *adenovirus* infection. It was observed that transcription of the E1A inducible E$_4$ gene utilizing wild-type *adenovirus* was induced 15-fold in the presence of cAMP treatment. The level of induction of E$_4$ mRNAs was only fourfold when utilizing E1A viral mutants. These investigators concluded that although no changes were observed in the levels of E1A protein during the course of induction, preexisting E1A protein acts in synergy with events triggered by cAMP to induce transcription of the viral early genes. Although the studies described in this section point to the functional importance of the CRE consensus sequence in the expression of the cAMP-responsive and E1A-inducible promoters, the mechanism of cAMP- and E1A-mediated events is not yet understood.

IDENTIFICATION OF THE CELLULAR PROTEIN FACTORS THAT INTERACT WITH THE RAT SOMATOSTATIN CRE ELEMENT

In vitro, protein-DNA-binding assays such as DNase I footprinting and gel retardation assays (7, 25, 46) have been utilized for the identification, characterization, and purification of cellular transactivator proteins. The success of these in vitro assays is based on the property that most transactivator proteins possess: high affinity and sequence-specific binding to defined regions of DNA. DNase I footprint assays can be used to identify regions of a radiolabeled DNA fragment that are protected from DNase I digestion because of the sequence-specific binding of protein factors. DNase I footprint assays utilizing the radiolabeled somatostatin promoter DNA as a probe and cell extracts from PC12 (31), CA-77 (3), or HeLa (24, 28) cells have shown that the −55 to −35 region of the somatostatin promoter, which harbors the CRE, is protected from DNase I digestion. Gel retardation assays have also been used to identify factor(s) binding to the CRE-containing region of the rat somatostatin gene (3). A radiolabeled DNA fragment containing the CRE element of the somatostatin promoter was utilized as a probe and allowed to interact in vitro with extracts prepared from various cell lines or tissues. The DNA/protein complexes were analyzed on low ionic strength polyacrylamide gels. Three sequence-specific DNA/protein complexes have been identified in extracts of many different cell types. These complexes show competitive binding to other CRE-consensus sequences, but do not compete for binding with fragments derived from a variety of other DNAs including the β-globin promoter, major late promoter, or upstream sequences of the somatostatin promoter. The activities forming the three sequence-specific complexes are chromatographically separable, which suggests that distinct entities are responsible for the formation of the three sequence-specific complexes (3). Similar observations are reported in the study by Hardy & Shenk (18), who utilized HeLa cell extracts fractionated on an ion exchange column. These fractions were measured by the gel retardation assay with the *adenovirus* E$_4$ CRE-like element and the somatostatin CRE as probes. Also, Cortes et al (9) observed multiple CRE-binding activities after chromatographic fractionation of HeLa extracts. These activities were assayed both by in vitro DNA-protein assays using the E$_4$ and somatostatin CRE elements and functional in vitro transcription assays.

Although the gel retardation and DNase I footprinting assays have implicated the CRE consensus in sequence-specific binding of cellular protein factor(s), the direct involvement of the CRE in the formation of these sequence-specific complexes has been determined by in vitro methylation interference assays (3). It was shown that the G residues within the TGACG-TCA core element come into direct contact with the protein factor(s) forming the DNA/protein complexes. Synthetic oligonucleotides containing point mutations of the G residues within the TGACGTCA palindrome fail to compete for binding in vitro. Similar methylation interference data have been reported by Green's laboratory (28), utilizing the early *adenovirus* promoter E_4, somatostatin, and other CRE-containing promoters.

PURIFICATION OF A CRE-BINDING 43-kd PROTEIN (CREB)

Purification to apparent homogeneity of a number of sequence-specific DNA-binding proteins has been achieved by use of conventional chromatography in combination with a sequence-specific DNA-affinity chromatography step. Kadonaga & Tjian (25) reported the development of a sequence-specific DNA-affinity column for the purification of the transcription factor SP1. The DNA-affinity column was constructed by coupling multimeric units of dou-ble-stranded synthetic oligonucleotides containing the binding site of interest to cyanogen bromide-activated sepharose. An alternative method for con-structing a high capacity DNA-affinity column involves the incorporation of biotinylated nucleotides into the ends of concatemerized DNA (4). The biotinylated DNA is subsequently bound by avidin, which has been im-mobilized on agarose.

In the last two years, a number of laboratories have employed CRE-sequence-specific affinity chromatography for the purification of CRE-binding cellular transcription factors. Purification of a 43-kd protein from PC12 extracts by a somatostatin CRE-sequence-specific affinity column was initially reported by Montminy & Bilezikjian (31). This 43-kd protein, re-ferred to as CREB for CRE-binding, protects the -55 to -32 region of the somatostatin promoter from DNase I digestion. Zhu et al (55) reported the purification of a 43-kd protein from rat brain extracts by employing ion exchange chromatography for the fractionation of three CRE-binding activi-ties followed by two cycles of DNA-affinity chromatography of the major CRE-binding fractions. This 43-kd protein was purified to an apparent single band on SDS gels. It similarly binds in a sequence-specific manner to the somatostatin CRE-containing promoter fragment as shown by Southwestern blots and DNase I footprints.

A 45-kd protein has also been purified by Hurst & Jones from HeLa cell extracts (24). These investigators used the sequences from the E1A-inducible *adenovirus* E_3 promoter for constructing the sequence-specific DNA-affinity chromatography column.

To elucidate the relationship between the proteins purified by CRE-affinity chromatography utilizing the CRE-consensus sequence of cAMP-responsive or E1A-inducible genes, Lin & Green (28) employed UV crosslinking experiments to attach the labeled CRE DNA covalently to the bound protein. The covalent DNA-protein complex was analyzed by SDS PAGE electrophoresis. These experiments demonstrated that a common 45-kd polypeptide was capable of interacting with both E1A and cAMP-inducible promoters. The 45-kd polypeptide binding to the *adenovirus* E1A-inducible promoters that contain CRE-like sequences is referred to as ATF (adenovirus transcription factor). The UV crosslinking results suggest that a common 43–45-kd protein, ATF/CREB, is involved in the activation of E1A-inducible or cAMP-inducible sets of genes that respond to different induction signals.

Hai et al (17) reported the purification of a series of polypeptides that migrate as 43 and 47-kda proteins by CRE-affinity chromatography utilizing CRE-like sequences from the *adenovirus* E_4 promoter. These polypeptides represent a family of proteins that are related by DNA-binding specificity and immunoreactivity. This family of immunologically related functions includes multiple forms of ATF and AP1. AP1, activator protein 1, has been shown to mediate phorbol ester action (27). The recognition sequence of AP1 is similar, but not identical, to the ATF-binding site (the AP1-binding site is $GTGAGT_A^CA$, whereas ATF is $TGA\underline{C}GT_A^CA$). The immunological cross-reactivity and similar DNA-binding specificity between ATF and AP1 suggests that these proteins contain similar amino acid sequences and may have originated from a common ancestral gene.

TRANSCRIPTIONAL ACTIVITY OF CREB

Although the 43-kd protein has been purified to apparent homogeneity by a number of laboratories (24, 31, 55) and has been shown to bind specifically to cAMP-responsive elements, a functional in vitro transcription assay is essential to show that the 43-kd protein is the somatostatin gene transactivator. Andrisani et al (4) developed a functional in vitro transcription assay for the rat somatostatin promoter. HeLa cell nuclear extracts were prepared according to Shapiro et al (43). Transcription from the somatostatin promoter was monitored by linking it to the bacterial CAT gene. In addition, the *adenovirus* major late promoter (MLP) was similarly fused to the CAT structural gene. This MLP-CAT construct served as an internal control in the in vitro transcription assays. Transcripts initiated from the somatostatin and MLP promoters were detected by a primer extension analysis.

The transcriptional activity of the 43-kd protein was examined in in vitro transcription assays after the endogenous CRE-binding activities were depleted from the HeLa cell extracts (4). This was accomplished by passing the transcriptionally active extract through a CRE-oligonucleotide avidin column.

While the depleted extract was unable to transcribe the somatostatin promoter, transcription from the MLP promoter, which served as an internal control, was unaffected. Addition of the purified 43-kd protein restored transcription to the somatostatin promoter, thus proving that the 43-kd protein is the somatostatin gene transactivator.

ACTION OF CREB/ATF

The mechanism of action of eukaryotic transactivator proteins is largely unknown. With the availability of purified CREB/ATF protein and the establishment of CREB/ATF-dependent in vitro transcription systems, a number of questions pertaining to the action of CREB/ATF are beginning to be addressed.

What is the Role of CREB/ATF in the Interaction with the Transcriptional Complex?

The transcriptional complex is composed of RNA polymerase II and a number of common transcription factors, such as TFIID, TFIIB, and TFIIE, which must be assembled in an ordered manner into a functional complex for initiation to occur (38, 39, 42). Early studies have shown that the TATAA box and cap site are necessary and sufficient for accurate transcription initiation. Subsequent studies (19) suggest that upstream activating sequences and their associated factors increase the rate of transcription probably by facilitating the association of the common transcription factors under conditions where these interactions are rate-limiting.

The studies by Horikoshi et al (23) and Hai et al (16) have addressed this question by utilizing the ATF purified protein and the *adenovirus* E_4 promoter. DNase I footprint studies showed that the ATF protein interacts with the TATA box binding factor, TFIID, and this interaction facilitates the formation of the initiation complex (23). Functional in vitro transcription assays conducted with the ATF-dependent E_4 promoter showed that ATF acts prior to initiation of transcription, during the first rate-limiting step referred to as the template-commitment step (16). These data suggest that ATF and TFIID initially bind to the promoter to form the template-committed complex, and this interaction promotes the binding of factors TFIIE, TFIIB, and RNA polymerase II.

How Does CREB Bind to DNA?

The somatostatin promoter CRE element, TGAC|GTCA, is a perfect palindrome. In prokaryotes, numerous transcription factors bind to palindromes as dimers; the monomers have reduced DNA binding affinity and transcriptional activity (36).

The functional importance of the somatostatin promoter palindromic CRE sequence was studied by constructing SST-CAT plasmids containing 0, ½, or 1 CRE (54). The response of these constructs to forskolin induction was examined by transient expression assays in PC12 cells. Forskolin, a post-receptor activator of adenylyl cyclase, induces transcription of 1 CRE-containing SST-CAT plasmid by 14-fold in PC12 cells, whereas the constructs containing no CRE or ½ CRE were induced two and threefold, respectively. These results point to the functional importance of the palindrome in somatostatin gene transcription and suggest that the 43-kd CREB protein may act as a dimer.

How Does CREB Become Activated by cAMP Triggered Events?

The purified 43-kd CREB protein is an excellent substrate for the cAMP-dependent protein kinase A in vitro (54, 55). Phosphorylation takes place on serine residues, as shown by phosphoamino acid analysis (54, 55). In addition, phosphorylation of CREB protein occurs in vivo (31). This phosphorylation is stimulated three to fourfold in PC12 cells treated with forskolin, and grown in the presence of ^{32}P-orthophosphate. Phosphorylation does not alter the binding affinity of the 43-kd CREB protein for the CRE, however. Extracts prepared from forskolin-treated cells do not display increased CRE-binding affinity as shown for the cAMP-responsive α-hCG promoter (10). These data suggest that phosphorylation may influence the transcription activation potential of CREB.

Yamamoto et al (54) added the catalytic subunit of the cAMP-dependent kinase A to in vitro transcription reactions with extracts isolated from PC12 cells. A 20-fold induction in the transcription directed from the somatostatin promoter was observed, which suggests that cAMP-dependent protein kinase A acts directly on the CREB protein.

A model proposed by Hanson & colleagues (40) on the mechanism of cAMP-stimulated transcription is diagrammed in Figure 1.

CLONING OF THE cAMP-RESPONSIVE DNA-BINDING PROTEIN

Isolation of cDNA clones encoding DNA-binding proteins can be achieved via several independent screening routes. One approach utilizes synthetic oligonucleotide probes deduced from the amino acid sequence obtained from the purified protein. Although this is a biochemically sound approach, difficulties can be encountered with low yields of the purified transactivator proteins. Also, the purified proteins often have blocked NH$_2$-termini; thus

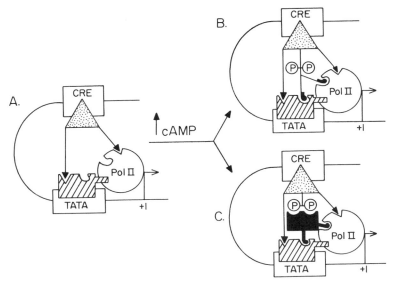

Figure 1 Model for cAMP regulation of gene transcription. (*A*) The CRE-binding protein *(stippled triangle)* binds to the CRE-consensus sequence. This binding stimulates basal transcription by interacting with proximal promoter elements such as the TATAA box binding factor TFIID *(diagonally lined box)* and/or RNA polymerase II. Elevation of cAMP levels induces phosphorylation of the CRE-binding protein, which further stimulates transcription by at least two general mechanisms (*B and C*). (*B*) Phosphorylated CREB recruits more transcription factors and/or increases the interaction between these factors. (*C*) Phosphorylated CREB interacts with a non-DNA binding protein *(solid box)*, which allows the formation of a higher order protein complex. Figure 1 reproduced with permission from Roesler et al (40)

internal peptides must be generated from the protein that in turn must be isolated and sequenced.

Alternatively, antibodies raised against the purified protein or to synthetic peptides can be utilized as a screening tool in λgtll expression libraries. Relatively large amounts of protein, however, are also necessary for producing antibodies.

Yet another approach, which is uniquely applicable to the isolation of cDNAs encoding sequence-specific DNA-binding proteins, is based on the renaturability and sequence-specific DNA-binding characteristics of this class of proteins. λgtll libraries expressing hybrid β-galactosidase fusion proteins are screened with ligated DNA probes containing the binding site of interest (48, 52). This technique has been successfully utilized for the isolation of a number of cDNAs encoding DNA-binding proteins (22, 48, 52).

Habener's laboratory reported the first isolation of a CREB-cDNA clone (22). This clone was obtained by screening a placental λgtll library for the expression of specific CRE-binding protein(s) and utilizing a CRE-consensus sequence as the radioactive probe. The isolated cDNA clone encodes a protein of 326 amino acids (MW = 35,044) and displays sequence-specific CRE-binding properties. It also belongs to a class of proteins that contain the structural motif referred to as a leucine zipper (26). This class of proteins, which includes myc, fos, C/EBP, GCN4, and c-jun, contains an array of leucine residues spaced with a periodicity of seven amino acid residues in a predicted amphipathic α-helix. The leucine side chains extending from one α-helix interdigitate with those displayed from a similar α-helix of a second polypeptide, which facilitates dimerization. Computer analysis of sequence similarity between the 35,000 CRE-binding protein and c-jun revealed a single region of 61% amino acid identity located at the carboxy-terminal end of the protein. These regions of similarity are located adjacent to the leucine zipper regions of the protein and constitute the basic domain. It has been suggested that the similarity of amino acid sequence in this domain may reflect the fact that these proteins have similar palindromic binding domains; TGACGTCA for CRE-binding protein vs TGAGTCA for c-jun.

Montminy's laboratory reported the isolation of a CREB-encoding cDNA from a rat PC12 λgt11 library (13). This cDNA clone was isolated utilizing oligonucleotide probes that were synthesized from amino acid sequence information obtained from tryptic peptide fragments of the purified 43-kd CREB protein. The predicted amino acid sequence of the human (22) and rat (13) CREB cDNA clones are quite similar. The predicted mass of the CREB protein encoded by the rat cDNA clone is 37 kd. The difference in the molecular weight between the deduced amino acid sequence derived from the cloned human and rat CREB cDNAs, 35 kd and 37 kd, respectively, and the purified 43-kd CREB protein has not been resolved. Post-translational modifications, such as phosphorylation and glycosylation, may account for some of this apparent difference. Montminy et al (13) noted several sites within the CREB molecule that might serve as potential sites of phosphorylation by the cAMP-dependent kinase A, kinase C, and casein kinase II. The functional significance of these sites in the activity and regulation of the CREB protein will obviously constitute an exciting area for future study.

The availability of the CREB cDNA clones should provide the tools necessary to increase our understanding of the structure/function of the CREB molecule in regulating somatostatin gene transcription. These observations are likely to reflect on our understanding of the entire family of cAMP-regulated genes.

SUMMARY

Since the cloning of the somatostatin cDNA and gene, the efforts of a number of laboratories have contributed to the understanding of somatostatin gene expression and regulation. A genetic element located approximately 40 nucleotides upstream from the somatostatin mRNA cap site is important in the expression and cAMP-induced transcription of this neuropeptide gene. The identification of this genetic element has enabled the identification, purification, and cloning of a new class of proteins: the somatostatin gene transactivator named CREB. The availability of cloned CREB will permit studies designed to understand not only the mechanism of somatostatin gene expression and regulation, but also the pathway of signal transduction triggered by cAMP-stimulated events.

NOTE ADDED IN PROOF   The cDNA sequence encoding a different CRE-binding protein named CRE-BP1 has been reported by Maekawa et al (29a). The human CRE-BP1 clone encodes a 54.5-kd protein, and it is distinct from the CREB clones isolated by Habener et al (22) and Gonzalez et al (13).

ACKNOWLEDGMENTS

This work was supported in part by grants from the National Institutes of Health. This is Journal Paper No. 12,031 from the Agricultural Experimentation Station, Purdue University.

Literature Cited

1. Andrews, P. C., Dixon, J. E. 1981. Isolation and structure of a peptide hormone predicted from an mRNA sequence: a second somatostatin from the catfish pancreas. *J. Biol. Chem.* 256:8267–70
2. Andrisani, O. M., Hayes, T. E., Roos, B., Dixon, J. E. 1987. Identification of the promoter sequences involved in the cell specific expression of the rat somatostatin gene. *Nucleic Acids Res.* 15:5715–28
3. Andrisani, O. M., Pot, D. A., Zhu, Z., Dixon, J. E. 1988. Three sequence-specific DNA protein complexes are formed with the same promoter element essential for expression of the rat somatostatin gene. *Mol. Cell. Biol.* 8:1947–56
4. Andrisani, O. M., Zhu, Z., Pot, D. A., Dixon, J. E. 1989. In vitro transcription directed from the somatostatin promoter is dependent upon a purified 43 kda DNA-binding protein. *Proc. Natl. Acad. Sci. USA* 86:2181–85
5. Aron, D. C., Muszynski, M., Birnbaum, R., Sabo, S., Roos, B. 1981. Somatostatin elaboration by monolayer cell cultures derived from transplantable rat medullary thyroid carcinoma: synergistic stimulatory effects of glucagon and calcium. *Endocrinology* 109:1830–34

6. Berk, A. J. 1986. *Adenovirus* promoters and E1A transactivation. *Annu. Rev. Genet.* 20:45–79
7. Carthew, R. W., Chodosh, L. A., Sharp, P. A. 1985. An RNA polymerase II transcription factor binds to an upstream element in the *adenovirus* major late promoter. *Cell* 43:439–48
8. Comb, M., Birnberg, N. C., Seasholtz, A., Herbert, E., Goodman, H. M. 1986. A cyclic AMP- and phorbol ester-inducible DNA element. *Nature* 323:353–56
9. Cortes, P., Buckbinder, L., Leza, A. M., Rak, N., Hearing, P., et al. 1988. EivF, a factor required for transcription of the *Adenovirus* EIV promoter binds to an element involved in E1A-dependent activation and cAMP induction. *Genes Dev.* 2:975–90
10. Delegeane, A. M., Ferland, L. H., Mellon, P. L. 1987. Tissue-specific enhancer of the human glycoprotein hormone α-subunit gene: dependence on cyclic-AMP inducible elements. *Mol. Cell. Biol.* 7:3994–4002
11. Engel, D. A., Hardy, S., Shenk, T. 1988. cAMP Acts in synergy with E1A protein to activate transcription of the *Adenovirus* early genes E_4 and E1A. *Genes Dev.* 2:1517–28
12. Funckes, C. L., Minth, C. D., Deschenes, R., Magazin, M., Tavianini,

M. A., et al. 1983. Cloning and characterization of a mRNA-encoding rat preprosomatostatin. *J. Biol. Chem.* 258:8781–87

13. Gonzalez, G. A., Yamamoto, K. K., Fischer, W. H., Karr, D., Menzel, P., et al. 1989. A cluster of phosphorylation sites on the cyclic AMP-regulated nuclear factor CREB predicted by its sequence. *Nature* 337:749–52

14. Goodman, R. H., Aron, D. C., Roos, B. A. 1983. Rat preprosomatostatin: structure and processing by microsomal membranes. *J. Biol. Chem.* 258:5570–73

15. Goodman, R. H., Jacobs, J. W., Chin, W. W., Lund, P. K., Dee, P. C., Habener, J. F. 1980. Somatostatin-28 encoded in a cloned cDNA obtained from a rat medullary thyroid carcinoma. *Proc. Natl. Acad. Sci. USA* 77:5869–73

16. Hai, T., Horikoshi, M., Roeder, R. G., Green, M. R. 1988. Analysis of the role of the transcription factor ATF in the assembly of a functional preinitiation complex. *Cell* 54:1043–51

17. Hai, T., Liu, F., Allegretto, E. A., Karin, M., Green, M. 1988. A family of immunologically related transcription factors that includes multiple forms of ATF and AP-1. *Genes Dev.* 2:1216–25

18. Hardy, S., Shenk, T. 1988. Adenoviral control regions activated by E1A and the cAMP response element bind to the same factor. *Proc. Natl. Acad. Sci. USA* 85:4171–75

19. Hawley, D. K., Roeder, R. G. 1987. Functional steps in transcription initiation and reinitiation from the major late promoter in a HeLa nuclear extract. *J. Biol. Chem.* 262:3452–61

20. Hayes, T. E., Dixon, J. E. 1985. Z-DNA in the rat somatostatin gene. *J. Biol. Chem.* 260:8145–56

21. Hobart, P., Crawford, R., Shen, L.-P., Pictet, R., Rutter, W. J. 1980. Cloning and sequence analysis of cDNAs encoding two distinct somatostatin precursors found in the endocrine pancreas of anglerfish. *Nature* 288:137–41

22. Hoeffler, J. P., Meyer, T. E., Yun, Y., Jameson, L. J., Habener, J. F. 1988. Cyclic AMP-responsive DNA-binding protein: structure based on a cloned placental cDNA. *Science* 242:1430–33

23. Horikoshi, M., Hai, T., Liu, Y. S., Green, M. R., Roeder, R. G. 1988. Transcription factor ATF interacts with the TATA factor to facilitate establishment of a preinitiation complex. *Cell* 54:1033–42

24. Hurst, H. C., Jones, N. C. 1987. Identification of factors that interact with

the E1A-inducible *Adenovirus* E₃ promoter. *Genes Dev.* 1:1132–46

25. Kadonaga, J. T., Tjian, R. 1986. Affinity purification of sequence-specific DNA binding proteins. *Proc. Natl. Acad. Sci. USA* 83:5889–93

26. Landschulz, W. H., Johnson, P. F., McKnight, S. L. 1988. The leucine zipper: a hypothetical structure common to a new class of DNA binding proteins. *Science* 240:1759–64

27. Lee, W., Mitchell, P., Tjian, R. 1987. Purified transcription factor AP-1 interacts with TPA-inducible enhancer elements. *Cell* 49:741–52

28. Lin, Y. S., Green, M. R. 1988. Interaction of a common cellular transcription factor, ATF, with regulatory elements in both E1A and cyclic AMP-inducible promoters. *Proc. Natl. Acad. Sci. USA* 85:3396–3400

29. Magazin, M., Minth, C. D., Funckes, C. L., Deschenes, R., Tavianini, M. A., Dixon, J. E. 1982. Sequence of a cDNA encoding pancreatic preprosomatostatin-22. *Proc. Natl. Acad. Sci. USA* 79:5152–56

29a. Maekawa, T., Sakura, H., Kanei-Ishii, C., Sado, T., Yoshimura, T., et al. 1989. Leucine zipper structure of the protein CRE-BP1 binding to cyclic AMP response element in brain. *EMBO J.* 8:2023–28

30. Minth, C. D., Taylor, W. L., Magazin, M., Tavianini, M. A., Collier, K., et al. 1982. The structure of cloned DNA complementary to catfish pancreatic somatostatin-14. *J. Biol. Chem.* 257:10372–77

31. Montminy, M. R., Bilezikjian, L. M. 1987. Binding of a nuclear protein to the cyclic-AMP response element of the somatostatin gene. *Nature* 328:175–78

32. Montminy, M. R., Goodman, R. H., Horovitch, S. J., Habener, J. F. 1984. Primary structure of a gene encoding rat preprosomatostatin. *Proc. Natl. Acad. Sci. USA* 81:3337–40

33. Montminy, M. R., Low, M. J., Tapia-Arancibia, L., Reichlin, S., Mandel, G., Goodman, R. D. 1986. Cyclic AMP regulates somatostatin mRNA accumulation in primary diencephalic cultures and in transfected fibroblast cells. *J. Neurosci.* 6:1171–76

34. Montminy, M. R., Sevarino, K. A., Wagner, J. A., Mandel, G., Goodman, R. H. 1986. Identification of a cyclic-AMP-responsive element within the rat somatostatin gene. *Proc. Natl. Acad. Sci. USA* 83:6682–86

35. Oyama, H., Bradshaw, R. A., Bates, O. J., Permutt, A. 1980. Amino acid se-

quence of catfish pancreatic somatostatin I. *J. Biol. Chem.* 255:2251–54

36. Ptashne, M. 1987. *A Genetic Switch.* Cambridge, MA: Cell Press & Blackwell Sci. 2nd ed.

37. Reichlin, S. 1983. Somatostatin. *New Engl. J. Med.* 309:1495–1501

38. Reinberg, D., Horikoshi, M., Roeder, R. G. 1987. Factors involved in specific transcription in mammalian RNA polymerase II. *J. Biol. Chem.* 262:3322–30

39. Reinberg, D., Roeder, R. G. 1987. Factors involved in specific transcription in mammalian RNA polymerase II. *J. Biol. Chem.* 262:3331–37

40. Roesler, W. J., Vandenbark, G. R., Hanson, R. W. 1988. Cyclic AMP and the induction of eukaryotic gene transcription. *J. Biol. Chem.* 263:9063–66

41. Sassone-Corsi, P. 1988. Cyclic-AMP induction of early *Adenovirus* promoters involves sequences required for E1A trans-activation. *Proc. Natl. Acad. Sci. USA* 85:7192–96

42. Sawadogo, M., Roeder, R. G. 1985. Interaction of a gene specific transcription factor with the *adenovirus* major late promoter upstream of the TATA box region. *Cell* 43:165–76

43. Shapiro, D. J., Sharp, P. A., Wahli, W. W., Keller, M. J. 1988. A high-efficiency HeLa cell nuclear transcription extract. *DNA* 7:47–55

44. Shen, L.-P., Pictet, R. L., Rutter, W. J. 1982. Human somatostatin I: sequence of the cDNA. *Proc. Natl. Acad. Sci. USA* 79:4575–79

45. Shen, L.-P., Rutter, W. J. 1984. Sequence of the human somatostatin I gene. *Science* 224:168–71

46. Siebenlist, U., Gilbert, W. 1980. Contacts between E. coli RNA polymerase and an early promoter of phage T$_7$. *Proc. Natl. Acad. Sci. USA* 77:122–26

47. Silver, B. J., Bokar, J. A., Virgin, J. B., Vallen, E. A., Milsted, A., Nilson, J. H. 1987. Cyclic AMP regulation of the human glycoprotein hormone α-subunit gene is mediated by an 18-base-pair element. *Proc. Natl. Acad. Sci. USA* 84:2198–2202

48. Singh, H., LeBowitz, J. H., Baldwin, A. S. Jr., Sharp, P. A. 1988. Molecular cloning of an enhancer binding protein: isolation by screening of an expression library with a recognition site DNA. *Cell* 52:415–23

49. Tavianini, M. A., Hayes, T. E., Magazin, M. D., Minth, C. D., Dixon, J. E. 1984. Isolation, characterization, and DNA-sequence of the rat somatostatin gene. *J. Biol. Chem.* 259:11798–11803

50. Taylor, W. L., Collier, K. J., Deschenes, R. J., Weith, H. L., Dixon, J. E. 1981. Sequence analysis of a cDNA coding for a pancreatic precursor to somatostatin. *Proc. Natl. Acad. Sci. USA* 78:6694–98

51. Vale, W., Rivier, C., Brown, M. 1977. Regulatory peptides of the hypothalamus. *Annu. Rev. Physiol.* 39:473–527

52. Vinson, C. R., LaMarco, K. L., Johnson, P. F., Landschulz, W. H., McKnight, S. L. 1988. In situ detection of sequence-specific DNA binding activity specified by a recombinant bacteriophage. *Genes Dev.* 2:801–6

53. Wynshaw-Boris, A., Gross Lugo, T., Short, J. M., Fournier, R. E. K., Hanson, R. W. 1984. Identification of a cAMP regulatory region in the gene for rat cytosolic phosphoenolpyruvate carboxykinase (GTP). *J. Biol. Chem.* 259:12161–69

54. Yamamoto, K. K., Gonzalez, G. A., Biggs, W. H. III, Montminy, M. R. 1988. Phosphorylation-induced binding and transcription efficacy of nuclear factor CREB. *Nature* 334:494–98

55. Zhu, Z., Andrisani, O. M., Pot, D. A., Dixon, J. E. 1989. Purification and characterization of a 43 kda transcription factor required for rat somatostatin gene expression. *J. Biol. Chem.* 264:6550–56

Annu. Rev. Physiol. 1990. 52:807–21

REGULATION OF INHIBIN SYNTHESIS IN THE RAT OVARY

Teresa K. Woodruff and Kelly E. Mayo

Department of Biochemistry, Molecular Biology and Cell Biology, Northwestern University, Evanston, Illinois 60208

KEY WORDS: follicle-stimulating hormone, activin, pregnancy, estrous cycle, reproduction

INTRODUCTION

The fundamental structure of the mammalian ovary is the follicle. Cells of the follicle, principally granulosa and theca cells, produce hormones and provide information necessary for the onset of puberty, for control of the reproductive cycle, and for the maintenance of pregnancy. Complex interactions involving pituitary hormones, such as follicle-stimulating hormone (FSH), gonadal steroids, such as estradiol, and gonadal polypeptides, such as inhibin, are required to support development of the rapidly proliferating follicle and to coordinate signaling pathways within the reproductive axis (13, 20, 56). Inappropriate alterations in hormone synthesis or secretion within the hypothalamic-pituitary-ovarian axis result in anovulatory, senescent, or disease states (17, 39, 70).

Inhibin has been recognized for some time to be a key hormone for the appropriate regulation of pituitary FSH secretion (14, 32, 42, 66, 67), although its biological role in reproductive processes is not completely understood. With recent advances in the characterization of the inhibin proteins and their genes, questions regarding the expression and regulation of ovarian inhibin during the reproductive lifespan of the animal are now being investigated. The development of the inhibin concept, the characterization of the inhibin protein, and the description of its biological activities have all been

0066-4278/90/0315-0807$02.00

the subject of recent reviews (13, 15, 35, 68, 74, 84). This review will focus on the regulation of inhibin production in the female rat during the estrous cycle and during pregnancy. Before examining these endocrine states, we will briefly consider the characteristics of the inhibin family of hormones and their expression in gonadal and extragonadal tissues.

STRUCTURE AND EXPRESSION OF RAT INHIBIN

Structure and Function of Inhibin and Related Hormones

Inhibin is a disulfide-linked heterodimer, consisting of an α chain and one of two highly homologous β chains designated β_A and β_B (36, 49, 58, 61). The α chain is an 18-kd peptide and the β chains are 14-kd peptides, which lead to the formation of a 32-kd α-β dimer in most species. Inhibin A (α-β_A) and inhibin B (α-β_B) (see reference 5 for nomenclature) act on the anterior pituitary to selectively suppress FSH biosynthesis and release (8, 24, 44, 86). A second gonadal hormone, activin, is formed by the dimerization of the inhibin β chains (37, 75). Activin A (β_A-β_A) and activin AB (β_A-β_B) stimulate FSH synthesis and secretion from anterior pituitary cells in culture and act as functional antagonists to inhibin. Combinatorial assembly of the α, β_A, and β_B chains therefore generates multiple hormonal activities able to regulate the pituitary-gonadal axis (73). Activin also has biological activities outside the reproductive system; these will be considered in the following section.

Molecular cloning of inhibin α and β subunit cDNAs from several mammalian species indicates that each of the protein subunits is encoded by a distinct gene, that these genes and the proteins they encode are structurally related to one another, and that the mature inhibin chains reside at the carboxyl-terminus of much larger precursor proteins that undergo proteolytic processing (22, 26, 38, 41, 82). Analysis of inhibin cDNA clones also reveals a surprising structural similarity between the β chains of inhibin (activin) and transforming growth factor-β (TGFβ), a molecule with diverse effects on cellular proliferation and differentiation (38, 40). Like activin, TGFβ can stimulate the secretion of FSH from anterior pituitary cells in culture (85). TGFβ and activin represent early examples of an emerging gene family, which also include mammalian Mullerian inhibiting substance genes (9), the *Drosophila* pattern formation gene decapentaplegic (53), the *Xenopus* gene *VG1,* which encodes a protein involved in mesodermal induction (77), and three related human genes encoding bone morphogens BMP-2, BMP-2A, and BMP-3 (83). This suggests that the hormones of the inhibin family, particularly the activins, may play a role in differentiation and development unrelated to their reproductive function.

Gonadal and Extragonadal Expression of Inhibin Genes

Inhibin was originally isolated from follicular fluid, and the gonads are clearly the primary source of circulating inhibin. Ovariectomy dramatically decreases serum inhibin as measured by bioassay or radioimmunoassay (33, 57, 62), and inhibin bioactivity and protein have been localized to the ovarian granulosa cell (2, 21, 45). All of the inhibin mRNAs are expressed in the ovary, although there is about 10-fold more α than β_A or β_B mRNA (38, 82). Bicsak & coworkers have used biosynthetic labeling of cultured granulosa cells to show that the excess α-subunit protein exists predominantly in the precursor form and is stored intracellulary in addition to being secreted (2). The observed excess in α-subunit expression suggests that the β subunit is likely to be rate-limiting for inhibin production, and that α-β heterodimers are likely to predominate over β-β dimers in the ovary. In the male, the inhibin mRNAs are also predominantly expressed in the testes, although testicular expression declines following the onset of spermatogenesis (24a, 31, 47). Inhibin is made by the testicular sertoli cells (45, 50), while activin is secreted by interstitial cells (34). Although this review will focus on the endocrine actions of inhibin, both inhibin and activin may also have paracrine functions in intragonadal signaling (30).

Because the ovary is a complex tissue, in situ hybridization has been a powerful tool for examining inhibin gene expression at the cellular level. This technique is outlined briefly in Figure 1, which shows several examples of inhibin β_A mRNA localization in both gonadal (ovary) and extragonadal (placenta and brain) tissues. In the ovary, the inhibin mRNAs are predominantly localized to the granulosa cell layer of healthy developing follicles, although the α mRNA is expressed at low levels elsewhere (46, 79). Ovarian expression will be considered in greater detail in a subsequent section.

A comprehensive survey of rat tissues by RNA hybridization has been reported by Meunier & coworkers (47). They observed that the α, β_A, and β_B mRNAs were expressed in a variety of tissues at differing ratios. The finding that the inhibin subunit mRNAs are widely expressed in nonreproductive tissues is intriguing and is consistent with roles for the inhibin and activin proteins outside the reproductive axis. Inhibin and activin expression has been further examined in several nongonadal tissues including the brain, pituitary, bone marrow, placenta, and adrenal. In the brain, inhibin α, β_A and β_B mRNAs were all detected by solution hybridization (47). The β_A subunit has been immunologically localized to neuronal fibers and cell bodies in the caudal medulla (64). The data shown in Figure 1 suggest that the protein is synthesized in this region, in that cell bodies predominantly localized in the nucleus of the solitary tract express the β_A mRNA. Some of these β_A-

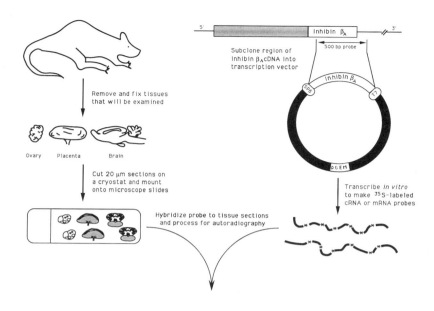

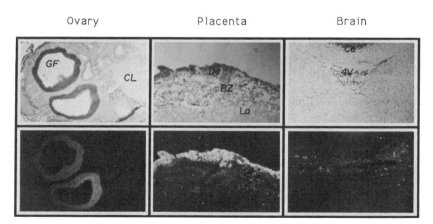

Figure 1 Localization of inhibin β_A-subunit mRNA in diverse cells types using in situ hybridization. The upper portion of the figure shows a schematic diagram of how tissues and probe are prepared for hybridization. The bottom portion of the figure shows localization of the β_A mRNA in ovary, placenta, and brain. The upper photograph in each case is a brightfield photomicrograph of a hemotoxylin-eosin (ovary and placenta) or cresyl violet (brain) stained section. The bottom photograph in each case is an identical field viewed under darkfield optics so that the silver grains indicative of inhibin β_A hybridization can be observed. Hybridization is seen in a mature ovarian follicle from a proestrous animal, in the decidual layer of the term placenta, and in neuronal cell bodies located predominantly in the nucleus of the solitary tract. Abbreviations are GC= Graafian follicle, CL= corpus luteum, De= decidua, BZ= basal zone, La= labyrinth, Ce= cerebellum, and 4V= fourth ventricle.

producing neurons send projections to hypothalamic magnocellular regions involved in oxytocin synthesis and therefore may participate in the modulation of oxytocin secretion (64). The α-subunit protein does not appear to be expressed in these cell groups.

The pituitary is also a site of inhibin or activin expression. The α-and β_B-subunit mRNAs, but not the β_A mRNA, are found in pituitary, and the α and β_B proteins have been localized to gonadotropes using immunocytochemistry. The expression of these subunits in the pituitary is influenced by estrogen (60). Since the anterior pituitary represents the major target for inhibin action, the presence of the α and β_B subunits in gonadotropes suggests possible paracrine or autocrine roles for inhibin or activin in regulating pituitary function. The inhibin α-subunit mRNA is also quite highly expressed in the adrenal cortex, thus suggesting a possible role in the regulation of corticosteroid production (10).

One of the more unexpected sources of extragonadal expression of an inhibin gene is in the bone marrow. Bone marrow appears to express only the β_A mRNA and is therefore likely to produce activin (47). Eto & coworkers have described the characterization of a factor that induces differentiation of a erythroleukemic cell line; this factor was subsequently shown to be identical to activin (23, 51). The biological activities of both highly purified and recombinant inhibin and activin in the hematopoietic system have been examined. Activin has been shown to induce erythroid differentiation, hemoglobin accumulation, and bone marrow colony formation, while inhibin antagonizes this function (4, 64a, 87). The mechanism by which the inhibin subunits exert their broad-ranging biological effects in these tissues has not been fully established, but the emerging evidence suggests that inhibin and activin are active outside the reproductive axis as important regulators of cellular differentiation.

Regulation of Inhibin Production by Granulosa Cells

Granulosa cells are affected by a spectrum of hormonal stimuli and respond based on their maturational status. The regulation of inhibin secretion by steroid and polypeptide hormones has been examined in primary rat granulosa cells by using either hybridization to measure inhibin mRNA within the cells or radioimmunoassay to measure inhibin protein in the culture medium. The levels of secreted inhibin and of inhibin mRNA are positively regulated by FSH in granulosa cell cultures, consistent with in vivo data that indicate that FSH is an important regulator of inhibin gene expression. (3, 69, 82, 86, 89). In addition, FSH directly increases the transcription rates of the inhibin α and β_A genes in primary granulosa cells, as demonstrated by in vitro nuclear run-on transcription assays (T. Woodruff, K. Mayo, unpublished). Luteinizing hormone (LH) stimulates inhibin production only after induction of its receptor with FSH (3, 72). Pharmacologic agents that act to enhance cellular cAMP levels also stimulate inhibin production by granulosa cells, which suggests that the effect of FSH and LH on inhibin production is cAMP-mediated (3, 69).

Many other peptide hormones modulate inhibin production by granulosa cells. Gonadotropin-releasing hormone (GnRH) attenuates the inducing effects of FSH on inhibin α mRNA accumulation and inhibits FSH-stimulated inhibin secretion in this system (3, 82), consistent with its actions in inhibiting granulosa cell differentiation (29). Vasoactive intestinal peptide, somatomedin C, insulin, and TGFβ have all been reported to increase inhibin production, while epidermal growth factor appears to be a negative regulator (3, 69, 88, 89). Steroid hormones by themselves seem to have little effect on inhibin secretion in this system, although androgens and corticosteroids have been reported to modulate FSH-induced inhibin secretion (69, 72).

REGULATION OF OVARIAN INHIBIN AS A FUNCTION OF REPRODUCTIVE STATUS

Inhibin Expression and Follicular Development During the Estrous Cycle

The reproductive cycle of the female rat is characterized by dynamic changes in serum steroid and gonadotropin levels as well as in follicular development. These changes are coordinated, in part, by alterations in the expression of ovarian inhibin (65). Folliculogenesis is a complex process that involves the growth and death of follicles, the formation of corpora lutea, and the appropriate production of steroid and polypeptide hormones by cells of the follicle (56). Inhibin synthesis is modulated as the follicle matures, a process that can be followed by examining inhibin production during the rat estrous cycle using in vitro bioassay (19), radioimmunoassay (28, 59a), or RNA hybridization approaches (46, 79).

The initiation of expression of the inhibin subunit mRNAs in the antral follicle occurs in two steps. On the morning of estrous, follicles are recruited that have the potential to ovulate four days later (the ovulatory pool). The α-subunit mRNA is found at low levels in follicles prior to their recruitment into this ovulatory pool (11, 46). These small antral follicles have previously been selected from the primordial pool to begin development. The initiator of this developmental pathway, as well as the role of independent α-subunit mRNA expression in these follicles, is unknown; perhaps the free α chain serves a paracrine or autocrine function in directing the subsequent ability of the follicle to enter the ovulatory pool. Once follicles have been recruited by the secondary FSH surge on the morning of estrous, these larger follicles (350 μm diameter) express the α-inhibin mRNA at higher levels and also initiate expression of the inhibin β_A mRNA. The increase in inhibin mRNA observed in newly recruited follicles on the morning of estrous is paralleled by an increase in serum inhibin, which leads eventually to the decline of FSH to basal levels (28). These changes in inhibin gene expression observed on the morning of estrous are likely to be controlled by the secondary FSH surge. This has been demonstrated in unilaterally ovariectomized (ULO) animals, in which there is a transient rise in serum FSH following removal of one ovary that leads to a compensatory follicular recruitment in the remaining ovary (6, 78). This ULO-induced rise in FSH leads to elevated expression of the inhibin mRNAs in these newly recruited follicles within 24 hr of surgery (11).

The follicles that are initially recruited on the morning of estrous do not all continue in the ovulatory tract. Approximately half of the follicles undergo a process of selective degeneration known as atresia (52). The atretic follicles, like the prerecruited follicles, express the α-and β_A-subunit mRNAs divergently (46, 80). Both mRNAs are dramatically reduced in the earliest stage of histologically identifiable atresia; the β_A mRNA is essentially undetectable in these follicles, while the α mRNA remains in low abundance until the later stages of atresia. The divergent expression of the inhibin subunit mRNAs in atretic and prerecruited follicles is intriguing. Firstly, it in part explains the observation that there is a 10-fold excess of α to β_A mRNA in whole ovarian RNA (38, 82), while in mature follicles examined by in situ hybridization the α and β_A mRNAs appear to be expressed at similar levels; the large pool of nonrecruited follicles presumably contributes substantially to the observed excess in α mRNA. Secondly, it suggests that production of the β_A subunit may be rate-limiting for inhibin heterodimer assembly in ovarian follicles. Lastly, it provides evidence for independent regulation of expression of the inhibin α and β_A genes.

Those follicles that escape atresia and continue to develop progressively increase in size (from 350 to 500 μm diameter) and also accumulate high levels of the inhibin mRNAs (46, 79). Likewise, serum inhibin levels rise during this time (28, 59a). Follicular development and enhanced inhibin expression are presumably under the influence of basal serum FSH. In support of this idea, inhibin mRNA levels increase in follicles that are progressing through the estrous cycle when FSH is transiently elevated following unilateral ovariectomy (11). The accumulation of the inhibin mRNAs in follicles of the ovulatory pool reaches a peak late in the afternoon of proestrous in Sprague-Dawley rats maintained on a 14 : 10 light : dark cycle. The reason for this large rise in inhibin levels on proestrus is unknown, but it may be that inhibin plays a role in synchronizing the subsequent preovulatory FSH surge. The preovulatory LH and FSH surges occur during the early evening of proestrous, and this elevation in gonadotropin levels stimulates mature follicles to initiate events that will lead to ovulation and subsequent luteinization.

Following the primary gonadotropin surges, inhibin gene expression is down-regulated, and the inhibin mRNAs are dramatically decreased in stimulated follicles by late in the evening of proestrus. Serum inhibin levels also decline during the proestrous to estrous transition (28, 59a). This decrease in inhibin expression appears to require the primary gonadotropin surges, since inhibin mRNAs remain elevated in mature follicles if the gonadotropin surges are blocked with a GnRH antagonist (57a, 81). This decrease in inhibin is postulated to allow serum FSH to remain elevated into the morning of estrous (secondary FSH surge), which serves to recruit a new crop of follicles that begin to produce inhibin, as outlined above. Meunier & coworkers have observed that in another strain of animals maintained under different lighting conditions the β_A subunit mRNA is turned off as described above, but that expression is reinitiated prior to ovulation, at a time when the α mRNA is not expressed (46). They suggest that activin is formed in these follicles and that it might function to enhance the secondary FSH surge.

Following ovulation and luteinization, inhibin mRNAs remain low in the newly formed corpus luteum. There is no detectable β_A mRNA in the corpus luteum (46, 79, Figure 1), although the α mRNA continues to be expressed at low levels (12, 46). The α-subunit protein has been immunocytochemically localized in the corpus luteum, which suggests that the protein may remain stable there after synthesis has diminished (45, 46).

The primary and secondary FSH surges are clearly independent with respect to the role inhibin plays in their generation. The primary FSH surge is GnRH-dependent, occurs despite elevated inhibin expression, and results in a subsequent decline of inhibin mRNA expression. The secondary FSH surge is GnRH-independent, occurs only when inhibin gene expression is turned off, and results in an enhanced expression of the inhibin subunit mRNAs in newly recruited follicles. Maintenance of the estrous cycle is therefore critically dependent on precise interplay between inhibin production in the ovary and FSH secretion from the pituitary. These relationships between pituitary FSH secretion and ovarian inhibin production at various points in follicular matura-tion are schematically depicted in Figure 2.

Inhibin Expression During the Fertile Cycle

Pregnancy is a unique endocrine state in which maternal cyclicity is replaced by a relatively quiescent period of gonadotropin secretion and follicular development (27). Maternal hormones in part direct the development of the fetal endocrine system. Moreover, the placenta provides a novel source of hormones that may act on both maternal and fetal targets. The pattern of inhibin expression in the maternal ovary during gestation is similar to that seen in the cyclic ovary; inhibin α, β_A, and β_B mRNAs are localized to granulosa cells of healthy antral follicles and diminish in the atretic follicles

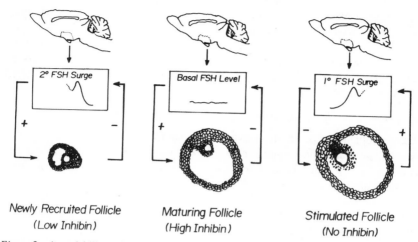

Figure 2   A model illustrating interactions between pituitary FSH secretion and ovarian inhibin production as a function of the maturational status of the follicle. Stimulatory effects are indicated by (+) and inhibitory effects by (–). In early follicular development FSH stimulates inhibin production, but in mature follicles the primary gonadotropin surges signal a rapid decline in inhibin gene expression.

characteristic of early pregnancy. The number of inhibin-expressing follicles is elevated early in pregnancy, falls to a mid-gestational nadir as a result of atresia, and rebounds to increase dramatically in late gestation as follicles that will ovulate following parturition mature (T. Woodruff et al, submitted). Following the postpartum ovulation, few hybridizing follicles are observed. Inhibin activity in ovarian venous plasma mirrors these changes in inhibin mRNA expression (71). Although the corpus luteum becomes functional for progesterone production, no expression of the inhibin mRNAs is observed in the corpora of pregnancy (T. Woodruff et al, submitted).

The fetal-placental unit develops following implantation of the blastocyst on day 5 or 6 of pregnancy in the rat. In addition to secreting hormones important in maternal endocrine regulation, the placenta produces a variety of factors that participate in the establishment of the fetal endocrine system. The role of inhibin in this process is not well understood, but inhibin and/or activin do appear to be placental hormones (1). Although the physiologic role of placental inhibin has not been examined in the rat, human placental extracts can decrease pituitary FSH secretion in a dose-dependent manner (43), and placental inhibin influences the production of chorionic gonadotropin in human placental primary cultures (54). We have localized inhibin α and β_A mRNAs to the cytotrophoblast cells in human placenta; these cells also express GnRH mRNA and peptide (T. K. Woodruff, K. E. Mayo, unpublished; 48), corticotropin-releasing factor (55), and somatostatin (76), thus suggesting that in the human inhibin is produced in cells that participate in directing endocrine aspects of early growth and development. Interestingly, the β_A mRNA is highly expressed in the rat placenta (47) while the α mRNA is nearly undetectable. The β_A mRNA is localized to the maternally-derived decidual cell layer (see Figure 1), which suggests that activin may be secreted from these cells.

Inhibin and the Immature and Senescent Animal

The establishment of adult reproductive cyclicity is preceded by a period of relative pituitary non-responsiveness during which FSH levels rise and fall and profiles of inhibin secretion change. Inhibin is produced in the pre-pubertal animal, and stimulation of immature animals with pregnant mares' serum gonadotropin results in elevated immunoreactive inhibin and inhibin α mRNA, which suggests that its synthesis is FSH-regulated (12, 33). Rivier & Vale have observed that from days 5 through 20 after birth serum inhibin and FSH levels rise simultaneously, but that at day 21 serum FSH levels decline while serum inhibin levels abruptly rise (59). Sander & coworkers have also demonstrated a progressive increase in the levels of bioactive inhibin in ovarian venous plasma during development (63). The inhibin produced by the immature animal plays a physiologic role in FSH regulation only after day 10. When an inhibin antiserum was infused into immature animals on days 10, 20, and 30 after birth, a significant elevation in serum FSH was found only on days 20 and 30 (59).

As the animal ages, regular estrous cycles are replaced first by irregular cycles and ultimately by an anestrous state. Accompanying these changes are ovarian follicular exhaustion and an impairment in the appropriate regulation of FSH synthesis and release (7). A larger percentage of follicles do not ovulate and continue to produce high levels of estradiol (25). Serum FSH levels become elevated and there is an increased duration of the estrous cycle (18). Moreover, the anterior pituitary becomes less sensitive to the negative influence of inhibin. DePaolo has examined the levels of bioactive inhibin as the adult female ages (16), and found that bioactive inhibin levels pro-gressively decline. Reproductive senescence can be characterized as a de-terioration of the influence of ovarian inhibin on the pituitary, which leads to an increase in serum FSH and, ultimately, to follicular exhaustion.

SUMMARY

The lifespan of the female rodent is characterized by dynamic changes in the hormonal regulation of the reproductive axis. From the time ovarian follicular growth is initiated in peripubertal animals, through recruitment, ovulation and luteinization during the estrous cycle, to the quiescent follicular development of pregnancy, and ultimately to follicular exhaustion, tremendous changes in follicular architecture, hormonal responsiveness, steroid secretion, and inhibin and activin synthesis occur. Similar changes in both the biosynthetic functions and hormonal responsiveness of the pituitary are likely to occur. Some of the information on inhibin expression during the reproductive lifespan of the rat reviewed here is summarized in a schematic fashion in Figure 3, which presents changes in serum FSH, ovarian inhibin production, and follicular development during different reproductive states. From recent observations regarding ovarian inhibin expression as a function of reproductive status, a partial picture of the complex interactions between steroid and peptide hormones necessary to maintain reproductive cyclicity in mammals is beginning to emerge. Study of the inhibin gene family and of other FSH-regulatory hormones is likely to further enhance our understanding of both normal reproductive processes and of reproductive disorders.

ACKNOWLEDGMENTS

Work from K. E. M.'s laboratory was supported by National Institutes of Health grants NS-24439 and HD-21921 and by the Chicago Community Trust Searle Scholars Program.

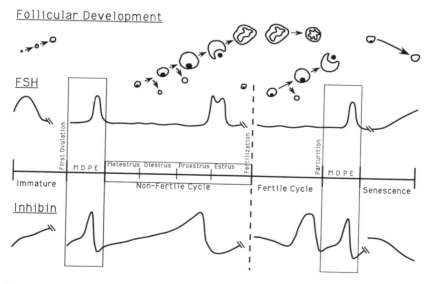

Figure 3 Changes in follicular development, FSH secretion, and inhibin production during the reproductive lifespan of the rat. A central time-line indicates periods of early development, reproductive cyclicity, pregnancy, and senescence. The repeated shaded regions indicate the four day rat estrous cycle, which is expanded in the central portion of the figure. The process of follicular atresia and maturation, ovulation, and luteinization are shown schematically at the top of the figure.

Literature Cited

1. Bandivdekar, A. H., Vijayalakshmi, S., Jaswaney, V. L., Sheth, A. R. 1981. Inhibin in human placenta. *Indian J. Exper. Biol.* 19:744–45
2. Bicsak, T. A., Cajender, S. B., Vale, W., Hseuh, A. J. W. 1988. Inhibin: studies of stored and secreted forms by biosynthetic labeling and immunodetection in cultured rat granulosa cells. *Endocrinology* 122:741–48
3. Bicsak, T., Tucker, E., Cappel, S., Vaughan, J., Rivier, J., et al. 1986. Hormonal regulation of granulosa cell inhibin biosynthesis. *Endocrinology* 119:2711–19
4. Bronxmeyer, H., Lu, L., Cooper, S., Schwall, R., Mason, A., Nikolics, K. 1988. Selective and indirect modulation of human multipotential and erythroid hematopoietic progenitor cell proliferation by recombinant human activin and inhibin. *Proc. Natl. Acad. Sci. USA* 85:9052–6
5. Burger, H., Igarashi, M. 1988. Inhibin: Definition and nomenclature, including related substances. *Endocrinology* 122:1701–2
6. Butcher, H. 1977. Changes in gonadotropins and steroids associated with unilateral ovariectomy of the rat. *Endocrinology* 101:830–40
7. Butcher, R., Page, R. 1981. Role of the aging ovary in cessation of reproduction. In *Dynamics of ovarian function*, ed. N. Schwartz, M. Hunzicker-Dunn. pp. 253–71. New York: Raven
8. Campen, C. A., Vale, W. 1988. Interaction between purified ovine inhibin and steroids on the release of gonadotropins from cultured rat pituitary cells. *Endocrinology* 123:1320–28
9. Cate, R., Mattaliano, R. J., Hession, C., Tizard, R., Farber, N. M., et al. 1986. Isolation of the bovine and human genes for muellerian inhibiting substance and expression of the human gene in animal cells. *Cell* 45:685–98
10. Crawford, R. J., Hammond, V. E., Evans, B. A., Coghan, J. P., Haralambidis, J., et al. 1987. α-Inhibin gene expression occurs in the ovine adrenal cortex, and is regulated by adrenocorticotropin. *Mol. Endocrinol.* 1:699–706
11. D'Agostino, J., Woodruff, T., Mayo, K., Schwartz, N. 1989. Unilateral ovariectomy increases inhibin mRNA levels in newly recruited follicles. *Endocrinology* 124:310–17
12. Davis, S. R., Dench, F., Nikolaidis, I., Clements, J. A., Forage, R. G., et al.

1986. Inhibin A-subunit gene expression in the ovaries of immature female rats is stimulated by pregnant mares serum gonadotrophin. *Biochem. Biophy. Res. Comm.* 138:1191–95
13. De Jong, F. 1988. Inhibin. *Physiol. Rev.* 68:555–607
14. De Jong, F. H., Sharpe, R. M. 1976. Evidence for inhibin-like activity in bovine follicular fluid. *Nature* 263:71–72
15. de Kretser, D., Robertson, D., Risbridger, G., Hedger, M., McLachlan, R., et al. 1988. Inhibin and related peptides. In *Progress in Endocrinology*, ed. H. Imura, K. Shizume, S. Yoshida, 1:13–23. Amsterdam: Excerpta Med.
16. DePaolo, L. 1987. Age associated increases in serum follicle-stimulating hormone levels on estrus are accompanied by a reduction in the ovarian secretion of inhibin. *Exper. Aging Res.* 13:3–7
17. DePaolo, L., Anderson, L., Hirshfield, A. 1981. Possible existence of a long-loop feedback system between FSH and inhibin in female rats. *Am. J. Physiol.* 240:E544–49
18. DePaolo, L., Chappel, S. 1986. Alterations in the secretion and production of follicle-stimulating hormone precede age-related lengthening of estrous cycles in the rat. *Endocrinology* 118:1127–33
19. DePaolo, L., Shander, V. D., Wise, P. M., Barraclough, C. A., Channing, C. P. 1979. Identification of inhibin-like activity in ovarian venous plasma of rats during the estrous cycle. *Endocrinology* 105:647–54
20. Dorrington, J., Armstrong, D. 1979. Effects of FSH on gonadal functions. *Recent Prog. Horm. Res.* 35:301–42
21. Erikson, G., Hsueh, A. 1978. Secretion of "inhibin" by rat granulosa cells in vitro. *Endocrinology* 103:1960–63
22. Esch, F., Shimasaki, S., Cooksey, D., Mercado, M., Mason, A., et al. 1987. Complementary deoxyribonucleic acid (cDNA) cloning and DNA sequence analysis of rat ovarian inhibins. *Molec. Endocrinol.* 1:388–96
23. Eto, Y., Tsuji, T., Takazawa, M., Takamo, S., Yokogawa, Y., Shibai, J. 1987. Purification and characterization of erythroid differentiation factor (EDF) isolated from human leukemia cell line THP1. *Biochem. Biophys. Res. Comm.* 142:1095–1103
24. Farnworth, P., Robertson, D., de Kretser, D., Burger, H. 1988. Effects of 31 kilodalton bovine inhibin on follicle-

stimulating hormone and luteinizing hormone in rat pituitary cells in vitro: actions under basal conditions. *Endocrinology* 122:207–13

24a. Feng, Z.-M., Bardin, W. C., Chen, C.-L. C. 1989. Characterization and regulation of testicular inhibin β-subunit mRNA. *Mol. Endocrinol.* 3:939–48

25. Finch, C., Felicio, L., Mobbs, C., Nelson, J. 1984. Ovarian and steroidal influences on neuroendocrine aging processes in female rodents. *Endocr. Rev.* 5:467–97

26. Forage, R. G., Ring, J. M., Brown, R. W., McInerney, B. V., Cobon, G. S., et al. 1986. Cloning and sequence analysis of cDNA species coding for the two subunits of inhibin from bovine follicular fluid. *Proc. Natl. Acad. Sci. USA* 83:3091–95

27. Greenwald, G. 1966. Ovarian follicular development and pituitary FSH and LH content in the pregnant rat. *Endocrinology* 79:572–578

28. Hasegawa, Y., Miyamoto, K., Igarashi, M., Yanake, T., Sasaki, K., Iwamura, S. 1987. Changes in serum concentrations of inhibin during the estrous cycle of the rat, pig, and cow. In *Inhibin:Non-Steroidal Regulation of FSH Secretion,* ed. J. Burger, D. deKretser, J. Findlay, M. Igarashi. 42:119–33. New York: Raven

29. Hseuh, A. J. W., Adashi, E., Jones, P. B. C., Welsh, T. 1984. Hormonal regulation of differentiation of cultured ovarian granulosa cells. *Endocr. Rev.* 5:76–127

30. Hseuh, A. J. W., Dahl, K. D., Vaughan, J., Tucker, E., Rivier, J., et al. 1987. Heterodimers and homodimers of inhibin subunits have different paracrine action in the modulation of luteinizing hormone-stimulated androgen biosynthesis. *Proc. Natl. Acad. Sci. USA* 84:5082–86

31. Keinan, D., Madigan, M. B., Bardin, W., Chen, C.-L. C. 1989. Expression and regulation of testicular inhibin α-subunit gene *in vivo* and *in vitro. Molec. Endocrinol.* 3:29–35

32. Klinefelter, H. F., Reifenstein, E. C., Albright, F. 1942. Syndrome characterized by gynecomastia, aspermatogenesis without a-lydigism, and increased excretion of follicle-stimulating hormone. *J. Clin. Endocrinol.* 2:615–27

33. Lee, V., McMaster, J., Quigg, H., Leversha, L. 1982. Ovarian and circulating inhibin levels in immature female rats treated with gonadotropin and after castration. *Endocrinology* 111:1849–54

34. Lee, W., Mason, A. J., Schwall, R., Szonyi, E., Mather, J. 1989. Secretion of activin by interstitial cells in the testes. *Science* 243:396–98

35. Ling, N., Ueno, N., Ying, S.-Y. Esch, R., Shimasaki, S., et al. 1988. Inhibins and activins. In *Vitamins and Hormones,* ed. G. Aurbach, D. McCormick. pp. 1–46. San Diego: Academic

36. Ling, N., Ying, S.-Y. Ueno, N., Esch, F., Denoroy, L., Guillemin, R. 1985. Isolation and partial characterization of a Mr 32,000 protein with inhibin activity from porcine ovarian follicular fluid. *Proc. Natl. Acad. Sci. USA* 82:7217–21

37. Ling, N., Ying, S.-Y., Ueno, N., Shimasali, S., Esch, F., et al. 1986. Pituitary FSH is released by a heterodimer of the β subunits from the two forms of inhibin. *Nature* 321:779–82

38. Mason, A., Hayflick, J., Ling, J., Esch, F., Ueno, N., et al. 1985. Complimentary DNA sequences of ovarian follicular fluid inhibin show precursor structure and homolgy with transforming growth factor-β. *Nature* 318:659–63

39. Mason, A., Pitts, S., Nikolics, K., Szonyi, E., Wilcox, J., et al. 1986. The hypogonadal mouse: reproductive functions restored by gene therapy. *Science* 234:1372–78

40. Massague, J. 1987. The TGF-β family of growth and differentiation factors. *Cell* 49:437–38

41. Mayo, K., Cerelli, G., Spiess, J., Rivier, J., Rosenfeld, M., et al. 1986. Inhibin A-subunit cDNAs from porcine ovary and human placenta. *Proc. Natl. Acad. Sci. USA* 83:5849–53

42. McCullagh, D. R. 1932. Dual endocrine activity of the testes. *Science* 76:19–20

43. McLachlan, R., Healy, C., Robertson, D., Burger, H., de Kretser, D. 1986. The human placenta: a novel source of inhibin. *Biochem. Biophys. Res. Commun.* 140:485–90

44. Mercer, J. E., Clements, J. A., Funder, J. W., Clarke, I. J. 1987. Rapid and specific lowering of pituitary FSH β mRNA levels by inhibin. *Mol. Cell. Endocrinol.* 53:251–54

45. Merchenthaler, I., Culler, M. D., Petrusz, P., Negro-Villar, A. 1987. Immunocytochemical localization of inhibin in rat and human reproductive tissues. *Mol. Cell. Endocrinol.* 54:239–43

46. Meunier, H., Cajander, S., Roberts, V., Rivier, C., Sawchenko, P., et al. 1988. Rapid changes in the expression of inhibin α- β_A- and β_B-subunits in ovarian cell types during the rat estrous cycle. *Molec. Endocrinol.* 2:1352–63

47. Meunier, H., Rivier, C., Evans, R.,
Vale, W. 1988. Gonadal and ex-
tragonadal expression of inhibin α-, β_A,-
and β_B-subunits in various tissues predicts diverse functions. *Proc. Natl.
Acad. Sci. USA* 85:247–51
48. Miyake, A., Sakumoto, T., Aono, T.,
Kawamura, Y., Maeda, T., Kurachi, K.
1982. Changes in luteinizing hormone-
releasing hormone in human placenta
throughout pregnancy. *Obstet. Gynecol.*
60:444
49. Miyamoto, K., Hasegawa, Y., Fukuda,
M., Nomura, M., Igarashi, M., et al.
1985. Isolation of porcine follicular fluid
inhibin of about 32 kDA. *Biochem. Biophys. Res. Commun.* 129:396–403
50. Morris, P. L., Vale, W., Cappel, S.,
Bardin, W. 1988. Inhibin production by
primary sertoli cell-enriched cultures:
regulation by follicle-stimulating hormone, androgens, and epidermal growth
factor. *Endocrinology* 122:717–25
51. Murata, M., Eto, Y., Shibai, H., Sakai,
M., Muramatsu, M. 1988.
Erythrodifferentiation factor is encoded
by the same mRNA as that of the inhibin
β_A chain. *Proc. Natl. Acad. Sci. USA*
85:2434–38
52. Osman, P. 1985. Rate and course of
atresia during follicular development in
the adult cyclic rat. *J. Reprod. Fertil.*
73:261–70
53. Padgett, R., Johnston, D., Gelbart, W.
1987. A transcript from a drosophila pattern gene predicts a protein homologous
to the transforming growth factor β
family. *Nature* 325:81–84
54. Petraglia, F., Sawchenko, P., Lim, A.,
Rivier, J., Vale, W. 1987. Localization,
secretion, and action of inhibin in human
placenta. *Science* 237:187–89
55. Petraglia, F., Sawchenko, P., Rivier, J.,
Vale, W. 1987. Evidence for local
stimulation of ACTH secretion by
corticotropin-releasing factor in human
placenta. *Nature* 328:717–19
56. Richards, J. 1988. Maturation of ovarian
follicles: actions and interactions of
pituitary and ovarian hormones on follicular cell differentiation. *Physiol. Rev.*
60:51–89
57. Rivier, C., Rivier, J., Vale, W. 1986.
Inhibin-mediated feedback control of
follicle-stimulating hormone secretion in
the female rat. *Science* 234:205–8
57a. Rivier, C., Roberts, V., Vale, W.
1989. Possible role of luteinizing hormone and follicle stimulating hormone
in modulating inhibin secretion and expression during the estrous cycle of the
rat. *Endocrinology* 125:876–82
58. Rivier, J., Spiess, J., McClintock, R.,

Vaughan, J., Vale, W. 1985. Purification and partial characterization of inhibin from porcine follicular fluid.
Biochem. Biophys. Res. Comm. 133:
120–27
59. Rivier, C., Vale, W. 1987. Inhibin:
measurement and role in the immature
female rat. *Endocrinology* 120:1688–
90
59a. Rivier, C., Vale, W. 1989. Im-
munoneutralization of endogenous inhibin modifies hormone secretion and
ovulation rate in the rat. *Endocrinology*
125:152–57
60. Roberts, V., Meunier, H., Vaughan, J.,
Rivier, J., Rivier, C., et al. 1989. Production and regulation of inhibin subunits in pituitary gonadotropes. *Endocrinology* 124:552–54
61. Robertson, D. M., Foulds, L. M.,
Leversha, L., Morgan, F. J., Hearn, M.
T. W., et al. 1985. Isolation of inhibin
from bovine follicular fluid. *Biochem.
Biophys. Res. Comm.* 126:220–26
62. Robertson, D. M., Hayward, S., Irby,
D., Jacobsen, J., Clarke, L., et al. 1988.
Radioimmunoassay of rat serum inhibin:
changes after PMSG stimulation and
gonadectomy. *Mol. Cell. Endocrinol.*
58:1–8
63. Sander, H., Meijs-Roelofs, A., Kramer,
P., van Leeuwen, E. 1985. Inhibin-like
activity in ovarian homogenates of pre-
pubertal female rats and its physiological significance. *J. Endocrinol.* 107:
251–57
64. Sawchenko, P., Plotsky, P., Pfeiffer,
S., Cunningham, E., Vaughan, J., et al.
1988. Inhibin β in central neural pathways involved in the control of oxytocin
secretion. *Nature* 334:615–17
64a. Schwall, R., Schmelzer, C. H., Mat-
suyama, E., Mason, A. 1989. Multiple actions of recombinant activin-A *in
vivo*. *Endocrinology* 125:1420–23
65. Schwartz, N. 1982. Role of ovarian inhibin in regulating FSH secretion in the
female rat. In *Intraovarian Control
Mechanisms*, ed. C. Channing, S. Segal. pp. 15–36. New York: Plenum
66. Schwartz, N. B., Channing, C. P. 1977.
Evidence for ovarian "inhibin": suppression of the secondary rise in serum
follicle stimulating hormone levels in
proestrous rats by injection of porcine
follicular fluid. *Proc. Natl. Acad. Sci.
USA* 74:5721–24
67. Steinberger, A., Steinberger, E. 1976.
Secretion of an FSH-inhibiting factor by
cultured Sertoli cells. *Endocrinology*
99:918–21
68. Steinberger, A., Ward, D. N. 1988. Inhibin. In *The Physiology of Reproduc-*

tion, ed. E. Knobil, J. Neil et al. pp. 567–83. New York: Raven

69. Suzuki, S., Miyamoto, K., Hasegawa, Y., Abe, Y., Ave, Y., et al. 1987. Regulation of inhibin production by rat granulosa cells. *Mol. Cell. Endocrinol.* 54:185–95

70. Tanabe, K., Gagliano, P., Channing, C. P., Nakamura, Y., Yoshimura, Y., et al. 1983. Levels of inhibin-F activity and steroids in human follicular fluid from normal women and women with polycystic ovarian disease. *J. Clin. Endocrinol. Met.* 57:24–31

71. Taya, K., Kimura, J., Sasamoto, S. 1984. Inhibin activity in ovarian venous plasma during pregnancy, pseudopregnancy and lactation in the rat. *Endocrinol. Jpn.* 31:427–33

72. Tsonis, C., Hillier, S., Baird, D. 1987. Production of inhibin bioactivity by human granulosa-lutein cells: stimulation by LH and testosterone in vitro. *J. Endocrinol.* 112:R11–14

73. Tsonis, C. G., Sharpe, R. M. 1986. Dual gonadal control of follicle-stimulating hormone. *Nature* 321:724–25

74. Vale, W., Rivier, C., Hsueh, A., Campen, C., Meunier, H., et al. 1988. Chemical and biological characterization of the inhibin family of protein hormones. *Recent Prog. Horm. Res.* 44:1–34

75. Vale, W., Rivier, J., Vaughan, J., McClintock, R., Corrigan, A., et al. 1986. Purification and characterization of an FSH-releasing protein from porcine ovarian follicular fluid. *Nature* 321:776–79

76. Watkins, W., Yen, S. 1980. Somatostatin in cytotrophoblast of the immature human placenta: localization by immunoperoxidase cytochemistry. *J. Clin. Endocrinol. Metab.* 5:969–71

77. Weeks, D., Melton, D. 1987. A maternal mRNA localized to the vegetal hemisphere in xenopus eggs codes for a growth factor related to TGFβ. *Cell* 51:861–67

78. Welschen, R., Dullaart, J., deJong, F. 1978. Interrelationships between circulating levels of estradiol-17β, progesterone, FSH and LH immediately after unilateral ovariectomy in the cyclic rat. *Biol. Reprod.* 18:421–27

79. Woodruff, T., D'Agostino, J., Schwartz, N., Mayo, K. 1988. Dynamic changes in inhibin messenger RNAs in rat ovarian follicles during the reproductive cycle. *Science* 239:1296–99

80. Woodruff, T., D'Agostino, J., Schwartz, N., Mayo, K. 1989. Modulation of rat inhibin mRNAs in preovulatory and atretic follicles. In *Growth Factors and the Ovary*, ed. A. N. Hirshfield. pp. 291–95. New York: Plenum

81. Woodruff, T., D'Agostino, J., Schwartz, N., Mayo, K. 1989. Decreased inhibin gene expression in preovulatory follicles requires the primary gonadotropin surges. *Endocrinology* 124:2193–99

82. Woodruff, T., Meunier, H., Jones, P., Hsueh, A., Mayo, K. 1987. Rat inhibin: molecular cloning of α and β subunit complementary deoxyribonucleic acids and expression in the ovary. *Mol. Endocrinol.* 1:561–68

83. Wozney, J. M., Rosen, V., Celeste, A. J., Mitsock, L. M., Whitters, M. J., et al. 1988. Novel regulators of bone formation: molecular clones and activities. *Science* 242:1528–34

84. Ying, S.-Y. 1988. Inhibins, activins, and follistatins: gonadal proteins modulating the secretion of follicle-stimulating hormone. *Endocr. Rev.* 9:267–93

85. Ying, S.-Y., Becker, A., Baird, A., Ling, N., Ueno, N., et al. 1986. Type beta transforming growth factor (TGFβ) is a potent stimulator of the basal secretion of follicle-stimulating hormone (FSH) in a pituitary monolayer system. *Biochem. Biophys. Res. Comm.* 135:950–56

86. Ying, S.-Y., Czvik, J., Becher, A., Ling, N., Ueno, N., Guillemin, R. 1987. Secretion of follicle-stimulating hormone and production of inhibin are reciprocally related. *Proc. Natl. Acad. Sci. USA* 84:4631–35

87. Yu, J., Shao, L., Lemas, V., Yu, A., Vaughan, J., et al. 1987. Importance of FSH-releasing protein and inhibin in erythrodifferentiation. *Nature* 330:765–67

88. Zhiwen, Z., Carson, R., Herington, A., Findlay, J., Burger, H. 1987. Regulation of ovarian granulosa cell inhibin by epidermal and transforming growth factors in vitro. *J. Clin. Invest.* 10:36 (Suppl. 4)

89. Zhiwen, Z., Carson, R., Herington, A., Lee, V., Burger, H. 1987. Follicle-stimulating hormone and somatomedin-c stimulate inhibin production by rat granulosa cells in vitro. *Endocrinology* 120:1633–38

Annu. Rev. Physiol. 1990. 52:823–40

GENE REGULATION BY RECEPTORS BINDING LIPID-SOLUBLE SUBSTANCES

Cary Weinberger

Laboratory of Cell Biology, National Institute of Mental Health, Bethesda, Maryland 20892

David J. Bradley

Laboratory of Cell Biology, National Institute of Mental Health and Howard Hughes Medical Institute, Bethesda, Maryland 20892

KEY WORDS: steroid hormones, transcriptional regulation, glucocorticoid receptor, signal transduction, receptor evolution

INTRODUCTION

The model for estrogen action proposed by Jensen & Gorski more than twenty years ago has served as a unifying theory to explain regulation of gene expression by many steroid hormones (34, 48). Each hormone triggers an allosteric change in a specific receptor protein converting it from a low affinity DNA-binding state to one with relatively higher affinity for DNA elements in the vicinities of target genes. This tighter DNA binding interaction is thought to catalyze the assembly of transcriptional complexes at nearby sites and activate target cell gene expression (111). Despite extensive characterization of the receptor proteins and their target DNA sequences, our knowledge of how the activated receptor initiates transcription from hormone-responsive genes is still incomplete (for other reviews see 5, 14, 24).

Recent identification of several steroid hormone receptor genes has helped to uncover a large family of nuclear receptor or ligand-dependent transcription

823

0066-4278/90/0315-0823$02.00

factors (24). Substantial structural homology among steroid receptors has facilitated the isolation of related receptors activated by many different classes of fat-soluble substances including thyroid hormones and retinoids. The common structural thread linking these hormones is that most are simple, terpenoid-like, non-saponifiable lipids. One of the significant questions arising from the identification of multiple receptors binding this extraordinarily diverse array of chemical signals is how a lipid-based system for coordinating physiologic responses evolved in eukaryotes. In this review we will discuss the structural and functional relationships of some of these lipophilic ligand-dependent nuclear receptors, their presumptive evolution from a primordial receptor gene, and how their continued study may help elucidate novel hormone systems.

MORPHOGENETIC AND HOMEOSTATIC LIPOPHILIC LIGANDS

Animal growth and development are primarily coordinated by regulating gene transcription (20). In general, the DNA complement in every cell is identical and must be selectively activated to generate the cell specialization found in different organs. During early animal development, cell lineages dictate the differentiation patterns of embryonic cells (97). Cell fates are determined by the temporal expression of transcriptional factors such as *Drosophila* homeotic gene products, which regulate the synthesis of proteins specifying cell identity (46). Overlapping this transcriptional control network, circulating lipophilic chemical signals in the animal modulate gene expression programs by their exclusive interactions with target cell intracellular receptors. Shifting hormone concentrations may result in dramatic developmental or cellular metabolic changes. Thus a plastic system precisely regulates the synthesis of proteins involved in cellular metabolism and differentiation.

Many of these hormones and vitamins relate information about the external milieu including changing temperatures and nutrient availability while others help to initiate specific developmental programs. Although most are secreted from various endocrine glands, many such as the fat-soluble vitamins A and D are taken up by the animal along with foodstuffs and may serve to induce enzymes required to metabolize these plant nutrients.

In contrast to cell surface receptors that bind hydrophilic molecules like epinephrine (10, 61), ligand-dependent transcription factors are activated by small (around 500 daltons) lipophilic compounds including steroid hormones, vitamin A and D, and thyroid hormones. Members of this particular class of transcription factors are often referred to as nuclear receptors because the active hormone-receptor complex is found in the nucleus (34, 48). Insect hormones, such as ecdysteroids that trigger molting, are also thought to bind and activate receptors in this (i.e. nuclear receptor) family (4). Their induction of chromosomal puffs in *Drosophila* salivary glands provided some of the first evidence that hormones specifically regulated RNA transcription (17). Inhibitors of RNA and protein synthesis clearly demonstrated that steroid hormones affect gene expression at the level of primary transcription (85).

These chemical signals perform specific physiologic tasks at different stages of development. In addition, the same molecule may play decidedly distinct roles in different species. For example, thyroid hormones are required for metamorphosis in amphibians and mediate thermoregulation in vertebrates (75, 90). Disparate functions for retinoids, in vision and limb bud development, also mark the multiple roles played by many of these compounds (88).

Besides their important roles in development, changes in concentrations of lipophilic ligands maintain homeostasis by initiating new protein synthesis (111). Differential affinities of the glucocorticoid and mineralocorticoid receptors for glucocorticoids establish a dynamic sensitivity range for reacting to variable steroid levels (2, 27). Through precise regulation of gene expression, glucocorticoids and other lipophilic ligands communicate information about environmental situations to target cells containing their receptor proteins.

A RECEPTOR FAMILY BINDING LIPID-SOLUBLE HORMONES AND VITAMINS

A significant hurdle to elucidating the mechanism of receptor-mediated transcriptional activation was the purification of sufficient quantities of receptor protein typically found at levels <5000 binding sites per cell. Radiolabeled steroid hormones were invaluable reagents in this context (53, 96, 109). Once purified, discrete receptor functions were identified (9, 94). Studies of mouse T-lymphocyte mutants resistant to glucocorticoid's cytolytic effects uncovered receptors defective in two functional properties—DNA and hormone binding (110, 112). Hormone-receptor complexes regulate target gene expression by binding to short *cis*-acting DNA sequences called hormone-responsive elements (HREs) in the vicinities of target genes (15). Like enhancer elements, HREs function in a position- and orientation-independent fashion, even when placed thousands of base pairs from the start of primary RNA synthesis (54).

Identification of Receptor Genes

Genes encoding the glucocorticoid (GR), estrogen (ER), progesterone (PR), and vitamin D receptors were identified using specific antibodies generated with purified receptor preparations (18, 37, 68, 71, 104) from cDNA expression libraries. We will focus our discussion on the GR although similar conclusions were reached with other receptors. Mapping of the glucocorticoid receptor domains on the primary amino acid sequence determined from cDNA clones was aided by several observations. (see Figure 1 for general nuclear receptor structural configuration).

First, partial proteolytic mapping of purified rat glucocorticoid receptor established its division into discrete binding domains for hormone and DNA (9, 94). Antibodies recognizing another region delimited an immunogenic domain. The boundaries of this domain were established in the GR amino terminus by identification of overlapping cDNA clones from an expression library (104). Secondly, two forms of the human GR were identified encoding proteins of 777 and 742 amino acids that, when expressed from the cDNAs in vitro, either bound or failed to bind glucocorticoids, respectively (43). Since the molecular differences were found at their extreme carboxyl termini, a

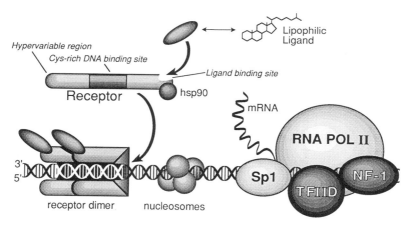

Figure 1 Model for gene regulation by lipid-soluble hormone-activated receptor proteins. The variety of lipids activating gene expression are represented by a terpenoid-like molecule with a cholesterol carbon skeleton here symbolized as an ovoid. Untransformed receptor is depicted as an elongated cylinder with a band of cysteine residues in the central portion forming the cysteine-rich DNA binding site (DBS) and a ligand binding site (LBS) found in the carboxyl terminus, while the activated, hormone-bound form assumes a more folded U-shape. All nuclear receptors maintain the same relative positions for the DBS and LBS when receptor amino acid comparisons are made. A hypervariable amino terminus of varying residue length is also indicated.

Hormonal induction of gene expression is initiated by ligand binding which may release receptor from interactions with proteins such as hsp90. Simultaneously, the receptor undergoes a conformational change inducing its dimerization, whereby it becomes more tightly bound to hormone response elements (white helix) that catalyze transcriptional complex assembly consisting of such factors as TATA box-binding factor (TFIID), CCAAT-binding factor (NF-1) and Sp1, along with RNA polymerase II. Activated receptor may also influence the phasing of nucleosomes to ultimately potentiate transcriptional initiation.

hormone binding domain was localized here. Last, amino acid comparisons of the human GR and the *Xenopus* transcription factor IIIA revealed surprising structural homology in repeated cysteine-rich fingers tandemly arranged in each of the polypeptides (72). Duplicated cysteine-rich fingers uncovered in all steroid receptor genes were proposed to coordinate zinc atoms, and they were thought to be essential for DNA binding (72, 105). This zinc finger motif is common to many other transcription factors including yeast GAL4, ADR1, adenovirus E1A, and the *trans*-acting factor Sp1 (7, 25, 50).

Receptor Homologies

Comparison of glucocorticoid and estrogen receptor sequences with other proteins revealed their relationship to the v-erb-A oncogene product of the avian erythroblastosis virus (37, 105). Approximately 40% amino acid identity was found in the cysteine-rich zinc finger region while only 17% similarity was seen in the carboxyl termini. This finding prompted the isolation of two cellular erb-A cDNAs, which were found to encode thyroid hormone receptors (91, 106). An extended family of ligand-dependent transcription factors derived from a primordial gene was strongly suggested by identification of receptors binding molecules as distinct as thyroid hormone and cortisol.

Radiolabeled DNA sequences (DNA fragments or consensus oligonucleotide probes) from the conserved putative DNA binding domains of nuclear receptor cDNAs were used to identify, under conditions of lowered hybridization stringency, cDNAs encoding mineralocorticoid and androgen receptors (3, 16, 62). A host of other putative receptor cDNAs have recently been isolated by these non-stringent hybridization methods. They are called orphan receptors because their corresponding ligands have, as yet, not been identified. The growing list of orphan receptors includes human estrogen receptor-related and human erb-A-related receptors (30, 73). One of these erb-A related proteins, ear-3, is the human correlate of COUP factor, which was biochemically purified by its ability to activate the chicken ovalbumin gene (101a). The existence of orphan receptors implies that many lipophilic substances, not previously recognized as hormones, may regulate gene expression via nuclear receptors.

NUCLEAR RECEPTOR MODULAR DOMAINS

Receptor Mutagenesis

Functional properties of steroid receptors have been examined by cotransfecting receptor-deficient eukaryotic cells in culture with two plasmid DNAs, one encoding a nuclear receptor and the other containing the corresponding hormone-response element linked to a heterologous reporter gene such as chloramphenicol acetyltransferase whose product is easily assayed (28, 35,

89). In this cotransfection system, exogenous hormone addition to cells activates the receptor, which then stimulates expression of the reporter gene. Using this assay, the effects of amino acid insertions and deletions on receptor function were then determined and compared with the domain assignments based on the predicted GR amino acid sequence and proteolytic mapping studies (9, 28, 60, 89, 105).

Mutations in the cysteine-rich region abolished transcriptional activation but left hormone binding intact, whereas small mutations in the carboxyl terminus abolished hormone binding and *trans*-activation. Larger deletions in the carboxyl terminus produced mutant receptors capable of activating gene expression regardless of whether hormone was present or not (33, 42, 70). These constitutively-active receptors implied that the carboxyl terminus masked the DNA binding region until hormone interaction changed the receptor conformation and exposed the cysteine-rich domain.

The amino termini or hypervariable regions of nuclear receptors are the least conserved regions and may exert gene selectivity properties (24). Mutations in the GR amino terminus produce molecules binding DNA and hormone normally, but with markedly suppressed transcriptional-activating functions (28). Furthermore, two forms of the progesterone receptor that differ in their amino termini are thought to differentially activate gene expression (99). These two receptors differ by length variations at the amino terminus, presumably directed by alternative initiation codon usage. Comparable variations in subtypes of the thyroid hormone and retinoic acid receptors may produce differences in their target gene specificity (8, 40, 98).

These mutational studies have predicted that receptor DNA and hormone binding domains might function independently of one another. GR or progesterone receptor polypeptide fragments comprising the cysteine-rich regions expressed in bacteria are sufficient for DNA binding activity (23, 30). Two zinc atoms are specifically required, presumably to coordinate four cysteine residues per finger region (26). Hormone binding activity may also be reconstituted in bacteria as carboxy-terminal receptor regions downstream of the conserved glycine-methionine in the DNA binding domain.

Functional Domains as Cassettes

Exchanging and scrambling various receptor domains has demonstrated the modular nature of nuclear receptors. Replacement of the entire hGR DNA binding domain with the corresponding hER region produced a chimeric receptor capable of activating transcription from a glucocorticoid response element (GRE) in response to estradiol (35). This method, called finger swapping, has been used to identify the ligands for orphan receptors. For example, the retinoic acid receptor was recognized by substituting the DNA binding domain of an orphan receptor with the corresponding GR domain. The resulting hybrid receptor effectively activated transcription from a GRE only in the presence of retinoids (29, 80). These results, as well as those of the constitutively-active receptors, support the model that hormone binding exposes the linked DNA binding region as a prerequisite for the assembly of the transcriptional initiation complex.

Swapping the ER and GR DNA-binding domains with DNA-binding regions from the yeast transcription factor, GAL4, or the prokaryotic transcriptional regulator, LEXA, converted the target gene specificity of the chimeric receptors (32, 41, 102). Combining zinc fingers from two different receptors indicates that the first finger directs the receptor specificity for a given hormone response element and therefore helps establish target gene discrimination (36). Remarkably, site-directed mutagenesis converting three amino acids just downstream of the first finger in the ER to the corresponding GR residues is sufficient to activate a glucocorticoid response element (64).

Modularity of nuclear receptors is underlined by experiments rearranging the GR carboxyl terminus to upstream receptor regions as well as fusing this domain to heterologous proteins such as the adenovirus transcriptional activator E1A (41, 81). Both configurations of scrambled proteins are hormone-responsive and their functions are repressed without regard to the structural organization of the fusion polypeptide. This reveals the positional flexibility of receptor functional domains, but also contradicts the contention that the hormone binding region simply unmasks the DNA binding domain upon hormone binding.

Analysis of other GR mutants indicates that the amino terminus codes for an acidic amino acid-containing polypeptide domain (τ1) that significantly enhances transcription (28, 33). It can be transferred to other nuclear receptors endowing them with greater transcriptional activity (98). If τ1 is tandemly added to a given receptor in more than one copy, the transcriptional response is even greater (41). Another acidic region of the hGR (τ2) between amino acids 526 and 555, in the so-called hinge region between the DNA and hormone binding domains, also activates transcription (41). The complete range of amino acid domains that will mimic this action has not been established, but a synthetic amphipathic α-helix derived from studies with the yeast activator protein GAL4 also enhances transcriptional activity (63). One tentative conclusion is that these nonconserved, negatively charged residues may be required for induction by interactions with a repeated sequence in RNA polymerase II (95).

TRANSCRIPTIONAL ACTIVATION

Receptor Dimerization and Allosteric Changes

One of the most challenging problems in lipid-activated transcriptional regulation is understanding the dynamic receptor structural changes accompanying hormone binding (6, 21, 39, 103, 108). Following hormone binding, receptors bind to their respective response elements as dimers (Figure 1). Receptor dimerization is critical for tight binding to corresponding hormone responsive elements, and deletion of the hormone binding domain reduces receptor affinity for HREs (59, 100). Translocation of activated receptor from the cytoplasm into the nucleus may be more suggestive of its increased affinity for target DNA sequences, because a variety of receptor antibodies show the hormone-naive receptor to be localized in the nucleus by immunohistochemistry (55, 107). In addition, studies with progesterone receptor indicate that hormone binding shifts the kinetics of the receptor/DNA association reaction (92).

A short amino acid sequence in the GR just downstream of the finger regions and another in the hormone binding domain are partly responsible for activated receptor migration into the nucleus (82). Interactions with other proteins have also been postulated to inhibit receptor from binding its target DNA elements (Figure 1). The abundant cytosolic heat shock protein hsp90 binds many different receptor proteins and, in particular, the GR carboxy-terminal hormone binding domain (49, 86).

Similarly, RU486, a potent antiglucocorticoid, induces GR translocation but this complex fails to *trans*-activate (38). Comparisons of GR sedimentation values in the presence of agonists or RU486 show that the antihormone stabilizes the 8S (pre-hormone binding) receptor form and prevents transformation to the 4S species. The estrogen antagonist hydroxytamoxifen and the agonist diethylstilbestrol also induce stable complex formation of ER with its DNA element (59). This binding complex is slightly altered in gel mobility when compared with that formed using estradiol, which indicates that these synthetic hormones may have trapped the receptor in an intermediate stage of conformation similar to the GR mutant that binds DNA but does not *trans*-activate (41, 59). Experiments with antiestrogens and ER-specific antibodies also provide evidence for a conformational change following hormone binding (67).

Uncoupling DNA-Binding and Transcriptional Activation

Boundaries for the DNA binding and transcriptional activating domains of nuclear receptors have been more difficult to segregate compared to those of other transcription factors such as Sp1 (50). Although most receptor DNA binding mutants cannot be uncoupled from transcription, one hGR mutant in the cysteine-rich region that converts a lysine to a glycine is capable of binding DNA, but not activating transcription (41). Another deletion mutant, removing most of the carboxy-terminal hormone binding region, also binds DNA but does not *trans*-activate (33, 89). Ostensibly, the mutations may have fixed the receptors in functionally intermediate stages that may be similar to that conformation induced by tamoxifen and diethylstilbestrol (59).

One particularly interesting GR mutant, nt^i (nuclear transfer increase), derived from mouse lymphoma cells that are normally killed by nanomolar concentrations of dexamethasone, possesses a higher affinity for DNA compared with the wild-type receptor (110). This receptor variant lacks the entire GR amino terminus and does not function in the dexamethasone-mediated lymphocytolysis assay. Its inactivity is mysterious in view of the graded transcriptional response in the cotransfection assay directed by in vitro mutagenized, amino-terminally deleted receptors (28), but may relate to the nonphysiologic levels of receptors and HREs expressed in transiently transfected cells overwhelming the transcriptional apparatus.

Hormone Response Elements and Chromatin

Identification of the binding and transcriptional-inducing DNA elements from various regions of hormone-responsive genes has permitted the identification of DNA sequence requirements necessary for characteristic receptor function. A DNA sequence within the mouse mammary tumor virus long terminal repeat confers hormone inducibility on physically linked heterologous genes (15). Other HREs have been characterized including those for thyroid hormones and estrogen (31, 56). Many of these response elements, such as that for the tyrosine aminotransferase (TAT) gene, are located several thousand base pairs away from the start of transcriptional initiation (47).

As described above, each nuclear receptor binds discrete DNA elements in vicinities of responsive genes. Characterization of many other glucocorticoid-inducible genes, for instance, has permitted the resolution of a consensus sequence, 5'-TGTTCT-3', through which glucocorticoid, progesterone, androgen, and mineralocorticoid receptors bind and activate gene expression (12, 13, 77). In addition, both the thyroid hormone and retinoic acid receptors can activate a thyroid hormone DNA response element (101). Although overlapping regulation by each may be demonstrated in cell culture, the physiologic significance of these interactions in vivo are questionable in view of the numerous nonproductive receptor binding sites (57).

In addition to the nuclear receptors, faithful control of RNA synthesis requires many polypeptide factors interacting with discrete DNA elements found upstream of initiation sites (Figure 1). In vivo footprinting experiments indicate that the GR is catalytically required to recruit *trans*-acting factors such as NF-1 and TATA box-binding (TFIID) proteins to their respective DNA sites following hormone administration (19). It is also thought that the activated receptor induces a phasing of nucleosomes near hormone-responsive gene elements (79, 87, 113). Correlation of DNAase I hypersensitive sites with this nucleoprotein reorganization may imply a receptor-induced torsional unwinding, ultimately affecting the binding capacities of other transcriptional factors near target genes. The ability to express a functional estrogen receptor and nearly full-length GR molecules in yeast suggests that the components involved in transcriptional initiation are probably conserved evolutionarily (69, 93).

Receptor-Mediated Repression

The functional duality of nuclear receptors (activation or inhibition of gene transcription) is shown by glucocorticoid-mediated repression of transcription from the proopiomelanocortin gene (22). Upstream DNA elements conferring dexamethasone-mediated repression have been identified in this gene and for another repression element in the α-subunit gene for human chorionic gonadotropin (1). Human GR mutants were analyzed for their abilities to repress α gene transcription (76). The amino terminal domain is not required for *trans*-repression—deletion of $\tau 1$ generated a more potent repressor, which demonstrated a reciprocal role for this region when compared with activation. In addition, the lysine-to-glycine substitution mutant that uncoupled DNA binding and positive *trans*-activation (41) retained normal repressor function. Preservation of the DNA binding domain was essential for the maintenance of repression functions (76). When the GR hormone binding region was either deleted or substituted by β-galactosidase coding information, repression function was not affected (76). Repression may also be explained by competition of the activated receptor with other transcriptional factors for specific binding sites like the CCAAT box (1, 76). An analogous situation may exist for a variant thyroid hormone receptor containing an altered carboxyl terminus that does not bind hormone—it inhibits transcription of thyroid hormone-responsive genes in cell culture when expressed with normal receptor forms in the presence of thyroid hormone (58).

RECEPTOR EVOLUTION

Evolution of the lipid-activated nuclear receptor genes from an ancestral gene can be postulated on the basis of the sequence conservation in various domains, particularly the DNA binding region (24). Presently, the nuclear receptor gene family can be classified into two subfamilies based on sequence homology: (*a*) the adrenocorticosteroid receptors, including those binding glucocorticoids, mineralocorticoids, progestins, and androgens and (*b*) erb-A related genes including thyroid hormone, retinoic acid, and vitamin D receptors. The distinction is based on the observation that the hormone binding regions for the members of the adrenocorticosteroid receptor family are more closely related than those for the erb-A related receptors. Additionally, since the adrenocorticosteroid receptors activate a GRE, whereas the retinoic acid and thyroid hormone receptors recognize a consensus thyroid hormone response element (31, 101), this criterion supports the branched division of the nuclear receptor family.

Receptor zinc finger domains are each encoded by distinct exons for the mineralocorticoid, progesterone, estrogen, and vitamin D receptors (3, 44, 45, 84). This finding supports a model whereby these sequences had duplicated and transposed to different chromosomal regions whereupon promoter elements and regulated hormone binding domains were linked in single transcription units. Distinctive hypervariable regions for each receptor may signify that transposition of DNA binding regions near promoter elements represented one of the first events required to assemble proteins with generalized DNA binding functions. Subsequent recruitment of other repressor elements (hormone binding domains) would have converted these DNA binding proteins into hormonally regulated transcription factors.

Discovery of linked thyroid hormone and retinoic acid receptor genes at two different genomic sites indicates that gene duplication and later chromosomal rearrangements may have played important roles in the evolution of these receptors (8). Notably, variant thyroid hormone and glucocorticoid receptors containing altered carboxy-terminal and amino-terminal regions generated by alternative splicing of a primary transcript may represent evolutionary forces currently at work (43, 58).

Evolutionary Determinants

In higher metazoans, increased tissue specialization demands sophisticated signaling networks. An assortment of chemical signals underly the physiologic and behavioral plasticities required to meet these challenges. Elevated basal metabolic rates by thyroid hormone during periods of reduced ambient temperature marks one instance where sensory transduction and hormonal regulatory mechanisms may have played critical means for animal survival.

During the course of animal development, variable environmental situations may have led to searches for new food types. Over long periods, animal foraging of particular plant species may have dictated the elevated synthesis of new proteins to aid metabolism of the nutrients found in these flora. Compounds like xanthophylls, carotenes, phytols, or tocols present in different plants could have served as subtle signals to augment the production of enzymes to meet this metabolic requirement. The competitive success of animal species fostered by the inheritance of these newly generated transcriptional factors would have guaranteed their transmission in the germline.

Other compounds, besides steroid and thyroid hormones, may interact with specific nuclear receptors. Tetrachlorodibenzodioxin or dioxin, a potent tumor promoter representing a class of compounds that includes carcinogens and drugs, activates a single presumptive nuclear receptor protein to stimulate transcription of P450 genes that are responsible for drug detoxification (83). Biochemical characterization of the dioxin receptor suggests that it is related to this class of lipid-activated transcriptional factors. Isolation of its gene may expedite the identification of an endogenous hormone serving to activate the dioxin receptor.

Other Potential Fat-Soluble Hormones

The diversity of substances interacting with members of the nuclear receptor family coupled with the rapidly expanding list of orphan receptors contributes to the ongoing search for their candidate ligands. Chemical composition is doubtlessly the most important criterion to assess whether a particular compound activates a nuclear receptor-like molecule. In general, compounds that have been shown to trigger these receptors are low molecular weight (<500 daltons), neutral lipophilic fats circulating in the animal at nanomolar concentrations. Reports by groups studying vitamin E action have noted its concentration in the cell nucleus following administration of its labeled derivative to rats, and even its binding to intracellular proteins (78). The lipophilic chemical structure of vitamin E and its regulation of xanthine oxidase suggest that tocopherols also bind specific nuclear receptors (11). Likewise, vitamin K may analogously activate a specific nuclear receptor by its structural similarity to vitamin E.

Oxygenated sterols have been documented to inhibit transcription of multiple enzymes and proteins involved in cholesterol biosynthesis (51). These cholesterol derivatives bind to cytosolic proteins with hierarchies of affinities that match their abilities to repress 5-hydroxymethyl-3-glutaryl CoA reductase activity, a typically regulated gene product (52). Because of their chemical similarity to steroid hormones, oxygenated sterols may bind to nuclear receptor-like molecules to regulate networks of genes participating in cholesterol metabolism.

Lower eukaryotes must also adjust biochemical pathways to meet variable growth conditions. DIF-1, a lipid-soluble compound, is required to turn on specific gene expression programs for stalk cell differentiation during fruiting body formation in *Dictyostelium discoideum* (74). Chemical analysis of this morphogenetic signal indicates its terpenoid relationship to the family of lipophilic ligands activating nuclear receptors, although no cellular binding components have yet been identified.

Other compounds operating by similar mechanisms could include plant hormones such as abscisic acid and gibberellins. Abscisic acid activates genes in a time-dependent fashion that is marked by the accumulation of specific RNA transcripts (66). The brassinosteroids, or plant hormones that are related to ecdysone, also regulate many cellular growth properties (65). They are physiologically active at nanomolar concentrations and their biological effects are inhibited by actinomycin D and cycloheximide just as are steroid hormones. Therefore, receptors for these substances may be identified by lowered stringency hybridization methods using consensus DNA probes from the conserved DNA binding region of various receptor genes.

FUTURE CHALLENGES

In order to learn more about the transcriptional activation event catalyzed by nuclear receptors, an important goal would be to reconstitute hormone-responsive in vitro transcription systems. These will help to define the hormone-induced receptor allosteric change as well as the other components in the transcriptional initiation complex, which includes RNA polymerase II, other transcription factors, and new hormonally responsive genes in nucleo-protein complexes. Purified receptors will also be invaluable for X-ray crystallographic studies to describe the precise three-dimensional configuration of amino acids in their DNA and hormone binding sites.

Perhaps the greatest challenge in nuclear receptor biology is the identification of ligands for the growing number of orphan receptors. The likely choices for potential binding substances need only be governed by the criteria that they are small and lipid-soluble. Among the candidate ligands that may bind nuclear receptor-like molecules are dioxin, tocopherol, 25-hydroxy-cholesterol, ecdysteroids, gibberellins, and possibly prostaglandins. Chimeric receptors could be constructed containing the GR DNA-binding region linked to the orphan receptor ligand binding domain and activated with batteries of lipophilic chemicals as accomplished for the retinoic acid receptor.

The assortment of lipids known to activate transcriptional proteins such as steroid hormone receptors has stimulated a great deal of excitement in the fields of endocrinology and human genetics. Hope for the future includes the prospect of identifying many novel lipid-soluble compounds regulating cellular biochemical pathways. Undoubtedly, their discovery will reveal new areas of physiologic control that will be of enormous pharmacological and therapeutic importance.

Literature Cited

1. Akerbloom, I. E. Slater, E. S., Beato, M., Baxter, J. D., Mellon, P. L. 1988. Negative regulation by glucocorticoids through interference with a cAMP-responsive enhancer. *Science* 241:350–53

2. Arriza, J. L., Simerly, R. B., Swanson, L. W., Evans, R. M. 1988. The neuronal mineralocorticoid receptor as a mediator of glucocorticoid response. *Neuron* 1:887–900

3. Arriza, J. L., Weinberger, C., Cerelli, G., Glaser, T. M., Handelin, B. L., 1987. Cloning of human mineralocorticoid receptor complementary DNA: structural and functional kinship with the glucocorticoid receptor. *Science* 237:268–75

4. Ashburner, M. 1980. Chromosomal action of ecdysone. *Nature* 285:435–36

5. Beato, M. 1989. Gene regulation by steroid hormones. *Cell* 56:335–44

6. Becker, P. B., Gloss, B., Schmid, W., Strahle, U., Schutz, G. 1986. In vivo protein-DNA interaction in a glucocorticoid response element require the presence of the hormone. *Nature* 324:686–88

7. Berg, J. M. 1986. Potential metal-binding domains in nucleic acid binding proteins. *Science* 232:485–87

8. Brand, N., Petkovich, M., Krust, A., Chambon, P., de The, H., et al. 1988. Identification of a second human retinoic acid receptor. *Nature* 332:850–53

9. Carlstedt-Duke, J., Okret, S., Wrange,

O., Gustafsson, J.-A. 1982. Immunochemical analysis of the glucocorticoid receptor: Identification of a third domain separate from the steroid-binding and DNA-binding domains. *Proc. Natl. Acad. Sci. USA* 79:4260–64

10. Carpenter, G. 1987. Receptors for epidermal growth factor and other polypeptide mitogens. *Annu. Rev. Biochem.* 56:881–914

11. Catignani, G. L., Chytil, F., Darby, W. J. 1974. Vitamin E deficiency: immunochemical evidence for increased accumulation of liver xanthine oxidase. *Proc. Natl. Acad. Sci. USA* 71:1966–68

12. Cato, A. C. B., Henderson, D., Ponta, H. 1987. The hormone response element of the mouse mammary tumor virus DNA mediates the progestin and androgen induction of transcription in the proviral long terminal repeat region. *EMBO J.* 6:363–68

13. Chalepakis, G., Arnemann, J., Slater, E., Bruller, H.-J., Gross, B., Beato, M. 1988. Differential gene activation by glucocorticoids and progestins through the hormone regulatory element of mouse mammary tumor virus. *Cell* 53:371–82

14. Chambon, P., Dierich, A., Gaub, M. P., Jakowiev, S., Jonstra, J., et al. 1984. Promoter elements of genes coding for proteins and modulation of transcription by oestrogens and progesterone. In *Recent Progress in Hormone Research,* ed. R. O. Greep. 40:1–42. New York: Academic

15. Chandler, V. L., Maler, B. A., Yamamoto, K. R. 1983. DNA sequences bound specifically by glucocorticoid receptor in vitro render a heterologous promoter hormone responsive in vivo. *Cell* 33:489–99

16. Chang, C., Kokontis, J., Liao, S. 1988. Molecular cloning of human and rat complementary DNA encoding androgen receptors. *Science* 240:324–26

17. Clever, U., Karlson, P. 1960. Induktion von Puff-Veranderungen in Speicheldrusenchromosomen von Chironomus tentans durch Ecdysone. *Exp. Cell Res.* 20:623–26

18. Conneely, O. M., Sullivan, W. P., Toft, D. O., Birnbaumer, M., Cook, R. G., et al. 1986. Molecular cloning of the chicken progesterone receptor. *Science* 233:767–70

19. Cordingley, M. G., Riegel, A. T., Hager, G. L. 1987. Steroid-dependent interaction of transcription factors with the inducible promoter of mouse mammary tumor virus in vivo. *Cell* 48:261–70

20. Darnell, J. 1982. Variety in the level of gene control in eukaryotic cells. *Nature* 297:365–71

21. Denis, M., Poellinger, L., Wikstrom, A. C., Gustafsson, J.-A. 1988. Requirement of hormone for thermal conversion of the glucocorticoid receptor to a DNA-binding state. *Nature* 333:686–88

22. Drouin, J., Charron, J., Gagner, J. P., Jeannotte, L., Nemer, M., et al. 1987. The pro-opiomelanocortin gene: a model for negative regulation of transcription by glucocorticoids. *J. Cell. Biochem.* 35:293–304

23. Eul, J., Meyer, M. E., Tora, L., Bocquel, M. T., Quirin-Stricker, C., et al. 1989. Expression of active hormone and DNA binding domains of the chicken progesterone receptor in E. coli. *EMBO J.* 8:83–90

24. Evans, R. M. 1988. The steroid and thyroid hormone receptor superfamily. *Science* 240:889–95

25. Evans, R. M., Hollenberg, S. M. 1988. Zinc fingers: guilt by association. *Cell* 52:1–3

26. Freedman, L. P., Luisi, B. F., Korszun, Z. R., Basavappa, R., Sigler, P. B., Yamamoto, K. R. 1988. The function and structure of the metal coordination sites within the glucocorticoid receptor DNA binding domain. *Nature* 334:543–46

27. Funder, J. W., Shepard, K. 1987. Adrenocortical steroids and the brain. *Annu. Rev. Phys.* 49:397–411

28. Giguere, V., Hollenberg, S. M., Rosenfeld, M. G., Evans, R. M. (1986). Functional domains of the human glucocorticoid receptor. *Cell* 46:645–52

29. Giguere, V., Ong, E. S., Segui, P., Evans, R. M. 1987. Identification of a receptor for the morphogen retinoic acid. *Nature* 330:624–29

30. Giguere, V., Yang, N., Segui, P., Evans, R. M. 1988. Identification of a new class of steroid hormone receptors. *Nature* 331:91–94

31. Glass, C. K., Holloway, J. M., Devary, O. V., Rosenfeld, M. G. 1988. The thyroid hormone receptor binds with opposite transcriptional effects to a common sequence motif in thyroid hormone and estrogen response elements. *Cell* 54:313–23

32. Godowski, P. J., Picard, D., Yamamoto, K. R. 1988. Signal transduction and transcriptional regulation by glucocorticoid receptor-lexA fusion proteins. *Science* 241:812–16

33. Godwoski, P. J., Rusconi, S., Miesfeld, R., Yamamoto, K. R. 1987. Glucocorticoid receptor mutants that are con-

stitutive activators of transcriptional enhancement. *Nature* 325:365–368

34. Gorski, J., Taft, D. O., Shyamala, G., Smith, D., Notides, A. 1968. Hormone receptors: Studies on the interactions of estrogens with the uterus. *Recent Progr. Horm. Res.* 24:45–72

35. Green, S., Chambon, P. 1986. Oestradiol induction of a glucocorticoid-responsive gene by a chimaeric receptor. *Nature* 325:75–78

36. Green, S., Kumar, V., Theulaz, I., Wahli, W., Chambon, P. 1988. The N-terminal DNA-binding 'zinc finger' of the oestrogen and glucocorticoid receptors determines target gene specificity. *EMBO J.* 7:3037–44

37. Green, S., Walter, P., Kumar, V., Krust, A., Bonert, J.-M., et al. 1986. Human oestrogen receptor cDNA: sequence, expression and homology to v-erb-A. *Nature* 320:134–39

38. Groyer, A., Schweizer-Groyer, G., Cadpond, F., Mariller, M., Baulieu, E.-E. 1987. Antiglucocorticosteroid effects suggest why steroid hormone is required for receptors to bind DNA in vivo but not in vitro. *Nature* 328:624–26

39. Guiochon-Mantel, A., Loosfelt, H., Ragot, T., Bailly, A., Atger, M., et al. 1988. Receptors bound to antiprogestin form abortive complexes with hormone responsive elements. *Nature* 336:695–98

40. Hodin, R. A., Lazar, M. A., Wintman, B. I., Darling, D. S., Koenig, R. J., et al. 1989. Identification of a thyroid hormone receptor that is pituitary-specific. *Science* 244:76–79

41. Hollenberg, S. M., Evans, R. M. 1988. Multiple and cooperative transactivation domains of the human glucocorticoid receptor. *Cell* 55:899–906

42. Hollenberg, S. M., Giguere, V., Segui, P., Evans, R. M. 1987. Colocalization of DNA-binding and transcriptional activation functions in the human glucocorticoid receptor. *Cell* 49:39–46

43. Hollenberg, S. M., Weinberger, C., Ong, E. S., Cerelli, G., Oro, A., et al. 1985. Primary structure and expression of a functional human glucocorticoid receptor cDNA. *Nature* 318:635–41

44. Huckaby, C. S., Conneely, O. M., Beattie, W. G., Dobson, A. D. W., Tsai, M.-J., O'Malley, B. W. 1987. Structure of the chromosomal chicken progesterone receptor gene. *Proc. Natl. Acad. Sci. USA* 84:8380–84

45. Hughes, M. R., Malloy, P. J., Kieback, D. G., Kesterson, R. A., Pike, J. W. et al. 1988. Point mutations in the human vitamin D receptor gene associated with

hypocalcemic rickets. *Science* 242: 1702–5

46. Ingham, P. W. 1989. The molecular genetics of embryonic pattern formation in *Drosophila. Nature* 335:25–34

47. Jantzen, H.-M., Strahle, U., Gloss, B., Stewart, F., Schmid, W., et al. 1987. Cooperativity of glucocorticoid response elements located far upstream of the tyrosine aminotransferase gene. *Cell* 49:29–38

48. Jensen, E. V., Suzuki, T., Kawashima, T., Stumpf, W. E., Jungblut, P. W., De Sombre, E. R. 1968. A two step mechanism for the interaction of estradiol with rat uterus. *Proc. Natl. Acad. Sci. USA* 59:632–38

49. Joab, I., Radanyi, C., Renoir, M., Buchou, T., Catelli, M.-G., et al. 1984. Common non-hormone binding component in non-transformed chick oviduct receptors of four steroid hormones. *Nature* 308:850–53

50. Kadonaga, J. T., Courey, A. J., Ladika, J., Tjian, R. 1988. Distinct regions of Sp1 modulate DNA binding and transcriptional activation. *Science* 242:1566–70

51. Kandutsch, A. A., Chen, H. W. 1975. Regulation of sterol synthesis in cultured cells by oxygenated derivatives of cholesterol. *J. Cell Physiol.* 85:415–24

52. Kandutsch, A. A., Thompson, E. B. 1980. Cytosolic proteins that bind oxygenated sterols. *J. Biol. Chem.* 255:10813–26

53. Katzenellenbogen, J. A., Carlson, K. E., Heiman, D. F., Robertson, D. W., Wei, L. L., Katzenellenbogen, B. S. 1983. Efficient and highly selective covalent labeling of the estrogen receptor with [³H] tamoxifen aziridine. *J. Biol. Chem.* 258:3487–95

54. Khoury, G., Gruss, P. 1983. Enhancer elements. *Cell* 33:313–14

55. King, W. J., Greene, G. L. 1984. Monoclonal antibodies localize estrogen receptor in the nuclei of target cells. *Nature* 307:745–47

56. Klein-Hitpass, L., Ryffel, G. U., Heitlinger, E., Cato, A. C. B. 1988. A 13 bp palindrome is a functional estrogen-responsive element and interacts specifically with estrogen receptor. *Nucl. Acids. Res.* 16:647–63

57. Klock, G., Strahle, U., Schutz, G. 1987. Oestrogen and glucocorticoid responsive elements are closely related but distinct. *Nature* 329:734–36

58. Koenig, R. J., Lazar, M. A., Hodin, R. A., Brent, G. A., Larsen, P. R., et al. 1989. Inhibition of thyroid hormone action by a non-hormone binding c-erb-A

protein generated by alternative mRNA splicing. *Nature* 337:659–61

59. Kumar, V., Chambon, P. 1988. The estrogen receptor binds tightly to its responsive element as a ligand-induced homodimer. *Cell* 55:145–55

60. Kumar, V., Green, S., Staub, A., Chambon, P. 1986. Localisation of the oestradiol-binding and putative DNA-binding domains of the human oestrogen receptor. *EMBO J.* 5:2231–36

61. Lefkowitz, R. J. 1987. Molecular and regulatory properties of adrenergic receptors. *Rec. Prog. Horm. Res.* 43:469–97

62. Lubahn, D. B., Joseph, D. R., Sullivan, P. M., Willard, H. F., French, F. S., Wilson, E. M. 1988. Cloning of human androgen receptor complementary DNA and localization to the X chromosome. *Science* 240:327–30

63. Ma, J., Ptashne, M. 1987. A new class of yeast transcriptional activators. *Cell* 51:113–19

64. Mader, S., Kumar, V., de Verneuil, H., Chambon, P. 1989. Three amino acids of the oestrogen receptor are essential to its ability to distinguish an oestrogen from a glucocorticoid-responsive element. *Nature* 338:271–74

65. Mandava, N. B. 1988. Plant growth-promoting brassinosteroids. *Annu. Rev. Plant Mol. Biol.* 39:23–52

66. Marcotte, W. R. Jr., Bayley, C. C., Quatrano, R. S. 1988. Regulation of a wheat promoter by abscisic acid in rice protoplasts. *Nature* 335:454–57

67. Martin, P. M., Berthois, Y., Jensen, E. V. 1988. Binding of antiestrogens exposes an occult antigenic determinant in the human estrogen receptor. *Proc. Natl. Acad. Sci. USA* 85:2533–37

68. McDonnell, D. P., Manglesdorf, D. J., Pike, J. W., Haussler, M. R., O'Malley, B. W. 1987. Molecular cloning of cDNA encoding the avian receptor for vitamin D. *Science* 235:1214–17

69. Metzger, D., White, J. H., Chambon, P. 1988. The human oestrogen receptor functions in yeast. *Nature* 334:31–36

70. Miesfeld, R., Godowski, P. J., Maler, B. A., Yamamoto, K. R. 1987. Glucocorticoid receptor mutants that define a small region sufficient for enhancer activation. *Science* 236:423–27

71. Miesfeld, R., Okret, S., Wikstrom, A.-C., Wrange, O., Gustafsson, J.-A., Yamamoto, K. R. 1984. Characterization of a steroid hormone receptor gene and mRNA in wild-type and mutant cells. *Nature* 312:779–81

72. Miller, J., McLachlan, A. D., Klug, A. 1985. Repetitive zinc-binding domains

in the protein transcription factor IIIA from *Xenopus* oocytes. *EMBO J.* 4:1609–14

73. Miyajima, N., Kadowaki, U., Fukushige, S., Shimizu, S., Semba, K., et al. 1988. Identification of two novel members of erbA superfamily by molecular cloning: the gene products of the two are highly related to each other. *Nucl. Acids. Res.* 16:11057-74

74. Morris, H. R., Taylor, G. W., Masento, M. S., Jermyn, K. A., Kay, R. R. 1987. Chemical structure of the morphogen differentiation inducing factor from *Dictyostelium discoideum. Nature* 328:811–14

75. Oppenheimer, J. H., Schwartz, H. L., Mariash, C. N., Kinlaw, W. B., Wong, N. C. W., Freake, H. C. 1987. Advances in our understanding of thyroid hormone action at the cellular level. *Endocr. Rev.* 8:288–388

76. Oro, A. E., Hollenberg, S. M., Evans, R. M. 1988. Transcriptional inhibition by a glucocorticoid receptor-β-galactosidase fusion protein. *Cell* 55:1109–14

77. Otten, A. D., Sanders, M. M., McKnight, G. S. 1988. The MMTV LTR promoter is induced by progesterone and dihydrotestosterone but not by estrogen. *Mol. Endocrinol.* 2:143–47

78. Patnaik, R. N., Nair, P. P. 1977. Studies on the binding of d-α-tocopherol to rat liver nuclei. *Arch. Biochem. Biophys.* 178:333–41

79. Perlmann, T., Wrange, O. 1988. Specific glucocorticoid receptor binding to DNA reconstituted in a nucleosome. *EMBO J.* 7:3073–79

80. Petkovich, M., Brand, N. J., Krust, A., Chambon, P. 1987. A human retinoic acid receptor which belongs to the family of nuclear receptors. *Nature* 330:444–50

81. Picard, D., Salser, S. J., Yamamoto, K. R. 1988. A movable and regulable inactivation function within the steroid binding domain of the glucocorticoid receptor. *Cell* 54:1073–80

82. Picard, D., Yamamoto, K. R. 1987. Two signals mediate hormone-dependent nuclear localization of the glucocorticoid receptor. *EMBO J.* 6:3333–40

83. Poland, A., Glover, E., Ebetino, F. H., Kende, A. S. 1986. Photoaffinity labeling of the Ah receptor. *J. Biol. Chem.* 261:6352–65

84. Ponglikitmongkol, M., Green, S., Chambon, P. 1988. Genomic organization of the human estrogen receptor gene. *EMBO J.* 7:3385–88

85. Porter, G. A., Bogoroch, R., Edelman, I. S. 1964. On the mechanism of action of aldosterone on sodium transport: the role of RNA synthesis. *Proc. Natl. Acad. Sci. USA* 52:1326–33

86. Pratt, W. B., Jolly, D. J., Pratt, D. V., Hollenberg, S. M., Giguere, V., et al. 1988. A region in the steroid binding domain determines formation of the non-DNA-binding, 9S glucocorticoid receptor complex. *J. Biol. Chem.* 263:267–73

87. Richard-Foy, H., Hager, G. L. 1987. Sequence-specific positioning of nucleosomes over the steroid-inducible MMTV promoter. *EMBO J.* 6:2321–28

88. Robertson, M. 1987. Towards a biochemistry of morphogenesis. *Nature* 330:420–21

89. Rusconi, S., Yamamoto, K. R. 1987. Functional dissection of the hormone and DNA binding activities of the glucocorticoid receptor. *EMBO J.* 6:1309–15

90. Samuels, H. H., Forman, B. M., Horowitz, Z. D., Ye, Z.-S. 1988. Regulation of gene expression by thyroid hormone. *J. Clin. Invest.* 81:957–67

91. Sap, J., Munoz, A., Damm, K., Goldberg, Y., Ghysdael, J., et al. 1986. The c-erb-A protein is a high-affinity receptor for thyroid hormone. *Nature* 324:635–40

92. Schauer, M., Chalepakis, G., Willmann, T., Beato, M. 1989. Binding of hormone accelerates the kinetics of glucocorticoid and progesterone receptor binding to DNA. *Proc. Natl. Acad. Sci. USA* 80:1123–27

93. Schena, M., Yamamoto, K. R. 1988. Mammalian glucocorticoid receptor derivatives enhance transcription in yeast. *Science* 241:965–67

94. Sherman, M. R., Pickering, L. A., Rollwagen, F. M., Miller, L. K. 1978. Mero-receptors: proteolytic fragments of receptors containing the steroid-binding site. *Fed. Proc.* 37:167–73

95. Sigler, P. B. 1988. Acid blobs and negative noodles. *Nature* 333:185–88

96. Simons, S. S., Thompson, E. B. 1981. Dexamethasone 21-mesylate: An affinity label of glucocorticoid receptors from rat hepatoma tissue culture cells. *Proc. Natl. Acad. Sci. USA* 78:3541–45

97. Slack, J. M. W. 1983. Morphogenetic gradients—past and present. *Trends Biochem. Sci.* 12:200–4

98. Thompson, C. C., Evans, R. M. 1989. Trans-activation by thyroid hormone receptors: functional parallels with steroid hormone receptors. *Proc. Natl. Acad. Sci. USA* 86:3494–98

99. Tora, L., Gronemeyer, H., Turcotte, B., Gaub, M.-P., Chambon, P. 1988. The N-terminal region of the chicken progesterone receptor specifies target gene activation. *Nature* 333:185–88

100. Tsai, S. Y., Carlstedt-Duke, J., Weigel, N. L., Dahlman, K., Gustafsson, J.-A., et al. 1988. Molecular interactions of steroid hormone receptor with its enhancer element: evidence for receptor dimer formation. *Cell* 55:361–69

101. Umesono, K., Giguere, V., Glass, C. K., Rosenfeld, M. G., Evans, R. M. 1988. Retinoic acid and thyroid hormone induce gene expression through a common responsive element. *Nature* 336:262–65

101a. Wang, L.-H., Tsai, S. Y., Cook, R. G., Beattie, W. G., Tsai, M.-J., O'Malley, B. W. 1989. COUP transcription factor is a member of the steroid receptor superfamily. *Nature* 340:163–66

102. Webster, N., Jin, J. R., Green, S., Hollis, M., Chambon, P. 1988. The yeast UAS$_G$ is a transcriptional enhancer in human HeLa cells in the presence of the GAL4 trans-activator. *Cell* 52:169–78

103. Webster, N., Green, S., Jin, J. R., Chambon, P. 1988. The hormone-binding domains of the estrogen and glucocorticoid receptors contain an inducible transcription activation function. *Cell* 54:199–207

104. Weinberger, C., Hollenberg, S. M., Ong, E. S., Harmon, J. M., Brower, S. T., et al. 1985. Identification of human glucocorticoid receptor complementary DNA by epitope selection. *Science* 228:740–42

105. Weinberger, C., Hollenberg, S. M., Rosenfeld, M. G., Evans, R. M. 1985. Domain structure of the human glucocorticoid receptor and homology with the viral erb-A oncogene product. *Nature* 318:670–72

106. Weinberger, C., Thompson, C. C., Ong, E. S., Lebo, R., Gruol, D. J., Evans, R. M. 1986. The c-erb-A gene encodes a thyroid hormone receptor. *Nature* 324:641–46

107. Welshons, W. V., Lieberman, M. E., Gorski, J. 1984. Nuclear localization of unoccupied estrogen receptors. *Nature* 307:747–49

108. Willmann, T., Beato, M. 1986. Steroid-free glucocorticoid receptor binds specifically to mouse mammary tumor virus DNA. *Nature* 324:688–91

109. Wrange, O., Okret, S., Radojcic, M., Carlstedt-Duke, J., Gustafsson, J.-A. 1984. Characterization of the purified activated glucocorticoid receptor from rat liver cytosol. *J. Biol. Chem.* 259:4534–41

110. Yamamoto, K. R., Gehring, U., Stamp-

fer, M. R., Sibley, C. 1976. Genetic approaches to steroid hormone action. *Rec. Prog. Hormone Res.* 32:3–32

111. Yamamoto, K. R. 1985. Steroid receptor regulated transcription of specific genes and gene networks. *Annu. Rev. Genet.* 19:209–52

112. Yamamoto, K. R., Stampfer, M. R., Tomkins, G. M. 1974. Receptors from glucocorticoid-sensitive lymphoma cells and two classes of insensitive clones: physical and DNA-binding properties. *Proc. Natl. Acad. Sci. USA* 71:3901–5

113. Zaret, K. S., Yamamoto, K. R. 1984. Reversible and persistent changes in chromatin structure accompany activation of a glucocorticoid-dependent enhancer element. *Cell* 38:29–38

Annu. Rev. Physiol. 1990. 52:841–51

REVERSE GENETICS USING TRANSGENIC MICE

Carlisle P. Landel, Shizhong Chen, and Glen A. Evans

Molecular Genetics Laboratory, The Salk Institute for Biological Studies, La Jolla, California 92037

KEY WORDS: toxigenes, cell ablation, Thy-1, homologous recombination, embryo injection

INTRODUCTION

Genetics provides a powerful tool for the analysis of development. Prokaryotes and lower eukaryotes that are amenable to genetic analysis have provided useful model systems for the dissection of complex physiologic processes. Traditional genetic analysis utilizing these organisms involves the creation of mutations that are selected on the basis of phenotype and used to understand the nature of the underlying genotype. This type of mutational genetics as applied to mammals and higher eukaryotes has been severely limited because of the difficulty in obtaining sufficient mutants for complete developmental analysis. In recent years, however, the use of transgenic organisms, in which pseudo-mutations are implanted in the germline through micromanipulation, has suggested a genetic approach in which the traditional logic is reversed. In this reverse genetic approach, a genotype is designed and constructed in vitro and implanted in the mouse germline by microinjection or by transfection into embryonic stem cells. The resulting transgenic animals often display a phenotype dependent on the particular design of the mutated gene. This reverse genetic approach allows a designed genotype to be used to discover the resulting phenotype and is particularly applicable to the analysis of mammalian development. Using transgenic technology, mutations can be produced to result in (*a*) aberrant expression of otherwise normal genes, (*b*) targeted ablation of cell populations, and (*c*) insertional inactivation of genes by homologous recombination.

0066-4278/90/0315-0841$02.00

MUTATIONS THAT RESULT IN ABERRANT GENE EXPRESSION

Mutations that are likely to provide important information of developmental significance may result from the introduction of genes containing various tissue-specific regulatory elements that can redirect the tissue-specific expression of normal gene products. This type of reverse genetic genotype places the expression of a normal gene under the control of regulatory elements that will alter the temporal or spatial regulation of gene expression. One example, which is now widely used, is the expression of oncogenes under the control of tissue-specific promoters to induce malignant transformation in the target tissue (21).

A second approach is to express a gene of unknown function or developmental significance according to an altered developmental program. In this method the resulting phenotype may suggest how the gene product functions in normal development. The Thy-1 glycoprotein is a 25-kd cell surface protein that is an important lineage marker in mouse T lymphocytes. The protein sequence suggests that the Thy-1 antigen gene, immunoglobulin genes, and other immunoglobulin-superfamily genes evolved from a common primordial gene, and its conservation of expression in vertebrates and some invertebrates suggests a functional importance. In spite of much speculation, however, the function of the Thy-1 antigen is unknown. Thy-1 is expressed on mature T lymphocytes, thymocytes, hematopoietic stem cells, and most central neurons, and its expression can be induced on activated B lymphocytes by treatment with interleukin-4. Since antibodies reacting and crosslinking the Thy-1 antigen induce T cell receptor-mediated activation of T cells, Thy-1 is thought to play a role in T cell or progenitor cell activation and maturation.

Reverse genetics was used to determine if Thy-1 might be important for lymphocyte activation or maturation through an attempt to alter the normal pattern of Thy-1 expression in transgenic mice (5, 16). A hybrid Thy-1 gene was constructed in which the immunoglobulin heavy chain enhancer was inserted into a large intron located downstream of the Thy-1 promoter region. Transgenic mice were produced by microinjecting the normal and altered Thy-1 gene into isolated mouse embryos and several founder animals were obtained. Transgenic animals carrying the normal Thy-1 gene expressed the gene at physiologic levels on thymocytes and in the brain, with slightly lower levels on splenic T cells. Animals carrying the Thy-1/Eμ construction also expressed Thy-1 on the surface of mature B lymphocytes and pre-B cells as judged by the coexpression of the B cell surface antigen B220. In addition to the expression of Thy-1 on B lymphocytes, over 80% of bone marrow cells expressed Thy-1, as compared to 7% or less Thy-1$^+$ cells in normal bone marrow. These transgenic mice developed a pre-B cell nonmalignant hyperplasia of the bone marrow and lymph nodes where the predominant cell types express surface characteristics of both T and B lymphocytes and are similar in many ways to the naturally occurring *lpr/lpr* mutant mouse.

Further analysis suggests that the presence of Thy-1 on the surface of pre-B cells induces rapid proliferation in vivo and in long-term bone marrow cultures. These data tend to suggest that Thy-1 may be involved in a signal transducing mechanism for the regulation of growth and expansion of lymphocyte progenitors in response to a lymphokine or other growth factor, or cell-cell interaction. Redirecting the expression of a gene to an inappropriate tissue in transgenic mice, then, can yield a phenotype that is extremely informative when dissecting the function of a new gene product. This approach is dependent upon understanding the regulation of tissue-specific gene expression and the availability of appropriate controlling elements.

MUTATIONS THAT RESULT IN PROGRAMMED CELL DEATH

Programmed cell death is an important aspect of mammalian development and occurs as a critical aspect of development of the mammalian nervous and immune systems. A few rare naturally occurring mutations have been discovered that result in premature or inappropriately timed cell death and subsequent developmental abnormalities. The past few years have seen the development of techniques for targeted cell ablation in transgenic animals by the expression of toxic gene products in a tissue-specific or developmentally stage-specific manner (for reviews, see 1, 8). This strategy involves the construction of "toxigenes" where a tissue-specific regulatory sequence is used to drive the expression of a gene encoding a toxic polypeptide. Initially silent, when activated at the appropriate developmental stage, expression of the toxin in the target cell induces cell suicide. This technique has proven useful for the investigation of developmental lineages, in determining the significance of cell-cell interactions in development, and in examining the functions of individual cell types.

Two toxic polypeptides have been used for cell ablation studies: diptheria toxin and ricin. Diptheria toxin is a single 62-kd polypeptide produced by the *tox* gene carried by lysogenic corynephage of pathogenic strains of *Corynebacterium diptheriae,* which is responsible for human diptheria. It consists of two separable domains, a 22-kd A subunit and a 40-kb B subunit, which together account for the high level of toxicity for most mammalian cells. The B subunit binds to the cell surface and mediates internalization of the A subunit. When inserted into the cytoplasm, the A subunit catalyzes the ADP-ribosylation of elongation factor 2, which results in an immediate cessation of protein synthesis and rapid cell death. Ricin is a toxic lectin produced by the castor bean *Ricinus communis* and exists as a heterodimer with noncovalently linked A and B subunits analogous to those of diptheria toxin. The B subunit contains a cell surface binding domain that recognizes surface galactose and induces internalization of the A subunit where it catalyzes the cleavage of the adenosine at position 4365 from the phosphodiester backbone of the 28S rRNA. Inactivation of the ribosomal 28S RNA leads to the cessation of protein synthesis and rapid cell death.

The construction of toxigenes requires in vitro genetic engineering of natural toxin genes. First, the coding sequence must be altered such that only a single toxic A subunit is made (18). Ricin is produced as a single nontoxic propeptide from which the A and B subunits are cleaved by proteolysis. The leader polypeptide must be removed to prevent secretion and allow cytoplasmic expression of the toxigene. Finally, suitable 3' and 5' flanking sequences, including restriction sites for insertion of appropriate regulatory sequences, must be included.

The initial demonstration of this technique used the 205 base pair 5' flanking region of the pancreatic elastase gene fused to the diptheria toxin A subunit toxigene (DT-A). Elastase is an important digestive protease produced exclusively by the acinar cells of the pancreas and represents one of the major protein products of differentiated pancreatic acinar cells. Transgenic mice were produced carrying the pancreas-specific toxigene by direct microinjection into isolated embryos (20). Expression of this toxigene at an early stage of embryogenesis would be expected to eliminate, at the very least, cells that are committed to differentiation into exocrine pancreatic cells by virtue of the early expression of elastase. As a result of these initial studies, seven of 24 founder transgenic animals carrying the elastase-DT-A toxin developed normally with the exception of severe abnormalities of the pancreas. The expression of this gene construct was associated with a severe reduction in the number of islet and ductal cells and a virtual absence of exocrine cells. Ablation of the pancrease at an early stage of development led to early death of the animals, making survival and derivation of a strain of transgenic mice for further study difficult.

Toxigenes have been used effectively for the analysis of development of the crystallin lens in transgenic mice through the development of DT-A and ricin A (R-A) vectors. Crystallins are produced by developing lens fiber cells and are encoded by a large multigene family. The genes encoding the major forms of crystallins, α, β, and γ, are differentially regulated during lens morphogenesis and produced by terminally differentiated lens fiber cells in large quantities. In the case of both the αA-crystallin gene and the γ2-crystallin gene, 5' flanking sequences and promoters appear to contain the majority of regulatory signals for precise temporal and spatial coordination of gene expression. Moreover, alterations in differentiation pathways and elimination of lens precursor cells do not affect viability or breeding potential of resulting transgenic mice so that strains may be established through breeding. Breitman et al (4) constructed transgenic mice in which the $\gamma2$-crystallin promoter directed the expression of DT-A in transgenic mice. Similarly, Landel et al (15) expressed the R-A toxigene from an αA-crystallin promoter and derived strains with well-defined abnormalities of lens development. Both αA crystallin-R-A and $\gamma2$ crystallin-DT-A mice demonstrate a profound microphthalmia characterized by fluid filled vesicles replacing much of the normal adult lens. Transgenic mice expressing the $\gamma2$-crystallin/DT-A toxigene demonstrated lens abnormalities whose severity varied among both different strains and individuals within a single strain ranging from cataracts and mild structural abnormalities to near destruction of the lens. The αA-crystallin/ricin animals demonstrated lens abnormalities and, in addition, a malformation and abnormal development of the neural retina. In addition, these animals produced ectopic lens fiber cells suggestive of a transdetermination of neural retina to lens.

Toxigene expression using pituitary-specific regulatory signals has been useful for clarifying some aspects of cell determination in the developing anterior pituitary. The precise lineage relationship between growth hormone-producing somatotropes and prolactin-producing lactotropes is unknown. A 310 bp 5' flanking sequence of the rat growth hormone gene is sufficient to direct expression to somatotropes and their immediate progenitors and has been used to direct cell ablation using a toxigene construction (2). Fusion of the growth hormone promoter with the DT-A toxigene resulted in three of 21 founder mice that lacked detectable levels of circulating growth hormone and demonstrated impaired growth. These animals had a nearly complete absence of somatotropes in the pituitary. In the transgenic pituitary, the 200,000 somatotropes were reduced in number to an average of 10 cells. Since earlier evidence had suggested that a rare population of pituitary producing cells both growth hormone and prolactin represented a common progenitor of somatotropes and lactotropes, examination of pituitaries from these transgenic animals could be used to test this hypothesis. Accompanying the absence of somatotropes was a severe decrease in the number of lactotropes, which suggested a developmental relationship between the two. The authors also noted rare islands of growth hormone producing cells, however, which suggested that some cells apparently escaped the expression or effects of the toxigene in the ablated pituitary.

An alternate approach to the expression of substances that are toxic is the targeted expression of genes that are not of themselves toxic, but which can metabolize drugs to toxic substances. The use of sensitizing genes rather than toxic genes may allow the production of viable animals where targeted ablation may be carried out in a tissue or cell type that is critical for normal development or survival. The herpes virus thymidine kinase (HSV-tk) is not harmful to most terminally differentiated cells and is widely used as a selective marker in tissue culture studies. Nucleoside analogues that have been developed for viral chemotherapy can be converted by the viral thymidine kinase to toxic metabolites. Acyclovir, FIAU [1-(2-deoxy-2-fluoro-β-D-arabinofuranosyl)-5-iodouracil], gancyclovir, and related drugs are relatively non-toxic to mammalian cells at low doses but block the replication of herpes virus (9). These drugs are not metabolized by mammalian thymidine kinases, but are phosphorylated by HSV-tk to nucleoside monophosphates, which can be further metabolized to nucleoside triphosphates by host enzymes, which leads to an inhibition of DNA synthesis. Transgenic mice have been generated in which the HSV-tk gene is expressed in a cell type specific manner, and in which cell ablation occurs after treating the animals with these drugs (3, 3a, 10).

A fusion of the HSV-tk gene with the immunoglobulin kappa light chain promoter and immunoglobulin heavy chain enhancer was used to generate transgenic mice. These regulatory elements direct gene expression in lymphoid cells of spleen, thymus, bone marrow, and lymph nodes in transgenic mice. Founder animals were derived that express detectable HSV-tk activity in spleen and thymus and low or undetectable activity in most other tissues. Upon treatment of these animals with gancyclovir, a dramatic reduction in the number of hematopoietic cells was seen that was directly related to the drug level in the blood. Severe atrophy of the spleen and lymph nodes was seen, which reduced the number of lymphoid cells to 15% of normal. Cell populations in the thymus were reduced to 2% of the normal number of thymocytes, with a virtual absence of the cortex and an extremely hypocellular medulla. Removal of the drug allowed almost complete repopulation of most lymphoid lineages, which indicated that nondividing progenitor cells were essentially not affected (10). Thymidine kinase obliteration was also directed to the anterior pituitary (3a). HSV-tk was placed under the control of the growth hormone (GH) or prolactin (Prl) promoter to ablate somatotropes and lactotropes, respectively. Treatment of the GH-HSV-tk mice with FIAU resulted in dwarf mice that essentially lacked both somatotropes and lactotropes, again suggesting that these cells share a common progenitor. Removal of the drug allowed repopulation of both cell types, which indicates that stem cells persist in the adult animal. Treatment of the Prl-HSV-tk mice with FIAU had no effect, thus indicating that Prl expression and lactotrope differentiation are post-mitotic events. Unlike DT-A or R-A toxigenes that inhibit protein synthesis, the thymidine kinase obliteration technique inhibits DNA synthesis, and thus ablation depends almost entirely on cell division in the target tissue. This approach is most applicable to tissues where cells are dividing rapidly through the adult life of the animal, as in the immune system.

MUTATIONS THAT MODEL HUMAN DISEASES

Transgenic animals that display phenotypes similar to human disorders may be useful for dissecting pathogenesis, for defining gene function, and for testing modalities of therapeutic intervention. The generation of animal models for human disease has taken several approaches including the insertion of genes encoding mouse homologs of human dominant mutations into the mouse germline in attempts to create a mouse analogue of a human disorder; the insertion of a human gene carrying a dominant mutation as a transgene to express a visible phenotype; and the insertion of the gene from a pathogenic virus into the mouse germline to simulate the pathogenesis associated with infection.

Osteogenesis imperfecta (OI) type 2 is a autosomal dominant disorder caused by the substitution of a single glycine residue in the triple helix of the α1-procollagen gene COLIAI. This substitution in a repeating Gly-X-Y structure alters the molecule so that collagen assembly is affected and results in abnormalities of bone formation. A similar phenotype was induced in a transgenic mouse strain by performing in vitro mutagenesis on the mouse homolog of the human α1 procollagen gene to induce the same amino acid substitution. The mutated gene was then used to produce transgenic mice by microinjection into isolated mouse embryos (23). All of the resulting transgenic animals died shortly after birth due to severe developmental defects in the formation of the skeleton. Analysis of these mice for the mutant procollagen demonstrated that expression of the mutation gene at levels as low as 10% of normal was sufficient to disrupt bone formation and lead to death. This suggests that the defective protein inhibits collagen assembly rather than forming a less stable molecule that is susceptible to degradation or altered secretion. In addition, this study demonstrates that human disorders may be modeled using transgenic animals by engineering suitable mutations in vitro.

Dycaico et al (7) used a human gene carrying a dominant mutant allele to create an animal model for the neonatal hepatitis of human α_1-antitrypsin deficiency. α_1-antitrypsin is a serum protein that inhibits trypsin, elastase, thrombin, and other serine proteases and prevents destruction of alveolar walls which, in the absence of a normal functioning enzyme, leads to emphysema. Associated with this disorder induced by the Z allele is hepatitis caused by failure of the abnormal α_1-antitrypsin to be correctly transported across the endoplasmic reticulum. About 15% of neonates that are homozygous for this allele develop hepatitis and obstructive jaundice and cirrhosis, presumably associated with defects in protein transport. The mutant human Z allele was used for the construction of transgenic mice and the resultant founders expressed human α_1-antitrypsin at approximately the same levels as found in humans. The transgenic animals also accumulated the mutant protein in the liver and, presumably because of faulty transport, developed hepatitis similar to that seen in human neonates. Thus these animals provide an appropriate model system for a dominant human disorder by expressing the human allele.

Various viral pathogens exist whose range is limited to humans and whose pathogenesis is poorly understood. One use of reverse genetics using transgenic mice is to create models of pathogenesis induced by these viruses by directly inserting all or part of the viral genome into transgenic mice, thus bypassing many restrictions in host range of the virus, which prevent the use of animal models. JC virus (JCV) is a human papovavirus that induces a multifocal leukoencephalopathy in humans characterized by chronic demyelination of nerves. Expression of the JCV early region after insertion into the genome of transgenic mice induces a similar disease state involving widespread demyelination and neurological symptoms similar to the natural mouse mutations *jimpy* and *quaking* (22, 25). The phenotype of these mice suggests that the expression of JCV T antigen arrests the maturation of oligodendrocytes and inhibits myelin production. Human T-lymphotropic virus type 1 (HTLV-1) is suspected to be a causative agent of adult T-cell leukemia and has been associated with neurologic disorders such as spastic paraperesis and multiple sclerosis. The *tat* gene of this virus encodes a transactivator of viral and host gene expression. Mice transgenic for the HTLV-1 *tat* gene express the gene product at high levels in nervous tissue. These animals develop tumors reminiscent of von Recklinghausen's neurofibromatosis in muscle and in the thymus, which results in thymic depletion and growth retardation (12, 19). The host range of human immunodeficiency virus HIV is limited to humans and chimpanzees, but it causes acquired immunodeficiency syndrome only in humans. Models for the disease are being sought via the production of mice transgenic for part or all of the HIV genome. Transgenic mice carrying the HIV *tat* gene develop a syndrome similar to Kaposi's sarcoma, which is seen as the initial manifestation of AIDS in about 25% of patients and which eventually develops in about 50% of all patients. Since the HIV *tat* gene is a transactivator of transcription, like the HTLV-1 *tat* gene, these data suggest that the HIV *tat* gene may directly induce the malignancies seen in AIDS patients through the activation of endogenous proto-oncogenes. HIV itself can not infect mice, as mice do not produce the HIV receptor CD4. In fact, HIV will not infect murine cells transfected with the CD4 gene and producing the protein on their surface appears to block viral internalization. To circumvent this block and infect mice directly, mice were made transgenic for the HIV genome (17, 26). These mice produce an infectious virus, develop a syndrome that mimics many of the symptoms of AIDS, and die at 25 days of age.

MUTATIONS THAT ELIMINATE THE EXPRESSION OF GENES

Most reverse genetic mutations involve the gain of function or aberrant gene expression and simulate natural dominant mutations. The process of chromosomal insertion after injection of DNA into the embryo, however, will involve random insertional inactivation of endogenous genes. About 15% of these insertions may result in a visible phenotype (usually embryonic lethal) when bred to homozygosity. At a low but detectable frequency, however, homologous recombination of exogenous DNA into the mammalian genome takes place. Homologous recombination resulting in an insertional inactivation mutation provides a technology for producing recessive mutations in transgenic mice.

Gene inactivation involves the construction of an artificial gene such that insertion by homologous recombination will inactivate the endogenous gene. Transformation of embryonic stem (ES) cell cultures with this construction followed by screening for the desired insertional event can result in inactivation of the endogenous gene carried by one chromosome. After amplification of the transfected ES cell line, ES cells are injected into isolated blastocysts and following reimplantation will result in chimeric animals where the ES cells contribute to most somatic and germ cells. If germ cell chimerism is obtained, the animals may be bred to obtain the desired insertional mutation in a homozygous state.

This approach of targeted mutagenesis has been used to inactivate the gene encoding the hypoxanthine-guanine phosphoribosyl transferase (HPRT) carried on the X chromosome of mice. Insertional inactivation was accomplished by infection with a retrovirus and selection of ES cell clones that grow in HAT selective medium (14). When used to produce chimeric animals through blastocyst injection, animals with an inactive HPRT gene were produced. Targeted mutagenesis by homologous recombination has also been used to produce HPRT⁻ chimeras (6, 11, 24).

For most genes, a positive selection for gene inactivation is not available or easily derived. In these cases, a selection system can be included in the targeting vector, or ES cells in which homologous recombination has taken place can be rapidly screened using the polymerase chain reaction (PCR). The construction used for insertion is prepared to contain unique sequences, such as the neomycin/kanamycin phosphotransferase of tn9 (neoʳ), and to potentially interrupt expression of a gene after homologous insertion. The presence of neoʳ allows cells containing a transfected gene to be selected by growth in the neomycin analogue geneticin (G418). For rapid screening, PCR primers are chosen so that only those ES cells in which homologous integration has occurred will demonstrate an appropriately sized amplified fragment. Since PCR reactions can be automated, screening thousands of colonies to identify the appropriate insertion is now possible.

Targeted mutagenesis has been used to create insertional inactivation mutations of the Hox1.1, Hox1.2, and En-2 genes (13, 27). Since these genes are related to genes of *Drosophila* that are important for the control of development, the availability of mice with targeted mutations at these loci will provide important insights into the control of mammalian development.

CONCLUSIONS

Traditional genetics depends on the creation of new mutations or the identification of naturally occurring mutations based on their phenotype. The detailed study of phenotype then allows the discovery and characterization of the mutant genotype and an eventual understanding of the underlying biology. In non-traditional or reverse genetics, the logic of experimentation proceeds backwards. One may now conceive of a possible genotype, prepare the genotype in the laboratory, and implant it into the mammalian genome to reveal the resulting phenotype. The advent of reverse genetics allows the creation of a wide variety of mutations that could not easily be obtained using traditional genetics and, with continued technical development and refinement, promises to greatly expand our understanding of mammalian biology.

Literature Cited

1. Beddington, R. S. P. 1988. Toxigenics: strategic cell death in the embryo. *Trends Genet.* 4:1–2
2. Behringer, R. R., Mathews, L. S., Palmiter, R. D., Brinster, R. L. 1988. Dwarf mice produced by genetic ablation of growth hormone-expressing cells. *Genes Devel.* 2:453–61
3. Borrelli, E., Heyman, R., Hsi, M., Evans, R. M. 1988. Targeting of an inducible toxic phenotype in animal cells. *Proc. Natl. Acad. Sci. USA* 85:7572–76
3a. Borelli, E., Heyman, R. A., Arias, C., Sawchenko, P. E., Evans, R. M. 1989. Transgenic mice with inducible dwarfism. *Nature* 339:538–41
4. Breitman, M. L., Clapoff, S., Rossant, J., Tsui, L.-C., Glode, L. M., et al. 1987. Genetic ablation: Targeted expression of a toxin gene causes microphthalmia in transgenic mice. *Science* 238:1563–65
5. Chen, S., Botteri, F., van der Putten, H., Landel, C. P., Evans, G. A. 1987. A lymphoproliferative abnormality associated with inappropriate expression of the Thy-1 antigen in transgenic mice. *Cell* 51:7–19
6. Doetschman, T., Maeda, N., Smithies, O. 1988. Targeted mutation of the *Hprt* gene in mouse embryonic stem cells. *Proc. Natl. Acad. Sci. USA* 85:8583–87
7. Dycaico, M. J., Grant, S. G. N., Felts, K., Nichols, W. S., Geller, S. A., et al. 1988. Neonatal hepatitis induced by α₁-antitrypsin: A transgenic mouse model. *Science* 242:1409–12
8. Evans, G. A. 1989. Dissecting mouse development with toxigenics. *Genes Devel.* 3:259–63
9. Furman, P. A., McGujirt, P. V., Keller, P. M., Fyfe, J. A., Elion, G. B. 1980. Inhibition by acyclovir of cell growth and DNA synthesis of cells biochemically transformed with herpes virus genetic information. *Virology* 102:420–30
10. Heyman, R. A., Borrelli, E., Lesley, J., Anderson, D., Richmond, D. D., et al. 1989. Thymidine kinase obliteration (TKO): creation of transgenic mice with controlled immune-deficiency. *Proc. Natl. Acad. Sci. USA*, 86:2698–702

11. Hooper, M., Hardy, K., Handyside, A., Hunter, S., Monk, M. 1987. HPRT-deficient (Lesch-Nyhan) mouse embryos derived from germline colonization by cultured cells. *Nature* 326:292–95

12. Hinrichs, S. H., Nerenberg, M., Reynolds, R. K., Khoury, G., Jay, G. 1987. A transgenic mouse model for human neurofibromatosis. *Science* 237:1340–43

13. Joyner, A. L., Skarnes, W. C., Rossant, J. 1989. Production of a mutation in mouse *En-2* gene by homologous recombination in embryonic stem cells. *Nature* 338:153–56

14. Kuehn, M. R., Bradley, A., Robertson, E. J., Evans, M. J. 1987. A potential animal model for Lesch-Nyan syndrome through introduction of HPRT mutations into mice. *Nature* 326:295–98

15. Landel, C. P., Zhao, J., Bok, D., Evans, G. A. 1988. Lens-specific expression of recombinant ricin induces developmental defects in the eyes of transgenic mice. *Genes Devel.* 2:1168–78

16. Landel, C. P., Chen, S., Botteri, F., van der Putten, H., Evans, G. A. 1989. Hematopoietic abnormalities induced by ectopic expression of the Thy-1 antigen in trangenic mice. In *Gene Transfer and Gene Therapy*, ed. I. Verma, R. Mulligan, A. Beaudet, pp. 179–88. New York: Liss

17. Leonard, J. M., Abramczuk, J. W., Pezen, D. S., Rutledge, R., Belcher, J. H., et al. 1988. Development of disease and virus recovery in transgenic mice containing HIV proviral DNA. *Science* 242:1665–70

18. Maxwell, I. H., Maxwell, F., Glode, L. M. 1986. Regulated expression of a diphtheria toxin A-chain gene transfected into human cancer cells: a possible strategy for inducing cancer cell suicide. *Cancer Res.* 46:4660–64

19. Nerenberg, M., Hinrichs, S. H., Reynolds, R. K., Khoury, G., Jay, G. 1987. The *tat* gene of human T-lymphotropic virus type 1 induces mesenchymal tumors in transgenic mice. *Science* 237:1324–29

20. Palmiter, R. D., Behringer, R. R., Quaife, C. J., Maxwell, F., Maxwell, I. H., Brinster, R. L. 1987. Cell lineage ablation in transgenic mice by cell-specific expression of a toxin gene. *Cell* 50:435–43

21. Rassoulzadegan, M., Cuzin, F. 1987. "Sub-threshold neoplastic states" created in transgenic mice. *Oncogene Res* 1:1–6

22. Small, J. A., Scangos, G. A., Cork, L., Jay, G., Khoury, G. 1986. The early region of human papavovirus JC induces dysmyelination in transgenic mice. *Cell* 46:13–18

23. Stacey, A., Bateman, F., Choi, T., Mascara, T., Cole, W., Jaenisch, R. 1988. Perinatal lethal osteogenesis imperfecta in transgenic mice bearing an engineered mutant pro-α1(I) collagen gene. *Nature* 332:131–36

24. Thomas, K. R., Capecchi, M. R. 1987. Site-directed mutagenesis by gene targeting in mouse embryo-derived stem cells. *Cell* 51:503–12

25. Trapp, B. D., Small, J. A., Pulley, M., Khoury, G., Scangos, G. A. 1988. Dysmyelination in transgenic mice containing JC virus early region. *Ann. Neurol.* 23:38–48

26. Vogel, J., Hinrichs, S. H., Reynolds, R. K., Luciw, P. A., Jay, G. 1988. The HIV *tat* gene induces dermal lesions resembling Kaposi's sarcoma in transgenic mice. *Nature* 335:606–11

27. Zimmer, A., Gruss, P. 1989. Production of chimaeric mice containing embryonic stem (ES) cells carrying a homoeobox *Hox 1.1* allele mutated by homologous recombination. *Nature* 338:150–53

SPECIAL TOPIC: CAGED COMPOUNDS IN CELLULAR PHYSIOLOGY

Jack H. Kaplan, Section Editor

Department of Physiology, University of Pennsylvania, Philadelphia, Pennsylvania 19104-6085

INTRODUCTION

This special topic section contains three chapters dealing with different aspects of the application of caged compounds in cellular physiology.

The general approach employed in the photo-activated release of caged compounds is illustrated in the following scheme: where a protected or chemically modified moiety is cleaved by light to release the previously caged substance. Most applications of this approach since the introduction of caged cAMP, caged ATP, caged ADP, and caged P_i have also employed the 2-nitrobenzyl chromophore illustrated in this scheme. Currently the photo-chemical release of caged substrates has been applied to cAMP, ATP, ADP, P_i, GTP, GTPγS, cGMP, and neurotransmitters including carbachol, glycine, glutamine, gaba, Ca^{2+}, Mg^{2+}, H^+, BAPTA, phenylephrine, and so on. Over the last decade, several informative reviews have appeared on various aspects of this field including synthetic and mechanistic aspects (5), applications in cellular physiology (1, 3, 4, 7), and applications to studies of active transport mechanisms (2).

The increasing application of this approach, using a variety of caged molecules in different physiologic systems, has been encouraged by other parallel technical advances. These include the patch-clamp methodology where electrical measurements can be made at the single cell or even single-channel level. This approach can now be combined with the enhanced kinetic resolution of the photorelease technique to produce rapid concentration changes in the micro-environment of a channel without mixing delays or solution-changing complications. The advances made in imaging and measur-

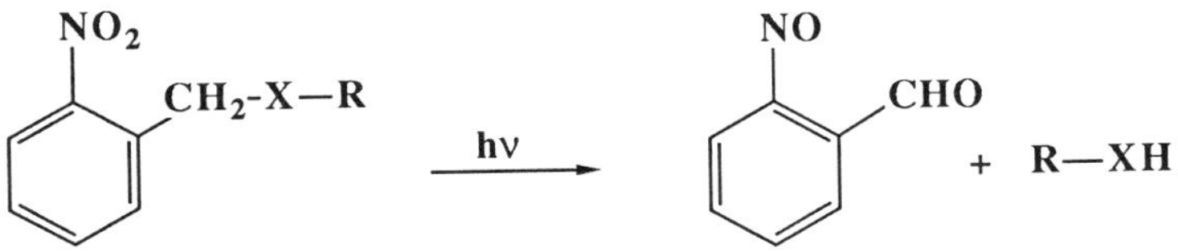

Figure 1 Generalized photochemical release of a caged substrate (R-XH) X = phosphate, carboxylate, ether, amine, amide or phenol.

ing cellular electrolytes at the single-cell level, pioneered by Tsien & colleagues (8), now can be used to monitor the results of rapid concentration jumps in substrate, messenger, or ion concentrations with sub-msec time resolution and sub-cellular spatial resolution. A recent novel and imaginative application of the photoactivation approach has been utilized to photorelease a fluorescent reporter molecule in a localized fashion. This approach, a reverse of the more familiar fluorescence recovery after photo-bleaching (FRAP), was used to examine at the single-cell level the flux of tubulin in kinetochore microtubules during mitosis (6).

Until now all the phosphate-containing substrates employed in enzyme activation via photoactivation have required caging of each substrate. This has led to the use of caged ATP, ADP, GTP, cGMP, and others. Since many if not all of these enzymes need Mg^{2+} as a co-factor, however, and since DM-nitrophen can be used as a caged Mg^{2+}, perhaps DM-nitrophen can be used as a more general photoactivating molecule for many enzyme systems.

Among the more interesting areas for future research is the application of photo-cleaved substrates or photo-released Mg^{2+} in studies of crystalline proteins. The ability to "add" substrates or ligands to crystalline enzymes via a non-disruptive procedure raises the possibility of obtaining diffraction patterns from the same protein crystals in different conformations. The next step would be to time resolve such crystal diffraction studies.

The three articles in this section review specific areas in which the photorelease approach has already yielded interesting results. It is fitting that two of these articles deal with muscle studies, since it is this area that has benefited mostly from photorelease methodologies. The first review by the Drs. Somlyo discusses uses that have been made of caged technology to examine a variety of aspects of the complex problem of regulation of smooth muscle contraction. The second article by Homsher and Millar deals with striated muscle where the details of the relation between cross-bridge cycle structures and biochemical changes have begun to be approached in a single preparation. These studies form the beginning of an approach where biochemical information hitherto obtainable only on isolated elements of the disrupted contractile system can now be studied in a situation closer to the in vivo state. The final chapter deals with the recent work on developing molecules that will serve as caged divalent cations. The divalent cations Ca^{2+} and Mg^{2+} play such a central role in physiologic processes that considerable effort has been made to produce molecules that will serve as a caged Ca or caged Mg. Some successes in this area have recently been achieved and the advantages and limitations of the currently available approaches are discussed in a variety of physiologic applications.

Literature Cited

1. Gurney, A. M., Lester, H. A. 1987. Light-flash physiology with synthetic compounds. *Physiol. Rev.* 67:583–617
2. Kaplan, J. H. 1986. Caged ATP as a tool in active transport research. In *Optical Methods in Cell Physiology (Soc. Gen. Physiol. Ser.),* ed. P. De Weer, B. Salzberg pp. 385–96. New York: Wiley
3. Kaplan, J. H., Somlyo, A. P. 1989. Flash photolysis of caged compounds: new tools for cellular physiology. *Trends Neurosci.* 12:54–59
4. Lester, H. A., Nerbonne, J. M. 1982. Physiological and pharmacological manipulations with light flashes. *Annu. Rev. Biophys. Bioenerg.* 11:151–75
5. McCray, J. A., Trentham, D. R. 1989. Properties and uses of photoreactive caged compounds. *Annu. Rev. Biophys. Chem.* 18:239–70
6. Mitchison, T. N. 1989. Polewards microtubule flux in the mitotic spindle: evidence from photoactivation of fluorescence. *J. Cell Biol.* 109:637–57
7. Nerbonne, J. M. 1986. Design and application of photolabile intracellular probes. See Ref. 2, pp. 417–45
8. Tsien, R. Y. 1989. Fluorescent probes of cell signalling. *Annu. Rev. Neurosci.* 12:207–53

Annu. Rev. Physiol. 1990. 52:857–74

FLASH PHOTOLYSIS STUDIES OF EXCITATION-CONTRACTION COUPLING, REGULATION, AND CONTRACTION IN SMOOTH MUSCLE

Andrew P. Somlyo and Avril V. Somlyo

Department of Physiology, University of Virginia Health Sciences Center, Box 449, Charlottesville, Virginia 22908

KEY WORDS: caged compounds, muscle physiology, contraction delays, muscle agonist-receptors, pharmacomechanical coupling

INTRODUCTION

The binding of an excitatory transmitter to its receptor on smooth muscle leads to contraction through the combined mechanisms of excitation-contraction coupling, contractile regulation, and crossbridge cycling (reviewed in 6, 23, 63, 68). Typical smooth muscle preparations consist of numerous cells with large surface/volume ratios and with geometries complicated by tortuous extracellular spaces lined with proteins. In such preparations, but even in single cells, the interpretation of any phenomenon evoked by the addition of a diffusible transmitter, messenger, or substrate is greatly complicated by diffusional delays. Photolysis of caged compounds overcomes such diffusional delays and, although still in its infancy, the application of this method to the study of excitation-contraction coupling,

857

contractile regulation, and contraction in smooth muscle, has already produced valuable new information.

The term "caged compound" was introduced to denote caged ATP (40), an ATP molecule that was rendered inaccessible as a substrate to the Na, K-ATPase by esterifying its terminal phosphate with a photolabile nitrobenzyl group. This general strategy of caging with a photolabile group has since been successfully applied to a number of adenine and guanine nucleotides, inositol 1, 4, 5 trisphosphate, and other compounds, particularly since a single step method of caging the substrate became available (77, 78). Photolysis of such a caged compound yields (within ms) an active compound instantaneously accessible to its ligand and a nitroso-ketone "leaving" group. The structure and photochemistry of these and other types of caged compounds have been reviewed elsewhere (20, 41, 47). The general concept underlying their design is to produce an inactive compound that can be diffused to and equilibrated at its site of action "at leisure", and then activated, within micro/milliseconds, by a light flash. Alternatively, an active photolabile compound, such as a dihydropyridine calcium-entry blocker, can be inactivated by flash photolysis. A recent novel approach called fluorescence photoactivation and dissipation allows one to produce foci of fluorescence within a cell and track the movement of the fluorescent molecules of interest. This technique is based on the removal, through photolysis, of the quenching effect of the photosensitive groups that were covalently attached to fluorescent compounds (81).

A recent and significant improvement in the application of caged compounds has been their introduction into cells permeabilized with staphylococcal alpha-toxin or with the saponin ester beta-escin. Smooth muscles (10, 42) and other cells (1) exposed to toxin become permeable to low molecular weight ($M_r \leq 1,000$ dalton) solutes while retaining high molecular weight compounds, including enzymes and calmodulin. Permeabilization with beta-escin creates larger holes that are permeable to calmodulin ($M_r = 17,000$ dalton). Since the majority of caged compounds are charged molecules, they generally do not penetrate the plasma membranes, and in earlier studies they had to be introduced into mechanically (skeletal) or saponin (smooth) skinned muscle fibers (18, 25, 71, 79). These methods led to the loss of a number of regulatory substances, soluble enzymes and others and, in the case of smooth muscle, uncoupled excitatory (e.g. alpha-adrenergic, muscarinic) receptors. Permeabilization with either alpha-toxin or beta-escin does not uncouple these receptors (42, 43) and permits the exploration of the effects of caged compounds under more nearly physiologic conditions. The caged compounds that we have thus far introduced into alpha-toxin and/or beta-escin permeabilized smooth muscles include caged ATP, GTPγS, and inositol 1, 4, 5 trisphosphate (InsP3).

EXCITATION-CONTRACTION COUPLING AND THE LATENCY OF ACTIVATION: THE USE OF CAGED InsP$_3$ AND CAGED PHENYLEPHRINE

Electromechanical coupling and pharmacomechanical coupling are the major modalities of excitation-contraction coupling in smooth muscle (69, 73 reviewed in 70). Electromechanical coupling is mediated by changes in surface membrane potential: the influx of Ca^{2+} through voltage gated channels, depolarization induced Ca^{2+} release, or the inhibition of these Ca^{2+} movements by hyperpolarization. Pharmacomechanical coupling is also mediated primarily by agonist-induced Ca^{2+} release or Ca^{2+} influx through ligand gated or second messenger gated channels (reviewed in 70, 76). According to its original definition (73), however, pharmacomechanical coupling may also include a component that modulates the sensitivity of the regulatory-contractile apparatus to Ca^{2+}.

The main applications of caged compounds to the study of excitation-contraction coupling in smooth muscle have been directed to pharmacomechanical coupling: Ca^{2+} release and, most recently, modulation of Ca^{2+} sensitivity. The major source of intracellular Ca^{2+} released by pharmacomechanical coupling is the sarcoplasmic reticulum (SR), although there may be another small nonmitochondrial, InsP$_3$-insensitive and GTPγS-sensitive compartment in some smooth muscles (44). Caged compounds have been particularly useful in exploring the kinetics and thus the mechanism of pharmacomechanical Ca^{2+} release from the SR. The rapid force development by smooth muscle responding to release of InsP$_3$ by photolysis from caged InsP$_3$ provides strong evidence of the role of InsP$_3$ as a physiologic messenger of pharmacomechanical Ca^{2+} release (70, 79).

The time elapsed (delay or latency) between excitation of the surface membrane and contraction is related to the mechanism of excitation-contraction coupling. Long, temperature-sensitive latencies are considered characteristic of chemical transmission, while short latencies, such as observed in fast striated muscles (48), are thought to be suggestive, though not diagnostic, of mechanical or electrical coupling mechanisms. Early evidence (5) revealed a very long (1 s at 39°C) delay between stimulation of excitatory (adrenergic) nerves and contraction of (rabbit pulmonary artery) smooth muscle, but did not resolve the question whether or not this was due to diffusional delays preceding the binding of the agonist to its receptor or to post-receptor events. With current technology, the latency can be separated into two components: the first, between binding of an agonist to its receptor and the rise in cytoplasmic Ca^{2+}, and a second, between the rise of Ca^{2+} and contraction. In the case of modulation of Ca^{2+}-sensitivity by an agonist, the relevant delay is the one between agonist-receptor interaction and the change in force.

The latency between agonist-receptor interaction and force-development has been explored with caged phenylephrine (70). The long (1.5±0.26 s at 20°C) interval between photolysis of this compound (Figure 1) and its high Q_{10} (2.7) are consistent with a chemical mechanism, presumably the hydrolysis of phosphatidylinositol biphosphate (PIP_2) to yield $InsP_3$ as the Ca^{2+}-releasing messenger (4). The relative contributions of Ca^{2+} influx or Ca^{2+} release to such agonist-induced contractions remain to be quantitated, but the results clearly show that neither of these processes is initiated by phenylephrine on a very fast (i.e.: ms) time scale. Two technical aspects of these experiments should be noted. First, it was necessary to use relatively high (50 μM) concentrations of caged phenylephrine in order to reach threshold con-

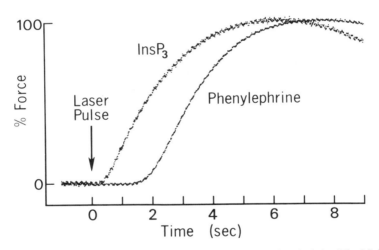

Figure 1 Two force transients recorded after photolysis of caged phenylephrine (50 μM) in an intact muscle strip and caged Ins(1,4,5)P_3 in a permeabilized muscle strip of guinea-pig portal vein at 20°C. A 50 ns laser pulse at 347 nm is indicated by the arrow. The peak force and $t_{1/2}$ to peak force for Ins(1,4,5)P_3 and phenylephrine were 177 μN, 1.4 s and 205 μN, 1.4 s, respectively. The lag phase preceding force development was 0.4 s for Ins (1,4,5)P_3 and 1.8 s for phenylephrine. The intact strip used for the caged phenylephrine experiment had been treated with 6-hydroxy-dopamine for 20 min to produce adrenergic denervation. This experiment was done in the presence of 143 mM potassium to depolarize the cell membrane. The Ins(1,4,5)P_3 response was obtained in a muscle strip permeabilized with 50 μg ml^{-1} saponin for 15 min and calcium loaded for 5 min at pCa6.6, 1 mM EGTA, followed by a 2 min wash in 0 calcium containing 1 mM EGTA solution, and subsequent incubation with 10 μM caged Ins(1,4,5)P_3 (esterified on the P^5 position) in a solution containing 0.1 mM EGTA and 90 μM calmodulin for 3 min before the laser flash. Approximately 10% Ins(1,4,5)P_3 and phenylephrine were released from the caged precursors (from reference 70).

centration sufficiently fast, given the rather slow dark reactions of this caged compound. Control experiments with (uncaged) phenylephrine jumps showed similar results, however, indicating that the long delay was not due to slow dark reactions or to an alpha-adrenergic antagonist action of the caged compound itself. Second, the experiments were done in high K^+ depolarizing solution to prevent activation of the surface membrane by the laser pulse itself. Under these conditions the responses were completely blocked by an alpha-adrenergic antagonist. Considering the high Q_{10} of the delay of contractions initiated by photolysis of caged phenylephrine, the increase in InsP$_3$ found after 500 ms in trachealis smooth muscle neurally stimulated at 37°C (49) is consistent with the time course of contraction induced by photorelease of caged agonist.

Excitatory receptors in smooth muscle (44), as in other systems (for review, 9), are coupled by G proteins to phospholipase C. Pharmacomechanical Ca^{2+} release can be directly evoked with nonhydrolyzable analogues of GTP, such as GTPγS (44, 45). The delay between the application of GTPγS and Ca^{2+} release and the physiologic response is rate-limited by the off-rate of GDP from the G proteins (e.g. 8, 9), however, and can be longer than the physiologic delay that is shortened through acceleration of the GDP off-rate by agonists. Therefore, the delays observed following the addition of GTPγS to permeabilized smooth muscle are longer than normally seen following the application of an agonist to intact muscle. Subthreshold concentrations of an agonist to accelerate the exchange of GTPγS for GDP on G protein would be expected to shorten the delay following photolysis of GTPγS.

Ca^{2+} is thought to be released through InsP$_3$-sensitive SR channels that are specifically blocked by heparin (14, 44, 45). The opening of channels, as contrasted to the operation of active transport systems and carriers, is generally thought to be associated with faster kinetics and less likely to require gating times of tens of msec. The upper limit of the delay between photorelease of high concentrations (up to about 50 μM) of released InsP$_3$ and the rise in Ca^{2+} measured with Fluo 3 (39, 50) in guinea pig portal vein smooth muscle (in the presence of 2 mM AMPPCP and the absence of ATP), is approximately 30 ms (K. Horiuti, A. V. Somlyo, D. R. Trentham, et al, in preparation). Longer delays were found at low InsP$_3$ concentrations. The delays were shortened by ATP and also by its nonhydrolyzable analogue AMPPCP, although both the delay and rate of release were very much depressed in the absence of nucleotides. InsP$_3$-induced Ca^{2+} release is reported to be absolutely dependent on ATP or one of its nonhydrolyzable analogues in cultured smooth muscle cells (64), but not in taenia caeci (33) or in basophilic leukemic cells (47a). These results suggest that the adenine nucleotides play a role other than as phosphate donors in modulating the InsP$_3$-gated channel. An InsP$_3$-gated channel could open with delay if, for example, the InsP$_3$

receptor at rest was not free, but occupied by an inactive compound, perhaps ATP or an InsP₃ metabolite. In such a case, the off-rate of this compound could rate-limit the on-rate of InsP₃ to its receptor and cause a delay in Ca^{2+} release. Alternatively, the delay in basophilic leukemia cells has been attributed (47a) to the kinetics of binding of multiple InsP₃ molecules thought to be required for opening Ca^{2+} channels.

Approximately 0.3–0.5 s (at 22°C) of the delay between activation, whether electromechanical or pharmacomechanical, and force is due to steps following the increase in $[Ca^{2+}]_i$. In contrast to Ca^{2+} release, the delay in force development following photolysis of caged InsP₃ (Figure 2) is relatively long (about 0.5±0.12 s at 22°C) and has a low Q_{10} (70). There is a similar (about 0.2–0.3 s at 22°C) delay between the rise in $[Ca^{2+}]_i$ and contraction in spontaneously active or electrically stimulated intact smooth muscle (29, 83). Similar latencies were found between photolysis of caged ATP and force initiated from the rigor state in the presence of Ca^{2+} (31). This delay was shorter, by nearly an order of magnitude, when ATP was released by photolysis into the myofilament lattice under conditions where the myosin light chains were prephosphorylated by treatment with ATPγS or the phosphatase inhibitor okadaic acid (31). In intact smooth muscle, there is also a close temporal relationship between myosin light chain phosphorylation

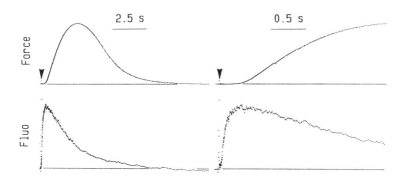

Figure 2 Ca^{2+} transients upon photolysis of caged InsP₃ in guinea pig ileum. The muscle strip was mounted in a 0.3 mm i.d. quartz capillary. One end of the muscle was attached to a force transducer via a tungsten wire and the other end attached to a tungsten wire anchored to the inner wall of the capillary tube. The muscle was permeabilized with staphylococcal alpha-toxin, the sarcoplasmic reticulum loaded with calcium by incubation at pCa6.3, 10 mM EGTA for 10 min, followed by rapid removal of Ca and EGTA and subsequent exposure to 30 μM caged InsP₃ (with the nitrobenzyl group on the P5 position) and 10 μM Fluo 3 at 25°C for 3 min, before photolysis with the 2 ms UV light from the flash lamp, indicated by the arrowhead. Approximately 15% of the caged InsP₃ was photolyzed. The force and Ca^{2+} (Fluo) responses are shown on a slow and fast time base. Note the delay of 350 and 30 ms for the force and Ca^{2+} transients, respectively (from K. Horiuti, et al, in preparation).

and stiffness (37). In view of the short delay between light chain phosphorylation and the mechanical events, the longer latencies between the rise in Ca^{2+} and contraction have been ascribed variously to prephosphorylation reactions between Ca^{2+}, calmodulin, and myosin light chain kinase (71, 83), a mechanical effect of series elastic elements, and to the kinetics of the (minimally) two-step reaction of myosin light chain phosphorylation and attachment of crossbridges into force-generating states (31).

CONTRACTILE REGULATION: CONTRACTION KINETICS OF PHASIC AND TONIC SMOOTH MUSCLES AND THE MODULATION OF Ca^{2+} SENSITIVITY

The primary regulatory mechanism of smooth muscle contraction is phosphorylation of myosin light chain (LC_{20}) by myosin light chain kinase that is activated by its regulatory subunit, Ca^{2+}-calmodulin, as the result of an increase in cytoplasmic Ca^{2+} (reviewed in 23, 58). Phosphorylation of LC_{20}, usually in response to an increase in $[Ca^{2+}]_i$ above its resting value (80–140 nM; reviewed in 66), is sufficient for the activation of myosin ATPase by actin (35). Relaxation, according to this mechanism, results from dephosphorylation of LC_{20} by myosin light chain phosphatases (21, 30, 59), usually, though not always, as a result of a decline in $[Ca^{2+}]_i$. The possibility of secondary, perhaps thin filament-associated, mechanisms of regulation (reviewed in 38) is outside the scope of this presentation, as decisive evidence of the physiologic role of such a mechanism has yet to be obtained, and its operation has not been explored with caged compounds.

The fact that myosin light chain phosphorylation is the major mechanism initiating smooth muscle contraction raises the question whether this process, rather than the kinetics of the crossbridge cycle, limits the rate of contraction under physiologic conditions. Related questions concern the manner in which myosin light chain phosphorylation may also be regulated by factors other than $[Ca^{2+}]_i$ and how variations in the regulatory mechanism contribute to the phasic or tonic properties (27, 28, 69) of smooth muscle. Activation of permeabilized smooth muscles through photolysis of caged ATP was particularly useful in answering some of these questions, as it was necessary to eliminate the effects of diffusion of ATP, required both as a phosphate donor for myosin phosphorylation and as a substrate of actomyosin ATPase.

The initiation of contraction from rigor, in the presence of maximally activating concentrations of Ca^{2+}-calmodulin, represented the condition in which phosphorylation of myosin LC_{20} was a prerequisite for contraction: force development under these conditions occurred at a rate similar to that observed in intact smooth muscles (Figure 3; 31, 71). In contrast, photolysis of caged ATP could turn on the already phosphorylated crossbridges without

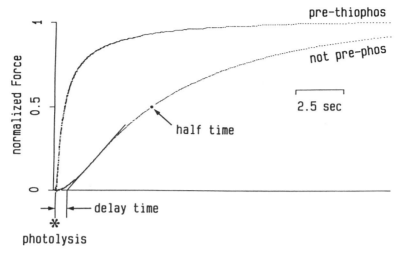

Figure 3   Kinetics of contraction initiated by flash photolysis of caged ATP in trachealis smooth muscle. In the upper trace the myosin light chains were pre-thiophosphorylated with ATPγS. In the lower trace the muscle had not been pre-phosphorylated before photolysis. Each force record was normalized to its amplitude of response. An HPLC analysis revealed that the amount of liberated ATP was (mM) 1.4 in the pre-phosphorylated and 1.5 in the non-phosphorylated muscle. The asterisk indicates the 2 ms pulse of UV light from the flash lamp (data from reference 31).

the intervening steps of phosphorylation in smooth muscles that, prior to photolysis, were thiophosphorylated with ATPγS or maintained with the phosphatase inhibitor okadaic acid (75), in a normally phosphorylated (with ATP) state during rigor. Under the latter conditions, force development was several times faster than when contraction was initiated in non-phosphorylated muscles, which indicates that myosin light chain phosphorylation is usually slower than crossbridge turnover and limits the rate of the force development.

Force development, initiated by photolysis of caged ATP, is faster in phasic than in tonic smooth muscles, regardless of whether the muscles are unphosphorylated or prephosphorylated before releasing ATP (31). These findings suggest that both the regulatory and the contractile apparatus are slower in tonic than in phasic smooth muscles. Differences in the maximum shortening velocity have also been found in intact smooth muscles (55). Whether such differences in mechanical properties are expressions of different myosin isozymes (13, 16), as suggested by recent observations (24), is yet to be established (74).

Mechanisms other than a change in cytoplasmic Ca^{2+} can also regulate smooth muscle contraction. This conclusion is supported by several lines of evidence. The force/Ca^{2+} ratio is higher during agonist-induced than high K^+-induced contractions (7, 26, 52, 57, 61), and the relationship between the $[Ca^{2+}]_i$ transient and force can diverge during a K^+ contraction (27, 28); in tonic smooth muscle, following its initial increase, $[Ca^{2+}_i]$ declines, while force continues to rise over a 30 min period. In contrast, in phasic smooth muscle the phasic decline in force is greater than would be predicted on the basis of the fall in $[Ca^{2+}]_i$ (27, 28). That such phasic fall in force need not be due to changes in $[Ca^{2+}]_i$ is also shown by the similarly phasic response of (ileum) smooth muscle (permeabilized with alpha toxin) to "clamped", submaximally activating concentrations of Ca^{2+} (42, 67). Inhibition of myosin light chain phosphatase converts such phasic contractions to more tonic ones (67). These findings suggest that, at least in some smooth muscles, phasic contractile properties and modulation of Ca^{2+} sensitivity may be the consequence of regulated of myosin light chain phosphatase(s) activity. According to this model, desensitization (27) of the regulatory/contractile apparatus of phasic smooth muscles to Ca^{2+} reflects regulated changes in the myosin light chain kinase/phosphatase activity ratio, most probably because of regulation of phosphatase. While this hypothesis will require considerable testing, it is supported by the very rapid and transient phosphorylation of phasic guinea pig ileum smooth muscle during K^+ contractions (28).

Sensitization to Ca^{2+}, observed in permeabilized smooth muscle, provides further evidence of the existence of regulatory mechanisms other than, or in addition to, changes in $[Ca^{2+}]_i$. Muscarinic (42, 43) and alpha-adrenergic (42, 43, 54) agonists in the presence of GTP or GTPγS and GTPγS itself (Figure 4 and 17, 42, 43) can markedly increase the contractile response to a given submaximal level of Ca^{2+}. In view of the sensitizing action of GTPγS and of the inhibition of the sensitizing effects of agonists and GTPγS by GDPβS, it is probable that sensitization is mediated by G protein (s). The question currently investigated is whether this G protein(s) is identical with or dissimilar to the G_P thought to couple agonists to phospholipase C.

The possible role of kinase C in sensitizing smooth muscle to $[Ca^{2+}]_i$ (e.g. 36, 60; briefly reviewed in 66) remains to be clarified. Evidence supporting such a mechanism is based on the increased Ca^{2+} sensitivity evoked by stimulators of kinase C, phorbol ester, and phosphatydil serine and by its inhibition by H7, a moderately specific kinase C inhibitor. The effects of these compounds on intact smooth muscle are complex and may or may not be associated with changes in cytoplasmic Ca^{2+} (reviewed in 66), due to a variety of effects, including some on receptor-effector coupling (3a, 36). Even in permeabilized smooth muscles, the Ca^{2+}-sensitizing action of phorbol esters has been variably reported to be associated with (56) or uncorrelated with (12) myosin light chain phosphorylation. Interestingly, in the sole study in which the effect of (brain) kinase C on permeabilized muscle

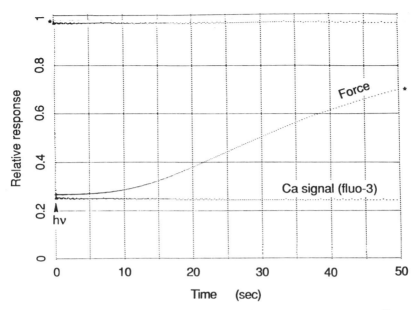

Figure 4 Modulation of force by GTPγS at constant Ca^{2+}. Force development and Ca^{2+} were monitored in a small strip of portal vein, mounted in a 0.3 mm i.d. quartz capillary, permeabilized with alpha-toxin, incubated with 77 μM caged GTPγS, 50 μM Fluo-3, pCa6.3, 10 mM EGTA, for 3 min prior to photolysis with a 2 msec pulse (arrowhead) of 360 nm light from a flash lamp. Note the approximately 10 sec delay before force rises and that there is no detectable change in Ca^{2+}. (From Ref. 72).

was studied, this effect was relaxation (34), rather than contraction. This is consistent with the inhibitory effect of phosphorylation of the kinase C sites on smooth muscle myosin (53). In view of this, the possibility arises that some of the effects of phorbol esters may be unrelated to protein phosphorylation, or that the effects observed are due to phosphorylation of proteins other than myosin. Finally, in view of the very slow time course of contractions induced by phorbol esters, there does not appear to be an urgent need for the use of caged compounds to explore their effects in smooth muscle.

MECHANISM OF CONTRACTION: CROSSBRIDGE CYCLE, COOPERATIVITY, AND FORCE DEVELOPMENT BY DETACHMENT OF NEGATIVELY STRAINED CROSSBRIDGES

Caged compounds have been particularly valuable in relating the biochemical kinetics of myosin ATPase to the mechanical transients of the crossbridge cycle in striated muscle (e.g. 18, 19, reviewed in 25). The rapid and synchronous manner in which photolysis of caged ATP provides the substrate to crossbridges has proven similarly useful in studies of smooth muscle. In addition to revealing the kinetics of crossbridge detachment and attachment into force-developing states, the use of caged ATP also provides unexpected evidence of cooperativity among crossbridges and of force development due to the detachment of negatively strained crossbridges.

Rigor is a state mechanically characterized by increased stiffness, in which myosin crossbridges are bound to actin in the absence of ATP. The existence of rigor in smooth muscle, inferred some 20 years ago (69), was clearly established by demonstrating that crossbridges present on myosin filaments in smooth muscle (65) assume, in the absence of ATP, an "arrowhead" configuration typical of rigor (71). The structural change in rigor, also detected in the X-ray pattern (3), is associated with the appearance of rigor stiffness and force (2, 71).

According to the crossbridge cycle mechanism of contraction, the initial step of the cycle following the binding of ATP to the rigor bridge is the detachment of myosin from actin. This is followed by ATP hydrolysis, attachment, transition to force-generating state(s), product release, and detachment. Photolysis of caged ATP permitted the precise measurement of the rapid phase of detachment and the detection of the somewhat complicated kinetics of relaxation from rigor (71). One of the major conclusions to emerge from this study was that the detachment rate, approximately $10^5 M^{-1} s^{-1}$, was too fast to be rate-limiting the ATPase cycle. Thus in the presence of physiologic, millimolar concentrations of ATP, detachment would occur at a rate of approximately $100 \ s^{-1}$, compared to the total hydrolysis rate of approximately $1-2 \ s^{-1}$ (62). This detachment rate, however, is one order of magnitude slower than in solution ($10^6 M^{-1} s^{-1}$) (46), as it is in striated muscle (18), which suggests a mechanochemical effect (strain dependence) of organized (filamentous) actin and myosin on the chemical cycle. In the presence of Ca^{2+}, the rapid phase of detachment is followed by force development (Figure 5) at a rate determined by the existing state of phosphorylation (see above). Photolysis of caged ATP in the absence of Ca^{2+} revealed a second, slower phase of detachment (Figure 5). Based on analogy with striated muscle (18), it is likely that this slow phase of detachment or bump represents the reattachment of initially detached crossbridges. If so, the biochemical scheme of the crossbridge cycle (25) suggests that the addition of inorganic phosphate (P_i) will drive crossbridges into the detached or more weakly bound (15) states, thus reducing the probability of cooperative reattachment. The addition of P_i to muscles prior to photolysis markedly accelerates relaxation (2) by reducing the slow phase of detachment or bump (71). This and the effect of mechanical manipulations [releasing or restretch-

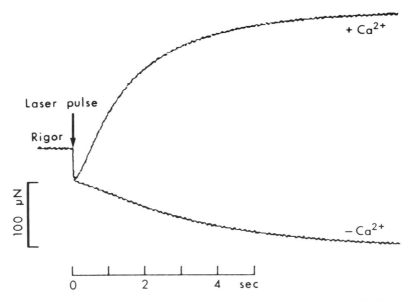

Figure 5   Two superimposed tension transients after liberation of ATP by photolysis of caged ATP in the presence ($+Ca^{2+}$) and absence ($-Ca^{2+}$) of Ca^{2+}. The muscle was stretched by 1% of its length before liberation of ATP. Both transients show a similar initial rapid fall in force caused by the detachment of rigor crossbridges by the released ATP. In the absence of Ca^{2+}, after the rapid detachment, the transient has a complex shape with a plateau of ~400 ms, followed by a slow fall to the relaxed baseline (from reference 71).

ing the muscles prior to photolysis; (71)] support the notion that the slow phase of detachment and the bump, accentuated in prereleased muscles (figure 8 in 71), are due to reattachment of previously detached crossbridges. The fact that crossbridges can reattach in the absence of Ca^{2+} and, consequently, in the absence of myosin light chain phosphorylation, implies the reattachment of nonphosphorylated crossbridges. Cooperativity (82) can support such reattachment and cause contraction in the absence of Ca^{2+}, at ATP concentration lower than the concentration of myosin heads in rigor. Under these conditions, the cooperative effect of rigor bridges facilitates the reattachment of bridges detached by micromolar ATP into force-generating states. Photolysis of micromolar quantities of ATP in smooth muscles in rigor revealed the existence of such cooperative contractions, which could be up to 40% of maximal Ca^{2+}-activated force (71). The use of CTP confirmed that this was not because of myosin being phosphorylated by a Ca^{2+}-insensitive kinase produced as the result of partial proteolysis (35, 80). CTP is a substrate for the myosin ATPase, but is not a phosphate donor in the myosin light chain kinase reaction (11). Nevertheless, in the absence of Ca^{2+}, photolysis of caged CTP, like that of caged ATP, caused bumps during detachment and contractions at micromolar concentrations. Therefore, the evidence for cooperative attachment of crossbridges in smooth muscle appears reasonably strong. Based on these findings and on the similar effects of P_i on the bump and relaxation, we have suggested (71) that the latch state (22) of high force/low phosphorylated myosin LC_{20} ratio may possibly reflect cooperative attachment of dephosphorylated crossbridges; in intact smooth muscle the cooperative action is thought to be mediated not by rigor, but by attached, phosphorylated crossbridges. This hypothesis is also compatible with the length-dependence of force maintenance at low levels of phosphorylation (51). The absence of latch at long ($1.4L_O$) lengths (L_O = optimal length for force development), and presumably reduced filament overlap, could be due to an insufficient number of attached and phosphorylated crossbridges available for cooperativity and/or to negative strain-dependence of cooperative reattachment.

In his 1957 model of contraction, Huxley (32) proposed that crossbridges can bear negative strain: the detachment of negatively strained crossbridges could result in force development (19, 32). If smooth muscles in rigor are prereleased to place negative strain on crossbridges, photolysis of caged ATP causes a very rapid early phase of force development (figure 11 in 71), coinciding with a fall in stiffness. The early, rapid contraction is significantly faster than the attachment rates, and it is thought to reflect force development caused by the detachment of negatively strained crossbridges.

SUMMARY AND CONCLUSION

1. Flash photolysis of caged compounds of phenylephrine, inositol 1, 4, 5 trisphosphate ($InsP_3$), GTPγS, ATP, and CTP has been successfully used to study excitation-contraction coupling, contractile regulation, and contraction in smooth muscle. Major processes explored with this method were (*a*) the delay between agonist-receptor interaction and contraction and between the rise in $InsP_3$, Ca^{2+} release and contraction; (*b*) the effect of myosin light chain phosphorylation on the rate of force development and the respective contributions of phosphorylation and crossbridge kinetics to differences between phasic and tonic smooth muscles; (*c*) the kinetics of the crossbridge cycle. We have also reviewed recent results obtained by other methods and bearing on the mechanisms of pharmacomechanical Ca^{2+} release and modulation of the Ca^{2+} sensitivity of the regulatory/contractile apparatus.

2. The long delay (1.5 s at 22°C) following activation of alpha$_1$-adrenergic receptors through photolysis of caged phenylephrine and the high Q_{10} of this process are consistent with the hypothesis that activation of phospholipase C is the major mechanism of alpha-adrenergic pharmacomechanical Ca^{2+} release.

3. The delay between photolysis of caged InsP$_3$ and Ca^{2+} release is short: 30 ms or less, while the latency of contraction is significant (0.3–0.5 s at 22°C) and similar to the lag between the rise in [Ca^{2+}]$_i$ and force development in intact smooth muscles. The latency of contraction following photolysis of caged ATP in permeabilized muscles in rigor, in the presence of Ca^{2+} and calmodulin, is similar, about 0.2–0.5 s at 22°C.

4. In muscles in which the myosin light chains are maintained in a phosphorylated state during rigor, photolysis of caged ATP initiates contractions with a short delay (10 ms or less). This result and those summarized above (2 and 3) suggest that the major portion of the delay between agonist-receptor interaction and contraction is due to activation of phospholipase C and InsP$_3$ production, and about 0.2–0.5 s of the delay (22°C) can be ascribed to prephosphorylation reactions between Ca^{2+}, calmodulin, and myosin light chain kinase, and/or to mechanical processes, or to the chemical kinetics of two-step reactions.

5. Force development from rigor, initiated by photolysis of caged ATP in the presence of Ca^{2+}-calmodulin, is rate-limited by myosin light chain phosphorylation; it is significantly accelerated if the myosin light chains are already phosphorylated prior to photolysis.

6. The rate of force development is faster in phasic than in tonic smooth muscles, whether contraction is initiated by photolysis of caged ATP in muscles that are unphosphorylated or prephosphorylated. This result suggests that the rate-limiting processes of both the regulatory and of the contractile mechanisms maybe quantitatively different in the two types of smooth muscle.

7. Evidence obtained with Ca^{2+} indicators in intact smooth muscles and in smooth muscles permeabilized by staphylococcal alpha-toxin or beta-escin indicates the existence of mechanisms mediated by G protein(s) that can modulate the Ca^{2+} sensitivity of the regulatory/contractile apparatus. Permeabilization with these methods has also been useful for the introduction of caged compounds into cells in which receptors remain coupled to their effectors. Sensitization of permeabilized smooth muscle to Ca^{2+} by photolysis of caged GTPγS has a very long (10–15 s) delay.

8. The detachment rate of crossbridges from the rigor state, measured following photolysis of caged ATP, is approximately 10^5M^{-1}S^{-1}; this rate is too fast to be rate limiting the crossbridge cycle.

9. A slow component of relaxation following crossbridge detachment, observed following photolysis of either caged ATP or caged CTP, is attributed to reattachment of unphosphorylated crossbridges through cooperativity of the remaining, attached rigor bridges. It is suggested that the state of high force/low phosphorylation observed during tonic force maintenance in intact smooth muscles (latch) may be due to similar reattachment of dephosphorylated cross bridges through the cooperative

action of remaining phosphorylated bridges. The existence of cooperativity in smooth muscles in rigor is revealed through the contractions evoked by photolytic release of micromolar concentrations of caged ATP or caged CTP into smooth muscles in rigor.

10. A very rapid phase of contraction, observed in the absence of Ca^{2+} in smooth muscles that were mechanically released during rigor in order to negatively strain crossbridges, is attributed to force development caused by the detachment of negatively strained bridges.

ACKNOWLEDGMENTS

The authors' research was supported by National Institutes of Health Grant H215835 to the Pennsylvania Muscle Institute. We thank Ms. Ruby Raines and Mrs. Betty Ferguson for preparation of the manuscript and Ms. Mary Alice Spina for illustrations.

Literature Cited

1. Ahnert-Hilger, G., Mach, W., Fohr, K. J., Gratzl, M. 1989. Poration by alpha-toxin and streptolysin O: An approach to analyze intracellular processes. In *Methods Cell Biol.* 31:63–90

2. Arner, A., Goody, R. S., Rapp, G., Ruegg, J. C. 1987. Relaxation of chemically skinned guinea pig taenia coli smooth muscle from rigor by photolytic release of adenosine-5'-triphosphate. *J. Muscle Res. Cell Motil.* 8:377–85

3. Arner, A., Malmqvist, U., Wray, J. S. 1988. X-ray diffraction and electron microscopy of living and skinned recto-coccygeus muscles of the rabbit. In *Sarcomeric and Nonsarcomeric Muscle: Basic and Applied Research Prospects for the 90s*, ed. U. Carraro, pp. 699–704. Padua: Unipress

3a. Baba, K., Baron, C. B., Coburn, R. F. 1989. Phorbol ester effects on coupling mechanisms during cholinergic contraction of swine tracheal smooth muscle. *J. Physiol.* 412:23–42

4. Berridge, M. J. 1988. Inositol lipids and calcium signalling. *Proc. R. Soc. London Ser. B* 234:359–78

5. Bevan, J. A., Verity, M. A. 1966. Post ganglionic sympathetic delay in vascular smooth muscle. *J. Pharmacol. Exp. Ther.* 152:221–30

6. Bohr, D. F., Somlyo, A. P., Sparks, H. V. Jr., eds. 1980. *Handbook of Physiology: The Cardiovascular System*, Vol. II. Bethesda, MD: Am. Physiol. Soc.

7. Bradley, A. B., Morgan, K. G. 1987. Alterations in cytoplasmic calcium sensitivity during porcine coronary artery contractions as detected by aequorin. *J. Physiol.* 385:437–48

8. Breitweiser, G. E., Szabo, G. 1988. Mechanism of muscarinic receptor-induced K^+ channel activation as revealed by hydrolysis-resistant GTP analogues. *J. Gen. Physiol.* 91:469–93

9. Casey, P. J., Gilman, A. G. 1988. G-protein involvement in receptor-effector coupling. *J. Biol. Chem.* 263:2577–80

10. Cassidy, P., Hoar, P. E., Kerrick, W. G. 1979. Irreversible thiophosphorylation and activation of tension in functionally skinned rabbit ileum strips by [^{35}S]ATP S. *J. Biol. Chem.* 254:11148–53

11. Cassidy, P., Kerrick, W. G. L. 1982. Superprecipitation of gizzard actomyosin, and tension in gizzard muscle skinned fibers in the presence of nucleotides other than ATP. *Biochim. Biophys. Acta* 705:63–69

12. Chatterjee, M., Tejada, M. 1986. Phorbol ester-induced contraction in chemically skinned vascular smooth muscle. *Am. J. Physiol.* 251:C356–61

13. Eddinger, T., Murphy, R. A. 1988. Two smooth muscle myosin heavy chains differ in their light meromyosin fragment. *Biochemistry* 27:3807–11

14. Ehrlich, B. E., Watras, J. 1988. Inositol 1, 4, 5-trisphosphate activates a channel from smooth muscle sarcoplasmic reticulum. *Nature* 336:583–86

15. Eisenberg, E., Hill, T. L. 1985. Muscle contraction and free energy transduction in biological systems. *Science* 227:999–1006

16. Erdödi, F., Bárány, M., Bárány, K. 1987. Myosin light chain isoforms and their phosphorylation in arterial smooth muscle. *Circ. Res.* 61:898–903

17. Fujiwara, T., Itoh, T., Kubota, Y., Kuriyama, H. 1989. Effects of guanosine nucleotides on skinned smooth muscle tissue of the rabbit mesenteric artery. *J. Physiol.* 408:535–47

18. Goldman, Y. E., Hibberd, M. G., Trentham, D. R. 1984. Relaxation of rabbit psoas muscle fibers from rigor by photochemical generation of adenosine 5'-triphosphate. *J. Physiol.* 354:577–604

19. Goldman, Y. E., McCray, J. A., Vallette, D. P. 1988. Cross-bridges in rigor fibres of rabbit psoas muscle support negative forces. *J. Physiol.* 398:P72

20. Gurney, A. M., Lester, H. A. 1987. Light-flash physiology with synthetic photosensitive compounds. *Physiol. Rev.* 67:583–617

21. Haeberle, J. R., Hathaway, D. R., DePaoli-Roach, A. A. 1985 Dephosphorylation of myosin by the catalytic subunit of a type-2 phosphatase produces relaxation of chemically skinned uterine smooth muscle. *J. Biol. Chem.* 260:9965–68

22. Hai, C. M., Murphy, R. A. 1988. Cross-bridge phosphorylation and regulation of latch state in smooth muscle. *Am. J. Physiol.* 254 (Cell Physiol.): C99–C106

23. Hartshorne, D. J. 1987. Biochemistry of the contractile process in smooth muscle. In *Physiology of the Gastrointestinal Tract*, ed. L. R. Johnson, pp. 423–82. New York: Raven. 2nd ed.

24. Helper, D. J., Lash, J. A., Hathaway, D. R. 1988. Distribution of isoelectric variants of the 17,000-dalton myosin light chain in mammalian smooth muscle. *J. Biol. Chem.* 263:15748–53

25. Hibberd, M. G., Trentham, D. R. 1986. Relationships between chemical and mechanical events during muscular contraction. *Annu. Rev. Biophys. Biophys. Chem.* 15:119–61

26. Himpens, B., Casteels, R. 1987. Measurement by Quin2 of changes of the intracellular calcium concentration in strips of the rabbit ear artery and of the guinea-pig ileum. *Pflügers Arch.* 408: 32–37

27. Himpens, B., Matthijs, G., Somlyo, A. P. 1989. Desensitization to cytoplasmic Ca^{2+} and Ca^{2+} sensitivities of guinea-pig ileum and rabbit pulmonary artery smooth muscle. *J. Physiol.* 413:489–503

28. Himpens, B., Matthijs, G., Somlyo, A. V., Butler, T., Somlyo, A. P. 1988. Cytoplasmic free calcium, myosin light chain phosphorylation and force in phasic and tonic smooth muscle. *J. Gen. Physiol.* 92:713–29

29. Himpens, B., Somlyo, A. P. 1988. Free calcium and force transients during depolarization and pharmacomechanical coupling in guinea pig smooth muscle. *J. Physiol.* 395:507–29

30. Hoar, P. E., Pato, M., Kerrick, W. G. L. 1985. Myosin light chain phosphatase. Effect on the activation and relaxation of gizzard smooth muscle skinned fibers. *J. Biol. Chem.* 260:8760–64

31. Horiuti, K., Somlyo, A. V., Goldman, Y. E., Somlyo, A. P. 1989. Kinetics of contraction initiated by flash photolysis of caged adenosine trisphosphate in tonic and phasic smooth muscles. *J. Gen. Physiol.* 94:769–81

32. Huxley, A. F. 1957. Muscle structure and theories of contraction. *Prog. Biophys. Biophys. Chem.* 7:255–318

33. Iino, M. 1987. Calcium dependent inositol trisphosphate-induced calcium release in the guinea-pig taenia caeci. *Biochem. Biophys. Res. Commun.* 142: 47–52

34. Inagaki, M., Yokokura, H., Itoh, T., Kanmura, Y., Kuriyama, H., Hidaka, H. 1987. Purified rabbit brain protein kinase C relaxes skinned vascular smooth muscle and phosphorylates myosin light chain. *Arch. Biochem. Biophys.* 254:136–41

35. Itoh, T., Ikebe, M., Kargacin, G. J., Hartshorne, D. J., Kemp, B. E., Fay, F. S. 1989. Effects of modulators of myosin light-chain kinase activity in single smooth muscle cells. *Nature* 338:164–67

36. Itoh, T., Kuboto, Y., Kuriyama, H. 1988. Effects of a phorbol ester on acetylcholine-induced Ca^{2+} mobilization and contraction in the porcine coronary artery. *J. Physiol.* 397:401–19

37. Kamm, K. E., Stull, J. T. 1986. Activation of smooth muscle contraction: relation between myosin phosphorylation and stiffness. *Science* 232:80–82

38. Kamm, K. E., Stull, J. T. 1989. Regulation of smooth muscle contractile elements by second messengers. *Annu. Rev. Physiol.* 51:299–313

39. Kao, J. P. Y., Harootunian, A. T., Tsien, R. Y. 1989. Photochemically generated cytosolic calcium pulses and their detection by Fluo-3. *J. Biol. Chem.* 264:8179–84

40. Kaplan, J. H., Forbush, B. III, Hoffman, J. F. 1978. Rapid photolytic release of adenosine 5'-trisphosphate from a protected analogue: utilization by the Na:K pump of human red blood cell ghosts. *Biochemistry* 17:1929–35

41. Kaplan, J. H., Somlyo, A. P. 1989. Flash photolysis of caged compounds:

new tools for cellular physiology. *Trends Neurosci.* 12:54–59

42. Kitazawa, T., Kobayashi, S., Horiuti, K., Somlyo, A. V., Somlyo, A. P. 1989. Receptor coupled, permeabilized smooth muscle: Role of the phosphatidylinositol cascade, G-proteins and modulation of the contractile response to Ca^{2+}. *J. Biol. Chem.* 264:5339–42

43. Kobayashi, S., Kitazawa, T., Somlyo, A. V., Somlyo, A. P. 1989. Cytosolic heparin inhibits muscarinic and alpha-adrenergic Ca^{2+} release in smooth muscle: Physiological role of inositol 1, 4, 5'-trisphosphate in pharmacomechanical coupling. *J. Biol. Chem.* 264:17997–18004

44. Kobayashi, S., Somlyo, A. P., Somlyo, A. V. 1988. Guanine nucleotide and inositol 1, 4, 5' trisphosphate-induced calcium release in rabbit main pulmonary artery. *J. Physiol.* 403:601–19

45. Kobayashi, S., Somlyo, A. V., Somlyo, A. P. 1988. Heparin inhibits the inositol 1, 4, 5-trisphosphate-dependent, but not the independent, calcium release induced by guanine nucleotide in vascular smooth muscle. *Biochem. Biophys. Res. Commun.* 153:625–31

46. Marston, S. B., Taylor, E. W. 1980. Comparison of the myosin and actomyosin ATPase mechanisms of the four types of vertebrate muscles. *J. Mol. Biol.* 139:573–600

47. McCray, J. A., Trentham, D. R. 1989. Properties and uses of photoreactive caged compounds. *Annu. Rev. Biophys. Biophys. Chem.* 18:239–70

47a. Meyer, T., Holowka, D., Stryer, L. 1988. Highly cooperative opening of calcium channels by inositol 1, 4, 5-trisphosphate. *Science* 240:653–55

48. Miledi, R., Parker, I., Zhu, P. H. 1982. Calcium transients evoked by action potentials in frog twitch muscle fibres. *J. Physiol.* 333:655–79

49. Miller-Hance, W. C., Miller, J. R., Wells, J. N., Stull, J. T., Kamm, K. E. 1988. Biochemical events associated with activation of smooth muscle contraction. *J. Biol. Chem.* 263:13979–82

50. Minta, A., Kao, J. P. Y., Tsien, R. Y. 1989. Fluorescent indicators for cytosolic calcium based on rhodamine and fluorescein chromophores. *J. Biol. Chem.* 264:8171–78

51. Moreland, R. S., Moreland, S., Murphy, R. A. 1988. Dependence of stress on length, Ca^{2+}, and myosin phosphorylation in skinned smooth muscle. *Am. J. Physiol.* 255:C473–78

52. Morgan, J. P., Morgan, K. G. 1984. Stimulus-specific patterns of in-

tracellular calcium levels in smooth muscle of ferret portal vein. *J. Physiol.* 351:155–67

53. Nishikawa, M., Sellers, J. R., Adelstein, R. S., Hidaka, H. 1984. Protein kinase C modulates in vitro phosphorylation of the smooth muscle heavy meromyosin by myosin light chain kinase. *J. Biol. Chem.* 259:8808–14.

54. Nishimura, J., Kolber, M., van Breemen, C. 1988. Norepinephrine and GTPγS increase myofilament Ca^{2+} sensitivity in alpha-toxin permeabilized arterial smooth muscle. *Biochem. Biophys. Res. Commun.* 157:677–683

55. Paul, R. J., Doerman, G., Zeugner, C., Ruegg, J. C. 1983. The dependence of unloaded shortening velocity on Ca^{2+}, calmodulin, and duration of contraction in "chemically skinned" smooth muscle. *Circ. Res.* 53:342–51

56. Rembold, C. M., Murphy, R. A. 1988. $[Ca^{2+}]$-dependent myosin phosphorylation in phorbol diester stimulated smooth muscle contraction. *Am. J. Physiol.* 255:C719–23

57. Rembold, C. M., Murphy, R. A. 1988. Myoplasmic $[Ca^{2+}]$ determines myosin phosphorylation in agonist stimulated swine arterial smooth muscle. *Circ. Res.* 63:593–603

58. Ruegg, J. C. 1986. *Calcium in Muscle Activation: A Comparative Approach,* ed. D. S. Farner, W. Burggren, S. Ishii, K. Johansen, H. Langer, G. Neuweiler, D. J. Randall, 19: New York: Springer-Verlag. 300 pp.

59. Ruegg, J. C., DiSalvo, J., Paul, R. J. 1982. Soluble relaxation factor from vascular smooth muscle: a myosin light chain phosphatase? *Biochem. Biophys. Res. Commun.* 106:1126–33

60. Ruzycky, A. L., Morgan, K. G. 1989. Involvement of the protein-kinase C system in calcium-force relationships in ferret aorta. *Br. J. Pharmacol.* 97:391–400

61. Sato, K., Ozaki, H., Karaki, H. 1988. Changes in cytosolic calcium level in vascular smooth muscle measured simultaneously with contraction using fluorescent calcium indicator fura-2. *J. Pharmacol. Exp. Ther.* 246:294–300

62. Sellers, J. R. 1985. Mechanism of the phosphorylation-dependent regulation of smooth muscle heavy meromyosin. *J. Biol. Chem.* 260:15815–19

63. Siegman, M. J., Somlyo, A. P., Stephens, N. L., eds. 1987. *Progress in Clinical and Biological Research: Regulation and Contraction of Smooth Muscle.* 245:1–507. New York: Liss

64. Smith, J. B., Smith, L. S., Higgins, B.

L. 1985. Temperature and nucleotide dependence of calcium release by myoinositol 1,4,5-trisphosphate in cultured vascular smooth muscle cells. *J. Biol. Chem.* 160:14413–16

65. Somlyo, A. P., Devine, C. E., Somlyo, A. V., Rice, R. V. 1973. Filament organization in vertebrate smooth muscle. *Philos. Trans. R. Soc. London Ser. B* 265:223–96

66. Somlyo, A. P., Himpens, B. 1989. Cell calcium and its regulation in smooth muscle. *FASEB J.* 3:2266–76

67. Somlyo, A. P., Kitazawa, T., Himpens, B., Matthijs, G., Horiuti, K., et al. 1989. Modulation of Ca^{2+}-sensitivity and of the time course of contraction in smooth muscle: A major role of protein phosphatases? *Advances in Protein Phosphatases,* ed. W. Merlevede, J. DiSalvo, 5:181–95. Belgium: Leuven Univ. Press

68. Somlyo, A. P., Somlyo, A. V. 1986. Smooth muscle structure and function. In *The Heart and Cardiovascular System,* ed. H. A. Fozzard, E. Haber, R. B. Jennings, A. M. Katz, H. E. Morgan, 2:845–64. New York: Raven. 915 pp.

69. Somlyo, A. P., Somlyo, A. V. 1968. Vascular smooth muscle: I. Normal structure, pathology, biochemistry, and biophysics. *Pharmacol. Rev.* 20:197–272

70. Somlyo, A. P., Walker, J. W., Goldman, Y. E., Trentham, D. R., Kobayashi, S., et al. 1988. Inositol trisphosphate, calcium and muscle contraction. *Philos. Trans. R. Soc. London Ser. B* 320:399–414

71. Somlyo, A. V., Goldman, Y. E., Fujimori, T., Bond, M., Trentham, D. R., Somlyo, A. P. 1988. Crossbridge kinetics, cooperativity and negatively strained crossbridges in vertebrate smooth muscle: a laser flash photolysis study. *J. Gen. Physiol.* 91:165–92

72. Somlyo, A. V., Kitazawa, T., Horiuti, K., Kobayashi, S., Trentham, D. R., Somlyo, A. P. 1989. Heparin-sensitive inositol trisphosphate signaling and the role of G-Proteins in Ca^{2+}-release and contractile regulation in smooth muscle. In *Frontiers in Smooth Muscle Research—Emil Bozler International Symposium,* ed. N. Sperelakis. New York: Liss. In press

73. Somlyo, A. V., Somlyo, A. P. 1968. Electromechanical and pharmacomechanical coupling in vascular smooth muscle. *J. Pharmacol. Exp. Ther.* 159:129–45

74. Sparrow, M. P., Arner, A., Mohammad, M. A., Hellstrand, P., Ruegg, J. C. 1987. Isoforms of myosin in smooth muscle. See Ref. 63, pp. 67–79

74a. Supattapone, S., Danoff, S. K., Theibert, A., Joseph, S. K., Steiner, J., Snyder, S. H. 1988. Cyclic AMP-dependent phosphorylation of a brain inositol trisphosphate receptor decreases its release of calcium. *Proc. Natl. Acad. Sci. USA* 85:8747–50

75. Takai, A., Bialojan, C., Troschka, M., Ruegg, J. C. 1987. Smooth muscle myosin phosphatase inhibition and force enhancement of black sponge toxin. *FEBS Lett.* 217:81–84

76. van Breemen, C., Saida, K. 1989. Cellular mechanisms regulating $[Ca^{2+}]_i$ smooth muscle. *Annul. Rev. Physiol.* 51:315–29

77. Walker, J. W., Fenney, J., Trentham, D. R. 1989. Photolabile precursors of inositol phosphates. Preparation and properties of 1-(2-nitrophenyl) ethyl esters of myo-inositol 1,4,5-trisphosphate. *Biochemistry* 28:3272–80

78. Walker, J. W., Reid, G. P., Trentham, D. R. 1989. Synthesis and properties of caged compounds. *Methods Enzymol.* 172:288–301

79. Walker, J. W., Somlyo, A. V., Goldman, Y. E., Somlyo, A. P., Trentham, D. R. 1987. Kinetics of smooth and skeletal muscle activation by laser pulse photolysis of caged inositol 1,4,5-trisphosphate. *Nature* 327:249–52

80. Walsh, M. P., Bridenbaugh, R., Hartshorne, D. J., Kerrick, W. G. L. 1982. Phosphorylation-dependent-activated tension in skinned gizzard muscle fibers in the absence of Ca^{2+}. *J. Biol. Chem.* 257:5987–90

81. Ware, B. R., Bruen, K. L. J., Cummings, R. T., Rurukawa, R. H., Krafft, G. A. 1986. In *Applications of Fluorescence in the Biomedical Sciences,* ed. D. L. Taylor, A. A. Wagoner, F. Lanni, R. F. Murphy, R. R. Birge, pp. 141–57. New York: Liss. 658 pp.

82. Weber, A., Murray, J. M. 1973. Molecular control mechanisms in muscle contraction. *Physiol. Rev.* 53:612–73

83. Yagi, S., Becker, P. L., Fay, F. S. 1988. Relationship between force and Ca^{2+} concentration in smooth muscle as revealed by measurements on single cells. *Proc. Natl. Acad. Sci. USA* 85:4109–13

Annu. Rev. Physiol. 1990. 52:875–96

CAGED COMPOUNDS AND STRIATED MUSCLE CONTRACTION

Earl Homsher and Neil C. Millar

Department of Physiology, School of Medicine, and the Jerry Lewis Neuromuscular Research Center, University of California at Los Angeles, Los Angeles, California 90024

KEY WORDS: photorelease, excitation-contraction coupling, actomyosin kinetics, caged calcium, caged nucleotides

INTRODUCTION

This review summarizes recent work using caged compounds for the study of muscular contraction. We focus on what flash photolysis has taught us about the reaction mechanism and regulation of the actomyosin system of the intact fiber lattice, both during force generation and shortening. An excellent series of complementary reviews is available to the interested reader. The reviews of Lester & Nerbonne (71), Gurney & Lester (50), and McCray & Trentham (75) describe the theory, synthesis, photolysis, and use of caged compounds in detail. For those interested in the crossbridge mechanism, the reviews of Hibberd & Trentham (55) and Goldman (42) include many of the caged experiments, and other topics in muscle contraction are covered by the reviews of Cooke (18), Brenner (14), Homsher (58), and Thomas (94).

The development of caged ATP by Kaplan et al (66) led to its first use in the study of muscle contraction in 1982 (43). Progress from 1982 to 1986 was relatively slow for two reasons. First, the synthesis and purification of caged compounds was slow (several weeks) and the yield was low (ca. 25%). Second, the production of a rapid and uniform photolysis of the caged compounds required the use of an expensive (ca. \$40,000) laser. In the past 3–4 years, however, two developments have occurred that should make these techniques available to most experimenters. First was the development of a

875

0066-4278/90-0315-0875\$02.00

simple and rapid (1–3 day) synthesis and purification technique for caged phosphate-containing moieties with high yield (100). Second was the development of a relatively inexpensive flash lamp system (82). This produces ~20–50 mJ in the wavelength range of 320–350 nm in a 500 μs flash, which is sufficient for many studies on striated muscle cells up to 1 cm in length. The general availability of these techniques should expedite progress.

THE ACTOMYOSIN ATPase IN SOLUTION

The reaction model shown in Figure 1 (38) has evolved from both transient and steady-state studies using solution biochemistry of the myosin subfragment 1 (S1) and acto-S1 ATPase. The ATPase pathway for both S1 and acto-S1 involves four basic steps: ATP binding, ATP hydrolysis, phosphate release, and ADP release. This view is an oversimplification, since steps one, three, and four, at least for S1 (95), are known to consist of two steps: the formation of a collision complex and a protein isomerization. The unique feature of the model in Figure 1 is that S1 binds to actin in two steps, first forming attached state I (designated A-M) and then isomerizing to attached state II (designated AM). Evidence for these two attached states comes from measurements of light scattering (which monitors the attachment step from S1 to state I) and of fluorescence of a pyrene label bound to actin (which monitors the isomerization step to state II) in equilibrium and pressure relaxation studies (17, 39). The attachment step is a rapid equilibrium $(k_{+1} > 1000 \ M^{-1}s^{-1}, \ K_I = 10^3\text{-}10^4 \ M^{-1})$, which is relatively independent of the presence of bound nucleotide. The equilibrium constant for the transition from attached state I to attached state II (K_{II}) is sensitive to ionic strength, pressure, and bound nucleotide. Values for these equilibrium constants and for the overall binding constant for actin $[K_{eq} = K_I(1 + K_{II})]$ under different conditions have been measured by Geeves (39) and Eisenberg (90, 91). In the absence of nucleotide or in the presence of ADP or AMPPNP, the equilibrium lies in the direction of attached state II $(K_{eq} = 10^6\text{-}10^8 \ M^{-1}, \ K_{II} = 10\text{-}10^2)$. When the bound nucleotide is ATP, ADP.P_i, or ATP γS, the equilibrium lies in the direction of attached state I $(K_{eq} \ M = 10^3\text{-}10^4 \ M^{-1}, \ K_{II} < 1)$. The predominantly populated states at each stage of the ATPase cycle at 20°C, 0.1 M KCl are indicated by solid boxes in Figure 1, and species that may be significantly populated as well are shown in dashed boxes. As the ATP hydrolysis cycle proceeds, S1 alternates between two states: one (AM) in which S1 is tightly bound, and one (A-M) in which S1 is in equilibrium with actin.

The difference in actin binding constants has led to the unfortunate appellation of "strongly" bound crossbridges for those in attached state II and "weakly" bound crossbridges for those in attached state I. This nomenclature unintentionally carries implications for crossbridge function that are not

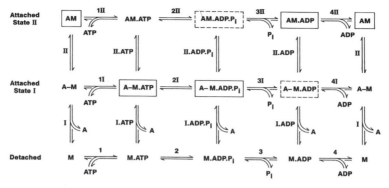

Figure 1   The Acto-S1 ATPase mechanism (based on reference 38). The bottom row shows the ATPase pathway of myosin S1 (*M*) in the absence of actin *(steps labeled 1,2,3, and 4)*. The middle row shows the ATPase pathway of acto-S1 in attached state I *(steps labeled 1I,2I,3I, and 4I)*, and the top row shows the acto-S1 ATPase pathway in attached state II *(steps labeled 1II,2II,3II, and 4II)*. In the vertical direction, actin binding to form attached state I is referred to as step I, and the isomerization to form-attached state II is referred to as step II, with the nucleotide bound to S1 (ATP, ADP, ADP.P$_i$) also indicated. By convention the forward reaction direction is from left to right and from bottom to top. k_{+1II} is the rate of ATP binding to AM and $k_{-I \cdot ATP}$ is the rate of actin release from A-M.ATP.

necessarily true. A better characterization would be that crossbridges whose K_{eq} is $>10^6$ M^{-1} spend a much greater fraction of their lifetime in attached state II than in attached state I or detached, while those whose K_{eq} is $<10^3$ M^{-1} spend a greater share of their time in attached state I or in the detached state.

The equilibrium constant between attached states I and II is sensitive to ionic strength; as ionic strength is increased K_{II} declines markedly, and the fraction of time an S1 molecule spends attached to actin progressively decreases (39). Thus to achieve a high degree of association, solution studies of the acto-S1 ATPase are usually performed under nonphysiologic conditions, at low ionic strength (i.e. 5 mM and usually at 15°C), or by using cross-linked acto-S1. Care must be taken when extrapolating to physiologic conditions. In the absence of actin, S1 hydrolyses ATP very slowly, and at low ionic strength, the turnover number (i.e. k_{cat} = ATPase steady-state rate/total S1 concentration) is 0.05 s^{-1}. This is accelerated at least 100-fold by actin (25); thus for cross-linked acto-S1, K_{cat} = 10 s^{-1} (these values are not significantly different at 0.1 M KCl) (11). The details of the acto-S1 ATPase are as follows:

1. ATP binding to S1 alone is fast and essentially irreversible (k_{+1} = 10^6–10^7 M^{-1}s^{-1}, K_1 = 10^{11} M^{-1}) (95). Acto-S1 exists in attached state II in the absence of nucleotide (K_{eq} = 10^8 M^{-1}) (17, 68). ATP binds to acto-S1

with an apparent association rate constant (k_a) of 2×10^6 $M^{-1}s^{-1}$ and produces a rapid and complete dissociation at 0.1 M ionic strength (to M.ATP), or partial dissociation at low ionic strength and high actin concentrations (to A-M.ATP and M.ATP). The dissociation step itself is a fast equilibrium ($K_{I.ATP} = 10^4$ M^{-1}), and the maximum rate of dissociation is controlled by step II ($K_{II.ATP} = 10^{-3}$, $k_{-I.ATP} \geq 5000s^{-1}$) (76).

2. The ATP hydrolysis step by S1 alone is rapid ($k_{+2} = 140$ s^{-1}) and reversible ($K_2 = 10$) at 0.1 M ionic strength and 20°C (5, 95). This step is very sensitive to temperature and ionic strength, so that at low ionic strength where comparisons with acto-S1 are possible, the values for S1 are $k_{+2} = 19$ s^{-1}, $K_2 = 2.2$ (12). The equivalent values with acto-S1 are $k_{+2} = 50$ s^{-1}, $K_2 = 1.5$, and $k_{+2I} = 40$ s^{-1}, $K_{2I} = 0.4$ for non-cross-linked acto-S1 (84) and $k_{+2I} = 23$ s^{-1}, $K_{2I} = 1.3$ for cross-linked acto-S1 (11). Thus the ATP hydrolysis step appears to be similar whether it occurs on an attached or a detached state. The hydrolysis step on AM.ATP (k_{+2II}) has not been measured, but should not have significant flux since the intermediate AM.ATP has a very short lifetime (76). Both M.ATP and M.ADP.P$_i$ are in rapid equilibrium with their actin-bound counterparts ($K_{I.ATP} = K_{I.ADP.P_i} = 10^4$ M^{-1}), so these states can attach and detach many times on the time scale of an ATP turnover.

3. The equilibrium constant of the phosphate release step lies to the right for both S1 and acto-S1. For S1, $K_3 = 0.1$ M (95), and although it has not been measured directly for acto-S1, detailed balance indicates that the dissociation constant for phosphate from A-M.ADP.P$_i$ ($K_d = K_{II.ADP.Pi}.K_{3II}$ or $K_{3I}.K_{II.ADP}$) is >100 M (38). For S1 alone, phosphate release (or more properly the isomerization preceding phosphate release) is the rate-limiting step of the ATPase cycle ($k_{+3} = 0.05$ s^{-1}); thus in the absence of actin, M.ADP.P$_i$ is the predominant steady-state complex (95). Although the rate of phosphate release from acto-S1 has not been measured and the rate-limiting step of the acto-S1 ATPase is not known with certainty, it appears (at least at low ionic strength) that the hydrolysis step is rate limiting, and therefore the rate constant of P$_i$ release from A-M.ADP.P$_i$ must be > 50 s^{-1} (11, 84).

4. The ^{32}P-exchange experiments of Sleep & Hutton (88) first indicated that there were two acto-S1.ADP states. The one formed on adding ADP to acto-S1 ($K_d = 200$ μM) is unable to bind P$_i$, while there is a second state formed during ATP turnover that can bind P$_i$. These two states may correspond respectively to AM.ADP and A-MADP in Figure 1 (although the binding constants of P$_i$ to these states are not known), or possibly the state formed by adding ADP to acto-S1 may not be part of the ATPase pathway at all. The rate of ADP release from S1 alone (k_{+4}) is 2 s^{-1} while the rates with acto-S1 are >500 s^{-1} from AM.ADP (k_{+4II}) and 2 s^{-1} from

A-M.ADP (k_{+4I}) (37, 87). Thus actin accelerates ADP release from attached state II, but not attached state I. As the products are released, the binding between actin and S1 becomes progressively tighter $[K_{II.ADP.P_i}<0.1, K_{II.ADP} = 100,$ and $K_{II} = 10^4$ (37, 39)].

THE ACTOMYOSIN ATPase IN FIBERS

Transient Kinetic Studies in Muscle Fibers

A sine qua non of the transient kinetic approach is the ability to rapidly (ca. 1 ms) and completely mix the reactants while monitoring the subsequent time course of markers of the reaction. Direct application of transient kinetic techniques to single demembranated fibers is limited because the muscle fiber diameter (50–100 μm) precludes rapid mixing of the fiber lattice contents with the bathing solution by diffusion in times less than several hundred milliseconds. This problem is overcome by allowing an inert precursor (the caged compound) to diffuse into the fiber and then suddenly releasing the active molecule (e.g. ATP or Ca^{2+}) throughout the fiber with an intense pulse of near UV light. The time course of a variety of mechanical, structural, or chemical parameters can then be measured and a reaction mechanism inferred. The transient kinetic studies of S1 and acto-S1 have furnished an experimental blueprint to follow in fiber work.

Rapid photogeneration of the reactant is essential to the success of this approach, and Table 1 lists some of the caged compounds used in the study of muscle with their half-times for product photogeneration. The rate of photorelease of nucleotides is sensitive to pH [a fall of 1 pH unit increases the rate of ATP generation by about tenfold (75)], temperature [the rate of ATP release has a Q_{10} of 2.2 (6)], and ionic strength [the rate of ATP release declines 10% for a 100 mM rise in ionic strength (75)]. The photolysis reaction also generates protons (therefore the solution should be heavily buffered) and the leaving group, nitrosoacetophenone. The nitrosoacetophenone reacts with -SH groups (ca. $3.5 \times 10^3 \ M^{-1}s^{-1}$) so ca. 10 mM DTT or glutathione is required to protect the SH groups of proteins (66, 75, 100). Despite reports that caged ATP is inert (239, 74), recent evidence indicates that caged ATP can bind to myosin (21a). If this is true, then the dissociation of caged ATP from the protein could limit the rate of photolytic product (ATP) binding to the protein, and the rate of the measured reaction would be underestimated.

Two fundamental questions remain about contracting muscle: (1) Is the solution ATPase mechanism the same as that occurring in a contracting fiber? One might expect the mechanism to be different since fibers contain a specific geometric arrangement of the contractile proteins in a fiber lattice, together with other regulatory and structural proteins. This means that reactions that are second order in solution may be first order in the fiber (57). (2) Do

Table 1 Halftimes for photolysis of caged compounds

Caged compound	Product	$t_{1/2}$ (halftime in ms)*
Caged ATP	ATP	8.00[a]
Caged ADP	ADP	8.70[b]
Caged AMP	AMP	3.50[a]
Caged P_i	P_i	<0.01[a]
S-caged ATPγS	ATPγS	20.00[a]
O-caged ATPγS	ATPγS	7.00[a]
Caged IP_3	IP_3	2.50–4.00[c]
DM-nitrophen	Ca^{2+}	0.15[d]
Nitr-5	Ca^{2+}	0.20[e]
Caged BAPTA	BAPTA	<1.00[f]

*conditions: ca. 20°C, pH7.1.
[a]Data from reference 100; [b]pH7.6., data from J. McCray, personal communication; [c]data from reference 99; [d]data from reference 65; [e]data from reference 96; [f]data from reference 28.

mechanical constraints (force or displacement) modify specific reaction rate constants? The reasons for believing that muscle shortening or lengthening affects rate constants include the following observations: (*a*) muscle force and stiffness are functions of muscle shortening velocity (35, 64, 103); (*b*) the rates of enthalpy production (heat + work) and ATP hydrolysis of the muscle vary with shortening velocity (58, 103); (*c*) the rate of ATP hydrolysis, force, and shortening velocity are modulated by calcium concentration, and calcium binding to troponin is modulated by the number of crossbridges attached to the thin filament (13, 14, 63, 67, 69).

In addition to these observations, thermodynamic considerations indicate that the rate constants of force-exerting step(s) must be affected by strain (57). The free energy content of a nonforce-producing crossbridge (whether detached or weakly attached) is independent of strain. On the other hand, a crossbridge that is generating force is strained, and its free energy content will be greater the more strained it is. This means that the change in free energy (Δ G) in the transition from the nonforce-producing state to the force-producing state will depend on strain and with it the K_{eq} for the transition. Specifically, if strain is increased (by imposing a load on a fiber), then the force-generating reaction will tend to be driven backwards, and K_{eq} will decrease. If strain is decreased (by allowing the fiber to shorten), then K_{eq} will increase. A change in the equilibrium constant must be reflected in changes in either or both the forward and reverse rate constants (since $K_{eq} = k_+/k_-$). Furthermore, since the periodicity of actin and myosin binding sites on the filaments differ, a fiber will contain crossbridges under a range of strains and therefore with a range of rate constants for the force-producing steps. Thus any measurement of a force-generating rate constant made in a fiber will represent some weighted average with contributions of different rates from different crossbridge strains. This situation is fundamentally different from the situation in solution where all S1 molecules can be considered identical (under zero strain).

ATP Binding and Crossbridge Detachment

The initial experiments performed on this topic were those of Goldman & his colleagues (43–45). The experiment begins with a demembranated muscle fiber equilibrated in a rigor solution containing caged ATP (pCa >8 at 20°C). Muscle fiber force and stiffness are continuously monitored, and following the photogeneration of 500 μM ATP, muscle force falls as seen in Figure 2 *(left)*. There are two phases to the tension change. The first phase lasts 10–30 ms and depends on the ATP concentration and on the initial rigor tension (varied by stretching or releasing the fiber immediately before the flash). At high initial tensions the force falls rapidly during this phase, while at lower initial tensions the force remains constant or even increases. This is followed by a second phase in which tension falls to zero over several hundred milliseconds. The rate of the second phase is independent of initial tension and ATP concentration. In-phase high frequency stiffness, which is roughly proportional to the number of attached crossbridges, declines monotonically following photogeneration of ATP in the absence of calcium.

Similar measurements have been made in the presence of Ca^{2+} (pCa 4.5) with the results shown in Figure 2 *(right)*. In this case, during the first phase force falls or remains the same, and in the second phase force increases until

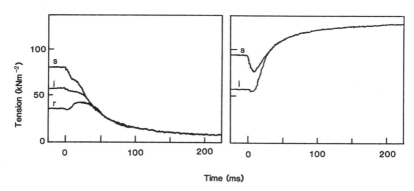

Figure 2   Tension transients initiated by photolysis of caged ATP. A single glycerinated rabbit psoas fiber was initially in rigor in a solution containing 5 mM caged ATP at 20°C, pH7.1, 200 mM ionic strength with pCa 9 *(left)* or pCa 4.5 *(right)*. At time zero a 30 mJ laser flash released about 500 μM ATP. The records are labeled *i* (isometric), *s* (1% prestretch 0.5 s before the flash), and *r* (1% release 0.5 s before the flash).

full isometric force is developed. The initial phase is similar in duration to that in the absence of calcium, and the rate force generation in the second phase is 80–100 s^{-1} at 20°C. As in the absence of Ca^{2+}, the initial phase is dependent on [ATP] while the second phase is not. In-phase stiffness declines as it does in the absence of calcium, but in this case it is balanced by a rise in out-of-phase (or quadrature stiffness), which is taken as indicating the number of attached and cycling crossbridges (44, 45).

Goldman et al (45) have shown that the behavior in Figure 2 can be explained by a model in which there is cooperative crossbridge binding to the thin filament. After ATP generation, crossbridges detach but can then immediately reattach and proceed to generate force even in the absence of Ca^{2+} because the thin filament is still switched on by the remaining attached crossbridges (13). It is assumed that crossbridges will always reattach to the nearest actin; thus there will be an increase in tension if the initial tension was low, or a decrease in tension if the initial tension was high. The mechanism of the second phase in the absence of calcium is complex, but probably includes crossbridges detaching by the reversal of the force-generating step as well as others continuing through the ATPase cycle before detaching. Modeling yields an apparent ATP binding constant to rigor crossbridges of 10^5–10^6 M^{-1}s^{-1}, in good agreement with the solution biochemical results. Similar behavior has been observed in muscle fibers from frog (32), rabbit soleus (105), insect (80, 81, 83, 104), and in cardiac muscle (8) and smooth muscle (89).

The interpretation above is supported by X-ray diffraction, birefringence, and ATP analogue studies at pCa>8. Poole et al (81) find that the intensity of the 1,1 equatorial reflections in rabbit psoas fibers shows a 60–70% decline in the first 5–10 ms following caged ATP photolysis. This is then followed by slow decline in intensity, like the slow decline in force. If the intensity of the equatorials is proportional to the number of attached crossbridges (14), then the rate of the fast phase yields an apparent ATP binding constant of 10^6 M^{-1}s^{-1}, and the amplitude of the slow phase suggests that 30–40% of the rigor crossbridges reattach after ATP binding. Poole et al (81) also find that the rate of the equatorial signal change with soleus fibers is exactly the same as with psoas, although the tension changes are much slower. They conclude that the rate of ATP binding and crossbridge detachment in these two fiber types is the same, in agreement with solution data (87).

Measurement of muscle fiber birefringence (which increases on crossbridges attachment to the thin filament) also shows (following ATP photogeneration in a rigor fiber) a fast initial decrease ($t_{1/2} = 10$–20 ms at 15°C) followed by a slower decrease ($t_{1/2} = 200$–400 ms) that parallels force decline (30, 62). In fibers whose troponin C (TnC) is dansylated, the TnC fluorescence is proportional to the extent to which the fiber is activated, either by Ca^{2+} or rigor linkages. Following photogeneration of ATP in fibers in rigor, the fluorescence signal decays as a single phase at a rate identical to the slow phase of tension decline (52). Finally, Dantzig et al (24) have examined the rate of crossbridge detachment following the photolysis of caged ATPγS. They find that, as in solution biochemistry studies (49, 77), the second order rate constant for nucleotide binding and crossbridge dissociation produced by ATPγS is about five times slower than that produced by ATP.

Thus available evidence is consistent with the conclusions that (*a*) in the fiber ATP binds rapidly to the crossbridge and produces crossbridge detachment; (*b*) this detachment is much faster than the turnover number and thus is not rate limiting; and (*c*) a cooperative mechanism allows transient force generation even in the absence of Ca^{2+}.

ATP Hydrolysis in the Fiber Lattice

Like the experiments on crossbridge dissociation in the fiber, measurements of the rate and equilibrium constants for the ATP cleavage step use an approach analogous to that of solution biochemistry. For this, Ferenczi et al (29) incubated muscle fibers in a caged ^{3}H-ATP solution, flashed the fibers and, at various times following photolysis, freeze-clamped the fibers and measured the amount of ATP, ADP, AMP, and caged ATP in the fiber extract. In these and subsequent experiments (8, 27, 31), fibers were flashed while suspended in air so that evaporative cooling of the fiber reduced the temperature to ~10–12°C (27). These "flash and smash" studies show the following salient features:

1. ATP splitting occurs in a biphasic fashion: a rapid (ca. 60 s^{-1} at 10°C) ATP hydrolysis (the P_i burst) followed by a slower steady-state rate that gives a turnover number of <0.1 s^{-1} at pCa >8 and 1.9 s^{-1} at pCa 4.5. This turnover number at pCa 4.5 is similar to that measured using other techniques and less than that of the fully actin-activated S1 ATPase (42). The rate of the P_i burst is greater than the rate of force rise in the presence of calcium (ca. 24 s^{-1} at 10°C, pCa 4.5) or the rate of force decline in the absence of calcium (ca. 10 s^{-1} at 10°C, pCa8), which indicates that the ATP hydrolysis step precedes crossbridge attachment. Further, since the turnover number (1.9 s^{-1}) is less than the rate of crossbridge attachment, the rate-limiting step must occur after crossbridge attachment. It is not clear whether there is a real difference between this and cross-linked acto-S1 in solution (where there is no P_i burst and the rate-limiting step is probably ATP cleavage), since the fiber experiment was performed at 0.2 M ionic strength, and the in vitro measurements have only been made at low ionic strength (11). The cleavage step is very sensitive to ionic

strength, and the rate-limiting step may be different in a solution (or gel) of acto-S1 at 0.2 M ionic strength.

2. The P_i burst size is dependent on the conditions of the measurement. (*a*) In the absence of myofilament overlap (sarcomere length >3.6 μm), the amplitude of the P_i burst (0.7 mol P_i/mol S1) is consistent with that observed using S1 (5, 72). (*b*) At full filament overlap in the absence of Ca^{2+} (pCa >8), the burst size increases to 1.1 mol P_i/mol S1. This increase is explained by the cooperativity hypothesis of Goldman et al (45). Because a fraction of crossbridges can reattach and exert force prior to complete deactivation of the thin filaments, some of the reattached S1 molecules can pass through a complete actin-activated ATP hydrolysis cycle, in addition to the initial P_i burst. (*c*) In the presence of Ca^{2+} at full overlap, the burst size increases to ~ 1.3 mol P_i/mol S1. This increase may be the result of work performed during the internal shortening that occurs during force development. The amount of work performed during the force development equals ca. 2–4 mJ/g of muscle (103). Thus an addition-al ATP hydrolysis will occur amounting to 0.4–0.8 mol P_i/mol S1 beyond the P_i burst at zero overlap (0.7 mol P_i/mol S1).

3. The equilibrium constant for ATP hydrolysis has been measured by photogeneration of sub-stoichiometric amounts of ^{3}H-ATP in the fiber (^{3}H-ATP $<$ the fiber S1 content, 200 μM). The measured ratio of ^{3}H-ADP/[3]H.ATP several hundred milliseconds after the flash will correspond to k_{+2}/k_{-2}. Ferenczi & Spencer (31) found this ratio was ca. 6. As $k_{+2}+k_{-2}$ was 60 s^{-1}, they concluded that $k_{+2} = 50$ s^{-1} and k_{-2} was 10 s^{-1}. Using a cold chase technique, Ferenczi (27) has also estimated the rate of ATP release (k_{-1}) from crossbridges (M.ATP, A-M.ATP, and AM.ATP) as 13 s^{-1}.The nature of the assumptions made in this type of experiment (complete binding of ^{3}H-ATP and the absence of significant product release) overestimates the rate. Nevertheless, this rate constant is in line with the solution studies of acto-S1 (41).

Phosphate Release

Thus far we have seen that the ATP binding, crossbridge detachment, and ATP hydrolysis steps in fibers are similar to those in solution. The phosphate release step, however, is clearly different. The addition of inorganic phosphate to fibers is known to reduce isometric force and stiffness, and the dependence of this effect upon P_i concentration gives a dissociation constant (K_d) for P_i of ~ 10 mM (19). This is 10^4 times tighter than estimates of K_d in solution (100 M), and suggests that in fibers at physiologic P_i concentrations this step is close to equilibrium. Other steady-state studies have shown that P_i does not significantly reduce maximal shortening velocity (19) and only mildly depresses the steady-state rate of ATP hydrolysis in isometrically contracting muscle fibers (67, 102). Further, ^{18}O exchange experiments indicate that P_i binds to the AM.ADP crossbridge (102).

The first transient kinetic experiments relating to P_i release were those of Hibberd et al (54), who repeated the caged ATP experiments described above, but in the presence of physiologic concentrations of inorganic P_i (0–25 mM). They found that the presence of P_i had little effect on the initial crossbridge detachment (i.e. the initial convergence of force), but in the absence of Ca^{2+}, P_i markedly accelerated the final relaxation rate (from 20 s^{-1} to 60 s^{-1} in 10 mM P_i), and in the presence of Ca^{2+} it accelerated the rate of force production (from 80 s^{-1} to 140 s^{-1} in 10 mM P_i). To explain these results Hibberd et al proposed that force production accompanies P_i release. This means that the observed rate of force production is given by the sum of the forward and reverse rate constants for P_i release ($k_+ + k_-[P_i]$), and the extent of force production will be governed by the equilibrium constant for P_i release. Thus in the presence of Ca^{2+}, as $[P_i]$ increases the rate of force development will increase, but because the equilibrium is shifted to the left, total isometric force will decline. In the absence of Ca^{2+}, $[P_i]$ accelerates the second (slow) rate of force decline by accelerating the reversal of the force generating step. This hypothesis is consistent with the observed rates of force decline and rise following ATP photogeneration, and the reduction in isometric force as $[P_i]$ rises (44, 45).

A direct transient kinetic technique for studying the phosphate release step involves the use of caged phosphate. This approach is an example of a perturbation technique in which a system is first allowed to come to a steady-state and is then suddenly perturbed. The approach to the new steady-state, or the return to the pre-existing steady-state, is observed and analyzed by methods analogous to those used in solution relaxation studies (51). The perturbation technique is also the basis for the classic studies of Ford et al (very rapid changes in muscle length) (34–36), as well as the more recent temperature jump (47) and pressure jump studies (40) on contracting fibers. In the caged P_i experiments a muscle fiber is activated in a solution containing caged P_i and allowed to reach a steady-state isometric force, whereupon P_i is rapidly photogenerated within the fiber lattice. This sudden increase in P_i produces an exponential decline in force as shown in Figure 3. Analyses of the P_i-induced decline in force (the "P_i transient") have led to the following observations and conclusions:

1. Control experiments have shown that the tension decline is not evoked by photolysis of caged ATP or caged AMP (70) and that the amplitude of the P_i transient is dependent on sarcomere overlap, but its rate is not. The effect is therefore specifically due to P_i binding to crossbridges (22).
2. The rate and extent of force decline is paralleled by a similar decline in

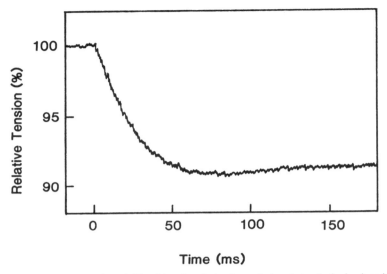

Figure 3 Tension transients initiated by photolysis of caged phosphate. A single glycerinated rabbit psoas fiber was contracting isometrically in a solution containing 5 mM caged P_i at 10°C, pH7.1, 200 mM ionic strength, pCa4.5. At time zero a 50 mJ laser flash released about 1 mM P_i.

muscle stiffness (21), which suggests that the decline in force is associated with crossbridge detachment.

3. The rate at which force declines with $\sim$ 1mM P_i is 30 s^{-1} at 10°C and $\sim$120 s^{-1} at 20°C (21, 22, 59; J. Dantzig et al, in preparation). These rates are in good agreement with the data and interpretation of Hibberd et al (54). A comparable though slower decline in force has been observed in rabbit slow fibers (60a).

4. The rate of the P_i transient increases as $[P_i]$ increases. The increase is not linear, but approaches an asymptote. This suggests that phosphate release is a two-step process, an initial protein isomerization step, producing force, that is followed by the release of P_i (J. Dantzig et al, in preparation).

5. The rate of the P_i transient increases with shortening velocity (59). In these experiments a rabbit psoas muscle fiber is fully activated and then allowed to shorten at a fixed velocity. During isovelocity shortening, force declines to a steady-state value, at which point P_i is photogenerated in the fiber lattice. Such experiments (at 10°C) show that the rate of the P_i transient increases linearly with shortening velocity from 30 s^{-1} (isometric) to 96 s^{-1} at 15% of V_{max}. Extrapolation to V_{max} suggests that the P_i transient rate would be ca. 500 s^{-1}. These data indicate that in a muscle fiber, the P_i release step is highly strain-dependent. Thermodynamics indicate that as the strain on the crossbridge falls (as in shortening) K_{eq} must rise, either by

an increase in the rate of the force-generating step or a fall in the rate of reversal of the force step. Since the rate of the P_i transient increases during shortening, the rate of the force-generating step probably increases during shortening.

These data, therefore, strongly support the idea that the production of force by the muscle is intimately related to the P_i release step.

ADP Release

Following force generation there must be a step (or steps) that controls the lifetime of the attached crossbridge, and the rate of this step must depend on whether or not the muscle is shortening. In a fiber contracting isometrically, the lifetime of the attached state should be long to minimize the ATP consumption. If the muscle is shortening, however, the lifetime must be reduced, otherwise the attached crossbridges would inhibit shortening and power output. In a muscle shortening near V_{max}, geometric constraints suggest that crossbridges remain attached for 1–2 ms (93). In solution it has been shown that the rate of ADP release from attached state I is slow (2 s^{-1}), but from state II is fast (>500 s^{-1}; 37). This is consistent with the observation by Siemankowski et al (87) that the rate of ADP dissociation from acto-S1 in solution (AM.ADP in Figure 1) is correlated with the maximum shortening velocity of muscles over a wide range of velocities.

Once again the caged ATP experiments provide a basis for studying the effect of ADP in fibers. Goldman's laboratory (20, 23) has shown that the initial phase of the force decline from rigor tension following photogeneration of ATP (both in the presence and absence of Ca^{2+}) is substantially slowed by the presence of 100 μM ADP, from ~60 s^{-1} to 30 s^{-1} (55). Thus ATP binding and crossbridge detachment are affected by ADP dissociation and rebinding, but the conditions of this experiment do not permit an estimate of the rates. However, Ferenczi et al (29) found that the presence of 2 mM ADP in a fiber initially in rigor did not greatly affect the rate of ATP cleavage following its photogeneration from caged ATP; thus the rate of ADP dissociation must be >20 s^{-1}. When there was no filament overlap, the same authors reported that the rate of ATP cleavage was reduced to ~13 s^{-1}, so the rate of ADP release from a detached crossbridge is slow.

When ADP is photogenerated in muscle fibers in rigor, the rigor force is reduced at a rate, and to an extent, that is dependent on ADP concentration (92). At saturating concentrations of ADP ($K_d = 45$ μM), the rigor force is reduced by 15%. In perturbation experiments in which ADP was photogenerated during isometric contraction, force rose at a rate of 10 s^{-1} and was independent of ADP concentration (70). This behavior can be explained by

ADP binding to rigor crossbridges to form a force-generating state that is not part of the usual ATPase cycle.

A more promising approach for studing the kinetics of ADP release in contracting fibers is the use of the fluorescent ATP analogue 3' (2')-O-(N-methyl) anthraniloyl-ATP (Mant-ATP). Mant-ATP is hydrolyzed in a fashion similar to ATP and supports force development and shortening. Its fluorescence increases on binding to myosin; thus by monitoring fiber fluorescence, ADP release can be monitored. Ferenczi et al (33) have shown that following photogeneration of 500 μM ATP in a rigor fiber containing Mant-ADP, both tension and fluorescence declined at a slow rate (1.8 s^{-1}), similar to the slow rate seen in solution.

These studies on ADP release do not yet form a clear pattern, and more studies will be necessary to properly characterize this important step.

EXCITATION CONTRACTION COUPLING

We have seen that a fiber can be activated from rigor by photogeneration of ATP, but this is a different process from physiologic activation of a relaxed living fiber. The former involves ATP binding to rigor crossbridges followed by ATP cleavage and then force generation, while the latter involves release of Ca^{2+} from the sacroplasmic reticulum (SR), binding of Ca^{2+} to troponin on the thin filament, and movement of tropomyosin before force can be generated. In addition to the involvement of different biochemical steps, the two methods of activation are associated with different experimental problems. Activation of relaxed fibers can be very non-uniform and yield slow rates of force rise because of compliance and internal shortening; whereas activation of a fiber from rigor may tend to produce a faster rate of force rise because the fiber is much stiffer prior to force development.

Calcium Regulation of Contraction

According to the steric blocking model, tropomyosin (Tm) blocks the myosin binding site on actin, and calcium binding to troponin (Tn) relieves this blocking (53, 61). Work in Eisenberg's group (15, 16), however, suggests that in regulated acto-S1 in solution and in glycerinated muscle fibers at low ionic strength, calcium regulates the ATPase and the rate of force production, respectively, without affecting actomyosin association. They concluded that Ca^{2+}/Tn/Tm does not control crossbridge attachment, but rather regulates the weak to strong force generating transition [corresponding to P_i release in the model of Stein et al (25, 90)]. This second hypothesis is really a refinement of the first, since tropomyosin (in the absence of Ca^{2+}) permits weak binding (perhaps a single point of attachment) (15), but blocks the structural change that leads to both accelerated product release and tight binding (perhaps more than one point of attachment). This is emphasized by studies that show that when a relaxed (pCa 9) fiber in ATPγS is suddenly exposed to a solution at pCa 4.5, in-phase stiffness rises, but no force is developed (24).

The predominant intermediates in relaxed muscle are M.ADP.P_i and A-M.ADP.P_i in rapid equilibrium. Figure 1 indicates that following Ca^{2+} activation the force-generating transition to AM.ADP can occur by two pathways, each composed of two steps. Ca^{2+} could potentially regulate either the state I to state II isomerization, or P_i release itself. Preliminary studies with caged P_i (60) indicate that the P_i transient rate is independent of $[Ca^{2+}]$, which suggests that calcium regulates the state I to state II transition. These data alone are not yet sufficiently complete to identify the regulatory step, however.

Another way to study Ca^{2+} regulation is to activate a relaxed muscle by photolysis of caged calcium. Two forms of caged calcium are currently available, both based on calcium chelators whose affinity for calcium is reduced by photolysis. The first developed was nitr-5, a BAPTA derivative, which is highly specific for Ca^{2+} and whose K_A for calcium (6.7×10^6 M^{-1}) decreases 40-fold on photolysis (96). The second is DM-nitrophen, an analogue of EDTA, whose K_a (5×10^8 M^{-1}) decreases by a factor of 10^5 on photolysis; thus it releases much more Ca^{2+} for a given amount of light energy than nitr-5. DM-nitrophen also binds Mg^{2+} (K_a $4 \times 10^5 M^{-1}$) (65), however, which necessitates altering the solution's Mg^{2+} content, and this in turn can affect physiologic function.

In the first study of muscle activation using caged calcium, calcium was photogenerated from nitr-5 in a relaxed frog skeletal muscle fiber (5 mM ATP, pCa>8, 13°C). Force rose with a $t_{1/2}$ of 40 ms, which is similar to that seen in living frog sartorius muscles (2, 3). When frog fibers were activated from rigor at pCa 4 by the photogeneration of ATP, or from rigor at pCa 8 by the simultaneous photogeneration of ATP and Ca^{2+}, force rose with a $t_{1/2}$ of about 20 ms. Ashley et al (3) concluded that the longer time required for force generation following calcium photogeneration was a consequence of the time needed to activate the thin filament by calcium binding or by conformational changes in the troponin-tropomyosin complex. Similar observations and conclusions were made using rabbit muscle fibers (4) at 15°C.

Different observations have been made using DM-nitrophen in glycerinated rabbit fibers. In this case, at 20–25°C, the rate of force rise following Ca^{2+} liberation in relaxed fibers (pCa>7, $t_{1/2} = 10$–22 ms) is slightly faster than that following ATP liberation in rigor fibers (pCa 4, $t_{1/2} = 15$–22 ms) (1, 7, 46, 79). A 1–2 ms lag precedes the rise in force following calcium release, while the lag is somewhat longer (3–5 ms) following photogeneration of ATP. At 10–12°C these differences are clearer: the lag with ATP (25 ms) is much longer than that with Ca^{2+} (2 ms), and the rate of tension rise with ATP ($t_{1/2}$

= 60 ms) is two times slower than with Ca^{2+} ($t_{1/2}$ = 25 ms) (79). The longer lag with ATP is related to its slower photogeneration, but at 10°C it may also reflect the temperature sensitivity of the ATP hydrolysis step, which is bypassed using caged Ca^{2+}. These data suggest that the differences reported in Ashley et al (2–4) are less related to processes occurring at the troponin-tropomyosin complex and more related to technical differences in the experiments.

Other signals have been used to identify the sequence of events leading to force generation. Both stiffness and X-ray diffraction measurements following muscle activation by calcium photogeneration from DM-nitrophen indicate that crossbridge attachment precedes tension development. At 22°C muscle fiber stiffness (attachment of crossbridges) leads force generation by ~5 ms (1, 7). At 20°C, Poole et al (79) find that the rate of the 1,1 equatorial signal ($t_{1/2}$ = 10–15 ms) is slightly faster than the rate of tension rise ($t_{1/2}$ = 15–20 ms). At 10°C the halftime of the 1,1 equatorial signal is again 10–15 ms while the halftime of the tension rise has increased to 30–40 ms. The change in equatorial reflections is indicative of a shift of crossbridge mass away from the thick filament that typically accompanies activation of the muscle (18, 61) and appears to monitor the initial crossbridge attachment process into nonforce-generating states. Calcium binding to troponin has been measured using fluorescently labeled troponin to monitor the changes in absorption dichroism that report calcium binding (1). Following photogeneration of calcium from DM-nitrophen at 22°C, the increase in absorption dichroism is complete 10 ms after the flash, meaning that calcium binding to troponin is complete before tension has risen to half its maximum value.

Taken together these data indicate that calcium binding and troponin-tropomyosin conformational changes are not rate-limiting steps in the development of force, and they suggest the following sequence of events at 20°C: calcium photogeneration ($t_{1/2}$ = 0.15 ms), calcium binding to troponin ($t_{1/2}$ < 2 ms), crossbridge attachment measured by stiffness or X-ray diffraction ($t_{1/2}$ = 6–15 ms), and tension development ($t_{1/2}$ = 11–22 ms).

Control of Calcium Release

The mechanism by which t-tubule depolarization induces release of Ca^{2+} from the terminal cisternae of the sarcoplasmic reticulum (SR) has been a mystery for years. Both electrical (73, 86) and chemical (10, 26) mechanisms have been suggested. Development of the concept that inositol 1,4,5-triphosphate (IP_3) regulates calcium release from the endoplasmic reticulum in a variety of cells (9) was soon followed by published evidence (97, 98) that IP_3 could both release Ca^{2+} from isolated skeletal SR and initiate contraction in muscle fibers whose sarcolemma was disrupted. Thus IP_3 might be the chemical mediator between t-tubule depolarization and Ca^{2+} release from the

SR. The notion of a chemical mediator fits nicely with the well-known delay between the action potential and the beginning of contraction, the latent period (56, 85).

Three lines of evidence must be developed before the IP_3 hypothesis can be accepted. (*a*) The enzymes necessary for IP_3 synthesis, release, and degradation must exist in an appropriate amounts. (*b*) IP_3 must be released during the latent period. This would most easily be established in studies of a skeletal muscle whose latent period is of long duration (60–90 ms); e.g. tortoise rectus femoris at 0°C (56). (*c*) Application of IP_3 in appropriate amount and location in the muscle fiber must produce a physiologic calcium release. This is the area in which caged compounds are most useful because release is rapid, can be quantitative and, by focusing the light, can be localized. Walker et al (101) have tested the IP_3 hypothesis for skeletal muscle by photogenerating IP_3 in saponin-treated skeletal muscle fibers. They find that although force generation is often initiated by photogeneration of IP_3, the rate of force development is 1000 times slower than the normal activation process, and they argue that it is unlikely that IP_3 is the E-C coupling messenger in skeletal muscle. The experiment is not conclusive, however, because measurement of isometric force development is not the most sensitive or precise test of this hypothesis. Like glycerinated fibers, saponin-treated fibers are probably non-uniform along their length and may lose cofactors during the saponin treatment. In compliant relaxed fibers, a non-uniform release of Ca^{2+} could produce a slow rise in force. Thus measurements using Ca^{2+}-sensitive probes or IP_3 photolysis at specific visualized sarcomeres should provide a more definitive test of the hypothesis.

Regardless of whether or not IP_3 is the E-C coupling mediator, caged moieties will be useful in testing such hypotheses.

CONCLUSIONS

The application of caged compounds to the study of muscle contraction has resulted in a major advance in our understanding of the molecular mechanism of force generation. It has been shown that the ATPase mechanism in the fiber is qualitatively the same as that of acto-S1 in solution. Specific steps in the fiber are quantitatively different, however, in that they exhibit strain dependence. In particular, the product release steps are perhaps the most important and least well understood parts of the ATPase mechanism.

There are also several additional approaches using caged compounds that could be exploited in the near future. (*a*) The flash and smash technique could be used to measure the time course of ATP hydrolysis in single fibers during shortening and lengthening contractions to characterize the ATPase rate and efficiency of contraction. This should help to solve some of the outstanding problems in muscle energetics. (*b*) Many of the experiments described in this review could be repeated using caged ATP analogues. to better define the relationship between specific steps and mechanical behavior. (*c*) Different reporter signals besides force and stiffness are already being measured. Spectroscopic probes in fibers provide the best comparison with solution studies, and work has already started using fluorescent ATP analogues and fluorescently labeled TnC. It would also be particularly informative to observe pyrene fluorescence from actin in a contracting fiber. (*d*) The mechanism of muscular activation and relaxation should be investigated in detail using both caged calcium and caged calcium-chelators (28).

ACKNOWLEDGMENTS

The authors are grateful to Kelly Frawley for help in the preparation of the manuscript, to Gert Rapp, Roger S. Goody, Michael Geeves, David Trentham, and Yale Goldman for discussion of the manuscript, and to the National Institutes of Health (AR 30988) and the Muscular Dystrophy Association for research support.

Literature Cited

1. Allen, T., Barsotti, R. J., Gordon, A. M., Kaplan, J. H., Goldman, Y. E. 1989. Structural changes in TNC during activation of skinned psoas fibers by laser photolysis of caged Ca. *Biophys. J.* 55:9A

2. Ashley, C. C., Barsotti, R. J., Ferenczi, M. A., Lea, T. J., Mulligan, I. P. 1987. Fast activation of skinned muscle fibres from the frog by photolysis of caged calcium. *J. Physiol.* 394:24P

3. Ashley, C. C., Barsotti, R. J., Ferenczi, M. A., Lea, T. J., Mulligan, I. P. 1988. Thin filament activation by photolysis of caged-calcium in skinned muscle fibers from the frog. *Biophys. J.* 53:564A

4. Ashley, C. C., Barsotti, R. J., Ferenczi, M. A., Lea, T. J., Mulligan, I. P., Tsien, R. Y. 1987. Caged-calcium photolysis activates demembranated muscle fibres from the rabbit. *J. Physiol.* 390:144P

5. Bagshaw, C. R., Trentham, D. R. 1973. The reversibility of adenosine triphosphate cleavage by myosin. *Biochem. J.* 133:323–28

6. Barabas, K., Keszthelyi, L. 1984. Temperature dependence of ATP release from "caged" ATP. *Acta Biochim. Biophys. Acad. Sci. Hung.* 19:305–9

7. Barsotti, R. J., Ellis-Davies, G., Kaplan, J. H., Goldman, Y. E. 1989. Kinetics of skeletal muscle fiber activation by photolysis of DM-Nitrophen

(caged Ca^{2+}) and caged ATP. *Biophys. J.* 55:10A

8. Barsotti, R. J., Ferenczi, M. A. 1988. Kinetics of ATP hydrolysis and tension production in skinned cardiac muscle of the guinea pig. *J. Biol. Chem.* 263: 16750–16756

9. Berridge, M. J., Irvine, R. F. 1984. Inositol trisphosphate, a novel second messenger in cellular signal transduction. *Nature* 312:315–21

10. Bianchi, C. P. 1968. *Cell Calcium.* New York: Appleton-Century-Crofts

11. Biosca, J. A., Travers, F., Barman, T. E., Audmard, E., Kassab, R. 1985. Transient kinetics of ATP hydrolysis by covalently cross-linked actomyosin complex by the rapid flow-quench method. *Biochemistry* 24:3814–20

12. Biosca, J. A., Travers, F., Hillaire, D., Barman, T. E. 1984. Cryoenzymic studies on S1: Perturbation of an enzyme reaction by temperature and solvent. *Biochemistry* 23:1947–55

13. Bremel, R. D., Weber, A. 1972. A cooperation within actin filament in vertebrate skeletal muscle. *Nature* 238:97–101

14. Brenner, B. 1987. Mechanical and structural approaches to correlation of cross-bridge action in muscle with actomyosin ATPase in solution. *Annu. Rev. Physiol.* 49:655–72

15. Brenner, B., Schoenberg, M., Chalo-

vich, J. M., Greene, L. E., Eisenberg, E. 1982. Evidence for crossbridge attachment in relaxed muscle at low ionic strength. *Proc. Natl. Acad. Sci. USA* 79:88–91

16. Chalovich, J. M., Eisenberg, E. 1982. Inhibition of actomyosin ATPase activity by troponin without blocking binding of myosin to actin. *J. Biol. Chem.* 257:2432–37

17. Coates, J. H., Criddle, A. H., Geeves, M. A. 1985. Pressure-relaxation studies of pyrene-labeled actin and myosin S1 from rabbit skeletal muscle. *Biochem. J.* 232:351–56

18. Cooke, R. 1986. The mechanism of muscle contraction. *CRC Crit. Rev. Biochem.* 21:53–118

19. Cooke, R., Pate, E. 1985. The effects of ADP and phosphate on the contraction of muscle fibers. *Biophys. J.* 48:789–98

20. Dantzig, J. A., Goldman, Y. E. 1989. Photolysis of caged ATP in muscle fibers with negatively strained crossbridges indicates that relaxation in the presence of MgADP is highly strain dependent. *Biophys. J.* 55:260A

21. Dantzig, J. A., Goldman, Y. E. 1989. Tension and stiffness decline following photolysis of caged phosphate within actively contracting glycerol-extracted fibers of rabbit psoas muscle. *Biophys. J.* 55:11A

21a. Dantzig, J. A., Goldman, Y. E., Luttman, M. L., Trentham, D. R., Woodward, S. K. A. 1989. Binding of caged ATP diastereoisomers to rigor crossbridges in glycerol extracted fibers of rabbit psoas muscle. *J. Physiol.* 419:64P

22. Dantzig, J. A., Lacktis, J. W., Homsher, E., Goldman, Y. E. 1987. Mechanical transients initiated by photolysis of caged P_i during active skeletal muscle contractions. *Biophys. J.* 51:3A

23. Dantzig, J. A., Trentham, D. R., Goldman, Y. E. 1986. Kinetics of activation of skeletal muscle fibers by photolysis of caged ATP in the presence of MgADP. *Biophys. J.* 49:268A

24. Dantzig, J. A., Walker, J. W., Trentham, D. R., Goldman, Y. E. 1988. Relaxation of muscle fibers with adenosine 5'-[γ-thio]triphosphate (ATP[γS]) and by laser photolysis of caged ATP[γS]: evidence for Ca^{2+}-dependent affinity of rapidly detaching zero-force cross-bridges. *Proc. Natl. Acad. Sci. USA* 85:6716–20

25. Eisenberg, E., Hill, T. L. 1985. Muscle contraction and free energy transduction in biological systems. *Science* 227:999–1006

26. Endo, M., Tanaka, M., Ogawa, Y. 1970. Calcium induced release of calcium from the sarcoplasmic reticulum of skinned muscle fibers. *Nature* 228:34–36

27. Ferenczi, M. A. 1986. Phosphate burst in permeable muscle fibers of the rabbit. *Biophys. J.* 50:471–77

28. Ferenczi, M. A., Goldman, Y. E., Trentham, D. R. 1989. Relaxation of permeabilized, isolated muscle fibers of the rabbit by rapid chelation of Ca^{2+}-ions through laser pulse photolysis of 'caged BAPTA.' *J. Physiol.* 419:163P

29. Ferenczi, M. A., Homsher, E., Trentham, D. R. 1984. The kinetics of magnesium adenosine triphosphate cleavage in skinned muscle fibres of the rabbit. *J. Physiol.* 352:575–99

30. Ferenczi, M. A., Irving, M., Peckham, M. 1986. Birefringence transients during relaxation of demembranated rabbit muscle fibres from rigor following laser flash photolysis of caged-ATP. *J. Physiol.* 381:86P

31. Ferenczi, M. A., Spencer, I. C. 1988. The elementary steps of the actomyosin ATPase in muscle fibres studied with caged-ATP. *Adv. Exp. Med. Biol.* 226:181–88

32. Ferenczi, M. A., Stienen, G. J. M. 1987. Force relaxation is skinned fast fibres of the iliofibularis muscle of *Xenopus laevis* by photolysis of caged ATP. *J. Physiol.* 398:73P

33. Ferenczi, M. A., Woodward, S. K. A., Eccleston, J. F. 1989. The rate of Mant-ADP release from cross-bridges of single skeletal muscle fibers. *Biophys. J.* 55:441A

34. Ford, L. E., Huxley, A. F., Simmons, R. M. 1977. Tension responses to sudden length change in stimulated frog muscle fibres near slack length. *J. Physiol.* 269:441–515

35. Ford, L. E., Huxley, A. F., Simmons, R. M. 1985. Tension transients during steady state shortening of frog muscle fibres. *J. Physiol.* 361:131–50

36. Ford, L. E., Huxley, A. F., Simmons, R. M. 1986. Tension transients during the rise of tetanic tension in frog muscle fibers. *J. Physiol.* 372:595–609

37. Geeves, M. A. 1989. The dynamic interaction between actin and myosin S1 in the presence of ADP. *Biochemistry* 28:5864–71

38. Geeves, M. A., Goody, R. S., Gutfreund, H. 1984. Kinetics of acto-S1 interactions as a guide to a model for the crossbridge cycle. *J. Muscle Res. Cell Motil.* 5:351–61

39. Geeves, M. A., Jeffries, T. E. 1988. The effect of nucleotide upon a specific isomerization of actomyosin S1. *Biochem. J.* 256:41–46

40. Geeves, M. A., Ranatunga, K. W. 1987. Tension responses to increased hydrostatic pressure in glycerinated rabbit psoas muscle fibres. *Proc. R. Soc. London Ser. B* 232:217–26

41. Geeves, M. A., Trentham, D. R. 1982. Protein-bound ATP: Properties of a key intermediate of the S1 ATPase from rabbit skeletal muscle. *Biochemistry* 21: 2782–89

42. Goldman, Y. E. 1987. Kinetics of the actomyosin ATPase in muscle fibers. *Annu. Rev. Physiol.* 49:637–54

43. Goldman, Y. E.., Hibberd, M. G., McCray, J. A., Trentham, D. R. 1982. Relaxation of muscle fibres by photolysis of caged ATP. *Nature* 300:701–5

44. Goldman, Y. E., Hibberd, M. G., Trentham, D. R. 1984. Relaxation of rabbit psoas muscle fibres from rigor by photochemical generation of adenosine-5'-triphosphate. *J. Physiol.* 354:577–604

45. Goldman, Y. E., Hibberd, M. G., Trentham, D. R. 1984. Initiation of active contraction by photogeneration of adenosine-5'-triphosphate in rabbit psoas muscle fibres. *J. Physiol.* 354:605–24

46. Goldman, Y. E., Kaplan, J. H. 1988. Activation of skeletal muscle fibers by photolysis of DM-nitrophen, a new caged Ca^{2+}. *Biophys. J.* 53:25A

47. Goldman, Y. E., McCray, J. A., Ranatunga, K. W. 1987. Transient tension changes initiated by laser temperature jumps in rabbit psoas muscle fibres. *J. Physiol.* 92:71–95

48. Deleted in proof

49. Goody, R. S., Hofmann, W. 1980. Stereochemical aspects of the interaction of myosin and actomyosin with nucleotides. *J. Muscle Res. Cell Motil.* 1:101–15

50. Gurney, A. M., Lester, H. A. 1987. Light-flash physiology with synthetic photosensitive compounds. *Physiol. Rev.* 67(2):583–617

51. Gutfreund, H. 1975. *Enzymes: Physical Principles.* London: Wiley. 242 pp.

52. Güth, K., Rensland, H., Goody, R. S., Potter, J. D. 1989. The TnCDANZ fluorescence intensity transient after flash photolysis of caged ATP. *Biophys. J.* 55:92A

53. Haselgrove, J. C. 1972. X-ray evidence for a conformational change in the actin-containing filaments of vertebrate striated muscle. *Cold Spring Harbor Symp. Quant. Biol.* 37:341–52

54. Hibberd, M. G., Dantzig, J. A., Trentham, D. R., Goldman, Y. E. 1985. Phosphate release and force generation in skeletal muscle fibers. *Science* 228: 1317–19

55. Hibberd, M. G., Trentham, D. R. 1986. Relationships between chemical and mechanical events during muscular contraction. *Annu. Rev. Biophys. Chem.* 15:119–61

56. Hill, A. V. 1950. Does heat production precede mechanical response in muscular contraction. *Proc. R. Soc. London Ser. B* 137:268–73

57. Hill, T. L. 1978. A theoretical formalism for the sliding filament model of contraction of striated muscle. *Prog. Biophys. Mol. Biol.* 28:267–340

58. Homsher, E. 1987. Muscle enthalpy production and its relationship to actomyosin ATPase. *Annu. Rev. Physiol.* 49:673–90

59. Homsher, E., Lacktis, J. 1988. The effect of shortening on the phosphate release step of the actomyosin ATPase mechanism. *Biophys. J.* 53:564A

60. Homsher, E., Lacktis. J. 1989. The effect of calcium concentration on the phosphate release step of the actomyosin ATPase mechanism. *Biophys. J.* 55: 261A

60a. Homsher, E., Millar, N. C. 1989. Tension transients induced by photolysis of caged phosphate in glycerinated rabbit soleus muscle fibers. *J. Physiol.* 419: 65P

61. Huxley, H. E. 1972. Structural changes in the actin-and myosin-containing filaments during contraction. *Cold Spring Harbor Symp. Quant. Biol.* 37:361–76

62. Irving, M., Peckham, M., Ferenczi, M. A. 1986. Birefringence as a probe of crossbridge orientation in demembranated muscle fibres. *Adv. Exp. Med. Biol.* 226:299–306

63. Julian, F. J., Moss, R. L. 1981. Effects of calcium and ionic strength on shortening velocity and tension development in frog skinned muscle fibers. *J. Physiol.* 311:179–99

64. Julian, F. J., Sollins, M. R. 1975. Variation of muscle stiffness with force at increasing speeds of shortening. *J. Gen. Physiol.* 66:287–302

65. Kaplan, J. H., Ellis-Davies, G. C. R. 1988. Photolabile chelators for the rapid photorelease of divalent cations. *Proc. Natl. Acad. Sci. USA* 85:6571–75

66. Kaplan, J. H., Forbush, B. III, Hoffman, J. F. 1978. Rapid photolytic release of adenosine 5'-triphosphate from a protected analogue: utilization by the Na:K pump of human red blood cell ghosts. *Biochemistry* 17:1929–35

67. Kawai, M., Guth, K., Winnikes, K., Haist, C., Ruegg, J. C. 1987. The effect of inorganic phosphate on ATP hydroly-

sis rate and the tension transients in chemically skinned rabbit psoas fibers. *Pflügers Arch.* 408:1–9

68. Konrad, M., Goody, R. S. 1982. Kinetics and thermodynamic properties of the ternary complex between F-actin, myosin S1 and AMPPNP. *Eur. J. Biochem.* 128:547–55

69. Kushmerick, M. S., Kramer, B. 1982. Force and ATPase rate in skinned skeletal muscle fibers. *Fed. Proc.* 41:2232–37

70. Lacktis, J. W., Homsher, E. 1987. The force response to photogenerated ADP in isometrically contracting glycerinated rabbit psoas muscle fibers. *Biophys. J.* 51:475A

71. Lester, H. A., Nerbonne, J. M. 1982. Physiological and pharmacological manipulations with light flashes. *Annu. Rev. Biophys. Bioeng.* 11:151–75

72. Lymn, R. W., Taylor, E. W. 1971. Mechanisms of adenosine triphosphate hydrolysis by actomyosin. *Biochemistry* 10:4617–24

73. Mathias, R. T., Levis, R. A., Eisenberg, R. S. 1980. Electrical models of excitation-contraction coupling and charge movement in skeletal muscle. *J. Gen. Physiol.* 76:1–31

74. McCray, J. A., Herbette, L., Kihara, T., Trentham, D. R. 1980. A new approach to time-resolved studies of ATP-requiring biological systems: laser flash photolysis of caged ATP. *Proc. Natl. Acad. Sci.* 77(12):7237–41

75. McCray, J. A., Trentham, D. R. 1989. Properties and uses of photoreactive caged compounds. *Annu. Rev. Biophys. Chem.* 18:239–70

76. Millar, N. C., Geeves, M. A. 1983. The limiting rate step of the ATP-mediated dissociation of actin from rabbit skeletal muscle myosin S1. *FEBS Lett.* 160:141–48

77. Millar, N. C., Geeves, M. A. 1988. Protein fluorescence changes associated with ATP and ATP γ S binding to skeletal muscle myosin subfragment 1 and actomyosin subfragment 1. *Biochem. J.* 249:735–43

78. Mornet, D., Bertrand, R., Pantel, P., Audemard, E., Kassab, R. 1981. Structure of the actin-myosin interface. *Nature* 292:301–6

79. Poole, K. J. V., Kaplan, J. H., Maéda, Y., Rapp, G., Goody, R. S. 1989. Dynamic tension and x-ray measurements on activation of rabbit psoas muscle using caged-calcium. *Biophys. J.* 55:12A

80. Poole, K. J. V., Rapp, G., Maéda, Y., Goody, R. S. 1988. Synchrotron radiation studies on insect flight muscle. *Top. Curr. Chem.* 147:1–29

81. Poole, K. J. V., Rapp, G., Maéda, Y., Goody, R. S. 1988. The time course of changes in the equatorial diffraction patterns from different muscle types on photolysis of caged-ATP. *Adv. Exp. Med. Biol.* 226:391–404

82. Rapp, G., Güth, K. 1988. A low cost high intensity flash devise for photolysis experiments. *Pflügers Arch.* 411:200–3

83. Rapp, G., Poole, K. J. V., Maéda, Y., Güth, K., Hendrix, J., Goody, R. S. 1986. Time-resolved structural studies on insect flight muscle after photolysis of caged-ATP. *Biophys. J.* 50:993–97

84. Rosenfeld, S. S., Taylor, E. W. 1984. The ATPase mechanism of skeletal and smooth muscle acto-subfragment 1. *J. Biol. Chem.* 259:11908–11919

85. Sandow, A. 1944. General properties of latency relaxation. *J. Cell. Comp. Physiol.* 24:221–56

86. Schneider, M. F., Chandler, W. K. 1973. Voltage dependent charge movement in skeletal muscle: a possible step in excitation contraction coupling. *Nature* 242:244–46

87. Siemankowski, R. F., Wiseman, M. O., White, H. D. 1985. ADP dissociation from actomyosin S1 is sufficiently slow to limit the unloaded shortening velocity in vertebrate muscle. *Proc. Natl. Acad. Sci. USA* 82:658–62

88. Sleep, J. A., Hutton, R. L. 1980. Exchange between inorganic phosphate and ATP in the medium by acto-S1. *Biochemistry* 19:1276–83

89. Somlyo, A. V., Goldman, Y. E., Fujimori, T., Bond, M., Trentham, D. R., Somlyo, A. P. 1988. Cross-bridge kinetics, cooperativity and negatively strained cross-bridges in vertebrate smooth muscle. A laser-flash photolysis study. *J. Gen. Physiol.* 91:165–92

90. Stein, L. A., Chock, P. B., Eisenberg, E. 1981. Mechanism of the actomyosin ATPase: effect of actin on the ATP hydrolysis step. *Proc. Natl. Acad. Sci. USA* 78:1346–50

91. Stein, L. A., Schwartz, R. P., Chock, P. B., Eisenberg, E. 1979. Mechanism of the actomyosin ATPase: Evidence that ATP hydrolysis can occur without dissociation of the actomyosin complex. *Biochemistry* 18:3895–3909

92. Tanner, J. W., Vallette, D. P., Thomas, D. D., Goldman, Y. E. 1989. Dichroic absorption and rigor force transients initiated by photolysis of caged ADP in fluorescent-labeled muscle fibers. *Biophys. J.* 55:9A

93. Taylor, E. W., Lymn, R. W. 1972. En-

zyme kinetics and the mechanism of muscle contraction. In *Muscle Biology*, Vol. 1, ed. R. G. Cassens. New York: Dekker

94. Thomas, D. D. 1987. Spectroscopic probes of muscle cross-bridge rotation. *Annu. Rev. Physiol.* 49:691–709

95. Trentham, D. R., Eccleston, J., Bagshaw, C. R. 1976. Kinetic analysis of ATPase mechanisms. *Q. Rev. Biophys.* 9:217–81

96. Tsien, R. Y., Zucker, R. S. 1986. Control of cytoplasmic calcium with photolable tetracarboxylate 2-nitrobenzhydrol chelators. *Biophys. J.* 50:843–53

97. Vergara, J., Tsien, R. Y., Delay, M. 1985. Inositol 1,4,5-trisphosphate: a possible chemical link in excitation-contraction coupling in muscle. *Proc. Natl. Acad. Sci. USA* 82:6352–56

98. Volpe, P., Salviati, G., DiVirgilio, F., Pozzan, F. 1985. Inositol 1,4,5-trisphosphate induces calcium release from sarcoplasmic reticulum of skeletal muscle. *Nature* 316:347–49

99. Walker, J. W., Feeney, J., Trentham, D. R. 1989. Photolabile precursors of inositol phosphates. Preparation and properties of 1-(2-nitrophenyl) ethyl esters of myo-inositol 1,4,5-trisphosphate. *Biochemistry* 28:3272–80

100. Walker, J. W., Reid, G. P., McCray, J. A., Trentham, D. R. 1988. Photolabile

1-(2-nitrophenyl)ethyl phosphate esters of adenine nucleotide analogues. Synthesis and mechanism of photolysis. *J. Am. Chem. Soc.* 110:7170–77

101. Walker, J. W., Somlyo, A. V., Goldman, Y. E., Somlyo, A. P., Trentham, D. R. 1987. Kinetics of smooth and skeletal muscle activation by laser pulse photolysis of caged inositol 1,4,5-trisphosphate. *Nature* 327:249–52

102. Webb, M. R., Hibberd, M. G., Goldman, Y. E., Trentham, D. R. 1986. Oxygen exchange between P_i in the medium and water during ATP hydrolysis mediated by skinned fibers from rabbit skeletal muscle. Evidence for P_i binding to a force-generating state. *J. Biol. Chem.* 261:15557–15564

103. Woledge, R. C., Curtin, N. A., Homsher, E. 1985. *Energetic Aspects of Muscle Contraction*. London: Academic. 359 pp.

104. Yamakawa, M., Güth, K., Hibberd, M. G., Goldman, Y. E. 1985. Relaxation of insect asynchronous flight muscle by photolysis of caged ATP. *Biophys. J.* 47:288A

105. Yamakawa, M., Ranatunga, K. W., Goldman, Y. E. 1986. Relaxation and initiation of active contraction of rabbit soleus muscle fibers by caged ATP photolysis. *Biophys. J.* 49:10A

Annu. Rev. Physiol. 1990. 52:897–914

PHOTOCHEMICAL MANIPULATION OF DIVALENT CATION LEVELS

Jack H. Kaplan

Department of Physiology, University of Pennsylvania, Philadelphia, Pennsylvania 19104-6085

KEY WORDS: caged calcium, caged magnesium, photorelease techniques, light-sensitive chelation, photoactivation

INTRODUCTION

The first description of photo-cleavable or caged compounds that might be of interest to cellular physiologists was of caged cAMP(12) and of caged ATP, ADP, and P_i (24). It seemed likely that this methodology could be applied to a wide range of substrates and transmitters. An obvious candidate for photoregulation was the concentration of free divalent cations, especially Ca^{2+}, which plays a central role in many cellular processes. In principle the strategies are obvious; in order to produce increases in free $[Ca^{2+}]$, it is necessary to design a Ca^{2+} chelator, the affinity of which decreases dramatically on photolysis. In order to lower $[Ca^{2+}]$, the affinity of a light-sensitive chelator should increase following illumination. An early approach to this problem employed a photo-isomerization strategy rather than photo-cleavage (8). This technique was based on the earlier work in which photo-isomerizable acetylcholine analogues were synthesized to probe the kinetics of acetylcholine-gated channel opening (7). This approach was exploited by Lester & colleagues (27) in a series of studies with a variety of $cis \rightleftharpoons trans$ photo-isomerizable agonists. The application of this strategy to metal ion chelation has so far met with limited success in providing useful compounds for biological studies. The light-sensitive chelation of Zn^{2+} ions has been described using 4,4'-bis(α-iminodiacetic acid)azotoluene (structure I in Figure 1), where photoactivation of the $trans \rightarrow cis$ isomerization produces a

897

0066-4278/90/0315-0897$02.00

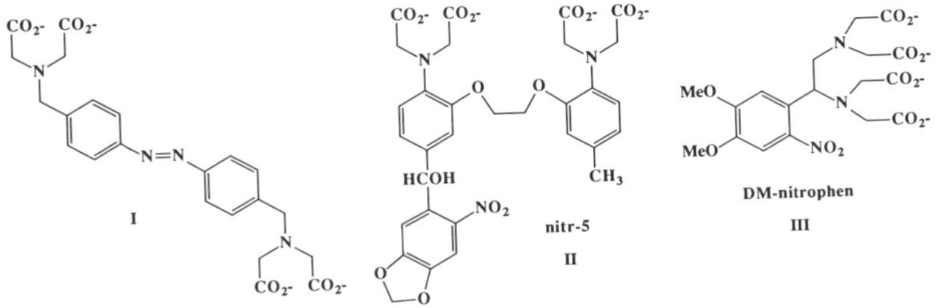

Figure 1   Structures of photolabile chelators for divalent cations.

nonplanar Zn^{2+} chelator from a planar molecule that did not chelate Zn^{2+} ions (8).

The requirements for a light-sensitive Ca^{2+} chelator that is useful in biological studies are straight-forward. Some of the requirements are already met by employing similar photochemistry to that used earlier with other caged compounds, while other needs arise from the specific requirement that generally holds for resting $[Ca^{2+}]$ and for saturating $[Ca^{2+}]$ in mediating cell physiologic responses. Thus for a caged Ca^{2+}, the affinity prior to photolysis should be lower than 0.1 μM, and after photolysis the photoproducts should ideally not bind Ca^{2+} at all (i.e. the K_d should be greater than $10^{-3}M$). The photochemical conversion should take place with a reasonably high quantum yield (the quantum yield for P_i release from caged P_i is 0.54, for example see Reference 24), and in order to be useful in most physiologic processes, the Ca^{2+} release process should be complete in $< 10^{-3}$ sec. In order to avoid photo damage to tissues, it is also preferable to activate the process with illumination at wavelengths > 300 nm; thus the chromophores (2-nitrobenzyl-derived moieties) used in the caged cAMP and caged ATP molecules fulfill this requirement. Furthermore the toxicity of photoproducts should be minimal or, if significant avoidable by the use of buffers or protecting reagents, such as glutathione or DTT, used in sodium pump and muscle contraction studies where ATPase activity or tension development is initiated by photolysis of caged nucleotides (17, 24). The requirements for a compound that lowers the free $[Ca^{2+}]$, a caged chelator, are similar with a photo-generated increase in Ca^{2+} affinity from $K_d > 10^{-5}M$ to one with $K_d < 10^{-7}M$. In most physiologic situations, it is necessary to be able to regulate $[Ca^{2+}]$ in the ranges of $10^{-7}M$ to $10^{-5}M$ without greatly affecting $[Mg^{2+}]$, which in most cells is around $10^{-3}M$. Thus a Ca^{2+}-selective chelator should preferentially bind Ca^{2+} rather than Mg^{2+} with a selectivity of at least 10^4-fold.

During the last five years considerable progress has been made in achieving these goals. There now exists two different approaches for a rapid photo-generated increase in $[Ca^{2+}]$, both based on the 2-nitrobenzyl chromophores, but having significant differences in their mechanisms and characteristics. There are also now two approaches to the photo-dependent decrease in $[Ca^{2+}]$. One of these molecules is simply a 2-nitrobenzyl mono-ester of BAPTA, which photoreleases BAPTA and is thus a caged chelator (15). The other is called diazo-2 and is based on principles similar to the nitr-2 type of molecule, where photolysis alters the nature of electron-withdrawing substituents, and on photolysis the affinity for Ca^{2+} is elevated and free $[Ca^{2+}]$ falls (2). There are as yet no other published reports on the characterization and application of these compounds or other candidates to lower $[M^{2+}]$.

The basis of these approaches will be the subject of this review. The properties of the molecules employed will be discussed with a focus on the caged divalent cations where $[M^{2+}]$ is increased on photolysis. In addition, the mechanism of Ca^{2+} release and the rates involved and a series of illustrative examples will be described that indicate some of the ways in which these new tools have already found application. A comparison will also be made of these approaches and the advantages and disadvantages of each considered.

CAGED $[M^{2+}]$ PHOTO-REGULATED INCREASE IN $[M^{2+}]$

The application of photorelease techniques to the problem of generating a rapid jump in free $[M^{2+}]$ has been achieved in the last few years. Two types of molecules have been employed. This section will deal with the most readily (commercially) available of these types, nitr-5 and DM-nitrophen. Each of these molecules provides an effective approach to a caged Ca^{2+}. Nitr-5 is highly specific for Ca^{2+} while DM-nitrophen has been used as a caged Ca^{2+} and a caged Mg^{2+}. The modus operandi for achieving the increase in M^{2+} is different for each molecule.

Nitr-5

A series of Ca^{2+}-selective chelators incorporating photo-sensitive 2-nitrobenzhydrol moieties were described and characterized in 1988 by Adams et al (1). These were a logical development of a series of compounds based on the aromatic (assumed) homologue of EGTA, BAPTA, previously described by Tsien (36). Electron-withdrawing or electron-donating groups attached to one of the aromatic rings of BAPTA were known to respectively lower or raise the affinity for Ca^{2+}. These effects are readily accounted for from well-known substituent effects encountered throughout organic chemistry. Tsien & colleagues realized that the photochemical generation of an electron-withdrawing substituent would produce the desired fall in affinity for Ca^{2+} ions needed for a caged Ca^{2+} molecule. The changes involved in such a process are shown in Figure 2, for Ca^{2+} chelation by nitr-5. The chemistry involved employs the intramolecular redox reaction where a 2-nitrobenzyl moiety is converted to a 2-nitroso structure with the associated cleavage at the benzylic carbon. In the case of nitr-5 (for structure see Figure 1), water is ejected and a ketone residue (electron-withdrawing) replaces the original alcohol (1). A scheme showing these transformations appears in Figure 2. The application of other members of this group, nitr-2 and nitr-7, had been described prior to the description of their synthesis and characterization (20). For reasons of greater difficulty in synthesis (nitr-7) or slowness in release rate (nitr-2), nitr-5 has been selected for further application and is the most readily available (from Calbiochem).

Nitr-5 has many of the advantages associated with the parent compound of this series, BAPTA. It shows high selectivity for Ca^{2+} over Mg^{2+} (about 10^5-fold), and above pH7 it shows little pH dependence in its chelation properties (1). Nitr-5 shows Ca^{2+}-dependent absorbance changes below 300 nm; thus the Ca^{2+} binding constants could be measured from spectra at varied free $[Ca^{2+}]$. The absorption spectra in the area of photolytic excitation (>300 nm) is dominated by the contribution from the nitrobenzyl chromophore and changes very little on titration with Ca^{2+}. On photolysis at 365 nm, the dissociation constant for the nitr-5-Ca^{2+} complex changes from 0.15 μM to 6μM, a 40-fold change. Since both nitr-5 complexed with Ca^{2+} and free nitr-5 are photo-sensitive, it is possible to determine the quantum yield for each process separately. The quantum yield for nitr-5-Ca^{2+} photolysis is 0.035 and for the nitr-5 molecule is 0.012. Flash photolysis kinetics of nitr-5 were also reported, and Ca^{2+} release takes place at rates of about 3000 s^{-1} (1). Thus nitr-5 has many of the desirable properties of a caged Ca compound that might be useful in studies of cellular processes. This series of compounds suffers from some disadvantages, however, so the ideal caged Ca^{2+} compound is not yet in hand.

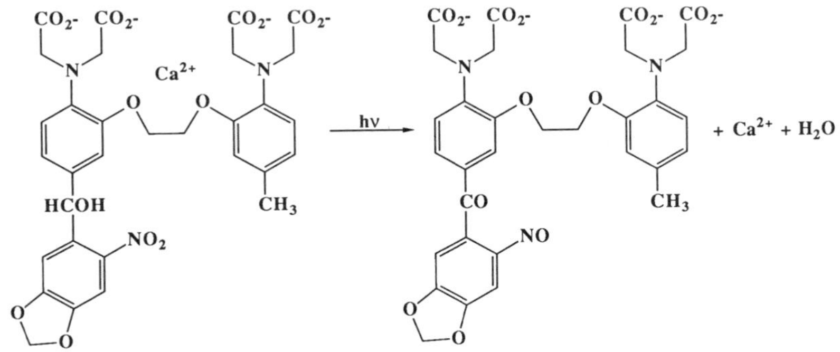

Figure 2   Photochemical release of Ca^{2+} with nitr-5.

One shortcoming of nitr-5 is its affinity for Ca^{2+} before photolysis. The disassociation constant is about 150 nM under conditions of physiologic ionic strength. Thus if resting $[Ca^{2+}]$ is to be maintained at around 100 nM, only a fraction of the total nitr-5 used has bound Ca^{2+} to be released on photolysis. Bearing in mind the rather low quantum efficiency of photolysis, many uncomplexed (and unphotolyzed) nitr-5 molecules could be available to buffer free Ca^{2+} released by photolysis of nitr-5-Ca^{2+} complexes. If the affinity of nitr-5 for Ca^{2+} was higher, lower nitr-5:nitr-5-Ca^{2+} ratios could be employed to obtain appropriately low free $[Ca^{2+}]$, and thus photorelease would be more efficient.

Many of the new tools available to study cellular physiologic processes are capable of further refinement. Nitr-5 falls into this category since it would be advantageous to have a tighter binding of Ca^{2+}, a higher quantum efficiency, and a greater change in affinity on photolysis. However, nitr-5 has already been used successfully in a variety of experimental situations.

Physiologic Applications of Nitr-5

Most applications of nitr-5 so far have employed the caged Ca^{2+} approach in the context of cellular neurophysiology: studying Ca^{2+} involvement in synaptic transmission or Ca^{2+} effects on ion channel activity. In non-excitable cells, studies have been performed on the effects of photo-released Ca^{2+} on K channels and on second messenger activation in fibroblasts. Some use of nitr-5 is beginning to be made in examining the regulation of muscle contraction by photo-releasing Ca^{2+} in skinned fibers.

The communication between neurons at synapses via transmitter secretion has recently been examined in two separate studies using nitr-5. In one of the studies, the involvement of presynaptic membrane potential in triggering transmitter release was examined (40). Two alternate hypotheses had previously been proposed and were examined experimentally. One hypothesis suggests that pre-synaptic action potentials trigger transmitter release by the entry of Ca^{2+} into presynaptic terminals through voltage-dependent Ca^{2+} channels. Ca^{2+} acts at high local concentrations at release sites near channel mouths to cause neurosecretion. The alternate hypothesis proposes that in addition to elevating presynaptic Ca^{2+}, presynaptic potential modulates transmitter release by a direct action. The availability of a caged Ca^{2+} together with voltage-clamped synaptic preparation enabled the investigators to independently vary $[Ca^{2+}]$ at a fixed voltage or voltage at fixed $[Ca^{2+}]$. Using nitr-5 in three-day-old B5-B19 neuron pairs from the buccal ganglia of the fresh water snail *Helisoma trivolvis*, Zucker & Hayden (40) showed that transmitter release occurred if presynaptic Ca^{2+} levels were elevated to the μM range, and that presynaptic voltage had no direct effect on neurosecretion. These experiments were performed using the whole-cell patch-clamp technique to monitor inhibitory post-synaptic current (ipsc) in B19. The nitr-5 loaded with Ca^{2+} was introduced into B5, the presynaptic neuron, using a second whole-cell patch-pipette. Prior to the use of the photorelease technique, it was extremely difficult to examine separately the effects of depolarization and Ca^{2+} entry, since the two events were tightly linked. The post-synaptic effects of Ca^{2+} were examined in a study conducted in rat brain hippocampal slices by Malenka et al (28). Long-term potentiation (LTP) of synaptic transmission in vertebrate brain is a cellular model for learning and memory. The phenomenon is that brief repetitive activation of excitatory synapses in the hippocampus results in an increase in synaptic strength that lasts for many hours. The role of post-synaptic Ca^{2+} in triggering LTP was examined recently and included the application of nitr-5 as a caged Ca^{2+}. In neurons, Ca^{2+} passes through a type of ligand-gated ion channel linked to the N-methyl-D-aspartate (NMDA) subtype of a glutamate receptor. The induction of LTP requires NMDA receptor activation. It has been suggested that Ca^{2+} entering through these channels acts as a second messenger to trigger LTP. The studies of Malenka et al were designed to examine the basis for such an hypothesis. Two of the three types of experiments performed employed nitr-5. CA1 pyramidal cells were filled with Ca^{2+}-loaded nitr-5 following impalement. Photolysis of Ca^{2+}-loaded nitr-5 produced a large increase in the amplitude and initial slope of the excitatory post-synaptic potential (EPSP), without a change in input resistance. Photolysis of intracellular nitr-5 not loaded with Ca^{2+} had no effect on synaptic transmission, which indicated that the release of Ca^{2+} from loaded nitr-5 was responsible for the EPSP enhancement. The enhancement lasted from 20 to 70 min but this period is of unknown significance because of the uncertainties in the stability of the elevated Ca^{2+} level in the face of cell buffers and extrusion mechanisms. The increase in EPSP after photolysis of Ca^{2+} loaded nitr-5 provided the "first direct demonstration that a rise in postsynaptic intracellular $[Ca^{2+}]$ is sufficient to enhance synaptic transmission" (28). In a second series of experiments, nitr-5 was used merely as an alternate (and more effective) EGTA to demonstrate that intracellular chelation of Ca^{2+} abolished LTP. Further experiments by Malenka et al (28) showed that blocking the rise in $[Ca^{2+}]$ by buffering with intracellular nitr-5 or by inhibiting Ca^{2+} influx with a large membrane depolarization led to block of potentiation. Interestingly, both studies (18, 40) relied on neither a firm knowledge of the level of Ca^{2+} in the cell following photolysis, nor the fact that the release of Ca^{2+} from nitr-5 Ca after photolysis is rapid. In these studies, photolysis times of 25 s or longer were used. In the study of LTP a significant question remaining is how long is the light-activated elevation of $[Ca^{2+}]$ maintained, and how does this relate to the duration of the LTP. The authors point out that the resolution of this problem awaits the development of a completely reversible Ca^{2+} chelator

(28). Though this may help, some progress might be made either by employing a caged chelator to lower $[Ca^{2+}]$ photochemically or by monitoring the $[Ca^{2+}]$ using one of the newer indicators, (Fluo-3 for example) described by Kao et al (22) and discussed below.

Earlier work in *Aplysia* central neurons and in rat sympathetic neurons employed nitr-5 or other members of the nitr series. Studies performed with nitr-2 in *Aplysia* central neurons suggested that the rather slow release rate (dark reaction 5 s^{-1}) would compromise the usefulness of nitr-2 (37). These studies did show, however, that UV activation of an intracellular light-sensitive chelator resulted in activation of membrane currents. Subsequent work using nitr-5 in *Aplysia* pace-maker neurons was able to characterize the activation of Ca^{2+}-activated K and nonspecific cation currents on photorelease of intracellular Ca^{2+} (26). An attempt was made in this work to monitor $[Ca^{2+}]$ with arsenazo III and to compare the effectiveness of nitr-5 and nitr-7. Nitr-5 was shown overall to be a more useful caged Ca^{2+} molecule. It is apparent in this work (26) and in the previous study on *Aplysia* (37) that there was considerable spatial inhomogeneity of the $[Ca^{2+}]$ in the cell following photolysis. The activation of a K current by photochemically generated increases of $[Ca^{2+}]$ was studied in rat sympathetic neurons by Gurney et al (20). Nitr-5 or the related compounds nitr-2 or nitr-7, complexed with Ca^{2+}, were introduced into sympathetic ganglion cells by dialysis from a patch-pipette electrode in the whole-cell, voltage-clamp mode. Light flashes released Ca^{2+} and activated a K^+ current. The authors suggest that their data show that the Ca^{2+}-activated apamine-sensitive K channel opens within a few msec after Ca^{2+} is elevated at the membrane surface. Significant questions remain, however, regarding the quantitation of the control and regulation of $[Ca^{2+}]$ in this preparation. The authors suggest that it will also be useful to combine the photorelease of Ca with techniques of measuring intracellular $[Ca^{2+}]$. This has recently been reported by Kao et al (22) who used Fluo-3 (31) to detect light-generated Ca^{2+}-pulses in fibroblasts and lymphocytes. The fluorescent indicator was loaded into these cells by using the acetoxyester technique or by microinjection into fibroblasts of Fluo-3 itself along with nitr-5. This technique seems to be particularly promising for following the increases in intracellular $[Ca^{2+}]$ obtained by photolysis of nitr-5 or DM-nitrophen (22). Fluo-3 is shown to permit continuous monitoring of $[Ca^{2+}]$ without interfering with the use of UV-sensitive caged compounds. The intensity of the Fluo-3 signal was employed in a study of Ca^{2+} oscillations in fibroblasts (21). These oscillations in intracellular $[Ca^{2+}]$ are produced by depolarizations of REF 52 cells and treatment with a variety of agents (bombesin, vasopressin, ATP) that produce a single transient rise in $[Ca^{2+}]$ in cells at the normal resting membrane potential. The effects of changes in intracellular $[Ca^{2+}]$ were examined in those cells using photolysis of nitr-5 (to increase Ca^{2+}, diazo-2 to decrease Ca^{2+} and caged InsP$_3$). It was shown that extracellular Ca^{2+} was necessary to produce the oscillations; the Ca^{2+} content of intracellular stores is probably an important factor. It is interesting that increasing intracellular [Ca^{2+}] by photolysis of nitr-5 had a different effect than did stimulating the increase with caged InsP$_3$ (21).

Nitr-5 has also been used in studies of muscle contraction. The time-course of activation following photolysis of nitr-5-Ca^{2+} complex in skinned psoas fibers was compared to the activation following photolysis of caged ATP (4). These and similar studies (5) are discussed in detail in the article by Homsher and Millar (this volume).

DM-Nitrophen

A new class of photolabile chelators for the rapid release of divalent cations were described by Ellis-Davies & Kaplan in 1988 (11), and the properties of the most readily (and now commercially from Calbiochem) available member of the series were subsequently reported (23). The basis for this approach comes from, on the one hand, our familiarity with the extremely tight binding that tetracarboxylate chelators (such as EGTA or EDTA) exhibit with divalent cations and, on the other hand, our awareness that dicarboxylates are rather poor chelators of divalent cations. Indeed, the dissociation constants, at neutral pH, for Ca^{2+} differ by about five orders of magnitude (10^{-8} M vs 10^{-3} M). Thus it was realized that if a tetracarboxylate molecule could be designed that on photochemical activation would cleave into two dicarboxylate chelators, a binding constant difference of some five orders of magnitude would ensure that chelated Ca^{2+} would be photoreleased after photolysis. The obvious candidates for such chemistry were 2-nitrophenyl compounds and were based on earlier experience with caged ATP. Synthesis was achieved of members of this class of compounds based upon EGTA and EDTA. The EDTA-based molecule is DM-nitrophen (for structure, see Figure 1). The EGTA-based molecule, unfortunately, had a K_d for Ca^{2+} prior to photolysis of about 25 μM, which is too low to be useful in most physiologic situations (although at elevated pH, this compound may also be useful).

The affinity of DM-nitrophen for Ca^{2+} ions at neutral pH (7.2) and normal ionic strength (0.15 M) was estimated to be about 5×10^{-9} M. This was determined by combining the use of Ca^{2+}-sensitive electrodes with the small decrease in the absorption spectrum of DM-nitrophen, which takes place on Ca^{2+} binding. By using a competitive binding procedure, the affinity for Mg^{2+} was estimated to be 2.5×10^{-6} M (23).

Exposure of solutions of DM-nitrophen to ultra-violet light of wavelengths greater than 320 nm results in characteristic changes in the absorption spectrum. If the affinity for Ca^{2+} is measured before and after complete photolysis, a change is observed from 5×10^{-9} M to about 3×10^{-3} M. If such photolyses are carried out in a (transparent) NMR tube containing a solution of DM-nitrophen in D_2O, the spectrum of DM-nitrophen prior to illumination is replaced by a spectrum composed of the sum of the spectra of iminodiacetic acid and the nitro-aryl-substituted iminodiacetic acid products shown in Figure 3 (G. Ellis-Davies, J. Kaplan, unpublished). Thus photolysis proceeds as expected to release Ca^{2+} via the cleavage of DM-nitrophen into two di-carboxylate molecules (see Figure 3). The quantum yield for the photorelease of Ca^{2+} from the DM-nitrophen-Ca^{2+} complex is 0.18.

The likely intermediate steps in the photolysis of DM-nitrophen-Ca^{2+} are shown in Figure 4. This sequence of intermediates is similar to the pathway previously described for caged ATP (39). Following that work, attempts have been made to measure the rate of release of Ca^{2+} and compare it to the breakdown of DM-nitrophen. As with caged ATP, after the initial photo-chemical activation a photochromic intermediate is generated (probably the aci-nitro intermediate in Figure 4), which decays at a characteristic rate. At pH7 the half-time for this decay was about three msec following the photoactivation of caged ATP, and the decay of this intermediate occurred at the same rate as the appearance of free ATP (29). For DM-nitrophen at pH7 the half-time for this decay was about 50–200 μsec (16, J. McCray, et al, manuscript in preparation).

In contrast to caged ATP, which shows a large pH dependence in the rate of decay of the (presumed) aci-nitro intermediate (one order of magnitude slower per unit increase in pH), there is only a slight pH dependence in the photolysis of DM-nitrophen. The faster rate of decay of the intermediate of DM-nitrophen is similar to the rate of decay of the caged acetylcholine agonists described previously (30, 38). The photolysis of these latter two compounds, DM-nitrophen and the acetylcholine agonists, involves the cleavage of a C-N bond, while caged ATP, which is significantly slower, involves the cleavage of a C-O bond.

Attempts were also made to measure the rate of release of Ca^{2+} more directly, where use was made of a metallochromic indicator antipyrylazo III. Following a laser light flash, cleavage of DM-nitrophen-Ca^{2+} in the presence of antipyrylazo III resulted in the rapid release of Ca^{2+} and an increase in the absorbance at 650 nm. The half-time for such a mono-exponential rise was

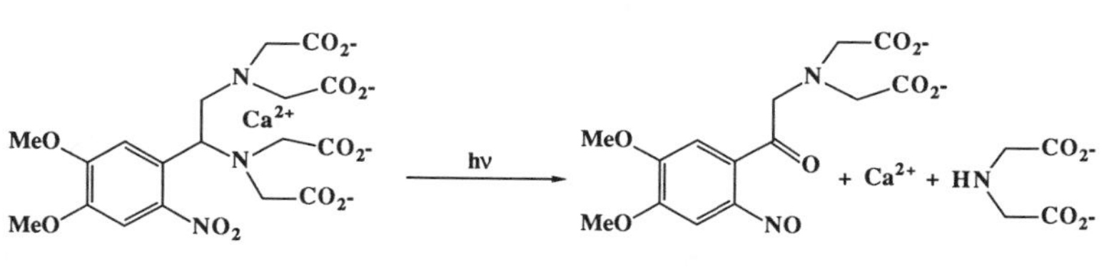

Figure 3   Photochemical release of Ca^{2+} with DM-nitrophen.

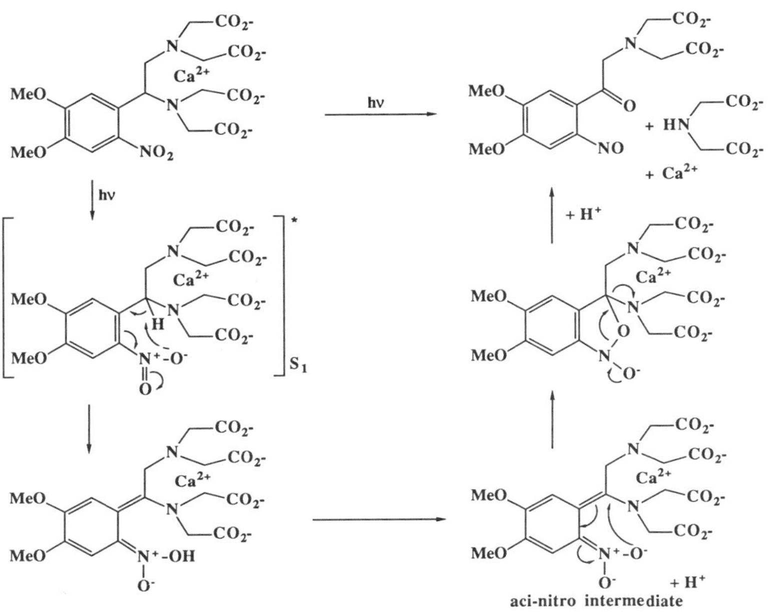

Figure 4 Photochemical reaction mechanism of DM-nitrophen-Ca^{2+} photolysis.

about 200 μsec (16). Previous studies employing temperature-jump relaxation techniques to antipyrylazo III-Ca^{2+} equilibria had identified a relaxation time of around 180 μsec (35). Thus at the moment it is not known whether this measurement of the rate of release of Ca^{2+} from DM-nitrophen is accurately reported by the antipyrylazo III absorbance data, or whether a more rapid release of Ca^{2+} occurs that is limited by the slower response-time of the indicator.

An interesting side product of the studies with metallochromic indicators was the observation that the kinetic profile of the increase in $[Ca^{2+}]$ depended upon the ratio of total $[Ca^{2+}]$ to [DM-nitrophen]. If DM-nitrophen is present in large excess (i.e. the ratio of DM-nitrophen to Ca^{2+} is 2:1), then a transient rise in $[Ca^{2+}]$ occurs, and a pulse is seen. If there is very little free DM-nitrophen (the ratio is now close to 1:1), then a step increase in $[Ca^{2+}]$ is observed. Most likely when DM-nitrophen is in large excess, photo-released Ca^{2+} can rebind to unphotolyzed free chelators. In the protocol described above, with antipyrylazo III, a pulse of $[Ca^{2+}]$ is seen that peaks in about 300 μsec and decays to base-line over the subsequent several msec. Thus by altering the ratio of DM-nitrophen to Ca^{2+}, it may be possible to generate either transient pulses in $[Ca^{2+}]$ or step increases in $[Ca^{2+}]$. These different profiles may mimic different cellular [Ca^{2+}] changes that actually occur in various physiologic situations. Similar effects might not be encountered with the nitr-5 series since the association rates between the chelators and the cations are probably faster in BAPTA-based than EDTA-based chelators.

Physiologic Applications of DM-Nitrophen

Experimental studies using DM-nitrophen as a source of free divalent cations have utilized the photorelease of Ca^{2+} in muscle and non-muscle systems. DM-nitrophen has also been used as a photolabile source of [Mg^{2+}] jumps in studies of the mechanism of the cation-activated ATPases (ion pumps).

Applications of DM-nitrophen as a caged Ca^{2+} in non-muscle cells have focused on resolving either temporal or sided effects of Ca^{2+} on ion channels. The first study used dorsal root ganglion (drg) neurons to investigate the effects of Ca^{2+} on cation currents through Ca^{2+} channels (32). Primary cultures of chick drg neurons were voltage-clamped with the whole-cell patch-clamp technique. The cells were dialyzed internally with solutions of low (10^{-8} M) Ca^{2+} buffered by DM-nitrophen or EGTA. Using the appropriate cocktail of channel blockers for various Na- or K- selective channels, it is possible to show that in the absence of Ca^{2+} or at low [Ca^{2+}], the Ca^{2+} channels pass a Na$^+$ current. Photolysis of the intracellular or extracellular DM-nitrophen-Ca^{2+} complex rapidly elevated [Ca^{2+}]. The kinetics of the inactivation of the currents through the Ca^{2+} channels were compared in several situations. These were (a) when Ca^{2+} ions were the main charge carrier; (b) when Na$^+$ ions were the main charge carrier. The effects of rapid increases in [Ca^{2+}] at the inner or outer aspects of the Ca^{2+} channel could be examined in each of these situations. Several points emerged from these studies (32). The photo-regulated increase in [Ca^{2+}] from 10^{-8} M to about 50 μM resulted in inactivation of the currents, but the kinetics of the change depended on the valence of the permeating cation. When Ca^{2+} or Ba^{2+} ions were the charge carrier, the currents inactivated with a time constant (τ) of about seven msec. When Na$^+$ was the charge carrier, τ was about 0.4 msec, and the block was more complete if the [Ca^{2+}] increase occurred at the extracellular surface.

The authors speculated that their data implied that Ca^{2+} channels may exist in either of two major conformational states; the Ca^{2+} or Na$^+$ conducting forms. Alternatively, if the channel conformation is not greatly altered by the permeating ion, then Ca^{2+}-induced inactivation occurs at a site closely associated with an internal permeation site. In these studies estimates were made of the amount of Ca^{2+} released in the cells by photolysis of droplets of extracted cytoplasm from the drg neurons. Estimates of 50 to 80 μM [Ca^{2+}] following a light pulse were obtained. Several points should be noted with respect to these studies: first, evidently the response times of the currents were slower than the estimated half-times for Ca^{2+} release from DM-nitrophen; thus we can be reasonably sure that the effects reported are not limited by the kinetics of Ca^{2+} release; second, in order to simplify the experimental situation, these studies were performed in the complete absence of Mg^{2+}.

The modulation of cardiac Ca^{2+} channel selectivity has also been studied (33). In these experiments amphibian heart was selected since this tissue is insensitive to the absence of Mg^{2+} in the extracellular medium. In frog heart, if the extracellular medium also contains very little (μM) Ca^{2+}, the cardiac action potentials have extremely long duration with extended depolarized plateau phases; as $[Ca^{2+}]$ is elevated the action potential shortens. Experiments were performed with strips of voltage-clamped frog ventricle, using the single sucrose gap technique, and the effects of photoreleased extracellular Ca^{2+} were studied on action potential shape, membrane current, and tension development. The extent of the rise in $[Ca^{2+}]$ in the extracellular space (but not the kinetics of the rise) was measured using Ca^{2+}-selective microelectrodes. Rapid elevation of $[Ca^{2+}]$ from about 5 to 100 μM following a single light flash quickly altered the permeability of the Ca^{2+} channel. The conductance to Na^+ ions was blocked in <500 μsec; although the $[Ca^{2+}]$ rose rapidly to produce this effect, there was a delay of some 60–80 msec before contraction of the ventricle strip was activated. These studies support the idea that the major route by which the Ca^{2+} necessary for contraction reaches the contractile apparatus in amphibian heart is via Ca^{2+} channels in the plasma membrane.

Although an obvious candidate for study using this approach is one of the many Ca^{2+}-activated K channels, as yet no studies have been performed with DM-nitrophen. The flux equivalent of the activation of conductance of one of these type of channels (the Gardos channel) was described following photolysis of intracellular DM-nitrophen-Ca^{2+} in resealed human red cell ghosts (23).

DM-nitrophen as a caged Ca^{2+} has been used in many studies relating to the mechanism of activation of muscle contraction. A more detailed discussion of the mechanism of striated muscle contraction is referred to in the review by Homsher & Millar in this volume. DM-nitrophen has been used to initiate contraction following photorelease of Ca^{2+} in single-skinned fibers using laser flash photolysis (18) or in fiber bundles using a photoflash lamp (34). The readout of the consequences of photoreleased Ca^{2+} in the fibers has included tension, both the kinetics and level (6, 10, 18), diffraction data [to several msec resolution (10, 34)], stiffness (6, 18), and changes in absorption dichroism of fluorescently labeled troponin (3). A limitation in all of these studies so far is a precise knowledge of the kinetics and amplitude of the change in $[Ca^{2+}]$ in the fiber following the light flash. Although it is possible to devise chemical methods to determine how much Ca^{2+} was released in a fiber, such methods inevitably give a volume-averaged measure of $[Ca^{2+}]$ in the entire irradiated sample. This includes the entire fiber myoplasm and the irradiated extracellular solution. In the future, perhaps appropriate Ca^{2+}-sensitive optical signals could be measured that might yield better estimates of $[Ca^{2+}]$ in skinned fibers isolated in oil prior to photolysis, so that the only irradiated solution of DM-nitrophen is within the fiber.

DM-nitrophen has been used as a caged Mg^{2+} in two sets of studies of the Na,K-ATPase or Na pump. In the first of these studies an extrinsic dye yielded rapidly changing fluorescent signals associated with enzyme turnover. When the enzyme turnover was initiated with photo-released Mg from DM-nitrophen-Mg^{2+}, the kinetics of the signal were the same as when turnover was initiated with caged ATP (25).

Recently, an interesting new experimental approach for studying ion pumps has been developed (13). This has combined electrical measurements of pump currents generated from membrane vesicles or patches adsorbed to black lipid membranes with the application of photo-cleaved substrates (initially caged ATP) to initiate and synchronize turnover of the adsorbed pump molecules (13). Initial observations of the currents generated on photo-initiation of sodium pump turnover using caged ATP produced a transient current described by two sequential rate constants (9, 14). In addition to difficulties in assigning either of these rate constants to a specific step in the pump cycle, it was also not clear if either of these (the rising or falling phase) was limited by the rate of ATP release from caged ATP (the half-time for this process is about three msec at pH7). The sodium pump, like other ion-activated ATPases, requires Mg as well as ATP for phosphorylation and turnover; thus it was also possible, in principle, to initiate current transients with a caged Mg in the presence of ATP. The release rate for Mg^{2+} from DM-nitrophen was assumed to be similar to Ca^{2+}, as similar photochromic intermediates have been observed in both cases (16). At pH7, the Mg^{2+} release rate is about one order of magnitude faster than the release rate for ATP from caged ATP (16). At higher pH values, this difference is more dramatic as ATP release is slowed by one order of magnitude per unit increase in pH (29) while the photocleavage of DM-nitrophen shows very little pH dependence (16; J. McCray et al, manuscript in preparation). Recent studies (P. De Weer et al, manuscript in preparation) have shown that the transient currents obtained by photo-releasing Mg to initiate Na pump turnover show identical kinetics to those obtained previously with caged ATP. Thus the earlier reports using caged ATP do not reflect rate limitations because of ATP release from caged ATP, but faithfully follow the rate of electrogenic steps in the pump cycle.

COMPARISON OF NITR-5 AND DM-NITROPHEN

In Table 1 most of the salient properties of nitr-5 and DM-nitrophen are collected. An examination of these values reveals some of the advantages and disadvantages of each of these molecules. In terms of Ca^{2+} affinity prior to photolysis, clearly DM-nitrophen has a considerable advantage; in order to buffer $[Ca^{2+}]$ below likely threshold values, the ratio of free DM-nitrophen:Ca-DM-nitrophen would be lower than the same ratio using nitr-5, so that more of the absorbed incident illumination would productively cleave bound chelator (and release Ca^{2+}) rather than cleave unloaded chelator. The considerably higher quantum yield for DM-nitrophen also will produce more efficient Ca^{2+} photorelease. A considerable advantage of nitr-5, however, is in its selectivity for Ca^{2+} over Mg^{2+}. Since the K_d for Mg^{2+} is close to 10 mM, while its K_d for Ca^{2+} is 150 nM, there will be very little chelation of Mg by nitr-5 in the concentration range where it effectively buffers $[Ca^{2+}]$. Although DM-nitrophen binds Ca^{2+} more tightly than Mg^{2+}, since the K_d for Mg^{2+} is in the micromolar range, DM-nitrophen will chelate significant quantities of Mg under physiologic conditions. It is possible to generate a membrane-permeable nitr-5 by utilizing the tetra-acetoxymethyl ester. Following hydrolysis of the esters (by endogenous esterases) after permeation into the cell, nitr-5 could buffer endogenous or added (using an ionophore) Ca^{2+} to below threshold levels (possibly the ratio nitr-5:Ca^{2+} could make subsequent photorelease relatively inefficient because of the K_d for Ca^{2+}). If the same techniques were used with a similar ester of DM-nitrophen under physiologic conditions, the photolabile chelator would also act as a caged Mg. It should be borne in mind that the tetra-ester of DM-nitrophen would also be expected to be less permeable than nitr-5 because of the higher pK of the EDTA-derived amino residues.

Just as the chelation of Mg can be a complication in certain physiologic situations, in others it can be exploited. As discussed above, DM-nitrophen has been employed as a caged Mg^{2+} molecule and recently the binding constant for Ba^{2+} has also been characterized (19). Undoubtedly DM-nitrophen will be a generic caged divalent cation source (M^{2+}) appropriate for the divalent cations for which EDTA itself is an efficient chelator. Indeed the same expectation applies to polyvalent cations that are bound by EDTA, but in this case, the binding by the dicarboxyl photoproducts might play a larger role.

Aside from considerations of selectivity, affinity, quantum yield, and so on, it is clear that the most significant difference between nitr-5 and DM-nitrophen is in the extent to which the chelator affinity changes on illumination. It might be possible through judicious use of novel substituents to increase the change of affinity seen with nitr-5. It seems unlikely, however, that the 40-fold change can be increased sufficiently to compete with the five orders of magnitude change observed with DM-nitrophen. This exceedingly large change comes about because of the fragmentation of the chelation center on photo-cleavage of DM-nitrophen. It seems more likely that applying the

SUBJECT INDEX

A

Abscisic acid
  cellular growth properties
    and, 834
Acetylcholine
  atrial membrane
    hyperpolarization and,
    200
  cardiac calcium ion channels
    and, 263-65
  cardiac potassium ion chan-
    nels and, 294
  endothelial cytoplasmic cal-
    cium concentration and,
    663
  endothelial secretion of, 661
  potassium ion channels and,
    218
Acetylcholine receptor
  myoblast fusion and, 689
Acid-base balance
  atrial natriuretic factor and,
    704
  regulation of
    amphibious invertebrates
      and, 69-71
Acinar cells
  permeabilized
    amylase secretion by, 354
  synaptophysin in, 649
Acquired immunodeficiency syndrome (AIDS), 848
ACTH
  cortisol secretion in teleosts
    and, 50
Actin
  myosin binding site on
    tropomyosin and, 888
  neutrophil locomotion and,
    373
Actin-binding proteins
  adrenal chromaffin granule
    membranes and, 651
Actinomycin D
  brassinosteroids and, 834
Actomyosin ATPase
  in muscle fibers, 879-88
  in solution, 876-79
Acyclovir
  toxicity of, 846
Adenosine
  cardiac calcium ion channels
    and, 263-65
  cardiac potassium ion chan-
    nels and, 294
  neuronal calcium ion channels
    and, 246
  potassium ion channels and,
    218

Adenosine diphosphate (ADP)
  calcium ion release in
    platelets and, 434
  endothelial cytoplasmic cal-
    cium concentration and,
    663
  inositol phosphate formation
    and, 662
  release in muscle fibers, 887-
    88
Adenosine triphosphate (ATP)
  endothelial cytoplasmic cal-
    cium concentration and,
    663
  endothelial secretion of, 661
  exocytosis and, 596-99
  formation by oxidative
    phosphorylation, 524-26
  hydrolysis in muscle fibers,
    883-84
  inositol phosphate formation
    and, 662
  prostaglandin secretion and,
    665
  stimulus-secretion coupling
    and, 596
Adenovirus transcriptional activator E1A, 829
Adenylate cyclase
  cardiac calcium ion channels
    and, 263-65
  endothelial, 664
  potassium ion channels and,
    229-31
  respiratory cyclase and, 150-
    51
Adipocytes
  digitonin-permeabilized
    adenylate cyclase activity
      in, 356
ADP
  See Adenosine diphosphate
Adrenal chromaffin cells
  calmodulin and, 653
  exocytosis from, 600-1
  permeabilized
    catecholamine release and,
    355-56
  protein III in, 652
  secretory vesicles of
    exocytosis of, 614-18
  synaptophysin in, 649
Adrenal chromaffin granule
  membranes
    actin-binding proteins associ-
      ated with, 651
Adrenal chromaffin granules
  annexins and, 653-54
Adrenaline
  See Epinephrine

β-Adrenergic agents
  respiratory cilia and, 150
α-Adrenergic agonists
  amino acid incorporation in
    hepatocytes and, 581
  osmoregulation in freshwater
    teleosts and, 48-49
β-Adrenergic agonists
  teleost osmoregulation and,
    50
Adrenocorticosteroid receptors
  hormone binding regions of,
    832
Adrenoreceptors
  calcium ion influx into
    myocardium and, 552-53
Adult T-cell leukemia
  human T-lymphotropic virus
    type 1 and, 848
AIDS
  See Acquired immunodeficiency
    syndrome
Air
  amphibious invertebrate gas
    exchange in, 63-65
Airway epithelia
  electrolyte transport by, 115-
    16
Airways
  immunoglobulin secretion in,
    177-92
Albumin
  hyperoncotic
    atrial natriuretic peptide-
      induced natriuresis
      and, 751
  serous cell, 102
Aldose reductase
  sorbitol biosynthesis and,
    733
Aldosterone
  biosynthesis of
    atrial natriuretic factor and,
    702
  secretion of
    atriopeptin and, 45
Allopurinol
  myocardial infarction and,
    498-99
  myocardial ischemia and,
    564-65
Amiloride
  sodium transport in neutro-
    phils and, 368
Amphibians
  oxyntic cells of
    electrical properties of,
    309-11
Androgens
  inhibin production and, 812

ANF
   See Atrial natriuretic factor
Angiogenesis
   endothelium-derived vasoac-
      tive agents and, 661
Angioplasty
   ischemic cardiac injury and,
      488
Angiotensin II
   amino acid incorporation in
      hepatocytes and, 581
   atrial natriuretic factor and,
      702
   cardiac calcium ion channels
      and, 267
   drinking reflex and, 49-50
   voltage-dependent calcium ion
      channels and, 281-82
Annelids
   calcium-containing concretions
      in, 88
Annexins
   adrenal chromaffin granules
      and, 653-54
   exocytosis and, 620
ANP
   See Atrial natriuretic peptide
Anthracene-9-carboxylic acid
   chloride ion secretion and,
      118
Antibodies
   G proteins and, 225-26
Antigens
   inhaled
      fate of, 184-86
Antileukoprotease
   serous cell, 101
Antioxidants
   ischemic cardiac injury and,
      493-95
Antipsychotics
   cell recovery mechanisms
      and, 32-33
Antitrypsin deficiency
   animal model for, 847
Apical membranes
   chloride ion channels of
      regulation of, 118-27
Aquatic animals
   calcium metabolism in, 77-89
Arachidonic acid
   calcium ion channels and,
      279-80
   sequestered calcium ion
      mobilization and, 581
   sodium transport in neut-
      rophils and, 367
Arginine vasotocin
   osmoregulation in freshwater
      teleosts and, 48
Arrhythmias
   reperfusion

ischemic cardiac injury
   and, 488-89
Atherogenesis
   endothelium and, 662
ATP
   See Adenosine triphosphate
Atrial natriuretic factor (ANF),
      699-705
   cardiac calcium ion channels
      and, 263-65
   renal circulation and, 699-701
   renal solute excretion and,
      702-5
   segmental tubular transport
      and, 701-2
Atrial natriuretic peptide (ANP),
      747-57
   actions along collecting duct,
      749-51
   cortical collecting duct
      sodium and water
      reabsorption and, 751-53
   inner medullary collecting
      duct and, 753-57
   renal actions of, 748-49
Atriopeptin
   fish osmoregulation and, 43-
      55
   physiologic effects in mam-
      mals, 44-45
   secretion in mammals
      control of, 46
Avian erythroblastosis virus
   v-erb-A oncogen product of,
      827
Axonemes
   respiratory ciliary, 138-44
Azidemethemoglobin, 21-22

B

Baclofen
   calcium ion currents and, 277
Bacteria
   membrane permeability in
      toluene and, 348-49
Bacteriotoxins
   cardiac calcium ion channels
      and, 265
BALT
   See Bronchial-associated lym-
      phoid tissue
Band 3 protein
   anion transport in erythrocytes
      and, 391-93
Benzamil
   sodium ion efflux in neut-
      rophils and, 366
Benzimidazoles
   gastric H,K-ATPase inhibition
      and, 337

Benzothiazepines
   neuronal calcium ion channels
      and, 251
Beta blockers
   ischemic cardiac injury and,
      488
Beta-escin
   cell permeabilization and, 858
Betaine
   renal metabolism and trans-
      port of, 735-37
Bezafibrate,
   sickle cell anemia and, 19
BHK cells
   permeabilization of
      hypertonic solutions and,
      350-51
Birds
   eggs of
      calcification of, 83
Blood coagulation
   annexins and, 620
   endothelium and, 661
Bohr effect, 12
Bradykinin
   chloride ion channels and,
      130
   endothelial cytoplasmic cal-
      cium concentration and,
      663
   inositol phosphate formation
      and, 662
   prostaglandin secretion and,
      665
   serous cells and, 105
   voltage-dependent calcium ion
      channels and, 279
Brain development
   POU-domain regulatory genes
      and, 782-86
Brassinosteroids
   cellular growth properties
      and, 834
8-Bromo-adenosine 3',5'-cyclic
      monophosphate
   pepsinogen secretion and,
      352-53
Bronchial-associated lymphoid
      tissue (BALT)
   function of, 184-86
   secretory immune response in
      generation of, 186-87
Bronchial secretions
   immunoglobulins in, 181-83
Bumetanide
   chloride ion transport in HL-
      60 cells and, 383
Bunyaviruses
   fusion reactions of, 676
BW 755C
   myocardial infarct size and,
      569

C

Caffeine
  calcium ion discharge in
    platelets and, 438
Caged compounds
  crossbridge cycle and, 866-69
  excitation-contraction coupling
    and, 859-63
  striated muscle contraction
    and, 875-92
Caged divalent cations, 897-912
Calcification
  mechanism of, 83-86
Calcium
  carbonic acid buffer system
    and, 80
  cytosolic
    elevation of, 663
  inorganic salts of
    solubility in water of, 78-
    80
  intracellular mobilization of
    inositol trisphosphate and,
    351-52
  metabolism in aquatic an-
    imals, 77-89
  potassium ion channels in
    lymphocytes and, 419-20
  regulation of muscle contrac-
    tion and, 888-90
  release from sarcoplasmic re-
    ticulum
    t-tubule depolarization and,
    890-91
Calcium carbonate
  as buffer, 86-87
  in invertebrates, 81
  solubility of, 78
  Calcium chloride
    solubility of, 78
Calcium ion channels
  endothelial, 663-64
  G protein gating of, 205-8
  G proteins modulating, 275-88
  inhibition of, 276-81
  L-type
    dihydropyridine receptors
      and, 261-63
    proteases and, 263
  mitogen-activated
    lymphocytes and, 422-24
  myoblast fusion and, 689
  neuronal, 243-44
  neurotransmitters and, 245-
    47
Calcium ion currents
  neuronal
    G proteins and, 247-51
Calcium ionophore A23187
  neutrophil degranulation and,
    374

Calcium ion overload
  mechanisms in reperfused
    ischemic myocardium,
    543-55
Calcium ions
  affinity for DM-nitrophen,
    904
  cell recovery mechanisms
    and, 27-39
  entry into platelets, 439-44
  intracellular
    model for manipulation of,
      579-80
  intramitochondrial enzymes
    sensitive to, 453-57
  platelet activation and, 431-32
  protein synthesis and, 577-87
  transport in neutrophils, 371-
    75
Calcium ion transport systems
  sarcolemmal
    perturbations of, 544-55
Calcium phosphate
  as buffer, 86-87
Calcium signaling
  in platelets, 431-45
Calcium sulfate
  solubility of, 78
Caldesmon
  adrenal chromaffin granule
    membranes and, 651
Calmodulin
  adrenal chromaffin cells and,
    653
  cell recovery mechanisms
    and, 32-33
  intracellular calcium and,
    467
  protein phosphorylation and,
    35-36
Calpactin
  adrenal chromaffin granules
    and, 653
Carbachol
  potassium ion channels and,
    228
Carbamyl phosphate synthetase
  intramitochondrial enzymes
    and, 457
Carbon dioxide
  properties in water and air,
    61-62
  reactions with hemoglobin, 1-
    23
Carbonic acid buffer system
  calcium and, 80
Carboxylic acid analogues
  chloride ion secretion and,
    118
Carcinus maenas axons
  hypoosmotically stressed
    cytochalasin B and, 34

Cardiac cells
  L-type calcium ion currents in
    regulation of, 257-68
Cardiac energetics
  load and length regulation of,
    505-18
Cardiac myocytes
  calcium ion channels in, 244
  potassium ion channels in
    muscarinic activation of,
    295-96
  voltage-dependent calcium ion
    channels in
    stimulation of, 283-84
Cardiac peptide hormone
  fish osmoregulation and, 43-
    55
Catalase
  as antioxidant, 495
  myocardial reperfusion injury
    and, 563
Catecholamines
  calcium ion influx into
    myocardium and, 552-53
  free radical generation and,
    490
  release of
    exocytotic, 591
    permeabilized adrenal chro-
      maffin cells and, 355-
      56
Cell death
  programmed
    mutations causing, 843-46
Cells
  regulatory volume decrease
    in, 400-5
  regulatory volume increase in,
    405-11
Cellular fusion reactions, 687-90
Cellular physiology
  caged compounds in, 853-55
Cell volume recovery
  calcium ion-activated, 27-39
Central nervous system
  atriopeptin and, 45
Cetiedil
  cell volume regulation in
    leukocytes and, 402
Charybdotoxin
  calcium ion-activated potas-
    sium channels and, 128
  cell volume regulation in
    leukocytes and, 403
  potassium ion channels in
    lymphocytes and, 417
Chemical stress
  calcium ion-dependent protein
    synthesis and, 586-87
Chemotactic factor
  Sodium/hydrogen exchange in
    leukocytes and, 407

sodium transport in neutrophils and, 367-68
Chlamydomonas
  exocytosis in, 612
Chloramines
  function of, 564
Chloride ion channels
  activation by cyclic AMP-dependent protein kinase, 120-21
  activation by hypotonic bathing solution, 126-27
  activation by protein kinase C, 121-23
  activation in excised, cell-free membrane patches, 119-20
  apical membrane identification of, 118-19
  inactivation by protein kinase C, 123-25
  in lymphocytes, 420-21
Chloride ions
  exchange in leukocytes, 382-83
2-Chloroadenosine
  calcium ion currents and, 277
Chlorpromazine
  cell recovery mechanisms and, 32-33
  cell volume regulation in leukocytes and, 402
  potassium ion channels in lymphocytes and, 417
Cholate
  gastric H,K-ATPase solubilization and, 333
Cholecystokinin
  pepsinogen secretion and, 352-53
Cholera toxin
  cardiac calcium ion channels and, 265
Cholesterol
  biosynthesis of oxygenated sterols and, 834
Cholinergic agents
  respiratory cilia and, 150
Chromatin
  hormone-responsive genes and, 831-32
Chromobindin A
  adrenal chromaffin granules and, 654
Cilia
  respiratory
    axonemal basis of motility of, 140-44
    mechanosensitivity of, 149-50
    movement and coordination of, 146-47
    mucus transport by, 145-46

physiology of, 137-52
  structure and function of, 138-44
  water transport by, 144-45
Cirrhosis
  atrial natriuretic factor and, 705
Clofibric acid
  sickle cell anemia and, 19
Collagen
  calcium ion release in platelets and, 434
  endothelial secretion of, 661
Collagen fibers
  assembly of urea and, 727
Complement system
  myocardial ischemic injury and, 569-70
Congestive heart failure
  atrial natriuretic factor and, 705
Conotoxin
  calcium ion channels and, 244
Coronaviruses
  fusion reactions of, 676
Cortical collecting duct
  sodium and water reabsorption in
    mechanisms of, 751-52
  water and sodium transport in atrial natriuretic peptide and, 752-53
Corticosteroids
  inhibin production and, 812
Cortisol
  secretion of atriopeptin and, 45
Crabs
  land
    ion conservation in, 72-73
CRE-binding 43-kd protein
  action of, 800-1
  purification of, 798-99
  transcriptional activity of, 799-800
Crossbridge cycle
  caged compounds and, 866-69
Crustaceans
  calcium-containing concretions in, 88
α-Cyano-4-hydroxycannimate
  anion exchange in neutrophils and, 384
  chloride ion transport in neutrophils and, 383
Cyclic AMP
  amylase secretion and, 354
  calcium-activated calmodulin and, 35

calcium ion entry into platelets and, 444
calcium ion sequestration in platelets and, 436-37
cardiac potassium ion channels and, 300
CRE-binding 43-kd protein and, 801-3
neuronal calcium ion channels and, 248
protein synthesis and, 584-85
respiratory cilia and, 150
serous cells and, 106-7
voltage-dependent calcium ion channels and, 282
Cyclic GMP
  calcium ion entry into platelets and, 444
  calcium ion sequestration in platelets and, 436-37
  cardiac calcium ion channels and, 267
Cycloheximide
  brassinosteroids and, 834
  protein synthesis and, 582
Cystic fibrosis
  epithelial hydroelectrolytic exchange system and, 165
Cytochalasin B
  cell recovery and, 34
  exocytosis from neutrophils and, 599
  neutrophil degranulation and, 370
Cytochalasin D
  Noetia red blood cells and, 34
Cytochrome b561
  large dense-core vesicles and, 630
  regulated exocytosis from neurons and, 629
Cytochrome c oxidase
  cytochrome c oxidation and, 533-34
Cytoskeleton
  hypoosmotic stress and, 34-35
  peripheral exocytosis and, 640

D

Dantroline
  calcium ion discharge in platelets and, 438
Dehydration stress
  amphibious invertebrates and, 71-72
Dehydrogenases
  intramitochondrial metabolism and, 453-56

Deoxyhemoglboin S
    aggregation in sickle cell
        anemia
    compunds preventing, 19
Deoxyhemoglobin
    stereochemistroy of hemes in,
        5-8
Detergents
    plasma membrane per-
        meabilization and, 346-
        47
Dextran sulfate
    plasma membrane permeabil-
        ity and, 350
Diacylglycerol
    calcium ion influx into
        myocardium and, 553
    formation of, 662-63
    potassium ion channels and,
        232-33
    protein kinase C activation
        and, 279
Dictyostelium discoideum
    fruiting body formation in
        stalk cell differentiation
        during, 834
Diethylstilbestrol
    estrogen receptor and, 830
Digitonin
    plasma membrane per-
        meabilization and, 346-
        47
Dihydropyridine receptors
    L-type calcium ion channels
        and, 261-63
Dihydropyridines
    neuronal calcium ion channels
        and, 251
    potassium ion channels in
        lymphocytes and, 417
Diltiazem
    cell volume regulation in
        leukocytes and, 403
    neuronal calcium ion channels
        and, 251
    potassium ion channels in
        lymphocytes and, 417
Dioxin receptor
    lipid-activated transcriptional
        factors and, 833-34
Diphenylamine-2-carboxylate
    chloride ion secretion and,
        118
Diphenylbutylpiperidines
    cell recovery mechanisms
        and, 32-33
2,3-Diphosphoglycerate
    β-chains in T-structure and,
        11
Diphtheria toxin
    cell ablation studies and, 843-
        44

Divalent cations
    photochemical manipulation
        of, 897-912
    photolabile chelators for, 898-
        99
    DM-nitrophen, 904-7
    nitr-5 compared, 909-12
    physiologic applications of,
        907-9
DNA
    CRE-binding 43-kd protein
        binding to, 800-1
Donnan equilibrium
    mucus hydration and, 163-66
Dopamine
    calcium ion currents and, 277
    potassium ion channels and,
        218
Dopamine β-hydroxylase
    large dense-core vesicles and,
        630
Drug detoxification
    nuclear receptor protein and,
        833
Dynein
    structure and mechanochemis-
        try of, 139

E

Edeine
    protein synthesis inhibition
        by, 582
EDTA
    enterocyte permeability and,
        349-50
Ehrlich ascites tumor cells
    permeability of
        dextran sulfate and, 350
Elasmobranchs
    osmoregulation in
        atriopeptin and, 47
        hormonal control of, 50
Electrolytes
    transport by airway epithelia,
        115-16
Electron transport chain
    oxygen and, 525
Elongation factor 2
    reticulocyte protein synthesis
        and, 583
Embryological development
    urea and, 727
Emulgen
    gastric H,K-ATPase
        solubilization and, 333
Endocrine cells
    microvesicle population of
        small synaptic vesicles and,
        631-33
    synaptophysin in, 649

voltage-dependent calcium ion
    channels in
        inhibition of, 276-81
        stimulation of, 281-83
Endoglycosidase F
    gastric H,K-ATPase and, 323
Endonexin I
    adrenal chromaffin granules
        and, 653
Endoplasmic fusion reactions,
    688-89
Endothelial cell growth factor
    inositol phosphate formation
        and, 662
Endothelial cells
    adenylate and guanylate cyc-
        lases of, 664
    calcium ion channels in, 663-
        64
    myocardial reperfusion injury
        and, 570-71
    potassium ion channels in,
        664
    vascular
        stimulus-secretion coupling
            in, 661-69
Endothelin
    endothelial secretion of, 661
Endothelium
    secretory functions of, 661-
        62
Endothelium-derived relaxing
    factor
    endothelial secretion of, 661
    stimulus-secretion coupling
        and, 666-67
Endotoxicosis
    intracellular calcium mobiliza-
        tion and, 351-52
Eosin-5-isothiocyanate
    anion exchange in neutrophils
        and, 384
Eosinophils
    exocytosis from, 600
Epidermal growth factor
    inhibin production and, 812
Epinephrine
    calcium ion release in
        platelets and, 434
Epithelia
    airway
        electrolyte transport by,
            115-16
        ion transport pathways in,
            315-17
Epithelial cells
    ciliated
        mechanism of ciliary re-
            sponse and, 148-52
Erythrocytes
    anion transport in
        band 3 protein and, 391-93

Estrogen receptor
  antiestrogens and, 830
  genes encoding, 825
  homologies of, 827
  receptor zinc finger domains
    and, 833
Ethacrynic acid
  chloride ion transport in neu-
    trophils and, 383
Euryhaline teleosts
  osmoregulation in
    atriopeptin and, 47
Excitation-contraction coupling,
  888-91
  caged compounds and, 859-63
Exocrine cells
  synaptophysin in, 649
Exocrine glands
  acid secretion by
    epithelial and cellular
      morphology of, 308
Exocytosis, 607-21
  adenosine triphosphate mod-
    ulating, 596-99
  early steps in, 610-11
  electrophysiologic assays of,
    612-13
  G proteins and, 591-603
  mediators of, 620
  mucin, 168-72
  regulated in neurons, 625-41
  secretory vesicle-associated
    proteins and, 647-56
  sites of
    specializations near, 611-12
  time-resolved, 613-20
Exocytotic membrane fusion
  properties of, 608-10
Exoplasmic fusion reactions,
  689-90

F

FADH
  oxidative phosphorylation
    and, 531-33
Fatty acids
  calcium ion channels and,
    279-80
Fibronectin
  endothelial secretion of, 661
Fibronectin receptor
  myoblast fusion and, 689-90
Filipin
  plasma membrane permeabil-
    ity and, 350
Fish atriopeptin, 43-55
Fish osmoregulation
  cardiac peptide hormone and,
    43-55
  hormonal control of, 48-50
Flash photolysis
  smooth muscle and, 857-71

Flufenamate
  anion exchange in neutrophils
    and, 384
FMRF-amide
  neuronal calcium ion channels
    and, 250
Fodrin
  adrenal chromaffin granule
    membranes and, 651
Follicle-stimulating hormone
  (FSH)
  secretion of
    inhibin and, 807
Forskolin
  calcium ion entry into
    platelets and, 444
  cardiac potassium ion chan-
    nels and, 300
  insulin secretion and, 355
  pepsinogen secretion and,
    352-53
Free radicals
  myocardial ischemia and,
    487-500
  oxygen-derived
    sources of, 563-65
    sources of, 489-90
Freshwater teleosts
  osmoregulation in
    atriopeptin and, 46
    hormonal control of, 48-49
FSH
  See Follicle-stimulating hor-
    mone
Fura-2
  calcium ion release in
    platelets and, 435
Furosemide
  chloride ion transport in neu-
    trophils and, 383
  potassium transport in neutro-
    phils and, 367

G

GABA
  See Gamma-aminobutyric acid
GALT
  See Gut-associated lymphoid
    tissue
Gamma-aminobutyric acid
  (GABA)
  calcium ion currents and, 277
  neuronal calcium ion channels
    and, 246
  potassium ion channels and,
    218
Gancyclovir
  toxicity of, 846
Gap junctions
  exocytotic membrane fusion
    and, 610
Gardos effect, 367

Gastric epithelia
  ion transport pathways in,
    315-17
Gastric H,K-ATPase, 321-39
  catalytic and transport func-
    tion of, 327-38
  catalytic subunit of
    primary sequence of, 323-
      24
  conformational structure of,
    326-27
  inhibitors of, 337-38
  molecular organization of,
    322-23
  regulation of, 334-37
  secondary structure of, 325-26
  solubilization and reconstitu-
    tion of, 333-34
Gastric juice
  secretion of
    membrane fusion in oxyntic
      cells and, 308
Gastric mucosa
  stimulus-secretion coupling
    events in, 352-54
Gastric secretory cells
  polarity of, 312-13
Gastrointestinal cells
  stimulus-secretion coupling
    events in, 351-55
Gecarcinus lateralis
  hydromineral balance in, 72
Gene expression
  mutations causing, 842-43
  mutations eliminating, 849-
    50
Genetics
  reverse, 841-50
Gene transcription
  animal growth and develop-
    ment and, 824-25
GH3 cells
  intracellular calcium ion ma-
    nipulation and, 579-80
Gibberellins
  cellular growth properties
    and, 834
Glomerular filtration rate
  atrial natriuretic factor and,
    699-700
  atrial natriuretic peptide and,
    748-49
Glucagon
  cardiac calcium ion channels
    and, 263-65
  teleost osmoregulation and,
    50
Glucocorticoid receptor
  genes encoding, 825-27
  homologies of, 827
  RU486 and, 830
Glucocorticoids
  atriopeptin secretion and, 46

Glucose
  sorbitol biosynthesis and, 733
Glucose-insulin-potassium
  ischemic cardiac injury and,
    488
Glycerophosphorylcholine
  renal metabolism and trans-
    port of, 737-38
Goblet cells
  secretion and mucogenesis
    and, 157-73
  structure and function of,
    166-72
Gonadotropin-releasing hormone
  inhibin production and, 812
G proteins
  calcium ion channel ligand
    binding sites and, 251-
    52
  calcium ion channel modula-
    tion and, 275-88
  calcium ion channels and,
    205-8
  cardiac L-type calcium ion
    currents and, 257-68
  cardiac potassium ion chan-
    nels and, 293-302
  exocytosis and, 591-603, 639
  ionic channels and, 197-208
  muscarinic atrial potassium
    ion channels and, 199-
    203
  neuronal calcium ion currents
    and, 247-51
  neuronal potassium ion chan-
    nels and, 204-5
  neuronal potassium ion cur-
    rents and, 215-34
  phospholipase C activity in
    neutrophils and, 356
  potassium ion channels and,
    222-33
  potassium ion channels in
    pituitary cells and, 203-4
  presence in nerve cells, 223-
    24
Gramicidin
  calcium ion discharge in
    platelets and, 438
Granulocyte-macrophage colony
  stimulating factor
  ion movements in neutrophils
    and, 376-77
Granulosa cells
  inhibin production by
    regulation of, 811-12
Growth factors
  stimulus-secretion coupling
    and, 668
Growth hormone gene expression
  development patterns of
    determinants of, 774-76

GTP-binding proteins
  exocytosis and, 655
Guanine nucleotides
  calcium ion currents and,
    277-78
Guanylate cyclase
  endothelial, 664
Gut-associated lymphoid tissue
  (GALT)
  IgA-secreting cells and, 186-
    87

H

Haemophilus pneumoniae
  secretory IgA and, 179
Heart
  calcium ion transients in,
    467-82
  mitochondrial respiration in
    control of, 523-38
  mitochondria of
    calcium ion transport sys-
      tem of, 451-62
  potassium ion channel regula-
    tion in
    G proteins and, 293-302
Heart cells
  L-type calcium ion currents in
    regulation of, 257-68
Helper T cells
  mucosal lymphoid tissues
    and, 187-90
Heme pockets
  residues in
    directed mutagenesis of,
      15-19
Hemes
  stereochemistry in hemoglo-
    bins, 5-8
Hemocyanin
  calcium binding to, 79
Hemoglobin
  as drug receptor, 19-23
  human
    reactions with oxygen and
      carbon monoxide, 1-23
    respiratory function and,
      14-15
    structures of, 3-4
Hemopoietic colony stimulating
  factors
  stimulus-secretion coupling
    and, 668
Hepatitis
  neonatal
    animal model for, 847
Hepatocytes
  membrane permeability in
    toluene and, 348-49
Herpesviruses
  fusion reactions of, 676

Herpesvirus thymidine kinase,
  845-46
Histamine
  cardiac calcium ion channels
    and, 263-65
  endothelial cytoplasmic cal-
    cium concentration and,
    663
  inositol phosphate formation
    and, 662
  prostaglandin secretion and,
    665
  secretion of
    calcium ion concentrations
      and, 356-57
  serous cells and, 105
  tissue plasminogen activator
    secretion and, 668
HIV
  See Human immunodeficiency
    virus
HL-60 cells
  anion exchange in
    pH and, 386-87
    substrate selectivity of,
      385-86
  anion transport in, 381-94
  exocytosis from, 599-600
Hormones
  lipid-soluble
    receptor family binding,
      825-27
  potassium ion channels and,
    218
HTLV-1
  See Human T-lymphotropic
    virus type 1
Human disease
  mutations modeling, 847-
    48
Human immunodeficiency virus
  (HIV)
  fusion reactions of, 676
  host range of, 848
Human T-lymphotropic virus
  type 1 (HTLV-1)
  adult T-cell leukemia and,
    848
Hyaluronidase
  ischemic cardiac injury and,
    488
Hydrogen ions
  transport in neutrophils, 375-
    76
Hydrogen peroxide
  function of, 564
Hydroxyapatite
  in vertebrate bone, 81-82
Hydroxyl anion
  function of, 564
8-Hydroxyquinoline
  calcium ion-dependent protein
    synthesis and, 586-87

Hydroxytamoxifen
  estrogen receptor and, 830
5-Hydroxytryptamine
  See Serotonin
Hypertension
  atrial natriuretic factor and,
    705
Hypochlorous acid
  function of, 564
Hypoosmotic stress
  cellular swelling and, 27
  cytoskeleton and, 34-35

I

Ibuprofen
  myocardial protective effect
    of, 569
Immotile cilia syndrome, 137
Immune exclusion
  secretory IgA and, 181
Immunoglobulin A
  secretory
    immune exclusion and, 181
    immunochemical features
      of, 178-83
    serous cell, 101
Immunoglobulin E
  in bronchoalveolar lavage
    fluid, 182
Immunoglobulin G
  bronchial mucosa and, 182-83
Immunoglobulins
  in bronchial secretions, 181-
    83
  secretion in airways, 177-92
Inflammatory response
  endothelium and, 662
Influenza virus hemagglutinin
  fusion-associated con-
    formational changes in,
    685
  fusion peptides of, 681-84
Inhibin
  production by granulosa cells
    regulation of, 811-12
  reproductive status and, 812-
    16
  structure and function of, 808
  synthesis in rat ovary
    regulation of, 807-17
Inhibin genes
  gonadal and extragonadal ex-
    pression of, 809-11
Inner medullary collecting duct
  sodium and water transport in
    atrial natriuretic peptide
      and, 753-57
Inositol phosphates
  calcium ion discharge in
    platelets and, 436
  formation of, 662-63

Inositol trisphosphate
  caged
    excitation-contraction cou-
      pling and, 859-63
  calcium ion influx into
    myocardium and, 553
  intracellular calcium mobiliza-
    tion and, 351
  potassium ion channels and,
    232
Insulin
  inhibin production and, 812
  secretion of
    glucose-induced, 354-55
Insulin-secreting cells
  exocytosis from, 601-2
Interleukin-1
  endothelium and, 662
  neutrophil adhesion to en-
    dothelial cells and, 571
Interleukin-2
  cell volume regulation in
    leukocytes and, 403
Intravascular thrombosis
  endothelial regulation of, 661
Invertebrates
  amphibious
    acid-base balance regulation
      in, 69-71
    dehydration stress and, 71-
      72
  calcium carbonate in, 81
  intertidal
    aerobic vs anaerobic
      metabolism in air-
        exposed, 63-65
  marine
    control of calcium in, 88-
      89
    respiratory and ionic regula-
      tion in, 61-73
Ion channels
  G proteins and, 197-208
  in oxyntic cells, 313-15
  in parietal cells, 315
  See also specific type
Ionomycin
  potassium ion channels in
    macrophages and, 420
Ion pumps
  DM-nitrophen and, 909
Ischemic heart disease
  free radicals and, 487-500
Isoproterenol
  chloride ion channels and,
    130
  respiratory cilia and, 150

K

Kidney
  atrial natriuretic factor and,
    699-705

atriopeptin and, 45
  See also associated structures
Kinases
  secretory vesicle, 651-52

L

La Crosse virus spike glycopro-
    tein
  fusion-associated con-
    formational changes in,
    685
Lactoferrin
  serous cell, 100-1
Lactotrophs
  appearance during develop-
    ment, 773-74
  pit-1 expression in
    ontogeny of, 780-82
Land crabs
  ion conservation in, 72-73
Large dense-core vesicles
  biogenesis of, 635-36
  distribution in neurons, 636-
    37
  exocytosis of, 637-38
    mechanisms of, 638-40
  membrane composition of,
    630-31
  regulated exocytosis from
    neurons and, 629-30
α-Latrotoxin
  exocytosis of small synaptic
    vesicles and, 637
Leukemia
  adult T-cell
    human T-lymphotropic
      virus type 1 and, 848
Leukocytes
  anion exchange in, 381-94
  cell volume regulation in,
    399-412
  free radical generation and,
    490
  ion movements in, 363-64
  regulatory volume decrease
    in, 400-5
  regulatory volume increase in,
    405-11
  volume regulation in
    significance of, 411-12
Leukotriene B4
  neutrophil activation during
    myocardial ischemia and,
    568
  sodium transport in neutro-
    phils and, 367
Lipid bilayers
  fusion of, 610
Lipids
  viral fusion reactions and,
    677

Lipocortin
  adrenal chromaffin granules
    and, 653
Lipophilic ligands
  morphogenetic and homeosta-
    tic, 824-25
Liver
  stimulus-secretion coupling
    events in, 351-52
Loop of Henle
  atrial natriuretic factor and,
    701-2
LR30
  sickle cell anemia and, 19-21
Lungs
  secretory immunity of, 177-92
  generation of, 183-90
Luteinizing hormone-releasing
  hormone
  voltage-dependent calcium ion
    channels and, 282
Lymphocytes
  calcium ion channels in
    mitogen-activated, 422-24
  chloride ion channels in, 420-
    21
  migratory patterns of, 191-92
  potassium ion channels in
    calcium-activated, 419-20
    voltage-gated, 417-19
  transmembrane ion fluxes in,
    415-24
Lymphokines
  mucosal lymphoid tissue hel-
    per T cells and, 187-88
Lysolecithin
  plasma membrane per-
    meabilization and, 346-
    47
Lysozyme
  serous cell, 99-100

M

Macrophages
  potassium ion channels in
    ionomycin and, 420
Mammalian cells
  protein synthesis in
    calcium-dependent regula-
      tion of, 577-87
Mammalian ventricle
  calcium ion transients in
    dissection of, 472-81
  cytoplasmic calcium ions in,
    467-82
Mammals
  atriopeptin secretion in
    control of, 46
  brain development in
    POU-domain regulatory
      genes and, 782-86

drinking reflex in
  angiotensin II and, 49
parietal cells of
  electrical properties of,
    311-12
  physiologic effects of
    atriopeptin in, 44-45
Mast cells
  exocytosis and, 593-99
  secretory vesicles of
    exocytosis of, 614-18
Mellitin
  inositol phosphate formation
    and, 662
Membrane attack complex
  ischemic myocardium and,
    570
Membrane fusion reactions
  viral, 675-78
Membrane permeabilization
  secretory cells investigated
    by, 594
Membrane potential
  calcium ion discharge in
    platelets and, 438
Metabolic alkalosis
  atrial natriuretic factor and,
    704
Microfilaments
  catecholamine release and,
    356
Microtubules
  axonemal, 138-39
Mineralocorticoid receptor
  receptor zinc finger domains
    and, 833
Mineralocorticoids
  atriopeptin secretion and, 46
Mitochondria
  cardiac
    calcium ion transport sys-
      tem of, 451-62
    membrane permeability in
      toluene and, 348-49
    total calcium in
      measurement of, 458
Mitogens
  calcium ion channels in lym-
    phocytes and, 422-24
  endothelial secretion of, 661
  Sodium/hydrogen ion ex-
    change in leukocytes
    and, 407
MK-473
  anion exchange in neutrophils
    and, 384
Molluscs
  calcium-containing concretions
    in, 88
  eggs of
    calcification of, 83
Mouse mammary tumor virus
  fusion reactions of, 676

Mucin exocytosis, 168-72
Mucin polymer
  structure and properties of,
    162-63
Mucociliary clearance
  cellular functions involved in,
    158
Mucociliary transport, 137-52
Mucoproteins
  in gastric juice, 308
Mucus
  pathology of, 165-66
  respiratory
    disulfide-bonded network
      model and, 159-60
    entangled-network model
      and, 160-62
    macromolecular conforma-
      tion of, 158-62
  transport by respiratory cilia,
    145-46
Mucus hydration
  Donnan equilibrium and, 163-
    66
Multiple sclerosis
  human T-lymphotropic virus
    type 1 and, 848
Muscle
  contraction of
    calcium regulation of, 888-
      90
    load and length effects on,
      509-13
    nitr-5 and, 904
    urea and, 727
  See also Smooth muscle; Stri-
    ated muscle
Muscle fibers
  actomyosin ATPase in, 879-
    88
  adenosine diphosphate release
    in, 887-88
  adenosine triphosphate hydro-
    lysis in, 883-84
  phosphate release in, 884-
    87
Mutagenesis
  targeted, 849-50
Mutations
  aberrant gene expression and,
    842-43
  gene expression eliminated
    by, 849-50
  modeling human diseases,
    847-48
  programmed cell death and,
    843-46
Mycophenolic acid
  endogenous GTP and, 596
Myocardial infarction
  measurement of
    tetrazolium staining and,
      491-92

xanthine oxidase inhibitors
and, 498-99
Myocardial ischemia
free radicals and, 487-500
Myocardial reperfusion injury
chemotactic factors and, 569-
70
endothelial cell and, 570-71
inhibition of neutrophil adhesion and, 572
leukocyte-mediated
modulation of, 561-73
neutrophil cell surface glycoproteins and, 571-72
reactive oxygen metabolites
and, 565-68
Myocardium
isolate linear
energetics of, 507-9
reperfused ischemic
calcium ion overload and,
543-55
ventricular
energetics of, 506-7
Myoglobin
carbon monoxide orientations
in, 18
Myo-inositol
physiologic functions of, 742
renal metabolism and transport of, 732-33
Myosin
neutrophil locomotion and,
373

N

NADH
oxidative phosphorylation
and, 531-33
NAP-taurine
anion exchange in neutrophils
and, 384
NEM-sensitive factor
exocytosis and, 620
Neonatal hepatitis
animal model for, 847
Nephron
cell volume regulation in,
761-70
Nephrosis
atrial natriuretic factor and,
705
Nerve cells
G proteins present in, 223-24
Neurofibromatosis
animal model for, 848
Neuromodulators
regulated secretion of
pathways of, 640-41
Neuronal cells
voltage-dependent calcium ion
channels in

inhibition of, 276-81
Neuronal synapses
exocytosis at, 611
Neurons
calcium ion channels in, 244
function of
calcium ion channels and,
243-44
potassium currents in
G proteins and, 215-34
potassium ion channels in
G protein gating of, 204-5
POU-domain gene expression
in, 786-87
regulated exocytosis from,
625-41
regulated secretion from
neuronal signaling and,
640-41
Neuropeptide Y
calcium ion currents and, 277
neuronal calcium ion channels
and, 246
Neurosecretory cells
exocytosis from, 600-1
Neurotransmitters
neuronal calcium ion channels
and, 245-47
regulated secretion of
pathways of, 640-41
synapsin I and, 652
Neutrophils
activation of
chemotactic stimuli and,
569-70
adherence-promoting cell surface glycoproteins of,
571-72
anion exchange in
pH and, 386-87
substrate selectivity of,
385-86
anion transport in, 381-94
calcium ion transport in, 371-
75
exocytosis from, 599
hydrogen ion transport in,
375-76
ion movements in
granulocyte-macrophage
colony stimulating fac-
tor and, 376-77
oxygen-derived free radicals
and, 563-64
phospholipase C activity in
G proteins and, 356
sodium and potassium ions
in, 365-71
as source of reactive oxygen
metabolites, 568-69
Newcastle-disease virus
plasma membrane permeability and, 349

Nifedipine
cell volume regulation in
leukocytes and, 403
neuronal calcium ion channels
and, 251
Niflumate
anion exchange in neutrophils
and, 384
Nigericin
chemotaxis in neutrophils
and, 369
Nitr-5, 899-901
DM-nitrophen compared, 909-
12
physiologic applications of,
901-4
5-Nitro-2-(3-phenylpropyl-
amino)-benzoate
chloride ion secretion and,
118
Nitroprusside
calcium ion entry into
platelets and, 444
platelet responses to agonists
and, 437
Noetia red blood cells
cell volume recovery by
cytochalasin D and, 34
Noradrenaline
See Norepinephrine
Norepinephrine
calcium ion currents and, 277
neuronal calcium ion channels
and, 246
potassium ion channels and,
218
Nuclear receptors, 823-35
dimerization and allosteric
changes in, 829-30
evolution of, 832-34
modular domains of, 827-29
transcriptional activation of,
829-32
DNA binding and, 830-31

O

n-Octylglucoside
gastric H,K-ATPase
solubilization and, 333
Ocypode quadrata
hydromineral balance in, 72
Oleoylacetylglycerol
calcium ion release in
platelets and, 435
Oligomycin
potassium transport in neutrophils and, 367
Omeprazole
gastric H,K-ATPase inhibition
and, 337-38

Opiates
  neuronal calcium ion channels
    and, 246
  potassium ion channels and,
    218
Opioid peptides
  calcium ion currents and,
    277
Organic solutes
  renal medullary
    distribution of, 729-31
    metabolism and transport
      of, 731-38
    physiologic significance of,
      738-43
    regulatory volume decrease
      and, 769-70
    regulatory volume increase
      and, 765
Orthomyxoviruses
  fusion reactions of, 676
Osmoregulation
  fish
    cardiac peptide hormone
      and, 43-55
    hormonal control of, 48-50
Osteogenesis imperfecta type 2
  animal model for, 847
Ouabain
  regulatory volume increase in
    leukocytes and, 406
  sodium ion efflux in neut-
    rophils and, 366
Oxidative phosphorylation
  adenosine triphosphate forma-
    tion by, 524-26
  regulation of, 526-31
Oxoacid dehydrogenase complex
  intramitochondrial enzymes
    and, 457
Oxygen
  electron transport chain and,
    525
  properties in water and air,
    61-62
  rate of myocardial respiration
    and, 534-36
  reactions with hemoglobin, 1-
    23
  reactive metabolites of
    myocardial reperfusion in-
      jury and, 565-68
    neutrophils and, 568-69
  reactive species of
    myocardial reperfusion in-
      jury and, 563-65
Oxygen-free radicals
  calcium ion overload in
    ischemic myocardium
    and, 553-54
Oxyhemoglobin
  stereochemistroy of hemes in,
    5-8

Oxyntic cells
  amphibian
    electrical properties of,
      309-11
    apical potassium ion per-
      meability in, 316
  ion channels in, 313-15
  ion transport in, 308-9
  patch-clamp studies of, 312-
    15
Oxypurinol
  myocardial infarction and,
    498-99

P

Pactamycin
  protein synthesis inhibition
    by, 582
Pancreas
  stimulus-secretion coupling
    events in, 354-55
Pancreatic islet cells
  synaptophysin in, 649
Paramecium
  exocytosis in, 611-12
Paramyxoviruses
  fusion reactions of, 676
Parathyroid cells
  exocytosis from, 601
Parathyroid hormone
  release of
    calcium ion concentrations
      and, 356
Parietal cells
  electrophysiology of, 307-17
  ion channels in, 315
  mammalian
    electrical properties of,
      311-12
  patch-clamp studies of, 312-
    15
Parotid cells
  exocytosis from, 602
Parotid gland
  acinar cells of
    synaptophysin in, 649
Pepsinogen
  in gastric juice, 308
  secretion of
    intracellular mechanisms of,
      352
Peptide α-amidase
  large dense-core vesicles and,
    630
Peroxidase
  serous cell, 101
Pertussis toxin
  calcium ion currents and,
    278
  cardiac calcium ion channels
    and, 265

G proteins and, 225
  voltage-dependent calcium ion
    channels and, 282
Peyer's patches
  IgA-secreting cells and, 186-
    87
pH
  anion exchange in neutrophils
    and, 386-87
  calcium ion mobilization in
    platelets and, 437-38
  viral fusion reactions and,
    676
Phenothiazines
  cell recovery mechanisms
    and, 32-33
  cell volume regulation in
    leukocytes and, 402
Phentolamine
  intracellular calcium mobiliza-
    tion and, 352
Phenylakylamine D600
  neuronal calcium ion channels
    and, 251
Phenylephrine
  caged
    excitation-contraction cou-
      pling and, 859-63
  Purkinje fiber automaticity and,
    301
Phorbol 12-myristate
  sodium transport in neut-
    rophils and, 367
Phorbol esters
  amylase secretion and,
    354
  neuronal calcium ion channels
    and, 248-49
  protein synthesis and, 584-
    85
Phorbol myristate acetate
  calcium ion release in
    platelets and, 435
Phosphate
  release in muscle fibers, 884-
    87
Phosphoinositidase
  activation of, 662-63
  prostaglandin formation and,
    665-66
Phospholipase A2
  annexins and, 620
  potassium ion channels and,
    233
Phospholipase C
  activity in neutrophils
    G proteins and, 356
  adrenal chromaffin granules
    and, 654
  neuronal calcium ion channels
    and, 248-49
  potassium ion channels and,
    231-33

Phospholipases
  calcium ion overload in
    ischemic myocardium
    and, 554-55
  voltage-dependent calcium ion
    channels and, 282-83
Phosphoproteins
  secretory vesicle, 651-52
Phosphorylation
  cardiac L-type calcium ion
    currents and, 257-68
Pimozide
  cell recovery mechanisms
    and, 32-33
Pituitary cells
  potassium ion channels in
    G protein pathway to, 203-
    4
  synaptophysin in, 649
Pituitary specific transcription
    factor, 776-79
  expression of
    ontogeny of, 780-82
Plant glycosides
  cell permeabilization by, 591
Plasma membrane
  permeabilization of, 346-51
Plasminogen activator inhibitor
  endothelium and, 661
Platelet-activating factor
  calcium ion release in
    platelets and, 434
  endothelium and, 662
  neutrophil activation during
    myocardial ischemia and,
    568
  sodium transport in neutro-
    phils and, 367
Platelet adhesion proteins
  endothelial secretion of, 661
Platelet-derived growth factor
  stimulus-secretion coupling
    and, 668
Platelets
  calcium ion entry into, 439-
    44
  calcium signaling in, 431-45
  exocytosis from, 599
  ionic gradients in, 432-34
Polymyxin B
  neuronal calcium ion channels
    and, 248-49
Polysaccharide
  serous cells and, 102-3
Potassium ion channels
  calcium-activated
    lymphocytes and, 419-20
  cardiac
    G protein mediated regula-
      tion of, 293-302
  endothelial, 664
  identification of, 28

muscarinic atrial
  G protein gating of, 199-
    203
neuronal
  G protein gating of, 204-5
  G proteins and, 215-34
  transmitters closing, 219-22
  transmitters opening, 218-
    19
in pituitary cells
  G protein pathway to, 203-
    4
secretagogue-induced activa-
    tion of, 130-32
voltage-gated
  lymphocytes and, 417-19
Potassium ions
  in neutrophils, 365-71
POU-domain protein recognition
    sites, 779-80
POU-domain regulatory genes
  mammalian brain development
    and, 782-86
Presynaptic membrane potential
  transmitter release and, 901-4
Progesterone receptor
  genes encoding, 825
  receptor zinc finger domains
    and, 833
Prolactin
  osmoregulation in freshwater
    teleosts and, 48
Prolactin gene expression
  development patterns of
    determinants of, 774-76
Proline rich proteins
  serous cell, 101-2
Proopiomelanocortin gene
  transcription of
    repression of, 832
Propranolol
  intracellular calcium mobiliza-
    tion and, 352
  respiratory cilia and, 150
Prostacyclin
  endothelial secretion of, 661
Prostaglandin receptor
  serous cells and, 105
Prostaglandins
  free radical generation and,
    490
  stimulus-secretion coupling
    and, 664-66
Proteases
  L-type calcium ion channels
    and, 263
Protein III
  adrenal chromaffin cells and,
    652
Protein kinase
  calcium ion currents and,
    278-80

cyclic AMP-dependent
  chloride ion channel activa-
    tion by, 120-21
Protein kinase C
  adrenal chromaffin granules
    and, 654
  calcium ion currents and,
    279
  calcium ion entry into
    platelets and, 443-44
  catecholamine release and,
    356
  chloride channel activation
    by, 121-23
  chloride channel inactivation
    by, 12325
  internal calcium ion release in
    platelets and, 437
  neuronal calcium ion channels
    and, 248-49
  volume regulation in leuko-
    cytes and, 408
Protein phosphorylation
  calcium-activated calmodulin
    and, 35-36
Proteins
  secretory vesicle-associated
    exocytosis and, 647-56
  serous cell, 99-102
  viral membrane fusion, 678-
    86
  See also specific type
Protein synthesis
  amino acid incorporation in,
    580-81
  calcium ion-dependent, 577-
    87
    thermal and chemical stress
      and, 586-87
  chronic depletion of seques-
    tered calcium ions and,
    584-86
  in reticulocytes, 583-84
  translational phase of, 581-
    83
Protozoa
  exocytosis in, 611-12
Proximal tubule, 709-23
  atrial natriuretic factor and,
    701
  osmotic water permeability
    of, 710-13
  transepithelial osmolality dif-
    ferences and, 713-17
  water flow across
    pathways of, 717-23
Purkinje fibers
  automaticity of
    phenylephrine and, 301
Pyruvate carboxylase
  intramitochondrial enzymes
    and, 457

Q

Quinidine
  potassium transport in neutrophils and, 367
Quinine
  cell volume regulation in leukocytes and, 402
  potassium ion channels in lymphocytes and, 417
  potassium transport in neutrophils and, 367

R

Rat ovary
  inhibin synthesis in regulation of, 807-17
Receptor genes
  identification of, 825-27
Receptors
  dimerization and allosteric changes in, 829-30
  evolution of, 832-34
  homologies of, 827
  mutagenesis of, 827-28
  transcriptional activation of, 829-32
  DNA binding and, 830-31
Rectin
  elasmobranch osmoregulation and, 50
Renal medullary organic solutes
  metabolism and transport of, 731-38
  physiologic significance of, 738-43
  regulation of, 727-43
  regulatory volume decrease and, 769-70
  regulatory volume increase and, 765
Renin
  biosynthesis of
    atrial natriuretic factor and, 702
Renin-angiotensin system
  atriopeptin and, 45
Reperfusion arrhythmias
  ischemic cardiac injury and, 488-89
Reproductive cycle
  ovarian inhibin and, 812-16
Reptiles
  eggs of
    calcification of, 83
Respiration
  abnormal hemoglobins and, 14-15
Respiratory cilia
  mechanosensitivity of, 149-50

motility of
  axonemal basis of, 140-44
  movement and coordination of, 146-47
  mucus transport by, 145-46
  structure and function of, 138-44
  water transport by, 144-45
Respiratory mucus
  disulfide-bonded network model and, 159-60
  entangled-network model and, 160-62
  macromolecular conformation of, 158-62
  pathology of, 165-66
Respiratory tract
  mucociliary transport in, 137-52
Reticulocytes
  protein synthesis in, 583-84
Retinoic acid receptor
  thyroid hormone response element and, 832
Retroviruses
  fusion reactions of, 676
Reverse genetics, 841-50
Rhabdoviruses
  fusion reactions of, 676
Ribavirin
  endogenous GTP and, 596
Ricin
  cell ablation studies and, 843-44
RU486
  glucocorticoid receptor and, 830
Ruthenium red
  calcium ion uptake into mitochondria and, 459-60
Ryanodine
  calcium ion discharge in platelets and, 439

S

Saponin
  plasma membrane permeabilization and, 346-47
Sarcolemma
  calcium ion pumps of, 551-52
  perturbations of, 544-55
Sarcoplasmic reticulum
  calcium ion transients in heart and, 477
  calcium release from
    t-tubule depolarization and, 890-91
SCH 28080
  gastric H,K-ATPase inhibition and, 338

Seawater elasmobranchs
  osmoregulation in
    atriopeptin and, 47
    hormonal control of, 50
Seawater teleosts
  osmoregulation in
    atriopeptin and, 46-47
    hormonal control of, 49-50
Second messengers
  calcium ion entry into platelets and, 442
  potassium ion channels and, 229-33
Secretory epithelia
  ion transport pathways in, 315-17
Secretory IgA
  immune exclusion and, 181
  immunochemical features of, 178-83
  serous cell, 101
Secretory IgA deficiency, 181-82
Secretory vesicles
  cytoskeletal proteins of, 650-51
  phosphoproteins and kinases of, 651-52
  proteins binding to, 649-55
  regulated exocytosis from neurons and, 626
  time-resolved exocytosis of, 613-20
Sendai virus
  fusion reactions of, 677
  plasma membrane permeability and, 349
Serotonin
  calcium ion currents and, 277
  calcium ion release in platelets and, 434
  potassium ion channels and, 218
  respiratory cilia and, 150
Serous cells, 97-108
  cyclic AMP and, 106-7
  distribution and appearance of, 98-99
  high molecular weight glycoconguates of, 102-4
  injured airways and, 107-8
  proteins of, 99-102
  secretion from
    regulation of, 104-7
Sickle cell anemia
  aggregation of deoxyhemoglobin S in
    compounds preventing, 19
Sindbis virus spike glycoprotein
  fusion-associated conformational changes in, 685

Skeletal calcium salts
  physiologic buffering and, 86-
    87
Skeletal myocytes
  voltage-dependent calcium ion
    channels in
    stimulation of, 283-84
Sliding microtubule model
  respiratory cilia motility and,
    140-41
Small synaptic vesicles
  biogenesis of, 633-35
  distribution in neurons, 636-
    37
  endocrine cells and, 631-
    33
  exocytosis of, 637-38
  mechanisms of, 638-40
  membrane composition of,
    630-31
  regulated exocytosis from
    neurons and, 626-29
Smooth muscle
  contraction of
    crossbridge cycle mech-
      anism of, 866-69
    regulation of, 863-66
  vascular
    atriopeptin and, 44
Sodium
  reabsorption of
    atrial natriuretic peptide
      and, 750-51
    cortical collecting duct and,
      751-52
    inner medullary collecting
      duct and, 753
Sodium arsenite
  calcium ion-dependent protein
    synthesis and, 586-87
Sodium chloride
  concentration in renal medul-
    la, 728
Sodium ions
  in neutrophils, 365-71
Sodium-potassium pump
  cardiac muscle cells and,
    548
  DM-nitrophen and, 909
  sodium ion efflux in neut-
    rophils and, 366
Sodium pump
  DM-nitrophen and, 909
Somatomedin C
  inhibin production and, 812
Somatostatin
  neuronal calcium ion channels
    and, 246
  osmoregulation in freshwater
    teleosts and, 48-49
  potassium ion channels and,
    218

Somatostatin CRE element
  cellular protein factors and,
    797-98
Somatostatin gene regulation,
    793-804
Somatostatin gene transcription
  cis-acting element and, 794-
    96
Somatotrophs
  appearance during develop-
    ment, 773-74
  pit-1 expression in
    ontogeny of, 780-82
Sorbitol
  physiologic functions of, 742-
    43
  renal metabolism and trans-
    port of, 733-35
Spastic paraperesis
  human T-lymphotropic virus
    type 1 and, 848
Staphylococcal α-toxin
  cell permeabilization by, 591
Staurosporine
  neuronal calcium ion channels
    and, 248-49
Steroid hormone receptor
  functional properties of, 827-
    28
Steroid hormones
  inhibin production and, 812
  ligand-dependent transcription
    factors and, 824-25
Sterols
  oxygenated
    cholesterol biosynthesis
      and, 834
Stilbenes
  anion exchange in neutrophils
    and, 383
Stimulus-secretion coupling,
    345-57
  adenosine triphosphate and,
    596
  mechanisms of, 664-68
  in vascular endothelial cells,
    661-69
Stomach
  endocrine cells of
    synaptophysin in, 649
Strepolysin-O
  cell permeabilization by, 591
Streptococcus pneumoniae
  secretory IgA and, 179
Striated muscle
  contraction of
    caged compounds and, 875-
      92
Substance P
  endothelial secretion of, 661
Superoxide anion
  function of, 564

Superoxide dismutase
  as antioxidant, 495
  myocardial reperfusion injury
    and, 563
  plasma half-life of, 497-98
  tetrazolium staining and, 496
Switch point hypothesis
  respiratory cilia motility and,
    141-44
Synapsin I
  neurotransmitter release and,
    652
  regulated exocytosis from
    neurons and, 627-28
  synaptic vesicles and, 651-52
  vesicle-cytoskeletal in-
    teractions and, 650
Synapsin II
  regulated exocytosis from
    neurons and, 627-28
Synaptic-like microvesicles
  synaptophysin and, 631-33
Synaptobrevin
  distribution of, 649
  regulated exocytosis from
    neurons and, 628-29
Synaptophysin
  exocytosis and, 620
  regulated exocytosis from
    neurons and, 628
  synaptic-like microvesicles
    and, 631-33
  transmembrane domains of,
    648-49
Syncytium formation
  viral fusion reactions and,
    676
Synexin
  exocytosis and, 620

T

T cells
  helper
    mucosal lymphoid tissues
      and, 187-90
Teleosts
  osmoregulation in
    atriopeptin and, 46-47
    hormonal control of, 48-
      50
12-O-Tetradecanoylphorbol-13-
    acetate
  insulin secretion and, 355
Tetrahymena
  exocytosis in, 611-12
Tetrazolium staining
  measurement of myocardial
    infarction and, 491-92
  superoxide dismutase and,
    496

Thermal stress
  calcium ion-dependent protein synthesis and, 586-87
Thrombin
  calcium ion discharge in platelets and, 438
  endothelial cytoplasmic calcium concentration and, 663
  inositol phosphate formation and, 662
  internal calcium ion discharged by, 435
  prostaglandin secretion and, 665
  tissue plasminogen activator secretion and, 668
Thrombolytic agents
  ischemic cardiac injury and, 488
Thrombosis
  intravascular
    endothelial regulation of, 661
Thrombospondin
  endothelial secretion of, 661
Thromboxane A2
  calcium ion release in platelets and, 434
Thyroid gland
  C cells of
    synaptophysin in, 649
Thyroid hormone receptor
  thyroid hormone response element and, 832
Thyroid hormones
  atriopeptin secretion and, 46
  ligand-dependent transcription factors and, 824-25
Thyrotrophs
  pit-1 expression in ontogeny of, 780-82
Thyrotropin-releasing hormone
  voltage-dependent calcium ion channels and, 282
Tissue plasminogen activator (TPA)
  endothelium and, 661
  stimulus-secretion coupling and, 668
TNF
  See Tumor necrosis factor
Togaviruses
  fusion reactions of, 676
Toluene
  plasma membrane permeabilization and, 348-49
Toxigenes, 843-46

TPA
  See Tissue plasminogen activator
Tracheobronchial tree
  serous cells of, 98
Transgenic mice
  reverse genetics and, 841-50
Transient fusion pore model
  exocytosis and, 639-40
Trematodes
  calcium-containing concretions in, 88
Trifluoperazine
  catecholamine release and, 355
  cell recovery mechanisms and, 32-33
  cell volume regulation in leukocytes and, 402
  potassium ion channels in lymphocytes and, 417
  sodium transport in neutrophils and, 368
Tropomyosin
  adrenal chromaffin granule membranes and, 651
  myosin binding site on actin and, 888
Troponin
  myosin binding site on actin and, 888
Troponin C
  intracellular calcium and, 467
Troponin C calcium binding
  cardiac muscle and, 511-12
T-tubule depolarization
  calcium release from sarcoplasmic reticulum and, 890-91
Tumor necrosis factor (TNF)
  neutrophil adhesion to endothelial cells and, 571
Tumor promoters
  Na+/H+ exchange in leukocytes and, 407
Turtle
  anoxic hibernation in, 87
Tyrosine kinase
  annexins and, 620

U

Urea
  protein and enzyme function and, 727
Urotensin II
  osmoregulation in freshwater teleosts and, 48-49

V

Valinomycin
  chemotaxis in neutrophils and, 369
Vanadate
  gastric H,K-ATPase inhibition and, 337
Vascular smooth muscle
  atriopeptin and, 44
Vasoactive intestinal peptide (VIP)
  elasmobranch osmoregulation and, 50
  inhibin production and, 812
  teleost osmoregulation and, 50
Vasomotor tone
  endothelium-derived vasoactive agents and, 661
Vasopressin
  amino acid incorporation in hepatocytes and, 581
  calcium ion release in platelets and, 434
Ventricular myocardium
  energetics of, 506-7
Verapamil
  cell volume regulation in leukocytes and, 403
  potassium ion channels in lymphocytes and, 417
Vertebrate bone
  crystalline bone in, 81-82
Vesicle-binding proteins
  calcium-dependent, 652-64
VIP
  See Vasoactive intestinal peptide
Viral chemotherapy
  toxicity of, 846
Viral membrane fusion proteins, 678-86
  conformation changes in, 684-86
  fusion peptides and, 680-84
  hydrophobic interactions of, 686
  oligomeric structures of, 679
  processing/activation of, 679-80
Viral membrane fusion reactions, 675-78
  site of, 686-87
Vitamin A
  ligand-dependent transcription factors and, 824-25
Vitamin D
  ligand-dependent transcription factors and, 824-25

Vitamin D receptor
  genes encoding, 825
  receptor zinc finger domains
    and, 833
Vitamins
  lipid-soluble
    receptor family binding,
      825-27
Von Recklinghausen's neurofi-
    bromatosis
  animal model for,
    848
Von Willebrand factor
  endothelial secretion of,
    661
  stimulus-secretion coupling
    and, 667

W

Water
  amphibious invertebrate gas
    exchange in, 63-65
  reabsorption of
    atrial natriuretic peptide
      and, 750-51
    cortical collecting duct and,
      751-52
    inner medullary collecting
      duct and, 753
  transport by respiratory cilia,
    144-45
Worms
  eggs of
    calcification of, 83

X

Xanthine oxidase
  oxygen-derived free radicals
    and, 564-65
Xanthine oxidase inhibi-
    tors
  myocardial infarction and,
    498-99

Y

Yeast
  membrane permeability in
    toluene and, 348-49

CUMULATIVE INDEXES

CONTRIBUTING AUTHORS, VOLUMES 48–52

A

Acker, H., 51:835–44
Agnew, W. S., 51:401–18
Aickin, C. C., 48:349–61
Al-Awqati, Q., 48:153–61
Albert, V. R., 52: 773–91
Almers, W., 52:607–24
Alvarez, O., 51:385–99
Andrews, W. V., 48:495–514
Andrisani, O. M., 52:793–806
Arendshorst, W. J., 49:295–317
Arieli, A., 51:543–59
Aronin, N., 48:537–50
Aronson, P. S., 51:419–41
Astumian, R. D., 50:273–90
Autelitano, D. J., 51:715–26

B

Balaban, R. S., 52:523–42,
  52:727–46
Baldwin, S. A., 51:459–71
Banchero, N., 49:465–76
Barajas, L., 51:67–80
Bartles, J. R., 51:755–70
Basbaum, C. B., 52:97–113
Baskin, D. G., 49:335–47
Bassingthwaighte, J. B.,
  48:321–34
Bauer, C., 51:845–56
Bean, B. P., 51:367–84
Bell, P. D., 49:275–93
Berger, F. G., 51:51–65
Betz, A. L., 48:241–50
Beyer, C., 49:349–64
Bibb, J. A., 52:381–97
Bidani, A., 50:639–52, 653–67
Birnbaumer, L., 52:197–213
Björklund, A. B., 48:447–59
Blair, R. W., 50:607–22
Blasdel, G., 51:561–81
Blum, M., 51:715–26
Bolanowski, M. A., 51:203–15
Boron, W., 48:377–88
Boulant, J. A., 48:639–54
Boveris, A., 48:703–20
Bradley, D., 52:823–40
Brenner, B., 49:655–72
Briggs, J. P., 49:251–73
Brostrom, C. O., 52:577–90
Brostrom, M. A., 52:577–90
Brown, A. M., 52:197–213
Brown, D., 51:771–84
Brown, D., 52:215–42
Brutsaert, D. L., 51:263–73

Buddington, R. K., 51:601–19
Burgoyne, R. D., 52:647–59
Burnstein, K. L., 51:683–99
Burton, H. W., 49:439–51
Busa, W. B., 48:389–402

C

Cadenas, E., 48:703–20
Cahalan, M. D., 52:415–30
Calaresu, F. R., 50:511–24
Calder, W. A., 49:107–20
Cameron, J. N., 52:77–95
Campbell, G. R., 48:295–306
Campbell, J. H., 48:295–306
Cantley, L. C., 50:207–23
Carlson, B. M., 49:439–51
Caron, M. G., 51:203–15
Carruthers, A., 50:257–71
Catterall, W. A., 50:395–406
Cereijido, M., 51:785–95
Chance, B., 48:703–20; 51:813–
  34
Chasis, J. A., 49:237–48
Chen, R., 52:773–91
Chen, S., 52:841–51
Chien, S., 49:177–92
Chilian, W. M., 49:477–87
Chua, B. H. L., 49:533–43
Cidlowski, J. A., 51:683–99
Clark, W. G., 48:613–24
Coburn, R. F., 49:573–82
Cogan, M. G., 52:669–708
Cohen, F. S., 48:163–74
Cohen, L., 51:527–41
Collins, S., 51:203–15
Conn, P. M., 48:495–514
Contreras, R. G., 51:785–95
Cooper, G., 49:501–18
Cooper, G., 52:505–22
Coslovsky, R., 48:537–50
Crandall, E. D., 50:639–52
Crapo, J. D., 48:721–31
Crenshaw, E. B., 52:773–91
Cross, N. L., 48:191–200

D

D'Amore, P. A., 49:453–64
Daniele, R. P., 52:177–95
De Camilli, P., 52:625–45
De Pont, J. J. H. H. M.,
  49:87–103
de Rouffignac, C., 50:123–40
De Weer, P., 50:225–41
Dean, J. B., 48:639–54

Demarest, J. R., 52:301–19
Denton, R. M., 52:451–66
Deuticke, B., 49:221–35
Diamond, J. M., 51:125–41;
  51:601–19
Dixon, J. E., 52:793–806
Dodgson, S. J., 50:669–94
Dolphin, A., 52:243–55
Donowitz, M., 48:135–50
Dorsa, D. M., 49:335–47
Downey, J. M., 52:487–504
Dratz, E. A., 49:765–91
DuBose, T. D. Jr., 50:653–67
Dufau, M. L., 50:483–508
Dunham, B., 48:335–45
Dussault, J. H., 49:321–34

E

Edelman, G. M., 48:417–30
Eipper, B. A., 50:333–44
Elalouf, J.-M., 50:123–40
Ellenberger, H. H., 50:593–606
Elsholtz, H. P., 52:773–91
Evans, D. H., 52:46–60
Evans, G. A., 52:841–51
Evans, R. M., 48:431–46

F

Fagius, J., 50:565–76
Faulkner, J. A., 49:439–51
Feder, H. H., 49:349–64
Feldman, J. L., 50:593–606
Ferraris, R. P., 51:125–41
Figlewicz, D. P., 49:335–47;
  49:383–95
Fine, L. G., 51:19–32
Finkbeiner, W., 52:97–113
Finkelstein, A., 48:163–74
Fisher, D. A., 51:67–80
Foreman, R. D., 50:607–22
Forman, B. M., 51:623–39
Forman, H. J., 48:669–80
Foskett, J. K, 52:399–414
Foster, K. A., 51:229–44
Franco, M., 49:275–93
Frankel, H. L., 50:577–92
Freeman, B., 48:693–702
Fricker, L. D., 50:309–21
Fridovich, I., 48:693–702
Frostig, R. D., 51:543–59
Fuller, R. S., 50:345–62
Funder, J. W., 49:397–411

G

Gabella, G., 49:583–94
Gadsby, D. C., 50:225–41
Gage, F. H., 48:447–59
Galla, J. H., 50:141–58
Gallacher, D. V., 50:65–80
Gardner, J. D., 48:103–17
Gelato, M. C., 48:569–92
Gerard, R. D., 51:245–62
Gershengorn, M. C., 48:515–26
Giebisch, G., 50:97–110
Goldman, Y. E., 49:637–54
Goldstein, G. W., 48:241–50
Gomperts, B. D., 52:591–606
Gonzalez-Marsical, L., 51:785–95
Gordon, C. J., 48:595–612
Gordon, E. E., 49:533–43
Gorospe, W. C., 48:495–514
Green, R., 50:97–110
Greger, R., 50:111–22
Grinstein, S., 52:399–414
Grinvald, A., 51:543–59
Gros, G., 50:669–94
Guggino, W. B., 52:761–72

H

Haas, M., 51:443–57
Haest, C. W. M., 49:221–35
Hai, C., 51:285–98
Handler, J. S., 51:729–40
Hansen, J., 48:495–514
Harris, C., 48:495–514
Havel, R. J., 48:119–34
Hazeki, O., 51:813–34
He, X., 52:773–91
Heath, J. E., 48:595–612
Hedin, L., 50:441–63
Heineman, F., 52:523–42
Henderson, A. H., 52:661–74
Henderson, P. J. F., 51:459–71
Hersey, S. J., 52:345–61
Hescheler, J., 52:257–74, 52:275–92
Heusner, A. A., 49:121–33
Hildesheim, R., 51:543–59
Höpp, H., 51:527–41
Hochmuth, R. M., 49:209–19
Holz, R. W., 48:175–89
Homsher, E., 49:673–90
Homsher, E., 52:875–96
Hopfer, U., 49:51–67
Horowitz, Z. D., 51:623–39
Houston, D. S., 48:307–20
Howard, G., 51:701–14
Howlett, T. A., 48:527–36
Hruby, D. E., 50:323–32
Hubbard, A. L., 51:755–70
Huckle, W. R., 48:495–514
Hurley, J. B., 49:793–812

Huttner, W. B., 50:363–76
Huxley, A., 50:1–16

I

Ingraham, H. A., 52:773–91
Inman, R., 49:163–75
Ishihara, A., 49:163–75

J

Jänig, W., 50:525–39
Jacobson, K., 49:163–75
Jaffe, L. A., 48:191–200
Jahn, R., 52:6225–45
Jamieson, D., 48:703–20
Jan, L. Y., 50:379–93
Jany, B., 52:97–113
Jensen, F. B., 50:161–79
Jensen, R. T., 48:103–17
Jones, D. P., 48:33–50

K

Kaback, H. R., 50:243–56
Kalia, M. P., 49:595–609
Kamm, K. E., 51:299–313
Kapiloff, M. S., 52:773–91
Kaplan, J. H., 52:897–914
Kaplowitz, N., 51:161–76
Karsch, F. J., 49:365–82
Kedes, L. H., 51:179–88
Keyes, P. L., 50:465–82
Kira, Y., 49:533–43
Klocke, R. A., 50:625–37
Kreisberg, J. I., 48:51–71
Kuijpers, G. A. J., 49:87–103
Kurtz, A., 51:845–56

L

Labarca, P., 51:385–99
Lacour, F., 49:383–95
Lakatta, E. G., 49:519–31
Landel, C. P., 52:841–51
Latorre, R. R., 51:385–99
Leeman, S. E., 48:537–50
Lefkowitz, R. J., 51:203–15
Lewis, R. S., 52:415–30
Liebman, P. A., 49:765–91
Liedtke, C. M., 49:51–67; 51:143–60
Lieke, E. E., 51:543–59
Lipton, J. M., 48:613–24
London, J., 51:527–41
Loo, D. D. F., 52:307–19
Lucchesi, B. R., 52:561–76
Luke, R. G., 50:141–58
Lundberg, J. M., 49:557–72
Lundblad, J. R., 51:715–26

M

Machen, T. E., 49:19–33
Mains, R. E., 50:333–44

Manahan, D. T., 51:585–600
Mangalam, H. J., 52:773–91
Marcus, M. L., 49:477–87
Maren, T. H., 50:695–717
Mathias, C. J., 50:577–92
Mayo, K. E., 48:431–46
Mayo, K. E., 52:807–21
McArdle, C. A., 48:495–514
McCall, R. B., 50:553–64
McCann, J., 52:115–35
McCormack, J., 52:451–66
McDermott, P. J., 49:533–43
Meidell, R. S., 51:245–62
Meisler, M. H., 51:701–14
Melchior, D. L., 50:257–71
Mendley, S. R., 51:33–50
Merriam, G. R., 48:569–92
Millar, N. C., 52:875–96
Miller, V. M., 48:307–20
Molski, T. F., 52:365–79
Monck, J. R., 51:107–24
Montrose-Rafizadeh, C., 52:761–72
Moolenaar, W. H., 48:363–76
Morgan, H. E., 49:533–43
Morkin, E., 49:545–54
Muallem, S., 51:83–105
Murphy, R. A., 51:275–83; 51:285–98

N

Navar, L. G., 49:275–93
Newby, A. C., 52:661–74
Nioka, S., 51:813–34
Nishi, S., 50:541–51
Norman, J., 51:19–32

O

Oberhauser, A., 51:385–99
Ookhtens, M., 51:161–76
Otero, A. S., 52:293–305
Owen, W. G., 49:743–64

P

Papazian, D. M., 50:379–93
Pappenheimer, J. R., 49:1–15
Paradiso, A. M., 49:19–33
Parker, K. R., 49:765–91
Parsegian, V. A., 48:201–12
Patel, Y. C., 48:551–68
Paul, R. J., 51:331–49
Perez, A., 52:345–61
Perutz, M. F., 52:1–25
Petersen, O. H., 50:65–80
Peterson, C. J., 49:533–43
Phillips, M. I., 49:413–35
Pierce, S. K., 52:27–42
Plotsky, P. M., 48:475–94
Politis, A. D., 52:27–42
Polosa, C., 50:541–51

Porte, D., 49:335–47; 49:383–95
Post, R., 51:1–15
Prosser, C. L., 48:1–6
Pryor, W. A., 48:657–68
Pugh, E. N., 49:715–41
Putney, J. W. Jr., 48:75–88

Q

Quinn, S., 50:409–26

R

Rabon, E., 52:321–44
Rakowski, R. F., 50:225–41
Rand, R. P., 48:201–12
Rees, L. H., 48:527–36
Reuben, M. A., 52:321–44
Reuss, L., 49:35–49
Richards, J. S., 50:441–63
Riggs, A. F., 50:181–204
Rink, T. J., 52:431–49
Rivier, C. L., 48:475–94
Roberts, J. L., 51:0–0
Robishaw, J., 51:229–44
Rodriguez-Boulan, E. J., 51:741–54
Rories, C., 51:653–81
Rosenfeld, G. M., 48:431–46
Rosenfeld, M. G., 52:773–91
Rosenthal, W., 52:275–92
Ross, W. N., 51:491–506
Roth, M. G., 51:797–810
Rubanyi, G. M., 48:307–20
Rudnick, G., 48:403–13
Ruel, J., 49:321–34
Russo, L. A., 49:533–43
Ryan, U. S., 48:263–77

S

Sage, S. O., 52:431–49
Saida, K., 51:315–29
Salas, P. J. I., 51:741–54
Salido, E. C., 51:67–80
Salzberg, B. M., 51:507–26
Samuels, H. H., 51:623–39
Sanders, M. J., 48:89–101
Sant'Ambrogio, G., 49:611–27
Saria, A., 49:557–72
Satir, P., 52:137–55
Schafer, J. A., 52:709–26
Scharschmidt, B. F., 49:69–85
Schatzmann, H. J., 51:473–85
Schild, L., 50:97–110
Schildmeyer, L. A., 49:489–99
Schimerlik, M. I., 51:217–40
Schnermann, J., 49:251–73
Schultz, G., 52:275–92
Schwartz, G. J., 48:153–61
Schwarz, T. L., 50:379–93

Schwertz, D. W., 48:51–71
Seidel, C. L., 49:489–99
Sha'afi, R. I., 52:365–79
Sheppard, K., 49:397–411
Shepro, D., 48:335–45
Shohet, S. B., 49:237–48
Simchowitz, L., 52:381–97
Simionescu, M., 48:279–93
Simionescu, N., 48:279–93
Simpson, E. R., 50:427–40
Simpson, P. C., 51:189–202
Sipols, A., 49:383–95
Sleigh, M. A., 52:137–55
Sleight, R. G., 49:193–208
Smith, L. L., 48:681–92
Smith, W. L., 48:251–62
Snyder, S. H., 48:461–71
Soll, A. H., 48:89–101
Soltoff, S. P., 48:9–31; 50:207–23
Somlyo, A. P., 52:857–74
Somlyo, A. V., 52:857–74
Sparks, H. V. Jr., 48:321–34
Spelsberg, T. C., 51:653–81
Spray, D. C., 47:281–304; 48:625–38
Srikant, C. B., 48:551–68
Staley, D., 48:495–514
Steinbach, J. H., 51:353–65
Sterne, R. E., 50:345–62
Sternini, C., 50:81–93
Stieger, B., 51:755–70
Stoddard, J. S., 49:35–49
Stolz, A., 51:161–76
Stull, J. T., 51:299–313
Swanson, L. W., 52:773–91
Szabo, G., 52:293–305

T

Taché, Y., 50:19–39
Takikawa, H., 51:161–76
Tamura, M., 51:813–34
Tani, M., 52:543–59
Taylor, C. R., 49:135–46
Tempel, B. L., 50:379–93
Thomas, D. D., 49:691–709
Thomas, G., 50:323–32
Thomas, M. J., 48:669–80
Thompson, R. W., 49:453–64
Thorne, B. A., 50:323–32
Thorner, J., 50:345–62
Timpe, L. C., 50:379–93
Toback, F. G., 51:33–50
Trautwein, W., 52:257–74; 52:275–92
Treacy, M. N., 52:773–91
Trimmer, J. S., 51:401–18
Troyer, D. A., 48:51–71
Truchot, J. P., 52:61–76
Ts'o, D. Y., 51:543–59
Tsong, T. Y., 50:273–90

V

van Breemen, C., 51:315–29
Van Dyke, R. W., 49:69–85
Vanhoutte, P. M., 48:307–20
Venkatachalam, M. A., 48:51–71
Verdugo, P., 52:157–76
Vonderhaar, B. K., 51:641–52

W

Wade, J. B., 48:213–23
Wade, R., 51:179–88
Wallin, B. G., 50:565–76
Walsh, J. H., 50:41–63
Waterman, M. R., 50:427–40
Watson, G., 51:51–65
Watson, P. A., 49:533–43
Waugh, R. E., 49:209–19
Weber, R. E., 50:161–79
Weibel, E. R., 49:147–59
Weinberger, C., 52:823–40
Welsh, M. J., 48:135–50
Welsh, M. J., 52:115–35
White, J. M., 52:675–97
Wier, W. G., 52:567–85
Williams, G. H., 50:409–26
Williams, J. A., 46:361–75; 48:225–38
Williamson, J., 51:107–24
Wiltbank, M. C., 50:465–82
Wittenberg, B. A., 51:857–78
Wittenberg, J. B., 51:857–78
Wolfe, L. S., 41:669–84
Wolff, S., 52:727–46
Woodruff, T. K., 52:807–21
Woods, S. C., 49:335–47; 49:383–95
Wright, E. M., 46:417–33; 47:127–42
Wright, S. H., 51:585–600
Wu, J., 51:527–41

X

Xiao, C., 51:527–41

Y

Yardley, C. P., 50:511–24
Ye, Z., 51:623–39
Yingst, D. R., 50:291–303
Yoshimura, M., 50:541–51

Z

Zěcević, D., 51:527–41
Zeidel, M. L., 52:747–59
Zimmerberg, J., 48:163–74
Ziska, S. E., 51:641–52

CHAPTER TITLES, VOLUMES 48–52

ACID-BASE REGULATION
Intracellular pH Regulation by Vertebrate
  Muscle   C. C. Aickin   48:349–61
Effects of Growth Factors on Intracellular pH
  Regulation   W. H. Moolenaar   48:363–76
Intracellular pH Regulation in Epithelial Cells   W. F. Boron   48:377–88
Mechanisms and Consequences of
  pH-Mediated Cell Regulation   W. B. Busa   48:389–402
ATP-Driven H$^+$ Pumping into Intracellular
  Organelles   G. Rudnick   48:403–13

CAGED COMPOUNDS IN CELLULAR PHYSIOLOGY
Flash Photolysis Studies of
  Excitation-Contraction Coupling Regulation,
  and Contraction in Smooth Muscle   A. P. Somlyo, A. V. Somlyo   52:857–74
Caged Compounds and Striated Muscle
  Contraction   E. Homsher, N. C. Millar   52:875–96
Photochemical Manipulation of Divalent
  Cation Levels   J. H. Kaplan   52:897–914

CARDIOVASCULAR PHYSIOLOGY
Specialized Properties and Solute Transport in
  Brain Capillaries   A. L. Betz, G. W. Goldstein   48:241–50
Prostaglandin Biosynthesis and Its
  Compartmentation in Vascular Smooth
  Muscle and Endothelial Cells   W. L. Smith   48:251–62
Metabolic Activity of Pulmonary Endothelium   U. S. Ryan   48:263–77
Functions of the Endothelial Cell Surface   M. Simionescu, N. Simionescu   48:279–93
Endothelial Cell Influences on Vascular
  Smooth Muscle Phenotype   J. H. Campbell, G. R. Campbell   48:295–306
Modulation of Vascular Smooth Muscle
  Contraction by the Endothelium   P. M. Vanhoutte, G. M. Rubanyi, V. M. Miller, D. S. Houston   48:307–20
Indicator Dilution Estimation of Capillary
  Endothelial Transport   J. B. Bassingthwaighte, H. V. Sparks, Jr.   48:321–34
Endothelial Cell Metabolism of Biogenic
  Amines   D. Shepro, B. Dunham   48:335–45
Microcirculatory Adaptation to Skeletal
  Muscle Transplantation   H. W. Burton, B. M. Carlson, J. A. Faulkner   49:439–51
Mechanisms of Angiogenesis   P. A. D'Amore, R. W. Thompson   49:453–64
Cardiovascular Responses to Chronic Hypoxia   N. Banchero   49:465–76
Coronary Vascular Adaptations to Myocardial
  Hypertrophy   W. M. Chilian, M. L. Marcus   49:477–87
Vascular Smooth Muscle Adaptation to
  Increased Load   C. L. Seidel, L. A. Schildmeyer   49:489–99
Cardiocyte Adaptation to Chronically Altered
  Load   G. Cooper, IV   49:501–18
Cardiac Muscle Changes in Senescence   E. G. Lakatta   49:519–31

Biochemical Mechanisms of Cardiac
  Hypertrophy   H. E. Morgan, E. E. Gordon, Y.
                                                Kira, B. H. L. Chua, L. A.
                                                Russo, C. J. Peterson, P. J.
                                                McDermott, P. A. Watson   49:533–43
Chronic Adaptations in Contractile Proteins:
  Genetic Regulation   E. Morkin   49:545–54
Medullary Basal Sympathetic Tone   F. R. Calaresu, C. P. Yardley   50:511–24
Pre- and Postganglionic Vasoconstrictor
  Neurons: Differentiation, Types, and
  Discharge Properties   W. Jänig   50:525–39
Electrophysiological Properties of Sympathetic
  Preganglionic Neurons   C. Polosa, M. Yoshimura,
                                                S. Nishi   50:541–51
Effects of Putative Neurotransmitters on
  Sympathetic Preganglionic Neurons   R. B. McCall   50:553–64
Peripheral Sympathetic Neural Activity in
  Conscious Humans   B. G. Wallin, J. Fagius   50:565–76
Cardiovascular Control in Spinal Man   C. J. Mathias, H. L. Frankel   50:577–92
Central Coordination of Respiratory and
  Cardiovascular Control in Mammals   J. L. Feldman, H. H. Ellenberger 50:593–606
Central Organization of Sympathetic
  Cardiovascular Response to Pain   R. D. Foreman, R. W. Blair   50:607–22
Developmental Regulation of Contractile
  Protein Genes   R. Wade, L. H. Kedes   51:179–88
Proto-Oncogenes and Cardiac Hypertrophy   P. C. Simpson   51:189–202
Genetic Regulation of Beta-Adrenergic
  Receptors   S. Collins, M. A. Bolanowski,
                                                M. G. Caron, R. J. Lefkowitz   51:203–15
Structure and Regulation of Muscarinic
  Receptors   M. I. Schimerlik   51:217–27
Role of G Proteins in the Regulation of the
  Cardiovascular System   J. Robishaw, K. A. Foster   51:229–44
Regulation of Tissue Plasminogen Activator
  Expression   R. D. Gerard, R. S. Meidell   51:245–62
The Endocardium   D. L. Brutsaert   51:263–73
Ca^{2+} as a Second Messenger within
  Mitochondria of the Heart and Other
  Tissues   J. McCormack, R. M. Denton   52:451–66
Cytoplasmic $[Ca^{2+}]_i$ in Mammalian Ventricle:
  Dynamic Control by Cellular Processes   W. G. Wier   52:467–85
Free Radical and Their Involvement during
  Long-Term Myocardial Ischemia and
  Reperfusion   J. M. Downey   52:487–504
Load and Length Regulation of Cardiac
  Energetics   G. Cooper, IV   52:505–22
Control of Mitochondrial Respiration in the
  Heart In Vivo   F. Heineman, R. S. Balaban   52:523–42
Mechanisms of Calcium^{2+} Overload in
  Reperfused Ischemic Myocardium   M. Tani   52:543–59
Modulation of Leukocyte Mediated
  Myocardial Reperfusion Injury   B. R. Lucchesi   52:561–76
Calcium Dependent Regulation of Protein
  Synthesis in Intact Mammalian Cells   C. O. Brostrom, M. A. Brostrom 52:577–90

CELL AND MOLECULAR PHYSIOLOGY
  Regulation of Transepithelial H^+ Transport by
    Exocytosis and Endocytosis   G. J. Schwartz, Q. Al-Awqati   48:153–61
  Osmotic Swelling of Vesicles   A. Finkelstein, J. Zimmerberg,
                                                F. S. Cohen   48:163–74
  The Role of Osmotic Forces in Exocytosis
    from Adrenal Chromaffin Cells   R. W. Holz   48:175–89
  Electrical Regulation of Sperm-Egg Fusion   L. A. Jaffe, N. L. Cross   48:191–200
  Mimicry and Mechanism in Phospholipid
    Models of Membrane Fusion   R. P. Rand, V. A. Parsegian   48:201–12

Role of Membrane Fusion in Hormonal Regulation of Epithelial Transport	J. B. Wade	48:213–23
Regulation of Membrane Fusion in Secretory Exocytosis	R. C. De Lisle, J. A. Williams	48:225–38
Lateral Diffusion of Proteins in Membranes	K. Jacobson, A. Ishihara, R. Inman	49:163–75
Red Cell Deformability and Its Relevance to Blood Flow	S. Chien	49:177–92
Intracellular Lipid Transport in Eukaryotes	R. G. Sleight	49:193–208
Erythrocyte Membrane Elasticity and Viscosity	R. M. Hochmuth, R. E. Waugh	49:209–19
Lipid Modulation of Transport Proteins in Vertebrate Cell Membranes	B. Deuticke, C. W. M. Haest	49:221–35
Red Cell Biochemical Anatomy and Membrane Properties	J. A. Chasis, S. B. Shohet	49:237–48
Mitogens and Ion Fluxes	S. P. Soltoff, L. C. Cantley	50:207–23
Voltage Dependence of the Na-K Pump	P. De Weer, D. C. Gadsby, R. F. Rakowski	50:225–41
Site-Directed Mutagenesis and Ion-Gradient Driven Active Transport: On the Path of the Proton	H. R. Kaback	50:243–56
Effect of Lipid Environment on Membrane Transport: The Human Erythrocyte Sugar Transport Protein/Lipid Bilayer System	D. L. Melchior, A. Carruthers	50:257–71
Electroconformational Coupling: How Membrane-Bound ATPase Transduces Energy From Dynamic Electric Fields	T. Y. Tsong, R. D. Astumian	50:273–90
Modulation of the Na,K-ATPase by Ca and Intracellular Proteins	D. R. Yingst	50:291–303
Structural and Functional Diversity in Vertebrate Skeletal Muscle	J. H. Steinbach	51:353–65
Classes of Calcium Channels in Vertebrate Cells	B. P. Bean	51:367–84
Varieties of Calcium-Activated Potassium Channels	R. R. Latorre, A. Oberhauser, P. Labarca, O. Alvarez	51:385–99
Molecular Diversity of Voltage-Sensitive Na Channels	J. S. Trimmer, W.S. Agnew	51:401–18
Anion Exchangers and Stilbene-Sensitive Transport Processes in Epithelia	P. S. Aronson	51:419–41
Properties and Diversity of (Na–+K–Cl) Cotransporters	M. Haas	51:443–57
Homologies Between Sugar Transporters from Lower Eukaryotes and Prokaryotes	S. A. Baldwin, P. J. F. Henderson	51:459–71
The Calcium Pump of the Surface Membrane and of the Sarcoplasmic	H. J. Schatzmann	51:473–85
G_E: A GTP-Binding Protein Mediating Exocytosis	B. D. Gomperts	52:591–606
Exocytosis	W. Almers	52:607–24
Pathways to Regulated Exocytosis in Neurons	P. De Camilli, R. Jahn	52:625–45
Secretory Vesicle-Associated Proteins and Their Role in Exocytosis	R. D. Burgoyne	52:647–59
Stimulus-Secretion Coupling in Vascular Endothelial Cells	A. C. Newby, A. H. Henderson	52:661–74
Viral and Cellular Membrane Fusion Proteins Proteins	J. M. White	52:675–97

CELL BIOLOGICAL APPROACHES TO BRAIN FUNCTION

Cell Adhesion Molecules in Neural Histogenesis	G. M. Edelman	48:417–30
Genes Encoding Mammalian Neuroendocrine Peptides: Strategies	K. E. Mayo, R. M. Evans, G. M. Rosenfeld	48:431–46
Neural Grafting in the Aged Rat Brain	F. H. Gage, A. Björklund	48:447–59
Neuronal Receptors	S. H. Snyder	48:461–71

COMPARATIVE PHYSIOLOGY

Integration and Central Processing in
Temperature Regulation   C. J. Gordon, J. E. Heath   48:595–612
Neurotransmitters in Temperature Control   J. M. Lipton, W. G. Clark   48:613–24
Cutaneous Temperature Receptors   D. C. Spray   48:625–38
Temperature Receptors in the Central Nervous
System   J. A. Boulant, J. B. Dean   48:639–54
Scaling Energetics of Homeothermic
Vertebrates: An Operational Allometry   W. A. Calder III   49:107–20
What Does the Power Function Reveal About
Structure and Function in Animals of
Different Size?   A. A. Heusner   49:121–33
Structural and Functional Limits to Oxidative
Metabolism: Insights from Scaling   C. R. Taylor   49:135–46
Scaling of Structural and Functional Variables
in the Respiratory System   E. R. Weibel   49:147–59
Functional Adaptations in Hemoglobins from
Ectothermic Vertebrates   R. E. Weber, F. B. Jensen   50:161–79
The Bohr Effect   A. F. Riggs   50:181–204
Integumental Nutrient Uptake by Aquatic
Organisms   S. H. Wright, D. T. Manahan   51:585–600
Ontogenetic Development of Intestinal
Nutrient Transporters   R. K. Buddington, J. M. Diamond   51:601–19
Ca^{2+}-Activated Cell Volume Recovery
Mechanisms   S. K. Pierce, A. D. Politis   52:27–42
An Emerging Role for a Cardiac Peptide
Hormone in Fish Osmoregulation   D. H. Evans   52:43–60
Respiratory and Ionic Regulation in
Invertebrates Exposed to both Water and
Air   J. Truchot   52:61–76
Unusual Aspects of Calcium Metabolism in
Aquatic Animals   J. N. Cameron   52:77–95

CONTRACTION IN SMOOTH MUSCLE CELLS

Ca^{2+} Crossbridge Phosphorylation, and
Contraction   C. Hai, R. A. Murphy   51:285–98
Regulation of Smooth Muscle Contractile
Elements by Second Messengers   K. E. Kamm, J. T. Stull   51:299–313
Cellular Mechanisms Regulating Smooth
Muscle Contraction   C. van Breemen, K. Saida   51:315–29
Smooth Muscle Energetics   R. J. Paul   51:331–49

ENDOCRINOLOGY

Mediation by Corticotropin Releasing Factor
(CRF) of Adenohypophysial Hormone
Secretion   C. L. Rivier, P. M. Plotsky   48:475–94
Mechanism of Action of Gonadotropin
Releasing Hormone   P. M. Conn, D. Staley, C. Harris,
                                              W. V. Andrews, W. C. Gorospe,
                                              C. A. McArdle, W. R. Huckle   48:495–514
Mechanism of Thyrotropin Releasing
Hormone Stimulation of Pituitary Hormone
Secretion   M. C. Gershengorn   48:515–26
Endogenous Opioid Peptides and
Hypothalamo-Pituitary Function   T. A. Howlett, L. H. Rees   48:527–36
Substance P and Neurotensin   N. Aronin, R. Coslovsky,
                                              S. E. Leeman   48:537–50
Somatostatin Mediation of Adenohypophysial
Secretion   Y. C. Patel, C. B. Srikant   48:551–68
Growth Hormone Releasing Hormone   M. C. Gelato, G. R. Merriam   48:569–92
Thyroid Hormones and Brain Development   J. H. Dussault, J. Ruel   49:321–34
Insulin in the Brain   D. G. Baskin, D. P. Figlewicz,
                                              S. C. Woods, D. Porte, Jr.,
                                              D. M. Dorsa   49:335–47

Sex Steroids and Afferent Input: Their Roles
  in Brain Sexual Differentiation   C. Beyer, H. H. Feder   49:349–64
Central Actions of Ovarian Steroids in the
  Feedback Regulation of Pulsatile Secretion
  of Luteinizing Hormone   F. J. Karsch   49:365–82
Gastroenteropancreatic Peptides and the
  Central Nervous System   D. P. Figlewicz, F. Lacour,
                                                     A. Sipols, D. Porte, Jr.,
                                                     S. C. Woods   49:383–95
Adrenocortical Steriods and the Brain   J. W. Funder, K. Sheppard   49:397–411
Functions of Angiotensin in the Central
  Nervous System   M. I. Phillips   49:413–38
Regulation of Aldosterone Secretion   S. Quinn, G. H. Williams   50:409–26
Regulation of the Synthesis of Steroidogenic
  Enzymes in Adrenal Cortical Cells by
  ACTH   E. R. Simpson, M. R. Waterman   50:427–40
Molecular Aspects of Hormone Action in
  Ovarian Follicular Development, Ovulation,
  and Luteinization   J. S. Richards, L. Hedin   50:441–63
Endocrine Regulation of the Corpus Luteum   P. L. Keyes, M. C. Wiltbank   50:465–82
Endocrine Regulation and Communicating
  Functions of the Leydig Cell   M. L. Dufau   50:483–508
A Family of POU-Domain and PIT-1
  Tissue-Specific Transcription Factors
  in Pituitary and Neuroendocrine
  Development   H. A. Ingraham, V. R. Albert,
                                                     R. Chen, E. B. Crenshaw, III,
                                                     H. P. Elsholtz, X. He, M.
                                                     S. Kapiloff, H. J. Mangalam,
                                                     L. W. Swanson, M. N. Treacy,
                                                     M. G. Rosenfeld   52:773–91
Somatostatin Gene Expression   O. M. Andrisani, J. E. Dixon   52:793–806
Regulation of Inhibin Synthesis in the Rat
  Ovary   T. K. Woodruff, K. E. Mayo   52:807–21
Gene Regulation by Receptors Binding
  Lipid-Soluble Substances   C. Weinberger, D. Bradley   52:823–40
Reverse Genetics Using Transgenic Mice   C. P. Landel, S. Chen,
                                                     G. A. Evans   52:841–51

GAP JUNCTIONS
Regulation of Gene Expression by Thyroid
  Hormone   H. H. Samuels, B. M. Forman,
                                                     Z. D. Horowitz, Z. Ye   51:623–39
Hormonal Regulation of Milk Protein Gene
  Expression   B. K. Vonderhaar, S. E. Ziska   51:641–52
Ovarian Steroid Action on Gene Expression:
  Mechanisms and Models   C. Rories, T. C. Spelsberg   51:653–81
Regulation of Gene Expression by
  Glucocorticoids   K. L. Burnstein, J. A. Cidlowski   51:683–99
Effects of Insulin on Gene Transcription   M. H. Meisler, G. Howard   51:701–14
Hormonal Regulation of POMC Gene
  Expression   D. J. Autelitano, J. R. Lundblad,
                                                     M. Blum, J. L. Roberts   51:715–26

GASTROINTESTINAL PHYSIOLOGY
Identification of Cellular Activation
  Mechanisms Associated with Salivary
  Secretion   J. W. Putney, Jr.   48:75–88
Characterization of Receptors Regulating
  Secretory Function in the Fundic Mucosa   M. J. Sanders, A. H. Soll   48:89–101
Receptors and Cell Activation Associated with
  Pancreatic Enzyme Secretion   J. D. Gardner, R. T. Jensen   48:103–117
Functional Activities of Hepatic Lipoprotein
  Receptors   R. J. Havel   48:119–34

Ca²⁺ and Cyclic AMP in Regulation of
Intestinal Na, K, and Cl Transport   M. Donowitz, M. J. Welsh   48:135–50
Regulation of Intracellular pH in the Stomach T. E. Machen, A. M. Paradiso   49:19–33
Role of H⁺ and HCO₃⁻ in Salt Transport in
Gallbladder Epithelium   L. Reuss, J. S. Stoddard   49:35–49
Proton and Bicarbonate Transport Mechanisms
in the Intestine   U. Hopfer, C. M. Liedtke   49:51–67
Proton Transport by Hepatocyte Organelles
and Isolated Membrane Vesicles   B. F. Scharschmidt, R. W. Van
                                              Dyke   49:69–85
Role of Proton and Bicarbonate Transport in
Pancreatic Cell Function   G. A. J. Kuijpers,
                                              J. J. H. H. M. De Pont   49:87–103
CNS Peptides and Regulation of Gastric Acid
Secretion   Y. Taché   50:19–39
Peptides as Regulators of Gastric Acid
Secretion   J. H. Walsh   50:41–63
Electrophysiology of Pancreatic and Salivary
Acinar Cells   O. H. Petersen, D. V. Gallacher   50:65–80
Structural and Chemical Organization of the
Myenteric Plexus   C. Sternini   50:81–93
Calcium Transport Pathways of Pancreatic
Acinar Cells   S. Muallem   51:83–105
Hormone Effects on Cellular Ca2+ Fluxes   J. Williamson, J. R. Monck   51:107–24
Specific Regulation of Intestinal Nutrient
Transporters by their Dietary Substrates   R. P. Ferraris, J. Diamond   51:125–41
Regulation of Chloride Transport in Epithelia C. M. Liedtke   51:143–60
The Role of Cytoplasmic Proteins in Hepatic
Bile Acid Transport   A. Stolz, H. Takikawa,
                                              M. Ookhtens, N. Kaplowitz   51:161–76
Electrophysiology of the Parietal Cell   J. R. Demarest, D. D. F. Loo   52:307–19
The Mechanism and Structure of the Gastric
H,K-ATPase   E. Rabon, M. A. Reuben   52:321–44
Permeable Cell Models in Stimulus-Secretion
Coupling   S. J. Hersey, A. Perez   52:345–61

GENETIC ANALYSIS OF VOLTAGE-SENSITIVE ION CHANNELS
Genetic Analysis of Ion Channels in
Vertebrates   W. A. Catterall   50:395–406
Ion Channels in Drosophila   D. M. Papazian, T. L. Schwarz,
                                              B. L. Tempel, L. C. Timpe,
                                              L. Y. Jan   50:379–93

ION MOVEMENTS IN LEUKOCYTES
Role of Ion Movements in Neutrophil
Activation   R. I. Sha'afi, T. F. Molski   52:365–79
Functional Analysis of the Modes of Anion
Transport in Neutrophils and HL-60 Cells   L. Simchowitz, J. A. Bibb   52:381–97
Ionic Mechanisms of Cell Volume Regulation
in Leukocytes   S. Grinstein, S. K. Foskett   52:399–414
Ion Channels and Signal Transduction in
Lymphocytes   R. S. Lewis, M. D. Cahalan   52:415–30
Calcium Signaling in Human Platelets   T. J. Rink, S. O. Sage   52:431–49

MOLECULAR MECHANISM OF MUSCLE CONTRACTION
Kinetics of the Actomyosin ATPase in
Muscle Fibers   Y. E. Goldman   49:637–54
Mechanical and Structural Approaches to
Correlation of Cross-Bridge Action in
Muscle with Actomyosin ATPase in
Solution   B. Brenner   49:655–72
Muscle Enthalpy Production and Its
Relationship to Actomyosin ATPase   E. Homsher   49:673–90

Spectroscopic Probes of Muscle Cross-Bridge
Rotation   D. D. Thomas   49:691–709

NEUROPHYSIOLOGY
Ionic Channels and Their Regulation by G
Protein Subunits   A. M. Brown, L. Birnbaumer   52:197–213
G Proteins and Potassium Currents in
Neurons   D. A. Brown   52:215–42
G Protein Modulation of Calcium Currents in
Neurons   A. C. Dolphin   52:243–55
Regulation of Cardiac L-Type Calcium
Current by Phosphorylation and G Proteins W. Trautwein, J. Hescheler   52:257–74
Role of G Proteins in Calcium Channel
Modulation   G. Schultz, W. Rosenthal,
                                        J. Hescheler, W. Trautwein   52:275–92
G Proteins Mediated Regulation of K⁺
Channels in Heart   G. Szabo, A. S. Otero   52:293–305

OPTICAL APPROACHES TO NEURON FUNCTIONS
Changes in Intracellular Calcium During
Neuron Activity   L. L. Cohen   51:487–90
Changes in Intracellular Calcium During
Neuron Activity   W. N. Ross   51:491–506
Optical Recording of Voltage Changes in
Nerve Terminals and in Fine Neuronal
Processes   B. M. Salzberg   51:507–26
Optical Measurement of Action Potential
Activity in Invertebrate Ganglia   L. Cohen, H. Höpp, J. Wu, C.
                                        Xiao, J. London, D. Zečević   51:527–541
Optical Imaging of Cortical Activity:
Real-Time Imaging Using Extrinsic
Dye-Signals and Imaging Based on Slow
Intrinsic Signals   E. E. Lieke, R. D. Frostig,
                                        A. Arieli, D. Y. Ts'o, R.
                                        Hildesheim, A. Grinvald   51:543–59
Optical Monitoring of In Vivo Cortical
Activity: Measurements with High Spatial
Resolution   G. Blasdel   51:561–81

PHOTOTRANSDUCTION IN VERTEBRATES
The Nature and Identity of the Internal
Excitational Transmitter of Vertebrate
Phototransduction   E. N. Pugh, Jr.   49:715–41
Ionic Conductances in Rod Photoreceptors W. G. Owen   49:743–64
The Molecular Mechanism of Visual
Excitation and Its Relation to the Structure
and Composition of the Rod Outer Segment P. A. Liebman, K. R. Parker,
                                        E. A. Dratz   49:765–91
Molecular Properties of the cGMP Cascade of
Vertebrate Photoreceptors   J. B. Hurley   49:793–812

POLARITY
Biogenesis of Endogenous Plasma Membrane
Proteins in Epithelial Cells   A. L. Hubbard, B. Stieger,
                                        J. R. Bartles   51:755–70
Development and Alteration of Polarity   M. Cereijido, R. G. Contreras,
                                        L. Gonzalez-Marsical   51:785–95
External and Internal Signals for Surface
Molecular Polarization   E. J. Rodriguez-Boulan,
                                        P. J. I. Salas   51:741–54
Molecular Biological Approaches to Protein
Sorting   M. G. Roth   51:797–810

Overview of Epithelial Polarity   J. S. Handler   51:729–40
Vesicle Recycling and Cell-Specific Function
  in Kidney Epithelial Cells   D. Brown   51:771–84

PREFATORY CHAPTERS
The Making of a Comparative Physiologist   C. L. Prosser   48:1–6
A Silver Spoon   J. R. Pappenheimer   49:1–15
Prefatory Chapter: Muscular Contraction   A. Huxley   50:1–16
Seeds of Na,K-ATPase   R. Post   51:1–15
Mechanisms Regulating the Reactions of
  Human Hemoglobin with Oxygen and
  Carbonmonoxide   M. F. Perutz   52:1–25

RECOMBINANT DNA TO STUDY NEUROPEPTIDE PROCESSING
Carboxypeptidase E   L. D. Fricker   50:309–21
Gene Transfer Techniques to Study
  Neuropeptide Processing   G. Thomas, B. A. Thorne,
    D. E. Hruby   50:323/-32
Peptide α-Amidation   B. A. Eipper, R. E. Mains   50:333–44
Enzymes Required for Yeast Prohormone
  Processing   R. S. Fuller, R. E. Sterne,
    J. Thorner   50:345–62
Tyrosine Sulfation and the Secretory Pathway   W. B. Huttner   50:363–76

RENAL AND ELECTROLYTE PHYSIOLOGY
ATP and the Regulation of Renal Cell
  Function   S. P. Soltoff   48:9–31
Renal Metabolism During Normoxia,
  Hypoxia, and Ischemic Injury   D. P. Jones   48:33–50
Inositol Phospholipid Metabolism in the
  Kidney   D. A. Troyer, D. W. Schwertz,
    J. I. Kreisberg, M. A.
    Venkatachalam   48:51–71
The Tubuloglomerular Feedback Mechanism:
  Functional and Biochemical Aspects   J. P. Briggs, J. Schnermann   49:251–73
Calcium as a Mediator of Tubuloglomerular
  Feedback   P. D. Bell, M. Franco, L. G. Navar   49:275–93
Altered Reactivity of Tubuloglomerular
  Feedback   W. J. Arendshorst   49:295–317
Chloride Transport in the Proximal Renal
  Tubule   L. Schild, R. Green, G. Giebisch   50:97–110
Chloride Transport in Thick Ascending Limb,
  Distal Convolution, and Collecting Duct   R. Greger   50:111–22
Hormonal Regulation of Chloride Transport in
  the Proximal and Distal Nephron   C. de Rouffignac, J.-M. Elalouf   50:123–40
Chloride Transport and Disorders of
  Acid-Base Balance   J. H. Galla, R. G. Luke   50:141–58
Cellular Events in Renal Hypertrophy   L. G. Fine, J. Norman   51:19–32
Autocrine and Paracrine Regulation of Kidney
  Epithelial Cell Growth   S. R. Mendley, F. G. Toback   51:33–50
Androgen-Regulated Gene Expression   F. G. Berger, G. Watson   51:51–65
Epidermal Growth Factor and the Kidney   D. A. Fisher, E. C. Salido,
    L. Barajas   51:67–80
Renal Effects of Atrial Natriuretic Factor   M. G. Cogan   52:669–708
Transepithelial Osmolality Differences,
  Hydraulic Conductivities, and Volume
  Absorption in the Proximal Tubule   J. A. Schafer   52:709–26
Regulation of the Predominant Renal
  Medullary Organic Solutes in Vivo   S. Wolff, R. S. Balaban   52:727–46
Renal Action of Atrial Natriuretic Peptide:
  Regulation of Collecting Duct Sodium and
  Water Transport   M. L. Zeidel   52:747–59
Cell Volume Regulation in the Nephron   C. Montrose-Rafizadeh,
    W. B. Guggino   52:761–72

RESPIRATORY PHYSIOLOGY

Oxy-Radicals and Related Species	W. A. Pryor	48:657–68
Oxidant Production and Bactericidal Activity in Phagocytes	H. J. Forman, M. J. Thomas	48:669–80
The Response of the Lung to Foreign Compounds That Produce Free Radicals	L. L. Smith	48:681–92
Antioxidant Defenses in the Lung	I. Fridovich, B. Freeman	48:693–702
The Relation of Free Radical Production to Hyperoxia	D. Jamieson, B. Chance, E. Cadenas, A. Boveris	48:703–20
Morphologic Changes in Pulmonary Oxygen Toxicity	J. D. Crapo	48:721–31
Polypeptide-Containing Neurons in Airway Smooth Muscle	J. M. Lundberg, A. Saria	49:557–72
Peripheral Airway Ganglia	R. F. Coburn	49:573–82
Innervation of Airway Smooth Muscle: Fine Structure	G. Gabella	49:583–94
Organization of Central Control of Airways	M. P. Kalia	49:595–609
Nervous Receptors of the Tracheobronchial Tree	G. Sant'Ambrogio	49:611–27
Velocity of CO_2 Exchange in Blood	R. A. Klocke	50:625–37
Velocity of CO_2 Exchanges in the Lungs	A. Bidani, E. D. Crandall	50:639–52
Kinetics of CO_2 Exchange in the Kidney	T. D. DuBose, Jr., A. Bidani	50:653–67
Velocity of CO_2 Exchange in Muscle and Liver	G. Gros, S. J. Dodgson	50:669–94
The Kinetics of HCO_3 Synthesis Related to Fluid Secretion, pH Control, and CO_2 Elimination	T. H. Maren	50:695–717
In Vivo Study of Tissue Oxidative Metabolism Using Nuclear Magnetic Resonance and Optical Spectroscopy	M. Tamura, O. Hazeki, S. Nioka, B. Chance	51:813–34
P_{O2} Chemoreception in Arterial Chemoreceptors	H. Acker	51:835–44
Oxygen Sensing in the Kidney and its Relation to Erythropoietin Production	C. Bauer, A. Kurtz	51:845–56
Transport of Oxygen in Muscle	B. A. Wittenberg, J. B. Wittenberg	51:857–78
The Serous Cell	C. B. Basbaum, B. Jany, W. Finkbeiner	52:97–113
Regulation of Cl^- and K^+ Channels in Airway Epithelium	J. McCann, M. J. Welsh	52:115–35
The Physiology of Cilia and Mucociliary Interactions	P. Satir, M. A. Sleigh	52:137–55
Goblet Cell Secretion and Mucogenesis	P. Verdugo	52:157–76
Immunoglobulin Secretion in the Airways	R. P. Daniele	52:177–95